W9-BUK-292

THE NEW PRESCRIPTION DRUG REFERENCE GUIDE

BY THE EDITORS OF
CONSUMER GUIDE®

Publications International, Ltd.

Louis Weber, C.E.O.
Publications International, Ltd.
7373 N. Cicero Ave.
Lincolnwood, IL 60646

Manufactured in the United States of America.

8 7 6 5 4 3 2

ISBN: 1-56173-298-2

Library of Congress Catalog Card Number: 91-65674

Drug consultants:
Donald Autio, M.S.
Deborah Harper Brown, Pharm.D.
Jerry Frazier, Pharm.D.
Maureen Garrity, B.S.
Cheryl Nunn, Pharm.D.
Ladia Cheng, Pharm.D.
Phillip Nowakowski, Pharm.D.

Contents

Introduction

The right drug for the right patient in the right dose by the right route at the right time. This rule sums up the decisions made when your doctor gives you a prescription. You've helped make those decisions by giving a complete medical history: You've informed your doctor of any previous allergic reactions you've suffered to drugs, foods, or dyes; of any other drugs you may be taking; of any chronic health problems you may have; and whether you are pregnant or breastfeeding an infant. Once you leave your doctor's office, prescription in hand, you have still more to do as a responsible patient.

You must know how to administer the medication you will be taking. You must understand and comply with your dosage schedule. You must know what to do should side effects occur. You must recognize the signals that indicate the need to call your doctor. All too often, patients leave their doctors' offices without a full understanding of the drug therapy they're about to start, with the result that they do not comply fully with their doctors' prescriptions. They may stop taking the medication too soon because it doesn't seem to work, or because they feel better, or because it causes bothersome side effects. They may take the drug improperly or at the wrong time or too often. They may continue drinking alcohol or taking other drugs, perhaps not even realizing that such products as cold pills, oral contraceptives (birth control pills), aspirin, and vitamins can affect the action of the newly prescribed drug. The end result may be that they do not get better; perhaps they will even get worse or suffer a dangerous overdose.

THE NEW PRESCRIPTION DRUG REFERENCE GUIDE provides the information that you need to take medications safely. Along with general information on reading a prescription and buying, storing, and using drugs, it provides an introduction to the action of drugs—how drugs work to stop infection, to lower blood pressure, or to relieve pain. It provides detailed information on hundreds of the most commonly prescribed drugs and several over-the-counter (nonprescription) products, including how to alleviate certain side effects, whether you should take the drug on an empty stomach or with meals, whether the drug is likely to affect your ability to drive a car, and whether you can substitute a generic drug for a prescribed brand-name medication. You will discover which side effects are common to some medications and which are danger signals that require immediate attention from your physician.

Of course, this book is not a substitute for consulting your doctor and pharmacist. They are your primary reference sources on the use of drugs. But to ensure that you receive the best health care possible, you, too, must be informed and knowledgeable about the drugs you use.

Filling Your Prescription

While you're having your prescription filled, you should make sure you understand what the drug is used for, your dosage schedule, how to store the medication properly, what kinds of precautions to take to prevent or reduce side effects, whether you should restrict your diet or drinking habits while taking the drug, which side effects are expected or unavoidable, and which side effects signal a need for a doctor's attention. Your first step in filling your prescription is reading what your doctor has written.

READING YOUR PRESCRIPTION

Prescriptions are not mysterious—they contain no secret messages. Many of the symbols and phrases doctors use on prescriptions are abbreviated Latin or Greek words; they are holdovers from the days when doctors actually wrote in Latin. For example, "gtt" comes from the Latin word *guttae*, which means drops, and "bid" is a shortened version of *bis in die*, which is Latin for twice a day.

You do not have to be a doctor, nurse, or pharmacist to read a prescription. You can (and should) learn how to read one yourself—after all, the prescription describes the drug you will be taking. You should understand what your doctor has written on the prescription blank to be sure that the label on the drug container you receive from your pharmacist coincides with your prescription.

The accompanying chart lists the most common prescription symbols and abbreviations. Use it as a guide to read the sample prescriptions that follow.

Common Abbreviations and Symbols Used in Writing Prescriptions

Abbreviation	Meaning	Derivation and Notes
aa	of each	*ana* (Greek)
ac	before meals	*ante cibum* (Latin)
AD	right ear	*auris dextra* (Latin)
AL	left ear	*auris laeva* (Latin)
AM	morning	*ante meridiem* (Latin)
AS	left ear	*auris sinistra* (Latin)
au	both ears	*auris* (Latin)
bid	twice a day	*bis in die* (Latin)
C	100	—
c	with	*cum* (Latin)
cap	capsule	—
cc or cm^3	cubic centimeter	30 cc equals one ounce
disp	dispense	—
dtd#	give this number	*dentur tales doses* (Latin)
ea	each	—
ext	for external use	—
gtt	drops	*guttae* (Latin)
gt	drop	*gutta* (Latin)
h	hour	*hora* (Latin)
hs	at bedtime	*hora somni* (Latin)
M ft	make	*misce fiat* (Latin)
mitt#	give this number	*mitte* (Latin)
ml	milliliter	30 ml equals one ounce (1 ml = 1 cc)
O	pint	*octarius* (Latin)
OD	right eye	*oculus dexter* (Latin)
OL	left eye	*oculus laevus* (Latin)
OS	left eye	*oculus sinister* (Latin)
OU	each eye	*oculus uterque* (Latin)
pc	after meals	*post cibum* (Latin)
PM	evening	*post meridiem* (Latin)
po	by mouth	*per os* (Latin)
prn	as needed	*pro re nata* (Latin)
q	every	*quaqua* (Latin)
qd	once a day; every day	*quaqua die* (Latin)
qid	four times a day	*quater in die* (Latin)
qod	every other day	—
s	without	*sine* (Latin)
sig	label as follows	*signa* (Latin)
sl	under the tongue	*sub lingua* (Latin)
SOB	shortness of breath	—
sol	solution	—
ss	half unit	*semis* (Latin)
stat	at once; first dose	*statim* (Latin)
susp	suspension	—
tab	tablet	—
tid	three times a day	*ter in die* (Latin)
top	apply topically	—
ung or ungt	ointment	*unguentum* (Latin)
UT	under the tongue	—
ut dict or UD	as directed	*ut dictum* (Latin)
x	times	—

The first sample prescription is for Darvon Compound-65 (Darvon cpd-65). The prescription tells the pharmacist to give you 24 capsules (#24), and it tells you to take one capsule (cap i) every four hours (q 4h) as needed (prn) for pain.

The prescription indicates that you may receive five refills (5x), that the label on the drug container should state the name of the drug (yes), and that the pharmacist may substitute (substitution) a less expensive equivalent product.

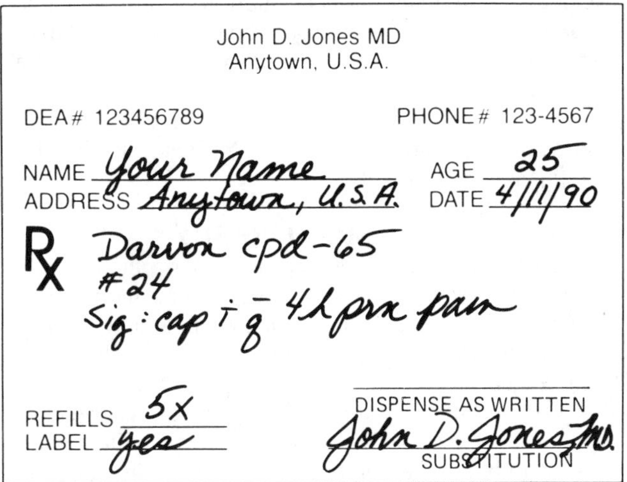
John D. Jones MD
Anytown, U.S.A.

DEA# 123456789 PHONE# 123-4567

NAME Your Name AGE 25
ADDRESS Anytown, U.S.A. DATE 4/11/90

Rx Darvon cpd-65
#24
Sig: cap i q 4h prn pain

REFILLS 5x
LABEL yes

DISPENSE AS WRITTEN
John D. Jones MD
SUBSTITUTION

Look at the second prescription. It shows that you will receive 100 (dtd C) tablets of Lanoxin, 0.125 mg. You will take three tablets at once (iii stat), then two (ii) tomorrow morning (AM), and one (i) every (q) morning (AM) thereafter with (c) orange juice (OJ). You will receive the specific brand noted (dispense as written), you may receive refills as needed (prn), and the name of the drug will be on the package (✓).

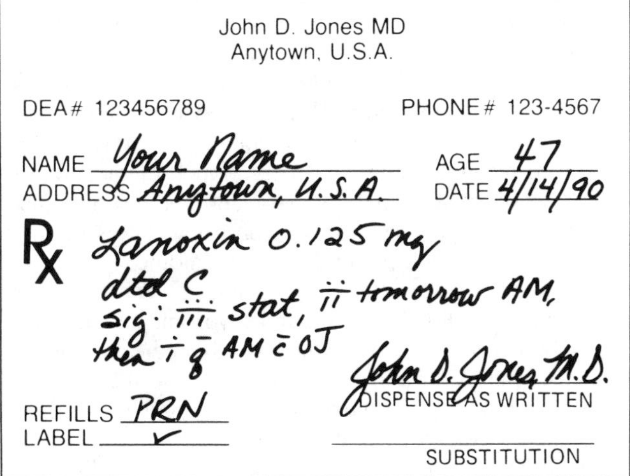
John D. Jones MD
Anytown, U.S.A.

DEA# 123456789 PHONE# 123-4567

NAME Your Name AGE 47
ADDRESS Anytown, U.S.A. DATE 4/14/90

Rx Lanoxin 0.125 mg
dtd C
Sig: iii stat, ii tomorrow AM,
then i q AM c OJ

John D. Jones M.D.
DISPENSE AS WRITTEN

REFILLS PRN
LABEL ✓

SUBSTITUTION

Do remember to check the label on the drug container. If the information on the label is not the same as on the prescription, question your pharmacist. Make sure you are receiving the right medication and the correct instructions for taking it.

TALKING TO YOUR PHARMACIST

Once you have read the prescription, its directions may seem clear enough, but will they seem clear when you get home? For example, the prescription for Darvon Compound-65 tells you to take one capsule every four hours as needed. How many capsules can you take each day—four, six, more? The phrase "as needed" is not clear, and unless you understand what it means, you don't know how much medication you can take per day. What if your prescription instructs you to take "one tablet four times a day"? What does four times a day mean? For some antibiotics, it may mean one tablet every six hours around the clock. For other medications, it may mean one tablet in the morning, one at noon, one in the early evening, and one at bedtime. For still others, it may mean one tablet every hour for the first four hours after you get up in the morning. Don't leave the pharmacy with unanswered questions; ask your pharmacist for an explanation of any confusing terms on your prescription.

Your pharmacist is a valuable resource in your health care. He or she should have a record of ALL the prescription drugs you receive, in order to detect any possible life-threatening drug interactions. It is, therefore, a good idea to purchase your medications through one pharmacy—choose one that maintains careful records.

The pharmacist will be able to tell you if your therapy may be affected by smoking tobacco, eating certain foods, or drinking alcohol, and if the drugs you are taking can cause drowsiness or nausea. He or she can tell you what to expect from the medication and about how long you will have to take it. Of course, people's treatments vary tremendously, but you should ask whether you will have to take medication for five to ten days (for example, to treat a mild respiratory infection) or for a few months (for example, to treat a kidney infection).

You should discuss with your pharmacist the possible side effects of your medication and ask for a description of symptoms. The pharmacist can tell you which side effects require prompt attention from your physician. For example, one of the major side effects of the drug phenylbutazone is the development of a blood disorder. Since a sore throat can be one of the early symptoms of a blood disorder, your pharmacist may instruct you to consult your physician if this symptom occurs.

Your pharmacist can also explain how to take your medicine. You need to know whether to take the drug before or after a meal or along with it. The timing of doses of a drug can make a big difference, and the effectiveness of each drug depends on following the directions for its use. Your pharmacist can tell you what is meant by the phrases "as needed," "as directed," and "take with fluid." For example, you may take water, but not milk, with some drugs. With other drugs, you should drink milk. Your pharmacist can also tell you how many refills you may have and whether you may need them.

OVER-THE-COUNTER DRUGS

Drugs that can be purchased without a prescription are referred to as over-the-counter (OTC) drugs. They are sold in a wide variety of settings, such as drugstores, grocery stores, and hotel lobbies. There are no legal requirements or limitations on who may buy or sell them.

Products sold OTC contain amounts of active ingredients considered to be safe for self-treatment by consumers when labeling instructions are followed.

Many people visit a doctor for ailments that can be treated effectively by taking nonprescription drugs. Actually, prescriptions are sometimes written for such drugs. Your pharmacist will be able to recommend appropriate use of OTC medications and preparations.

If your pharmacist recommends that you not take certain OTC drugs, follow the advice. OTC drugs may affect the way your body reacts to the prescription drugs you are taking. For instance, people taking tetracycline should avoid taking antacids or iron-containing products at the same time; their use should be separated by at least two hours. Antacids and iron interfere with the body's absorption of tetracycline, thereby decreasing its effectiveness. Be sure you know what you are taking. If you are unsure of the type or contents of your medications, ask your doctor or pharmacist.

GENERIC DRUGS

One way your pharmacist can help you save money is by dispensing generic drugs. "Generic" means not protected by trademark registration. The generic name of a drug is usually a shortened form of its chemical name. Any manufacturer can use the generic name when marketing a drug. For example, many manufacturers make a drug called tetracycline.

Usually, a manufacturer uses a trade name (or brand name) as well as a generic name for a drug. A trade name is registered, and only the manufacturer who holds the trademark can use the trade name when marketing a drug. For example, only Lederle Laboratories can call their tetracycline product Achromycin V, and only the Upjohn Company can use the trade name Panmycin for tetracycline. Most trade names are easy to remember, are capitalized in print, and usually include the registered symbol (®) after them. You should know the generic name and the trade name of every drug you are taking.

Many people think that drugs with trade names are made by large manufacturers and generic drugs are made by small manufacturers. But, in fact, a manufacturer may market large quantities of a drug under a brand name and may also sell the base chemical to several other companies, some of which sell the drug generically and some of which sell it under their own brand names. For example, the antibiotic ampicillin is the base for over 200 different products. However, all ampicillin is produced by only a few dozen drug companies.

Generic drugs are generally priced lower than their trademarked equivalents, largely because they are not as widely advertised. However, not every drug is available generically, and not every generic is significantly less expensive than its trademarked equivalent. Nevertheless, consumers may be able to save as much as 40 percent by purchasing a generic product. For example, 100 tablets of Inderal (40 mg) may cost \$22 to \$25. One hundred tablets of the generic equivalent product may cost about \$18—a savings of \$4 to \$7.

For certain drugs, however, it's inadvisable to "shop around" for a generic equivalent. Although the Food and Drug Administration has stated that there is no evidence to suspect serious differences between trade-name drugs and generic drugs, differences have been shown to exist between brands of certain drugs. The tablets or capsules from different manufacturers may not dissolve in the stomach at the same rate or to the same extent, because of variations in the way they are made or the fillers (nonactive ingredients) that are used. This is especially true for the various generic digoxin and phenytoin products. It is, therefore, important to discuss with your doctor or pharmacist the advantages or disadvantages of any particular generic product.

All states have some form of substitution law that allows pharmacists to fill prescriptions with the least expensive equivalent product. However, your doctor can authorize the use of a specific brand of medication by signing on the appropriate line or otherwise noting this on the prescription form (see the sample prescriptions on the previous page). You should be aware that certain patients can sometimes respond in different ways to various equivalent products, and your doctor may have good reasons for being specific. Discuss this with your doctor.

HOW MUCH TO BUY

On a prescription, your doctor specifies exactly how many tablets or capsules or how much liquid medication you will receive. But if you must take a drug for a long time, or if you are very sensitive to drugs, you may want to purchase a different quantity.

The amount of medication to buy depends on several factors. The most obvious is how much money you have or, for those who have a comprehensive insurance program, how much the insurance company will pay for each purchase. These factors may help you decide how much medication to buy, but you must also consider the kind of medication you will be taking (for example, how long it can be stored).

Medications to treat heart disease, high blood pressure, diabetes, or a thyroid condition may be purchased in large quantity. Patients with such chronic conditions take medication for prolonged periods. Chances are, they will pay less per tablet or capsule by purchasing large quantities of drugs. Generally, the price per dose decreases with the amount of the drug purchased. In other words, a drug that usually costs six cents per tablet may cost four or five cents per tablet if you buy 100 at a time.

Many doctors prescribe only a month's supply of drugs, even those drugs that will be taken for a long time. If you wish to buy more, check with your pharmacist. It is also important to make sure that you have enough medication on hand to cover vacation travel and long holidays. Serious side effects could occur if you miss even a few doses of such drugs as propranolol, prednisone, or clonidine.

If you have been plagued by annoying side effects or have had allergic reactions to some drugs, you may want to ask your pharmacist to dispense only enough medication on initial prescriptions for a few days or a week, so that you can determine how your body reacts to the drug. Pharmacists cannot take back prescription drugs once they have left the pharmacy. You may have to pay more per dose if the pharmacist gives you a small quantity of the drug, but at least you will not be paying for a supply of medication you cannot take. Be sure you can get the remainder of the prescribed amount of the drug if no serious or intolerable side effects occur. With some drugs, after you have received part of the intended amount, you cannot receive more without obtaining another prescription.

STORING YOUR DRUGS

Before you leave the pharmacy, find out how you should store your medication. If drugs are stored in containers that do not protect them from heat or moisture, they may lose potency.

All medications should be kept in their original containers. Different medications should NOT be mixed in one container, in order to prevent confusion about which drug is being taken. In addition, some drugs may lose their potency when stored with other medications. Never remove the label from the prescription vial. It contains your prescription number (for refills), the name of the medication, and directions for proper use.

You can safely store most prescription drugs at room temperature and out of direct sunlight. Even those drugs dispensed in colored bottles or containers that reflect light should be kept out of direct sunlight.

Some drugs require storage in the refrigerator; other medications should not be refrigerated. For example, some liquid cough suppressants thicken as they become cold and will not pour from the bottle. Some people keep nitroglycerin tablets in the refrigerator because they believe the drug will be more stable when kept cold. Nitroglycerin, however, should not be stored in the refrigerator.

Even if the label on your medication states "keep refrigerated," this does NOT mean you can keep the drug in the freezer. If frozen and thawed, coated tablets may crack, and some liquids may separate into layers that can't be remixed.

Many people keep prescription drugs and other medications in the bathroom medicine cabinet, but this is one of the WORST places to keep drugs. Small children can easily climb onto the sink and reach drugs stored above it. Also, the temperature and humidity changes in the bathroom may adversely affect the stability of prescription and nonprescription drugs.

It is required by law that all prescription medications for oral use be dispensed in childproof containers. If you find the container difficult to open AND if there are no small children in your home, you can request that your pharmacist dispense your medication in a nonchildproof container.

Definitions Used to Describe Storage Temperatures

Excessive Cold	Any temperature under 36°F (2°C)
Refrigerated	Any cold place where the temperature is between 36° and 46°F (2°-8°C)
Cool	Any temperature between 46° and 59°F (8°-15°C)
Room temperature	Temperature usually between 59° and 86°F (15°-30°C)
Excessive heat	Any temperature above 104°F (40°C)

KEEP ALL DRUGS AWAY FROM CHILDREN, and do not keep unused prescription drugs. Flush leftover medication down the toilet or pour it down the sink, and wash and destroy the empty container. Regularly clean out your medicine cabinet and discard all drugs you are no longer using and drugs that have expired (the expiration date is often listed on the prescription label). These drugs can be dangerous to your children, and you might be tempted to take them in the future if you develop similar symptoms. Similar symptoms may not be due to the same disease, and you may complicate your condition by taking the wrong drug.

If a child accidentally swallows medication or receives too much of a prescribed medication, IMMEDIATELY CALL YOUR LOCAL POISON CONTROL CENTER, A NEARBY EMERGENCY ROOM, OR YOUR DOCTOR for instructions and recommendations. These phone numbers should be written down in a readily accessible place. You should also keep a bottle of syrup of ipecac (available without a prescription) for each child under five years of age in your home (in case the poison control center or emergency room personnel or your doctor recommends that you induce vomiting in the child). Do not, however, use the syrup of ipecac unless instructed to do so by a health professional.

Administering Medication Correctly

You must use medicine correctly to obtain its full benefit. If you administer drugs improperly, you may not receive their full therapeutic effects. Furthermore, improper administration can be dangerous. Some drugs may become toxic if used incorrectly.

Before administering medications to children or elderly patients, ask your doctor for instructions. Children and older patients can be more sensitive to dosage amounts and side effects of medications.

LIQUIDS

Liquid medications are used in several different ways. Some are intended to be used externally on the skin; some are placed into the eye, ear, nose, or throat; still others may be taken internally. Before taking or using any liquid medication, look at the label to see if there are specific directions.

A suspension is a liquid product that contains particles that settle to the bottom of the container. It must be shaken before you use the medicine. If you don't shake it well each time, you may not get the correct amount of the active ingredient—as the amount of liquid remaining in the bottle becomes smaller, the drug becomes more concentrated. You will be getting more of the active ingredient with each dose. It may even reach toxic levels.

When opening the bottle, point it away from you. Some liquid medications build up pressure inside the bottle; the liquid could spurt out and stain your clothing. If the medication is for application to the skin, pour a small quantity onto a cotton pad or a piece of gauze. Do not use a large piece of cotton or gauze, since it will absorb the liquid and much will be wasted. Don't pour the medication into your cupped hand; you may spill some of it. If you're using it on only a small area, you can spread the medication with your finger or a cotton-tipped applicator. Never dip cotton-tipped applicators or pieces of cotton or gauze into the bottle; since this might contaminate the rest of the medication.

Liquid medications that are to be swallowed must be measured accurately. When your doctor prescribes one teaspoonful of medication, he or she is thinking of a 5-milliliter (ml) medical spoon. The teaspoons you have at home can hold anywhere from 2 to 10 ml of liquid. If you use one of these to measure your medication, you may get too little or too much drug with each dose. Ask your pharmacist for a medical teaspoon or one of the other plastic devices for accurately measuring liquid medications. Most of these cost only a few cents and are well worth their cost in ensuring accurate dosage. In addition, while many children balk at medication taken from a teaspoon, they often enjoy taking it from a "special" spoon.

CAPSULES, TABLETS, AND ORAL POWDERS

Many people find it hard to swallow a tablet or capsule. If tablets or capsules tend to catch in your throat, rinse your mouth with water, or at least wet your mouth, before attempting to take a tablet or capsule. Place the tablet or capsule on the back of your tongue, take a drink, and swallow. If it is too large, or still "sticks" in your throat, empty the capsule or crush the tablet into a spoon and mix it with applesauce, soup, or even chocolate syrup. But BE SURE TO CHECK WITH YOUR PHARMACIST BEFORE YOU DO SO. Some tablets and capsules should not be crushed or opened and must be swallowed whole—your pharmacist can tell you which ones they are.

If you have trouble swallowing a tablet or capsule and do not wish to mix the medication with food, ask your doctor to prescribe a liquid drug preparation or a chewable tablet instead, if one is available.

Occasionally, medications come in oral powder form (for example, cholestyramine and colestipol). Such medications should be carefully mixed with liquids, then swallowed. These medications should NOT be swallowed dry.

SUBLINGUAL TABLETS

Some drugs, such as nitroglycerin, are prepared as tablets that must be placed under the tongue. Such medications are more rapidly or more completely absorbed into the bloodstream from the lining of the mouth than they are from the stomach and intestinal tract.

To take a sublingual tablet properly, place the tablet under your tongue, close your mouth, and hold the saliva in your mouth and under your tongue as long as you can before swallowing (to allow the tablet to completely dissolve). If you have a bitter taste in your mouth after five minutes, the drug has not been completely absorbed. Wait at least five more minutes before drinking water. Drinking too soon may wash the medication into the stomach before it has been absorbed thoroughly. Do not smoke, eat, or chew gum while the medication is dissolving.

BUCCAL TABLETS

Some drugs, such as nitroglycerin, are prepared as tablets that must be placed under the lip or in the cheek. These products are designed to release a dose of the drug over a period of time.

To take a buccal tablet properly, place the tablet between the upper lip and gum (above the front teeth) or between the cheek and gum. If you eat or drink during the three to five hours that it takes for the tablet to dissolve, place the tablet between the upper lip and gum. Do not go to sleep with a tablet in your mouth because it could slip down your throat and cause choking. Do not use chewing tobacco when a tablet is in place.

EYE DROPS AND EYE OINTMENTS

Before administering eye drops or ointments, wash your hands. Then lie down or sit down, and tilt your head back.

Using your thumb and forefinger, gently and carefully pull your lower eyelid down to form a pouch. Hold the dropper close to your eyelid without touching it. Drop the prescribed amount of medicine into this pouch and slowly close your eyes. Try not to blink. Keep your eyes closed, and place one finger at the corner of the eye next to your nose for a minute or two, applying slight pressure (this is done to prevent loss of medication through the duct that drains fluid from the surface of the eye into the nose and throat). Then wipe away any excess with a clean tissue. Do not wash or wipe the dropper before replacing it in the bottle—you might accidentally contaminate the rest of the medication. Close the bottle tightly to keep out moisture.

To administer an eye ointment, squeeze a line of ointment in the prescribed amount into the pouch formed as for administering eye drops (avoid touching the tube to your eyelid), and close your eye. Roll your eye a few times to spread the ointment.

Be sure the drops or ointments you use are intended for use in the eye (all products manufactured for use in the eye must be sterilized to prevent eye infections). Also, check the expiration date on the label or container of the medication. Don't use a drug product after the specified date, and never use any eye product that has changed color. If you find that the medication contains particles that weren't there when you bought it, don't use it.

EAR DROPS

Ear drops must be administered so that they fill the ear canal. To administer ear drops properly, tilt your head to one side, turning the affected ear upward. Grasp the earlobe and gently pull it upward and back to straighten the ear canal. When administering ear drops to a child, GENTLY pull the child's earlobe downward and back. Fill the dropper and place the prescribed number of drops (usually a dropperful) into the ear, but be careful to avoid touching the sides or edge of the ear canal. The dropper can easily become contaminated by contact with the ear canal.

Keep the ear tilted upward for five to ten seconds while continuing to hold the earlobe. Your doctor may want you to gently insert a small wad of clean cotton into the ear to ensure that the drops do not escape. Do not wash or wipe the dropper after use; replace it in the bottle and tightly close the bottle to keep out moisture.

Before administering the medication, you may warm the bottle of ear drops by rolling the bottle back and forth between your hands to bring the solution to body temperature. DO NOT place the bottle in boiling water. The ear drops may become so hot that they will cause pain when placed in the ear. Also, boiling water can loosen or peel off the label and might even destroy the medication.

NOSE DROPS AND SPRAYS

Before using nose drops or sprays, gently blow your nose if you can. To administer nose drops, fill the dropper, tilt your head back, and place the prescribed number of drops into your nose. To prevent contamination of the rest of the medicine, do not touch the dropper to the nasal membranes. Keep your head tilted for five to ten seconds, and sniff gently two or three times.

Do not tilt your head back when using a nasal spray. Insert the sprayer into the nose, but try to avoid touching the inner nasal membranes. Sniff and squeeze the sprayer at the same time. Do not release your grip on the sprayer until you have withdrawn it from your nose (to prevent nasal mucus and bacteria from entering the plastic bottle and contaminating its contents). After you have sprayed the prescribed number of times in one or both nostrils, gently sniff two or three times.

Unless your doctor has told you otherwise, you should not use nose drops or sprays for more than two or three days at a time. If they have been prescribed for a longer period, do not administer nose drops or sprays from the same container for more than one week. Bacteria from your nose can easily enter the container and contaminate the solution. If you must take medication for more than a week, purchase a new container. NEVER allow anyone else to use your nose drops or spray.

RECTAL SUPPOSITORIES

Rectal suppositories are used to deliver various types of medication. They may be used as laxatives, sleeping aids, or tranquilizers or as preparations that are used to relieve the itching, swelling, and pain of hemorrhoids. Regardless of the reason for their use, all rectal suppositories are inserted in the same way.

In extremely hot weather, a suppository may become too soft to handle properly. If this happens, place the suppository in the refrigerator, in a glass of cool water, or under running cold water until it becomes firm. A few minutes is usually sufficient. Before inserting a suppository, remove any aluminum wrappings. Rubber finger coverings or disposable rubber gloves may be worn when inserting a suppository, but they are not necessary unless your fingernails are extremely long and sharp.

To insert a suppository, lie on your left side with your right knee bent. Push the suppository, pointed end first, into the rectum as far as is comfortable. You may feel like defecating, but lie still for a few minutes and try not to have a bowel movement for at least an hour. If you cannot insert a suppository, or if the process is painful, you can coat the suppository with a thin layer of petroleum jelly or mineral oil to make insertion easier.

Manufacturers of many suppositories that are used in the treatment of hemorrhoids suggest that the suppositories be stored in the refrigerator. Be sure to ask your pharmacist if the suppositories you have purchased should be stored in the refrigerator.

VAGINAL OINTMENTS AND CREAMS

Most vaginal products are packaged with complete instructions for use. If a woman is not sure how to administer vaginal medication, she should ask her pharmacist.

Before using any vaginal ointment or cream, read the directions. They will probably tell you to attach the applicator to the top of the tube and to squeeze the tube from the bottom until the applicator is completely filled. Then lie on your back with your knees drawn up. Hold the applicator horizontally or pointed slightly downward, and insert it into the vagina as far as it will go comfortably. Press the plunger down to empty the cream or ointment into the vagina. Withdraw the plunger and wash it in warm, soapy water. Rinse it thoroughly and allow it to dry completely. When the plunger is dry, return it to its original package.

VAGINAL TABLETS AND SUPPOSITORIES

Most packages of vaginal tablets or suppositories include complete directions for use, but you may wish to review these general instructions.

Remove any foil wrapping. Place the tablet or suppository in the applicator that is provided. Lie on your back with your knees drawn up. Hold the applicator horizontally or tilted slightly downward, and insert it into the vagina as far as it will comfortably go. Depress the plunger slowly to release the tablet or suppository into the vagina. Withdraw the applicator and wash it in warm, soapy water. Rinse it and let it dry completely. When the applicator is dry, return it to its package.

Unless your doctor has told you otherwise, do not douche two to three weeks before or after you use vaginal tablets or suppositories. Be sure to ask your doctor for specific recommendations on douching.

THROAT LOZENGES AND DISCS

Both lozenges and discs contain medication that is released in the mouth to soothe a sore throat, to reduce coughing, or to treat laryngitis. Neither should be chewed; they should be allowed to dissolve in the mouth. After the lozenge or disc has dissolved, try not to swallow or drink any fluids for a while.

THROAT SPRAYS

To administer a throat spray, open your mouth wide and spray the medication as far back as possible. Try not to swallow—hold the spray in your mouth as long as you can, and do not drink any fluids for several minutes. This gives the medication a greater opportunity to work. Swallowing a throat spray is not harmful, but if you find that your throat spray upsets your stomach, don't swallow it; simply spit the throat spray out.

TOPICAL OINTMENTS AND CREAMS

Most topical (used on the skin) ointments and creams exert only local effects—that is, they affect only the area on which they are applied. Most creams and ointments are expensive (especially steroid products, such as betamethasone valerate, fluocinolone, fluocinonide, hydrocortisone, and triamcinolone) and should be applied to the skin as thinly as possible. A thin layer is as effective as (but less costly than) a thick layer. Furthermore, some steroid-containing creams and ointments can cause toxic side effects if applied too heavily.

Before applying the medication, moisten the skin by immersing it in water or by dabbing the area with a clean, wet cloth. Blot the skin almost dry and apply the medication as directed. Gently massage it into the skin until the cream or ointment disappears. You should feel no greasiness after applying a cream. After an ointment is applied, the skin will feel slightly greasy.

If your doctor has not indicated whether you should receive a cream or an ointment, ask your pharmacist for the one you prefer. Creams are greaseless and do not stain your clothing. Creams are best to use on the scalp or other hairy areas of the body. However, if your skin is dry, ask for an ointment. Ointments help keep skin soft for a longer period.

If your doctor tells you to place a wrap on top of the skin after the cream or ointment has been applied, you may use a wrap of transparent plastic film like that used for wrapping food. A wrap holds the medication close to the skin and helps to keep the skin moist so that the drug can be absorbed. To use a wrap correctly, apply the cream or ointment as directed, then wrap the area with a layer of transparent plastic film. Follow your doctor's directions EXACTLY, and keep the wrap in place only as long as you are told to do so. If you keep a wrap on the skin too long, too much of the drug may be absorbed, which may lead to increased side effects. Do not use a wrap without your doctor's approval, and never use one on an oozing lesion.

AEROSOL SPRAYS

Many topical (applied to the skin) items are packaged as pressurized aerosol sprays. These sprays usually cost more than the cream or ointment form of the same medication. They are especially useful on very tender or hairy areas of the body, where it is difficult to apply a cream or ointment. Aerosols can provide a cooling effect on burns or rashes.

Before using an aerosol, shake the can to evenly disperse the particles of medication. Hold the container upright four to six inches from the skin. Press the nozzle for a few seconds, then release.

Never use an aerosol around the face or eyes. If your doctor tells you to use the spray on a part of your face, apply it to your hand and then rub it into the area. If you get it into your eyes or on a mucous membrane, it can be very painful; and it may even damage the eyes.

Aerosol sprays may feel cold when they are applied. If this sensation bothers you, ask your pharmacist or doctor whether another form of the same product is available.

TRANSDERMAL PATCHES

Transdermal patches allow controlled, continuous release of medication. They are convenient and easy to use. For best results, apply the patch to a hairless or clean-shaven area of skin, avoiding scars and wounds. Choose a site (such as the chest or upper arm) that is not subject to excessive movement. It is all right to bathe or shower with a patch in place. In the event that the patch becomes dislodged, discard and replace it. Replace a patch by applying a new unit in another spot. By doing this, you allow for uninterrupted drug therapy and minimal skin irritation.

If redness or irritation develops at the application site, consult your physician. Some people are sensitive to the materials used to make the patches.

Coping with Side Effects

Drugs have certain desirable effects—that's why they are taken. The desirable effects of a drug are known as the drug's activity or therapeutic effects. Drugs, however, have undesirable effects as well. Undesirable effects are called side effects, adverse reactions, or, in some cases, lethal effects. An adverse reaction is any undesirable effect of a drug. It can range from minor to toxic or lethal.

Even if you experience minor side effects, it is very important that you take your medication exactly as it was prescribed. You should take the full dose at the appropriate times throughout the day for the length of time prescribed by your doctor. Taking a lesser amount of medication to avoid side effects or because your condition appears to be improving is NOT appropriate. A smaller dose may not provide any benefit whatsoever; that is, half of the dose may not provide half of the therapeutic effects.

Some side effects are expected and unavoidable, but others may surprise the doctor as well as the patient. Unexpected reactions may be due to a person's individual response to the drug.

Side effects generally fall into one of two major groups—those that are obvious and those that cannot be detected without laboratory testing. Discussion between you and your doctor about your medication should not be restricted to easily recognized side effects; other, less obvious side effects may also be harmful.

If you know a particular side effect is expected from a particular drug, you can relax a little. Most expected side effects are temporary and need not cause alarm. You'll merely experience discomfort or inconvenience for a short time. For example, you may become drowsy after taking an antihistamine or develop a stuffy nose after taking reserpine or certain other drugs that lower blood pressure. Of course, if you find minor side effects especially bothersome, you should discuss them with your doctor, who may be able to prescribe another drug or at least assure you that the benefits of the drug far outweigh its side effects. Sometimes, side effects can be minimized or eliminated by changing your dosage schedule or taking the drug with meals. Be sure, however, to consult your doctor or pharmacist before making such a change.

Many side effects, however, signal a serious, perhaps dangerous, problem. If these side effects appear, you should consult your doctor immediately. The following discussion should help you determine whether your side effects require attention from your physician.

OBVIOUS SIDE EFFECTS

Some side effects are obvious to the patient; others can be discerned only through laboratory testing. We have divided our discussion according to the body parts affected by the side effects.

Ears

Although a few drugs may cause loss of hearing if taken in large quantities, hearing loss is uncommon. Drugs that are used to treat problems of the ear may cause dizziness, and many drugs produce tinnitus (a sensation of ringing, buzzing, thumping, or hollowness in the ears). Discuss with your doctor any persistent problem with your hearing or your ears.

Eyes

Blurred vision is a common side effect of many drugs. Medications such as digoxin may cause you to see a halo around a lighted object (a television screen or a traffic light), and other drugs may cause night blindness. Chlordiazepoxide and clidinium combination makes it difficult to judge distance accurately while driving and also makes the eyes sensitive to sunlight. While the effects on the eyes caused by digoxin are danger signs of toxicity, the effects caused by chlordiazepoxide and clidinium combination are to be expected. In any case, if any eye-related problems occur while you are taking medication, contact your physician.

Gastrointestinal System

The gastrointestinal system includes the mouth, esophagus, stomach, small and large intestines, and rectum. A side effect that affects the gastrointestinal system can be expected from almost any drug. Many drugs produce dry mouth, mouth sores, difficulty in swallowing, heartburn, nausea, vomiting, diarrhea, constipation, loss of appetite, or abnormal cramping. Other drugs cause bloating and gas, and some cause rectal itching.

Diarrhea can be expected after taking many drugs. Diarrhea caused by most drugs is temporary and self-limiting; that is, it should stop within three days. During this time, do not take any diarrhea remedy; drink liquids to replace the fluid you are losing. If the diarrhea lasts more than three days or is accompanied by fever, call your doctor.

Diarrhea sometimes signals a problem. For example, some antibiotics can cause severe diarrhea. When diarrhea is severe, the intestine may become ulcerated and begin to bleed. If you have severe diarrhea (diarrhea that lasts for several days, or stools that contain blood, pus, or mucus) while taking antibiotics, contact your doctor.

As a side effect of drug use, constipation is less serious and more common than diarrhea. It occurs when a drug slows down the activity of the bowel. Medications such as chlorpromazine and amitriptyline slow bowel activity. Constipation also occurs when drugs cause moisture to be absorbed from the bowel, resulting in a more solid stool. It may also occur if a drug acts on the nervous system to decrease nerve impulses to the intestine—an effect produced, for example, by methyldopa. Constipation produced by a drug can last several days. You may help relieve it by drinking eight to ten glasses of water a day, including more fiber in your diet, and getting plenty of exercise (unless your doctor directs you to do otherwise). Do not take laxatives unless your doctor directs you to do so. If constipation continues for more than three days, call your doctor.

Circulatory System

Drugs may speed up or slow down the heartbeat. If a drug slows the heartbeat, you may feel drowsy and tired or even dizzy. If a drug accelerates the heartbeat, you probably will experience palpitations (thumping in the chest). You may feel as though your heart is skipping a beat occasionally. For most people, none of these symptoms indicates a serious problem. However, if they occur frequently, consult your doctor, who may adjust your drug dosage or prescribe other medication.

Some drugs cause edema (fluid retention)—fluid from the blood collects outside the blood vessels. Ordinarily, edema is not serious. But if you are steadily gaining weight or have gained more than three pounds within a week, talk to your doctor.

Drugs may increase or decrease blood pressure. When blood pressure decreases, you may feel drowsy or tired; you may become dizzy, or even faint, especially when you rise suddenly from a sitting or reclining position. If a drug makes you dizzy or light-headed, sit or lie down for a while. To avoid light-headedness when you stand, contract and relax the muscles of your legs for a few moments before rising. Push one foot against the floor while raising the other foot slightly, alternating feet so that you are "pumping" your legs in a pedaling motion. Get up slowly, and be especially careful on stairs. When blood pressure increases, you may feel dizzy, have a headache or blurred vision, hear a ringing or buzzing in your ears, or experience frequent nosebleeds. If these symptoms occur, call your doctor.

Nervous System

Drugs that act on the nervous system may cause drowsiness or stimulation. If a drug causes drowsiness, you may become dizzy or your coordination may become impaired. If a drug causes stimulation, you may become nervous or have insomnia or tremors. Neither drowsiness nor stimulation is cause for concern for most people. When you are drowsy, however, you should be careful around machinery and should avoid driving. Some drugs cause throbbing headaches, and others produce tingling in the fingers or toes. If these symptoms don't disappear in a few days to a week, call your doctor.

Respiratory System

Side effects common to the respiratory system include stuffy nose, dry throat, shortness of breath, and slowed breathing. A stuffy nose and dry throat usually disappear several days after starting a medication. If these side effects are bothersome, you may use nose drops (consult your doctor first) or throat lozenges, or you may gargle with warm salt water to relieve them. Shortness of breath is a characteristic side effect of some drugs (for example, propranolol). If shortness of breath occurs frequently, check with your doctor. It may be a sign of a serious side effect, or you may simply be overexercising.

Skin

Skin reactions include rash, swelling, itching, and sweating. Itching, swelling, and rash frequently indicate a drug allergy. You should NOT continue to take a drug if you develop an allergy to it, but consult your doctor before stopping the drug.

Some drugs increase sweating; others decrease it. Drugs that decrease sweating may cause problems during exercise or hot weather when your body needs to sweat to reduce body temperature.

If you have a minor skin reaction not diagnosed as an allergy, ask your pharmacist for a soothing cream. Your pharmacist may also suggest that you take frequent baths or dust the sensitive area with a suitable powder.

Another type of skin reaction is photosensitivity (also called phototoxicity or sun toxicity)—that is, unusual sensitivity to the sun. Tetracyclines can cause photosensitivity. If, while taking such a drug, you are exposed to the sun for even a brief period of time (10 or 15 minutes), you may experience a severe sunburn. You do not have to stay indoors while taking these drugs, but you should be fully clothed while outside, and you should not remain in the sun too long. Furthermore, you should use a protective sunscreen while in the sun—ask your pharmacist to help you choose one. Since medications may remain in your bloodstream after you stop taking them, you should continue to follow these precautions for two days after treatment with these drugs has been completed.

SUBTLE SIDE EFFECTS

Some side effects are difficult to detect. You may not notice any symptoms at all, or you may notice only slight ones. Therefore, your doctor may want you to have periodic blood tests or eye examinations to ensure that no subtle damage is occurring to any of your organ systems while you are on certain medications.

Kidneys

If one of the side effects of a drug is to reduce the kidneys' ability to remove chemicals and other substances from the blood, these substances begin to accumulate in body tissues. Over a period of time, this accumulation may cause vague symptoms, such as swelling, fluid retention, nausea, headache, or weakness. Obvious symptoms, especially pain, are rare.

Liver

Drug-induced liver damage may result in fat accumulation within the liver. Since the liver is responsible for converting many drugs and body chemicals into compounds that can be eliminated by other organs of the body (kidneys, lungs, gastrointestinal tract), drug-induced liver damage can result in a buildup of these substances. Because liver damage may be quite advanced before it produces any symptoms, periodic blood tests of liver function are recommended during therapy with certain drugs.

Blood

A great many drugs affect the blood and the circulatory system but do not produce noticeable symptoms for some time. Some drugs decrease the number of red blood cells—the cells responsible for carrying oxygen and nutrients throughout the body. If you have too few red blood cells, you become anemic; you appear pale and feel tired, weak, dizzy, and perhaps hungry. Other drugs decrease the number of white blood cells—the cells responsible for combating infection. Having too few white blood cells increases susceptibility to infection and may prolong illness. If a sore throat or a fever begins after you start taking a drug and continues for a few days, you may have an infection and too few white blood cells to fight it. Call your doctor.

DRUG USE DURING PREGNANCY AND BREAST-FEEDING

Before taking ANY medication, it is very important to tell your doctor if you are pregnant (or planning to become pregnant) or are breast-feeding an infant. For most drugs, complete information on safety during pregnancy and while breast-feeding is lacking. This is not due to negligence or lack of concern on the part of regulatory agencies, but to the fact that it would be unethical to conduct drug experiments on pregnant and nursing women. With this in mind, you should discuss with your doctor the risks versus the benefits of taking any medications during pregnancy or while nursing an infant.

MANAGEMENT OF SIDE EFFECTS

Consult the drug profiles to determine whether the side effects you are experiencing are minor (relatively common and usually not serious) or major (symptoms that you should consult your doctor about). If your side effects are minor, you may be able to compensate for them (see the following table for suggestions). However, consult your doctor if you find minor side effects persistent or particularly bothersome.

If you experience any major side effects, contact your doctor immediately. Your dosage may need adjustment, or you may have developed a sensitivity to the drug. Your doctor may want you to switch to an alternative medication to treat your disorder. Never stop taking a prescribed medication unless you first discuss it with your doctor.

Common Minor Side Effects

Side Effect	Management
Constipation	Increase the amount of fiber in your diet; drink plenty of fluids*; exercise*
Decreased sweating	Avoid working or exercising in the sun or under warm conditions
Diarrhea	Drink lots of water to replace lost fluids; if diarrhea lasts longer than three days, call your doctor
Dizziness	Avoid operating machinery or driving a car
Drowsiness	Avoid operating machinery or driving a car
Dry mouth	Suck on candy or ice chips, or chew sugarless gum
Dry nose and throat	Use a humidifier or vaporizer
Fluid retention (mild)	Avoid adding salt to foods; keep legs raised, if possible
Headache	Remain quiet; take aspirin* or acetaminophen*
Insomnia	Take the last dose of the drug earlier in the day*; drink a glass of warm milk at bedtime; ask your doctor about an exercise program
Itching	Take frequent baths or showers, or use wet soaks
Nasal congestion	If necessary, use nose drops*
Palpitations (mild)	Rest often; avoid tension; do not drink coffee, tea, or cola; stop smoking
Upset stomach	Take the drug with milk or food*

***Consult your doctor first**

How Drugs Work

Prescription drugs fall into a number of groups according to the conditions for which they are prescribed. In the following pages, we will provide you with a better understanding of the types of medications that are prescribed for different medical conditions. We'll describe the intended actions of drugs and the therapeutic effects you can expect from various types of medications.

CARDIOVASCULAR DRUGS

Antianginals

Since the heart is a muscle that must work continuously, it requires a constant supply of nutrients and oxygen. The chest pain known as angina occurs when there is an insufficient supply of blood, and consequently of oxygen, to the heart. There are several types of antianginal drugs. These include vasodilators (nitroglycerin, isosorbide dinitrate), calcium channel blockers (diltiazem, nifedipine, verapamil), and beta blockers (acebutolol, atenolol, labetalol, metoprolol, nadolol, pindolol, propranolol, timolol). All of these drugs act by increasing the amount of oxygen that reaches the heart muscle.

Antiarrhythmics

If the heart does not beat rhythmically or smoothly (a condition called arrhythmia), its rate of contraction must be regulated. Antiarrhythmic drugs (disopyramide, mexiletine, procainamide, propranolol, tocainide, quinidine) prevent or alleviate cardiac arrhythmias by altering nerve impulses within the heart.

Antihypertensives

Briefly, high blood pressure is a condition in which the pressure of the blood against the walls of the blood vessels is higher than what is considered normal. High blood pressure, or hypertension, which can eventually cause damage to the brain, eyes, heart, or kidneys, is controllable. If a medication for high blood pressure has been prescribed, it is very important that you continue to take it regularly, even if you don't notice any symptoms of hypertension. If hypertension is controlled, other damage can be prevented. Drugs that counteract or reduce high blood pressure can effectively prolong a hypertensive patient's life.

Several different drug actions produce an antihypertensive effect. Some drugs block nerve impulses that cause arteries to constrict; others slow the heart rate and decrease its force of contraction; still others reduce the amount of a certain hormone (aldosterone) in the blood that causes blood pressure to rise. The effect of any of these is to reduce blood pressure. The mainstay of antihypertensive therapy is often a diuretic, a drug that reduces body fluids. Examples of additional antihypertensive drugs include clonidine, hydralazine, methyldopa, prazosin, and reserpine.

Diuretics

Diuretic drugs, such as chlorothiazide, chlorthalidone, furosemide, hydrochlorothiazide, methyclothiazide, and spironolactone, promote the loss of water and salt from the body (this is why they are sometimes called "water pills"). This loss of water and salt results in lowering of blood pressure. They also lower blood pressure by increasing the diameter of blood vessels. Because many antihypertensive drugs cause the body to retain salt and water, they are often used concurrently with diuretics. Most diuretics act directly on the kidneys, but there are different types of diuretics, each with different actions. Thus, therapy for high blood pressure can be individualized for each patient's needs.

Thiazide diuretics, such as chlorothiazide, chlorthalidone, hydrochlorothiazide, and methyclothiazide, are the most commonly prescribed water pills available today. They are generally well tolerated and can be taken once or twice a day. Since patients do not develop a tolerance to their antihypertensive effect, they can be taken for prolonged periods. However, a major drawback to thiazide diuretics is that they often deplete the body of potassium. This depletion can be compensated for with a potassium supplement. Potassium-rich foods and liquids, such as bananas, apricots, and orange juice, can also be used to help correct the potassium deficiency. Salt substitutes are another source of potassium. Your doctor will direct you as to which source of potassium, if any, is appropriate for you to use.

Loop diuretics, such as furosemide, act more vigorously than thiazide diuretics. (The term "loop" refers to the structures in the kidneys on which these medications act.) Loop diuretics promote more water loss but also deplete more potassium.

To remove excess water from the body but retain its store of potassium, manufacturers developed potassium-sparing diuretics. Drugs such as spironolactone, triamterene, and amiloride are effective in treating potassium loss, heart failure, and hypertension. Potassium-sparing diuretics are combined with thiazide diuretics in medications such as spironolactone and hydrochlorothiazide combination, triamterene and hydrochlorothiazide combination, and amiloride and hydrochlorothiazide combination. Such combinations enhance the antihypertensive effect and reduce the loss of potassium. They are now among the most commonly used antihypertensive agents.

Cardiac Glycosides

Cardiac glycosides include drugs that are derived from digitalis (for example, digoxin and digitoxin). This type of drug slows the rate of the heart but increases its force of contraction. Cardiac glycosides, therefore, act as both heart depressants and stimulants and may be used to regulate irregular heart rhythm or to increase the volume of blood pumped by the heart in heart failure.

Anticoagulants

Drugs that prevent blood clotting are called anticoagulants (blood thinners). Anticoagulants fall into two categories.

The first category contains only one drug, heparin. Heparin must be given by injection, so its use is generally restricted to hospitalized patients.

The second category includes oral anticoagulants, principally derivatives of the drug warfarin. Warfarin may be used in the treatment of conditions such as stroke, heart disease, and abnormal blood clotting. It is also used to prevent the movement of a clot, which could cause serious problems. It acts by preventing the liver from manufacturing the proteins responsible for blood clot formation.

Persons taking warfarin must avoid using many other drugs (including aspirin), because their interaction with the anticoagulant could cause internal bleeding. Patients taking warfarin should check with their pharmacist or physician before using any other medications, including over-the-counter products for coughs or colds. In addition, they must have their blood checked frequently by their physician to ensure that the drug is maintaining the correct degree of thinning.

Antihyperlipidemics

Drugs used to treat atherosclerosis (arteriosclerosis, or hardening of the arteries) act to reduce the serum (the liquified portion of blood) levels of cholesterol and triglycerides (fats), which form plaques (deposits) on the walls of arteries. Some antihyperlipidemics, such as cholestyramine and colestipol, bind to bile acids in the gastrointestinal tract, thereby decreasing the body's production of cholesterol. Clofibrate and probucol also decrease the body's production of cholesterol. Use of such drugs is generally recommended only after diet therapy and lifestyle changes have failed to lower blood lipids to desirable levels. Even then, diet therapy should be continued.

Vasodilators

Vasodilating drugs cause the blood vessels to dilate (widen). Some of the antihypertensive agents, such as hydralazine and prazosin, lower blood pressure by dilating the arteries or veins. Other vasodilators are used in the treatment of stroke and diseases characterized by poor circulation. Ergoloid mesylates, for example, are used to reduce the symptoms of senility by increasing blood flow to the brain.

Beta Blockers

Beta-blocking drugs block the response of the heart and blood vessels to nerve stimulation, thereby slowing the heart rate and reducing high blood pressure. They are used in the treatment of a wide range of diseases including angina, hypertension, migraine headaches, and arrhythmias. Propranolol and metoprolol are two examples of beta blockers.

Calcium Channel Blockers

Calcium channel blockers (diltiazem, nifedipine, verapamil) are used for the prevention of angina (chest pain). Verapamil is also useful in correcting certain arrhythmias (heartbeat irregularities) and lowering blood pressure. This group of drugs is thought to prevent angina and arrhythmias by blocking or slowing calcium flow into muscle cells, which results in vasodilation (widening of the blood vessels) and greater oxygen delivery to the heart muscle.

DRUGS FOR THE EARS

For an ear infection, a physician usually prescribes an antibiotic and a steroid, or a medication that contains a combination of these. The antibiotic attacks the infecting bacteria, and the steroid reduces the inflammation and pain. Often, a local anesthetic, such as benzocaine or lidocaine, may also be prescribed to relieve pain.

DRUGS FOR THE EYES

Almost all drugs that are used to treat eye problems can be used to treat disorders of other parts of the body as well.

Glaucoma is one of the major disorders of the eye, especially in people over 40 years of age, and results in increased pressure within the eyeball. Although glaucoma is sometimes treated surgically, pressure in the eye can usually be reduced, and blindness prevented, through use of eye drops. Two drugs frequently prescribed as eye drops are epinephrine and pilocarpine.

Pilocarpine is a cholinergic drug. Cholinergic drugs act by stimulating parasympathetic nerve endings. Stimulation of these nerve endings alters the activity of many organs throughout the body. For example, a cholinergic drug can cause the heart rate to decrease, intestinal activity to increase, and the bronchioles within the lungs to constrict. When used in the eyes, pilocarpine causes constriction of the pupils and increases the flow of aqueous humor (fluid) out of the eye, thereby reducing the pressure.

Epinephrine is a newer name for the body chemical called adrenaline. Epinephrine is secreted in the body when one must flee from danger, resist attack, or combat stress. Epinephrine has adrenergic properties, such as increasing the amount of sugar in the blood, accelerating the heartbeat, and dilating the pupils. The mechanism by which epinephrine lowers pressure within the eye is not completely understood, but it appears to involve both a decrease in the production of aqueous humor and an increase in the outflow of this fluid from the eye.

Antibiotics are used to treat bacterial eye infections. Steroids can also be used to treat noninfectious eye inflammations, as long as these medications are not used for too long a period of time. Pharmacists carefully monitor requests for eye drop refills, particularly for drops that contain steroids, and may refuse to refill such medication until you have revisited your doctor because these products can cause further eye problems with long-term use.

GASTROINTESTINAL DRUGS

Antinauseants

Antinauseants reduce the urge to vomit. One of the most effective antinauseants is the phenothiazine derivative prochlorperazine. This medication acts on the vomiting center in the brain. It is often administered rectally and usually alleviates nausea and vomiting within a few minutes to an hour. Antihistamines are also commonly used to prevent nausea and vomiting, especially when those symptoms are due to motion sickness. This type of medication may also work at the vomiting center in the brain.

Anticholinergics

Anticholinergic drugs—for example, dicyclomine—slow the action of the bowel and reduce the amount of stomach acid. Because these drugs slow the action of the bowel by relaxing the muscles and relieving spasms, they are said to have an antispasmodic action.

Antiulcer Medications

Antiulcer medications are prescribed to relieve symptoms and promote healing of peptic ulcers. The antisecretory ulcer medications cimetidine, famotidine, and ranitidine work by suppressing the production of excess stomach acid. Another antiulcer drug, sucralfate, works by forming a chemical barrier over an exposed ulcer (like a bandage) thereby protecting the ulcer from stomach acid. These drugs provide sustained relief from ulcer pain and promote healing.

Antidiarrheals

Diarrhea may be caused by many conditions, including influenza and ulcerative colitis, and can sometimes occur as a side effect of drug therapy. Narcotics and anticholinergics slow the action of the bowel and can thereby help alleviate diarrhea. A medication such as diphenoxylate and atropine contains both a narcotic and an anticholinergic.

HORMONES

A hormone is a substance produced and secreted by a gland. Hormones stimulate and regulate body functions. Hormone drugs are given to mimic the effects of naturally produced hormones.

Hormone drugs are prescribed to treat various conditions. Most often, they are used to replace naturally occuring hormones that are not being produced in amounts sufficient to regulate specific body functions. This category of medication also includes oral contraceptives and certain types of drugs that are used to combat inflammatory reactions.

Thyroid Drugs

Thyroid hormone was one of the first hormone drugs to be produced synthetically. Originally, thyroid preparations were made by drying and pulverizing the thyroid glands of animals and then forming them into tablets. Such preparations are still used today in the treatment of patients who have reduced levels of thyroid hormone production. However, a synthetic thyroid hormone (levothyroxine) is also available.

Antidiabetic Drugs

Insulin, which is secreted by the pancreas, regulates the level of glucose (a form of sugar) in the blood, as well as the metabolism of carbohydrates and fats. Insulin's counterpart, glucagon, stimulates the liver to release stored glucose. Both insulin and glucagon must be present in the right amounts to maintain proper blood sugar levels.

Treatment of diabetes mellitus (the condition in which the body is unable to produce and/or utilize insulin) may involve an adjustment of diet and/or the administration of insulin or oral antidiabetic drugs. Glucagon is given only in emergencies (for example, insulin shock, when blood sugar levels must be raised quickly).

Oral antidiabetic medications induce the pancreas to secrete more insulin by acting on small groups of cells within the pancreas that make and store insulin. Oral antidiabetic medications are prescribed for diabetic patients who are unable to regulate their blood sugar levels through diet modification alone. These medications cannot be used by patients who have insulin-dependent (juvenile-onset, or Type I) diabetes—their blood sugar levels can be controlled only with injections of insulin.

Steroids

The pituitary gland secretes adrenocorticotropic hormone (ACTH), which directs the adrenal glands to produce adrenocorticosteroids (for example, cortisone). Oral steroid preparations (for example, prednisone) may be used to treat inflammatory diseases such as arthritis or to treat poison ivy, hay fever, or insect bites. How these drugs relieve inflammation is currently unknown.

Steroids may also be applied to the skin to treat certain inflammatory skin conditions. Triamcinolone and the combination of fluocinonide, hydrocortisone, and iodochlorhydroxyquin are examples of steroid hormone creams or ointments.

Sex Hormones

Although the adrenal glands secrete small amounts of sex hormones, these hormones are produced mainly by the sex glands. Estrogens are the female hormones responsible for secondary sex characteristics such as development of the breasts and maintenance of the lining of the uterus. Testosterone (androgen) is the corresponding male hormone. It is responsible for secondary sex characteristics such as a beard, a deepened voice, and the maturation of external genitalia. Progesterone is also produced in females—it prepares the uterus for pregnancy.

Testosterone reduces elimination of protein from the body, thereby producing an increase in muscle size. Athletes sometimes take drugs called anabolic steroids (chemicals similar to testosterone) for this effect, but such use of these drugs is dangerous. Anabolic steroids can adversely affect the heart, nervous system, and kidneys.

Most oral contraceptives (birth control pills) combine estrogen and progesterone, but some contain only progesterone. The estrogen in birth control pills prevents egg production. Progesterone aids in preventing ovulation, alters the lining of the uterus, and thickens cervical mucus—processes that help to prevent conception and implantation. Oral contraceptives have many side effects, so their use should be discussed with a physician.

Conjugated estrogens are used as replacement therapy to treat symptoms of menopause in women whose bodies are no longer producing sufficient amounts of estrogen. Medroxyprogesterone is used to treat uterine bleeding and menstrual problems. It prevents uterine bleeding by inducing and maintaining a lining in the uterus that resembles the lining produced during pregnancy. In addition, it suppresses the release of the pituitary gland hormone that initiates ovulation.

ANTI-INFECTIVES

Antibiotics

Antibiotics are used to treat a wide variety of bacterial infections. They are usually derived from molds or are produced synthetically. Antibiotics inhibit the growth of bacteria by interfering with their production of certain biochemicals necessary to sustain life or by interfering with their ability to use available nutrients. The body's natural defenses then have a much easier time eliminating the infection.

When used properly, antibiotics are usually effective. To adequately treat an infection, antibiotics must be taken regularly for a specific period of time. If you do not take an antibiotic for the prescribed period, microorganisms resistant to the antibiotic are given the opportunity to continue growing, and your infection could recur. Aminoglycosides, cephalosporins, erythromycins, penicillins (including ampicillin and amoxicillin), and tetracyclines are examples of antibiotics.

Antibiotics do not counteract viruses, such as those causing the common cold, so their use in cold therapy is inappropriate.

Antivirals

Antiviral drugs are used to combat viral infections. An antiviral drug called acyclovir is being used in the management of herpes. Acyclovir reduces the reproduction of the herpes virus in initial outbreaks, lessens the number of recurring outbreaks, and speeds the healing of herpes blisters. However, this antiviral drug does not cure herpes.

Vaccines

Vaccines were used long before antibiotics became available. A vaccine contains weakened or dead disease-causing microorganisms or parts of such organisms, which activate the body's immune system to produce a natural defense against a particular disease (such as polio or measles). A vaccine may be used to alleviate or treat an infectious disease, but most commonly it is used to prevent a specific disease.

Other Anti-infectives

Drugs called anthelmintics are used to treat worm infestations. Fungal infections are treated with antifungals (such as nystatin)—drugs that destroy and prevent the growth of fungi.

A pediculicide is a drug used to treat a person infested with lice, and a scabicide is a preparation used to treat a person with scabies.

ANTINEOPLASTICS

Antineoplastic drugs are used in the treatment of cancer. Most of the drugs in this category prevent the growth of rapidly dividing cells, such as cancer cells. Antineoplastics are, without exception, extremely toxic and can cause serious side effects. But for many cancer victims, the benefits derived from chemotherapy with antineoplastic drugs far outweigh the risks involved.

TOPICAL DRUGS

Drugs are often applied topically (locally to the skin) to treat skin disorders with minimal systemic (throughout the body) side effects. Antibiotic creams or ointments are used to treat skin infections, and adrenocorticosteroids are used to treat inflammatory skin conditions. Another common dermatologic (skin) problem is acne. Acne can be—and often is—treated with over-the-counter drugs, but it sometimes requires prescription medication. Antibiotics such as tetracycline, erythromycin, or clindamycin are used orally or applied topically to slow the growth of the bacteria that play a role in the formation of acne pustules. Keratolytics (agents that soften the skin and cause the outer cells to slough off) are also sometimes prescribed.

Some drugs applied to the skin do have effects within the body. For example, nitroglycerin is absorbed into the bloodstream from ointment or patches placed on the skin. The absorbed nitroglycerin dilates blood vessels and prevents anginal pain. Clonidine, scopolamine, and estrogen are available as transdermal patches, also.

CENTRAL NERVOUS SYSTEM DRUGS

Sedatives

Medications used in the treatment of anxiety or insomnia selectively reduce activity in the central nervous system (brain and spinal cord). Drugs that have a calming effect include barbiturates, chlordiazepoxide, clorazepate, diazepam, doxepin, hydroxyzine, meprobamate, and oxazepam. Drugs to induce sleep in insomniacs include butabarbital, flurazepam, temazepam, and triazolam.

Tranquilizers

Major tranquilizers or antipsychotic agents are usually prescribed for patients with psychoses (certain types of mental disorders). These drugs calm certain areas of the brain but permit the rest of the brain to function normally. They act as a screen that allows transmission of some nerve impulses but restricts others. The drugs most frequently used are phenothiazines, such as chlorpromazine and thioridazine. Haloperidol, a butyrophenone, has the same effect as chlorpromazine.

Antidepressants

Tricyclic antidepressants (such as amitriptyline), tetracyclic antidepressants (such as maprotiline), and monoamine oxidase (MAO) inhibitors (such as phenelzine) are used to combat depression. Antidepressants are also used in the preventive treatment of migraine headaches, although the manner in which they help these headaches is not clearly understood.

Antidepressants may produce serious side effects, and they can interact with other drugs. MAO inhibitors can also interact with certain foods, resulting in dangerous increases in blood pressure. Therefore, they should be used very carefully.

Amphetamines

Amphetamines or adrenergic drugs are commonly used as anorectics (drugs used to reduce the appetite). These drugs temporarily quiet the part of the brain that causes hunger, but they also keep a person awake, speed up the heart, and raise blood pressure. After two to three weeks, these medications begin to lose their effectiveness as appetite suppressants.

Amphetamines stimulate most people, but they have the opposite effect on hyperkinetic children. Hyperkinesis (the condition of being highly overactive) is difficult to diagnose or define and requires a specialist to treat. When hyperkinetic children take amphetamines or the adrenergic drug methylphenidate, their activity slows down. Why amphetamines affect hyperkinetic children in this way is unknown. Most likely, they quiet these youngsters by selectively stimulating parts of the brain that ordinarily provide control of activity.

Anticonvulsants

Drugs such as phenytoin and phenobarbital are used to control seizures and other symptoms of epilepsy. They selectively reduce excessive stimulation in the brain.

Antiparkinsonism Agents

Parkinson's disease is a progressive disorder that is due to a chemical imbalance in the brain. Victims of Parkinson's disease have uncontrollable tremors, develop a characteristic stoop, and eventually become unable to walk. Drugs such as benztropine, trihexyphenidyl, levodopa, and bromocriptine are used to correct the chemical imbalance, thereby relieving the symptoms of the disease. Benztropine and trihexyphenidyl are also used to relieve tremors caused by other medications.

Analgesics

Pain is not a disease but a symptom. Drugs used to relieve pain are called analgesics. These drugs form a rather diverse group. We do not fully understand how most analgesics work. Whether they all act on the brain is not known. Analgesics fall into two categories; they may be either narcotic or nonnarcotic.

Narcotics are derived from the opium poppy. They act on the brain to cause deep analgesia and often drowsiness. Some narcotics relieve coughing spasms and are used in many cough syrups. Narcotics relieve pain and give the patient a feeling of well-being. They are also addictive. Manufacturers have attempted to produce nonaddictive synthetic narcotic derivatives but have not yet been successful.

Many nonnarcotic pain relievers are commonly used. Salicylates are the most commonly used pain relievers in the United States today. The most widely used salicylate is aspirin. While aspirin ordinarily does not require a prescription, many doctors may prescribe it to treat such diseases as arthritis.

The aspirin substitute acetaminophen may be used in place of aspirin to relieve pain. It does not, however, reduce inflammation (such as that caused by arthritis).

A number of analgesics contain codeine or other narcotics combined with nonnarcotic analgesics (such as aspirin or acetaminophen). These analgesics are not as potent as pure narcotics but are frequently as effective. Because these medications contain narcotics, they have potential for abuse and must be used with caution.

Anti-inflammatory Drugs

Inflammation is the body's response to injury. It causes swelling, pain, fever, redness, and itching. Aspirin is one of the most effective anti-inflammatory drugs. Other drugs, called nonsteroidal anti-inflammatory drugs (for example, fenoprofen, ibuprofen, indomethacin, naproxen, and tolmetin), relieve inflammation and may be more effective than aspirin in certain individuals. Steroids are also used to treat inflammatory diseases.

When sore muscles tense, they cause pain, inflammation, and spasm. Skeletal muscle relaxants (for example, orphenadrine, aspirin, and caffeine combination; meprobamate and aspirin combination; and chlorzoxazone and acetaminophen combination) can relieve these symptoms. Skeletal muscle relaxants are often given in combination with an anti-inflammatory drug such as aspirin. Some doctors, however, believe that aspirin and rest are better for alleviating the pain and inflammation of muscle strain than are skeletal muscle relaxants.

RESPIRATORY DRUGS

Antitussives

Antitussives control coughs. There are numerous over-the-counter (nonprescription) antitussives available—most of them contain dextromethorphan. Codeine is a narcotic antitussive that is an ingredient in many prescription cough medications. These cough syrups must be absorbed into the blood and must circulate and act on the brain before they relieve a cough; they do not "coat" the throat.

Expectorants

Expectorants are used to change a nonproductive cough to a productive one (one that brings up phlegm). Expectorants are supposed to increase the amount of mucus produced. However, drinking water or using a vaporizer or humidifier is probably more effective in increasing mucus production. Popular expectorant ingredients include ammonium chloride, guaifenesin, potassium guaiacolsulfonate, and terpin hydrate.

Decongestants

Decongestants constrict blood vessels in the nose and sinuses to open up air passages. They are available as oral preparations, nose drops, and nose sprays. Oral decongestants are slow-acting but do not interfere with production of mucus or movement of the cilia (special hair-like structures) of the respiratory tract. They can, however, increase blood pressure, so they should be used cautiously by patients with high blood pressure. Topical decongestants (nose drops or spray) provide almost immediate relief. They do not increase blood pressure as much as oral decongestants, but they do slow the movement of the cilia.

People who use these products may also develop a tolerance for them. Tolerance can be described as a need for ever-increasing dosages to achieve a beneficial effect. The additional disadvantage of developing tolerance is that the risk of side effects increases as the dosage increases. Consequently, topical decongestants should not be used for more than a few days at a time.

Bronchodilators

Bronchodilators (agents that open airways in the lungs) and agents that relax smooth-muscle tissue (such as that found in the lungs) are used to improve breathing. Theophylline and aminophylline are oral bronchodilators commonly used to relieve the symptoms of asthma and pulmonary emphysema. Albuterol and metaproterenol are inhalant bronchodilators, which act directly on the muscles of the bronchi (breathing tubes).

Antihistamines

Histamine is a body chemical that, when released in the body, typically causes swelling and itching. Antihistamines counteract these symptoms of allergy by blocking the effects of histamine. For mild respiratory allergies, such as hay fever, antihistamines can be used. Diphenhydramine and other antihistamines are relatively slow-acting. Severe allergic reactions sometimes require the use of epinephrine (which is not an antihistamine); in its injectable form, it is very fast-acting.

Some antihistamines are also used to prevent or treat the symptoms of motion sickness. Diphenhydramine and meclizine are examples of drugs used for this purpose.

VITAMINS AND MINERALS

Vitamins and minerals are chemical substances that are vital to the maintenance of normal body function. Most people obtain enough vitamins and minerals in their diet, but some people have vitamin deficiencies. Serious nutritional deficiencies lead to diseases such as pellagra and beriberi, which must be treated by a physician. People who have an inadequate or restricted diet, people who have certain disorders or debilitating illnesses, and women who are pregnant or breast-feeding are among those who may benefit from taking supplemental vitamins and minerals. However, even these people should consult a doctor to see if a true vitamin deficiency exists.

Drug Profiles

On the following pages are drug profiles for the most commonly prescribed drugs, as well as a few selected over-the-counter medications. These profiles are arranged alphabetically according to generic name.

A drug profile summarizes the most important information about a particular drug. By studying a drug profile, you will learn what to expect from your medication, when to be concerned about possible side effects, which drugs interact with the drug you are taking, and how to take the drug to achieve its maximum benefit. Each profile includes the following information:

generic name

The drugs profiled in this book are listed by generic names. You should know both the generic and the trade names of ALL of the medications you are taking. If you don't know the contents of your medication, check with your pharmacist.

BRAND NAMES (Manufacturers)
The most common trade names of each generic product are listed, along with the manufacturers' names. Not every available trade name is included, but as many as possible have been listed. "Various manufacturers" is listed for some of the generic names—this indicates that there are generic products available.

TYPE OF DRUG
The chemical or pharmacologic class or pharmacologic effect is listed for each generic drug.

INGREDIENTS
The components of each drug product are itemized. Many drugs contain several active chemical components; all are included under this category.

DOSAGE FORMS
The most common forms (for example, tablets, capsules, liquid, suppositories) of each profiled drug are listed, as well as the drug's alcohol content, if any. Strengths or concentrations are also provided.

STORAGE
Storage requirements for each of the dosage forms listed are discussed. These directions should be followed carefully, in order to ensure the potency of your medications.

USES

It is important that you understand why you are taking each of your medications. This section includes the most important and most common clinical uses for each drug profiled. Your doctor may prescribe a drug for a reason that does not appear in this list. The exclusion does not mean that your doctor has made an error. However, if the use for which you are taking a drug does not appear in this category and if you have any questions about why the drug was prescribed, consult your doctor. A description of how the drug is thought to work is also provided in this section.

TREATMENT

Instructions are provided on how to take each profiled medication in order to obtain its maximum benefit. Information can be found on whether the drug can be taken with food; how to apply the ointment, cream, ear drops, or eye drops; how to insert suppositories; and recommendations for what to do if you miss a dose of your medication.

SIDE EFFECTS

Minor. The most common and least serious reactions to a drug are listed in this section. Most of these side effects, if they occur, disappear in a day or two. Do not expect to experience these side effects; but if they occur and are particularly annoying, do not hesitate to seek medical advice.

Suggestions for preventing or relieving some of these side effects are also provided.

Major. Major side effects are less common than minor side effects, and you will probably never experience them. However, should any of the reactions listed in this section occur, you should call your doctor. These reactions indicate that something may be going wrong with your drug therapy. You may have developed an allergy to the drug, or some other problem could have occurred. If you experience a major side effect, it may be necessary to adjust your dosage or to substitute a different medication in your treatment. It is important to discuss this with your doctor.

Keep in mind that new side effects are being reported daily. If you experience a reaction that is bothersome or severe, consult your doctor immediately, even if the side effect is not listed.

INTERACTIONS

This section lists the medications (both prescription and over-the-counter drugs) and foods that can interact with the profiled drug. Certain drugs are safe when used alone but may cause serious reactions when taken in combination with other drugs or chemicals or with certain foods. A description of how the profiled drug interacts with other drugs or foods and what to expect if the two are taken together is also provided. Keep in mind that not all possible drug combinations have been tested. It is, therefore, important that your pharmacist and health care providers be aware of ALL of the drugs you are taking (both prescription and over-the-counter).

WARNINGS

This section lists the precautions necessary for safe use of the profiled drug. It provides information on drugs that should be avoided if you have had a previous allergic reaction or severe drug reaction, as well as information on the conditions or disease states that require close monitoring while this drug is being taken.

In this section you will also find out whether the profiled drug is likely to affect your driving ability, whether you are likely to become tolerant to its effects, if it is dangerous to stop taking the drug abruptly, and if you should discuss with your doctor stopping the drug before having surgery or any other medical or dental procedure.

Certain individuals are allergic to the color additive FD&C Yellow No. 5 (tartrazine). This section provides information on the tartrazine content of the various dosage forms.

Other information included in this category might concern supplemental therapy—for example, drinking extra fluids while treating a urinary tract infection or wearing cotton panties while treating a vaginal infection.

A discussion of the known risks of treatment with this drug during pregnancy or while breast-feeding an infant is provided. It should be kept in mind that for the majority of drugs available, the risks to a fetus or to a nursing infant are not known. Experiments are not usually conducted on pregnant women and infants (for ethical reasons). You should, therefore, discuss the risks and benefits of any particular drug therapy with your doctor if you are pregnant, are planning to become pregnant, or are nursing an infant.

Accurbron—see theophylline

Accutane—see isotretinoin

---

acebutolol

BRAND NAME (Manufacturer)
Sectral (Wyeth-Ayerst)
TYPE OF DRUG
Beta-adrenergic blocking agent
INGREDIENT
acebutolol
DOSAGE FORM
Capsules (200 mg and 400 mg)
STORAGE
Acebutolol should be stored at room temperature in a tightly closed container.

USES

Acebutolol is used to treat high blood pressure or irregular heartbeat. Acebutolol belongs to a group of medicines known as beta-adrenergic blocking agents or, more commonly, beta blockers. These drugs work by controlling impulses along certain nerve pathways.

TREATMENT

Acebutolol can be taken either on an empty stomach or with food or milk (as directed by your doctor). In order to become accustomed to taking this medication, try to take it at the same time(s) each day.

If you miss a dose of this medication, take the missed dose as soon as possible, unless it is almost time for your next dose. In that case, do not take the missed dose at all; just wait until the next scheduled dose. Do not double the next dose of the medication.

It is important to remember that acebutolol does not cure high blood pressure, but it will help to control the condition as long as you continue to take it.

SIDE EFFECTS

Minor. Abdominal pain, anxiety, constipation, diarrhea, dizziness, dry eyes, fatigue, gas, headache, heartburn, nausea, runny nose, sleeping problems, or vomiting. These side effects should disappear as your body adjusts to this medication.

If you are extra-sensitive to the cold, be sure to dress warmly during cold weather.

Plain, nonmedicated eye drops (artificial tears) may help to relieve eye dryness.

To relieve constipation, increase the amount of fiber in your diet (bran, fresh fruits and vegetables, salads, and whole-grain breads) unless your doctor directs you to do otherwise.

If you feel dizzy, sit or lie down for a while; get up slowly from a sitting or reclining position, and be careful on stairs.

Major. Tell your doctor about any side effects that are persistent or particularly bothersome. IT IS ESPECIALLY IMPORTANT TO TELL YOUR DOCTOR about chest pain; cold fingers or feet (due to decreased blood circulation to skin, fingers, and toes); confusion; cough; depression; fluid accumulation; hair loss; impotence; itching; muscle, joint, or back pain; numbness; rash; shortness of breath; sore throat; swelling of the feet; unusual bleeding or bruising; urination problems; visual disturbances or eye pain; or wheezing.

INTERACTIONS

Acebutolol may interact with other types of medications:

1. Indomethacin, other nonsteroidal anti-inflammatory agents, aspirin, or other salicylates may decrease the blood-pressure-lowering effects of beta blockers.

2. Concurrent use of beta blockers and calcium channel blockers (diltiazem, nifedipine, and verapamil) or disopyramide can lead to heart failure or very low blood pressure.

3. Side effects may also be increased if beta blockers are taken with digoxin, epinephrine, phenylephrine, phenylpropanolamine, phenothiazine tranquilizers, reserpine, clonidine, prazosin, or monoamine oxidase (MAO) inhibitors. At least 14 days should separate the use of a beta blocker and the use of an MAO inhibitor.

4. Beta blockers may antagonize (work against) the effects of theophylline, aminophylline, albuterol, isoproterenol, metaproterenol, and terbutaline.

5. Beta blockers can also interact with insulin or oral antidiabetic agents—raising or lowering blood sugar levels or masking the symptoms of low blood sugar.

6. The action of beta blockers may be increased if they are used with chlorpromazine, cimetidine, furosemide, hydralazine, or oral contraceptives (birth control pills), which could have a negative effect.

7. Alcohol, barbiturates, and rifampin can decrease blood concentrations of this drug, which can result in a decrease of effectiveness.

Before starting acebutolol, BE SURE TO TELL YOUR DOCTOR about any medications you are already taking, especially any of the medications listed above.

WARNINGS

Before starting this medication, it is important to tell your doctor about any unusual or allergic reactions you have had to any medications, especially to acebutolol or any other beta blocker (atenolol, betaxolol, carteolol, esmolol, labetalol, metoprolol, nadolol, penbutolol, pindolol, propranolol, timolol).

- Tell your doctor if you now have or if you have ever had asthma, bronchitis, diabetes mellitus, heart block, heart failure, kidney disease, liver disease, peripheral vascular disease (poor circulation in the fingers or toes), severe bradycardia (slowed heart rate), or thyroid disease.
- You may want to check your pulse while taking this medication. If your pulse is much slower than your usual rate (or if it is less than 50 beats per minute), check with your doctor. A pulse rate that is too slow may cause circulation problems.

• This medicine may affect your body's response to exercise. Ask your doctor what an appropriate amount of exercise would be for you, taking into account your medical condition.
• It is important that you do not stop taking this medicine without first checking with your doctor. Some conditions may become worse when the medicine is stopped suddenly, and the danger of a heart attack is increased in some patients. Your doctor may want you to gradually reduce the amount of medicine you take before stopping completely. Make sure that you have enough medicine on hand to last through vacations, holidays, and weekends.
• Before having surgery or any other medical or dental treatment, tell your physician or dentist that you are taking this medicine. Often, this medication will be discontinued 48 hours prior to any major surgery.
• While taking this medicine, do not use any over-the-counter (nonprescription) allergy, asthma, cough, cold, sinus, or diet preparation without first checking with your pharmacist or doctor. The combination of these medicines with a beta blocker can result in high blood pressure.
• Be sure to tell your doctor if you are pregnant. Although acebutolol appears to be safe in animals, studies in pregnant women have not been conducted. Also, tell your doctor if you are breast-feeding an infant. Small amounts of acebutolol may pass into human breast milk.

---

acetaminophen and codeine combination

BRAND NAMES (Manufacturers)
acetaminophen with codeine (various manufacturers)
Aceta with Codeine (Century)
Capital with Codeine (Carnrick)
Phenaphen-650 with Codeine (Robins)
Phenaphen with Codeine (Robins)
Tylenol with Codeine (McNeil)
Ty-tabs (Major)

TYPE OF DRUG
Analgesic combination

INGREDIENTS
acetaminophen and codeine

DOSAGE FORMS
Tablets (300 mg acetaminophen with 7.5 mg, 15 mg, 30 mg, or 60 mg codeine; 325 mg acetaminophen with 30 mg or 60 mg codeine; 650 mg acetaminophen with 30 mg codeine)
Capsules (325 mg acetaminophen with 15 mg, 30 mg, or 60 mg codeine)
Oral elixir (120 mg acetaminophen and 12 mg codeine per 5-ml spoonful, with 7% alcohol)
Note that on the label of the vial of tablets or capsules, the name of this drug is followed by a number. This number refers to the amount of codeine present (#1 contains 7.5 mg codeine, #2 has 15 mg codeine, #3 has 30 mg codeine, and #4 contains 60 mg codeine).

STORAGE
This medication should be stored at room temperature. It should never be frozen.

USES

Acetaminophen and codeine combination is used to relieve mild to severe pain (formulations with higher codeine contents are used to relieve more severe pain). Codeine is a narcotic analgesic that acts on the central nervous system (brain and spinal cord) to relieve pain.

TREATMENT

In order to avoid stomach upset, you can take this medication with food or milk.

This medication works most effectively if you take it at the onset of pain, rather than waiting until the pain becomes intense.

Measure the dose of the liquid form of this medication carefully with a specially designed 5-ml measuring spoon. An ordinary kitchen teaspoon is not accurate enough for measuring the dosage.

If you are taking this medication on a regular schedule and you miss a dose, take the missed dose as soon as possible, unless it is almost time for the next dose. In that case, don't take the missed dose at all; just return to your regular dosing schedule. Do not double the next dose.

SIDE EFFECTS

Minor. Constipation, dizziness, drowsiness, dry mouth, false sense of well-being, flushing, light-headedness, loss of appetite, nausea, painful or difficult urination, or sweating. These side effects should disappear as your body adjusts to the medication.

If you are constipated, increase the amount of fiber in your diet (fresh fruits and vegetables, salads, bran, and whole-grain breads), exercise, and drink more water (unless your doctor directs you to do otherwise).

To reduce mouth dryness, chew sugarless gum or suck on ice chips or hard candy.

If you feel dizzy or light-headed, sit or lie down for a while; get up slowly from a sitting or reclining position, and be careful on stairs.

Major. Tell your doctor about any side effects that are persistent or particularly bothersome. IT IS ESPECIALLY IMPORTANT TO TELL YOUR DOCTOR about anxiety, difficulty in breathing, excitation, fatigue, palpitations, rash, restlessness, sore throat and fever, tremors, unusual bleeding or bruising, weakness, or yellowing of the eyes or skin.

INTERACTIONS

This medication interacts with several other types of drugs:

1. Concurrent use with other central nervous system depressants (such as alcohol, antihistamines, barbiturates, benzodiazepine tranquilizers, muscle relaxants, and phenothiazine tranquilizers) or with tricyclic antidepressants can cause extreme drowsiness.

2. A monoamine oxidase (MAO) inhibitor taken within 14 days of this medication can lead to unpredictable and severe side effects.

3. Long-term use and high doses of the acetaminophen portion of this medication can increase the effects of oral anticoagulants (blood thinners, such as warfarin); this combination may lead to bleeding complications.

4. Anticonvulsants (antiseizure medications), barbiturates, and alcohol can increase the liver toxicity caused by large doses of the acetaminophen portion of this medication.

BE SURE TO TELL YOUR DOCTOR about any medications you are currently taking, especially any listed above.

WARNINGS

- Tell your doctor about unusual or allergic reactions you have had to any medications, especially to acetaminophen, codeine, or other narcotic analgesics (such as hydrocodone, hydromorphone, meperidine, methadone, morphine, oxycodone, and propoxyphene).
- Tell your doctor if you now have or if you have ever had an acute abdominal condition, asthma, a blood disorder, brain disease, colitis, epilepsy, gallstones or gallbladder disease, head injuries, heart disease, kidney disease, liver disease, lung disease, mental illness, prostate disease, thyroid disease, or urethral strictures.
- If this drug makes you dizzy or drowsy, do not take part in any activity that requires alertness, such as driving a car or operating potentially dangerous equipment.
- Before having surgery or any other medical or dental treatment, be sure to tell your doctor or dentist that you are taking this medication.
- Because this product contains codeine, it has the potential for abuse and must be used with caution. Usually, it should not be taken on a regular schedule for longer than ten days at a time. Tolerance develops quickly; do not increase the dosage or stop taking the drug abruptly unless you first consult your doctor. If you have been taking large amounts of this medication for long periods, you may experience a withdrawal reaction (diarrhea, excessive yawning, gooseflesh, irritability, muscle aches, nausea, runny nose, shivering, sleep disorders, stomach cramps, sweating, trembling, vomiting, or weakness). Your doctor may, therefore, want to reduce the dosage gradually.
- Because this product contains acetaminophen, additional drugs that contain acetaminophen should not be taken without your doctor's approval. Be sure to check the labels on over-the-counter pain, sinus, allergy, asthma, diet, cough, and cold products before you use them in order to see if they contain acetaminophen.
- Be sure to tell your doctor if you are pregnant. The effects of this medication during pregnancy have not been thoroughly studied in humans. Codeine used regularly in large doses during pregnancy can result in addiction of the fetus, leading to withdrawal symptoms (diarrhea, excessive crying, excessive yawning, irritability, fever, sneezing, tremors, or vomiting) at birth. Also, tell your doctor if you are breast-feeding an infant. Small amounts of this drug may pass into breast milk and cause drowsiness in the nursing infant.

---

acetaminophen and hydrocodone combination

BRAND NAMES (Manufacturers)

Amacodone (Trimen)
Bancap HC (Forest)
Co-Gesic (Central)
Dolacet (Hauck)
Duradyne DHC (Forest)
Hydrogesic (Edwards)
Hy-Phen (Ascher)
Lortab 5 (Russ)*
Norcet (Abana)*
T-Gesic (T.E. Williams)
Vicodin (Knoll)
Zydone (DuPont)
*Available in different strengths

TYPE OF DRUG

Analgesic combination

INGREDIENTS

acetaminophen and hydrocodone

DOSAGE FORMS

Tablets (500 mg acetaminophen with 2.5 mg, 5 mg, or 7.5 mg hydrocodone; 650 mg acetaminophen with 7.5 mg hydrocodone; 750 mg acetaminophen with 7.5 mg hydrocodone)
Capsules (500 mg acetaminophen with 5 mg hydrocodone)
Liquid (120 mg acetaminophen with 2.5 mg hydrocodone per 5-ml spoonful, with 7% alcohol)

STORAGE

Acetaminophen and hydrocodone combination tablets, capsules, and liquid should be stored at room temperature in tightly closed, light-resistant containers.

USES

This medication is used to relieve moderate to severe pain. Hydrocodone is a narcotic analgesic that acts on the central nervous system (brain and spinal cord) to relieve pain.

TREATMENT

To avoid stomach upset, take this drug with food or milk.

Each dose of the oral liquid form of this medication should be measured carefully with a specially designed 5-ml measuring spoon. An ordinary kitchen teaspoon is not accurate enough.

This medication works most effectively if you take it at the onset of pain, rather than waiting until the pain becomes intense.

If you are taking this medication on a regular schedule and you miss a dose, take the missed dose as soon as possible, unless it is almost time for your next dose. In that case, don't take the missed dose at all; just return to your regular dosing schedule. Do not double the next dose.

SIDE EFFECTS

Minor. Constipation, dizziness, dry mouth, false sense of well-being, flushing, light-headedness, loss of appetite, nausea, painful or difficult urination, or sweating. These side effects should disappear as your body adjusts to the medication.

If you are constipated, increase the amount of fiber in your diet (fresh fruits and vegetables, salads, bran, and whole-grain breads), exercise, and drink more water (unless your doctor directs you to do otherwise).

To reduce mouth dryness, chew sugarless gum or suck on ice chips or hard candy.

If you feel dizzy or light-headed, sit or lie down for a while; get up from a sitting or reclining position slowly, and be careful on stairs.

Major. Tell your doctor about any side effects that are persistent or particularly bothersome. IT IS ESPECIALLY IMPORTANT TO TELL YOUR DOCTOR about anxiety, difficulty in breathing, excitation, fatigue, palpitations, rash, restlessness, sore throat and fever, tremors, unusual bleeding or bruising, weakness, or yellowing of the eyes or skin.

INTERACTIONS

This medication interacts with several other types of drugs:

1. Concurrent use of this medication with other central nervous system depressants (such as alcohol, antihistamines, barbiturates, benzodiazepine tranquilizers, muscle relaxants, and phenothiazine tranquilizers) or with tricyclic antidepressants can cause extreme drowsiness.

2. A monoamine oxidase (MAO) inhibitor taken within 14 days of this drug can lead to unpredictable and severe side effects.

3. Long-term use and high doses of the acetaminophen portion of this medication can increase the effects of oral anticoagulants (blood thinners, such as warfarin); this combination may lead to bleeding complications.

4. Anticonvulsants (antiseizure medications), barbiturates, and alcohol can increase the liver toxicity caused by large doses of the acetaminophen portion of this medication.

BE SURE TO TELL YOUR DOCTOR about any medications you are currently taking, especially any of those listed above.

WARNINGS

- Tell your doctor about unusual or allergic reactions you have had to any medications, especially to acetaminophen, hydrocodone, or other narcotic analgesics (such as codeine, hydromorphone, meperidine, methadone, morphine, oxycodone, and propoxyphene).
- Tell your doctor if you now have or if you have ever had acute abdominal conditions, asthma, blood disorders, brain disease, colitis, epilepsy, gallstones or gallbladder disease, a head injury, heart disease, kidney disease, liver disease, lung disease, mental illness, prostate disease, thyroid disease, or urethral strictures.
- If this drug makes you dizzy or drowsy, do not take part in any activity that requires alertness, such as driving a car or operating potentially dangerous equipment.
- Before having surgery or any other medical or dental treatment, be sure to tell your doctor or dentist that you are taking this medication.
- Because this product contains hydrocodone, it has the potential for abuse and must be used with caution. Usually, it should not be taken on a regular schedule for longer than ten days at a time. Tolerance develops quickly; do not increase the dosage or stop taking the drug abruptly unless you first consult your doctor. If you have been taking large amounts of this medication for long periods, you may experience a withdrawal reaction (diarrhea, excessive yawning, gooseflesh, irritability, muscle aches, nausea, runny nose, shivering, sleep disorders, stomach cramps, sweating, trembling, vomiting, or weakness). Your doctor may, therefore, want to reduce the dosage gradually.
- Because this product contains acetaminophen, additional medications that contain acetaminophen should not be taken without your doctor's approval. Check the labels on over-the-counter (nonprescription) pain, sinus, allergy, asthma, diet, cough, and cold products to see if they contain acetaminophen.
- Be sure to tell your doctor if you are pregnant. The effects of this medication during pregnancy have not been thoroughly studied in humans. Regular use of hydrocodone in large doses during pregnancy can result in addiction of the fetus, leading to withdrawal symptoms (diarrhea, excessive crying, excessive yawning, fever, irritability, sneezing, tremors, or vomiting) at birth. Also, tell your doctor if you are breast-feeding an infant. Small amounts of this medication may pass into breast milk and cause excessive drowsiness in the nursing infant.

---

acetaminophen and oxycodone combination

BRAND NAMES (Manufacturers)
oxycodone hydrochloride with acetaminophen (various manufacturers)
Percocet (DuPont)
Tylox (McNeil)

TYPE OF DRUG
Analgesic combination

INGREDIENTS
acetaminophen and oxycodone

DOSAGE FORM
Tablets (325 mg acetaminophen with 5 mg oxycodone; 500 mg acetaminophen with 5 mg oxycodone)

STORAGE
Acetaminophen and oxycodone tablets should be stored at room temperature in a tightly closed container.

USES

Acetaminophen and oxycodone combination is used to relieve moderate to severe pain. Oxycodone is a narcotic analgesic that acts on the central nervous system (brain and spinal cord) to relieve pain.

TREATMENT

In order to avoid stomach upset, you can take this medication with food or milk.

This medication works most effectively if you take it at the onset of pain, rather than waiting until the pain becomes intense.

If you are taking this medication on a regular schedule and you miss a dose, take the missed dose as soon as possible, unless it is almost time for your next dose. In that case, don't take the missed dose at all; just return to your regular dosing schedule. Do not double the next dose.

SIDE EFFECTS

Minor. Constipation, dizziness, drowsiness, dry mouth, false sense of well-being, flushing, light-headedness, loss of appetite, nausea, painful or difficult urination, or sweating. These side effects should disappear as your body adjusts to the medication.

If you are constipated, increase the amount of fiber in your diet (fresh fruits and vegetables, salads, bran, and whole-grain breads), exercise, and drink more water (unless your doctor directs you to do otherwise).

To reduce mouth dryness, chew sugarless gum or suck on ice chips or hard candy.

If you feel dizzy or light-headed, sit or lie down for a while; get up from a sitting or reclining position slowly, and be careful on stairs.

Major. Tell your doctor about any side effects that are persistent or particularly bothersome. IT IS ESPECIALLY IMPORTANT TO TELL YOUR DOCTOR about anxiety, difficulty in breathing, excitation, fatigue, palpitations, rash, restlessness, sore throat and fever, tremors, unusual bleeding or bruising, weakness, or yellowing of the eyes or skin.

INTERACTIONS

This medication interacts with several other types of drugs:

1. Concurrent use of this medication with other central nervous system depressants (such as alcohol, antihistamines, barbiturates, benzodiazepine tranquilizers, muscle relaxants, and phenothiazine tranquilizers) or with tricyclic antidepressants can cause extreme drowsiness.

2. A monoamine oxidase (MAO) inhibitor taken within 14 days of this medication can lead to unpredictable and severe side effects.

3. Long-term use and high doses of the acetaminophen portion of this medication can increase the effects of oral anticoagulants (blood thinners, such as warfarin); this combination may lead to bleeding complications.

4. Anticonvulsants (antiseizure medications), barbiturates, and alcohol can increase the liver toxicity caused by large doses of the acetaminophen portion of this medication.

BE SURE TO TELL YOUR DOCTOR about any medications you are currently taking, especially any listed above.

WARNINGS

- Tell your doctor about unusual or allergic reactions you have had to any medications, especially to acetaminophen, oxycodone, or other narcotic analgesics (such as codeine, hydrocodone, hydromorphone, meperidine, methadone, morphine, and propoxyphene).
- Tell your doctor if you now have or if you have ever had an acute abdominal condition, asthma, blood disorders, brain disease, colitis, epilepsy, gallstones or gallbladder disease, head injuries, heart disease, kidney disease, liver disease, lung disease, mental illness, prostate disease, thyroid disease, or urethral strictures.
- If this drug makes you dizzy or drowsy, do not take part in any activity that requires alertness, such as driving a car or operating potentially dangerous equipment.
- Before having surgery or any other medical or dental treatment, be sure to tell your doctor or dentist that you are taking this medication.
- Because this product contains oxycodone, it has the potential for abuse and must be used with caution. Usually, it should not be taken on a regular schedule for longer than ten days at a time. Tolerance develops quickly; do not increase the dosage or stop taking the drug abruptly unless you first consult your doctor. If you have been taking large amounts of this medication for long periods, you may experience a withdrawal reaction (muscle aches, diarrhea, gooseflesh, runny nose, nausea, vomiting, shivering, trembling, stomach cramps, sleep disorders, irritability, weakness, excessive yawning, or sweating). Your doctor may, therefore, want to reduce the dosage gradually.
- Because this product contains acetaminophen, additional medications that contain acetaminophen should not be taken without your doctor's approval. Check the labels on over-the-counter (nonprescription) pain, sinus, allergy, asthma, diet, cough, and cold products to see if they contain acetaminophen.
- Be sure to tell your doctor if you are pregnant. The effects of this medication during pregnancy have not been thoroughly studied in humans. Oxycodone, used regularly in large doses during pregnancy, can result in addiction of the fetus, leading to withdrawal symptoms (irritability, excessive crying, tremors, fever, vomiting, diarrhea, sneezing, or excessive yawning) at birth. Also, tell your doctor if you are breast-feeding an infant. Small amounts of this medication may pass into breast milk and cause excessive drowsiness in the nursing infant.

---

acetaminophen and propoxyphene combination

BRAND NAMES (Manufacturers)

Darvocet-N 50 (Lilly)
Darvocet-N 100 (Lilly)
Dolene AP-65 (Lederle)
Genagesic (Goldline)
Propacet 100 (Lemmon)
propoxyphene hydrochloride with acetaminophen (various manufacturers)
Wygesic (Wyeth)

TYPE OF DRUG

Analgesic combination

INGREDIENTS

acetaminophen and propoxyphene

DOSAGE FORMS

Tablets (325 mg acetaminophen with 50 mg propoxyphene napsylate; 650 mg acetaminophen with 100 mg propoxyphene napsylate; 650 mg acetaminophen with 65 mg propoxyphene hydrochloride)
Capsules (650 mg acetaminophen with 65 mg propoxyphene hydrochloride)

STORAGE

Acetaminophen and propoxyphene combination tablets and capsules should be stored at room temperature in tightly closed containers.

USES

This medication is used to relieve moderate to severe pain. Propoxyphene is a narcotic analgesic that acts on the central nervous system (brain and spinal cord) to relieve pain.

TREATMENT

In order to avoid stomach upset, you can take this medication with food or milk.

This medication works most effectively if you take it at the onset of pain, rather than waiting until the pain becomes intense.

If you are taking this medication on a regular schedule and you miss a dose, take the missed dose as soon as possible, unless it is almost time for the next dose. In that case, don't take the missed dose at all; just return to your regular dosing schedule. Do not double the next dose.

SIDE EFFECTS

Minor. Constipation, dizziness, drowsiness, dry mouth, false sense of well-being, flushing, light-headedness, loss of appetite, nausea, painful or difficult urination, or sweating. These side effects should disappear as your body adjusts to the drug.

If you are constipated, increase the amount of fiber in your diet (fresh fruits and vegetables, salads, bran, and whole-grain breads), exercise, and drink more water (unless your doctor directs you to do otherwise).

To reduce mouth dryness, chew sugarless gum or suck on ice chips or hard candy.

If you feel dizzy or light-headed, sit or lie down for a while; get up from a sitting or lying position slowly, and be careful on stairs.

Major. Tell your doctor about any side effects that are persistent or particularly bothersome. IT IS ESPECIALLY IMPORTANT TO TELL YOUR DOCTOR about anxiety, difficulty in breathing, excitation, fatigue, palpitations, rash, restlessness, sore throat and fever, tremors, unusual bleeding or bruising, weakness, or yellowing of the eyes or skin.

INTERACTIONS

This medication interacts with several other types of drugs:

1. Concurrent use of this medication with other central nervous system depressants (such as alcohol, antihistamines, barbiturates, benzodiazepine tranquilizers, muscle relaxants, and phenothiazine tranquilizers) or with tricyclic antidepressants can cause extreme drowsiness.

2. A monoamine oxidase (MAO) inhibitor taken within 14 days of this medication can lead to unpredictable and severe side effects.

3. Long-term use and high doses of the acetaminophen portion of this medication can increase the effects of oral anticoagulants (blood thinners, such as warfarin); this combination may lead to bleeding complications.

4. Anticonvulsants (antiseizure medication), barbiturates, and alcohol can increase the liver toxicity caused by large doses of the acetaminophen portion of this medication.

5. The propoxyphene portion of this medication decreases the elimination of carbamazepine from the body, which can lead to an increase in side effects.

Before starting to take this medication, BE SURE TO TELL YOUR DOCTOR about any medications you are currently taking, especially any of those listed above.

WARNINGS

- Tell your doctor about unusual or allergic reactions you have had to any medications, especially to acetaminophen, propoxyphene, or other narcotic analgesics (such as codeine, hydrocodone, hydromorphone, meperidine, methadone, morphine, and oxycodone).
- Tell your doctor if you now have or if you have ever had an acute abdominal condition, asthma, a blood disorder, brain disease, colitis, epilepsy, gallstones or gallbladder disease, a head injury, heart disease, kidney disease, liver disease, lung disease, mental illness, prostate disease, thyroid disease, or urethral strictures.
- If this drug makes you dizzy or drowsy, do not take part in any activity that requires alertness, such as driving a car or operating potentially dangerous equipment.
- Before having surgery or any other medical or dental treatment, be sure to tell your doctor or dentist that you are taking this medication.
- Because this product contains propoxyphene, it has the potential for abuse and must be used with caution. Usually, it should not be taken on a regular schedule for longer than ten days at a time. Tolerance develops quickly; do not increase the dosage or stop taking the drug abruptly unless you first consult your doctor. If you have been taking large amounts of this medication for long periods, you may experience a withdrawal reaction (muscle aches, diarrhea, gooseflesh, runny nose, nausea, vomiting, shivering, trembling, stomach cramps, sleep disorders, irritability, weakness, excessive yawning, or sweating). Your doctor may, therefore, want to reduce the dosage gradually to prevent or minimize this response.
- Because this product contains acetaminophen, additional medications that contain acetaminophen should not be taken without your doctor's approval. Check the labels on over-the-counter (nonprescription) pain, sinus, allergy, asthma, diet, cough, and cold products to see if they contain acetaminophen.
- Be sure to tell your doctor if you are pregnant. The effects of this medication during pregnancy have not been thoroughly studied in humans. Propoxyphene used regularly in large doses during pregnancy can result in addiction of the fetus, leading to withdrawal symptoms (irritability, excessive crying, tremors, fever, vomiting, diarrhea, sneezing, or excessive yawning) at birth. Also, tell your doctor if you are breast-feeding an infant. Small amounts of this medication may pass into breast milk and cause excessive drowsiness in the nursing infant.

acetaminophen with codeine—see acetaminophen and codeine combination

Aceta with Codeine—see acetaminophen and codeine combination

---

acetazolamide

BRAND NAMES (Manufacturers)
acetazolamide (various manufacturers)
AK-Zol (Akorn)
Dazamide (Major)
Diamox (Lederle)
Diamox Sequels (Lederle)

TYPE OF DRUG
Carbonic anhydrase inhibitor

INGREDIENT
acetazolamide

DOSAGE FORMS
Tablets (125 mg and 250 mg)
Sustained-release capsules (500 mg)

STORAGE
Acetazolamide tablets and capsules should be stored at room temperature in tightly closed containers.

USES

This medication is used to treat glaucoma, epilepsy, and edema (fluid retention) and to prevent or treat the symptoms of mountain sickness. It is unclear exactly how acetazolamide works.

TREATMENT

In order to avoid stomach irritation, you can take acetazolamide with food or with a full glass of water or milk (unless your doctor directs you to do otherwise).

The sustained-release form of this medication should be swallowed whole. Chewing, crushing, or breaking these capsules destroys their sustained-release activity and possibly increases the side effects.

If you miss a dose of this medication, take the missed dose as soon as possible, unless it is almost time for the next dose. In that case, do not take the missed dose; just return to your regular dosing schedule. Do not double the next dose.

SIDE EFFECTS

Minor. Confusion, drowsiness, increased urination, loss of appetite, or a tingling feeling. These side effects should disappear as your body adjusts to the medication.

Major. Tell your doctor about any side effects that are persistent or particularly bothersome. IT IS ESPECIALLY IMPORTANT TO TELL YOUR DOCTOR about bloody or black, tarry stools; blurred vision; convulsions; difficult or painful urination; fever; rash; unusual bleeding or bruising; or yellowing of the eyes or skin.

INTERACTIONS

Acetazolamide interacts with other types of medications:

1. Acetazolamide can decrease the excretion through the kidneys of amphetamines, ephedrine, flecainide, mexiletine, pseudoephedrine, tocainide, and quinidine, which can lead to an increased risk of side effects with these medications. Acetazolamide can also increase the side effects (to the bones) of phenobarbital, phenytoin, and primidone.

2. Dosage adjustments of insulin or oral antidiabetic medications may be necessary when this medication is started.

3. The therapeutic benefits of methenamine, methotrexate, lithium, or large doses of aspirin may be decreased by acetazolamide.

Before starting to take acetazolamide tablets or capsules, BE SURE TO TELL YOUR DOCTOR about any medications that you are currently taking, especially any of the medications that are listed above.

WARNINGS

- Tell your doctor about unusual or allergic reactions you have had to any medications, especially to acetazolamide, methazolamide, sulfonamide antibiotics, diuretics (water pills), oral antidiabetics, dapsone, sulfone, or sulfoxone.
- Before starting to take this medication, be sure to tell your doctor if you now have or if you have ever had acidosis, Addison's disease (underactive adrenal gland), diabetes mellitus, electrolyte disorders, gout, kidney disease, or liver disease.
- If this drug makes you dizzy or drowsy, avoid taking part in any activity that requires alertness, such as driving a car or operating potentially dangerous equipment.
- Although several generic versions of this drug are available, you should not switch from one brand to another without your doctor's or pharmacist's approval. Not all of these products are equivalent.
- Tolerance to this drug can develop quickly. Check with your doctor if you feel this drug is losing effectiveness.
- Be sure to tell your doctor if you are pregnant. Although this drug appears to be safe in humans, birth defects have been reported in the offspring of animals that received large doses during pregnancy. Also, tell your doctor if you are breast-feeding an infant. It is not known whether acetazolamide passes into breast milk.

---

acetohexamide

BRAND NAME (Manufacturer)
Dymelor (Lilly)

TYPE OF DRUG
Oral antidiabetic

INGREDIENT
acetohexamide

DOSAGE FORM
Tablets (250 mg and 500 mg)

STORAGE
This medication should be stored at room temperature in a tightly closed container.

USES

Acetohexamide is used for the treatment of diabetes mellitus (sugar diabetes) that appears in adulthood and cannot be managed by control of diet alone. This type of diabetes is known as non-insulin-dependent diabetes (sometimes called maturity-onset or Type II diabetes). Acetohexamide lowers blood sugar by increasing the release of insulin from the pancreas.

TREATMENT

In order for this medication to work correctly, it must be taken as directed by your doctor. It is best to take this medicine at the same time each day in order to maintain a constant blood sugar level. It is important, therefore, to try not to miss any doses of this medication. If you do miss a dose, take it as soon as possible, unless it is almost time for the next dose. In that case, do not take the missed dose at all; just return to your regular dosing schedule. Do not double the next dose. Tell your doctor if you feel any side effects from missing a dose of this drug.

Diabetics who are taking oral antidiabetic medication may need to be switched to insulin if they develop diabetic coma, have a severe infection, are scheduled for major surgery, or become pregnant.

SIDE EFFECTS

Minor. Diarrhea, headache, heartburn, loss of appetite, nausea, vomiting, or stomach pain or discomfort. These side effects usually disappear during treatment, as your body adjusts to the medication.

Acetohexamide may increase your sensitivity to sunlight. It is, therefore, important to use caution during exposure to the sun. You may want to wear protective clothing and sunglasses. Use an effective sunscreen, and avoid exposure to sunlamps.

Major. If any of the side effects you experience are persistent or particularly bothersome, it is important to notify your doctor. IT IS ESPECIALLY IMPORTANT TO TELL YOUR DOCTOR about dark urine, fatigue, itching of the skin, light-colored stools, rash, sore throat and fever, unusual bleeding or bruising, or yellowing of the eyes or skin.

INTERACTIONS

Acetohexamide interacts with a number of other types of medications:

1. When combined with acetohexamide, chloramphenicol, fenfluramine, guanethidine, insulin, miconazole, monoamine oxidase (MAO) inhibitors, oxyphenbutazone, oxytetracycline, phenylbutazone, probenecid, aspirin or other salicylates, sulfinpyrazone, and sulfonamide antibiotics can lower blood sugar levels—sometimes to dangerously low levels.

2. When combined with acetohexamide, thyroid hormones, dextrothyroxine, epinephrine, phenytoin, thiazide diuretics (water pills), and cortisone-like medications (such as dexamethasone, hydrocortisone, and prednisone) can actually increase blood sugar levels—just what you are trying to avoid.

3. Rifampin can decrease the blood concentrations of acetohexamide, which can lead to a decrease in its effectiveness.

4. Oral antidiabetic medications can increase the effects of warfarin, which can lead to bleeding complications.

5. Beta-blocking medications (such as acebutolol, atenolol, labetalol, metoprolol, nadolol, pindolol, propranolol, and timolol) combined with acetohexamide can result in either high or low blood sugar levels. Beta blockers can also mask the symptoms of low blood sugar, which can be dangerous.

BE SURE TO TELL YOUR DOCTOR about any medications you are currently taking, especially any of those listed above.

WARNINGS

• It is important to tell your doctor if you have ever had an unusual or allergic reaction to this medicine or to any other medications, particularly acetazolamide, sulfonamide antibiotics, diuretics (water pills), and other oral antidiabetics.

• It is also important to tell your doctor if you now have or have ever had kidney disease, liver disease, severe infection, or thyroid disease.

• Follow the special diet that your doctor gave you. This is an important part of controlling your blood sugar and is necessary in order for this medicine to work properly.

• Avoid drinking alcoholic beverages while taking this medication (unless otherwise directed by your doctor). Some patients who take this medicine suffer nausea, vomiting, dizziness, stomach pain, pounding headache, sweating, and redness of the face and skin when they drink alcohol. Also, large amounts of alcohol can lower blood sugar to dangerously low levels.

• Be sure to tell your doctor or dentist that you are taking this medicine before having surgery or any other medical or dental treatment.

• Test for sugar in your urine as directed by your doctor. It is a convenient way to determine whether your diabetes is being controlled by this medicine.

• Eat or drink something containing sugar right away if you experience any symptoms of low blood sugar (anxiety, chills, cold sweats, cool or pale skin, drowsiness, excessive hunger, headache, nausea, nervousness, rapid heartbeat, shakiness, unusual tiredness, weakness). It is important that your family and friends know how to recognize the symptoms of low blood sugar and know what to do if they should observe any of these symptoms occuring in you.

Even if the symptoms of low blood sugar are corrected by eating or drinking sugar, it is important to contact your doctor as soon as possible after experiencing them. The blood-sugar-lowering effects of this medicine can last for hours, and the symptoms of low blood sugar may return during this period. Good sources of sugar are orange juice, corn syrup, honey, sugar cubes, and ordinary table sugar. You are at greatest risk of developing low blood sugar if you skip or delay meals, if you exercise more than usual, if you cannot eat because you are experiencing nausea or vomiting, or if you drink large amounts of alcoholic beverages.

• Be sure to tell your doctor if you are pregnant. Studies in animals have shown that this type of medicine can cause birth defects. Studies have not been conducted in humans, however. It is also important to tell your doctor if you are breast-feeding an infant. Small amounts of acetohexamide may pass into your breast milk.

Aches-N-Pain—see ibuprofen

Achromycin V—see tetracycline

Actagen-C Cough Syrup—see pseudoephedrine, triprolidine, and codeine combination

Acticort 100—see hydrocortisone (topical)

Actifed with Codeine—see pseudoephedrine, triprolidine, and codeine combination

---

acyclovir (topical)

BRAND NAME (Manufacturer)
Zovirax (Burroughs Wellcome)

TYPE OF DRUG
Antiviral

INGREDIENT
acyclovir

DOSAGE FORM
Ointment (5%)

STORAGE
Acyclovir ointment should be stored in a cool, dry place.

USES

Acyclovir is used to treat genital herpes and herpes infections of the skin. Acyclovir prevents the growth and multiplication of the *Herpes* virus. This drug does not cure a herpes infection, but may relieve the pain associated with the viral infection and may shorten its duration.

TREATMENT

Apply acyclovir as soon as possible after the symptoms of a herpes infection appear. Wash the infected area with soap and water, and allow it to dry. To avoid spreading the infection, use a rubber glove or a finger cot to apply the ointment. Apply enough acyclovir to cover the entire area of the infection.

Complete the full course of therapy (usually about ten days), even if your symptoms disappear before the end of this period.

If you miss a dose of this medication, apply the missed dose as soon as possible. However, if you do not remember until it is almost time for the next dose, do not apply the missed dose at all; just return to your regular dosing schedule. Do not use a double dose of the medication at the next application.

SIDE EFFECTS

Minor. You may experience temporary pain, burning, stinging, itching, or rash when this medication is applied. This sensation should disappear as your body adjusts to the medication.

Major. Tell your doctor about any side effects that are persistent or particularly bothersome.

INTERACTIONS

Acyclovir should not interact with other medications if it is used according to directions.

WARNINGS

- Tell your doctor about unusual or allergic reactions you have had to any medications, especially to acyclovir.
- Acyclovir ointment is intended for use on the skin only; it should not be used in or around the eyes.
- Try to avoid sexual activity while you have signs or symptoms of genital herpes; this medication does not prevent the transmission of herpes to other individuals, nor does it prevent recurrences.
- This medication has been prescribed for your current infection only. A subsequent infection, or one that someone else has, may require a different medication. Do not give your medicine to other people or use it to treat other infections, unless your doctor directs you to do so.
- Be sure to tell your doctor if you are pregnant. Although this drug appears to be safe in animals, studies in humans during pregnancy have not been conducted. Also, tell your doctor if you are breast-feeding an infant. It is not known whether acyclovir passes into breast milk.

Adalat—see nifedipine

Adapin—see doxepin

Adipex-P—see phentermine

Adipost—see phendimetrazine

Adphen—see phendimetrazine

Adsorbocarpine—see pilocarpine (ophthalmic)

Advil—see ibuprofen

Aerolate—see theophylline

Aeroseb-HC—see hydrocortisone (topical)

Akarpine—see pilocarpine (ophthalmic)

AK-Ramycin—see doxycycline

AK-Ratabs—see doxycycline

AK-Spore—see neomycin, polymyxin B, and bacitracin or gramicidin combination (ophthalmic)

AK-Spore H.C. Otic—see hydrocortisone, polymyxin B, and neomycin combination (otic)

AK-Sulf—see sodium sulfacetamide (ophthalmic)

AK-Sulf Forte—see sodium sulfacetamide (ophthalmic)

AK-Trol—see dexamethasone, neomycin sulfate, and polymyxin B combination (ophthalmic)

AK-Zol—see acetazolamide

Ala-Cort—see hydrocortisone (topical)

Ala-Quin—see hydrocortisone and iodochlorhydroxyquin combination (topical)

Ala-Scalp—see hydrocortisone (topical)

Alatone—see spironolactone

Alazide—see spironolactone and hydrochlorothiazide combination

Alazine—see hydralazine

---

albuterol

BRAND NAMES (Manufacturers)
Proventil (Schering)
Ventolin (Glaxo)

TYPE OF DRUG
Bronchodilator

INGREDIENT
albuterol

DOSAGE FORMS
Tablets (2 mg and 4 mg)
Inhalation aerosol (each spray delivers 90 mcg)
Oral syrup (2 mg per 5-ml spoonful)

STORAGE
Albuterol tablets and oral syrup should be stored at room temperature in a tightly closed, light-resistant container. The inhalation aerosol should be stored at room temperature away from excessive heat—the contents are pressurized and can explode if heated.

USES

Albuterol is used to relieve wheezing and shortness of breath caused by lung diseases such as asthma, bronchitis, and emphysema. This drug acts directly on the muscles of the bronchi (breathing tubes) to relieve bronchospasm (muscle contractions of the bronchi), which in turn reduces airway resistance and allows air to move more freely to and from the lungs.

TREATMENT

In order to lessen stomach upset, you can take albuterol tablets and oral syrup with food (unless your doctor directs you to do otherwise).

Each dose of oral syrup should be measured carefully with a 5-ml measuring spoon designed for that purpose. Ordinary kitchen teaspoons are not accurate enough.

The inhalation aerosol form of this medication is usually packaged with an instruction sheet. Read the directions carefully before using this medication. The container should be shaken well just before each use. The contents tend to settle on the bottom, so it is necessary to shake the bottle in order to distribute the ingredients evenly and equalize the doses. If more than one inhalation is necessary, wait at least one full minute between doses, in order to receive the full benefit of the first dose.

If you miss a dose of this medication and remember within an hour, take the missed dose immediately; then follow your regular dosing schedule for the next dose. If you miss the dose by more than an hour, just wait until the next scheduled dose. Do not double the dose.

SIDE EFFECTS

Minor. Anxiety, dizziness, flushing, headache, insomnia, irritability, loss of appetite, muscle cramps, nausea, nervousness, restlessness, sweating, tremors, vomiting, weakness, or dryness or irritation of the mouth or throat (from the inhalation aerosol). These side effects should disappear as your body adjusts to the medication.

To help prevent dryness or irritation of the mouth or throat, rinse your mouth with water after each dose of the inhalation aerosol.

In order to avoid difficulty in falling asleep, check with your doctor to see if you can take the last dose of this medication several hours before bedtime each day.

If you feel dizzy, sit or lie down for a while; get up from a sitting or reclining position slowly, and be careful on stairs.

Major. Tell your doctor about any side effects that are persistent or particularly bothersome. IT IS ESPECIALLY IMPORTANT TO TELL YOUR DOCTOR about chest pain, difficult or painful urination, itching, palpitations, or rash.

INTERACTIONS

Albuterol interacts with several other types of drugs:

1. The beta blockers (acebutolol, atenolol, labetalol, metoprolol, nadolol, pindolol, propranolol, timolol) antagonize (act against) this medication, decreasing its effectiveness.

2. Monoamine oxidase (MAO) inhibitors, tricyclic antidepressants, antihistamines, levothyroxine, and over-the-counter (nonprescription) cough, cold, asthma, allergy, diet, and sinus medications may increase the side effects of this medication.

3. There may be a change in the dosage requirements of insulin or oral antidiabetic medications when albuterol is started.

4. The blood-pressure-lowering effects of guanethidine may be decreased by this medication.

5. The use of albuterol with other bronchodilator drugs (either oral or inhalant drugs) can have additive side effects. Discuss this with your doctor.

BE SURE TO TELL YOUR DOCTOR about any medications you are currently taking, especially any listed above.

WARNINGS

- Tell your doctor about unusual or allergic reactions you have had to medications, especially to albuterol or any related drug (metaproterenol, terbutaline, amphetamines, ephedrine, epinephrine, isoproterenol, norepinephrine, phenylephrine, phenylpropanolamine, pseudoephedrine).
- Tell your doctor if you now have or if you have ever had diabetes mellitus, an enlarged prostate gland, epilepsy, glaucoma, heart disease, high blood pressure, or thyroid disease.
- This medication can cause dizziness. Your ability to perform tasks that require alertness, such as driving a car or operating potentially dangerous equipment, may be decreased. Appropriate caution should, therefore, be taken.
- Before having surgery or any other medical or dental treatment, be sure to tell the doctor or dentist that you are taking this medication.
- Do not exceed the recommended dosage of this medication; excessive use may lead to an increase in side effects or a loss of effectiveness.
- Avoid contact of the aerosol inhalation with your eyes.
- Do not puncture, break, or burn the aerosol container. The contents are under pressure and may explode.
- Contact your doctor if you do not respond to the usual dose of this medication. It may be a sign of worsening asthma, which may require additional therapy.
- Be sure to tell your doctor if you are pregnant. The effects of this medication during pregnancy have not been thoroughly studied in humans, but it has caused side effects in the offspring of animals that received large doses during pregnancy. Also, tell your doctor if you are breast-feeding an infant. It is not known whether albuterol passes into breast milk.

Aldactazide—see spironolactone and hydrochlorothiazide combination

Aldactone—see spironolactone

Aldomet—see methyldopa

Aldoril—see methyldopa and hydrochlorothiazide combination

Aller-chlor—see chlorpheniramine

Allerest 12-Hour—see phenylpropanolamine and chlorpheniramine combination

Allerfrin with Codeine—see pseudoephedrine, triprolidine, and codeine combination

Allergen—see antipyrine, benzocaine, oxyquinoline, and glycerin combination

AllerMax—see diphenhydramine

---

allopurinol

BRAND NAMES (Manufacturers)

allopurinol (various manufacturers)

Lopurin (Boots)
Zurinol (Major)
Zyloprim (Burroughs Wellcome)

TYPE OF DRUG

Antigout

INGREDIENT

allopurinol

DOSAGE FORM

Tablets (100 mg and 300 mg)

STORAGE

Allopurinol tablets should be stored at room temperature in a tightly closed container.

USES

This medication is used to treat gout and to lower blood uric acid levels. Allopurinol blocks the body's production of uric acid.

TREATMENT

In order to avoid stomach irritation, you can take allopurinol with food or with a full glass of water or milk. It may take at least a week before the full effects of this medication are observed.

Drink at least ten to 12 glasses (eight ounces each) of fluids per day while taking this medication in order to prevent the formation of kidney stones.

If you miss a dose of this medication, take the missed dose as soon as possible, unless it is almost time for the next dose. In that case, do not take the missed dose at all; just return to your regular dosing schedule. Do not double the next dose.

SIDE EFFECTS

Minor. Diarrhea, drowsiness, nausea, stomach upset, or vomiting. These side effects should disappear as your body adjusts to the medication.

Major. Tell your doctor about any side effects that are persistent or particularly bothersome. IT IS ESPECIALLY IMPORTANT TO TELL YOUR DOCTOR about blurred vision, chills, difficult or painful urination, fatigue, fever, loss of hair, muscle aches, numbness or tingling sensations, paleness, rash, sore throat, unusual bleeding or bruising, or yellowing of the eyes or skin.

INTERACTIONS

Allopurinol interacts with several other types of drugs:

1. Alcohol, diuretics (water pills), and pyrazinamide can increase blood uric acid levels, thus decreasing the effectiveness of allopurinol.

2. Allopurinol can increase the body store of iron salts, which can lead to iron toxicity.

3. When combined with allopurinol, ampicillin can increase the chance of skin rash; thiazide diuretics and captopril can increase the chance of allergic reactions; and cyclophosphamide can increase the chance of blood disorders. Allopurinol can also increase the blood levels and side effects of mercaptopurine, azathioprine, oral anticoagulants (blood thinners, such as warfarin), and theophylline.

4. Vitamin C can make the urine acidic, which can increase the risk of kidney stone formation with allopurinol.

Before starting to take allopurinol, BE SURE TO TELL YOUR DOCTOR about any medications you are currently taking, especially any of those listed above.

WARNINGS

- Tell your doctor about unusual or allergic reactions you have had to any medications, especially to allopurinol.
- Tell your doctor if you now have or if you have ever had blood disorders, kidney disease, or liver disease. Also, tell your doctor if you have a relative with idiopathic hemochromatosis (a disorder of iron metabolism).
- If this drug makes you dizzy or drowsy, do not take part in any activity that requires alertness, such as driving a car or operating potentially dangerous equipment.
- Be sure to tell your doctor if you are pregnant. Although this drug appears to be safe in animals, studies in pregnant women have not been conducted. Also, tell your doctor if you are breast-feeding an infant. It is not known whether allopurinol passes into breast milk.

Alphatrex—see betamethasone dipropionate

---

alprazolam

BRAND NAME (Manufacturer)

Xanax (Upjohn)

TYPE OF DRUG

Benzodiazepine sedative/hypnotic

INGREDIENT

alprazolam

DOSAGE FORM

Tablets (0.25 mg, 0.5 mg, and 1 mg)

STORAGE

This medication should be stored at room temperature in a tightly closed, light-resistant container.

USES

Alprazolam is prescribed to treat symptoms of anxiety and anxiety associated with depression. It is not clear exactly how this medicine works, but it may relieve anxiety by acting as a depressant of the central nervous system. This drug is currently used by many people to relieve nervousness. It is effective for this purpose for short periods, but it is important to try to remove the cause of the anxiety as well.

TREATMENT

This medication should be taken exactly as directed by your doctor. It can be taken with food or a full glass of water if stomach upset occurs. Do not take this medication with antacids, since they may retard its absorption from the gastrointestinal tract.

If you are taking this medication regularly and you miss a dose, take the missed dose immediately if you remember within an hour of the scheduled dose. If more than an hour has passed, skip the dose you missed and wait for the next scheduled dose. Do not double the dose.

SIDE EFFECTS

Minor. Bitter taste in mouth, constipation, diarrhea, dizziness, drowsiness (after a night's sleep), dry mouth, excessive salivation, fatigue, flushing, headache, heartburn, loss of appetite, nausea, nervousness, sweating, or vomiting. As your body adjusts to the medication, these side effects should disappear.

To relieve constipation, increase the amount of fiber in your diet (fresh fruits and vegetables, salads, bran, and whole-grain breads), exercise, and drink more water (unless your doctor directs you to do otherwise).

Dry mouth can be relieved by chewing sugarless gum or by sucking on ice chips.

If you feel dizzy, sit or lie down for a while; get up slowly from a sitting or reclining position, and be careful on stairs.

Major. Tell your doctor about any side effects that are persistent or particularly bothersome. IT IS ESPECIALLY IMPORTANT TO TELL YOUR DOCTOR about blurred or double vision, chest pain, severe depression, difficulty in urinating, fainting, falling, fever, hallucinations, joint pain, mouth sores, nightmares, palpitations, rash, shortness of breath, slurred speech, sore throat, uncoordinated movements, unusual excitement, unusual tiredness, or yellowing of the eyes or skin.

INTERACTIONS

Alprazolam interacts with several other types of medications:

1. To prevent oversedation, this drug should not be taken with alcohol, other sedative drugs, central nervous system depressants (such as antihistamines, barbiturates, muscle relaxants, pain medications, narcotics, medicines for seizures, and phenothiazine tranquilizers), or antidepressant medications.

2. This medication may decrease the effectiveness of carbamazepine, levodopa, and oral anticoagulants (blood thinners) and may increase the side effects of phenytoin.

3. Disulfiram, oral contraceptives (birth control pills), isoniazid, and cimetidine can increase the blood levels of alprazolam, which can lead to toxic effects.

4. Concurrent use of rifampin may decrease the effectiveness of alprazolam.

Before starting to take alprazolam, BE SURE TO TELL YOUR DOCTOR about any medications you are currently taking, especially any of those listed above.

WARNINGS

- Tell your doctor about unusual or allergic reactions you have had to any medications, especially to alprazolam or other benzodiazepine tranquilizers (such as chlordiazepoxide, clorazepate, diazepam, flurazepam, halazepam, lorazepam, oxazepam, prazepam, temazepam, or triazolam).
- Tell your doctor if you now have or if you have ever had liver disease, kidney disease, epilepsy, lung disease, myasthenia gravis, narrow-angle glaucoma, porphyria, mental depression, or mental illness.
- This medicine can cause drowsiness. Avoid tasks that require mental alertness, such as driving a car or using potentially dangerous equipment.
- This medication has the potential for abuse and must be used with caution. Tolerance may develop quickly; do not increase the dosage of the drug without first consulting your doctor. It is also important not to stop this drug suddenly if you have been taking it in large amounts or if you have used it for several weeks. Your doctor may want to reduce the dosage gradually.
- This is a safe drug when used properly. When it is combined with other sedative drugs or alcohol, however, serious side effects can develop.
- Be sure to tell your doctor if you are pregnant. This medicine may increase the chance of birth defects if it is taken during the first three months of pregnancy. In addition, too much use of this medicine during the last six months of pregnancy may result in addiction of the fetus—leading to withdrawal side effects in the newborn. Also, use of this medicine during the last weeks of pregnancy may cause drowsiness, slowed heartbeat, and breathing difficulties in the infant. Also, tell your doctor if you are breast-feeding an infant. This medicine can pass into breast milk and cause excessive drowsiness, slowed heartbeat, and breathing difficulties in nursing infants.

Alupent—see metaproterenol

Alzapam—see lorazepam

Amacodone—see acetaminophen and hydrocodone combination

---

amantadine

BRAND NAME (Manufacturer)
Symmetrel (DuPont)
TYPE OF DRUG
Antiparkinsonism agent and antiviral
INGREDIENT
amantadine
DOSAGE FORMS
Capsules (100 mg)
Oral syrup (50 mg per 5-ml spoonful)
STORAGE
Amantadine should be stored at room temperature (never frozen) in a tightly closed container.

USES

Amantadine is used to treat the symptoms of Parkinson's disease and to prevent or treat respiratory tract infections caused by influenza A virus. It is thought to relieve the symptoms of Parkinson's disease by increasing the levels of dopamine, an important chemical in the brain, which is lacking in these patients. Amantadine is also an antiviral agent that slows the growth of the influenza virus.

TREATMENT

Amantadine can be taken on an empty stomach or with food or milk.

Each dose of the oral syrup should be measured carefully with a specially designed 5-ml measuring spoon. An ordinary kitchen teaspoon is not accurate enough.

If you are taking amantadine to treat a viral infection, you should start taking it as soon as possible after exposure to the infection. Continue to take this medication for the entire time prescribed by your doctor (usually seven to 14 days), even if the symptoms of infection disappear before the end of that period. If you stop taking the drug too soon, the virus is given a chance to continue growing and the infection could recur.

Amantadine works best when the level of medicine in your bloodstream is kept constant. Therefore, take the doses at evenly spaced intervals day and night. For example, if you are to take two doses a day, the doses should be spaced 12 hours apart.

If you are taking amantadine to treat Parkinson's disease, you should know that the full effects of this medication may not become apparent for several weeks.

If you miss a dose of this medication, take the missed dose as soon as possible, unless it is almost time for the next dose. In that case, don't take the missed dose at all; just return to your regular dosing schedule. Do not double the next dose.

SIDE EFFECTS

Minor. Constipation, dizziness, dry mouth, fatigue, headache, insomnia, loss of appetite, nausea, or vomiting. These side effects should gradually disappear.

To relieve constipation, increase the amount of fiber in your diet (fresh fruits and vegetables, salads, bran, and whole-grain breads), exercise, and drink more water (unless your doctor directs you to do otherwise).

If you feel dizzy, sit or lie down for a while; get up slowly from a sitting or reclining position, and be careful on stairs.

To relieve mouth dryness, chew sugarless gum or suck on ice chips or hard candy.

Major. Tell your doctor about any side effects that are persistent or particularly bothersome. IT IS ESPECIALLY IMPORTANT TO TELL YOUR DOCTOR about anxiety, confusion, convulsions, depression, fluid retention, hallucinations, purplish-red spots on the skin, shortness of breath, skin rash, slurred speech, or visual disturbances.

INTERACTIONS

Amantadine interacts with several other types of drugs:

1. Concurrent use of amantadine and alcohol can lead to dizziness, fainting, and confusion.

2. Phenothiazine tranquilizers and tricyclic antidepressants in combination with amantadine can lead to confusion, hallucinations, and nightmares.

BE SURE TO TELL YOUR DOCTOR about any medications you are currently taking, especially any of those listed above.

WARNINGS

- Be sure to tell your doctor about unusual or allergic reactions you have had to any medications, especially to amantadine.
- Before starting to take amantadine, tell your doctor if you now have or if you have ever had epilepsy, heart or blood vessel disease, kidney disease, mental disorders, or stomach ulcers.
- If this drug makes you dizzy, avoid taking part in any activity that requires alertness, such as driving a car or operating potentially dangerous equipment.
- If you are taking amantadine to treat Parkinson's disease, do not stop taking the medication unless you first consult your doctor. Stopping the drug abruptly may lead to a worsening of the disease. Your doctor may, therefore, want to reduce your dosage gradually to prevent this from occurring. In addition, tolerance to the benefits of amantadine can develop in several months. If you notice a loss of effectiveness, CONTACT YOUR DOCTOR.
- Be sure to tell your doctor if you are pregnant. Although amantadine appears to be safe in humans, birth defects have been reported in the offspring of animals that received large doses during pregnancy. Also, tell your doctor if you are breast-feeding an infant. Small amounts of amantadine pass into breast milk and can cause side effects in the nursing infant.

Amaril D Spantab—see phenylpropanolamine, phenylephrine, chlorpheniramine, and phenyltoloxamine combination

Amen—see medroxyprogesterone

---

amiloride

BRAND NAMES (Manufacturers)
amiloride (various manufacturers)
Midamor (Merck Sharp & Dohme)

TYPE OF DRUG
Diuretic and antihypertensive

INGREDIENT
amiloride

DOSAGE FORM
Tablets (5 mg)

STORAGE
Amiloride should be stored at room temperature in a tightly closed container.

USES

Amiloride is prescribed to treat high blood pressure. It is also used to reduce fluid accumulation in the body caused by conditions such as heart failure, cirrhosis of the liver, kidney disease, and the long-term use of some medications. Amiloride reduces fluid accumulation by increasing the elimination of salt and water through the kidneys. It may also be used in combination with other diuretics to prevent potassium loss.

TREATMENT

To decrease stomach irritation, you can take amiloride with a glass of milk or with a meal (unless your doctor directs you to do otherwise). Try to take it at the same time every day. Avoid taking a dose after 6:00 P.M.; otherwise, you may have to get up during the night to urinate.

If you miss a dose of this medication, take the missed dose as soon as possible, unless it is almost time for the next one. In that case, do not take the missed dose at all; just wait until the next scheduled dose. Do not double the dose.

This medication does not cure high blood pressure, but it will help to control the condition as long as you continue to take it.

SIDE EFFECTS

Minor. Constipation, diarrhea, dizziness, dry mouth, gas, headache, heartburn, loss of appetite, nasal congestion, nausea, sleeping problems, stomach upset, or vomiting. These side effects should disappear as your body adjusts to the medication.

To relieve constipation, increase the amount of fiber in your diet (fresh fruits and vegetables, salads, bran, and whole-grain breads) and exercise more (unless your doctor directs you to do otherwise).

Dry mouth can be relieved by sucking on ice chips or a piece of hard candy or by chewing sugarless gum.

To avoid dizziness or light-headedness when you stand, contract and relax the muscles of your legs for a few moments before rising from a sitting position. Do this by alternately pushing one foot against the floor while raising the other foot slightly, so that you are "pumping" your legs in a pedaling motion.

Major. Tell your doctor about any side effects that are persistent or particularly bothersome. IT IS ESPECIALLY IMPORTANT TO TELL YOUR DOCTOR about anxiety; black, tarry stools; chest pain; confusion; cough; extreme tiredness or weakness; hair loss; impotence; itching; joint pain; mental depression; muscle aches; muscle cramps; nervousness; palpitations; rash; ringing in the ears; shakiness; shortness of breath; tingling in the fingers, lips, or toes; visual disturbances; or yellowing of the eyes or skin.

INTERACTIONS

Amiloride interacts with several other types of medications and certain foods:

1. Concurrent use of this medication with spironolactone, triamterene, potassium salts, low-salt milk, salt substitutes, captopril, enalapril, or laxatives may cause serious side effects from hyperkalemia (high levels of potassium in the blood). Check with your physician before using any of these medications or products.

2. Amiloride may increase the side effects of lithium and digoxin.

Before starting to take amiloride, BE SURE TO TELL YOUR DOCTOR about any medications you are currently taking, especially any of those listed above.

WARNINGS

- Be sure to tell your doctor if you have ever had unusual or allergic reactions to medications, especially to amiloride or any other diuretic.
- Tell your doctor if you now have or if you have ever had kidney disease or urination problems, hyperkalemia, diabetes mellitus, liver disease, or acidosis.
- Amiloride can cause hyperkalemia (high levels of potassium in the blood). Signs of hyperkalemia include palpitations (rapid or irregular heartbeat); confusion; numbness or tingling in your hands, feet, or lips; anxiety; or unusual tiredness or weakness. In order to avoid this problem, do not alter your diet and do not use salt substitutes unless you first consult your doctor.
- While taking this medication, limit your intake of alcoholic beverages in order to prevent dizziness and light-headedness.
- Do not take any over-the-counter (nonprescription) medication for weight control or for cough, cold, allergy, asthma, or sinus problems, unless you first check with your doctor.
- To prevent severe water loss (dehydration) while taking this medication, check with your doctor if you have any illness that causes severe or continuous nausea, vomiting, or diarrhea.
- Be sure to tell your doctor if you are pregnant. This drug crosses the placenta. Although this drug appears to be safe in animals, studies in humans have not been conducted. Also, tell your doctor if you are breast-feeding an infant. Small amounts of this drug pass into breast milk.

amiloride and hydrochlorothiazide combination

BRAND NAME (Manufacturer)
Moduretic (Merck Sharp & Dohme)
TYPE OF DRUG
Diuretic and antihypertensive
INGREDIENTS
amiloride and hydrochlorothiazide
DOSAGE FORM
Tablets (5 mg amiloride and 50 mg hydrochlorothiazide)
STORAGE
Amiloride and hydrochlorothiazide combination should be stored at room temperature in a tightly closed container.

USES

Amiloride and hydrochlorothiazide combination is prescribed to treat high blood pressure. It is also used to reduce fluid accumulation in the body caused by conditions such as heart failure, cirrhosis of the liver, kidney disease, and the long-term use of some medications. This medication reduces fluid accumulation by increasing the elimination of salt and water through the kidneys. Amiloride is combined with hydrochlorothiazide to prevent potassium loss from the body.

TREATMENT

To avoid stomach upset, you can take this medication with food or with a full glass of milk or water (unless your doctor directs you to do otherwise). Try to take it at the same time every day. Avoid taking a dose after 6:00 P.M.; otherwise, you may have to get up during the night to urinate.

If you miss a dose of this medication, take the missed dose as soon as possible, unless it is almost time for the next one. In that case, do not take the missed dose at all; just wait until the next scheduled dose. Do not double the dose.

This medication does not cure high blood pressure, but it will help to control the condition as long as you take it.

SIDE EFFECTS

Minor. Constipation, cramps, diarrhea, dizziness, drowsiness, headache, heartburn, loss of appetite, restlessness, or upset stomach. As your body adjusts to this medication, these side effects should disappear.

This medication can cause increased sensitivity to sunlight. Avoid prolonged exposure to sunlight and sunlamps, wear protective clothing, and use an effective sunscreen.

To relieve constipation, increase the amount of fiber in your diet (fresh fruits and vegetables, salads, bran, and whole-grain breads) and exercise more (unless your doctor directs you to do otherwise).

To avoid dizziness or light-headedness when you stand, contract and relax the muscles of your legs for a few moments before rising. Do this by alternately pushing one foot against the floor while raising the other foot slightly, so that you are "pumping" your legs in a pedaling motion.

Major. Tell your doctor about any side effects that are persistent or particularly bothersome. IT IS ESPECIALLY IMPORTANT TO TELL YOUR DOCTOR about anxiety; blurred vision; bruising; confusion; difficulty in breathing; dry mouth; excessive thirst; excessive weakness or tiredness; fever; impotence; itching; joint pain; mood changes; muscle spasms; nausea; nervousness; palpitations; skin rash; sore throat; tingling in your fingers, lips, or toes; unusual bleeding; vomiting; or yellowing of the eyes or skin.

INTERACTIONS

Amiloride and hydrochlorothiazide combination interacts with several other types of medications and certain foods:

1. Concurrent use with triamterene, spironolactone, potassium salts, low-salt milk, salt substitutes, captopril, enalapril, or laxatives can cause serious side effects from hyperkalemia (high levels of potassium in the blood).

2. This drug may decrease the effectiveness of oral anticoagulants, antigout medications, insulin, oral antidiabetic medicines, and methenamine.

3. Indomethacin may decrease the blood-pressure-lowering effects of this drug, which can be dangerous.

4. Fenfluramine may increase the blood-pressure-lowering effects of this drug, which can be dangerous.

5. Cholestyramine and colestipol can decrease the absorption of amiloride and hydrochlorothiazide from the gastrointestinal tract. Therefore, this drug should be taken one hour before or four hours after a dose of cholestyramine or colestipol.

6. The side effects of amphotericin B, calcium, cortisone and cortisone-like steroids (such as hydrocortisone, prednisone, and prednisolone), digoxin, digitalis, lithium, quinidine, sulfonamide antibiotics, and vitamin D may be increased when these drugs are taken concurrently with amiloride and hydrochlorothiazide.

BE SURE TO TELL YOUR DOCTOR about any medications you are currently taking, especially any of those listed above.

WARNINGS

- Tell your doctor about unusual or allergic reactions you have had to any medications, especially to amiloride, hydrochlorothiazide, or any other diuretic or to any sulfa drug, including acetazolamide, oral antidiabetic medications, or sulfonamide antibiotics.
- Tell your doctor if you now have or if you have ever had kidney disease or problems with urination, diabetes mellitus, gout, liver disease, asthma, pancreatic disease, systemic lupus erythematosus, acidosis, or hyperkalemia.
- This drug can occasionally cause potassium loss from the body. Signs of potassium loss include dry mouth, thirst, weakness, muscle pain or cramps, nausea, and vomiting. If you experience any of these symptoms, call your doctor.
- Amiloride can cause hyperkalemia (high levels of potassium in the blood). Signs of hyperkalemia include palpitations (rapid or irregular heartbeat); confusion; numbness or tingling in the hands, feet, or lips; anxiety; and unusual tiredness or weakness. In order to avoid this problem, do not alter your diet and do not use salt substitutes unless your doctor tells you to do so.
- While taking this medication, limit your intake of alcoholic beverages in order to prevent dizziness.
- Do not take any over-the-counter (nonprescription) medication for weight control or for cough, cold, asthma, allergy, or sinus problems unless you first check with your doctor.
- To prevent dehydration while taking this medication, check with your doctor if you have any illness that causes severe or continuous nausea, vomiting, or diarrhea.
- This drug can raise the blood sugar level in diabetic patients. Therefore, blood sugar levels should be monitored carefully with blood or urine tests when this drug is being taken.
- A doctor does not usually prescribe this drug or other "fixed-dose" products as the first choice in the treatment of high blood pressure. Usually the patient first receives each ingredient singly. If the response is adequate to the fixed dose contained in this product, it can then be substituted. The advantage of a combination product is increased convenience and (often) decreased cost.
- Be sure to tell your doctor if you are pregnant. Hydrochlorothiazide crosses the placenta and may cause adverse effects in the developing fetus. Also, tell your doctor if you are breast-feeding an infant. Small amounts of this drug pass into breast milk.

---

aminophylline

BRAND NAMES (Manufacturers)
aminophylline (various manufacturers)
Amoline (Major)
Phyllocontin (Purdue Frederick)
Somophyllin (Fisons)
Somophyllin-DF (Fisons)
Truphylline (G & W)

TYPE OF DRUG
Bronchodilator

INGREDIENT
aminophylline (theophylline as the ethylenediamine salt)

DOSAGE FORMS
Tablets (100 mg and 200 mg)
Controlled-release tablets (225 mg)
Oral liquid (105 mg per 5-ml spoonful)
Suppositories (250 mg and 500 mg)
Rectal solution (300 mg per 5 ml)

STORAGE
Aminophylline tablets, liquid, and rectal solution should be stored at room temperature in tightly closed containers. This medication should never be frozen. The suppositories should be stored in a cool place. They can be refrigerated if they become too soft.

USES

Aminophylline is prescribed to treat breathing problems (wheezing and shortness of breath) caused by asthma, bronchitis, or emphysema. It relaxes the smooth muscles of the bronchial airways (breathing tubes), thus opening the air passages to the lungs and allowing air to move in and out more easily.

TREATMENT

Aminophylline should be taken on an empty stomach, 30 to 60 minutes before a meal or two hours after a meal. If this medication causes stomach irritation, however, you can take it with food or with a full glass of water or milk (unless your doctor directs you to do otherwise).

Aminophylline works best when the level of the medication in your bloodstream is kept constant. It is best, therefore, to take it at evenly spaced intervals day and night. For example, if you are to take four doses a day, the doses should be spaced six hours apart.

The controlled-release tablets should be swallowed whole (if the tablet is scored for breaking, you can break it along these lines). Chewing, crushing, or crumbling the tablets destroys their sustained-release activity and possibly increases the side effects.

Doses of the oral liquid should be measured carefully with a 5-ml measuring spoon or a cup specially designed for that purpose. Ordinary kitchen spoons are not accurate enough.

To use the suppository form of this medication, remove the foil wrapper and moisten the suppository with water (if it is too soft to insert, refrigerate it for half an hour or run cold water over it before removing the wrapper). Lie on your left side with your right knee bent. Push the suppository into the rectum, pointed end first. Lie still for a few minutes. Try to avoid having a bowel movement for at least an hour after inserting the suppository. Aminophylline suppositories can be irritating to rectal tissue. Therefore, they should not be used for prolonged periods.

Aminophylline rectal solution is packaged with detailed patient instructions. Be sure to read the instructions before using this medication. If crystals appear in the solution, redissolve the crystals by partially immersing the bottle in warm water. The syringe should be washed after each application. To prevent rectal irritation, do not use this solution continuously for longer than 24 to 36 hours.

Try not to miss any doses of this medication. If you do miss a dose, take the missed dose as soon as possible, unless it is almost time for the next dose. In that case, do not take the missed dose at all; just return to your regular dosing schedule. Do not double the next dose of this medication unless your doctor has directed you to do so.

SIDE EFFECTS

Minor. Diarrhea, dizziness, feeling faint, flushing, headache, heartburn, increased urination, insomnia, irritability, loss of appetite, nausea, nervousness, stomach pain, or vomiting. These side effects should disappear as your body adjusts to the medication.

If you feel dizzy or light-headed, sit or lie down for a while; get up slowly from a sitting or reclining position, and be careful on stairs.

Major. Tell your doctor about any side effects that are persistent or particularly bothersome. IT IS ESPECIALLY IMPORTANT TO TELL YOUR DOCTOR about black, tarry stools; confusion; convulsions; difficulty in breathing; muscle twitches; palpitations; rash; severe abdominal pain; or unusual weakness.

INTERACTIONS

Aminophylline interacts with several other types of medications:

1. It can increase the effects (increased urination) of furosemide.

2. Reserpine in combination with aminophylline can cause a rapid heart rate.

3. Beta blockers (acebutolol, atenolol, labetalol, metoprolol, nadolol, pindolol, propranolol, timolol) can decrease the effectiveness of aminophylline.

4. Aminophylline can increase the side effects of the following products: over-the-counter (nonprescription) sinus, cough, cold, asthma, allergy, and diet preparations; digoxin; and oral anticoagulants (blood thinners, such as warfarin).

5. Aminophylline can decrease the effectiveness of phenytoin and lithium.

6. Phenobarbital, carbamazepine, and rifampin can increase the elimination of aminophylline from the body, thus decreasing its effectiveness.

7. Cimetidine, erythromycin, troleandomycin, oral contraceptives (birth control pills), allopurinol, and thiabendazole can decrease the elimination of aminophylline from the body, thus increasing its side effects.

8. Antidiarrheal medications prevent the absorption of aminophylline. Therefore, at least one hour should separate doses of these two types of medications.

Before starting to take aminophylline, BE SURE TO TELL YOUR DOCTOR about any of the medications you are currently taking, especially any of those listed above.

WARNINGS

- Tell your doctor about any unusual or allergic reactions you have had to medications, especially to aminophylline, theophylline, caffeine, dyphylline, oxtriphylline, or theobromine.
- Tell your doctor if you now have or if you have ever had an enlarged prostate gland, fibrocystic breast disease, heart disease, kidney disease, low or high blood pressure, liver disease, stomach ulcers, or thyroid disease.
- Cigarette or marijuana smoking may affect the action of this drug. Be sure to tell your doctor if you smoke. Also, do not suddenly stop smoking without informing your doctor.
- High fever, diarrhea, the flu, and influenza vaccinations can affect the action of this drug. You should tell your doctor about episodes of high fever or prolonged diarrhea. Before having any vaccinations, especially those to prevent the flu, tell your doctor that you are taking this medication.
- Avoid drinking large amounts of caffeine-containing beverages (coffee, cocoa, tea, and cola drinks) and avoid eating large amounts of chocolate. These products may increase the side effects of aminophylline.
- Do not change your diet without first consulting your doctor. Eating charbroiled foods or a high-protein, low-carbohydrate diet can affect the action of this drug.
- Before having surgery or other medical or dental treatment, tell your doctor or dentist you are taking this drug.
- Before taking any over-the-counter (nonprescription) asthma, allergy, cough, cold, sinus, or diet products, ask your doctor or pharmacist. These products may add to the side effects of aminophylline.
- Be sure to tell your doctor if you are pregnant. Although aminophylline appears to be safe during pregnancy, studies in humans have not been conducted. Birth defects have been observed in the offspring of animals that received large doses of this drug during pregnancy. Also, tell your doctor if you are breast-feeding an infant. Small amounts of aminophylline pass into breast milk and may cause irritability, fretfulness, or insomnia in nursing infants.

Amitril—see amitriptyline

---

amitriptyline

BRAND NAMES (Manufacturers)
Amitril (Warner Chilcott)
amitriptyline hydrochloride (various manufacturers)
Elavil (Merck Sharp & Dohme)
Endep (Roche)
TYPE OF DRUG
Tricyclic antidepressant
INGREDIENT
amitriptyline
DOSAGE FORM
Tablets (10 mg, 25 mg, 50 mg, 75 mg, 100 mg, and 150 mg)
STORAGE
Store at room temperature in a tightly closed container.

USES

Amitriptyline is used to relieve the symptoms of mental depression. This medication belongs to a group of drugs referred to as the tricyclic antidepressants. These medicines are thought to relieve depression by increasing the concentration of certain chemicals necessary for nerve transmission in the brain.

TREATMENT

This medication should be taken exactly as your doctor prescribes. It can be taken with water or with food to lessen the chance of stomach irritation, unless your doctor tells you to do otherwise.

The effects of therapy with this medication may not become apparent for two or three weeks.

If you miss a dose of this medication, take the missed dose as soon as possible, and then return to your regular dosing schedule. However, if the dose you missed was a once-a-day bedtime dose, do not take that dose in the morning; check with your doctor instead. If the dose is taken in the morning, it may cause some unwanted side effects. Never double the dose.

SIDE EFFECTS

Minor. Constipation, cramps, diarrhea, dizziness, drowsiness, dry mouth, fatigue, heartburn, loss of appetite, nausea, peculiar tastes in the mouth, restlessness, sweating, vomiting, weakness, or weight gain or loss. As your body adjusts to the medication, these side effects should disappear.

This medication may cause increased sensitivity to sunlight. You should, therefore, avoid prolonged exposure to sunlight and sunlamps. Wear protective clothing and use an effective sunscreen.

Amitriptyline may cause your urine to turn blue-green; this effect is harmless.

Dry mouth can be relieved by chewing sugarless gum or by sucking on ice chips or hard candy.

To relieve constipation, increase the amount of fiber in your diet (fresh fruits and vegetables, salads, bran, and whole-grain breads), exercise, and drink more water (unless your doctor directs you to do otherwise).

To avoid dizziness when you stand, contract and relax the muscles of your legs for a few moments before rising. Do this by alternately pushing one foot against the floor while raising the other foot slightly, so that you are "pumping" your legs in a pedaling motion.

Major. Tell your doctor about any side effects that are persistent or particularly bothersome. IT IS ESPECIALLY IMPORTANT TO TELL YOUR DOCTOR about agitation, anxiety, blurred vision, chest pain, confusion, convulsions, difficulty in urinating, enlarged or painful breasts (in both sexes), fainting, fever, fluid retention, hair loss, hallucinations, headaches, impotence, mood changes, mouth sores, nervousness, nightmares, numbness in the fingers or toes, palpitations, ringing in the ears, seizures, skin rash, sleep disorders, sore throat, tremors, uncoordinated movements or balance problems, unusual bleeding or bruising, or yellowing of the eyes or skin.

INTERACTIONS

Amitriptyline interacts with a number of other types of medications:

1. Extreme drowsiness can occur when this medicine is taken with central nervous system depressants (such as alcohol, antihistamines, barbiturates, benzodiazepine tranquilizers, muscle relaxants, narcotics, pain medications, phenothiazine tranquilizers, and sleeping medications) or with other antidepressants.

2. Amitriptyline may decrease the effectiveness of antiseizure medications and may block the blood-pressure-lowering effects of clonidine and guanethidine.

3. Oral contraceptives (birth control pills) or estrogen-containing drugs can increase the side effects and reduce the effectiveness of the tricyclic antidepressants (including amitriptyline).

4. Cimetidine can decrease the elimination of amitriptyline from the body, thus increasing the possibility of side effects.

5. Tricyclic antidepressants may increase the side effects of thyroid medication and of over-the-counter (nonprescription) cough, cold, allergy, asthma, sinus, and weight-control medications.

6. The concurrent use of tricyclic antidepressants and monoamine oxidase (MAO) inhibitors should be avoided because the combination may result in fever, convulsions, or high blood pressure. At least 14 days should separate the use of amitriptyline and the use of an MAO inhibitor.

Before starting to take amitriptyline, BE SURE TO TELL YOUR DOCTOR about any medications you are currently taking, especially any of those listed above.

WARNINGS

- Tell your doctor if you have had unusual or allergic reactions to medications, especially to amitriptyline or any of the other tricyclic antidepressants (imipramine, doxepin, trimipramine, amoxapine, protriptyline, desipramine, maprotiline, nortriptyline).
- Tell your doctor if you have a history of alcoholism, or if you have ever had asthma, high blood pressure, liver or kidney disease, heart disease, a heart attack, circulatory disease, stomach problems, intestinal problems, difficulty in urinating, enlarged prostate gland, epilepsy, glaucoma, thyroid disease, mental illness, or electroshock therapy.

• If this drug makes you dizzy or drowsy, do not take part in any activity that requires alertness, such as driving a car or operating potentially dangerous equipment.
• Before having surgery or other medical or dental treatment, tell your doctor or dentist you are taking this drug.
• Do not stop taking this drug suddenly. Abruptly stopping it can cause nausea, headache, stomach upset, fatigue, or a worsening of your condition. Your doctor may want to reduce the dosage gradually.
• The effects of this medication may last as long as seven days after you have stopped taking it, so continue to observe all precautions during that period.
• Be sure to tell your doctor if you are pregnant. Studies have not been done in humans; however, studies in animals have shown that this type of medication can cause side effects to the fetus when given to the mother in large doses during pregnancy. Also, tell your doctor if you are breast-feeding an infant. Small amounts of this drug can pass into breast milk and may cause unwanted side effects, such as irritability or sleeping problems, in nursing infants.

amitriptyline hydrochloride—see amitriptyline

Amoline—see aminophylline

---

amoxapine

BRAND NAME (Manufacturer)
Asendin (Lederle)
TYPE OF DRUG
Tricyclic antidepressant
INGREDIENT
amoxapine
DOSAGE FORM
Tablets (25 mg, 50 mg, 100 mg, and 150 mg)
STORAGE
This medication should be stored at room temperature in a tightly closed container.

USES

Amoxapine is used to relieve the symptoms of mental depression. This medication belongs to a group of drugs referred to as the tricyclic antidepressants. These medicines are thought to relieve depression by increasing the concentration of certain chemicals necessary for nerve transmission in the brain.

TREATMENT

This medication should be taken exactly as your doctor prescribes. It can be taken with water or with food to lessen the chance of stomach irritation, unless your doctor tells you to do otherwise.

If you miss a dose of this medication, take the missed dose as soon as possible, then return to your regular dosing schedule. However, if the dose you missed was a once-a-day bedtime dose, do not take that dose in the morning; check with your doctor instead. If the dose is taken in the morning, it may cause some unwanted side effects. Never double the dose.

SIDE EFFECTS

Minor. Constipation, cramps, diarrhea, dizziness, drowsiness, dry mouth, fatigue, heartburn, loss of appetite, nausea, peculiar tastes in the mouth, restlessness, sweating, vomiting, weakness, or weight gain or loss. As your body adjusts to the medication, these side effects should disappear.

This medication may cause increased sensitivity to sunlight. You should, therefore, avoid prolonged exposure to sunlight and sunlamps. Wear protective clothing, and use an effective sunscreen.

Dry mouth can be relieved by chewing sugarless gum or by sucking on ice chips or hard candy.

To relieve constipation, increase the amount of fiber (bran, salads, fresh vegetables and fruits, and whole-grain breads) in your diet, exercise, and drink more water (unless your doctor directs you to do otherwise).

To avoid dizziness or light-headedness when you stand, contract and relax the muscles of your legs for a few moments before rising. Do this by alternately pushing one foot against the floor while raising the other foot slightly, so that you are "pumping" your legs in a pedaling motion.

Major. Tell your doctor about any side effects that are persistent or particularly bothersome. IT IS ESPECIALLY IMPORTANT TO TELL YOUR DOCTOR about agitation, anxiety, blurred vision, chest pains, confusion, convulsions, difficulty in urinating, enlarged or painful breasts (in both sexes), fainting, fever, fluid retention, hair loss, hallucinations, headaches, impotence, mood changes, mouth sores, nervousness, nightmares, numbness in the fingers or toes, palpitations, ringing in the ears, seizures, skin rash, sleep disorders, sore throat, tremors, uncoordinated movements or balance problems, unusual bleeding, or yellowing of the eyes or skin.

INTERACTIONS

Amoxapine interacts with a number of other types of drugs:
1. Extreme drowsiness can occur when this medicine is taken with central nervous system depressants, including alcohol, antihistamines, barbiturates, benzodiazepine tranquilizers, muscle relaxants, narcotics, pain medications, phenothiazine tranquilizers, and sleeping medications, or with other antidepressants.
2. Amoxapine may decrease the effectiveness of antiseizure medications and may block the blood-pressure-lowering effects of clonidine and guanethidine.
3. Birth control pills or estrogen-containing drugs can increase the side effects and reduce the effectiveness of the tricyclic antidepressants (including amoxapine).
4. Cimetidine can decrease the elimination of amoxapine from the body, increasing the possibility of side effects.
5. Tricyclic antidepressants may increase the side effects of thyroid medication and over-the-counter (nonprescription) cough, cold, allergy, asthma, sinus, and diet medications.
6. The concurrent use of tricyclic antidepressants and monoamine oxidase (MAO) inhibitors should be avoided, because the combination may result in fever, convulsions, or high blood pressure. At least 14 days should separate the use of amoxapine and the use of an MAO inhibitor.

BE SURE TO TELL YOUR DOCTOR about any medications you are currently taking, especially any of those listed above.

WARNINGS

- Tell your doctor if you have had unusual or allergic reactions to medications, especially to amoxapine or any of the other tricyclic antidepressants (amitriptyline, imipramine, doxepin, trimipramine, protriptyline, desipramine, maprotiline, nortriptyline).
- Tell your doctor if you have a history of alcoholism, or if you now have or ever had asthma, high blood pressure, liver or kidney disease, heart disease, a heart attack, circulatory disease, stomach problems, intestinal problems, difficulty in urinating, enlarged prostate gland, epilepsy, glaucoma, thyroid disease, mental illness, or electroshock therapy.
- If this drug makes you dizzy or drowsy, do not take part in any activity that requires alertness, such as driving a car or operating potentially dangerous equipment.
- Before having surgery or other medical or dental treatment, tell your doctor or dentist you are taking this drug.
- Do not stop taking this drug suddenly. Abruptly stopping it can cause nausea, headache, stomach upset, fatigue, or a worsening of your condition. Your doctor may want to reduce the dosage gradually.
- The effects of this medication may last as long as seven days after you have stopped taking it, so continue to observe all precautions during that period.
- Be sure to tell your doctor if you are pregnant. Studies have not been done in humans; however, studies in animals have shown that this type of medication can cause side effects to the fetus when large doses are given to the mother during pregnancy. Also, tell your doctor if you are breast-feeding an infant. Small amounts of this drug can pass into breast milk and may cause unwanted effects, such as irritability or sleeping problems, in nursing infants.

---

amoxicillin

BRAND NAMES (Manufacturers)

amoxicillin (various manufacturers)
Amoxil (Beecham)
Larotid (Beecham)
Polymox (Bristol)
Trimox (Squibb)
Utimox (Parke-Davis)
Wymox (Wyeth)

TYPE OF DRUG

Antibiotic

INGREDIENT

amoxicillin

DOSAGE FORMS

Capsules (250 mg and 500 mg)
Chewable tablets (125 mg and 250 mg)
Oral suspension (125 mg and 250 mg per 5-ml spoonful)
Oral suspension drops (50 mg per ml)

STORAGE

Amoxicillin tablets and capsules should be stored at room temperature in tightly closed containers. The oral suspension should be stored in the refrigerator in a tightly closed container. Any unused portion of the suspension should be discarded after 14 days because the drug loses its potency after that time. This medication should never be frozen.

USES

Amoxicillin antibiotic is used to treat a wide variety of bacterial infections, including infections in the middle ear, in the upper and lower respiratory tracts, and in the urinary tract. Amoxicillin acts by severely injuring the cell walls of the infecting bacteria, thereby preventing them from growing and multiplying.

Amoxicillin kills susceptible bacteria but is not effective against viruses, parasites, or fungi.

TREATMENT

Amoxicillin can be taken either on an empty stomach or with food or milk (in order to prevent stomach upset).

The suspension form of this medication should be shaken well just before measuring each dose. The contents tend to settle on the bottom of the bottle, so it is necessary to shake the container to distribute the ingredients evenly and equalize the doses. Each dose should then be measured carefully with a specially designed 5-ml measuring spoon or the 1-ml dropper provided, as directed by your doctor or pharmacist. An ordinary kitchen teaspoon is not accurate enough for measuring your dosage of this medication.

It is important to continue to take this medication for the entire time prescribed by your doctor (usually seven to 14 days), even if the symptoms of infection disappear before the end of that period. If you stop taking the drug too soon, resistant bacteria are given the chance to continue growing, and the infection could recur.

Amoxicillin works best when the level of medicine in your bloodstream is kept constant. It is best, therefore, to take the doses at evenly spaced intervals day and night. For example, if you are to take three doses a day, the doses should be spaced eight hours apart.

If you miss a dose of this drug, take the missed dose immediately. However, if you don't remember to take the missed dose until it is almost time for your next dose, take it; space the next dose about halfway through the regular interval between doses; then return to your regular schedule. Do not skip any doses.

SIDE EFFECTS

Minor. Diarrhea, heartburn, nausea, or vomiting. These side effects should disappear as your body adjusts to the drug.

Major. Tell your doctor about any side effects that are persistent or particularly bothersome. IT IS ESPECIALLY IMPORTANT TO TELL YOUR DOCTOR about bloating, chills, cough, darkened tongue, difficulty in breathing, fever, irritation of the mouth, muscle aches, rash, rectal or vaginal itching, severe or bloody diarrhea, or sore throat. Also, if your symptoms of infection seem to be getting worse rather than improving, you should contact your doctor.

INTERACTIONS

Amoxicillin interacts with other types of medications:

1. Probenecid can increase the blood concentration of this medication.

2. Amoxicillin may decrease the effectiveness of oral contraceptives (birth control pills), and pregnancy could result. You should, therefore, use a different or additional form of birth control while taking this medication. Discuss this with your doctor.

3. The concurrent use of amoxicillin and allopurinol can increase the risk of developing a rash.

BE SURE TO TELL YOUR DOCTOR about any medications you are currently taking, especially any listed above.

WARNINGS

- Tell your doctor about unusual or allergic reactions you have had to any medications, especially to amoxicillin, ampicillin, or penicillin or to cephalosporin antibiotics, penicillamine, or griseofulvin.
- Tell your doctor if you now have or if you have ever had kidney disease, asthma, or allergies.
- This medication has been prescribed for your current infection only. Another infection later on, or one that someone else has, may require a different medicine. You should not give your medicine to other people or use it for other infections, unless your doctor specifically directs you to do so.
- Diabetics taking amoxicillin should know that this drug may cause a false-positive sugar reaction with a Clinitest urine glucose test. To avoid this problem while taking amoxicillin, you should switch to Clinistix or Tes-Tape to test your urine for sugar.
- Be sure to tell your doctor if you are pregnant. Although amoxicillin appears to be safe during pregnancy, extensive studies in humans have not been conducted. Also, tell your doctor if you are breast-feeding an infant. Small amounts of this medication pass into breast milk and may temporarily alter the bacterial balance in the intestinal tract of the nursing infant, resulting in diarrhea.

---

amoxicillin and clavulanic acid combination

BRAND NAME (Manufacturer)
Augmentin (Beecham)

TYPE OF DRUG
Antibiotic

INGREDIENTS
amoxicillin and clavulanic acid

DOSAGE FORMS
Tablets (500 mg amoxicillin and 125 mg clavulanic acid; 250 mg amoxicillin and 125 mg clavulanic acid)
Chewable tablets (125 mg amoxicillin and 31.25 mg clavulanic acid; 250 mg amoxicillin and 62.5 mg clavulanic acid)
Oral suspension (125 mg amoxicillin and 31.25 mg clavulanic acid per 5-ml spoonful; 250 mg amoxicillin and 62.5 mg clavulanic acid per 5-ml spoonful)

STORAGE
Amoxicillin and clavulanic acid tablets should be stored at room temperature in a tightly closed container. The oral suspension should be stored in the refrigerator in a tightly closed container. Any unused portion of the suspension should be discarded after ten days because the drug loses its potency after that time. This drug should never be frozen.

USES

Amoxicillin and clavulanic acid combination is used to treat a wide variety of bacterial infections, including infections of the middle ear, skin, sinuses, lower respiratory tract, and urinary tract. Amoxicillin is an antibiotic that acts by severely injuring the cell membranes of infecting bacteria, thereby preventing them from growing and multiplying. Clavulanic acid has no antibacterial activity. It acts to prevent the breakdown of amoxicillin in the body.

Amoxicillin and clavulanic acid combination kills susceptible bacteria, but it is not effective against viruses, parasites, or fungi.

TREATMENT

Amoxicillin and clavulanic acid combination can be taken either on an empty stomach or with food or milk (in order to prevent stomach upset).

The suspension form of this medication should be shaken well just before measuring each dose. The contents tend to settle on the bottom of the bottle, so it is necessary to shake the container to distribute the ingredients evenly and to equalize the doses. Each dose should then be measured carefully with a specially designed 5-ml measuring spoon. An ordinary kitchen teaspoon is not accurate enough.

It is important to continue to take this medication for the entire time prescribed by your doctor (usually seven to ten days), even if the symptoms of infection disappear before the end of that period. If you stop taking the drug too soon, resistant bacteria are given the chance to continue growing, and the infection could recur.

Amoxicillin and clavulanic acid combination works best when the level of medicine in your bloodstream is kept constant. It is best, therefore, to take the doses of this medication at evenly spaced intervals throughout the day and night. For example, if you are to take three doses a day, the doses should be spaced eight hours apart.

If you miss a dose of this medication, take the missed dose immediately. However, if you do not remember to take the missed dose until it is almost time for your next dose, take the missed dose; space the next dose about halfway through the regular interval between doses; and then return to your regular schedule. Try not to skip any doses.

SIDE EFFECTS

Minor. Abdominal discomfort, bloating, diarrhea, gas, headache, heartburn, nausea, or vomiting. These side effects should disappear as your body adjusts to this medication.

Major. Tell your doctor about any side effects that are persistent or particularly bothersome. IT IS ESPECIALLY IMPORTANT TO TELL YOUR DOCTOR about bloody or prolonged diarrhea, chills, cough, darkened tongue, difficulty in breathing, fever, irritation of the mouth, itching, muscle aches, rash, rectal or vaginal itching, sore throat, or unusual bleeding or bruising. Also, if your symptoms of infection seem to be getting worse rather than improving, you should contact your doctor.

INTERACTIONS

Amoxicillin and clavulanic acid can interact with several other types of medications:

1. Probenecid can increase the blood concentration of amoxicillin.

2. Amoxicillin may decrease the effectiveness of oral contraceptives (birth control pills), and pregnancy could result. You should, therefore, use a different or additional form of

birth control while taking this medication. Discuss this with your doctor.

3. Amoxicillin and clavulanic acid can increase the risk of side effects with disulfiram (Antabuse).

4. The risk of skin rash is increased when amoxicillin and allopurinol are taken concurrently.

Before starting this medication, BE SURE TO TELL YOUR DOCTOR about all of the medications you are currently taking, especially any of the medications listed above.

WARNINGS

- Tell your doctor about unusual or allergic reactions you have had to any medications, especially to amoxicillin, ampicillin, penicillin, cephalosporin antibiotics, penicillamine, griseofulvin, or clavulanic acid.
- Tell your doctor if you now have or if you have ever had allergies, asthma, kidney disease, or mononucleosis.
- This medication has been prescribed for your current infection only. A subsequent infection, or one that someone else has, may require a different medication. You should not give your medicine to other people or use it to treat other infections, unless your doctor specifically directs you to do so.
- Diabetics taking amoxicillin should know that this drug may cause a false-positive sugar reaction with a Clinitest urine glucose test. To avoid this problem while taking amoxicillin, you should switch to Clinistix or Tes-Tape to test your urine for sugar.
- Be sure to tell your doctor if you are pregnant. Although amoxicillin and clavulanic acid combination appears to be safe during pregnancy, studies in humans have not been conducted. Also, tell your doctor if you are breast-feeding an infant. Small amounts of this medication pass into breast milk and may cause diarrhea in the nursing infant.

Amoxil—see amoxicillin

---

amphetamine

BRAND NAME (Manufacturer)
Amphetamine Sulfate (Lannett)

TYPE OF DRUG
Amphetamine

INGREDIENT
amphetamine

DOSAGE FORM
Tablets (5 mg and 10 mg)

STORAGE
Store at room temperature in a tightly closed container.

USES

This medication is a central nervous system stimulant that increases mental alertness and decreases fatigue. It is used to treat narcolepsy (a disorder involving uncontrollable desires to sleep or actual sleep attacks that occur in a rapid and unpredictable manner) and abnormal behavioral syndrome in children (hyperkinetic syndrome or attention deficit disorder). The way this medication acts to control abnormal behavioral syndrome in children is not clearly understood.

Amphetamine is also used as an appetite suppressant during the first few weeks of dieting (while you are trying to establish new eating habits). It is thought to relieve hunger by altering nerve impulses to the appetite control center in the brain. Its effectiveness as an appetite suppressant lasts only for short periods (three to 12 weeks), however.

TREATMENT

In order to avoid stomach upset, you can take amphetamine with food or with a full glass of milk or water (unless your doctor directs you to do otherwise).

If this medication is being used to treat narcolepsy or abnormal behavioral syndrome in children, the first dose each day should be taken soon after awakening. Subsequent doses should be spaced at four- to six-hour intervals.

If this medication has been prescribed as a diet aid, it should be taken one hour before each meal.

In order to avoid difficulty in falling asleep, the last dose of this medication each day should be taken four to six hours before bedtime.

If you miss a dose of this medication, take the missed dose as soon as possible, unless it is almost time for your next dose. In that case, don't take the missed dose at all, just return to your regular dosing schedule. Do not double the next dose.

SIDE EFFECTS

Minor. Abdominal cramps, constipation, diarrhea, dizziness, dry mouth, false sense of well-being, insomnia, irritability, loss of appetite, nausea, overstimulation, restlessness, unpleasant taste in the mouth, or vomiting. These side effects should disappear as your body adjusts to the medication.

In order to prevent constipation while taking this medication, increase the amount of fiber in your diet (bran, fresh fruits and vegetables, salads, whole-grain cereals and breads), drink more water, and exercise more (unless your doctor directs you to do otherwise).

Dry mouth can be relieved by sucking on ice chips or a piece of hard candy or by chewing sugarless gum.

If you feel dizzy, sit or lie down for a while; get up from a sitting or lying position slowly, and be careful on stairs.

Major. Tell your doctor about any side effects that are persistent or particularly bothersome. IT IS ESPECIALLY IMPORTANT TO TELL YOUR DOCTOR about blurred vision, confusion, fatigue, headaches, impotence, mental depression, palpitations, rash, sweating, tightness in the chest, tremors, uncoordinated movements, or unusual bleeding or bruising.

INTERACTIONS

Amphetamine interacts with several other types of medications:

1. The concurrent use of amphetamine and a monoamine oxidase (MAO) inhibitor (isocarboxazid, pargyline, phenelzine, tranylcypromine) should be avoided, since the combination may result in convulsions or high fever. At least 14 days should separate the use of amphetamine and the use of an MAO inhibitor.

2. Barbiturate medications, phenothiazine tranquilizers (especially chlorpromazine), and tricyclic antidepressants can antagonize (act against) this medication.

3. Amphetamine can decrease the blood-pressure-lowering effects of antihypertensive medications (especially guanethi-

dine) and may alter insulin and oral antidiabetic medication dosage requirements in diabetic patients.
4. The side effects of other central nervous system stimulants, such as caffeine, over-the-counter (nonprescription) appetite suppressants, and cough, cold, allergy, asthma, or sinus preparations, may be increased by amphetamine.
5. Acetazolamide and sodium bicarbonate can decrease the elimination and prolong the duration of action of the amphetamines.

BE SURE TO TELL YOUR DOCTOR about any medications you are currently taking, especially any of those listed above.

WARNINGS

- Tell your doctor about unusual or allergic reactions you have had to any medications, especially to amphetamine or other central nervous system stimulants (albuterol, dextroamphetamine, ephedrine, epinephrine, isoproterenol, metaproterenol, norepinephrine, phenylephrine, phenylpropanolamine, pseudoephedrine, terbutaline).
- Tell your doctor if you have a history of drug abuse, or if you have ever had problems with agitation, diabetes mellitus, glaucoma, heart or blood vessel disease, high blood pressure, or thyroid disease.
- Amphetamine can mask the symptoms of extreme fatigue and can cause dizziness. Your ability to perform hazardous tasks, such as driving a car or operating potentially dangerous machinery, may be decreased. Appropriate caution should, therefore, be taken.
- Before having surgery or any other medical or dental treatment, be sure to tell your doctor or dentist that you are taking this medication.
- Amphetamine may be habit-forming when taken for long periods of time (both physical and psychological dependence can occur). Therefore, you should not increase the dose of this medication or take it for longer than 12 weeks unless you first consult your doctor. It is also important that you not stop taking this medication abruptly—fatigue, sleep disorders, mental depression, nausea, vomiting, stomach cramps, or pain can occur. Your doctor may, therefore, want to decrease the dose gradually in order to prevent these side effects.
- Be sure to tell your doctor if you are pregnant. Although studies have not been done in humans, some of the amphetamines have caused heart, brain, and biliary tract abnormalities in the fetuses of animals who received large doses of these drugs during pregnancy. Also, tell your doctor if you are breast-feeding an infant. Small amounts of this drug pass into breast milk.

Amphetamine Sulfate—see amphetamine

---

ampicillin

BRAND NAMES (Manufacturers)
D-Amp (Dunhall)
Omnipen (Wyeth)
Polycillin (Bristol)
Principen (Squibb)
Totacillin (Beecham)

TYPE OF DRUG
Antibiotic

INGREDIENT
ampicillin

DOSAGE FORMS
Capsules (250 mg and 500 mg)
Oral suspension (125 mg and 250 mg per 5-ml spoonful)
Oral suspension drops (100 mg per ml)

STORAGE
Ampicillin capsules should be stored at room temperature; ampicillin liquid suspension and drops should be refrigerated but should never be frozen. Do not keep any of these medications beyond the expiration date written on the container. All containers should be closed tightly to keep out moisture.

USES

Ampicillin is used to treat a wide variety of bacterial infections, including middle ear infections in children and infections of the respiratory, urinary, and gastrointestinal tracts. This type of antibiotic acts by severely injuring the cell walls of the infecting bacteria—thereby preventing them from growing and multiplying. Ampicillin kills susceptible bacteria but is not effective against viruses, parasites, or fungi.

TREATMENT

It is best to take ampicillin on an empty stomach (one hour before or two hours after a meal) with a full glass of water (not juice or soda pop).

If you have been prescribed the liquid suspension form of this drug, be sure to shake the bottle well. The contents tend to settle on the bottom of the bottle, so it is necessary to shake the container to distribute the ingredients evenly and equalize the doses. Be sure to use specially marked droppers or spoons to accurately measure the correct amount of liquid. Household teaspoons vary in size and may not give you the correct dosage.

Ampicillin works best when the level of medicine in your bloodstream is kept constant. It is, therefore, best to take the doses at evenly spaced intervals day and night. For example, if you are to take four doses a day, the doses should be spaced six hours apart.

If you miss a dose, take it as soon as possible. If it is already time for the next dose, take it; space the next two doses at half the normal time interval (for example, if you were supposed to take one tablet every six hours, take your next two doses every three hours); then resume your normal dosing schedule.

It is very important to continue to take this medication for the entire time prescribed by your doctor (usually ten days), even if the symptoms disappear before the end of that period. If you stop taking the drug too soon, resistant bacteria are given a chance to continue growing, and the infection could recur.

SIDE EFFECTS

Minor. Diarrhea, nausea, or vomiting. These side effects should disappear as your body adjusts to the medication.

Major. Tell your doctor about any side effects that are persistent or particularly bothersome. IT IS ESPECIALLY IMPORTANT TO TELL YOUR DOCTOR about darkened tongue, difficulty in breathing, fever, joint pain, mouth sores, rash, rectal or vaginal itching, severe or bloody diarrhea, or sore throat. Also, if your symptoms of infection seem to be getting worse rather than improving, you should contact your doctor.

INTERACTIONS

This drug interacts with other types of medications:

1. Ampicillin interacts with allopurinol, chloramphenicol, erythromycin, paromomycin, tetracycline, and troleandomycin.

2. Ampicillin may decrease the effectiveness of oral contraceptives (birth control pills), and pregnancy could result. You should, therefore, use a different or additional form of birth control while taking ampicillin.

BE SURE TO TELL YOUR DOCTOR about any medications you are currently taking, especially any of those listed above.

WARNINGS

- Tell your doctor about unusual or allergic reactions you have had to any medications, especially to ampicillin, amoxicillin, penicillin, cephalosporin antibiotics, penicillamine, or griseofulvin.
- Tell your doctor if you now have or if you have ever had liver disease, kidney disease, asthma, hay fever, or other allergies.
- This medication has been prescribed for your current infection only. Another infection later on, or one that someone else has, may require a different medicine. Do not give your medicine to other people or use it for other infections, unless your doctor directs you to do so.
- Diabetics taking ampicillin should know that this drug may cause a false-positive sugar reaction with a Clinitest urine glucose test. To avoid this problem while taking ampicillin, you should switch to Clinistix or Tes-Tape to test your urine for sugar.
- Be sure to tell your doctor if you are pregnant. Although ampicillin appears to be safe during pregnancy, extensive studies in humans have not been conducted. Also, tell your doctor if you are breast-feeding an infant. Small amounts of this medication pass into breast milk and may temporarily alter the bacterial balance in the intestinal tract of the nursing infant, resulting in diarrhea.

Anadrol-50—see oxymetholone

Anamine T.D.—see pseudoephedrine and chlorpheniramine combination

Anaprox—see naproxen

Anaprox DS—see naproxen

Android—see methyltestosterone

Anorex—see phendimetrazine

Ansaid—see flurbiprofen

Anspor—see cephradine

Antabuse—see disulfiram

antipyrine, benzocaine, oxyquinoline, and glycerin combination

BRAND NAMES (Manufacturers)
Allergen (Goldline)
Auralgan (Ayerst)
Auromid (Vangard)
Auroto Otic (Barre)
Earocol (Mallard)
Oto (Vortech)

TYPE OF DRUG
Otic analgesic and anesthetic

INGREDIENTS
antipyrine, benzocaine, oxyquinoline, and glycerin

DOSAGE FORM
Otic solution (5.4% antipyrine, 1.4% benzocaine, oxyquinoline in glycerin)

STORAGE
This medication should be stored at room temperature in a tightly closed container. If the solution changes color or consistency, do not use it any longer. Never add water to the solution; it may lose its effectiveness.

USES

Antipyrine, benzocaine, oxyquinoline, and glycerin combination is used to relieve congestion, pain, and inflammation caused by an ear infection. It can also be used to help remove excess wax from the ear. Antipyrine is an analgesic (pain-reliever); benzocaine is a local anesthetic (deadens the nerve endings); and glycerin provides a drying effect.

TREATMENT

For accuracy, and in order to avoid contamination, another person should administer the ear drops if possible.

If you want to warm the ear drops before administration, roll the bottle back and forth between your hands. DO NOT place the bottle in boiling water.

To administer, tilt the head to one side with the affected ear turned upward. Grasp the earlobe and gently pull it upward and back to straighten the ear canal. (If administering ear drops to a child, gently pull the earlobe downward and back.) Fill the dropper and place the prescribed number of drops into the ear. Be careful not to touch the dropper to the ear canal, since the dropper can easily become contaminated. Keep the ear tilted upward for about five minutes. Your doctor may want you to put a piece of cotton soaked with the drug into your ear to keep the drug from leaking out. In order to avoid contamination, DO NOT wash or wipe the dropper after use.

If you miss a dose, administer the drops as soon as possible, unless it is almost time for the next dose. In that case, do not use the missed dose at all; just return to your regular schedule.

SIDE EFFECTS

Minor. Burning or itching immediately upon application. The burning or itching should last for only a few minutes.

Major. Be sure to tell your doctor about any severe or persistent burning or itching.

INTERACTIONS

This medication should not interact with other medications as long as it is used according to directions.

WARNINGS

- Tell your doctor about any unusual or allergic reactions you have had to medications, especially to antipyrine, benzocaine, or any local anesthetic or to oxyquinoline or glycerin.
- Before taking this medication, tell your doctor if you have ever had a perforated eardrum or ear discharge.
- Be sure to tell your doctor if you are pregnant. The effects of antipyrine, benzocaine, oxyquinoline, and glycerin during pregnancy have not been studied. Also, tell your doctor if you are breast-feeding an infant. It is not known if this drug passes into human breast milk.

Antivert—see meclizine

Antivert/25—meclizine

Antivert/50—meclizine

Antrizine—see meclizine

Anturane—see sulfinpyrazone

Anucort—see hydrocortisone, benzyl benzoate, bismuth resorcin compound, bismuth subgallate, zinc oxide, and Peruvian balsam combination (topical)

Anumed HC—see hydrocortisone, benzyl benzoate, bismuth resorcin compound, bismuth subgallate, zinc oxide, and Peruvian balsam combination (topical)

Anusol HC—see hydrocortisone, benzyl benzoate, bismuth resorcin compound, bismuth subgallate, zinc oxide, and Peruvian balsam combination (topical)

Anxanil—see hydroxyzine

Apresoline—see hydralazine

Aquachloral Supprettes—see chloral hydrate

Aquaphyllin—see theophylline

Aquatensen—see methyclothiazide

Aristocort (systemic)—see triamcinolone (systemic)

Aristocort (topical)—see triamcinolone (topical)

Aristocort A—see triamcinolone (topical)

Armour Thyroid—see thyroid hormone

Artane—see trihexyphenidyl

Artane Sequels—see trihexyphenidyl

A.S.A. Enseals—see aspirin

Asbron G—see theophylline and guaifenesin combination

Asendin—see amoxapine

Asmalix—see theophylline

---

aspirin

BRAND NAMES (Manufacturers)

A.S.A. Enseals* (Lilly)
aspirin* (various manufacturers)
Bayer* (Glenbrook)
Bayer Children's* (Glenbrook)
Easprin (Parke-Davis)
Ecotrin* (Smith Kline)
Empirin* (Burroughs Wellcome)
Measurin* (Winthrop Pharmaceuticals)
ZORprin (Boots)
*Available over-the-counter (without a prescription)

TYPE OF DRUG

Analgesic and anti-inflammatory

INGREDIENT

aspirin

DOSAGE FORMS

Tablets (65 mg, 81 mg, 325 mg, and 500 mg)
Chewable tablets (81 mg)
Enteric-coated tablets (325 mg, 500 mg, 650 mg, and 975 mg)
Sustained-release tablets (650 mg and 800 mg)
Caplets (325 mg and 500 mg)
Suppositories (60 mg, 120 mg, 130 mg, 195 mg, 200 mg, 300 mg, 325 mg, 600 mg, 650 mg, and 1.2 g)

STORAGE

Store at room temperature in a tightly closed container. Moisture causes aspirin to decompose.

USES

Aspirin is used to treat mild to moderate pain, fever, and inflammatory conditions, such as rheumatic fever, rheumatoid arthritis, and osteoarthritis. Because it prevents the formation of blood clots, aspirin has also been shown to be effective in reducing the risk of transient ischemic attacks (small strokes) and to have a protective effect against heart attacks in men with angina (chest pain).

Aspirin is a useful medication that is utilized in the treatment of a wide variety of diseases. Because it is so common and so readily available, you may not think of it as "real medicine." This is a common misconception; aspirin certainly is "real medicine." If your doctor prescribes or recommends aspirin for your condition, it is for a good reason. FOLLOW YOUR DOCTOR'S DIRECTIONS CAREFULLY!

TREATMENT

To avoid stomach irritation, you should take aspirin with food or with a full glass of water or milk.

Chewable aspirin tablets may be chewed, dissolved in fluid, or swallowed whole.

Sustained-release or enteric-coated tablets should be swallowed whole. Crushing, chewing, or breaking these tablets destroys their sustained-release activity and increases side effects.

To use the suppository, remove the foil wrapper and moisten the suppository with water (if it is too soft to insert, refrigerate the suppository for half an hour or run cold water over it before you remove the wrapper). Lie on your left side with your right knee bent. Push the suppository into the rectum, pointed end first. Lie still for a few minutes. Avoid having a bowel movement for at least an hour to give the drug time to be absorbed.

If you are using aspirin to treat an inflammatory condition, it may take two or three weeks until the full benefits are observed.

If you are taking aspirin on a regular schedule and you miss a dose, take the missed dose as soon as possible, unless it is almost time for the next dose. In that case, do not take the missed dose at all; just return to your regular dosing schedule. Do not double the next dose.

SIDE EFFECTS

Minor. Heartburn, nausea, or vomiting. These side effects should disappear as your body adjusts to the medication.

Major. Tell your doctor about any side effects that are persistent or particularly bothersome. IT IS ESPECIALLY IMPORTANT TO TELL YOUR DOCTOR about any loss of hearing; bloody or black, tarry stools; confusion; difficult or painful urination; difficulty in breathing; dizziness; severe stomach pain; skin rash; or unusual weakness.

INTERACTIONS

Aspirin interacts with a number of other types of medications:

1. Aspirin can increase the effects of anticoagulants (blood thinners), such as warfarin, leading to bleeding complications.

2. The antigout effects of probenecid and sulfinpyrazone may be blocked by aspirin.

3. Aspirin can increase the gastrointestinal side effects of nonsteroidal anti-inflammatory drugs, alcohol, phenylbutazone, and adrenocorticosteroids (cortisone-like medicines).

4. Ammonium chloride, methionine, and furosemide can increase the side effects of aspirin.

5. Acetazolamide, methazolamide, antacids, and phenobarbital can decrease the effectiveness of aspirin.

6. Aspirin can increase the side effects of methotrexate, penicillin, thyroid hormone, phenytoin, sulfinpyrazone, naproxen, valproic acid, insulin, and oral antidiabetic medications.

7. It can decrease the effects of spironolactone.

Before starting to take aspirin, BE SURE TO TELL YOUR DOCTOR about any medications you are currently taking, especially any of those listed above.

WARNINGS

- Tell your doctor about unusual or allergic reactions you have had to any medications, especially to aspirin, methyl salicylate (oil of wintergreen), tartrazine, diclofenac, diflunisal, flurbiprofen, fenoprofen, ibuprofen, indomethacin, ketoprofen, meclofenamate, mefenamic acid, naproxen, piroxicam, sulindac, or tolmetin.
- Before starting to take aspirin, be sure to tell your doctor if you now have or if you have ever had asthma, bleeding disorders, congestive heart failure, diabetes, glucose-6-phosphate dehydrogenase (G6PD) deficiency, gout, hemophilia, high blood pressure, kidney disease, liver disease, nasal polyps, peptic ulcers, or thyroid disease.
- Before having surgery or any other medical or dental treatment, be sure to tell your doctor or dentist that you are taking aspirin. Aspirin is usually discontinued five to seven days before surgery, in order to prevent bleeding complications.
- The use of aspirin in children (about 16 years of age or less) with the flu or chicken pox has been associated with a rare, life-threatening condition called Reye's syndrome. Aspirin should, therefore, not be given to children with signs of an infection.
- Large doses of aspirin (greater than eight 325-mg tablets per day) can cause erroneous urine glucose test results. Diabetics should, therefore, check with their doctor before changing insulin doses while taking this medication.
- Additional medications that contain aspirin should not be taken without your doctor's approval. Be sure to check the labels on over-the-counter (nonprescription) pain, sinus, allergy, asthma, cough, and cold preparations to see if they contain aspirin.
- Be sure to tell your doctor if you are pregnant. Aspirin has been shown to cause birth defects in the offspring of animals that received large doses during pregnancy. Large doses of aspirin given to a pregnant woman close to term can prolong labor and cause bleeding complications in the mother and heart problems in the infant. Also, tell your doctor if you are breast-feeding an infant. Small amounts of aspirin pass into breast milk.

---

aspirin and codeine combination

BRAND NAME (Manufacturer)
Empirin with Codeine (Burroughs Wellcome)

TYPE OF DRUG
Analgesic combination

INGREDIENTS
aspirin and codeine

DOSAGE FORM
Tablets (325 mg aspirin with 15 mg, 30 mg, or 60 mg of codeine)

Note that on the label of the vial of tablets, the name of this drug is followed by a number. This number refers to the amount of codeine: #2 contains 1/4 grain (15 mg) codeine, #3 has 1/2 grain (30 mg) codeine, and #4 contains 1 grain (60 mg) codeine.

STORAGE
Aspirin and codeine combination tablets should be stored at room temperature in a tightly closed container. Care should be taken to prevent moisture from entering the container, as it will cause the aspirin in this product to decompose.

USES

This medication is used to relieve tension headaches and mild to severe pain. Codeine is a narcotic analgesic that acts on the central nervous system to relieve pain.

TREATMENT

In order to avoid stomach upset, you can take this medication with food or milk.

This medication works most effectively if you take it at the onset of pain, rather than waiting until the pain becomes intense.

If you are taking this medication on a regular schedule and you miss a dose, take the missed dose as soon as possible, unless it is almost time for your next dose. In that case, don't take the missed dose at all; just return to your regular dosing schedule. Do not double the next dose.

SIDE EFFECTS

Minor. Constipation, dizziness, drowsiness, dry mouth, false sense of well-being, flushing, indigestion, lightheadedness, loss of appetite, nausea, sweating, and vomiting. These side effects should disappear as your body adjusts to the medication.

If you are constipated, increase the amount of fiber in your diet (fresh fruits and vegetables, salads, bran, and wholegrain breads), drink more water, and exercise (unless your doctor directs you to do otherwise).

Chew sugarless gum or suck on ice chips or a piece of hard candy to reduce mouth dryness.

If you feel dizzy or light-headed, sit or lie down for a while; get up from a sitting or lying position slowly, and be careful on stairs.

Major. Tell your doctor about any side effects that are persistent or particularly bothersome. IT IS ESPECIALLY IMPORTANT TO TELL YOUR DOCTOR about severe abdominal pain; bloody or black, tarry stools; chest tightness; difficult or painful urination; difficulty in breathing; fatigue; itching; palpitations; rash; ringing in the ears; tremors; or yellowing of the eyes or skin.

INTERACTIONS

This medication interacts with several other types of drugs:

1. Concurrent use of it with other central nervous system depressants (such as alcohol, antihistamines, barbiturates, benzodiazepine tranquilizers, muscle relaxants, and phenothiazine tranquilizers) or with tricyclic antidepressants can cause extreme drowsiness.

2. The concurrent use of aspirin and codeine combination and monoamine oxidase (MAO) inhibitors should be avoided. At least 14 days should separate the use of aspirin and codeine combination and the use of an MAO inhibitor.

3. Alcohol and anti-inflammatory medication can increase the gastrointestinal side effects of this medication.

4. The side effects of anticoagulants (blood thinners, such as warfarin), oral antidiabetic agents, phenytoin, and methotrexate may be increased by the aspirin in this product.

5. Large doses of antacids increase the elimination of the aspirin portion of this medication from the body and decrease its effectiveness.

6. Aspirin may decrease the antigout effects of probenecid and sulfinpyrazone.

BE SURE TO TELL YOUR DOCTOR about any medications you are currently taking, especially any listed above.

WARNINGS

- Tell your doctor about unusual or allergic reactions you have had to medications, especially to aspirin, methyl salicylate (oil of wintergreen), diclofenac, diflunisal, flurbiprofen, fenoprofen, ibuprofen, indomethacin, ketoprofen, meclofenamate, mefenamic acid, naproxen, piroxicam, sulindac, and tolmetin or to codeine or other narcotic analgesics (such as hydrocodone, hydromorphone, meperidine, methadone, morphine, oxycodone, and propoxyphene).
- Tell your doctor if you now have or if you have ever had abdominal disease, Addison's disease, bleeding or blood disorders, brain disease, colitis, epilepsy, gallstones or gallbladder disease, head injuries, heart disease, hemophilia, kidney disease, liver disease, lung disease, peptic ulcers, porphyria, enlarged prostate gland, or thyroid disease.
- If this drug makes you dizzy or drowsy, do not take part in any activity that requires alertness, such as driving a car or operating potentially dangerous equipment.
- Before having surgery or any other medical or dental treatment, be sure to tell your doctor or dentist that you are taking this medication. Aspirin-containing medication is usually discontinued five to seven days before surgery, to prevent bleeding complications.
- The use of aspirin in children (about 16 years of age or less) with the flu or chicken pox has been associated with a rare, life-threatening condition called Reye's syndrome. Aspirin-containing products should, therefore, not be given to children with signs of infection.
- Because this drug contains codeine, it has the potential for abuse and must be used with caution. Usually, it should not be taken on a regular schedule for longer than ten days at a time. Tolerance develops quickly; do not increase the dosage or stop taking the drug abruptly, unless you first consult your doctor. If you have been taking large amounts of this medication for long periods, you may experience a withdrawal reaction (muscle aches, diarrhea, gooseflesh, runny nose, nausea, vomiting, shivering, trembling, stomach cramps, sleep disorders, irritability, weakness, excessive yawning, or sweating). Your doctor may, therefore, want to reduce the dosage gradually.
- Because this product contains aspirin, additional medications that contain aspirin should not be taken without your doctor's approval. Check the labels on over-the-counter (nonprescription) pain, sinus, allergy, asthma, cough, and cold products to see if they contain aspirin.
- Diabetic patients should be aware that large doses of aspirin (more than eight 325-mg tablets per day) may interfere with urine sugar testing. Diabetics should, therefore, check with their doctor before changing their insulin dose.
- Be sure to tell your doctor if you are pregnant. The effects of this medication during pregnancy have not been thoroughly studied in humans. Codeine, used regularly in large doses during pregnancy, may result in addiction of the fetus, leading to withdrawal symptoms (irritability, excessive crying, tremors, fever, vomiting, diarrhea, sneezing, or excessive yawning) at birth. Large amounts of aspirin taken close to the end of pregnancy may prolong labor and cause bleeding problems in the mother and heart problems in the newborn infant. Also, tell your doctor if you are breast-feeding an infant. Small amounts of this medication may pass into breast milk and cause excessive drowsiness in the nursing infant.

aspirin and meprobamate combination—see meprobamate and aspirin combination

aspirin and oxycodone combination

BRAND NAMES (Manufacturers)
Codoxy (Halsey)
oxycodone hydrochloride, oxycodone terephthalate, and aspirin (various manufacturers)
Percodan (DuPont)
Percodan-Demi (DuPont)

TYPE OF DRUG
Analgesic combination

INGREDIENTS
aspirin and oxycodone

DOSAGE FORM
Tablets (325 mg aspirin with 2.25 mg oxycodone hydrochloride and 0.19 mg oxycodone terephthalate; 325 mg aspirin with 4.5 mg oxycodone hydrochloride and 0.38 mg oxycodone terephthalate)

STORAGE
Store at room temperature in a tightly closed container. Moisture causes the aspirin in this product to decompose.

USES

This combination medication is used to relieve moderate to severe pain. Oxycodone is a narcotic analgesic that acts on the central nervous system to relieve pain.

TREATMENT

In order to avoid stomach upset, you can take this medication with food or milk.

This medication works most effectively if you take it at the onset of pain, rather than waiting until the pain becomes intense.

If you are taking this medication on a regular schedule and you miss a dose, take the missed dose as soon as possible, unless it is almost time for your next dose. In that case, don't take the missed dose at all; just return to your regular dosing schedule. Do not double the next dose.

SIDE EFFECTS

Minor. Constipation, dizziness, drowsiness, dry mouth, false sense of well-being, flushing, indigestion, lightheadedness, loss of appetite, nausea, sweating, or vomiting. These side effects should disappear as your body adjusts to the medication.

If you are constipated, increase the amount of fiber in your diet (fresh fruits and vegetables, salads, bran, and whole-grain breads), drink more water, and exercise (unless your doctor directs you to do otherwise).

Chew sugarless gum or suck on ice chips or a piece of hard candy to reduce mouth dryness.

If you feel dizzy, light-headed, or nauseated, sit or lie down for a while; get up from a sitting or lying position slowly, and be careful on stairs.

Major. Tell your doctor about any side effects that are persistent or particularly bothersome. IT IS ESPECIALLY IMPORTANT TO TELL YOUR DOCTOR about bloody or black, tarry stools; chest tightness; difficult or painful urination; difficulty in breathing; fatigue; itching; palpitations; rash; ringing in the ears; severe abdominal pain; tremors; or yellowing of the eyes or skin.

INTERACTIONS

This medication interacts with several other types of drugs:

1. Concurrent use of this medication with other central nervous system depressants (such as alcohol, antihistamines, barbiturates, benzodiazepine tranquilizers, muscle relaxants, and phenothiazine tranquilizers) or with tricyclic antidepressants can cause extreme drowsiness.

2. The concurrent use of aspirin and oxycodone combination and monoamine oxidase (MAO) inhibitors should be avoided. At least 14 days should separate the use of this drug and the use of an MAO inhibitor.

3. Alcohol and anti-inflammatory medications can increase the gastrointestinal side effects of this medication.

4. The side effects of anticoagulants (blood thinners, such as warfarin), oral antidiabetic agents, phenytoin, and methotrexate may be increased by the aspirin in this product.

5. Large doses of antacids increase the elimination of the aspirin portion of this medication from the body and decrease its effectiveness.

6. The aspirin portion of this medication may decrease the antigout effects of probenecid and sulfinpyrazone.

BE SURE TO TELL YOUR DOCTOR about any medications you are currently taking, especially any listed above.

WARNINGS

- Tell your doctor about unusual or allergic reactions you have had to medications, especially to aspirin, methyl salicylate (oil of wintergreen), diclofenac, diflunisal, flurbiprofen, fenoprofen, ibuprofen, indomethacin, ketoprofen, meclofenamate, mefenamic acid, naproxen, piroxicam, sulindac, or tolmetin or to oxycodone or other narcotic analgesics (such as codeine, hydrocodone, hydromorphone, meperidine, methadone, morphine, or propoxyphene).
- Tell your doctor if you now have or if you have ever had abdominal disease, Addison's disease, bleeding or blood disorders, brain disease, colitis, epilepsy, gallstones or gallbladder disease, head injuries, heart disease, hemophilia, kidney disease, liver disease, lung disease, peptic ulcers, porphyria, enlarged prostate gland, or thyroid disease.
- If this drug makes you dizzy or drowsy, do not take part in any activity that requires alertness, such as driving a car or operating potentially dangerous equipment.
- Before having surgery or any other medical or dental treatment, tell your doctor or dentist that you are taking this drug. Aspirin-containing medications are usually stopped five to seven days before surgery, in order to prevent complications.
- The use of aspirin in children (about 16 years of age or less) with the flu or chicken pox has been associated with a rare, life-threatening condition called Reye's syndrome. Aspirin-containing products should, therefore, not be given to children who have any signs of infection.
- Because this drug contains oxycodone, it has the potential for abuse and must be used with caution. Usually, it should not be taken on a regular schedule for longer than ten days at a time. Tolerance develops quickly; do not increase the dosage or stop taking the drug abruptly, unless you first consult your doctor. If you have been taking large amounts of this medication for long periods, you may experience a withdrawal reaction (muscle aches, diarrhea, gooseflesh, runny nose, nausea, vomiting, shivering, trembling, stomach cramps, sleep disorders, irritability, weakness, ex-

cessive yawning, or sweating). Your doctor may, therefore, want to reduce the dosage gradually to prevent or minimize this response.

• Because this product contains aspirin, additional medications that contain aspirin should not be taken without your doctor's approval. Check the labels on over-the-counter (nonprescription) pain, sinus, allergy, asthma, cough, and cold products to see if they contain aspirin.

• Diabetic patients should be aware that large doses of aspirin (more than eight 325-mg tablets per day) may interfere with urine sugar testing. Diabetics should, therefore, check with their doctor before changing their insulin dose.

• Be sure to tell your doctor if you are pregnant. The effects of this medication during pregnancy have not been thoroughly studied in humans. Oxycodone, used regularly in large doses during pregnancy, may result in addiction of the fetus, leading to withdrawal symptoms (irritability, excessive crying, tremors, fever, vomiting, diarrhea, sneezing, or excessive yawning) at birth. Large amounts of aspirin taken close to the end of pregnancy may prolong labor and cause bleeding problems in the mother and heart problems in the newborn infant. Also, tell your doctor if you are breast-feeding an infant. Small amounts of this medication may pass into breast milk and cause excessive drowsiness in the nursing infant.

---

aspirin, caffeine, and butalbital combination

BRAND NAMES (Manufacturers)

B-A-C (Mayrand)
butalbital with aspirin and caffeine (various manufacturers)
Fiorgen PF (Goldline)
Fiorinal (Sandoz)
Isollyl Improved (Rugby)
Lanorinal (Lannett)
Marnal (Vortech)

TYPE OF DRUG

Analgesic combination and sedative

INGREDIENTS

aspirin, caffeine, and butalbital

DOSAGE FORMS

Tablets (325 mg aspirin, 40 mg caffeine, and 50 mg butalbital; 650 mg aspirin, 40 mg caffeine, and 50 mg butalbital)
Capsules (325 mg aspirin, 40 mg caffeine, and 50 mg butalbital)

STORAGE

Aspirin, caffeine, and butalbital combination tablets and capsules should be stored at room temperature in tightly closed containers. Moisture causes the aspirin in this product to decompose.

USES

This combination medication is used to relieve tension headaches and mild to moderate pain. Butalbital belongs to a group of drugs known as barbiturates. The barbiturates act on the central nervous system (brain and spinal cord) to produce relaxation. Caffeine is a central nervous system stimulant. It constricts blood vessels in the head, which may help to relieve headaches.

TREATMENT

In order to avoid stomach upset, you can take this medication with food or milk.

This drug works most effectively if you take it at the onset of pain, rather than waiting until the pain is intense.

If you are taking this medication on a regular schedule and you miss a dose, take the missed dose as soon as possible, unless it is almost time for your next dose. In that case, don't take the missed dose at all; just return to your regular dosing schedule. Do not double the next dose.

SIDE EFFECTS

Minor. Dizziness, drowsiness, gas, loss of appetite, nausea, nervousness, sleeping disorders, or vomiting. These side effects should disappear as your body adjusts to the medication.

If you feel dizzy or light-headed, sit or lie down for a while; get up from a sitting or lying position slowly, and be careful on stairs.

Major. Tell your doctor about any side effects that are persistent or particularly bothersome. IT IS ESPECIALLY IMPORTANT TO TELL YOUR DOCTOR about bloody or black, tarry stools; chest tightness; confusion; difficult or painful urination; light-headedness; loss of coordination; palpitations; rash; ringing in the ears; shortness of breath; severe abdominal pain; sore throat and fever; or yellowing of the eyes or skin.

INTERACTIONS

This medication interacts with several other types of drugs:

1. Concurrent use of this medication with other central nervous system depressants (such as alcohol, antihistamines, barbiturates, benzodiazepine tranquilizers, muscle relaxants, and phenothiazine tranquilizers) or with tricyclic antidepressants can cause extreme drowsiness.

2. Alcohol and anti-inflammatory medications can increase the gastrointestinal side effects of this medication.

3. The side effects of anticoagulants (blood thinners, such as warfarin), oral antidiabetic agents, phenytoin, and methotrexate may be increased by the aspirin in this product.

4. Large doses of antacids increase the elimination of the aspirin portion of this medication from the body and decrease its effectiveness.

5. Aspirin may decrease the antigout effects of probenecid and sulfinpyrazone.

6. Butalbital can increase the elimination from the body of oral contraceptives (birth control pills), carbamazepine, adrenocorticosteroids (cortisone-like drugs), digoxin, doxycycline, tricyclic antidepressants, griseofulvin, metronidazole, theophylline, aminophylline, and quinidine, thereby decreasing the effectiveness of these medications.

7. The side effects of cyclophosphamide may be increased by butalbital.

BE SURE TO TELL YOUR DOCTOR about any medications you are currently taking, especially any of those listed above.

WARNINGS

• Tell your doctor about unusual or allergic reactions you have had to medications, especially to aspirin, methyl salicylate (oil of wintergreen), diclofenac, diflunisal, flurbiprofen, fenoprofen, ibuprofen, indomethacin, ketoprofen, meclofenamate, mefenamic acid, naproxen, piroxicam, sulindac, or tolmetin; to caffeine; or to butalbital or other barbiturates (such as phenobarbital, pentobarbital, or secobarbital).

• Tell your doctor if you now have or if you have ever had bleeding problems, blood disorders, diabetes mellitus, heart disease, hemophilia, hyperactivity, kidney disease, liver disease, mental depression, peptic ulcers, or thyroid disease.

• If this drug makes you dizzy or drowsy, do not take part in any activity that requires alertness, such as driving a car or operating potentially dangerous equipment.

• Before having surgery or any other medical or dental treatment, be sure to tell your doctor or dentist that you are taking this medication. Aspirin-containing medication is usually discontinued five to seven days before surgery to prevent bleeding complications.

• The use of aspirin in children (about 16 years of age or less) with the flu or chicken pox has been associated with a rare, life-threatening condition called Reye's syndrome. Aspirin-containing products should, therefore, not be given to children with signs of infection.

• Because this drug contains butalbital, it has the potential for abuse and must be used with caution. Tolerance develops quickly; do not increase the dosage or stop taking the drug abruptly, unless you first consult your doctor. If you have been taking large amounts of this medication for long periods, you may experience a withdrawal reaction (muscle aches, diarrhea, convulsions, sleep disorders, nervousness, irritability, or weakness). Your doctor may, therefore, want to reduce the dosage gradually.

• Because this product contains aspirin, additional medications that contain aspirin should not be taken without your physician's approval. Check the labels on over-the-counter (nonprescription) pain, sinus, allergy, asthma, cough, and cold products to see if they contain aspirin.

• You should not take more than six tablets or capsules of this drug in one day, unless your doctor specifically directs you to do so.

• Diabetic patients should be aware that large doses of aspirin (more than eight 325-mg tablets or capsules per day) may interfere with urine sugar testing. Diabetics should, therefore, check with their doctor before changing their insulin dose.

• Be sure to tell your doctor if you are pregnant. The effects of this medication during pregnancy have not been thoroughly studied in humans. Butalbital, used regularly in large doses during pregnancy, may result in addiction of the fetus, leading to withdrawal symptoms (irritability, excessive crying, tremors, fever, vomiting, diarrhea, sneezing, or excessive yawning) at birth. Large amounts of aspirin taken close to the end of pregnancy may prolong labor and cause bleeding problems in the mother and heart problems in the newborn infant. Also, tell your doctor if you are breast-feeding an infant. Small amounts of this medication may pass into breast milk and cause excessive drowsiness in the nursing infant.

---

aspirin, caffeine, and dihydrocodeine combination

BRAND NAME (Manufacturer)
Synalgos-DC (Ives)

TYPE OF DRUG
Analgesic combination

INGREDIENTS
aspirin, caffeine, and dihydrocodeine

DOSAGE FORM
Capsules (356.4 mg aspirin, 30 mg caffeine, and 16 mg dihydrocodeine)

STORAGE
This medication should be stored at room temperature in a tightly closed container. Moisture causes the aspirin in this product to decompose.

USES

Aspirin, caffeine, and dihydrocodeine combination is used to relieve mild to moderate pain. Dihydrocodeine is a narcotic analgesic that acts on the central nervous system (brain and spinal cord) to relieve pain. Caffeine is a central nervous system stimulant. It constricts the blood vessels in the head, which may help to relieve headaches.

TREATMENT

In order to avoid stomach upset, you can take this medication with food or milk.

This medication works most effectively if you take it at the onset of pain, rather than waiting until the pain becomes intense.

If you are taking this medication on a regular schedule and you miss a dose, take the missed dose as soon as possible, unless it is almost time for your next dose. In that case, don't take the missed dose at all; just return to your regular dosing schedule. Do not double the next dose.

SIDE EFFECTS

Minor. Constipation, dizziness, drowsiness, dry mouth, false sense of well-being, headache, indigestion, loss of appetite, nausea, nervousness, restlessness, sleep disorders, sweating, or vomiting. These side effects should disappear as your body adjusts to the medication.

If you are constipated, increase the amount of fiber in your diet (fresh fruits and vegetables, salads, bran, and whole-grain breads), drink more water, and exercise (unless your doctor directs you to do otherwise).

Chew sugarless gum or suck on ice chips or a piece of hard candy to reduce mouth dryness.

If you feel dizzy or light-headed, sit or lie down for a while; get up from a sitting or lying position slowly, and be careful on stairs.

Major. Tell your doctor about any side effects that are persistent or particularly bothersome. IT IS ESPECIALLY IMPORTANT TO TELL YOUR DOCTOR about black, tarry stools; blurred vision; chest tightness; difficult or painful urination; difficulty in breathing; fainting; itching; light-headedness; loss of coordination; palpitations; ringing in the ears; severe abdominal pain; skin rash; sore throat and fever; or unusual bleeding or bruising.

INTERACTIONS

This medication interacts with several other types of drugs:

1. Concurrent use of this medication with other central nervous system depressants (such as alcohol, antihistamines, barbiturates, benzodiazepine tranquilizers, muscle relaxants, and phenothiazine tranquilizers) or with tricyclic antidepressants can cause extreme drowsiness.

2. Concurrent use of this drug and monoamine oxidase (MAO) inhibitors should be avoided. At least 14 days should separate the use of aspirin, caffeine, and dihydrocodeine combination and the use of an MAO inhibitor.
3. Alcohol and anti-inflammatory medication can increase the gastrointestinal side effects of this medication.
4. The aspirin in this product may increase the side effects of anticoagulants (blood thinners, such as warfarin), oral antidiabetic agents, phenytoin, and methotrexate.
5. Large doses of antacids increase the elimination of the aspirin portion of this medication from the body and decrease its effectiveness.
6. The aspirin portion of this medication may decrease the antigout effects of probenecid and sulfinpyrazone.

BE SURE TO TELL YOUR DOCTOR about any medications that you are currently taking, especially any of the medications that are listed above.

WARNINGS

• Tell your doctor about unusual or allergic reactions you have had to medications, especially to aspirin, methyl salicylate (oil of wintergreen), diclofenac, diflunisal, flurbiprofen, fenoprofen, ibuprofen, indomethacin, ketoprofen, meclofenamate, mefenamic acid, naproxen, piroxicam, sulindac, or tolmetin; to dihydrocodeine or other narcotic analgesics (such as codeine, hydrocodone, hydromorphone, meperidine, methadone, morphine, oxycodone, and propoxyphene); or to caffeine.

• Tell your doctor if you now have or if you have ever had abdominal disease, Addison's disease, bleeding or blood disorders, brain disease, colitis, epilepsy, gallstones or gallbladder disease, head injuries, heart disease, hemophilia, kidney disease, liver disease, lung disease, peptic ulcers, prostate disease, or thyroid disease.

• If this drug makes you dizzy or drowsy, do not take part in any activity that requires alertness, such as driving a car or operating potentially dangerous equipment.

• Before having surgery or any other medical or dental treatment, be sure to tell your doctor or dentist that you are taking this medication. Aspirin-containing medication is usually discontinued five to seven days before surgery, to prevent bleeding complications.

• The use of aspirin in children (about 16 years of age or less) with the flu or chicken pox has been associated with a rare, life-threatening condition called Reye's syndrome. Aspirin-containing products should, therefore, not be given to children with signs of infection.

• Because this drug contains dihydrocodeine, it has the potential for abuse and must be used with caution. Usually, it should not be taken on a regular schedule for longer than ten days at a time. Tolerance develops quickly; do not increase the dosage or stop taking the drug abruptly, unless you first consult your doctor. If you have been taking large amounts of this medication for long periods, you may experience a withdrawal reaction (muscle aches, diarrhea, gooseflesh, runny nose, nausea, vomiting, shivering, trembling, stomach cramps, sleep disorders, irritability, weakness, excessive yawning, or sweating). Your doctor may, therefore, want to reduce the dosage gradually.

• Because this product contains aspirin, additional medications that contain aspirin should not be taken without your doctor's approval. Check the labels on over-the-counter (nonprescription) pain, sinus, allergy, asthma, cough, and cold products to see if they contain aspirin.

• Diabetics should be aware that large doses of aspirin (more than eight 325-mg tablets of aspirin per day) may interfere with urine sugar testing and should, therefore, check with their doctor before changing their insulin dose.

• Be sure to tell your doctor if you are pregnant. The effects of this medication during pregnancy have not been thoroughly studied in humans. Dihydrocodeine, used regularly in large doses during pregnancy, may result in addiction of the fetus, leading to withdrawal symptoms (irritability, excessive crying, tremors, fever, vomiting, diarrhea, sneezing, or excessive yawning) at birth. Large amounts of aspirin taken close to the end of pregnancy may prolong labor and cause bleeding problems in the mother and heart problems in the newborn infant. Also, tell your doctor if you are breast-feeding an infant. Small amounts of this medication may pass into breast milk and cause excessive drowsiness in the nursing infant.

---

aspirin, caffeine, and propoxyphene combination

BRAND NAMES (Manufacturers)
Darvon Compound-65 (Lilly)
Dolene Compound-65 (Lederle)
Doxaphene Compound (Major)
propoxyphene hydrochloride compound (various manufacturers)

TYPE OF DRUG
Analgesic combination

INGREDIENTS
aspirin, caffeine, and propoxyphene

DOSAGE FORM
Capsules (389 mg aspirin, 32.4 mg caffeine, and 32 mg propoxyphene; 389 mg aspirin, 32.4 mg caffeine, and 65 mg propoxyphene)

STORAGE
Aspirin, caffeine, and propoxyphene capsules should be stored at room temperature in a tightly closed container. Moisture causes the aspirin to decompose.

USES

Aspirin, caffeine, and propoxyphene combination is used to relieve mild to moderate pain. Propoxyphene is a narcotic analgesic that acts on the central nervous system (brain and spinal cord) to relieve pain. Caffeine is a central nervous system stimulant. It constricts blood vessels in the head, which may help to relieve headaches.

TREATMENT

In order to avoid stomach upset, you can take this medication with food or milk.

This medication works most effectively if you take it at the onset of pain, rather than waiting until the pain becomes intense.

If you are taking this medication on a regular schedule and you miss a dose, take the missed dose as soon as possible, unless it is almost time for your next dose. In that case, don't take the missed dose at all; just return to your regular dosing schedule. Do not double the next dose.

SIDE EFFECTS

Minor. Constipation, dizziness, drowsiness, dry mouth, false sense of well-being, flushing, indigestion, loss of appetite, nausea, sweating, or vomiting. These side effects should disappear as your body adjusts to the medication.

If you are constipated, increase the amount of fiber in your diet (fresh fruits and vegetables, salads, bran, and whole-grain breads), drink more water, and exercise (unless your doctor directs you to do otherwise).

If you feel dizzy or light-headed, sit or lie down for a while; get up from a sitting or lying position slowly, and be careful on stairs.

Major. Tell your doctor about any side effects that are persistent or particularly bothersome. IT IS ESPECIALLY IMPORTANT TO TELL YOUR DOCTOR about severe abdominal pain; bloody or black, tarry stools; chest tightness; difficult or painful urination; difficulty in breathing; fatigue; itching; light-headedness; palpitations; rash; ringing in the ears; tremors; or yellowing of the eyes or skin.

INTERACTIONS

This medication interacts with several other types of drugs:

1. Concurrent use of this medication with other central nervous system depressants (such as alcohol, antihistamines, barbiturates, benzodiazepine tranquilizers, muscle relaxants, or phenothiazine tranquilizers) or with tricyclic antidepressants can cause extreme drowsiness.

2. Concurrent use of this medication and monoamine oxidase (MAO) inhibitors should be avoided. At least 14 days should separate the use of aspirin, caffeine, and propoxyphene combination and the use of an MAO inhibitor.

3. Alcohol and anti-inflammatory medication can increase the gastrointestinal side effects of this medication.

4. The aspirin in this product may increase the side effects of anticoagulants (blood thinners, such as warfarin), oral antidiabetic agents, phenytoin, and methotrexate.

5. Large doses of antacids increase the elimination of the aspirin portion of this medication from the body and decrease its effectiveness.

6. The aspirin portion of this medication may decrease the antigout effects of probenecid and sulfinpyrazone.

7. The propoxyphene portion of this medication can decrease the elimination of carbamazepine from the body, which can lead to an increase in side effects.

BE SURE TO TELL YOUR DOCTOR about any medications you are currently taking, especially any listed above.

WARNINGS

- Tell your doctor about unusual or allergic reactions you have had to medications, especially to aspirin, methyl salicylate (oil of wintergreen), diclofenac, diflunisal, flurbiprofen, fenoprofen, ibuprofen, indomethacin, ketoprofen, meclofenamate, mefenamic acid, naproxen, piroxicam, sulindac, or tolmetin; to propoxyphene or other narcotic analgesics (such as codeine, hydrocodone, hydromorphone, meperidine, methadone, morphine, and oxycodone); or to caffeine.
- Tell your doctor if you now have or if you have ever had abdominal disease, Addison's disease, bleeding or blood disorders, brain disease, colitis, epilepsy, gallstones or gallbladder disease, head injuries, heart disease, hemophilia, kidney disease, liver disease, lung disease, peptic ulcer, prostate disease, or thyroid disease.
- If this drug makes you dizzy or drowsy, do not take part in any activity that requires alertness, such as driving a car or operating potentially dangerous equipment.
- Before having any surgery or other medical or dental treatment, be sure to tell your doctor or dentist that you are taking this medication. Aspirin-containing medication is usually discontinued five to seven days before surgery, to prevent bleeding complications.
- The use of aspirin in children (about 16 years of age or less) with the flu or chicken pox has been associated with a rare, life-threatening condition called Reye's syndrome. Aspirin-containing products should, therefore, not be given to children with signs of infection.
- Because this drug contains propoxyphene, it has the potential for abuse and must be used with caution. Usually, it should not be taken on a regular schedule for longer than ten days at a time. Tolerance develops quickly; do not increase the dosage or stop taking the drug abruptly, unless you first consult your doctor. If you have been taking large amounts of this medication for long periods, you may experience a withdrawal reaction (muscle aches, diarrhea, gooseflesh, runny nose, nausea, vomiting, shivering, trembling, stomach cramps, sleep disorders, irritability, weakness, excessive yawning, or sweating). Your doctor may, therefore, want to reduce the dosage gradually.
- Because this product contains aspirin, additional medications that contain aspirin should not be taken without your doctor's approval. Check the labels on over-the-counter (nonprescription) pain, sinus, allergy, asthma, cough, and cold products to see if they contain aspirin.
- You should not take more than six capsules of this drug in one day, unless your doctor specifically directs you to do so.
- Diabetics should be aware that large doses of aspirin (more than eight 325-mg tablets of aspirin per day) may interfere with urine sugar testing. Diabetics should, therefore, check with their doctor before changing their insulin dose.
- Be sure to tell your doctor if you are pregnant. The effects of this medication during pregnancy have not been thoroughly studied in humans. Propoxyphene, used regularly in large doses during pregnancy, may result in addiction of the fetus, leading to withdrawal symptoms (irritability, excessive crying, tremors, fever, vomiting, diarrhea, sneezing, or excessive yawning) at birth. Large amounts of aspirin taken close to the end of pregnancy may prolong labor and cause bleeding problems in the mother and heart problems in the newborn infant. Also, tell your doctor if you are breast-feeding an infant. Small amounts of this medication may pass into breast milk and cause excessive drowsiness in the nursing infant.

---

aspirin, caffeine, butalbital, and codeine combination

BRAND NAMES (Manufacturers)

B-A-C #3 (Mayrand)
Fiorinal with Codeine (Sandoz)

TYPE OF DRUG
Analgesic combination and sedative

INGREDIENTS
aspirin, caffeine, butalbital, and codeine

DOSAGE FORMS
Tablets (325 mg aspirin, 40 mg caffeine, 50 mg butalbital, and 30 mg codeine)

Capsules (325 mg aspirin, 40 mg caffeine, 50 mg butalbital, and 7.5 mg, 15 mg, or 30 mg codeine)

Note that on the label of the vial of tablets or capsules the name of this drug is followed by a number. This number refers to the amount of codeine present (#1 contains 7.5 mg codeine, #2 has 15 mg codeine, and #3 contains 30 mg codeine).

STORAGE
Aspirin, caffeine, butalbital, and codeine combination tablets and capsules should be stored at room temperature in tightly closed containers. Moisture causes the aspirin in this product to decompose.

USES
This combination medication is used to relieve tension headaches and mild to moderate pain. Codeine is a narcotic analgesic that acts on the central nervous system (brain and spinal cord) to relieve pain. Butalbital belongs to a group of drugs known as barbiturates. The barbiturates act on the central nervous system to produce relaxation. Caffeine is a central nervous system stimulant. It constricts blood vessels in the head, which may help to relieve headaches.

TREATMENT
In order to avoid stomach upset, you can take this medication with food or milk.

This medication works most effectively if you take it at the onset of pain, rather than waiting until the pain becomes intense.

If you are taking this medication on a regular schedule and you miss a dose, take the missed dose as soon as possible, unless it is almost time for your next dose. In that case, don't take the missed dose at all; just return to your regular dosing schedule. Do not double the next dose.

SIDE EFFECTS
Minor. Constipation, dizziness, drowsiness, flushing, headache, indigestion, loss of appetite, nausea, nervousness, sleep disorders, sweating, tiredness, or vomiting. These side effects should disappear as your body adjusts to the medication.

If you feel dizzy or light-headed, sit or lie down for a while; get up from a sitting or lying position slowly, and be careful on stairs.

If you are constipated, increase the amount of fiber in your diet (fresh fruits and vegetables, salads, bran, and whole-grain breads), drink more water, and exercise (unless your doctor directs you to do otherwise).

Major. Tell your doctor about any side effects that are persistent or particularly bothersome. IT IS ESPECIALLY IMPORTANT TO TELL YOUR DOCTOR about bloody or black, tarry stools; blurred vision; chest tightness; confusion; difficult or painful urination; loss of coordination; palpitations; rash; ringing in the ears; shortness of breath; severe abdominal pain; sore throat and fever; or yellowing of the eyes or skin.

INTERACTIONS
This combination medication interacts with several other types of drugs:

1. Concurrent use of this medication with other central nervous system depressants (such as alcohol, antihistamines, barbiturates, benzodiazepine tranquilizers, muscle relaxants, or phenothiazine tranquilizers) or with tricyclic antidepressants can cause extreme drowsiness.

2. Alcohol and anti-inflammatory medications can increase the gastrointestinal side effects of this medication.

3. The side effects of anticoagulants (blood thinners, such as warfarin), oral antidiabetic agents, phenytoin, and methotrexate may be increased by the aspirin in this product.

4. Large doses of antacids increase the elimination of the aspirin portion of this medication from the body and decrease its effectiveness.

5. Aspirin may decrease the antigout effects of probenecid and sulfinpyrazone.

6. Butalbital can increase the elimination from the body of oral contraceptives (birth control pills), carbamazepine, adrenocorticosteroids (cortisone-like drugs), digoxin, doxycycline, tricyclic antidepressants, griseofulvin, metronidazole, theophylline, aminophylline, and quinidine, thereby decreasing the effectiveness of these medications.

7. The side effects of cyclophosphamide may be increased by butalbital.

8. This medication may interact with monoamine oxidase (MAO) inhibitors.

BE SURE TO TELL YOUR DOCTOR about any medications you are currently taking, especially any of those listed above.

WARNINGS
- Tell your doctor about unusual or allergic reactions you have had to medications, especially to aspirin, methyl salicylate (oil of wintergreen), diclofenac, diflunisal, flurbiprofen, fenoprofen, ibuprofen, indomethacin, ketoprofen, meclofenamate, mefenamic acid, naproxen, piroxicam, sulindac, or tolmetin; to codeine or other narcotic analgesics (such as hydrocodone, hydromorphone, meperidine, methadone, morphine, oxycodone, and propoxyphene); to caffeine; or to butalbital or other barbiturates (such as phenobarbital, pentobarbital, and secobarbital).
- Tell your doctor if you now have or if you have ever had abdominal disease, Addison's disease, bleeding or blood disorders, brain disease, colitis, epilepsy, gallstones or gallbladder disease, head injuries, heart disease, hemophilia, kidney disease, liver disease, lung disease, peptic ulcers, porphyria, prostate disease, or thyroid disease.
- If this drug makes you dizzy or drowsy, do not take part in any activity that requires alertness, such as driving a car or operating potentially dangerous equipment.
- Before having surgery or any other medical or dental treatment, be sure to tell your doctor or dentist that you are taking this medication. Aspirin-containing medication is usually discontinued five to seven days before surgery, to prevent bleeding complications.
- The use of aspirin in children (about 16 years of age or less) with the flu or chicken pox has been associated with a rare, life-threatening condition called Reye's syndrome. Aspirin-containing products should, therefore, not be given to children with signs of infection.
- Because this drug contains codeine and butalbital, it has

the potential for abuse and must be used with caution. Usually, it should not be taken on a regular schedule for longer than ten days at a time. Tolerance develops quickly; do not increase the dosage or stop taking the drug abruptly, unless you first consult your doctor. If you have been taking large amounts of this medication for long periods, you may experience a withdrawal reaction (muscle aches, diarrhea, gooseflesh, runny nose, nausea, vomiting, shivering, trembling, stomach cramps, sleep disorders, irritability, weakness, excessive yawning, or sweating). Your doctor may, therefore, want to reduce the dosage gradually.

- Because this product contains aspirin, additional medications that contain aspirin should not be taken without your doctor's approval. Check the labels on over-the-counter (nonprescription) pain, sinus, allergy, asthma, cough, and cold products to see if they contain aspirin.
- You should not take more than six tablets or capsules of this drug in one day, unless your doctor specifically directs you to do so.
- Diabetic patients should be aware that large doses of aspirin (more than eight 325-mg tablets or capsules per day) may interfere with urine sugar testing. Diabetics should, therefore, check with their doctor before changing their insulin dose.
- Be sure to tell your doctor if you are pregnant. The effects of this medication during pregnancy have not been thoroughly studied in humans. Codeine and butalbital, used regularly in large doses during pregnancy, may result in addiction of the fetus, leading to withdrawal symptoms (irritability, excessive crying, tremors, fever, vomiting, diarrhea, sneezing, or excessive yawning) at birth. Large amounts of aspirin taken close to the end of pregnancy may prolong labor and cause bleeding problems in the mother and heart problems in the newborn infant. Also, tell your doctor if you are breast-feeding an infant. Small amounts of this medication may pass into breast milk and cause excessive drowsiness in the nursing infant.

---

astemizole

BRAND NAME (Manufacturer)
Hismanal (Janssen)
TYPE OF DRUG
Antihistamine
INGREDIENT
astemizole
DOSAGE FORM
Tablets (10 mg)
STORAGE
Store this medication in a tightly closed container in a cool, dry place, away from heat or direct light, and out of the reach of children.

USES

Astemizole is indicated for the treatment of the allergic symptoms of conditions such as hay fever or hives. It belongs to a group of drugs known as antihistamines, which act by blocking the action of histamine, a chemical that is released by the body during an allergic reaction. It may be useful in patients unable to tolerate side effects, such as sedation, that other antihistamines may produce.

TREATMENT

Astemizole should be taken only as needed, and the prescribed dose should not be exceeded.

Because food significantly impairs the absorption of this medication, the drug should be taken on an empty stomach, at least two hours after a meal. No additional food should be taken for at least an hour after a dose is taken.

It may take up to two days for astemizole to achieve its full therapeutic effect.

SIDE EFFECTS

Minor. Abdominal pain, diarrhea, drowsiness, dry mouth, gas, headache, increased appetite, nervousness, increased sensitivity to sunlight, or weight gain.

To relieve mouth dryness, chew sugarless gum or suck on ice chips or hard candy.

Major. Tell your doctor about any side effects that are persistent or particularly bothersome. It is ESPECIALLY IMPORTANT TO TELL YOUR DOCTOR about symptoms of a hypersensitivity reaction such as shortness of breath or rash.

INTERACTIONS

Although clinical studies with astemizole have not shown significant interactions with depressants, such as alcohol or diazepam, it is important to be aware of the possibility of interactions. BE SURE TO TELL YOUR DOCTOR about all medications you are taking before starting astemizole.

WARNINGS

- Tell your doctor about unusual or allergic reactions you have had to any medication, especially to astemizole.
- Although astemizole is a less-sedating antihistamine, some patients may be more sensitive to its effects. Until you are familiar with how astemizole affects you, be especially cautious in performing tasks that require alertness, such as driving a car or operating potentially dangerous machinery.
- Tell your physician of any known liver ailments. Patients with diseases of the liver may not eliminate astemizole as rapidly as those with normal liver function.
- Be sure to tell your doctor if you are pregnant or plan to become pregnant. The safety of astemizole in pregnant women has not been established. In animal studies in which administered doses of astemizole exceeded dosage levels used in humans, an increased incidence of low birth weight and risk of infant death was noted. Since breakdown products of the drug may remain in the body for up to four months after use, this fact should be taken into consideration if pregnancy is being planned.
- Because babies are more sensitive to the side effects of antihistamines, such as excitement or irritability, astemizole is not recommended in nursing mothers until its effects upon infants are more fully established.

Atarax—see hydroxyzine

---

atenolol

BRAND NAME (Manufacturer)
Tenormin (ICI Pharma)
TYPE OF DRUG
Beta-adrenergic blocking agent

INGREDIENT
atenolol
DOSAGE FORM
Tablets (50 mg and 100 mg)
STORAGE
Atenolol should be stored at room temperature in a tightly closed, light-resistant container.

USES

Atenolol is used to treat high blood pressure and angina (chest pain). It belongs to a group of medicines known as beta-adrenergic blocking agents or, more commonly, beta blockers. These drugs work by controlling impulses along certain nerve pathways.

TREATMENT

Atenolol can be taken with a glass of water, with meals, immediately following meals, or on an empty stomach, depending on your doctor's instructions. Try to take the medication at the same time(s) each day.

Try not to miss any doses of this medication. If you do miss a dose, take the missed dose as soon as possible. However, if the next scheduled dose is within eight hours (if you are taking this medicine only once a day) or within four hours (if you are taking this medicine more than once a day), do not take the missed dose at all; just return to your regular dosing schedule. Do not double the next dose.

It is important to remember that atenolol does not cure high blood pressure, but it will help to control the condition as long as you continue to take it.

SIDE EFFECTS

Minor. Anxiety; constipation; decreased sexual ability; diarrhea; difficulty in sleeping; drowsiness; dryness of the eyes, mouth, and skin; headache; nausea; nervousness; stomach discomfort; tiredness; or weakness. These side effects should disappear as your body adjusts to the medicine.

If you are extra-sensitive to the cold, be sure to dress warmly during cold weather.

To relieve constipation, increase the amount of fiber in your diet (fresh fruits and vegetables, salads, bran, and whole-grain breads), and drink more water (unless your doctor directs you to do otherwise).

Plain, nonmedicated eye drops (artificial tears) may help to relieve eye dryness.

Sucking on ice chips or chewing sugarless gum helps relieve mouth or throat dryness.

Major. Tell your doctor about any side effects that are persistent or particularly bothersome. IT IS ESPECIALLY IMPORTANT TO TELL YOUR DOCTOR about breathing difficulty or wheezing; cold hands or feet (due to decreased blood circulation to skin, fingers, and toes); confusion; dizziness; fever and sore throat; hair loss; hallucinations; lightheadedness; mental depression; nightmares; reduced alertness; skin rash; swelling of the ankles, feet, or lower legs; or unusual bleeding or bruising.

INTERACTIONS

Atenolol interacts with a number of other medications:

1. Indomethacin has been shown to decrease the blood-pressure-lowering effects of the beta blockers. This may also happen with aspirin or other salicylates.

2. Concurrent use of beta blockers and calcium channel blockers (diltiazem, nifedipine, verapamil) or disopyramide can possibly lead to heart failure or very low blood pressure.

3. Cimetidine and oral contraceptives (birth control pills) can increase the blood concentrations of beta blockers, which can result in greater side effects.

4. Side effects may also be increased when beta blockers are taken with clonidine, digoxin, epinephrine, phenylephrine, phenylpropanolamine, phenothiazine tranquilizers, prazosin, or monoamine oxidase (MAO) inhibitors. At least 14 days should separate the use of a beta blocker and the use of an MAO inhibitor.

5. Alcohol, barbiturates, and rifampin can decrease blood concentrations of atenolol, which can result in a decrease of effectiveness.

6. Beta blockers may antagonize (work against) the effects of theophylline, aminophylline, albuterol, isoproterenol, metaproterenol, and terbutaline.

7. Beta blockers can also interact with insulin or oral antidiabetic agents—raising or lowering blood sugar levels or masking the symptoms of low blood sugar.

8. The action of beta blockers may be increased if they are used with chlorpromazine, furosemide, or hydralazine, which may have a negative effect.

BE SURE TO TELL YOUR DOCTOR about any medications you are currently taking, especially any of those listed above.

WARNINGS

- Before starting to take this medication, it is important to tell your doctor if you have ever had unusual or allergic reactions to any beta blocker (acebutolol, atenolol, betaxolol, carteolol, esmolol, labetalol, metoprolol, nadolol, penbutolol, pindolol, propranolol, timolol).
- Tell your doctor if you now have or if you have ever had allergies, asthma, hay fever, eczema, slow heartbeat, bronchitis, diabetes mellitus, emphysema, heart or blood vessel disease, kidney disease, liver disease, thyroid disease, or poor circulation in the fingers or toes.
- You may want to check your pulse while taking this medication. If your pulse is much slower than your usual rate (or if it is less than 50 beats per minute), check with your doctor. A pulse rate that is too slow may cause circulation problems.
- Atenolol may affect your body's response to exercise. Make sure you discuss with your doctor a safe amount of exercise for your medical condition.
- It is important that you do not stop taking this medicine without first checking with your doctor. Some conditions may become worse when the medicine is stopped suddenly, and the danger of a heart attack is increased in some patients. Your doctor may want you to gradually reduce the amount of medicine you take before stopping completely. Make sure that you have enough medicine on hand to last through vacations, holidays, and weekends.
- Before having surgery or any other medical or dental treatment, tell the physician or dentist that you are taking this medicine. Often, this medication will be discontinued 48 hours prior to any major surgery.
- This medicine can cause dizziness, drowsiness, lightheadedness, or decreased alertness. Therefore, exercise caution while driving a car or using any potentially dangerous equipment.

• While taking this medicine, do not use any over-the-counter (nonprescription) asthma, allergy, cough, cold, sinus, or diet preparations unless you first check with your pharmacist or doctor. Some of these medicines can cause high blood pressure when taken at the same time as a beta blocker.

• Be sure to tell your doctor if you are pregnant. Animal studies have shown that some beta blockers can cause problems in pregnancy when used at very high doses. Adequate studies have not been done in humans, but there has been some association between beta blockers used during pregnancy and low birth weight, as well as breathing problems and slow heart rate in the newborn infants. However, other reports have shown no effects on newborn infants. Also, tell your doctor if you are breast-feeding an infant. Small amounts of atenolol may pass into breast milk.

---

atenolol and chlorthalidone combination

BRAND NAME (Manufacturer)
Tenoretic (ICI Pharma)

TYPE OF DRUG
Beta-adrenergic blocking agent and diuretic

INGREDIENTS
atenolol and chlorthalidone

DOSAGE FORM
Tablets (50 mg atenolol and 25 mg chlorthalidone; 100 mg atenolol and 25 mg chlorthalidone)

STORAGE
Atenolol and chlorthalidone combination tablets should be stored at room temperature in a tightly closed, light-resistant container. The tablets should be protected from moisture during storage.

USES

Atenolol and chlorthalidone combination is prescribed to treat high blood pressure. Chlorthalidone is a diuretic, which reduces fluid accumulation in the body by increasing the elimination of salt and water through the kidneys. Atenolol belongs to a group of medicines known as beta-adrenergic blocking agents or, more commonly, beta blockers. They work by controlling impulses along certain nerve pathways.

TREATMENT

This medication can be taken with a glass of water, with meals, immediately following meals, or on an empty stomach, depending on your doctor's instructions.

Try to take the medication at the same times(s) each day. Avoid taking a dose after 6:00 P.M.; otherwise, you may have to get up during the night to urinate.

If you miss a dose of this medication, take the missed dose as soon as possible, unless it is almost time for your next dose. In that case, do not take the missed dose at all; just wait until the next scheduled dose. Do not double the dose.

Atenolol and chlorthalidone combination does not cure high blood pressure, but it will help to control the condition as long as you continue to take it.

SIDE EFFECTS

Minor. Anxiety, constipation, cramps, decreased sexual ability, diarrhea, difficulty in sleeping, dizziness, drowsiness, dryness of the eyes and skin, gas, headache, heartburn, loss of appetite, nervousness, restlessness, stomach discomfort, sweating, or tiredness. These side effects should disappear as your body adjusts to the medication.

Chlorthalidone can cause increased sensitivity to sunlight. It is important, therefore, to avoid prolonged exposure to sunlight and sunlamps. Wear protective clothing and sunglasses, and use an effective sunscreen.

If you become extra-sensitive to the cold, be sure to dress warmly during cold weather.

Plain, nonmedicated eye drops (artificial tears) may help to relieve eye dryness.

To relieve constipation, increase the amount of fiber in your diet (fresh fruits and vegetables, salads, bran, and whole-grain breads) unless your doctor directs you to do otherwise.

Sucking on ice chips or chewing sugarless gum helps to relieve mouth and throat dryness.

To avoid dizziness or light-headedness when you stand, contract and relax the muscles of your legs for a few moments before rising. Do this by alternately pushing one foot against the floor while raising the other foot slightly, so that you are "pumping" your legs in a pedaling motion.

Major. Tell your doctor about any side effects that are persistent or particularly bothersome. IT IS ESPECIALLY IMPORTANT TO TELL YOUR DOCTOR about blurred vision, cold hands and feet (due to decreased blood circulation to skin, fingers, and toes), confusion, depression, difficulty in breathing, dry mouth, excessive thirst, excessive weakness, fever, hair loss, hallucinations, itching, joint pain, mood changes, muscle pain or spasms, nausea, nightmares, numbness or tingling in the fingers or toes, palpitations, rapid weight gain (three to five pounds within a week), reduced alertness, ringing in the ears, skin rash, sore throat, swelling, unusual bleeding or bruising, vomiting, or yellowing of the eyes or skin.

INTERACTIONS

Atenolol and chlorthalidone combination can interact with other types of medications:

1. Indomethacin, aspirin, and other salicylates may decrease the blood-pressure-lowering effects of beta blockers.

2. Concurrent use of atenolol and calcium channel blockers (diltiazem, nifedipine, verapamil) or disopyramide can lead to heart failure or very low blood pressure.

3. Cimetidine can increase blood levels of atenolol, resulting in greater side effects. Side effects may also be increased when atenolol is taken with clonidine, digoxin, epinephrine, phenylephrine, phenylpropanolamine, phenothiazine tranquilizers, prazosin, reserpine, oral contraceptives (birth control pills), or monoamine oxidase (MAO) inhibitors. At least 14 days should separate the use of atenolol and the use of an MAO inhibitor.

4. Atenolol can antagonize (act against) the effects of theophylline, aminophylline, albuterol, isoproterenol, metaproterenol, and terbutaline.

5. Alcohol, barbiturates, and rifampin can decrease blood levels of beta blockers, resulting in decreased effectiveness.

6. The action of beta blockers may be increased if they are

used with chlorpromazine, furosemide, or hydralazine, which may have a negative effect.
7. Atenolol and chlorthalidone can interact with insulin and oral antidiabetic agents—raising or lowering blood sugar levels and masking the symptoms of low blood sugar.
8. Chlorthalidone can decrease the effectiveness of oral anticoagulants (blood thinners, such as warfarin), antigout medications, and methenamine.
9. Fenfluramine may increase the blood-pressure-lowering effects of this drug, which can be dangerous.
10. Cholestyramine and colestipol can decrease the absorption of chlorthalidone from the gastrointestinal tract. Chlorthalidone should, therefore, be taken one hour before or four hours after a dose of cholestyramine or colestipol (if you have also been prescribed one of these medications).
11. Chlorthalidone may increase the side effects of amphotericin B, calcium supplements, cortisone-like steroids (such as cortisone, dexamethasone, hydrocortisone, prednisone, and prednisolone), digoxin, digitalis, lithium, quinidine, sulfonamide antibiotics, and vitamin D.

Before starting atenolol and chlorthalidone combination, BE SURE TO TELL YOUR DOCTOR about all of the medications you are currently taking, especially any of the ones listed above.

WARNINGS

• Tell your doctor about unusual or allergic reactions you have had to medications, especially to atenolol or any other beta blocker (acebutolol, betaxolol, carteolol, esmolol, labetalol, metoprolol, nadolol, penbutolol, pindolol, propranolol, timolol), to chlorthalidone or other diuretics (such as bendroflumethiazide, benzthiazide, chlorothiazide, cyclothiazide, hydrochlorothiazide, hydroflumethiazide, methyclothiazide, metolozone, polythiazide, quinethazone, trichlormethiazide, and furosemide), or to any sulfa drug, including oral antidiabetic medications and sulfonamide antibiotics.

• Tell your doctor if you now have or if you have ever had asthma, diabetes mellitus, heart disease, gout, kidney disease or problems with urination, liver disease, lung disease, pancreatitis, poor circulation in the fingers or toes, systemic lupus erythematosus, or thyroid disease.

• Chlorthalidone can cause potassium loss. Signs of potassium loss include dry mouth, thirst, weakness, muscle pain or cramps, nausea, and vomiting. If you experience any of these symptoms, call your doctor. To help prevent this problem, your doctor may have blood tests performed periodically to monitor your potassium levels. To help avoid potassium loss, take this medication with a glass of fresh or frozen orange juice or cranberry juice, or eat a banana every day. The use of a salt substitute also helps to prevent potassium loss. Do not change your diet, however, until you discuss it with your doctor. Too much potassium may also be dangerous.

• While taking this medication, limit your intake of alcohol in order to prevent dizziness and light-headedness.

• Do not take any over-the-counter (nonprescription) medication for weight control or for allergy, asthma, cough, cold, or sinus problems unless you first check with your doctor.

• To prevent severe water loss (dehydration) while taking this medication, check with your doctor if you have any illness that causes severe or continuous nausea, vomiting, or diarrhea.

• This medication can raise blood sugar levels in diabetic patients. Blood sugar should be monitored carefully with blood or urine tests when this medication is being taken.

• You may want to check your pulse while taking this medication. If your pulse is much slower than your usual rate (or if it is less than 50 beats per minute), check with your doctor; a pulse rate that slow may cause circulation problems.

• Atenolol can affect your body's response to exercise. Make sure that you ask your doctor what an appropriate amount of exercise would be for you, taking into account your medical condition.

• Before having surgery or any other medical or dental treatment, tell your doctor or dentist that you are taking this medicine. Often, this medication will be discontinued 48 hours prior to any major surgery.

• This medication can cause dizziness, drowsiness, lightheadedness, or decreased alertness. Therefore, exercise caution whenever driving a car or operating potentially dangerous equipment.

• A doctor does not usually prescribe a "fixed-dose" drug like this as the first choice in the treatment of high blood pressure. Usually the patient first receives each ingredient singly. If there is an adequate response to the fixed dose contained in this product, it can then be substituted. The advantage of a combination product is increased convenience and (often) decreased cost.

• It is important that you do not stop taking this medicine unless you first check with your doctor. Some conditions worsen when this medicine is stopped suddenly, and the danger of a heart attack is increased in some patients. Your doctor may, therefore, want you to gradually reduce the amount of medicine you take before stopping completely. Make sure that you have enough medicine on hand to last through vacations, holidays, and weekends.

• Be sure to tell your doctor if you are pregnant. Animal studies have shown that some beta blockers can cause problems in pregnancy when used at very high doses. Studies have not been conducted in humans, but there has been some association between use of beta blockers during pregnancy and low birth weight, as well as breathing problems and slow heart rate in newborn infants. However, other reports have shown no effects on newborn infants. Also, tell your doctor if you are breast-feeding an infant. Although problems in humans have not been reported, small amounts of this medication may pass into breast milk, so caution is warranted.

Ativan—see lorazepam

Atromid-S—see clofibrate

---

atropine, scopolamine, hyoscyamine, and phenobarbital combination

BRAND NAMES (Manufacturers)
Barophen (various manufacturers)
belladonna alkaloids with phenobarbital (various manufacturers)

Donnamor (H.L. Moore)
Donna-Sed (Vortech)
Donnatal (Robins)
Hyosophen (Rugby)
Kinesed (Stuart)
Malatal (Mallard)
Neoquess (Forest)
Relaxadon (Geneva Generics)
Spasmolin (various manufacturers)
Spasmophen (Lannett)
Spasquid (Geneva Generics)
Susano (Halsey)

TYPE OF DRUG
Anticholinergic and sedative

INGREDIENTS
atropine, scopolamine, hyoscyamine, and phenobarbital

DOSAGE FORMS
Tablets (0.0194 mg atropine, 0.0065 mg scopolamine, 0.1037 mg hyoscyamine, and 16.2 mg phenobarbital)
Capsules (0.0194 mg atropine, 0.0065 mg scopolamine, 0.1037 mg hyoscyamine, and 16.2 mg phenobarbital)
Oral elixir (0.0194 mg atropine, 0.0065 mg scopolamine, 0.1037 mg hyoscyamine, and 16.2 mg phenobarbital, with 23% alcohol)

STORAGE
The medication should be stored at room temperature (never frozen) in a tightly closed, light-resistant container.

USES
This medication is used to treat bed-wetting, lack of bladder control, motion sickness, premenstrual tension, and stomach and intestinal disorders.

Atropine, scopolamine, and hyoscyamine belong to a group of drugs known as belladonna alkaloids or anticholinergic agents. These drugs block certain nerve pathways, thereby slowing the gastrointestinal tract and decreasing urination. Phenobarbital is a sedative that acts directly on the brain to slow the activity of the nervous system.

TREATMENT
This medication should be taken 30 minutes to one hour before meals (unless your doctor directs you to do otherwise). In order to reduce stomach upset, you can take it with food or with a glass of water or milk.

At least one hour should separate doses of this drug and either antacids or antidiarrheal medications—they may prevent gastrointestinal absorption of this drug.

Measure the liquid form of this medication carefully with a specially designed 5-ml measuring spoon. An ordinary kitchen teaspoon is not accurate enough.

If you miss a dose, don't take the missed dose at all; just return to your regular dosing schedule. Don't double the next dose.

SIDE EFFECTS
Minor. Confusion; constipation; decreased sexual desire; dizziness; drowsiness; dry mouth, nose, and throat; headache; insomnia; loss of taste; muscle pain; nausea; nervousness; reduced sweating; sensitivity of eyes to sunlight; vomiting; or weakness. These side effects should disappear as your body adjusts to the medication.

If you are constipated, increase the amount of fiber in your diet (fresh fruits and vegetables, salads, bran, and whole-grain breads), exercise, and drink more water (unless your doctor directs you to do otherwise).

Chew sugarless gum or suck on ice chips or a piece of hard candy to reduce mouth dryness.

Wear sunglasses if your eyes become sensitive to light.

To avoid dizziness or light-headedness when you stand, contract and relax the muscles of your legs for a few moments before rising. Do this by pushing one foot against the floor while raising the other foot slightly, alternating feet so that you are "pumping" your legs in a pedaling motion.

Major. Tell your doctor about any side effects that are persistent or particularly bothersome. IT IS ESPECIALLY IMPORTANT TO TELL YOUR DOCTOR about blurred vision, difficulty in breathing, difficulty in urinating, hallucinations, hot and dry skin, palpitations, rash, slurred speech, sore throat, or yellowing of the eyes or skin.

INTERACTIONS
This medication interacts with several other types of drugs:

1. The belladonna alkaloids and phenobarbital can cause extreme drowsiness when combined with central nervous system depressants (such as alcohol, antihistamines, barbiturates, benzodiazepine tranquilizers, muscle relaxants, narcotics, and pain medications) or with tricyclic antidepressants.

2. Amantadine, antihistamines, haloperidol, monoamine oxidase (MAO) inhibitors, phenothiazine tranquilizers, procainamide, quinidine, and tricyclic antidepressants can increase the side effects of the belladonna alkaloids. At least 14 days should separate the use of this drug and the use of an MAO inhibitor.

3. Phenobarbital can increase the elimination and decrease the effectiveness of oral anticoagulants (blood thinners, such as warfarin), cortisone-like medications, digoxin, griseofulvin, doxycycline, metronidazole, phenytoin, and tricyclic antidepressants.

WARNINGS
• Tell your doctor about unusual or allergic reactions you have had to any medications, especially to atropine, scopolamine, hyoscyamine, phenobarbital, or to other barbiturates (such as butalbital, primidone, pentobarbital, and secobarbital).

• Tell your doctor if you now have or if you have ever had glaucoma, heart disease, hiatal hernia, high blood pressure, internal bleeding, kidney disease, liver disease, lung disease, myasthenia gravis, porphyria, enlarged prostate gland, obstructed bladder, obstructed intestine, ulcerative colitis, or thyroid disease.

• If this medication makes you dizzy or drowsy or blurs your vision, do not take part in any activity that requires alertness, such as driving a car or operating potentially dangerous equipment. Be careful on stairs, and avoid getting up from a lying or sitting position suddenly.

• This medication can decrease sweating and heat release from the body. Therefore, avoid getting overheated by strenuous exercise in hot weather, and avoid taking hot baths, showers, and saunas.

• Before having surgery or any other medical or dental treatment, tell the doctor or dentist that you are taking this drug.

• Be sure to tell your doctor if you are pregnant. This medication crosses the placenta. Phenobarbital given to the mother close to term can cause breathing problems and bleeding complications in the newborn infant. Also, tell your doctor if you are breast-feeding an infant. Small amounts of this medication pass into breast milk and may cause excessive drowsiness or irritability in the nursing infant.

Augmentin—see amoxicillin and clavulanic acid combination

Auralgan—see antipyrene, benzocaine, oxyquinoline, and glycerin combination

auranofin

BRAND NAME (Manufacturer)
Ridaura (Smith Kline & French)
TYPE OF DRUG
Antirheumatic
INGREDIENT
auranofin
DOSAGE FORM
Capsules (3 mg)
STORAGE
Auranofin should be stored at room temperature in a tightly closed container.

USES

Auranofin is a gold compound used to treat active rheumatoid arthritis. It is unclear how auranofin works to relieve the symptoms of rheumatoid arthritis.

TREATMENT

Auranofin can be taken either on an empty stomach or with food or milk (as directed by your doctor). It can be taken along with other antirheumatic medications.

The full effects of auranofin for the control of arthritis symptoms may not become apparent for several months. It is important to continue taking this medication until your doctor instructs you to do otherwise.

Auranofin is generally reserved for arthritis patients who have not responded to or did not tolerate other medications. It should be used in conjunction with, not in place of, a total treatment program, which can include diet, exercise, rest, and heat treatments.

If you miss a dose of this medication, take the missed dose as soon as possible, unless it is almost time for the next dose. In that case, do not take the missed dose at all; just wait until the next scheduled dose. Do not double the dose.

SIDE EFFECTS

Minor. Abdominal cramps, constipation, diarrhea, gas, heartburn, loss of appetite, nausea, or vomiting. As your body adjusts to auranofin, these effects should disappear.

To relieve constipation, increase the amount of fiber in your diet (fresh fruits and vegetables, salads, bran, and whole-grain breads), exercise, and drink more water (unless your doctor directs you to do otherwise).

Major. Tell your doctor about any side effects that are persistent or particularly bothersome. IT IS ESPECIALLY IMPORTANT TO TELL YOUR DOCTOR about black or tarry stools, blood in the urine, fever, gingivitis (inflammation of the gums), hair loss, itching, metallic taste, mouth sores, persistent diarrhea, rash, shortness of breath, tingling or pain in the fingers or toes, tongue sores, unusual bleeding or bruising, or yellowing of the skin or eyes.

INTERACTIONS

Auranofin can increase the blood concentration of phenytoin, which can increase the risk of side effects.

Before taking auranofin, BE SURE TO TELL YOUR DOCTOR about any medications you are currently taking, especially if you are taking phenytoin.

WARNINGS

- Tell your doctor about any unusual or allergic reactions you have had to any medications, especially to auranofin or injectable gold compounds (aurothioglucose or gold sodium thioglucose).
- Before taking auranofin, be sure to tell your doctor if you now have or if you have ever had blood disorders, bone marrow disease, inflammatory bowel disease (ulcerative colitis or Crohn's disease), kidney disease, liver disease, or rash.
- Regular blood and urine tests should be performed to assess possible side effects of auranofin. It is important for you to keep all your scheduled appointments in order to avoid possible complications.
- Tell your doctor if you are pregnant. Studies in pregnant women have not been performed. However, birth defects have occurred in the offspring of pregnant animals given large doses of auranofin. Also, tell your doctor if you are breast-feeding an infant. It is not yet known if auranofin passes into human breast milk, but it has been shown to pass into the milk of animals.

Auromid—see antipyrine, benzocaine, oxyquinoline, and glycerin combination

Auroto Otic—see antipyrine, benzocaine, oxyquinoline, and glycerin combination

Aventyl—see nortriptyline

Azaline—see sulfasalazine

azatadine

BRAND NAME (Manufacturer)
Optimine (Schering)
TYPE OF DRUG
Antihistamine
INGREDIENT
azatadine
DOSAGE FORM
Tablets (1 mg)
STORAGE
Store at room temperature in a tightly closed container.

USES

This medication belongs to a group of drugs known as antihistamines (antihistamines block the action of histamine, a chemical released by the body during an allergic reaction). It is, therefore, used to treat or prevent symptoms of allergy.

TREATMENT

To avoid stomach upset, you can take azatadine with food or with a full glass of milk or water (unless your doctor directs you to do otherwise).

If you miss a dose of this medication, take the missed dose as soon as possible, unless it is almost time for your next dose. In that case, don't take the missed dose at all; just return to your regular dosing schedule. Do not double the next dose.

SIDE EFFECTS

Minor. Confusion; constipation; diarrhea; difficult or painful urination; dizziness; dry mouth, throat, or nose; headache; irritability; loss of appetite; nausea; restlessness; ringing or buzzing in the ears; stomach upset; or unusual increase in sweating. These side effects should disappear as your body adjusts to the medication.

This medication can cause increased sensitivity to sunlight. It is, therefore, important to avoid prolonged exposure to sunlight and sunlamps. Wear protective clothing and use an effective sunscreen.

If you are constipated, increase the amount of fiber in your diet (fresh fruits and vegetables, salads, bran, and whole-grain breads), exercise, and drink more water (unless your doctor tells you not to do so).

Chew sugarless gum or suck on ice chips or a piece of hard candy to reduce mouth dryness.

If you feel dizzy or light-headed, sit or lie down for a while; get up from a sitting or lying position slowly, and be careful on stairs.

Major. Tell your doctor about any side effects that are persistent or particularly bothersome. IT IS ESPECIALLY IMPORTANT TO TELL YOUR DOCTOR about blurred vision, change in menstruation, clumsiness, feeling faint, fever, flushing of the face, hallucinations, palpitations, rash, sleeping disorders, seizures, shortness of breath, sore throat, tightness in the chest, unusual bleeding or bruising, or unusual tiredness.

INTERACTIONS

Azatadine interacts with other types of medications:

1. Concurrent use of it with other central nervous system depressants (such as alcohol, barbiturates, benzodiazepine tranquilizers, muscle relaxants, narcotics, pain medications, and phenothiazine tranquilizers) or with tricyclic antidepressants can cause extreme drowsiness.

2. Monoamine oxidase (MAO) inhibitors (isocarboxazid, pargyline, phenelzine, tranylcypromine) can increase the side effects of this medication. At least 14 days should separate use of this drug and use of an MAO inhibitor.

3. Azatadine can also decrease the activity of oral anticoagulants (blood thinners such as warfarin).

BE SURE TO TELL YOUR DOCTOR about any medications you are currently taking, especially any listed above.

WARNINGS

- Tell your doctor about unusual or allergic reactions you have had to medications, especially to azatadine or any other antihistamine (brompheniramine, carbinoxamine, chlorpheniramine, clemastine, cyproheptadine, dexchlorpheniramine, dimenhydrinate, dimethindene, diphenhydramine, diphenylpyraline, doxylamine, hydroxyzine, promethazine, pyrilamine, trimeprazine, tripelennamine, triprolidine).
- Tell your doctor if you now have or if you have ever had asthma, blood vessel disease, glaucoma, high blood pressure, kidney disease, peptic ulcers, enlarged prostate gland, or thyroid disease.
- Azatadine can cause drowsiness or dizziness. Your ability to perform tasks that require alertness, such as driving a car or operating potentially dangerous equipment, may be decreased. Appropriate caution should, therefore, be taken.
- Be sure to tell your doctor if you are pregnant. The effects of this medication during pregnancy have not been thoroughly studied in humans. Also, tell your doctor if you are breast-feeding an infant. Small amounts of azatadine pass into breast milk and may cause unusual excitement or irritability in nursing infants.

---

azathioprine

BRAND NAME (Manufacturer)
Imuran (Burroughs Wellcome)
TYPE OF DRUG
Immunosuppressant
INGREDIENT
azathioprine
DOSAGE FORM
Tablets (50 mg)
STORAGE
Azathioprine should be stored at room temperature in a tightly closed, light-resistant container.

USES

This medication is used to prevent rejection of kidney transplants and to control the symptoms of severe rheumatoid arthritis. It is not clear exactly how azathioprine works, but it is known to act on the body's immune system.

TREATMENT

In order to prevent nausea and vomiting, you can take azathioprine with food or after a meal (unless your doctor directs you to do otherwise).

Try not to miss any doses of this medication. If you do miss a dose, take the missed dose as soon as possible, unless it is almost time for the next scheduled dose. In that case, do not take the missed dose at all; just return to your regular dosing schedule. Do not double the next dose. If you miss more than one dose, CHECK WITH YOUR DOCTOR.

SIDE EFFECTS

Minor. Diarrhea, nausea, or vomiting. These side effects should disappear as your body adjusts to the medication.

Major. Tell your doctor about any side effects that are persistent or particularly bothersome. IT IS ESPECIALLY IMPORTANT TO TELL YOUR DOCTOR about darkened urine, fever, hair loss, joint pains, mouth sores, muscle aches, skin rash, sore throat, unusual bleeding or bruising, or yellowing of the eyes or skin.

INTERACTIONS

BE SURE TO TELL YOUR DOCTOR if you are already taking allopurinol. It can increase the blood levels of azathioprine, which can lead to serious side effects.

WARNINGS

- Be sure to tell your doctor about any unusual or allergic reactions that you have had to any medications, especially to azathioprine.
- Before starting to take this medication, be sure to tell your doctor if you now have or if you have ever had gout, kidney disease, liver disease, pancreatitis, or recurrent infections.
- Azathioprine is potent medicine. Your doctor will want to monitor your therapy carefully with blood tests, so that you take the least amount of the drug possible.
- Do not stop taking this medication unless you first check with your doctor. Stopping therapy with this drug abruptly may lead to a worsening of your condition. Your doctor may, therefore, want to start you on another drug before therapy with azathioprine is stopped.
- There is a chance that azathioprine may cause unwanted effects months or years later. These delayed effects may include certain types of cancer. Be sure to discuss these possible effects with your doctor.
- Azathioprine can increase your susceptibility to infections. It is, therefore, important to contact your doctor at the first sign of infection. Your dose of azathioprine may need to be adjusted.
- Be sure to tell your doctor if you are pregnant. Birth defects have been reported in the offspring of animals that received large doses of azathioprine during pregnancy. This drug also has the potential for producing birth defects in human offspring. Use of this drug is not recommended during pregnancy. There is a possibility that birth defects may occur in the offspring if either the male or female is using this drug at the time of conception. Use of birth control is recommended while taking this drug. Also, tell your doctor if you are breast-feeding an infant. It is not known whether azathioprine passes into breast milk.

Azo Gantanol—see sulfamethoxazole and phenazopyridine combination

Azo Gantrisin—see sulfisoxazole and phenazopyridine combination

Azolid—see phenylbutazone

Azo-Standard—see phenazopyridine

Azo-Sulfisoxazole—see sulfisoxazole and phenazopyridine combination

Azulfidine—see sulfasalazine

Azulfidine EN-tabs—see sulfasalazine

B-A-C—see aspirin, caffeine, and butalbital combination

B-A-C #3—see aspirin, caffeine, butalbital, and codeine combination

baclofen

BRAND NAME (Manufacturer)
Lioresal (Geigy)

TYPE OF DRUG
Muscle relaxant

INGREDIENT
baclofen

DOSAGE FORM
Tablets (10 mg and 20 mg)

STORAGE
Baclofen should be stored at room temperature in a tightly closed container.

USES

This medication is used to relieve muscle spasms. It is unclear exactly how baclofen works to relieve spasticity, but it is known that the drug acts on the central nervous system (brain and spinal cord).

TREATMENT

Baclofen can be taken either on an empty stomach or with food or a full glass of milk or water.

If you miss a dose of this medication and remember within an hour, take the missed dose immediately. If more than an hour has passed, do not take the missed dose at all; just return to your regular dosing schedule. Do not double the next dose.

SIDE EFFECTS

Minor. Abdominal pain, constipation, diarrhea, dizziness, drowsiness, dry mouth, fatigue, headache, insomnia, loss of appetite, nasal congestion, vomiting, or weight gain. These side effects should disappear as your body adjusts to the medication.

To relieve constipation, increase the amount of fiber in your diet (fresh fruits and vegetables, salads, bran, and whole-grain breads), exercise, and drink more water (unless your doctor directs you to do otherwise).

If you feel dizzy, sit or lie down for a while; get up slowly from a sitting or lying position, and be careful on stairs.

To relieve mouth dryness, chew sugarless gum or suck on ice chips or a piece of hard candy.

Major. Tell your doctor about any side effects that are persistent or particularly bothersome. IT IS ESPECIALLY IMPORTANT TO TELL YOUR DOCTOR about chest pain, confusion, convulsions, depression, fainting, false sense of well-being, hallucinations, muscle pain, palpitations, ringing in the ears, slurred speech, tremors, or visual disturbances.

INTERACTIONS

Baclofen interacts with several other types of medications:

1. Concurrent use of baclofen with other central nervous system depressants (such as alcohol, antihistamines, barbiturates, benzodiazepine tranquilizers, muscle relaxants, narcotics, pain medications, phenothiazine tranquilizers, and sleeping medicines) or with tricyclic antidepressants can lead to extreme drowsiness.

2. The dosage of oral antidiabetic medications may need to be altered when baclofen is started.

BE SURE TO TELL YOUR DOCTOR about any medications you are currently taking, especially any listed above.

WARNINGS

- Be sure to tell your doctor about any unusual or allergic reactions you have had to any drugs, especially to baclofen.
- Before starting to take baclofen, be sure to tell your doctor if you now have or if you have ever had diabetes mellitus, epilepsy, kidney disease, mental disorders, or a stroke.
- If this drug makes you dizzy or drowsy, avoid taking part in any activity that requires alertness, such as driving a car.
- Do not stop taking this medication unless you first check with your doctor. Stopping therapy with this medication abruptly can lead to hallucinations, nervousness, convulsions, and mood changes. Your doctor may, therefore, want to reduce your dosage gradually.
- Be sure to tell your doctor if you are pregnant. Although baclofen appears to be safe in humans, birth defects have been reported in the offspring of animals that received large doses of this drug during pregnancy. Also, tell your doctor if you are breast-feeding an infant. It is not known whether baclofen passes into breast milk.

Bactine Hydrocortisone—see hydrocortisone (topical)

Bactocill—see oxacillin

Bactrim—see sulfamethoxazole and trimethoprim combination

Bactrim DS—see sulfamethoxazole and trimethoprim combination

Bancap HC—see acetaminophen and hydrocodone combination

Banex-LA—see phenylpropanolamine and guaifenesin combination

Barbita—see phenobarbital

Baridium—see phenazopyridine

Barophen—see atropine, scopolamine, hyoscyamine, and phenobarbital combination

Bayer—see aspirin

Bayer Children's—see aspirin

Beepen-VK—see penicillin VK

Belix—see diphenhydramine

belladonna alkaloids with phenobarbital—see atropine, scopolamine, hyoscyamine, and phenobarbital combination

Benadryl—see diphenhydramine

Benadryl Kapseals—see diphenhydramine

bendroflumethiazide

BRAND NAME (Manufacturer)
Naturetin (Princeton)
TYPE OF DRUG
Diuretic and antihypertensive
INGREDIENT
bendroflumethiazide
DOSAGE FORM
Tablets (2.5 mg, 5 mg, and 10 mg)
STORAGE
This medication should be stored at room temperature in a tightly closed container.

USES

Bendroflumethiazide is prescribed to treat high blood pressure. It is also used to reduce fluid accumulation in the body caused by conditions such as heart failure, cirrhosis of the liver, kidney disease, and the long-term use of some medications. This medication reduces fluid accumulation by increasing the elimination of salt and water through the kidneys.

TREATMENT

To decrease stomach irritation, you can take this medication with a glass of milk or with a meal (unless your doctor directs you to do otherwise). Try to take it at the same time every day. Avoid taking a dose after 6:00 P.M.; otherwise, you may have to get up during the night to urinate.

If you miss a dose of this medication, take the missed dose as soon as possible, unless it is almost time for the next dose. In that case, do not take the missed dose at all; just wait until the next scheduled dose. Do not double the dose.

This medication does not cure high blood pressure, but it will help to control the condition as long as you continue to take it.

SIDE EFFECTS

Minor. Constipation, cramps, diarrhea, dizziness, drowsiness, headache, heartburn, loss of appetite, restlessness, or upset stomach. As your body adjusts to the medication, these side effects should disappear.

This medication can cause increased sensitivity to sunlight. It is, therefore, important to avoid prolonged exposure to sunlight and sunlamps. Wear protective clothing and use an effective sunscreen.

To relieve constipation, increase the amount of fiber in your diet (fresh fruits and vegetables, salads, bran, and whole-grain breads) and exercise more (unless your doctor directs you to do otherwise).

To avoid dizziness or light-headedness when you stand, contract and relax the muscles of your legs for a few moments before rising. Do this by pushing one foot against the floor while raising the other foot slightly, alternating feet so that you are "pumping" your legs in a pedaling motion.

Major. Tell your doctor about any side effects that are persistent or particularly bothersome. IT IS ESPECIALLY IMPORTANT TO TELL YOUR DOCTOR about blurred vision, confusion, difficulty in breathing, dry mouth, excessive thirst, excessive weakness, fever, itching, joint pain, mood changes, muscle pain or spasms, nausea, palpitations, skin rash, sore throat, tingling in the fingers or toes, unusual bleeding or bruising, vomiting, or yellowing of the eyes or skin.

INTERACTIONS

This drug interacts with several other drugs:

1. It may decrease the effectiveness of oral anticoagulants, antigout medications, insulin, oral antidiabetic medicines, and methenamine.

2. Fenfluramine can increase the blood-pressure-lowering effects of bendroflumethiazide (which can be dangerous).

3. Indomethacin can decrease the blood-pressure-lowering effects of bendroflumethiazide, thereby counteracting the desired effects.

4. Cholestyramine and colestipol decrease the absorption of this medication from the gastrointestinal tract. Bendroflumethiazide should, therefore, be taken one hour before or four hours after a dose of cholestyramine or colestipol (if you have also been prescribed one of these medications).

5. The side effects of amphotericin B, calcium, cortisone-like steroids (such as cortisone, dexamethasone, hydrocortisone, prednisone, and prednisolone), digoxin, digitalis, lithium, quinidine, sulfonamide antibiotics, and vitamin D may be increased by bendroflumethiazide.

BE SURE TO TELL YOUR DOCTOR about any medications you are currently taking, especially any of those listed above.

WARNINGS

- Tell your doctor about unusual or allergic reactions you have had to any medications, especially to diuretics or any other sulfa drugs, including oral antidiabetic medications or sulfonamide antibiotics.
- Before you start taking bendroflumethiazide, tell your doctor if you now have or if you have ever had kidney disease or problems with urination, diabetes mellitus, gout, liver disease, asthma, pancreatic disease, or systemic lupus erythematosus.
- Bendroflumethiazide can cause potassium loss. Signs of potassium loss include dry mouth, thirst, weakness, muscle pain or cramps, nausea, and vomiting. If you experience any of these symptoms, call your doctor. To help avoid potassium loss, take this drug with a glass of fresh or frozen orange juice or cranberry juice, or eat a banana every day. The use of a salt substitute also helps to prevent potassium loss. Do not change your diet or use a salt substitute, however, before discussing it with your doctor. Too much potassium can also be dangerous. Your doctor may want you to have blood tests performed periodically in order to monitor your potassium levels.
- Limit your intake of alcoholic beverages while taking this medication, in order to prevent dizziness and lightheadedness.
- If you have high blood pressure, do not take any over-the-counter (nonprescription) medications for weight control or for allergy, asthma, cough, cold, or sinus problems unless your doctor directs you to do so.
- To prevent dehydration (severe water loss) while taking this medication, check with your doctor if you have any illness that causes severe or continuous nausea, vomiting, or diarrhea.
- This medication can raise blood sugar in diabetic patients. Therefore, blood sugar levels should be carefully monitored by blood or urine tests when this medication is being taken.
- This product contains the color additive FD&C Yellow No. 5 (tartrazine), which can cause allergic-type reactions (rash, fainting, difficulty in breathing) in certain susceptible individuals.
- Be sure to tell your doctor if you are pregnant. Bendroflumethiazide can cross the placenta and may cause adverse effects in the developing fetus. Also, tell your doctor if you are breast-feeding an infant. Although problems in humans have not been reported, small amounts of this drug can pass into breast milk, so caution is warranted.

Benemid—see probenecid

Bentyl—see dicyclomine

Benylin Cough Syrup—see diphenhydramine

---

benzthiazide

BRAND NAMES (Manufacturers)
benzthiazide (various manufacturers)
Exna (Robins)
Hydrex (Trimen)
Marazide (Vortech)

TYPE OF DRUG
Diuretic and antihypertensive

INGREDIENT
benzthiazide

DOSAGE FORM
Tablets (50 mg)

STORAGE
This medication should be stored at room temperature in a tightly closed container.

USES

Benzthiazide is prescribed to treat high blood pressure. It is also used to reduce fluid accumulation in the body caused by conditions such as heart failure, cirrhosis of the liver, kidney disease, and the long-term use of some medications. This medication reduces fluid accumulation by increasing the elimination of sodium and water through the kidneys.

TREATMENT

To decrease stomach irritation, you can take this medication with a glass of milk or with a meal (unless your doctor directs you to do otherwise). Try to take it at the same time every day. Avoid taking a dose after 6:00 P.M.; otherwise, you may have to get up during the night to urinate.

If you miss a dose of this medication, take the missed dose as soon as possible, unless it is almost time for the next dose. In that case, do not take the missed dose at all; just wait until the next scheduled dose. Do not double the next dose.

This medication does not cure high blood pressure, but it will help to control the condition as long as you continue to take it.

SIDE EFFECTS

Minor. Constipation, cramps, diarrhea, dizziness, drowsiness, headache, heartburn, loss of appetite, restlessness, or upset stomach. These side effects should disappear as your body adjusts to the medication.

This medication can cause increased sensitivity to sunlight. It is, therefore, important to avoid prolonged exposure to sunlight and sunlamps. Wear protective clothing, and use an effective sunscreen.

To relieve constipation, increase the amount of fiber in your diet (fresh fruits and vegetables, salads, bran, and whole-grain cereals and breads) and exercise (unless your doctor directs you to do otherwise).

To avoid dizziness or light-headedness when you stand, contract and relax the muscles of your legs for a few moments before rising. Do this by pushing one foot against the floor while raising the other foot slightly, alternating feet so that you are "pumping" your legs in a pedaling motion.

Major. Tell your doctor about any side effects that are persistent or particularly bothersome. IT IS ESPECIALLY IMPORTANT TO TELL YOUR DOCTOR about blurred vision, confusion, difficulty in breathing, dry mouth, excessive thirst, excessive weakness, fever, itching, joint pain, mood changes, muscle pain or spasms, nausea, palpitations, skin rash, sore throat, tingling in the fingers or toes, unusual bleeding or bruising, vomiting, or yellowing of the eyes or skin.

INTERACTIONS

Benzthiazide interacts with several other types of medications:

1. It may decrease the effectiveness of oral anticoagulants, antigout medications, insulin, oral antidiabetic medicines, and methenamine.

2. Fenfluramine can increase the blood-pressure-lowering effects of benzthiazide, which can be dangerous.

3. Indomethacin can decrease the blood-pressure-lowering effects of benzthiazide, thereby counteracting the desired effects.

4. Cholestyramine and colestipol decrease the absorption of this medication from the gastrointestinal tract. Benzthiazide should, therefore, be taken one hour before or four hours after a dose of cholestyramine or colestipol (if you have also been prescribed one of these medications).

5. The side effects of amphotericin B, calcium, cortisone-like steroids (such as cortisone, dexamethasone, hydrocortisone, prednisone, and prednisolone), digoxin, digitalis, lithium, quinidine, sulfonamide antibiotics, and vitamin D may be increased by benzthiazide.

BE SURE TO TELL YOUR DOCTOR about any medications you are currently taking, especially any of those listed above.

WARNINGS

- Tell your doctor about unusual or allergic reactions you have had to any medications, especially to diuretics or any other sulfa drugs, including oral antidiabetic medications or sulfonamide antibiotics.
- Before you start taking benzthiazide, tell your doctor if you now have or if you have ever had kidney disease or problems with urination, diabetes mellitus, gout, liver disease, asthma, pancreatic disease, or systemic lupus erythematosus.
- Benzthiazide can cause potassium loss. Signs of potassium loss include dry mouth, thirst, weakness, muscle pain or cramps, nausea, and vomiting. If you experience any of these symptoms, call your doctor. To help avoid potassium loss, take this drug with a glass of fresh or frozen orange juice or cranberry juice, or eat a banana every day. The use of a salt substitute also helps to prevent potassium loss. Do not change your diet or take a salt substitute, however, before discussing it with your doctor. Too much potassium can also be dangerous. Your doctor may want to have blood tests performed periodically in order to monitor your potassium levels.
- Limit your intake of alcoholic beverages while taking this medication, in order to prevent dizziness and light-headedness.
- If you have high blood pressure, do not take any over-the-counter (nonprescription) medications for weight control or for allergy, asthma, cough, cold, or sinus problems unless your doctor directs you to do so.
- To prevent dehydration (severe water loss) while taking this medication, check with your doctor if you have any illness that causes severe or continuous nausea, vomiting, or diarrhea.
- This medication can raise blood sugar in diabetic patients. Therefore, blood sugar levels should be carefully monitored by blood or urine tests when this medication is being taken.
- Some of these products contain the color additive FD&C Yellow No. 5 (tartrazine), which can cause allergic-type reactions (wheezing, rash, fainting, difficulty in breathing) in certain susceptible individuals.
- Be sure to tell your doctor if you are pregnant. Benzthiazide can cross the placenta and may cause adverse effects in the developing fetus. Also, tell your doctor if you are breast-feeding an infant. Although problems in humans have not been reported, small amounts of this drug can pass into breast milk, so caution is warranted.

---

benztropine

BRAND NAMES (Manufacturers)

benztropine (various manufacturers)
Cogentin (Merck Sharp & Dohme)

TYPE OF DRUG

Anticholinergic and antiparkinsonism agent

INGREDIENT

benztropine

DOSAGE FORM

Tablets (0.5 mg, 1 mg, and 2 mg)

STORAGE

Benztropine tablets should be stored at room temperature in a tightly closed container.

USES

Benztropine is used to treat the symptoms of Parkinson's disease or to control the side effects of phenothiazine tranquilizers. It is not clearly understood how this medication works, but it is thought to act by balancing certain chemicals in the brain.

TREATMENT

In order to reduce stomach irritation, you can take benztropine tablets with food or just after a meal.

Antacids and antidiarrheal medicines prevent the absorption of this medication, so at least one hour should separate doses of benztropine and one of these medicines.

If you miss a dose of this medication, take the missed dose as soon as possible, unless it is within two hours of your next dose. In that case, don't take the missed dose at all; just return to your regular dosing schedule. Do not double the next dose.

SIDE EFFECTS

Minor. Bloating; blurred vision; constipation; dizziness; drowsiness; dry mouth, throat, and nose; false sense of well-being; headache; increased sensitivity of the eyes to light; muscle cramps; nausea; nervousness; reduced sweating; or weakness. These side effects should disappear as your body adjusts to the medication.

If you are constipated, increase the amount of fiber in your diet (fresh fruits and vegetables, salads, bran, and whole-grain breads), exercise, and drink more water (unless your doctor directs you to do otherwise).

Chew sugarless gum or suck on ice chips or a piece of hard candy to reduce mouth dryness.

Wear sunglasses if your eyes become sensitive to light.

To avoid dizziness and light-headedness when you stand, contract and relax the muscles of your legs for a few moments before rising. Do this by pushing one foot against the floor while raising the other foot slightly, alternating feet so that you are "pumping" your legs in a pedaling motion.

Major. Tell your doctor about any side effects that are persistent or particularly bothersome. IT IS ESPECIALLY IMPORTANT TO TELL YOUR DOCTOR about depression, difficulty sleeping, difficulty in urinating, hallucinations, involuntary muscle movements, loss of balance, memory loss, mood changes, numbness of the fingers, palpitations, or unusual excitement.

Some side effects may occur for a short time after discontinuing this drug. Consult your doctor if they become bothersome.

INTERACTIONS

Benztropine interacts with several other types of drugs:

1. It can cause extreme drowsiness when combined with alcohol or other central nervous system depressants (such as antihistamines, barbiturates, benzodiazepine tranquilizers, muscle relaxants, narcotics, and pain medications) or with tricyclic antidepressants.

2. Amantadine, antihistamines, haloperidol, monoamine oxidase (MAO) inhibitors, phenothiazine tranquilizers, procainamide, quinidine, and tricyclic antidepressants can increase the side effects of benztropine. At least 14 days should separate the use of this drug and the use of an MAO inhibitor.

Before starting to take this medication, BE SURE TO TELL YOUR DOCTOR about any medications you are currently taking, especially any of those listed above.

WARNINGS

- Tell your doctor about unusual or allergic reactions you have had to any medications, especially to benztropine.
- Tell your doctor if you now have or if you have ever had achalasia, glaucoma, heart disease, high blood pressure, kidney disease, liver disease, myasthenia gravis, blockage of the intestinal tract or urinary tract, enlarged prostate gland, stomach ulcers, or thyroid disease.
- If this drug makes you dizzy or drowsy, avoid any activity that requires alertness, such as driving or operating potentially dangerous equipment. Be careful on stairs, and avoid getting up suddenly from a lying or sitting position.
- This medication can decrease sweating and heat release from the body. You should, therefore, avoid getting overheated by strenuous exercise in hot weather and should avoid taking hot baths, showers, and saunas.
- Elderly patients are more sensitive to the effects of benztropine. Contact your doctor if confusion, disorientation, agitation, or hallucinations occur.
- Be sure to tell your doctor if you are pregnant. Extensive studies of the use of benztropine during pregnancy have not been conducted. Also, tell your doctor if you are breast-feeding an infant. Small amounts of this medication may pass into breast milk.

---

betamethasone (systemic)

BRAND NAME (Manufacturer)
Celestone (Schering)
TYPE OF DRUG
Adrenocorticosteroid hormone
INGREDIENT
betamethasone
DOSAGE FORMS
Tablets (0.6 mg)
Oral syrup (0.6 mg per 5-ml spoonful, with less than 1% alcohol)
STORAGE
Betamethasone should be stored at room temperature in a tightly closed container. Discard any outdated medication or any medication that is no longer needed.

USES

Your adrenal glands naturally produce certain cortisone-like chemicals. These chemicals are involved in various regulatory processes in the body (such as those involving fluid balance, temperature, and reaction to inflammation). Betamethasone belongs to a group of drugs known as adrenocorticosteroids (or cortisone-like medications). It is used to treat a variety of disorders, including endocrine and rheumatic disorders; asthma; blood diseases; certain cancers; eye disorders; gastrointestinal disturbances, such as ulcerative colitis; respiratory diseases; and inflammations such as arthritis, dermatitis, and poison ivy. How this drug acts to relieve these disorders is not completely understood.

TREATMENT

In order to prevent stomach irritation, you can take betamethasone with food or milk.

The oral syrup form of this medication should be measured carefully with a specially designed 5-ml measuring spoon. An ordinary kitchen teaspoon is not accurate enough.

If you are taking only one dose of this medication each day, try to take it before 9:00 A.M. This will mimic the body's normal production of this type of chemical.

It is important to try not to miss any doses of betamethasone. However, if you do miss a dose of this medication, follow these guidelines:

1. If you are taking it more than once a day, take the missed dose as soon as possible, and return to your regular schedule. If it is already time for the next dose, double the dose.

2. If you are taking this medication once a day, take the dose you missed as soon as possible, unless you don't remember until the next day. In that case, do not take the missed dose at all; just follow your regular schedule. Do not double the next dose.

3. If you are taking this drug every other day, take it as soon as you remember. If you missed the scheduled time by a whole day, take it when you remember; then skip a day before you take the next dose. Do not double the dose.

If you miss more than one dose of betamethasone, CONTACT YOUR DOCTOR.

SIDE EFFECTS

Minor. Dizziness, false sense of well-being, increased appetite, increased susceptibility to infections, increased sweating, indigestion, menstrual irregularities, muscle weakness, nausea, reddening of the skin on the face, restlessness, sleep disorders, or weight gain. These side effects should disappear as your body adjusts to the medication.

Major. Tell your doctor about any side effects that are persistent or particularly bothersome. IT IS ESPECIALLY IMPORTANT TO TELL YOUR DOCTOR about abdominal enlargement; acne or other skin problems; back or rib pain; bloody or black, tarry stools; blurred vision; convulsions; fever and sore throat; glaucoma; growth impairment (in children); headaches; impaired healing of wounds; increased thirst and urination; menstrual irregularities; mental depression; mood changes; muscle wasting; nightmares; peptic ulcers; puffiness of the face; rapid weight gain (three to five pounds within a week); rash; shortness of breath; thinning of the skin; unusual bleeding or bruising; or unusual weakness.

INTERACTIONS

Betamethasone interacts with several other types of drugs:

1. Alcohol, aspirin, and anti-inflammatory medications (diflunisal, ibuprofen, indomethacin, ketoprofen, mefenamic acid, meclofenamate, naproxen, piroxicam, sulindac, tolmetin) aggravate the stomach problems that are common with use of this medication.

2. The dosage of oral anticoagulants (blood thinners, such as warfarin), oral antidiabetic drugs, or insulin may need to be altered when this medication is started or stopped.

3. The loss of potassium caused by betamethasone can lead to serious side effects in individuals taking digoxin. Thiazide diuretics (water pills) can increase the potassium loss caused by betamethasone.

4. Phenobarbital, phenytoin, rifampin, and ephedrine can increase the elimination of betamethasone from the body, thereby decreasing its effectiveness.

5. Oral contraceptives (birth control pills) and estrogen-containing drugs may decrease the elimination of this drug from the body, which can lead to an increase in side effects.

6. Betamethasone can increase the elimination of aspirin and isoniazid, thereby decreasing the effectiveness of these two medications.

7. Cholestyramine and colestipol can chemically bind this medication in the stomach and gastrointestinal tract and prevent its absorption.

BE SURE TO TELL YOUR DOCTOR about any medications you are currently taking, especially any listed above.

WARNINGS

- Tell your doctor about unusual or allergic reactions you have had to any medications, especially to betamethasone or other adrenocorticosteroids (such as cortisone, dexamethasone, hydrocortisone, methylprednisolone, paramethasone, prednisolone, prednisone, and triamcinolone).
- Be sure to tell your doctor if you now have or if you have ever had bone disease, diabetes mellitus, emotional instability, glaucoma, fungal infections, heart disease, high blood pressure, high cholesterol levels, myasthenia gravis, peptic ulcers, osteoporosis, thyroid disease, tuberculosis, ulcerative colitis, kidney disease, or liver disease.
- To help avoid potassium loss while using this drug, take your dose with a glass of fresh or frozen orange juice, or eat a banana each day. The use of a salt substitute also helps to prevent potassium loss. Discuss this with your doctor.
- If you are using this medication for longer than a week, you may need to receive higher dosages if you are subjected to stress, such as serious infections, injury, or surgery. Discuss this with your doctor.
- If you have been taking this drug for more than a week, do not stop taking it suddenly. If it is stopped suddenly, you may experience abdominal or back pain, dizziness, fainting, fever, muscle or joint pain, nausea, vomiting, shortness of breath, or extreme weakness. Your doctor may, therefore, want to reduce the dosage gradually. Never increase the dose or take the drug for longer than the prescribed time, unless you first consult your doctor.
- While you are taking this drug, you should not be vaccinated or immunized. This medication decreases the effectiveness of vaccines and can lead to overwhelming infection if a live-virus vaccine is administered.
- Before having skin tests, surgery, or any other medical or dental treatment, be sure to tell your doctor or dentist that you are taking betamethasone.
- Because this drug can cause glaucoma and cataracts with long-term use, your doctor may want you to have your eyes examined by an ophthalmologist periodically during treatment.
- If you are taking this medication for prolonged periods, you should wear or carry an identification card or notice stating that you are taking an adrenocorticosteroid.
- This medication can raise blood sugar levels in diabetic patients. Blood sugar should, therefore, be monitored carefully with blood tests when this medication is being taken. If you notice a change in your blood sugar levels, contact your doctor.

• Be sure to tell your doctor if you are pregnant. This type of drug crosses the placenta. Although studies in humans have not been conducted, birth defects have been observed in the offspring of animals that were given large doses of this drug during pregnancy. Also, tell your doctor if you are breast-feeding an infant. Small amounts of this type of drug pass into breast milk and may cause growth suppression or a decrease in natural adrenocorticosteroid production in the nursing infant.

---

betamethasone dipropionate (topical)

BRAND NAMES (Manufacturers)
Alphatrex (Savage)
betamethasone dipropionate (various manufacturers)
Diprolene (Schering)
Diprosone (Schering)
TYPE OF DRUG
Adrenocorticosteroid hormone
INGREDIENT
betamethasone
DOSAGE FORMS
Ointment (0.05%)
Cream (0.05%)
Lotion (0.05%)
Aerosol (0.1%)
STORAGE
Betamethasone dipropionate ointment, cream, and lotion should be stored at room temperature in tightly closed containers. This medication should never be frozen.

The aerosol form of this medication is packaged under pressure. It should not be stored near heat or an open flame or in direct sunlight, and the container should never be punctured.

USES

Your adrenal glands naturally produce certain cortisone-like chemicals. These chemicals are involved in various regulatory processes in the body (such as those involving fluid balance, temperature, and reaction to inflammation). Betamethasone dipropionate belongs to a group of drugs known as adrenocorticosteroids (or cortisone-like medications). It is used to relieve the skin inflammation (redness, swelling, itching, and discomfort) associated with conditions such as dermatitis, eczema, and poison ivy. How betamethasone dipropionate acts to relieve these disorders is not completely understood.

TREATMENT

Before applying this medication, wash your hands. Then, unless your doctor gives you different instructions, gently wash the area of the skin where the medication is to be applied. With a clean towel, pat the area almost dry; it should be slightly damp when you put the medicine on.

If you are using the lotion form of this medication, shake it well before pouring it out. The contents tend to settle on the bottom of the bottle, so it is necessary to shake the container to distribute the ingredients evenly and equalize the doses.

Apply a small amount of the medication to the affected area in a thin layer. Do not bandage the area unless your doctor tells you to do so. If you are to apply an occlusive dressing (like kitchen plastic wrap), be sure you understand the instructions. Wash your hands again after application.

If you are using the aerosol spray form of this medication, shake the can in order to disperse the medication evenly. Hold the can upright, six to eight inches from the area to be sprayed, and spray the area for one to three seconds. DO NOT SMOKE while you are using the aerosol spray; the contents are under pressure and may explode when exposed to heat or flames.

Avoid applying this medication to areas with cuts or open wounds.

If you miss a dose of this medication, apply the dose as soon as possible, unless it is almost time for the next application. In that case, do not apply the missed dose; just return to your regular schedule. Do not put twice as much of the medication on your skin at the next application.

SIDE EFFECTS

Minor. Acne, burning sensation, itching, skin dryness, or rash.

If the affected area is extremely dry or scaling, the skin may be moistened before applying the medication by soaking in water or by applying water with a clean cloth. The ointment form is probably better for dry skin.

A mild, temporary stinging sensation may occur after this medication is applied. If this persists, contact your doctor.

Major. Tell your doctor about any side effects that are persistent or particularly bothersome. IT IS ESPECIALLY IMPORTANT TO TELL YOUR DOCTOR about blistering, increased hair growth, irritation of the affected area, loss of skin color, secondary infection in the area being treated, or thinning of the skin with easy bruising.

INTERACTIONS

This medication should not interact with any other medications as long as it is used according to directions.

WARNINGS

• Tell your doctor about unusual or allergic reactions you have had to any medications, especially to betamethasone dipropionate or any other adrenocorticosteroid (such as amcinonide, clocortolone, cortisone, desonide, desoximetasone, dexamethasone, diflorasone, flumethasone, fluocinolone, fluocinonide, fluorometholone, flurandrenolide, halcinonide, hydrocortisone, methylprednisolone, prednisolone, prednisone, and triamcinolone).

• Tell your doctor if you now have or if you have ever had blood vessel disease, chicken pox, diabetes mellitus, fungal infection, peptic ulcer, shingles, tuberculosis, tuberculosis of the skin, vaccinia, or any other type of infection, especially at the site currently being treated.

• If irritation develops while using this drug, immediately discontinue its use and notify your doctor.

• This product is not for use in the eyes or on mucous membranes; contact may result in side effects.

• Do not use this product with an occlusive wrap unless your doctor directs you to do so. Systemic absorption of this drug is increased if extensive areas of the body are treated, particularly if occlusive bandages are used. If it is necessary for you to use this drug under a wrap, follow your doctor's instructions exactly; do not leave the wrap in place longer than specified.

- If you are using this medication on a child's diaper area, do not put tight-fitting diapers or plastic pants on the child. This may lead to increased systemic absorption of the drug and a possible increase in side effects.
- Elderly patients and younger children have naturally thinner skin, and, therefore, betamethasone dipropionate is more likely to be absorbed. Be sure to report any adverse effects to your doctor.
- In order to avoid freezing skin tissue when using the aerosol form of betamethasone dipropionate, make sure that you do not spray for more than three seconds, and hold the container at least six inches from the skin.
- When using the aerosol form of this medication on the face, cover your eyes and do not inhale the spray.
- Use this medication only for your current condition. Do not use it for another problem later or give it to other people to use.
- Be sure to tell your doctor if you are pregnant. If large amounts of this drug are applied for prolonged periods, some of it will be absorbed and may cross the placenta. Although studies in humans have not been conducted, birth defects have been observed in the offspring of animals that were given large oral doses of this type of drug during pregnancy. Also, tell your doctor if you are breast-feeding an infant. If absorbed through the skin, small amounts of the drug pass into breast milk and may cause growth suppression or a decrease in natural adrenocorticosteroid production in the nursing infant.

---

betamethasone dipropionate and clotrimazole combination (topical)

BRAND NAME (Manufacturer)
Lotrisone (Schering)

TYPE OF DRUG
Adrenocorticosteroid hormone and antifungal

INGREDIENTS
betamethasone dipropionate and clotrimazole

DOSAGE FORM
Topical cream (0.05% betamethasone dipropionate and 1% clotrimazole)

STORAGE
This medication should be stored at room temperature (never frozen) in a tightly closed container. Discard any outdated or unneeded medication.

USES

Betamethasone dipropionate and clotrimazole combination is used to treat fungal infections of the skin. Clotrimazole is an antifungal agent that prevents the growth and multiplication of a wide range of fungi and yeast, including *Candida*. Betamethasone dipropionate belongs to a group of drugs known as adrenocorticosteroids (or cortisone-like medications). Your adrenal glands naturally produce certain cortisone-like chemicals. These chemicals are involved in various regulatory processes in the body. Betamethasone dipropionate is added to this combination to relieve skin inflammation (redness, swelling, itching, and discomfort).

TREATMENT

Before applying betamethasone dipropionate and clotrimazole combination, you should wash your hands. Then, unless your doctor tells you to do otherwise, cleanse the affected area with soap and water. Pat the skin with a clean towel until it is almost dry. Gently massage a small amount of the cream over the entire area that is affected and the skin immediately surrounding this area. Avoid applying the medication to areas with cuts or open wounds. Don't bandage or cover the area after applying the medication, unless your doctor instructs you to do so. Wash your hands again after application.

Improvement in your condition may not become apparent for as long as a week after you begin treatment with this drug. However, you should be sure to complete the full course of medication. If you stop using this drug too soon, resistant fungi are given a chance to continue growing, and the infection could recur. If your condition has not improved after four weeks, CONTACT YOUR DOCTOR. Clotrimazole may not be effective against the organism causing your infection.

If you miss a dose of this medication, apply the dose as soon as possible, unless it is almost time for the next application. In that case, do not apply the missed dose; just return to your regular schedule. Do not put twice as much of the medication on your skin at the next application.

SIDE EFFECTS

Minor. Acne and burning sensation. You may also experience some burning, itching, redness, or stinging when this drug is applied to the skin. These side effects should disappear as your body adjusts to this medication.

Major. Tell your doctor about any side effects that are persistent or particularly bothersome. IT IS ESPECIALLY IMPORTANT TO TELL YOUR DOCTOR about blistering, increased hair growth, irritation, loss of skin color, peeling of the skin, swelling, or thinning of the skin with easy bruising.

INTERACTIONS

Betamethasone dipropionate and clotrimazole combination should not interact with other medications as long as it is used according to directions.

WARNINGS

- Tell your doctor about unusual or allergic reactions you have had to any medications, especially to betamethasone dipropionate or other adrenocorticosteroids (amcinonide, clocortolone, cortisone, desonide, desoximetasone, dexamethasone, diflorasone, flumethasone, fluocinolone, fluocinonide, fluorometholone, flurandrenolide, halcinonide, hydrocortisone, methylprednisolone, prednisolone, prednisone, triamcinolone) or to clotrimazole.
- Tell your doctor if you now have or if you have ever had blood vessel disease, chicken pox, diabetes mellitus, fungal infection, peptic ulcers, pulmonary tuberculosis, shingles, tuberculosis of the skin, vaccinia, or any other type of infection, especially at the site being treated.

• If irritation develops while using this drug, immediately discontinue its use and notify your doctor.
• This product is not for use in the eyes or on mucous membranes; contact may result in side effects.
• Do not use this product with an occlusive wrap unless your doctor directs you to do so. Systemic absorption of this drug is increased if extensive areas of the body are treated, particularly if occlusive bandages are used. If it is necessary for you to use this drug under a wrap, follow your doctor's instructions exactly; do not leave the wrap in place longer than specified.
• If you are using this medication on a child's diaper area, do not put tight-fitting diapers or plastic pants on the child. This may lead to increased systemic absorption of the drug and a possible increase in side effects.
• Elderly patients and younger children have naturally thinner skin, and, therefore, the drug is more likely to be absorbed. Report any adverse effects to your doctor.
• This medication has been prescribed for your current infection only. A subsequent infection, or one that someone else has, may require a different medication. Therefore, you should not give your medicine to other people or use it for other infections, unless directed to do so by your doctor.
• In order to avoid reinfection, keep the affected area clean and dry, wear freshly laundered clothing, and avoid wearing tight-fitting clothes.
• Be sure to tell your doctor if you are pregnant. If large amounts of this drug are applied for prolonged periods, some of it will be absorbed and may cross the placenta. Although studies in humans have not been conducted, birth defects have been observed in the offspring of animals that were given large oral doses of adrenocorticosteroids during pregnancy. Also, tell your doctor if you are breast-feeding an infant. If absorbed through the skin, small amounts of this type of drug pass into breast milk and may cause growth suppression or a decrease in adrenocorticosteroid production in the nursing infant.

---

betamethasone valerate (topical)

BRAND NAMES (Manufacturers)
betamethasone valerate (various manufacturers)
Betatrex (Savage)
Beta-Val (Lemmon)
Valisone (Schering)
Valisone Reduced Strength (Schering)
TYPE OF DRUG
Adrenocorticosteroid hormone
INGREDIENT
betamethasone
DOSAGE FORMS
Cream (0.01% and 0.1%)
Ointment (0.1%)
Lotion (0.1%)
STORAGE
This medication should be stored at room temperature (never frozen) in a tightly closed container.

USES

Your adrenal glands naturally produce certain cortisone-like chemicals. These chemicals are involved in various regulatory processes in the body (such as those involving fluid balance, temperature, and reaction to inflammation). Betamethasone valerate belongs to a group of drugs known as adrenocorticosteroids (or cortisone-like medications). It is used to relieve the skin inflammation (redness, swelling, itching, and discomfort) associated with conditions such as dermatitis, eczema, and poison ivy. How this drug acts to relieve these disorders is not completely understood.

TREATMENT

Before applying this medication, wash your hands. Then, unless your doctor gives you different instructions, gently wash the area of the skin where the medication is to be applied. With a clean towel, pat the area almost dry; it should be slightly damp when you put the medicine on.

If you are using the lotion form of this drug, shake it well before pouring out the medicine. The contents tend to settle on the bottom of the bottle, so it is necessary to shake the container to distribute the ingredients evenly and equalize the doses.

Apply a small amount of the medication to the affected area in a thin layer. Avoid applying medication to cuts or open wounds. Do not bandage the area unless your doctor tells you to do so. If you are to apply an occlusive dressing (like kitchen plastic wrap), be sure you understand the instructions. Wash your hands again after application.

If you miss a dose of this medication, apply the dose as soon as possible, unless it is almost time for the next application. In that case, do not apply the missed dose; just return to your regular dosing schedule. Do not put twice as much on your skin at the next application.

SIDE EFFECTS

Minor. Acne, burning sensation, itching, rash, or skin dryness.

If the affected area is extremely dry or scaling, the skin may be moistened before applying the medication by soaking in water or by applying water with a clean cloth. The ointment form is probably better for dry skin.

A mild, temporary stinging sensation may occur after this medication is applied. If this persists, contact your doctor.

Major. Tell your doctor about any side effects that are persistent or particularly bothersome. IT IS ESPECIALLY IMPORTANT TO TELL YOUR DOCTOR about blistering, increased hair growth, irritation of the affected area, loss of skin color, secondary infection of the area being treated, or thinning of the skin with easy bruising.

INTERACTIONS

This medication should not interact with any other medications as long as it is used according to directions.

WARNINGS

• Tell your doctor about unusual or allergic reactions you have had to any medications, especially to betamethasone valerate or other adrenocorticosteroids (such as amcinonide, clocortolone, cortisone, desonide, desoximetasone, dexamethasone, diflorasone, flumethasone, fluocinolone, fluocinonide, fluorometholone, flurandrenolide, halcinonide, hydrocortisone, methylprednisolone, prednisolone, prednisone, and triamcinolone).

• Tell your doctor if you now have or if you have ever had blood vessel disease, chicken pox, diabetes mellitus, fungal infection, peptic ulcers, shingles, tuberculosis, tuberculosis of the skin, vaccinia, or any other type of infection, especially at the site currently being treated.

• If irritation develops while using this drug, immediately discontinue its use and notify your doctor.

• This product is not for use in the eyes or on mucous membranes; contact may result in side effects.

• Use this drug only for your current condition. Do not use it for another problem or give it to others to use.

• Do not use this product with an occlusive wrap unless your doctor directs you to do so. Systemic absorption of this drug is increased if extensive areas of the body are treated, particularly if occlusive bandages are used. If it is necessary for you to use this drug under a wrap, follow your doctor's instructions exactly; do not leave the wrap in place longer than specified.

• If you are using this medication on a child's diaper area, do not put tight-fitting diapers or plastic pants on the child. This may lead to increased systemic absorption of the drug and a possible increase in side effects.

• Elderly patients and younger children have naturally thinner skin, and, therefore, the drug is more likely to be absorbed. Report any adverse effects.

• Be sure to tell your doctor if you are pregnant. If large amounts of this drug are applied for prolonged periods, some of it will be absorbed and may cross the placenta. Although studies in humans have not been conducted, birth defects have been observed in the offspring of animals that were given large oral doses of this type of drug during pregnancy. Also, tell your doctor if you are breast-feeding an infant. If absorbed through the skin, small amounts of this type of drug pass into breast milk and may cause growth suppression or a decrease in natural adrenocorticosteroid production in the nursing infant.

Betapen-VK—see penicillin VK

Betatrex—see betamethasone valerate (topical)

Beta-Val—see betamethasone valerate (topical)

---

betaxolol (ophthalmic)

BRAND NAME (Manufacturer)
Betoptic (Alcon)

TYPE OF DRUG
Antiglaucoma ophthalmic solution

INGREDIENT
betaxolol

DOSAGE FORM
Ophthalmic drops (0.5% betaxolol)

STORAGE
Store at room temperature in a tightly closed container. Discard any outdated medication.

USES

Betaxolol is used to reduce pressure in the eye caused by glaucoma or other eye conditions. This medication belongs to a group of drugs known as beta blockers. When applied to the eye, betaxolol reduces pressure within the eye, perhaps by decreasing eye fluid (aqueous humor) production and by increasing the outflow of fluid from the eye.

TREATMENT

Wash your hands with soap and water before applying this drug. To avoid contamination of the drops, do not touch the tube portion of the dropper or let it touch your eye; do not wipe off or rinse the dropper after use.

To apply the drops, tilt your head back and pull down your lower eyelid with one hand to make a pouch below the eye. Drop the prescribed amount of medicine into this pouch and slowly close your eyes. Try not to blink. Keep your eyes closed, and place one finger at the corner of the eye next to your nose for a minute or two, applying slight pressure (this is done to prevent loss of medication into the nose and throat canal). Then wipe away any excess with a clean tissue. Since administering the drug is somewhat difficult, you may want to have someone else apply the drops for you.

If you miss a dose of this medication, apply the missed dose as soon as possible, then return to your regular dosing schedule. However, if it is almost time for the next dose, skip the dose you missed. Do not double the next dose.

SIDE EFFECTS

Minor. When you first apply this medication, it may sting or burn your eyes. This should stop in a few minutes. You may also notice sensitivity of your eyes to bright lights or sunlight. Wearing sunglasses and avoiding excessive exposure to sunlight may help relieve this sensitivity.

Major. Tell your doctor about any side effects that are persistent or particularly bothersome. IT IS ESPECIALLY IMPORTANT TO TELL YOUR DOCTOR about hives, irritation of the eye that lasts more than a few minutes after application, itching, or skin rash. Major side effects are rare when this product is used correctly. However, depression, fluid accumulation, insomnia, shortness of breath, or swelling of the feet may occur with this drug. If you have any of these symptoms, contact your doctor.

INTERACTIONS

Betaxolol may increase the side effects of reserpine and oral beta blockers. Before starting to take betaxolol, BE SURE TO TELL YOUR DOCTOR about any medications you are currently taking, especially any of those listed above.

WARNINGS

• Tell your doctor about unusual or allergic reactions you have had to any medications, especially to betaxolol or to any other beta blocker (acebutolol, atenolol, carteolol, esmolol, labetalol, metoprolol, nadolol, penbutolol, pindolol, propranolol, timolol).

• Before starting betaxolol, be sure to tell your doctor if you now have or if you have ever had asthma, diabetes mellitus, heart failure, lung disease, or thyroid disease.

• Before having surgery or any other medical or dental treatment, tell your doctor or dentist that you are taking this medication. Your doctor or dentist may want to gradually withdraw this medication prior to the procedure.

• Be sure to tell your doctor if you are pregnant. Although betaxolol appears to be safe in animals, studies in pregnant women have not been conducted. Also, tell your doctor if you are breast-feeding an infant. Small amounts of betaxolol will pass into breast milk.

---

betaxolol (systemic)

BRAND NAME (Manufacturer)
Kerlone (Searle)
TYPE OF DRUG
Beta-adrenergic blocking agent
INGREDIENT
betaxolol
DOSAGE FORM
Tablets (10 mg and 20 mg)
STORAGE
Betaxolol should be stored at room temperature in a tightly closed container.

USES

Betaxolol is prescribed for the treatment of high blood pressure. Betaxolol belongs to a group of medicines known as beta-adrenergic blocking agents or, more commonly, beta blockers. These drugs work by controlling impulses along certain nerve pathways.

TREATMENT

Betaxolol can be taken with a glass of water, with meals, immediately following meals, or on an empty stomach, depending on your doctor's instructions. Try to take the medication at the same time(s) each day.

Try not to miss any doses of this medication. If you do miss a dose of the medication, take the missed dose as soon as possible. However, if the next scheduled dose is within eight hours (if you are taking this medication only once a day) or within four hours (if you are taking this medication more than once a day), do not take the missed dose at all; just return to your regular dosing schedule. Do not double the next dose of the medication.

It is important to remember that betaxolol does not cure high blood pressure, but it will help to control the condition as long as you continue to take it.

SIDE EFFECTS

Minor. Decreased sexual ability, diarrhea, fatigue, headache, indigestion, or nausea. These side effects should diminish as your body adjusts to the medication.

Major. Tell your doctor about any side effects that are persistent or particularly bothersome. IT IS ESPECIALLY IMPORTANT TO TELL YOUR DOCTOR about breathing difficulty or wheezing; cold hands or feet due to decreased blood circulation to the skin, fingers, and toes; confusion; dizziness; fever and sore throat; hair loss; hallucinations; light-headedness; mental depression; nightmares; reduced alertness; skin rash; swelling of the ankles, feet, or lower legs; or unusual bleeding or bruising.

INTERACTIONS

Betaxolol interacts with a number of other types of medications:

1. Indomethacin, other nonsteroidal anti-inflammatory agents, aspirin, or other salicylates may decrease the blood-pressure-lowering effects of beta blockers.

2. Calcium channel blockers (nifedipine, verapamil, diltiazem, lisinopril) may be used with beta blockers such as betaxolol unless the patient has heart trouble. Very low blood pressure and heart failure have been observed in patients with impaired heart function who take beta blockers.

3. Side effects may also be increased if beta blockers are taken with epinephrine, phenylephrine, phenylpropanolamine, phenothiazine tranquilizers, reserpine, clonidine, prazosin, or monoamine oxidase (MAO) inhibitors. At least 14 days should separate the use of a beta blocker and the use of an MAO inhibitor.

4. Beta blockers may antagonize (work against) the effects of theophylline, aminophylline, albuterol, isoproterenol, metaproterenol, and terbutaline.

5. Beta blockers can also interact with insulin or oral antidiabetic agents—raising or lowering blood sugar levels or masking symptoms of low blood sugar.

6. The action of beta blockers may be increased if they are used with furosemide or hydralazine, which could have a negative effect.

7. Alcohol, barbiturates, and rifampin can decrease blood concentrations of this drug, which can result in a decrease in effectiveness.

8. If you are on both betaxolol and clonidine, and both of these medications are to be discontinued, it is recommended that the betaxolol be tapered off over several days before the gradual reduction of clonidine.

9. In patients who have congestive heart failure treated with digitalis glycosides (for example, digoxin or digitoxin), caution should be used as both betaxolol and digitalis products may slow heart conduction.

Before starting to take betaxolol, BE SURE TO TELL YOUR DOCTOR about any medications you are already taking, especially any of the medications listed above.

WARNINGS

• Tell your doctor about any unusual or allergic reactions you have had to any medications, especially to betaxolol or any other beta blocker (acebutolol, atenolol, carteolol, esmolol, labetolol, metoprolol, nadolol, penbutalol, pindolol, propranolol, timolol).

• Tell your doctor if you now have or if you have ever had asthma, bronchitis, diabetes mellitus, heart block, heart failure, kidney disease, liver disease, peripheral vascular disease (poor circulation in the fingers or toes), severe bradycardia (slowed heart rate), or thyroid disease.

• Betaxolol therapy may increase the risk of cardiac failure in some patients. Report any abnormal heart function to your doctor.

• Patients with severe bronchospastic disease (such as asthma) should, in general, not receive beta blockers. Inform your physician if you experience breathing difficulties.

• In diabetics, betaxolol may block some of the warning signs of low blood sugar (hypoglycemia), such as rapid pulse rate, but not others, such as dizziness or sweating.

• You may want to check your pulse while taking this drug. If your pulse is much slower than your usual rate (or if it is less than 50 beats per minute), check with your doctor. A pulse that is too slow may cause circulation problems.
• This medication may affect your body's response to exercise. Ask your doctor what an appropriate amount of exercise would be for you, taking into account your medical condition.
• It is important that you do not stop taking this medication without first checking with your doctor. Some conditions such as angina pectoris may become worse when the medication is stopped suddenly, and the danger of a heart attack is increased in some patients. Your doctor may want you to gradually reduce the amount of medication you take before stopping completely. Make sure that you have enough medication on hand to last through vacations, holidays, and weekends.
• Tell your doctor or dentist that you are taking this medication before having surgery or any other medical or dental treatment. Often, this medication will be discontinued 48 hours prior to any major surgery.
• While taking this medication, do not use any over-the-counter (nonprescription) allergy, asthma, cough, cold, sinus, or diet preparation without first checking with your doctor or pharmacist. The combination of these medications with a beta blocker can result in high blood pressure.
• Betaxolol may reduce intraocular pressure and give a misleading negative glaucoma test.
• Be sure to tell your doctor if you are pregnant. Animal studies have shown that some beta blockers can cause problems in pregnancy when used at very high doses. Adequate studies have not been conducted in humans, but there has been some association between beta blockers used during pregnancy and low birth weight, as well as breathing problems and slow heart rate in the newborn. Also, tell your doctor if you are breast-feeding an infant. Although this medication has not been shown to cause problems in breast-fed infants, some of the medication may pass into breast milk, so caution is warranted.
• The safety of this medication has not been established in children.

---

bethanechol

BRAND NAMES (Manufacturers)
bethanechol chloride (various manufacturers)
Duvoid (Norwich-Eaton)
Myotonachol (Glenwood)
Urabeth (Major)
Urecholine (Merck Sharp & Dohme)
TYPE OF DRUG
Cholinergic
INGREDIENT
bethanechol
DOSAGE FORM
Tablets (5 mg, 10 mg, 25 mg, and 50 mg)
STORAGE
Bethanechol should be stored at room temperature in a tightly closed container.

USES

Bethanechol is used to relieve retention of urine in the bladder. It acts on the nerves of the bladder to cause emptying.

TREATMENT

Bethanechol should be taken on an empty stomach one hour before or two hours after a meal. If it is taken soon after eating, nausea and vomiting may occur.

If you miss a dose and remember within an hour, take the missed dose immediately. If more than an hour has passed, do not take the missed dose at all; just return to your regular dosing schedule. Do not double the next dose.

SIDE EFFECTS

Minor. Abdominal cramps, belching, diarrhea, dizziness, excessive salivation, flushing of the skin, headache, nausea, sweating, or vomiting. These side effects should disappear as your body adjusts to the medication.

If you feel dizzy, sit or lie down for a while; get up slowly from a sitting or reclining position, and be careful on stairs.
Major. Tell your doctor about any side effects that are persistent or particularly bothersome. IT IS ESPECIALLY IMPORTANT TO TELL YOUR DOCTOR about chest pain, feeling faint, or shortness of breath.

INTERACTIONS

Bethanechol interacts with several other types of drugs:
1. Procainamide and quinidine can decrease the therapeutic effects of bethanechol.
2. Concurrent use of bethanechol and mecamylamine or trimethaphan can lead to a serious drop in blood pressure.

Before starting to take bethanechol, BE SURE TO TELL YOUR DOCTOR about any medications you are currently taking, especially any of those listed above.

WARNINGS

• Tell your doctor about unusual or allergic reactions you have had to any medications, especially to bethanechol.
• Before starting to take this medication, be sure to tell your doctor if you have ever had any of the following disorders: asthma, epilepsy, heart disease, high or low blood pressure, Parkinson's disease, stomach ulcers, thyroid disease, or an obstruction of the intestine or bladder.
• If this drug makes you dizzy, avoid taking part in any activity that requires alertness, such as driving a car or operating potentially dangerous equipment.
• Be sure to tell your doctor if you are pregnant. Although bethanechol appears to be safe during pregnancy, extensive studies in humans have not been conducted. Thus, bethanechol should only be administered during pregnancy if the benefits to the mother clearly outweigh potential risks to the fetus. Also, tell your doctor if you are breast-feeding. It is not known if small amounts of bethanechol pass into breast milk, so cautious use is warranted in nursing women.

bethanechol chloride—see bethanechol

Bethaprim DS—see sulfamethoxazole and trimethoprim combination

Betoptic—see betaxolol (ophthalmic)

Blanex—see chlorzoxazone and acetaminophen combination

Bleph-10—see sodium sulfacetamide (ophthalmic)

Blocadren—see timolol (systemic)

Bonine—see meclizine

Bontril PDM—see phendimetrazine

Bontril Slow-Release—see phendimetrazine

Brethaire—see terbutaline

Brethine—see terbutaline

Brevicon—see oral contraceptives

Brexin L.A.—see pseudoephedrine and chlorpheniramine combination

Bricanyl—see terbutaline

Bromatapp—see phenylpropanolamine, phenylephrine, and brompheniramine combination

---

bromocriptine

BRAND NAME (Manufacturer)
Parlodel (Sandoz)
Parlodel SnapTabs (Sandoz)
TYPE OF DRUG
Dopamine agonist and antiparkinsonism agent
INGREDIENT
bromocriptine
DOSAGE FORMS
Tablets (2.5 mg)
Capsules (5 mg)
STORAGE
Bromocriptine should be stored at room temperature in a tightly closed, light-resistant container.

USES

This medication is used to treat the symptoms of Parkinson's disease and to decrease milk production in women who choose not to breast-feed their infants. Bromocriptine relieves the symptoms of Parkinson's disease by replacing a chemical (dopamine) that is diminished in the brains of these patients. Bromocriptine prevents milk production by blocking the action of the responsible hormone (prolactin).

TREATMENT

In order to avoid stomach irritation during therapy with bromocriptine, you can take the medication with food or with a full glass of water or milk.

If you miss a dose of this medication and remember within four hours, take the missed dose immediately. If more than four hours have passed, do not take the missed dose at all; just return to your regular dosing schedule. Do not double the next dose.

SIDE EFFECTS

Minor. Abdominal pain, constipation, diarrhea, dizziness, drowsiness, fatigue, headache, insomnia, light-headedness, loss of appetite, nasal congestion, nausea, or vomiting. These should disappear as your body adjusts to the drug.

Dizziness or fainting may occur, especially following the first dose. It is best, therefore, to take the first dose while lying down. If you feel dizzy or light-headed with later doses, sit or lie down; get up slowly; and be careful on stairs.

To relieve constipation, increase the amount of fiber in your diet (fresh fruits and vegetables, salads, bran, and whole-grain breads), exercise, and drink more water (unless your doctor directs you to do otherwise).

Major. Tell your doctor about any side effects that are persistent or particularly bothersome. IT IS ESPECIALLY IMPORTANT TO REPORT ANY abnormal, involuntary movements; anxiety; confusion; convulsions; depression; difficulty in swallowing; fainting; fluid retention; hallucinations; nervousness; nightmares; skin rash; shortness of breath; tingling in the hands or feet; or visual disturbances.

INTERACTIONS

Bromocriptine interacts with several other medications:

1. Phenothiazine tranquilizers, methyldopa, haloperidol, metoclopramide, reserpine, and monoamine oxidase (MAO) inhibitors decrease the beneficial effects of bromocriptine.

2. Dosages of antihypertensive medications may require adjustment when bromocriptine is started.

Before starting to take bromocriptine, BE SURE TO TELL YOUR DOCTOR about any medications you are currently taking, especially any of those listed above.

WARNINGS

- Tell your doctor about unusual or allergic reactions you have had to any medications, especially to bromocriptine or ergotamine.
- Before starting this drug, tell your doctor if you now have or have ever had heart or blood vessel disease, kidney disease, liver disease, or mental disorders.
- If this drug makes you dizzy or drowsy, avoid tasks that require alertness, such as driving a car.
- Do not stop taking bromocriptine unless you first check with your doctor. Stopping the drug abruptly may lead to a worsening of your condition. Your doctor may want to reduce your dosage gradually to prevent this from occurring.
- Tell your doctor if you are pregnant. It is generally recommended that bromocriptine not be used during pregnancy because there have been reports of birth defects in both animals and humans whose mothers received the drug during pregnancy. Also, tell your doctor if you are breast-feeding. Bromocriptine blocks milk production.

Bromophen T.D.—see phenylpropanolamine, phenylephrine, and brompheniramine combination

Bromphen—see brompheniramine

---

brompheniramine

BRAND NAMES (Manufacturers)
Bromphen (various manufacturers)

brompheniramine maleate (various manufacturers)
Diamine T.D. (Major)
Dimetane* (Robins)
Dimetane Extentabs* (Robins)
Veltane (Lannett)
*Available over-the-counter (without a prescription)

TYPE OF DRUG
Antihistamine

INGREDIENT
brompheniramine

DOSAGE FORMS
Tablets (4 mg)
Sustained-release tablets (8 mg and 12 mg)
Oral elixir (2 mg per 5-ml spoonful, with 3% alcohol)

STORAGE
Brompheniramine tablets and oral elixir should be stored at room temperature in tightly closed containers.

USES

This medication belongs to a group of drugs known as antihistamines (antihistamines block the action of histamine, a chemical that is released by the body during an allergic reaction). Brompheniramine is used to treat or prevent symptoms of allergy.

TREATMENT

Stomach upset may occur with the use of this medicine. To avoid this side effect, you can take brompheniramine with food or with a full glass of milk or water (unless your doctor directs you to do otherwise).

The elixir form should be measured carefully with a specially designed 5-ml measuring spoon. An ordinary kitchen teaspoon is not accurate enough.

The sustained-release tablets should be swallowed whole. Breaking, chewing, or crushing them destroys their sustained-release activity and may increase side effects.

If you miss a dose, take the missed dose as soon as possible, unless it is almost time for your next dose. In that case, don't take the missed dose at all; just return to your regular dosing schedule. Do not double the next dose.

SIDE EFFECTS

Minor. Blurred vision; confusion; constipation; diarrhea; difficult or painful urination; dizziness; dry mouth, throat, or nose; headache; irritability; loss of appetite; nausea; restlessness; ringing or buzzing in the ears; stomach upset; or unusual increase in sweating. These side effects should disappear as your body adjusts to the medication.

This medication can cause increased sensitivity to sunlight. It is, therefore, important to avoid prolonged exposure to sunlight and sunlamps. Wear protective clothing, and use an effective sunscreen.

If you are constipated, increase the amount of fiber in your diet (fresh fruits and vegetables, salads, bran, and whole-grain breads), exercise, and drink more water (unless your doctor tells you not to do so.)

Chew sugarless gum, or suck on ice chips or a piece of hard candy to reduce mouth dryness.

If you feel dizzy or light-headed, sit or lie down for a while; get up slowly, and be careful on stairs.

Major. Tell your doctor about any side effects that are persistent or particularly bothersome. IT IS ESPECIALLY IMPORTANT TO TELL YOUR DOCTOR about a change in menstruation, clumsiness, feeling faint, flushing of the face, hallucinations, palpitations, rash, seizures, shortness of breath, sleeping disorders, sore throat or fever, tightness in the chest, unusual bleeding or bruising, or unusual tiredness or weakness.

INTERACTIONS

Brompheniramine interacts with several other drugs:

1. Concurrent use of it with central nervous system depressants (such as alcohol, barbiturates, benzodiazepine tranquilizers, muscle relaxants, narcotics, pain medications, and phenothiazine tranquilizers) or with tricyclic antidepressants can cause extreme drowsiness.

2. Monoamine oxidase (MAO) inhibitors (isocarboxazid, pargyline, phenelzine, tranylcypromine) can increase the side effects of this medication. At least 14 days should separate the use of this drug and the use of an MAO inhibitor.

3. Brompheniramine can decrease the activity of oral anticoagulants (blood thinners, such as warfarin).

BE SURE TO TELL YOUR DOCTOR about any medications you are currently taking, especially any listed above.

WARNINGS

- Tell your doctor about unusual or allergic reactions you have had to medications, especially to brompheniramine or to any other antihistamine (such as carbinoxamine, chlorpheniramine, clemastine, cyproheptadine, dexchlorpheniramine, dimenhydrinate, dimethindene, diphenhydramine, diphenylpyraline, doxylamine, hydroxyzine, promethazine, pyrilamine, terfenadine, trimeprazine, tripelennamine, and triprolidine).
- Tell your doctor if you now have or if you have ever had asthma, blood vessel disease, glaucoma, high blood pressure, kidney disease, peptic ulcers, enlarged prostate gland, or thyroid disease.
- Brompheniramine can cause drowsiness or dizziness. Your ability to perform tasks that require alertness, such as driving a car or operating potentially dangerous machinery, may be decreased. Appropriate caution should be taken.
- Be sure to tell your doctor if you are pregnant. The effects of this medication during pregnancy have not been thoroughly studied in humans. Also, tell your doctor if you are breast-feeding an infant. Small amounts of brompheniramine pass into breast milk and may cause unusual excitement or irritability in nursing infants.

brompheniramine maleate—see brompheniramine

brompheniramine, phenylephrine, and phenylpropanolamine—see phenylpropanolamine, phenylephrine, and brompheniramine combination

Bronchial—see theophylline and guaifenesin combination

bronkodyl—see theophylline

---

bumetanide

BRAND NAME (Manufacturer)
Bumex (Roche)

TYPE OF DRUG
Diuretic and antihypertensive
INGREDIENT
bumetanide
DOSAGE FORM
Tablets (0.5 mg, 1 mg, and 2 mg)
STORAGE
Bumetanide should be stored at room temperature in a tightly closed, light-resistant container.

USES
Bumetanide is prescribed to treat high blood pressure. It is also used to reduce fluid accumulation in the body caused by conditions such as heart failure, cirrhosis of the liver, kidney disease, and the long-term use of some medications. This medication reduces fluid accumulation by increasing the elimination of salt and water through the kidneys.

TREATMENT
To decrease stomach irritation, you can take this medication with a glass of milk or with a meal (unless your doctor directs you to do otherwise). Try to take it at the same time every day. Avoid taking a dose after 6:00 P.M.; otherwise you may have to get up during the night to urinate.

If you miss a dose of this medication, take the missed dose as soon as possible, unless it is almost time for the next one. In that case, do not take the missed dose at all; just wait until the next scheduled dose. Do not double the next dose.

This medication does not cure high blood pressure, but it will help to control the condition as long as you continue to take it.

SIDE EFFECTS
Minor. Blurred vision, constipation, cramps, diarrhea, dizziness, headache, loss of appetite, sore mouth, or stomach upset. As your body adjusts to the medication, these side effects should disappear.

This medication causes an increase in the amount of urine or frequency of urination when you first begin to take it. It may also cause you to have an unusual feeling of tiredness. These effects should lessen after several days.

This medication can cause increased sensitivity to sunlight. It is, therefore, important to avoid prolonged exposure to sunlight and sunlamps. Wear protective clothing, and use an effective sunscreen.

To relieve constipation, increase the amount of fiber in your diet (fresh fruits and vegetables, salads, bran, and whole-grain cereals and breads) and exercise (unless your doctor directs you to do otherwise).

To avoid dizziness or light-headedness when you stand, contract and relax the muscles of your legs for a few moments before rising. Do this by pushing one foot against the floor while raising the other foot slightly, alternating feet so that you are "pumping" your legs in a pedaling motion.

Major. Tell your doctor about any side effects that are persistent or particularly bothersome. IT IS ESPECIALLY IMPORTANT TO TELL YOUR DOCTOR about abdominal pain, confusion, difficulty in breathing, dry mouth, fainting, itching, joint pains, loss of appetite, mood changes, muscle pain and cramps, nausea, palpitations, rash, ringing in the ears, sore throat, thirst, tingling in the fingers and toes, unusual bleeding or bruising, vomiting, weakness, or yellowing of the eyes or skin.

INTERACTIONS
Bumetanide interacts with several other types of drugs:

1. It can increase the side effects of alcohol, barbiturates, narcotics, cephalosporin antibiotics, chloral hydrate, cortisone and cortisone-like steroids (such as dexamethasone, hydrocortisone, prednisone, and prednisolone), digoxin, digitalis, lithium, amphotericin B, cisplatin, mercaptopurine, and polymyxin B.

2. Probenecid and indomethacin may decrease the diuretic effectiveness of this medication.

Before taking bumetanide, BE SURE TO TELL YOUR DOCTOR about any medications you are currently taking, especially any of those listed above.

WARNINGS
- Tell your doctor about unusual or allergic reactions you have had to any medications, especially to bumetanide, other diuretics, or any other sulfa drugs, including oral antidiabetic medicines or sulfonamide antibiotics.
- Before you start taking this medication, tell your doctor if you now have or if you have ever had kidney disease or problems with urination, diabetes mellitus, gout, liver disease, or asthma.
- Bumetanide can cause potassium loss. Signs of potassium loss include dry mouth, thirst, weakness, muscle pain or cramps, nausea, and vomiting. If you experience any of these symptoms, call your doctor. Your doctor may want to have blood tests performed periodically in order to monitor your potassium levels. To help avoid potassium loss, take this medication with a glass of fresh or frozen orange or cranberry juice, or eat a banana every day. The use of a salt substitute also helps prevent potassium loss. Do not change your diet or use a salt substitute, however, before discussing it with your doctor. Too much potassium may also be dangerous.
- Before having surgery or any other medical or dental treatment, be sure to tell your doctor or dentist that you are taking bumetanide.
- In order to avoid dizziness or fainting while taking this medication, try not to stand for long periods of time; avoid drinking excessive amounts of alcohol; and avoid strenuous exercise in hot weather, as well as hot baths, showers, and saunas.
- If you have high blood pressure, do not take any over-the-counter (nonprescription) medication for weight control or for cough, cold, allergy, asthma, or sinus problems, unless you first check with your doctor.
- To prevent severe water loss (dehydration) while taking this medication, check with your doctor if you have any illness that causes severe or continuous nausea, vomiting, or diarrhea.
- This medication can raise blood sugar levels in diabetic patients. Therefore, blood sugar should be monitored carefully with blood or urine tests when this medication is being taken.
- Be sure to tell your doctor if you are pregnant. This drug crosses the placenta. Although studies in humans have not been conducted, adverse effects have been reported in the offspring of animals that were given large doses of this drug during pregnancy. Also, tell your doctor if you are breast-feeding an infant. Although problems in humans have not been reported, small amounts of this drug pass into breast milk.

Bumex—see bumetanide

bupropion

BRAND NAME (Manufacturer)
Wellbutrin (Burroughs Wellcome)
TYPE OF DRUG
Antidepressant
INGREDIENT
bupropion hydrochloride
DOSAGE FORM
Tablets (75 mg and 100 mg)
STORAGE
Store at room temperature in a tightly closed container.

USES

Bupropion is used to relieve the symptoms of mental depression. The exact mechanism of action of bupropion is unknown, but it is thought to relieve depression by altering the concentration of certain chemicals that are necessary for nerve transmission in the brain.

TREATMENT

It is important to take your medication on a regular schedule as recommended by your physician. If you miss a dose and the next regular dose should be taken in less than six hours, skip the missed dose and take the next dose at the regularly scheduled time. Never double the dose.

The effects of this medication may not become apparent for several weeks.

SIDE EFFECTS

Minor. Constipation, decreased appetite, decreased sexual ability, diarrhea, dizziness, dry mouth, excessive sweating, fatigue, headache, irregular heartbeat, insomnia, nausea, sedation, or vomiting. These side effects should decrease or disappear as your body adjusts to the medication.

To relieve constipation, increase the amount of fiber in your diet (fresh fruits and vegetables, salads, bran, and whole-grain breads), exercise, and drink more water (unless your doctor directs you to do otherwise).

To decrease dry mouth, chew sugarless gum or suck on ice chips or hard candy.

To avoid dizziness when you stand, contract and relax the muscles in your legs for a few moments before rising. Do this by pushing one foot against the floor while raising the other foot slightly, alternating feet so that you are "pumping" your legs in a pedaling motion.

Major. Tell your doctor about any side effects that are persistent or particularly bothersome. IT IS ESPECIALLY IMPORTANT TO TELL YOUR DOCTOR about agitation, blurred vision, movement disorders, rash, tremors, or seizures.

INTERACTIONS

1. Bupropion may decrease the effectiveness of carbamazepine, phenobarbital, or phenytoin, which may lead to increased seizures.
2. Bupropion can interact with monoamine oxidase (MAO) inhibitors. At least 14 days should separate the use of this drug and the use of an MAO inhibitor.
3. Bupropion may decrease the effectiveness of cimetidine.
4. Alcohol may increase the side effects of bupropion.

WARNINGS

- Tell your doctor about unusual or allergic reactions you have had to any medications, especially to bupropion.
- Tell your doctor if you now have or have ever had cataracts or vision problems, seizures or epilepsy, bulimia, anorexia nervosa, mania, or respiratory disorders.
- This medication may make you tired or drowsy or affect your thinking ability. You should not operate potentially dangerous equipment or drive an automobile until you know how this drug affects you.
- Do not stop taking this medication abruptly or increase the dose unless directed by your physician. Stopping abruptly or increasing your dose in large amounts can lead to increased side effects.
- Do not take any over-the-counter medication or new prescription drug without discussing it with your doctor or pharmacist. Many over-the-counter preparations and some prescription medications may interact with bupropion.
- Tell your doctor if you are pregnant. In high doses, bupropion has caused chromosomal changes in animals, but the effects in humans are unknown. Also, tell your doctor if you are breast-feeding an infant. This medication can pass into the breast milk and potentially lead to adverse effects in the infant.

BuSpar—see buspirone

buspirone

BRAND NAME (Manufacturer)
BuSpar (Bristol-Myers)
TYPE OF DRUG
Antianxiety agent
INGREDIENT
buspirone hydrochloride
DOSAGE FORM
Tablets (5 mg and 10 mg)
STORAGE
Buspirone should be stored at room temperature in a tightly closed container. Avoid exposure to high temperatures (greater than 86°F).

USES

Buspirone is prescribed to treat the symptoms of anxiety. It is not yet clear exactly how this medication works. Buspirone has been shown to be effective in relieving symptoms of anxiety, but it is important to try to remove the cause of the anxiety as well.

TREATMENT

Buspirone should be taken exactly as directed by your doctor. It can be taken with food or a full glass of water if stomach upset occurs.

If you are taking this drug regularly and miss a dose, take the missed dose immediately if you remember within an hour. If more time has passed, however, skip the dose you missed and wait for the next scheduled dose. Do not double the dose.

SIDE EFFECTS

Minor. Diarrhea, dizziness, excitement, fatigue, headache, light-headedness, nasal congestion, nausea, nervousness, sleeping problems, sweating, or weakness. These side effects should disappear as your body adjusts to this medication.

If you feel dizzy or light-headed, sit or lie down for a while; get up slowly from a sitting or reclining position, and be careful on stairs.

Major. Tell your doctor about any side effects that are persistent or particularly bothersome. IT IS ESPECIALLY IMPORTANT TO TELL YOUR DOCTOR about chest pain, confusion, feelings of anger, incoordination, muscle pain, numbness, rash, ringing in the ears, sore throat, tingling in your fingers or toes, or tremors.

INTERACTIONS

Although extensive studies have not yet been completed, buspirone may interact with several other medications.

To prevent oversedation, this drug should not be taken with alcohol or other central nervous system depressants (such as antihistamines, barbiturates, muscle relaxants, pain medicines, narcotics, medicines for seizures, phenothiazine tranquilizers, and antidepressants).

Before starting buspirone, BE SURE TO TELL YOUR DOCTOR about any medications you are currently taking, especially any of those listed above.

WARNINGS

- Before starting buspirone, be sure to tell your doctor about any unusual or allergic reactions you have had to any medications, especially to buspirone.
- Tell your doctor if you now have or if you have ever had kidney disease, liver disease, or psychiatric disorders.
- Until you experience how this medication affects you, do not drive a car or operate potentially dangerous machinery.
- Be sure to tell your doctor if you are pregnant. Although buspirone appears to be safe in animals, studies in pregnant women have not been conducted. Also, tell your doctor if you are breast-feeding an infant. Small amounts of buspirone have been shown to pass into the milk of animals.

---

busulfan

BRAND NAME (Manufacturer)
Myleran (Burroughs Wellcome)

TYPE OF DRUG
Antineoplastic (anticancer drug)

INGREDIENT
busulfan

DOSAGE FORM
Tablets (2 mg)

STORAGE
Busulfan should be stored at room temperature in a tightly closed container.

USES

Busulfan belongs to a group of drugs known as alkylating agents. It is used to treat leukemia. This medication works by binding to the rapidly growing cancer cells, preventing their multiplication and growth.

TREATMENT

Busulfan can be taken either on an empty stomach or with food or milk (as directed by your doctor).

The timing of the doses of this medication is important. Be sure you completely understand your doctor's instructions on how this medication should be taken.

If you miss a dose of this medication, do not take the missed dose at all; just return to your regular dosing schedule. Do not double the next dose.

SIDE EFFECTS

Minor. Diarrhea, dizziness, nausea, stomach upset, or vomiting. These side effects may disappear as your body adjusts to the medication. However, it is important to continue taking this medication despite any nausea or vomiting that may occur. Busulfan also causes hair loss, which is reversible when the medication is stopped.

If you feel dizzy, sit or lie down for a while; get up from a sitting or lying position slowly, and be careful on stairs.

Major. Be sure to tell your doctor about any side effects that are persistent or particularly bothersome. IT IS ESPECIALLY IMPORTANT TO TELL YOUR DOCTOR about blurred vision, breast enlargement (in both sexes), chills, confusion, cough, darkening of the skin, difficulty in breathing, dry skin, fatigue, fever, itching, joint pain, loss of appetite, menstrual irregularities, mouth sores, muscle weakness, skin rash, sore throat, unusual bleeding or bruising, weight loss, or yellowing of the eyes or skin.

INTERACTIONS

Busulfan can increase the blood levels of uric acid, which can block the effectiveness of antigout medications (allopurinol, probenecid, sulfinpyrazone).

Before starting to take busulfan, BE SURE TO TELL YOUR DOCTOR about any medications you are currently taking, especially any antigout medication.

WARNINGS

- Tell your doctor about unusual or allergic reactions you have had to any medications, especially to busulfan.
- Before starting to take this medication, be sure to tell your doctor if you now have or if you have ever had blood disorders, chronic or recurrent infections, gout, or kidney stones.
- You should not receive any immunizations or vaccinations while taking this medication. Busulfan blocks the effectiveness of the vaccine and may result in infection.
- It is important to drink plenty of fluids (up to two or three quarts each day) while taking this medication, in order to prevent uric acid kidney stones from developing.
- Busulfan can lower your platelet count, thereby decreasing your body's ability to form blood clots. You should, therefore, be especially careful while brushing your teeth, flossing, or using toothpicks, razors, or fingernail scissors. Try to avoid falls and other injuries.
- Before having surgery or other medical or dental treatment, tell your doctor or dentist you are taking this drug.
- Busulfan can decrease fertility in both men and women.
- Be sure to tell your doctor if you are pregnant. Birth defects have been reported in both animals and humans whose mothers received busulfan during pregnancy. The risks should be discussed with your doctor. Also, tell your doctor if you are breast-feeding an infant. It is not known whether busulfan passes into breast milk.

butalbital with aspirin and caffeine—see aspirin, caffeine, and butalbital combination

Butazolidin—see phenylbutazone

Byclomine—see dicyclomine

Bydramine Cough Syrup—see diphenhydramine

Cafergot—see ergotamine and caffeine combination

Cafetrate—see ergotamine and caffeine combination

Caladryl Hydrocortisone—see hydrocortisone (topical)

Calan—see verapamil

Calan SR—see verapamil

---

calcifediol

BRAND NAME (Manufacturer)
Calderol (Organon)
TYPE OF DRUG
Vitamin D analog
INGREDIENT
calcifediol (25-hydroxycholecalciferol)
DOSAGE FORM
Capsules (20 mcg and 50 mcg)
STORAGE
Calcifediol capsules should be stored at room temperature in a tightly closed, light-resistant container.

USES

Vitamin D is essential to many body systems, including bone structure, regulation of blood calcium levels, and heart and muscle contraction. Since vitamin D is activated in the kidneys, patients with chronic (long-term) kidney failure are unable to produce enough active vitamin D on their own. Calcifediol is one of the active forms of vitamin D. This medication is used to treat bone disease and hypocalcemia (low blood calcium levels) in patients on dialysis.

TREATMENT

Calcifediol can be taken either on an empty stomach or with food or milk (as directed by your doctor).

If you miss a dose of this medication, take the missed dose as soon as possible, unless it is almost time for the next dose. In that case, do not take the missed dose at all; just return to your regular dosing schedule. Do not double the next dose.

SIDE EFFECTS

Minor. None, at the dosages normally prescribed.
Major. The side effects associated with calcifediol therapy are usually the result of too much medication (vitamin D toxicity). Tell your doctor about any side effects that are persistent or particularly bothersome. IT IS ESPECIALLY IMPORTANT TO TELL YOUR DOCTOR about blurred vision, bone pain, constipation, dry mouth, headache, irritability, loss of appetite, mental disorders, metallic taste in the mouth, muscle pain, nausea, palpitations, runny nose, increased thirst, increased urination, vomiting, weakness, or weight loss.

INTERACTIONS

Calcifediol interacts with several types of medications:
1. The dosage of calcifediol may need to be altered if anticonvulsant medication (such as phenytoin, phenobarbital, and primidone) is started.
2. Cholestyramine, colestipol, and mineral oil can decrease the absorption of calcifediol from the gastrointestinal tract.

BE SURE TO TELL YOUR DOCTOR about any medications you are currently taking, especially any of those listed above.

WARNINGS

- Tell your doctor about unusual or allergic reactions you have had to any medications, especially to calcifediol, calcitriol, dihydrotachysterol, ergocalciferol, or vitamin D.
- Before starting to take this medication, be sure to tell your doctor if you now have or if you have ever had heart or blood vessel disease, hypercalcemia (high levels of calcium in the bloodstream), hyperphosphatemia (high levels of phosphate in the bloodstream), vitamin D intoxication, or sarcoidosis.
- Before taking over-the-counter products that contain calcium, phosphates, magnesium, or vitamin D, consult your doctor. These ingredients can increase the side effects of calcifediol.
- Be sure to tell your doctor if you are pregnant. Although calcifediol (in normal doses) appears to be safe during pregnancy, extensive studies in humans have not been conducted. Birth defects have been reported in the offspring of animals that received large doses of this medication during pregnancy. Also, tell your doctor if you are breast-feeding an infant. Small amounts of calcifediol pass into breast milk.

Calciferol—see ergocalciferol (vitamin D)

---

calcitriol

BRAND NAME (Manufacturer)
Rocaltrol (Roche)
TYPE OF DRUG
Vitamin D analog
INGREDIENT
calcitriol (1,25-dihydroxycholecalciferol)
DOSAGE FORM
Capsules (0.25 mcg and 0.5 mcg)
STORAGE
Calcitriol should be stored at room temperature in a tightly closed, light-resistant container.

USES

Vitamin D is essential to bone structure, regulation of blood calcium levels, and heart and muscle contraction. Since vitamin D is activated in the kidneys, patients with chronic kidney failure are unable to produce enough active vitamin D on their own. Calcitriol is one of the active forms of vitamin D. This drug is used to treat bone disease and hypocalcemia (low blood calcium levels) in dialysis patients.

TREATMENT

Calcitriol can be taken either on an empty stomach or with food or milk (as directed by your doctor).

If you miss a dose of this medication, take the missed dose as soon as possible, unless it is almost time for the next dose. In that case, do not take the missed dose at all; just return to your regular dosing schedule. Do not double the next dose.

SIDE EFFECTS

Minor. None, at the dosages normally prescribed.

Major. Side effects result from too much medication (vitamin D toxicity). Tell your doctor about any side effects that are persistent or particularly bothersome. IT IS ESPECIALLY IMPORTANT TO TELL YOUR DOCTOR about appetite loss, blurred vision, bone pain, constipation, dry mouth, headache, irritability, mental disorders, metallic taste, muscle pain, nausea, palpitations, runny nose, increased thirst, increased urination, vomiting, weakness, or weight loss.

INTERACTIONS

Calcitriol interacts with several types of medications:

1. The dosage of calcitriol may need to be adjusted if anticonvulsant medication (phenytoin, phenobarbital, or primidone) is started.

2. Cholestyramine, colestipol, and mineral oil can decrease the absorption of calcitriol from the gastrointestinal tract.

BE SURE TO TELL YOUR DOCTOR about any medications you are currently taking, especially any of those listed above.

WARNINGS

- Tell your doctor about unusual or allergic reactions you have had to any medications, especially to calcitriol, calcifediol, dihydrotachysterol, ergocalciferol, or vitamin D.
- Before starting to take this drug, tell your doctor if you have ever had heart or blood vessel disease, hypercalcemia (high levels of blood calcium), hyperphosphatemia (high levels of blood phosphate), vitamin D intoxication, or sarcoidosis.
- Before taking any over-the-counter (nonprescription) products that contain calcium, phosphates, magnesium, or vitamin D, check with your doctor. These ingredients can increase the side effects of calcitriol.
- Be sure to tell your doctor if you are pregnant. Although calcitriol appears to be safe during pregnancy in humans, birth defects have been reported in the offspring of animals that received large doses during pregnancy. Also, tell your doctor if you are breast-feeding an infant. Small amounts of calcitriol pass into breast milk.

CaldeCort Anti-Itch—see hydrocortisone (topical)

CaldeCort Light with Aloe—see hydrocortisone (topical)

Calderol—see calcifediol

Cam-ap-es—see hydralazine, hydrochlorothiazide, and reserpine combination

Capital with Codeine—see acetaminophen and codeine combination

Capoten—see captopril

Capozide—see captopril and hydrochlorothiazide

---

captopril

BRAND NAME (Manufacturer)
Capoten (Squibb)

TYPE OF DRUG
Antihypertensive

INGREDIENT
captopril

DOSAGE FORM
Tablets (12.5 mg, 25 mg, 50 mg, and 100 mg)

STORAGE
Captopril should be stored at room temperature in a tightly closed container.

USES

Captopril is used to treat high blood pressure and congestive heart failure. It is a vasodilator (it dilates the blood vessels) that acts by blocking the production of chemicals that may be responsible for constricting or narrowing blood vessels.

TREATMENT

To obtain maximum benefit from captopril, you should take it on an empty stomach one hour before meals. In order to become accustomed to taking this medication, try to take it at the same time(s) every day.

It may be several weeks before you notice the full effects of this medication.

If you miss a dose of this medication, take the missed dose as soon as possible, unless it is almost time for the next dose. In that case, do not take the missed dose at all; just wait until the next scheduled dose. Do not double the dose.

Captopril does not cure high blood pressure, but it will help to control the condition as long as you continue to take it.

SIDE EFFECTS

Minor. Abdominal pain, constipation, diarrhea, dizziness, dry mouth, fatigue, flushing, headache, insomnia, loss of taste, loss of appetite, nausea, or vomiting. These side effects should disappear as your body adjusts to the medication.

This medication can increase your sensitivity to sunlight. It is, therefore, important to avoid prolonged exposure to sunlight and sunlamps. Wear protective clothing and sunglasses, and use an effective sunscreen.

To relieve constipation, increase the amount of fiber in your diet (fresh fruits and vegetables, salads, bran, and whole-grain breads), exercise, and drink more water (unless your doctor directs you to do otherwise).

To relieve mouth dryness, suck on ice chips or a piece of hard candy or chew sugarless gum.

To avoid dizziness or light-headedness when you stand, contract and relax the muscles of your legs for a few moments before rising. Do this by pushing one foot against the floor while raising the other foot slightly, alternating feet so that you are "pumping" your legs in a pedaling motion.

Major. Tell your doctor about any side effects that are per-

sistent or particularly bothersome. IT IS ESPECIALLY IMPORTANT TO TELL YOUR DOCTOR about chest pain; chills; difficult or painful urination; fever; itching; mouth sores; palpitations; prolonged vomiting or diarrhea; rash; sore throat; swelling of the face, hands, or feet; tingling in the fingers or toes; unusual bleeding or bruising; or yellowing of the eyes or skin.

INTERACTIONS

Captopril interacts with several other types of medications:

1. Diuretics (water pills) and other antihypertensive medications can cause an excessive drop in blood pressure when combined with captopril (especially with the first dose).

2. The combination of captopril with spironolactone, triamterene, amiloride, potassium supplements, or salt substitutes can lead to hyperkalemia (dangerously high levels of potassium in the bloodstream).

3. Antineoplastic agents (anticancer drugs) or chloramphenicol can increase the bone marrow side effects of captopril.

4. Concurrent use of captopril and allopurinol can increase the risk of developing an allergic reaction.

5. Indomethacin can decrease the blood-pressure-lowering effects of captopril.

Before starting captopril, TELL YOUR DOCTOR about any drugs you are taking, especially any of those listed above.

WARNINGS

- Tell your doctor about any reactions you have had to medications, especially to captopril or enalapril.
- Tell your doctor if you now have or if you have ever had aortic stenosis, blood disorders, kidney disease, systemic lupus erythematosus, or a heart attack or stroke.
- Be careful—excessive perspiration, dehydration, or prolonged vomiting or diarrhea can lead to an excessive drop in blood pressure while you are taking this medication. Contact your doctor if you have any of these symptoms.
- Before having surgery or other medical or dental treatment, tell your doctor you are taking this drug.
- If you have high blood pressure, do not take any over-the-counter (nonprescription) medication for weight control, or for allergy, asthma, sinus, cough, or cold problems unless you first check with your doctor.
- Do not stop taking this medication unless you first consult your doctor. Stopping this drug abruptly may lead to a rise in blood pressure.
- Be sure to tell your doctor if you are pregnant. Although this drug appears to be safe in animals, extensive studies in humans during pregnancy have not been conducted. Also, tell your doctor if you are breast-feeding an infant. Small amounts of captopril pass into breast milk.

---

captopril and hydrochlorothiazide combination

BRAND NAME (Manufacturer)
Capozide (Squibb)

TYPE OF DRUG
Antihypertensive and diuretic

INGREDIENTS
captopril and hydrochlorothiazide

DOSAGE FORM
Tablets (25 mg captopril and 15 mg hydrochlorothiazide; 25 mg captopril and 25 mg hydrochlorothiazide; 50 mg captopril and 15 mg hydrochlorothiazide; 50 mg captopril and 25 mg hydrochlorothiazide)

STORAGE
Captopril and hydrochlorothiazide combination tablets should be stored at room temperature in a tightly closed container. This medication should be stored away from moisture and high heat (above 86°F).

USES

Captopril and hydrochlorothiazide combination is used to treat high blood pressure. Captopril is a vasodilator (it widens the blood vessels) that acts by blocking the production of chemicals that may be responsible for constricting blood vessels. Hydrochlorothiazide is a diuretic (water pill), which reduces body fluid accumulation by increasing the elimination of salt and water through the kidneys.

TREATMENT

To obtain the maximum benefit from this medication, take it on an empty stomach one hour before meals. In order to become accustomed to taking this medication, try to take it at the same time(s) every day.

Avoid taking a dose of this medication after 6:00 P.M.; otherwise, you may have to get up during the night to urinate.

It may be several weeks before you notice the full effects of this medication.

If you miss a dose of this medication, take the missed dose as soon as possible, unless it is almost time for the next dose. In that case, do not take the missed dose at all; just wait until the next scheduled dose. Do not double the dose.

Captopril and hydrochlorothiazide combination does not cure high blood pressure, but it will help to control the condition as long as you continue to take it.

SIDE EFFECTS

Minor. Abdominal pain, blurred vision, constipation, cramping, diarrhea, dizziness, fatigue, flushing, headache, insomnia, loss of appetite, or loss of taste. These side effects should disappear as your body adjusts to this medication.

Hydrochlorothiazide can increase your sensitivity to sunlight. It is, therefore, important to avoid prolonged exposure to sunlight and sunlamps. Wear protective clothing and sunglasses, and use an effective sunscreen.

To relieve constipation, increase the amount of fiber in your diet (fresh fruits and vegetables, salads, bran, and whole-grain breads) and exercise (unless your doctor directs you to do otherwise).

To relieve mouth dryness, suck on ice chips or hard candy or chew sugarless gum.

To avoid dizziness or light-headedness when you stand, contract and relax the muscles of your legs for a few moments before rising. Do this by alternately pushing one foot against the floor while raising the other foot slightly, so that you are "pumping" your legs in a pedaling motion.

Major. Tell your doctor about any side effects that are per-

sistent or particularly bothersome. IT IS ESPECIALLY IMPORTANT TO TELL YOUR DOCTOR about chest pain; chills; cough; difficult or painful urination; dry mouth; fever; hair loss; itching; mouth sores; muscle pain or cramps; nausea; palpitations; rash; shortness of breath; sore throat; swelling of the face, hands, or feet; thirst; tingling in the fingers or toes; unusual bleeding or bruising; vomiting; weakness; or yellowing of the eyes or skin.

INTERACTIONS

Captopril and hydrochlorothiazide combination can interact with several other types of medications:

1. The combination of captopril with spironolactone, triamterene, amiloride, potassium supplements, or salt substitutes can lead to hyperkalemia (dangerously high levels of potassium in the bloodstream).
2. Antineoplastic agents (anticancer drugs) and chloramphenicol can increase the bone marrow side effects of captopril.
3. Concurrent use of captopril and allopurinol can increase the risk of developing an allergic reaction.
4. Diuretics (water pills) and other antihypertensive medications can cause an excessive drop in blood pressure when combined with captopril (especially with the first dose).
5. Hydrochlorothiazide can decrease the effectiveness of oral anticoagulants, antigout medications, insulin, oral antidiabetic medicines, and methenamine.
6. Fenfluramine can increase the blood-pressure-lowering effects of hydrochlorothiazide (which can be dangerous).
7. Indomethacin can decrease the blood-pressure-lowering effects of captopril and hydrochlorothiazide, thereby counteracting the desired effects.
8. Cholestyramine and colestipol decrease the absorption of hydrochlorothiazide from the gastrointestinal tract. Hydrochlorothiazide should, therefore, be taken one hour before or four hours after a dose of cholestyramine or colestipol (if you have also been prescribed one of these drugs).
9. Hydrochlorothiazide may increase the side effects of amphotericin B, calcium supplements, cortisone and cortisone-like steroids (such as dexamethasone, hydrocortisone, prednisone, and prednisolone), digoxin, digitalis, lithium, quinidine, sulfonamide antibiotics, and vitamin D.

Before starting captopril and hydrochlorothiazide combination, BE SURE TO TELL YOUR DOCTOR about any medications you are currently taking, especially any listed above.

WARNINGS

• Tell your doctor about unusual or allergic reactions you have had to any medications, especially to captopril or to hydrochlorothiazide or other diuretics (such as bendroflumethiazide, benzthiazide, chlorothiazide, chlorthalidone, cyclothiazide, hydroflumethiazide, methyclothiazide, metolozone, polythiazide, quinethazone, trichlormethiazide, and furosemide) or to sulfa medications (oral antidiabetic medications or sulfonamide antibiotics).

• Tell your doctor if you have ever had aortic stenosis, blood disorders, diabetes mellitus, gout, kidney disease or problems with urination, liver disease, pancreatic disease, a heart attack, or systemic lupus erythematosus.

• Hydrochlorothiazide can cause potassium loss. Signs of potassium loss include dry mouth, thirst, weakness, muscle pain or cramps, nausea, and vomiting. If you experience any of these symptoms, call your doctor. To help prevent this problem, your doctor may have blood tests performed periodically to monitor your potassium levels. To help avoid potassium loss, take this medication with a glass of fresh or frozen orange juice or cranberry juice, or eat a banana every day. The use of a salt substitute also helps to prevent potassium loss. Do not change your diet or use a salt substitute, however, until you discuss it with your doctor. Too much potassium may also be dangerous.

• Limit your intake of alcoholic beverages while taking this medication, in order to prevent dizziness and lightheadedness.

• If you have high blood pressure, do not take any over-the-counter (nonprescription) medications for weight control or for allergy, asthma, cough, cold, or sinus problems, unless your doctor directs you to do so.

• To prevent dehydration (severe water loss) while taking this medication, check with your doctor if you have any illness that causes severe or continuous diarrhea, nausea, or vomiting.

• This medication can raise blood sugar levels in diabetic patients. Therefore, sugar levels should be carefully monitored with blood or urine tests when this medication is started.

• Before having surgery or any other medical or dental treatment, be sure to tell your doctor or dentist that you are taking this medication.

• This drug may cause dizziness. Use caution while driving or operating potentially dangerous machinery.

• A "fixed-dose" drug like this is not generally the first choice in the treatment of high blood pressure. Usually, the patient first receives each ingredient singly. If there is an adequate response to the fixed dose contained in this product, it can then be substituted. The advantage of a combination product is increased convenience and (often) decreased cost.

• Do not stop taking this medication unless you first consult your doctor. Stopping this drug abruptly may lead to a rise in blood pressure.

• Be sure to tell your doctor if you are pregnant. Although this drug combination appears to be safe in animals, studies in pregnant women have not been conducted. Hydrochlorothiazide can cause adverse effects in the newborn infant if it is given to the mother close to term. Also, tell your doctor if you are breast-feeding an infant. Although problems in humans have not been reported, small amounts of this drug can pass into breast milk, so caution is warranted.

Caquin—see hydrocortisone and iodochlorhydroxyquin combination (topical)

Carafate—see sucralfate

---

carbamazepine

BRAND NAMES (Manufacturers)

carbamazepine (various manufacturers)
Epitol (Lemmon)
Tegretol (Geigy)
Tegretol Chewable (Geigy)

TYPE OF DRUG
Anticonvulsant
INGREDIENT
carbamazepine
DOSAGE FORMS
Tablets (200 mg)
Chewable tablets (100 mg)
Oral suspension (100 mg per 5-ml spoonful)
STORAGE
Carbamazepine tablets and oral suspension should be stored at room temperature in tightly closed containers.

USES

This medication is used for the treatment of seizure disorders and for relief of neuralgia (nerve pain). The mechanism of carbamazepine's antiseizure activity is unknown, but it is not related to other anticonvulsants. Carbamazepine is not an ordinary pain reliever—it should not be used for minor aches or pains.

TREATMENT

Carbamazepine works best when the level of medicine in your bloodstream is kept constant. It is best, therefore, to take it at evenly spaced intervals day and night. For example, if you are to take four doses a day, the doses should be spaced six hours apart.

Try not to miss any doses of this medication. If you do miss a dose, take the missed dose as soon as possible, unless it is almost time for the next dose. In that case, do not take the missed dose at all; just return to your regular dosing schedule. Do not double the next dose unless your doctor directs you to do so. If you are taking carbamazepine for a seizure disorder and you miss two or more doses, be sure to contact your doctor.

SIDE EFFECTS

Minor. Agitation; blurred vision; confusion; constipation; diarrhea; dizziness; drowsiness; dry mouth; headache; loss of appetite; muscle or joint pain; nausea; restlessness; sweating; vomiting; or weakness. These side effects should disappear as your body adjusts to the medication.

This medication can increase your sensitivity to sunlight. It is, therefore, important to avoid prolonged exposure to sunlight and sunlamps. Wear protective clothing and sunglasses, and use an effective sunscreen.

To relieve constipation, increase the amount of fiber in your diet (fresh fruits and vegetables, salads, bran, and whole-grain breads), exercise, and drink more water (unless your doctor directs you to do otherwise).

To relieve mouth dryness, suck on ice chips or a piece of hard candy or chew sugarless gum.

If you feel dizzy or light-headed, sit or lie down for a while; get up slowly from a sitting or reclining position, and be careful on stairs.

Major. Be sure to tell your doctor about any side effects that are persistent or particularly bothersome. IT IS ESPECIALLY IMPORTANT FOR YOU TO TELL YOUR DOCTOR about abdominal pain, chills, depression, difficulty in breathing, difficulty in urinating, eye discomfort, fainting, fever, hair loss, hallucinations, impotence, loss of balance, mouth sores, nightmares, numbness or tingling sensations, palpitations, ringing in the ears, skin rash, sore throat, swelling of the hands and feet, twitching, unusual bleeding or bruising, or yellowing of the eyes or skin.

INTERACTIONS

Carbamazepine interacts with other types of medications:

1. Concurrent use of it with central nervous system depressants (such as alcohol, antihistamines, barbiturates, benzodiazepine tranquilizers, muscle relaxants, narcotics, pain medications, and phenothiazine tranquilizers) or with tricyclic antidepressants can cause extreme drowsiness.

2. Phenobarbital, phenytoin, and primidone can decrease blood levels and effectiveness of carbamazepine.

3. Isoniazid, propoxyphene, verapamil, cimetidine, troleandomycin, and erythromycin can increase the blood levels of carbamazepine, which can lead to increased side effects.

4. The combination of lithium and carbamazepine can lead to central nervous system side effects.

5. Carbamazepine can decrease the effectiveness of phenytoin, oral anticoagulants (blood thinners, such as warfarin), doxycycline, oral contraceptives (birth control pills), ethosuximide, valproic acid, aminophylline, and theophylline.

6. The use of carbamazepine within 14 days of the use of a monoamine oxidase (MAO) inhibitor can lead to serious side effects.

Before you start to take carbamazepine, BE SURE TO TELL YOUR DOCTOR about any medications you are currently taking, especially any of those listed above.

WARNINGS

- Tell your doctor about unusual or allergic reactions you have had to any medications, especially to carbamazepine or to tricyclic antidepressants (such as amitriptyline, desipramine, doxepin, imipramine, protriptyline, or nortriptyline).
- Tell your doctor if you now have or if you have ever had bone marrow depression, blood disorders, glaucoma, heart disease, kidney disease, or liver disease.
- Before having surgery or any other medical or dental treatment, be sure to tell your doctor or dentist that you are taking this medication.
- If this medication makes you dizzy or drowsy, do not take part in any activity that requires alertness, such as driving a car or operating potentially dangerous equipment.
- If you are taking this medication to control a seizure disorder, do not stop taking it suddenly. If you stop abruptly, you may experience uncontrollable seizures.
- Be sure to tell your doctor if you are pregnant. Birth defects have been reported more often in infants whose mothers have seizure disorders. It is unclear if the increased risk of birth defects is associated with the disorder or with the anticonvulsant medications, such as carbamazepine, that are used to treat the condition. The risks and benefits of treatment should be discussed with your doctor. Also, tell your doctor if you are breast-feeding an infant. Small amounts of carbamazepine pass into breast milk.

---

carbenicillin

BRAND NAME (Manufacturer)
Geocillin (Roerig)

TYPE OF DRUG
Antibiotic
INGREDIENT
carbenicillin indanyl sodium
DOSAGE FORM
Tablets (382 mg)
STORAGE
Store at room temperature in a tightly closed container.

USES

Carbenicillin is used to treat infections of the urinary tract and the prostate gland. It acts by severely injuring the cell walls of the infecting bacteria, thereby preventing them from growing and multiplying. Carbenicillin kills susceptible bacteria but is not effective against viruses, parasites, or fungi.

TREATMENT

Carbenicillin should be taken on an empty stomach or with a glass of water one hour before or two hours after a meal.

Carbenicillin works best when the level of medicine in your bloodstream is kept constant. It is best, therefore, to take the doses at evenly spaced intervals day and night. For example, if you are taking four doses a day, the doses should be spaced six hours apart.

If you miss a dose of this medication, take the missed dose immediately. However, if you do not remember to take the missed dose until it is almost time for your next dose, take it; space the following dose about halfway through the regular interval between doses; and then return to your regular schedule. Try not to skip any doses.

It is important to continue to take this medication for the entire time prescribed by your doctor (usually seven to 14 days), even if the symptoms of the infection disappear before the end of that period. If you stop taking the drug too soon, resistant bacteria are given the chance to continue growing, and the infection could recur.

SIDE EFFECTS

Minor. Diarrhea, heartburn, nausea, or vomiting. These side effects should disappear as your body adjusts to the medication.
Major. Tell your doctor about any side effects that are persistent or particularly bothersome. IT IS ESPECIALLY IMPORTANT TO TELL YOUR DOCTOR about bloating, chills, cough, darkened tongue, difficulty in breathing, fever, irritation of the mouth, muscle aches, rash, rectal or vaginal itching, severe diarrhea, or sore throat. Also, if your symptoms of infection seem to be getting worse rather than improving, you should contact your doctor.

INTERACTIONS

Carbenicillin interacts with other types of medications:
1. Probenecid can increase the blood concentrations and side effects of this medication.
2. Carbenicillin may decrease the effectiveness of oral contraceptives (birth control pills), and pregnancy could result. You should, therefore, use a different or additional form of birth control while taking this medication. Discuss this with your doctor.

BE SURE TO TELL YOUR DOCTOR about any medications you are currently taking, especially any listed above.

WARNINGS

- Tell your doctor about unusual or allergic reactions you have had to any drugs, especially to carbenicillin or penicillins or to cephalosporin antibiotics, penicillamine, or griseofulvin.
- Tell your doctor if you now have or if you have ever had kidney disease, asthma, or allergies.
- This medication has been prescribed for your current infection only. Another infection later on, or one that someone else has, may require a different medicine. You should not give your medicine to other people, or use it for other infections, unless your doctor specifically directs you to do so.
- Diabetics taking carbenicillin should know that this drug can cause a false-positive sugar reaction with a Clinitest urine glucose test. To avoid this problem, while taking carbenicillin you should switch to Clinistix or Tes-Tape to test your urine for sugar.
- Be sure to tell your doctor if you are pregnant. Although carbenicillin appears to be safe during pregnancy, extensive studies in humans have not been conducted. Also, tell your doctor if you are breast-feeding an infant. Small amounts of this medication pass into breast milk and may temporarily alter the bacterial balance in the intestinal tract of the nursing infant, resulting in diarrhea.

Carbodec—see pseudoephedrine and carbinoxamine combination

Carbodec DM—see pseudoephedrine, carbinoxamine, and dextromethorphan combination

Cardec DM—see pseudoephedrine, carbinoxamine, and dextromethorphan combination

Cardec-S—see pseudoephedrine and carbinoxamine combination

Cardioquin—see quinidine

Cardizem—see diltiazem

Cardizem SR—see diltiazem

---

carisoprodol

BRAND NAMES (Manufacturers)
carisoprodol (various manufacturers)
Rela (Schering)
Soma (Wallace)
Soprodol (Schein)
TYPE OF DRUG
Muscle relaxant
INGREDIENT
carisoprodol
DOSAGE FORM
Tablets (350 mg)
STORAGE
Carisoprodol should be stored at room temperature in a tightly closed container.

USES

This medication is used to relieve painful muscle conditions. It should be used in conjunction with rest, physical therapy, and other measures to alleviate discomfort. It is not clear exactly how carisoprodol works, but it is thought to act as a central nervous system depressant. It does not act directly on muscles.

TREATMENT

In order to avoid stomach irritation, you can take carisoprodol with food or with a full glass of water or milk (unless your doctor directs you to do otherwise).

If you miss a dose of this medication and remember within an hour, take the missed dose immediately. If more than an hour has passed, do not take the missed dose at all; just return to your regular dosing schedule. Do not double the next dose of this drug.

SIDE EFFECTS

Minor. Dizziness, drowsiness, headache, hiccups, insomnia, nausea, stomach pain, or vomiting. These side effects should disappear as your body adjusts to the medication.

If you feel dizzy, sit or lie down for a while; get up slowly from a sitting or reclining position, and be careful on stairs.

Major. Tell your doctor about any side effects that are persistent or particularly bothersome. IT IS ESPECIALLY IMPORTANT TO TELL YOUR DOCTOR about agitation, depression, fainting, irritability, loss of coordination, palpitations, or tremors.

INTERACTIONS

Carisoprodol interacts with several other types of medications: Concurrent use of it with other central nervous system depressants (such as alcohol, antihistamines, barbiturates, benzodiazepine tranquilizers, muscle relaxants, narcotics, pain medications, phenothiazine tranquilizers, and sleeping medications) or with tricyclic antidepressants can lead to extreme drowsiness.

BE SURE TO TELL YOUR DOCTOR about any medications you are currently taking, especially any of those listed above.

WARNINGS

- Tell your doctor about unusual or allergic reactions you have had to any medications, especially to carisoprodol, meprobamate, or tybamate.
- Before starting to take carisoprodol, tell your doctor if you now have or if you have ever had kidney disease, liver disease, or porphyria.
- If this drug makes you dizzy or drowsy, avoid taking part in any activity that requires alertness, such as driving a car or operating potentially dangerous equipment.
- Some of these products contain the color additive FD&C Yellow No. 5 (tartrazine), which can cause allergic-type reactions (rash, fainting, shortness of breath) in certain susceptible individuals.
- Carisoprodol has the potential for abuse and should be used with caution. Do not increase the dosage or stop taking the drug unless you first consult your doctor. If you have been taking carisoprodol for several months and you stop taking it abruptly, you could experience a withdrawal reaction. Your doctor may, therefore, want to decrease your dosage of the medication gradually.
- Be sure to tell your doctor if you are pregnant. Although carisoprodol appears to be safe during pregnancy, extensive studies have not been conducted in humans. Also, tell your doctor if you are breast-feeding an infant. This medication passes into breast milk and can cause excessive drowsiness and stomach upset in nursing infants.

Catapres—see clonidine

Catapres-TTS—see clonidine

Ceclor—see cefaclor

CeeNU—see lomustine

---

cefaclor

BRAND NAME (Manufacturer)
Ceclor (Lilly)
TYPE OF DRUG
Cephalosporin antibiotic
INGREDIENT
cefaclor
DOSAGE FORMS
Capsules (250 mg and 500 mg)
Oral suspension (125 mg, 187 mg, 250 mg, and 775 mg per 5-ml spoonful)
STORAGE
Cefaclor capsules should be stored at room temperature in a tightly closed container. The oral suspension form of this drug should be stored in the refrigerator in a tightly closed container. Any unused portion of the oral suspension should be discarded after 14 days because the drug loses its potency after that time. This medication should never be frozen.

USES

This medication is used to treat a wide variety of bacterial infections, including those of the middle ear, upper and lower respiratory tract, and urinary tract. This drug acts by severely injuring the cell walls of the infecting bacteria, thereby preventing them from growing and multiplying. Cefaclor kills susceptible bacteria, but it is not effective against viruses, parasites, or fungi.

TREATMENT

Cefaclor can be taken either on an empty stomach or with food or milk (in order to avoid an upset stomach).

The contents of the suspension form of cefaclor tend to settle on the bottom of the bottle, so it is necessary to shake the container well to distribute the ingredients evenly and equalize the doses. Each dose should then be measured carefully with a specially designed 5-ml measuring spoon or with the dropper provided. An ordinary kitchen teaspoon is not accurate enough.

Cephalosporin antibiotics work best when the level of medicine in your bloodstream is kept constant. It is best, therefore, to take the doses at evenly spaced intervals day and night. For example, if you are to take three doses a day, the doses should be spaced eight hours apart.

If you miss a dose of this medication, take the missed dose immediately. If you do not remember to take the missed dose until it is almost time for your next dose, take it; space the following dose halfway through the regular interval between doses; then return to your regular dosing schedule. Try not to skip any doses.

It is important to continue to take this medication for the entire time prescribed by your doctor (usually seven to 14 days), even if the symptoms disappear before the end of that period. If you stop taking this drug too soon, resistant bacteria are given a chance to continue growing, and the infection could recur.

SIDE EFFECTS

Minor. Abdominal pain, diarrhea, dizziness, fatigue, headache, heartburn, loss of appetite, nausea, or vomiting. These side effects should disappear as your body adjusts to the medication.

If you feel dizzy, sit or lie down for a while; get up slowly from a sitting or reclining position, and be careful on stairs.

Major. Tell your doctor about any side effects that are persistent or particularly bothersome. IT IS ESPECIALLY IMPORTANT TO TELL YOUR DOCTOR about darkened tongue, difficulty in breathing, fever, itching, joint pain, rash, rectal or vaginal itching, severe diarrhea (which can be watery or can contain pus or blood), sore mouth, stomach cramps, tingling in the hands or feet, or unusual bleeding or bruising. Also, if your symptoms of infection seem to be getting worse rather than improving, you should contact your doctor.

INTERACTIONS

Cefaclor interacts with several other types of medications:

1. Probenecid can increase the blood concentrations and side effects of this medication.

2. The side effects, especially effects on the kidneys, of furosemide, bumetanide, ethacrynic acid, colistin, vancomycin, polymyxin B, and aminoglycoside antibiotics can be increased by cefaclor.

BE SURE TO TELL YOUR DOCTOR about any medications you are currently taking, especially any listed above.

WARNINGS

• Tell your doctor about unusual or allergic reactions you have had to any medication, especially to cefaclor or other cephalosporin antibiotics (such as cefamandole, cephalexin, cephradine, cefadroxil, cefazolin, cefoperazone, cefotaxime, ceftizoxime, cephalothin, cephapirin, cefuroxime, and moxalactam) or to penicillin antibiotics.

• Tell your doctor if you now have or if you have ever had kidney disease.

• This medication has been prescribed for your current infection only. Another infection later on, or one that someone else has, may require a different medicine. You should not give your medication to other people or use it for other infections, unless your doctor specifically directs you to do so.

• Diabetics who are taking cefaclor should know that this medication can cause a false-positive sugar reaction with a Clinitest urine glucose test. To avoid this problem while taking cefaclor, you should switch to Clinistix or Tes-Tape to test your urine sugar content.

• Be sure to tell your doctor if you are pregnant. Although the cephalosporin antibiotics appear to be safe during pregnancy, extensive studies in humans have not been conducted. Also, tell your doctor if you are breast-feeding an infant. Small amounts of this medication pass into breast milk and may temporarily alter the bacterial balance in the intestinal tract of the nursing infant, resulting in diarrhea.

---

cefadroxil

BRAND NAMES (Manufacturers)

Duricef (Mead Johnson)
Ultracef (Bristol)

TYPE OF DRUG

Cephalosporin antibiotic

INGREDIENT

cefadroxil

DOSAGE FORMS

Tablets (1 g)
Capsules (500 mg)
Oral suspension (125 mg, 250 mg, and 500 mg per 5-ml spoonful)

STORAGE

Cefadroxil tablets and capsules should be stored at room temperature in tightly closed containers. The oral suspension form of this drug should be stored in the refrigerator in a tightly closed container. Any unused portion of the oral suspension should be discarded after 14 days because the drug loses its potency after that time. This medication should never be frozen.

USES

This medication is used to treat a wide variety of bacterial infections, including those of the middle ear, upper and lower respiratory tract, and urinary tract. This drug acts by severely injuring the cell walls of the infecting bacteria, thereby preventing them from growing and multiplying. Cefadroxil kills susceptible bacteria, but it is not effective against viruses, parasites, or fungi.

TREATMENT

You can take cefadroxil either on an empty stomach or, to avoid stomach upset, with food or milk.

The contents of the suspension form of cefadroxil tend to settle on the bottom of the bottle, so it is necessary to shake the container well to distribute the ingredients evenly and equalize the doses. Each dose should then be measured carefully with a specially designed 5-ml measuring spoon or with the dropper provided. An ordinary kitchen teaspoon is not accurate enough.

Cephalosporin antibiotics work best when the level of medicine in your bloodstream is kept constant. It is best, therefore, to take the doses at evenly spaced intervals day and night. For example, if you are to take two doses a day, the doses should be spaced 12 hours apart.

If you miss a dose of this medication, take the missed dose immediately. However, if you do not remember to take the missed dose until it is almost time for your next dose, take it;

space the following dose halfway through the regular interval between doses; then return to your regular schedule. Try not to skip any doses.

It is important to continue to take this medication for the entire time prescribed by your doctor (usually seven to 14 days), even if the symptoms disappear before the end of that period. If you stop taking this drug too soon, resistant bacteria are given a chance to continue growing, and the infection could recur.

SIDE EFFECTS

Minor. Abdominal pain, diarrhea, dizziness, fatigue, headache, heartburn, loss of appetite, nausea, or vomiting. These side effects should disappear as you adjust to the drug.

If you feel dizzy, sit or lie down for a while; get up slowly from a sitting or reclining position, and be careful on stairs.

Major. Tell your doctor about any side effects that are persistent or particularly bothersome. IT IS ESPECIALLY IMPORTANT TO TELL YOUR DOCTOR about darkened tongue, difficulty in breathing, fever, itching, joint pain, rash, rectal or vaginal itching, severe diarrhea (which can be watery, or contain pus or blood), sore mouth, stomach cramps, tingling in the hands or feet, or unusual bleeding or bruising. Also, if your symptoms of infection seem to be getting worse rather than improving, contact your doctor.

INTERACTIONS

Cefadroxil interacts with several other types of medications:

1. Probenecid can increase the blood concentrations and side effects of this medication.

2. The side effects, especially effects on the kidneys, of furosemide, bumetanide, ethacrynic acid, colistin, vancomycin, polymyxin B, and aminoglycoside antibiotics can be increased by cefadroxil.

Before you start to take this medication, BE SURE TO TELL YOUR DOCTOR about any medications you are currently taking, especially any of those listed above.

WARNINGS

- Tell your doctor about unusual or allergic reactions you have had to any medication, especially to cefadroxil or other cephalosporin antibiotics (such as cefamandole, cephalexin, cefaclor, cephradine, cefazolin, cefoperazone, cefotaxime, ceftizoxime, cephalothin, cephapirin, cefoxitin, cefuroxime, and moxalactam) or to penicillin antibiotics.
- Tell your doctor if you have ever had kidney disease.
- This medication has been prescribed for your current infection only. Another infection later on, or one that someone else has, may require a different medicine. You should not give your medication to other people or use it for other infections, unless so directed by your doctor.
- Diabetics taking cefadroxil should know that this drug can cause a false-positive sugar reaction with a Clinitest urine glucose test. To avoid this problem, switch to Clinistix or Tes-Tape to test your urine for sugar.
- Be sure to tell your doctor if you are pregnant. Although the cephalosporin antibiotics appear to be safe during pregnancy, extensive studies in humans have not been conducted. Also, tell your doctor if you are breast-feeding an infant. Small amounts of this medication pass into breast milk and may temporarily alter the bacterial balance in the intestinal tract of the nursing infant, resulting in diarrhea.

Celestone—see betamethasone (systemic)

Cena-K—see potassium chloride

Centrax—see prazepam

---

cephalexin

BRAND NAMES (Manufacturers)

Keflet (Dista)
Keflex (Dista)

TYPE OF DRUG

Cephalosporin antibiotic

INGREDIENT

cephalexin

DOSAGE FORMS

Tablets (250 mg, 500 mg, and 1 g)
Capsules (250 mg and 500 mg)
Oral suspension (125 mg and 250 mg per 5-ml spoonful)
Pediatric oral suspension (100 mg per ml)

STORAGE

Cephalexin tablets and capsules should be stored at room temperature in tightly closed containers. The oral suspension forms of this drug should be stored in the refrigerator in tightly closed containers. Any unused portion of the oral suspension should be discarded after 14 days because the drug loses its potency after that time. This medication should never be frozen.

USES

This medication is used to treat a wide variety of bacterial infections, including those of the middle ear, upper and lower respiratory tract, and urinary tract. This drug acts by severely injuring the cell walls of the infecting bacteria, thereby preventing them from growing and multiplying. Cephalexin kills susceptible bacteria, but it is not effective against viruses, parasites, or fungi.

TREATMENT

You can take cephalexin either on an empty stomach or, to avoid stomach upset, with food or milk.

The contents of the suspension form of cephalexin tend to settle on the bottom of the bottle, so it is necessary to shake the container well to distribute the ingredients evenly and equalize the doses. Each dose should then be measured carefully with a specially designed 5-ml measuring spoon or with the dropper provided. An ordinary kitchen teaspoon is not accurate enough.

Cephalosporin antibiotics work best when the level of medicine in your bloodstream is kept constant. It is best, therefore, to take your doses of this medication at evenly spaced intervals throughout the day and night. For example, if you are to take four doses of the medication a day, the doses should be spaced six hours apart.

If you miss a dose, take the missed dose immediately. However, if you do not remember to take the missed dose until it is almost time for your next dose, take it; space the following dose halfway through the regular interval between doses; then return to your regular schedule. Do not skip any doses.

It is important to continue to take this medication for the entire time prescribed by your doctor (usually seven to 14 days), even if the symptoms disappear before the end of that period. If you stop taking this drug too soon, resistant bacteria are given a chance to continue growing, and the infection could recur.

SIDE EFFECTS

Minor. Abdominal pain, diarrhea, dizziness, fatigue, headache, heartburn, loss of appetite, nausea, or vomiting. These side effects should disappear as your body adjusts to the medication.

If you feel dizzy, sit or lie down for a while; get up slowly from a sitting or reclining position, and be careful on stairs.

Major. Tell your doctor about any side effects that are persistent or particularly bothersome. IT IS ESPECIALLY IMPORTANT TO TELL YOUR DOCTOR about darkened tongue, difficulty in breathing, fever, itching, joint pain, rash, rectal or vaginal itching, severe diarrhea (which can be watery, or contain pus or blood), sore mouth, stomach cramps, tingling in the hands or feet, or unusual bleeding or bruising. Also, if your symptoms of infection seem to be getting worse rather than improving, you should contact your doctor.

INTERACTIONS

Cephalexin interacts with several other types of drugs:

1. Probenecid can increase the blood concentrations of this medication.

2. The side effects, especially effects on the kidneys, of furosemide, bumetanide, ethacrynic acid, colistin, vancomycin, polymyxin B, and aminoglycoside antibiotics can be increased by cephalexin.

BE SURE TO TELL YOUR DOCTOR about any medications you are currently taking, especially any of those listed above.

WARNINGS

• Tell your doctor about unusual or allergic reactions you have had to any medication, especially to cephalexin or other cephalosporin antibiotics (such as cefamandole, cephradine, cefaclor, cefadroxil, cefazolin, cefoperazone, cefotaxime, ceftizoxime, cephalothin, cephapirin, cefoxitin, cefuroxime, and moxalactam) or to penicillin antibiotics.

• Tell your doctor if you now have or if you have ever had kidney disease.

• This medication has been prescribed for your current infection only. Another infection later on, or one that someone else has, may require a different medicine. You should not give your medication to other people or use it for other infections, unless your doctor specifically directs you to do so.

• Diabetics taking cephalexin should know that this drug can cause a false-positive sugar reaction with a Clinitest urine glucose test. To avoid this problem while taking cephalexin, you should switch to Clinistix or Tes-Tape to test your urine for sugar.

• Be sure to tell your doctor if you are pregnant. Although the cephalosporin antibiotics appear to be safe during pregnancy, extensive studies in humans have not been conducted and cautious use is warranted. Also, tell your doctor if you are breast-feeding an infant. Small amounts of this medication pass into breast milk and may temporarily alter the bacterial balance in the intestinal tract of the nursing infant, resulting in diarrhea.

---

cephradine

BRAND NAMES (Manufacturers)

Anspor (Smith Kline & French)
Velosef (Squibb)

TYPE OF DRUG

Cephalosporin antibiotic

INGREDIENT

cephradine

DOSAGE FORMS

Capsules (250 mg and 500 mg)
Oral suspension (125 mg and 250 mg per 5-ml spoonful)

STORAGE

Cephradine capsules should be stored at room temperature in tightly closed containers. The oral suspension form of this drug should be stored in the refrigerator in a tightly closed container. Any unused portion of the oral suspension should be discarded after 14 days because the drug loses its potency after that time. This medication should never be frozen.

USES

This medication is used to treat a wide variety of bacterial infections, including those of the middle ear, upper and lower respiratory tract, and urinary tract. This drug acts by severely injuring the cell walls of the infecting bacteria, thereby preventing them from growing and multiplying. Cephradine kills susceptible bacteria, but it is not effective against viruses, parasites, or fungi.

TREATMENT

You can take cephradine either on an empty stomach or, in order to avoid an upset stomach, with food or milk.

The contents of the suspension form of cephradine tend to settle on the bottom of the bottle, so it is necessary to shake the container well to distribute the ingredients evenly and equalize the doses. Each dose should then be measured carefully with a specially designed 5-ml measuring spoon or with the dropper provided. An ordinary kitchen teaspoon is not accurate enough.

Cephalosporin antibiotics work best when the level of medicine in your bloodstream is kept constant. It is best, therefore, to take the doses at evenly spaced intervals day and night. For example, if you are to take four doses a day, the doses should be spaced six hours apart.

If you miss a dose of this medication, take the missed dose immediately. However, if you do not remember to take the missed dose until it is almost time for your next dose, take it; space the following dose halfway through the regular interval between doses; then return to your regular schedule. Try not to skip any doses.

It is important to continue to take this medication for the entire time prescribed by your doctor (usually seven to 14 days), even if the symptoms disappear before the end of that period. If you stop taking this drug too soon, resistant bacteria are given a chance to continue growing, and the infection could recur.

SIDE EFFECTS

Minor. Abdominal pain, diarrhea, dizziness, fatigue, headache, heartburn, loss of appetite, nausea, or vomiting. These side effects should disappear as your body adjusts to the medication.

If you feel dizzy, sit or lie down for a while; get up slowly from a sitting or reclining position, and be careful on stairs.

Major. Tell your doctor about any side effects that are persistent or particularly bothersome. IT IS ESPECIALLY IMPORTANT TO TELL YOUR DOCTOR about darkened tongue, difficulty in breathing, fever, itching, joint pain, rash, rectal or vaginal itching, severe diarrhea (which can be watery, or contain pus or blood), sore mouth, stomach cramps, tingling in the hands or feet, or unusual bleeding or bruising. Also, if your symptoms of infection seem to be getting worse rather than improving, you should contact your doctor.

INTERACTIONS

Cephradine interacts with several other types of medications:

1. Probenecid can increase the blood concentrations and side effects of this medication.

2. The side effects, especially effects on the kidneys, of furosemide, bumetanide, ethacrynic acid, colistin, vancomycin, polymyxin B, and aminoglycoside antibiotics can be increased by cephradine.

BE SURE TO TELL YOUR DOCTOR about any medications you are currently taking, especially any of the medications that are listed above.

WARNINGS

- Tell your doctor about unusual or allergic reactions you have had to any medication, especially to cephradine or other cephalosporin antibiotics (such as cefamandole, cephalexin, cefaclor, cefadroxil, cefazolin, cefoperazone, cefotaxime, ceftizoxime, cephalothin, cephapirin, cefoxitin, cefuroxime, and moxalactam) or to penicillin antibiotics.
- Tell your doctor if you now have or if you have ever had kidney disease.
- This medication has been prescribed for your current infection only. Another infection later on, or one that someone else has, may require a different medicine. You should not give your medication to other people or use it for other infections, unless your doctor specifically directs you to do so.
- Diabetics taking cephradine should know that this drug can cause a false-positive sugar reaction with a Clinitest urine glucose test. To avoid this problem while taking cephradine, you should switch to Clinistix or Tes-Tape to test your urine for sugar.
- Be sure to tell your doctor if you are pregnant. Although the cephalosporin antibiotics appear to be safe during pregnancy, extensive studies in humans have not been conducted. Also, tell your doctor if you are breast-feeding an infant. Small amounts of this medication pass into breast milk and may temporarily alter the bacterial balance in the intestinal tract of the nursing infant, resulting in diarrhea.

Cerespan—see papaverine

Cetacort—see hydrocortisone (topical)

Cetamide—see sodium sulfacetamide (ophthalmic)

Chenix—see chenodiol

---

chenodiol

BRAND NAME (Manufacturer)
Chenix (Reid-Rowell)

TYPE OF DRUG
Gallstone dissolver

INGREDIENT
chenodiol

DOSAGE FORM
Tablets (250 mg)

STORAGE
Chenodiol tablets should be stored at room temperature in a tightly closed container.

USES

This medication is used to dissolve gallstones in individuals who cannot tolerate surgery. Chenodiol is a naturally occurring bile acid that blocks the body's production of cholesterol. This action leads to gradual dissolution of cholesterol gallstones. It has no effect on calcified gallstones.

TREATMENT

In order to obtain the maximum benefit from this medication, you should take it with food or milk. It is important to continue taking this medication for the entire time prescribed by your doctor (usually six months to two years), even if your symptoms disappear. If you stop using this drug too soon, your symptoms could recur (the gallstones may not have completely dissolved).

If you miss a dose of this medication, take the missed dose as soon as possible, unless it is almost time for the next dose. In that case, do not take the missed dose at all; just return to your regular dosing schedule. Do not double the next dose.

SIDE EFFECTS

Minor. Constipation, diarrhea, gas, heartburn, loss of appetite, nausea, stomach cramps, or vomiting. These side effects should disappear as your body adjusts to the medication.

To relieve constipation, increase the amount of fiber in your diet (fresh fruits and vegetables, salads, bran, and whole-grain breads), exercise, and drink more water (unless your doctor directs you to do otherwise).

If diarrhea continues to be a problem, contact your doctor. Antidiarrheal medications may be effective for short periods, or your doctor may want to decrease your dose of chenodiol.

Major. Tell your doctor about any side effects that are persistent or particularly bothersome. IT IS ESPECIALLY IMPORTANT TO TELL YOUR DOCTOR about yellowing of the eyes or skin.

INTERACTIONS

Chenodiol interacts with other types of medications:

1. Cholestyramine, colestipol, and aluminum-containing antacids can decrease the absorption of chenodiol from the gastrointestinal tract.

2. Estrogen-containing drugs, oral contraceptives (birth control pills), probucol, and clofibrate can counteract the effectiveness of chenodiol.

Before you start to take this medication, BE SURE TO TELL YOUR DOCTOR about any medications you are currently taking, especially any of those listed above.

WARNINGS

- Tell your doctor about any unusual or allergic reactions you have had to medications, especially to chenodiol.
- Tell your doctor if you now have or if you have ever had biliary tract disease, blood vessel disease, colon cancer, inflammatory bowel disease, liver disease, or pancreatitis.
- Body weight and diet influence the formation and dissolution of gallstones. A high-fiber, low-fat diet and weight reduction are recommended to increase the effectiveness of chenodiol.
- Be sure to tell your doctor if you are pregnant. Although extensive studies in humans have not been conducted, this medication has caused birth defects in the offspring of animals that received large doses of it during pregnancy. Also, tell your doctor if you are breast-feeding. It is not known whether chenodiol passes into breast milk.

Cheracol—see codeine and guaifenesin combination

Cherapas—see hydralazine, hydrochlorothiazide, and reserpine combination

Chlorafed (Half-Strength)—see pseudoephedrine and chlorpheniramine combination

Chlorafed Timecelles—see pseudoephedrine and chlorpheniramine combination

chloral hydrate

BRAND NAMES (Manufacturers)
Aquachloral Supprettes (Webcon)
chloral hydrate (various manufacturers)
Noctec (Squibb)
TYPE OF DRUG
Sedative/hypnotic
INGREDIENT
chloral hydrate
DOSAGE FORMS
Capsules (250 mg and 500 mg)
Oral syrup (250 mg and 500 mg per 5-ml spoonful)
Suppositories (325 mg, 500 mg, and 650 mg)
STORAGE
Store at room temperature in a tightly closed, light-resistant container. This medication should never be frozen. The suppositories should be kept in the glass container in which they were dispensed.

USES

Chloral hydrate is used as a sleeping aid in the treatment of insomnia. Exactly how chloral hydrate works is not clearly understood, but it is known to be a central nervous system depressant.

TREATMENT

Chloral hydrate should be taken 15 to 30 minutes before bedtime.

In order to prevent stomach irritation, you should take chloral hydrate capsules with a full glass of water (unless your doctor directs you to do otherwise). The capsules should be swallowed whole to avoid their bad taste.

Each dose of the oral syrup should be measured carefully with a specially designed 5-ml measuring spoon. An ordinary kitchen teaspoon is not accurate enough. The syrup should then be mixed with at least one-half glass (four ounces) of a nonalcoholic beverage (to avoid stomach irritation and to mask the taste).

To insert the suppository form of this medication, first unwrap it and moisten it slightly with water (if the suppository is too soft, run cold water over it or refrigerate it for 30 minutes before you unwrap it). Lie down on your left side with your right knee bent. Push the suppository well into the rectum with your finger. Try to avoid having a bowel movement for at least an hour.

The use of this drug as a sleeping aid should be limited to two weeks. After that period, chloral hydrate loses its ability to induce and sustain sleep.

SIDE EFFECTS

Minor. Diarrhea, dizziness, drowsiness during the day, gas, headache, nausea, stomach irritation, unpleasant taste in the mouth, or vomiting. These side effects should disappear as your body adjusts to the medication.

If you feel dizzy or light-headed, sit or lie down for a while; get up slowly from a sitting or reclining position, and be careful on stairs.

Major. Tell your doctor about any side effects that are persistent or particularly bothersome. IT IS ESPECIALLY IMPORTANT TO TELL YOUR DOCTOR about confusion, difficulty in breathing, disorientation, excitation, fatigue, feeling faint, hallucinations, hives or itching, loss of coordination, nightmares, skin rash, or yellowing of the eyes or skin.

INTERACTIONS

Chloral hydrate interacts with a number of other types of medications:

1. Concurrent use of chloral hydrate with other central nervous system depressants (such as alcohol, barbiturates, benzodiazepine tranquilizers, muscle relaxants, narcotics, pain medications, phenothiazine tranquilizers, and other sleeping medications) or with tricyclic antidepressants can lead to extreme drowsiness.

2. Chloral hydrate can increase the effects of oral anticoagulants (blood thinners, such as warfarin), which can lead to bleeding complications.

BE SURE TO TELL YOUR DOCTOR about any medications you are currently taking, especially any listed above.

WARNINGS

- Tell your doctor about unusual or allergic reactions you have had to any medications, especially to chloral hydrate or to triclofos.
- Before starting to take this medication, be sure to tell your doctor if you now have or if you have ever had gastritis, heart disease, kidney disease, liver disease, or porphyria.

• If this drug makes you dizzy or drowsy, do not take part in any activity that requires alertness, such as driving a car.
• Some dosage forms of this drug contain the color additive FD&C Yellow No. 5 (tartrazine), which can cause allergic-type reactions (shortness of breath, fainting, rash) in susceptible individuals.
• This drug has the potential for abuse and must be used with caution. Tolerance develops quickly; do not increase the dosage or stop taking this drug unless you first consult your doctor. If you have been taking chloral hydrate for a long time or have been taking large doses, you may experience anxiety, muscle twitching, tremors, weakness, dizziness, nausea, vomiting, insomnia, or blurred vision when you stop taking it. Your doctor may, therefore, want to reduce your dosage gradually.
• Be sure to tell your doctor if you are pregnant. Although extensive studies in animals and humans have not been conducted, it is known that chloral hydrate crosses the placenta. If it is used for prolonged periods during the last three months of pregnancy, there is a chance that the infant will be born addicted to the medication and will experience a withdrawal reaction (convulsions and irritability) at birth. Also, tell your doctor if you are breast-feeding an infant. Small amounts of chloral hydrate pass into breast milk and may cause excessive drowsiness in the nursing infant.

---

chlorambucil

BRAND NAME (Manufacturer)
Leukeran (Burroughs Wellcome)
TYPE OF DRUG
Antineoplastic (anticancer drug)
INGREDIENT
chlorambucil
DOSAGE FORM
Tablets (2 mg)
STORAGE
Chlorambucil should be stored at room temperature in a tightly closed, light-resistant container.

USES

Chlorambucil belongs to a group of drugs known as alkylating agents. It is used to treat a variety of cancers. Chlorambucil works by binding to the rapidly growing cancer cells, preventing their multiplication and growth.

TREATMENT

Chlorambucil can be taken either on an empty stomach or with food or milk (as directed by your doctor).

The timing of the doses of this medication is important. Be sure you completely understand your doctor's instructions on how this medication should be taken.

If you miss a dose of this medication, take the missed dose as soon as possible, unless it is almost time for the next dose. In that case, do not take the missed dose at all; just return to your regular dosing schedule. Do not double the next dose.

SIDE EFFECTS

Minor. Nausea, stomach upset, or vomiting. These side effects may disappear as your body adjusts to this medication. It is important, however, to continue taking this medication despite any nausea and vomiting that may occur.

Chlorambucil can also cause hair loss, which is reversible when the medication is stopped.

Major. Tell your doctor about any side effects that are persistent or particularly bothersome. IT IS ESPECIALLY IMPORTANT TO TELL YOUR DOCTOR about chills, convulsions, difficulty in breathing, fever, itching, joint pain, menstrual irregularities, mouth sores, skin rash, sore throat, unusual bleeding or bruising, or yellowing of the eyes or skin.

INTERACTIONS

Chlorambucil can increase the blood levels of uric acid, which can block the effectiveness of antigout medications (allopurinol, probenecid, sulfinpyrazone).

BE SURE TO TELL YOUR DOCTOR about any medications you are currently taking, especially any listed above.

WARNINGS

• Tell your doctor about unusual or allergic reactions you have had to any drugs, especially to chlorambucil or melphalan.
• Before starting to take this medication, be sure to tell your doctor if you now have or if you have ever had blood disorders, chronic or recurrent infections, gout, or kidney stones.
• You should not receive any immunizations or vaccinations while taking this medication. Chlorambucil blocks the effectiveness of the vaccine and may lead to overwhelming infection if a live-virus vaccine is administered.
• While you are taking this medication, it is important that you drink plenty of fluids to prevent the formation of uric acid kidney stones.
• Chlorambucil can lower your platelet count, which can decrease your body's ability to form blood clots. You should, therefore, be especially careful while brushing your teeth, flossing, or using toothpicks, razors, or fingernail scissors. Try to avoid falls and other injuries. Before having any surgery or other medical or dental treatment, be sure that your doctor or dentist knows that you are taking this medication.
• Chlorambucil can decrease fertility in both sexes.
• Be sure to tell your doctor if you are pregnant. Birth defects have been reported in both animals and humans whose mothers received chlorambucil during pregnancy. The risks should be discussed with your doctor. Also, tell your doctor if you are breast-feeding an infant. It is not known whether or not chlorambucil passes into breast milk.

---

chloramphenicol (systemic)

BRAND NAMES (Manufacturers)
chloramphenicol (various manufacturers)
Chloromycetin Kapseals (Parke-Davis)
TYPE OF DRUG
Antibiotic
INGREDIENT
chloramphenicol
DOSAGE FORMS
Capsules (250 mg and 500 mg)
Oral suspension (150 mg per 5-ml spoonful)

STORAGE
Chloramphenicol capsules and oral suspension should be stored at room temperature in tightly closed, light-resistant containers. This medication should never be frozen.

USES
This medication is an antibiotic that is used to treat a wide variety of bacterial infections. It attaches to the bacteria and blocks their production of protein, thereby preventing their growth and multiplication. Chloramphenicol kills susceptible bacteria, but it is not effective against viruses, parasites, or fungi.

TREATMENT
Chloramphenicol is most effective if it is taken on an empty stomach one hour before or two hours after a meal.

The suspension form of this medication should be shaken well just before measuring each dose. The contents tend to settle on the bottom of the bottle, so it is necessary to shake the container to distribute the ingredients evenly and equalize the doses. Each dose should then be measured carefully with a specially designed 5-ml measuring spoon. An ordinary kitchen teaspoon is not accurate enough.

Chloramphenicol works best when the level of medicine in your bloodstream is kept constant. It is best, therefore, to take the doses at evenly spaced intervals day and night. For example, if you are to take four doses a day, the doses should be spaced six hours apart.

Try not to miss any doses of this medication. If you do miss a dose, take it as soon as you remember. However, if you do not remember to take the missed dose until it is almost time for your next dose, take the missed dose immediately; space the following dose about halfway through the regular interval between doses; then continue with your regular dosing schedule.

It is important to continue to take this medication for the entire time prescribed by your doctor (usually seven to 14 days), even if the symptoms disappear before the end of that period. If you stop taking the drug too soon, resistant bacteria are given a chance to continue growing, and the infection could recur.

SIDE EFFECTS
Minor. Diarrhea, headache, nausea, or vomiting. These side effects should disappear as your body adjusts to the medication.
Major. Tell your doctor about any side effects that are persistent or particularly bothersome. IT IS ESPECIALLY IMPORTANT TO TELL YOUR DOCTOR about confusion, depression, fever, itching, mouth sores, skin rash, sore throat, sores on the tongue, tingling sensations, unusual bleeding or bruising, or unusual weakness. Also, if the symptoms of your infection seem to be getting worse rather than improving, you should contact your doctor.

INTERACTIONS
Chloramphenicol interacts with several other drugs:
1. It can increase the blood levels of dicumarol, phenytoin, phenobarbital, tolbutamide, and chlorpropamide, thereby leading to an increase in side effects.
2. Chloramphenicol can reduce the effectiveness of iron, vitamin B_{12}, and cyclophosphamide.
3. The blood levels and side effects of chloramphenicol may be increased by acetaminophen and penicillin.
4. Concurrent use of chloramphenicol and antineoplastic drugs (anticancer medicines), colchicine, gold, oxyphenbutazone, penicillamine, or phenylbutazone can lead to an increase in side effects, especially to the bone marrow.

BE SURE TO TELL YOUR DOCTOR about any medications you are currently taking, especially any of those listed above.

WARNINGS
- Tell your doctor about unusual or allergic reactions you have had to any drugs, especially to chloramphenicol.
- Before starting to take this medication, tell your doctor if you now have or if you have ever had kidney disease, liver disease, or porphyria.
- Diabetic patients should know that chloramphenicol can cause false-positive readings with the Clinitest urine glucose test. Temporarily switching to Clinistix or Tes-Tape to monitor urine glucose levels avoids this problem.
- Chloramphenicol has been prescribed for your current infection only. Another infection later on, or one that someone else has, may require a different medicine. You should not give your medication to other people or use it for other infections, unless your doctor specifically directs you to do so.
- Be sure to tell your doctor if you are pregnant. Chloramphenicol crosses the placenta. Although it appears to be safe during the early stages of pregnancy, chloramphenicol can cause serious side effects in a newborn infant if it is given to the mother late in pregnancy. Also, tell your doctor if you are breast-feeding an infant. Small amounts of chloramphenicol pass into breast milk and can cause serious side effects in nursing infants.

Chlorate—see chlorpheniramine

---

chlordiazepoxide

BRAND NAMES (Manufacturers)
chlordiazepoxide hydrochloride (various manufacturers)
Libritabs (Roche)
Librium (Roche)
Lipoxide (Major)
Reposans-10 (Wesley)
TYPE OF DRUG
Benzodiazepine sedative/hypnotic
INGREDIENT
chlordiazepoxide
DOSAGE FORMS
Capsules (5 mg, 10 mg, and 25 mg)
Tablets (5 mg, 10 mg, and 25 mg)
STORAGE
This medication should be stored at room temperature in tightly closed, light-resistant containers.

USES
Chlordiazepoxide is prescribed to treat the symptoms of anxiety and alcohol withdrawal. It is not clear exactly how this medicine works, but it may relieve anxiety by acting as a

depressant of the central nervous system. Chlordiazepoxide is currently used by many people to relieve nervousness. It is effective for this purpose for short periods, but it is important to try to remove the cause of the anxiety as well.

TREATMENT

This medication should be taken exactly as directed by your doctor. It can be taken with food or a full glass of water if stomach upset occurs. Do not take this medication with a dose of antacids, since they may retard its absorption.

If you are taking this medication regularly and you miss a dose, take the missed dose immediately. If more than an hour has passed, however, skip the dose you missed and wait for the next scheduled dose. Do not double the dose.

SIDE EFFECTS

Minor. Bitter taste in the mouth, constipation, depression, diarrhea, dizziness, drowsiness (after a night's sleep), dry mouth, excessive salivation, fatigue, flushing, headache, heartburn, loss of appetite, nausea, nervousness, sweating, or vomiting. As your body adjusts to the medicine, these side effects should disappear.

To relieve constipation, increase the fiber in your diet (fresh fruits and vegetables, salads, bran, and whole-grain breads), exercise, and drink more water (unless your doctor instructs you to do otherwise).

Dry mouth can be relieved by chewing sugarless gum or by sucking on ice chips.

If you feel dizzy, sit or lie down for a while; get up slowly from a sitting or reclining position, and be careful on stairs.

Major. Tell your doctor about any side effects that are persistent or particularly bothersome. IT IS ESPECIALLY IMPORTANT TO TELL YOUR DOCTOR about blurred or double vision, chest pain, difficulty in urinating, fainting, falling, fever, hallucinations, joint pain, mouth sores, nightmares, palpitations, rash, severe depression, shortness of breath, slurred speech, sore throat, uncoordinated movements, unusual excitement, unusual tiredness, or yellowing of the eyes or skin.

INTERACTIONS

Chlordiazepoxide interacts with several other drugs:

1. To prevent oversedation, this drug should not be taken with alcohol, other sedative drugs, central nervous system depressants (such as antihistamines, barbiturates, muscle relaxants, pain medicines, narcotics, medicines for seizures, and phenothiazine tranquilizers), or antidepressants.
2. This medication may decrease the effectiveness of carbamazepine, levodopa, and oral anticoagulants (blood thinners) and may increase the effects of phenytoin.
3. Disulfiram, oral contraceptives (birth control pills), isoniazid, and cimetidine can increase the blood levels of chlordiazepoxide, which can lead to toxic effects.
4. Concurrent use of rifampin may decrease the effectiveness of chlordiazepoxide.

BE SURE TO TELL YOUR DOCTOR about any medications you are currently taking, especially any of the medications that are listed above.

WARNINGS

• Tell your doctor about unusual or allergic reactions you have had to any medications, especially to chlordiazepoxide or other benzodiazepine tranquilizers (such as alprazolam, clorazepate, diazepam, flurazepam, halazepam, lorazepam, oxazepam, prazepam, temazepam, and triazolam).

• Tell your doctor if you now have or if you have ever had liver disease, kidney disease, epilepsy, lung disease, myasthenia gravis, porphyria, mental depression, or mental illness.

• This medicine can cause drowsiness. Avoid tasks that require alertness, such as driving a car or operating potentially dangerous machinery.

• Before having surgery or any other medical or dental treatment, tell your doctor or dentist that you are taking this drug.

• This medication has the potential for abuse and must be used with caution. Tolerance may develop quickly; do not increase the dosage of the drug without first consulting your doctor. It is also important not to stop this drug suddenly if you have been taking it in large amounts or if you have used it for several weeks. Your doctor may want to reduce your dosage of this medication gradually.

• This is a safe drug when used properly. When it is combined with other sedative drugs or alcohol, however, serious side effects may develop.

• Be sure to tell your doctor if you are pregnant. This medicine may increase the chance of birth defects if it is taken during the first three months of pregnancy. In addition, too much use of this medicine during the last six months of pregnancy may lead to addiction of the fetus, resulting in withdrawal side effects in the newborn. Also, use of this medicine during the last weeks of pregnancy may cause excessive drowsiness, slowed heartbeat, and breathing difficulties in the infant. Tell your doctor if you are breast-feeding an infant. This medicine can pass into breast milk and cause excessive drowsiness, slowed heartbeat, and breathing difficulties in the nursing infant.

---

chlordiazepoxide and amitriptyline combination

BRAND NAME (Manufacturer)
Limbitrol (Roche)

TYPE OF DRUG
Benzodiazepine antianxiety and antidepressant

INGREDIENTS
chlordiazepoxide and amitriptyline

DOSAGE FORM
Tablets (5 mg chlordiazepoxide and 12.5 mg amitriptyline; 10 mg chlordiazepoxide and 25 mg amitriptyline)

STORAGE
Chlordiazepoxide and amitriptyline combination tablets should be stored at room temperature in a tightly closed, light-resistant container.

USES

Chlordiazepoxide and amitriptyline combination is used for the treatment of depression associated with anxiety. Amitriptyline belongs to a group of drugs referred to as tricyclic antidepressants. These medicines are thought to relieve depression by increasing the concentration of certain chemicals necessary for nerve transmission in the brain. It is not clear exactly how chlordiazepoxide works, but it may relieve anxiety by acting as a depressant of the central nervous system (brain and spinal cord).

TREATMENT

This medication should be taken exactly as your doctor prescribes. In order to avoid stomach upset, you can take it with food or with a full glass of milk or water (unless your doctor directs you to do otherwise). Do not take chlordiazepoxide and amitriptyline tablets with a dose of antacids—they retard absorption of this medication.

If you are taking this medication regularly and you miss a dose, take the missed dose as soon as possible, unless it is almost time for your next dose. In that case, do not take the missed dose at all; just return to your regular dosing schedule. Do not double the dose.

The benefits of therapy with this medication may not become apparent for two or three weeks.

SIDE EFFECTS

Minor. Agitation, anxiety, blurred vision, confusion, constipation, cramps, diarrhea, dizziness, drowsiness, dry mouth, fatigue, headache, heartburn, insomnia, loss of appetite, nausea, peculiar tastes in the mouth, restlessness, sweating, vomiting, weakness, or weight gain or loss. These side effects should disappear as your body adjusts to the medication.

This drug may cause increased sensitivity to sunlight, so avoid prolonged exposure to sunlight and sunlamps. Wear protective clothing and sunglasses, and use an effective sunscreen.

Amitriptyline may cause the urine to turn blue-green. This is a harmless effect.

Dry mouth can be relieved by chewing sugarless gum or by sucking on ice chips or a piece of hard candy.

To relieve constipation, increase the amount of fiber in your diet (fresh fruits and vegetables, salads, bran, whole-grain breads), exercise, and drink more water (unless your doctor directs you to do otherwise).

To avoid dizziness or light-headedness when you stand, contract and relax the muscles of your legs for a few moments before rising. Do this by pushing one foot against the floor while raising the other foot slightly, alternating feet so that you are "pumping" your legs in a pedaling motion.

Major. Tell your doctor about any side effects that are persistent or particularly bothersome. IT IS ESPECIALLY IMPORTANT TO TELL YOUR DOCTOR about chest tightness, convulsions, difficult or painful urination, enlarged or painful breasts (in both sexes), fainting, fever, fluid retention, hair loss, hallucinations, impotence, mood changes, mouth sores, nervousness, nightmares, numbness in the fingers or toes, palpitations, ringing in the ears, skin rash, sore throat, tremors, uncoordinated movements or balance problems, unusual bleeding or bruising, or yellowing of the eyes or skin.

INTERACTIONS

Chlordiazepoxide and amitriptyline combination interacts with several other types of medications:

1. Extreme drowsiness can occur when this medicine is taken with central nervous system depressants (such as alcohol, antihistamines, barbiturates, other benzodiazepine tranquilizers, muscle relaxants, narcotics, pain medications, phenothiazine tranquilizers, and sleeping medications) or with other antidepressants.

2. Amitriptyline may decrease the effectiveness of antiseizure medications and may block the blood-pressure-lowering effects of clonidine and guanethidine.

3. Estrogen-containing drugs and oral contraceptives (birth control pills) can increase the side effects and reduce the effectiveness of amitriptyline.

4. Amitriptyline may increase the side effects of thyroid medication and over-the-counter (nonprescription) cough, cold, allergy, asthma, sinus, and diet medications.

5. The concurrent use of amitriptyline and monoamine oxidase (MAO) inhibitors should be avoided because the combination may result in fever, convulsions, or high blood pressure. At least 14 days should separate the use of this drug and the use of an MAO inhibitor.

6. Chlordiazepoxide may decrease the effectiveness of carbamazepine, levodopa, and oral anticoagulants (blood thinners) and may increase the effects of phenytoin.

7. Disulfiram, oral contraceptives (birth control pills), isoniazid, and cimetidine can increase the blood levels of chlordiazepoxide, which could possibly lead to toxic effects.

8. Concurrent use of rifampin may decrease the effectiveness of chlordiazepoxide and amitriptyline.

9. Cimetidine can decrease the elimination of amitriptyline from the body, which can increase the possibility of side effects.

BE SURE TO TELL YOUR DOCTOR about any medications you are currently taking, especially any of the medications that are listed above.

WARNINGS

- Tell your doctor about unusual or allergic reactions you have had to any medications, especially to chlordiazepoxide or other benzodiazepine tranquilizers (such as alprazolam, clorazepate, diazepam, flurazepam, halazepam, lorazepam, oxazepam, prazepam, temazepam, and triazolam), or to amitriptyline or other tricyclic antidepressants (such as desipramine, imipramine, nortriptyline, or doxepin).
- Tell your doctor if you have a history of alcoholism or if you have ever had asthma, high blood pressure, liver or kidney disease, lung disease, myasthenia gravis, heart disease, a heart attack, circulatory disease, stomach problems, intestinal problems, difficulty in urinating, enlarged prostate gland, epilepsy, glaucoma, thyroid disease, mental illness, or electroshock therapy.
- If this drug makes you dizzy or drowsy, do not take part in any activity that requires alertness, such as driving a car or operating potentially dangerous equipment.
- Before having surgery or any other medical or dental treatment, be sure to tell your doctor or dentist that you are taking this medication.
- The effects of this medication may last as long as seven days after you have stopped taking it, so continue to observe all precautions during this period.
- This medication has the potential for abuse and must be used with caution. Tolerance develops quickly; do not increase the dosage of the drug unless you first consult your doctor. It is also important not to stop taking this drug sud-

denly, especially if it has been used in large amounts or has been used for longer than several weeks. Abruptly stopping this medication may cause nausea, headache, stomach upset, fatigue, or a worsening of your condition. Your doctor may want to reduce the dosage gradually.

• Be sure to tell your doctor if you are pregnant. Chlordiazepoxide may increase the chance of birth defects if it is taken during the first three months of pregnancy. In addition, too much use of this medication during the last six months of pregnancy may lead to addiction of the fetus, resulting in withdrawal symptoms in the newborn. Use of this medication during the last weeks of pregnancy may cause excessive drowsiness, slowed heartbeat, and breathing difficulties in the newborn infant. Also, tell your doctor if you are breastfeeding an infant. This medicine may pass into breast milk and cause excessive drowsiness, slowed heartbeat, breathing difficulty, and irritability in the nursing infant.

---

chlordiazepoxide and clidinium combination

BRAND NAMES (Manufacturers)
Clindex (Rugby)
Clinoxide (Geneva Generics)
Clipoxide (Schein)
Librax (Roche)
Lidox (Major)
Zebrax (Hauck)

TYPE OF DRUG
Benzodiazepine antianxiety and anticholinergic

INGREDIENTS
Chlordiazepoxide and clidinium

DOSAGE FORM
Capsules (5 mg chlordiazepoxide and 2.5 mg clidinium)

STORAGE
Chlordiazepoxide and clidinium combination capsules should be stored at room temperature in a tightly closed, light-resistant container.

USES

Chlordiazepoxide and clidinium combination is used in conjunction with other drugs to treat peptic ulcer or irritable bowel syndrome. Clidinium is an anticholinergic agent that slows the activity of the gastrointestinal tract and reduces the production of stomach acid. Chlordiazepoxide belongs to a group of drugs known as benzodiazepine tranquilizers. It is not clear exactly how chlordiazepoxide works, but it may relieve anxiety by acting as a depressant of the central nervous system (brain and spinal cord).

TREATMENT

You should take chlordiazepoxide and clidinium combination 30 to 60 minutes before meals. It can be taken with water or milk. Do not take it with antacids, since they may interfere with its absorption.

If you miss a dose, take the missed dose as soon as possible, unless it is almost time for your next dose. In that case, do not take the missed dose at all; just return to your regular dosing schedule. Do not double the next dose.

SIDE EFFECTS

Minor. Blurred vision, change in your sense of taste, confusion, constipation, decreased sweating, depression, diarrhea, dizziness, drowsiness, dry mouth, fatigue, headache, insomnia, nausea, or vomiting. These side effects should disappear as your body adjusts to the medication.

This medication can cause increased sensitivity to sunlight. You should, therefore, avoid prolonged exposure to sunlight and sunlamps. Wear protective clothing and sunglasses, and use an effective sunscreen.

Dry mouth can be relieved by chewing sugarless gum or by sucking on ice chips or a piece of hard candy.

To relieve constipation, increase the amount of fiber in your diet (fresh fruits and vegetables, salads, bran, and whole-grain breads), exercise, and drink more water (unless your doctor directs you to do otherwise).

To avoid dizziness or light-headedness when you stand, contract and relax the muscles of your legs for a few minutes before rising. Do this by pushing one foot against the floor while raising the other foot slightly, alternating feet so that you are "pumping" your legs in a pedaling motion.

Major. Tell your doctor about any side effects that are persistent or particularly bothersome. IT IS ESPECIALLY IMPORTANT TO TELL YOUR DOCTOR about decreased sexual ability, difficulty in breathing, difficult or painful urination, excitation, fluid retention, hallucinations, palpitations, rash, sore throat, uncoordinated movements, or yellowing of the eyes or skin.

INTERACTIONS

This medication interacts with several other types of drugs:

1. Extreme drowsiness can occur when this medicine is taken with other central nervous system depressants (such as alcohol, antihistamines, barbiturates, muscle relaxants, narcotics, pain medications, phenothiazine tranquilizers, and sleeping medications) or with tricyclic antidepressants.

2. Chlordiazepoxide can decrease the effectiveness of carbamazepine, levodopa, and oral anticoagulants (blood thinners) and may increase the effects of phenytoin.

3. Disulfiram, oral contraceptives (birth control pills), isoniazid, and cimetidine can increase the blood levels of chlordiazepoxide, which could possibly lead to toxic effects.

4. Concurrent use of rifampin may decrease the effectiveness of chlordiazepoxide and clidinium.

5. Amantadine, haloperidol, phenothiazine tranquilizers, procainamide, quinidine, and tricyclic antidepressants may increase the side effects of clidinium.

Before starting to take this medication, BE SURE TO TELL YOUR DOCTOR about any medications you are currently taking, especially any of those listed above.

WARNINGS

• Tell your doctor if you have ever had unusual or allergic reactions to any medications, especially to chlordiazepoxide or other benzodiazepine tranquilizers (such as alprazolam, clorazepate, diazepam, flurazepam, halazepam, lorazepam, oxazepam, prazepam, temazepam, and triazolam) or to clidinium.

• Tell your doctor if you now have or if you have ever had glaucoma, obstructed bladder or intestine, enlarged prostate gland, heart disease, lung disease, liver disease, kidney disease, ulcerative colitis, porphyria, high blood pressure, myasthenia gravis, epilepsy, thyroid disease, emotional instability, or hiatal hernia.

- This medication can decrease sweating and heat release from the body. You should, therefore, avoid becoming overheated by strenuous exercise in hot weather and should avoid taking hot baths, showers, and saunas.
- This medicine can cause drowsiness. Avoid tasks that require alertness, such as driving a car or operating potentially dangerous equipment.
- Before having surgery or any other medical or dental treatment, tell your doctor or dentist that you are taking this drug.
- This medication has the potential for abuse and must be used with caution. Tolerance develops quickly; do not increase the dosage unless you first consult your doctor. It is also important not to stop taking this drug suddenly if you have been using it in large amounts or for longer than several weeks. Your doctor may reduce the dosage gradually.
- This is a safe drug when used properly. When it is combined with other sedative drugs or alcohol, however, serious side effects may develop.
- Be sure to tell your doctor if you are pregnant. This medicine may increase the chance of birth defects if it is taken during the first three months of pregnancy. In addition, too much use of this medicine during the last six months of pregnancy may cause the baby to become dependent on it. This may result in withdrawal symptoms in the infant at birth. Use of this medicine during the last weeks of pregnancy may cause excessive drowsiness, slowed heartbeat, and breathing difficulties in the newborn infant. Also, tell your doctor if you are breast-feeding an infant. This medicine may pass into breast milk and cause excessive drowsiness, slowed heartbeat, and breathing difficulties in the nursing infant.

chlordiazepoxide hydrochloride—see chlordiazepoxide

---

chlorhexidine gluconate

BRAND NAME (Manufacturer)
Peridex (Procter & Gamble)

TYPE OF DRUG
Oral rinse

INGREDIENT
chlorhexidine as the gluconate salt

DOSAGE FORM
Solution (0.12%)

STORAGE
This product should be stored at room temperature in a tightly closed, light-resistant container. Chlorhexidine gluconate solution should not be frozen.

USES

Chlorhexidine gluconate solution is prescribed by dentists for the treatment of gingivitis. Gingivitis is a medical term for inflammation of the gums characterized by redness, swelling, and bleeding upon probing. Although it is unknown exactly how the product works, it is believed to eliminate bacteria, which can cause dental plaque. Dental plaque is one of several causes of gingivitis.

TREATMENT

Treatment with chlorhexidine gluconate solution should begin following a thorough cleaning of your teeth by your dental practitioner.

Measure 1/2 fluid ounce (as marked in the cap given with the product) of chlorhexidine gluconate solution, and swish in the mouth for at least 30 seconds. Do not dilute it in water or other liquids. It should be used full strength.

Do not swallow chlorhexidine gluconate solution following use. It should be expectorated (spit out) after rinsing the mouth.

SIDE EFFECTS

Minor. Irritation of the inside of the mouth can occur following use of this product. In addition, some patients may experience temporary taste disturbances. However, there have been no permanent taste disturbances reported with continued use of chlorhexidine.

Major. Tell your dentist about any side effects that are persistent or particularly bothersome. IT IS ESPECIALLY IMPORTANT TO TELL YOUR DENTIST about inflammation and swelling of the parotid salivary gland.

Chlorhexidine may cause staining of the teeth and tongue. This staining will be more noticeable in patients who have a heavy accumulation of plaque. Usually, this staining is temporary and can be easily removed from most tooth surfaces with dental cleaning. Rarely, some persons, especially those with plaque, will have permanent stains.

INTERACTIONS

There do not appear to be any significant drug interactions with this medication. However, you should make sure your dentist knows about all the medications you are taking.

WARNINGS

- Tell your doctor about any reactions you have had to any drugs, especially to chlorhexidine gluconate solution.
- Chlorhexidine gluconate solution has not been fully evaluated in children under the age of 18. Therefore, the product should not be used by children in this age group.
- To determine the effectiveness of chlorhexidine use, it is advisable to have dental checkups at least every six-months.
- Be sure to tell your dentist if you are pregnant or breast-feeding an infant. Studies have not yet determined the effects of using chlorhexidine in pregnant or nursing women or their babies. Therefore, use of this product during this time should be carefully considered.

Chlor-Niramine—see chlorpheniramine

Chlorofon-F—see chlorzoxazone and acetaminophen combination

Chloromycetin Kapseals—see chloramphenicol (systemic)

---

chlorothiazide

BRAND NAMES (Manufacturers)
chlorothiazide (various manufacturers)
Diachlor (Major)

Diurigen (Goldline)
Diuril (Merck Sharp & Dohme)

TYPE OF DRUG

Diuretic and antihypertensive

INGREDIENT

chlorothiazide

DOSAGE FORMS

Tablets (250 mg and 500 mg)
Oral suspension (250 mg per 5-ml spoonful; 0.5% alcohol)

STORAGE

Store at room temperature in a tightly closed container.

USES

Chlorothiazide is prescribed to treat high blood pressure. It is also used to reduce fluid accumulation in the body caused by conditions such as heart failure, cirrhosis of the liver, kidney disease, and the long-term use of some medications. It reduces fluid accumulation by increasing the elimination of salt and water through the kidneys.

TREATMENT

To decrease stomach irritation, you can take this medication with a glass of milk or with a meal (unless your doctor directs you to do otherwise). Try to take it at the same time every day. Avoid taking a dose after 6:00 P.M.; otherwise, you may have to get up during the night to urinate.

If you miss a dose of this medication, take the missed dose as soon as possible, unless it is almost time for the next dose. In that case, do not take the missed dose at all, just wait until the next scheduled dose. Do not double the dose.

This medication does not cure high blood pressure, but it will help to control the condition as long as you take it.

SIDE EFFECTS

Minor. Constipation, cramps, diarrhea, dizziness, drowsiness, headache, heartburn, loss of appetite, restlessness, or upset stomach. As your body adjusts to the medication, these side effects should disappear.

This medication can cause increased sensitivity to sunlight. Avoid prolonged exposure to sunlight or sunlamps. Wear protective clothing, and use effective sunscreen.

To relieve constipation, increase the amount of fiber in your diet (fresh fruits and vegetables, salads, bran, and whole-grain breads) and exercise (unless your doctor directs you to do otherwise).

To avoid dizziness or light-headedness when you stand, contract and relax the muscles of your legs for a few moments before rising. Do this by pushing one foot against the floor while raising the other foot slightly, alternating feet so that you are "pumping" your legs in a pedaling motion.

Major. Tell your doctor about any side effects that are persistent or particularly bothersome. IT IS ESPECIALLY IMPORTANT TO TELL YOUR DOCTOR about blurred vision, confusion, difficulty in breathing, dry mouth, excessive thirst, excessive weakness, fever, itching, joint pain, mood changes, muscle pains or spasms, nausea, palpitations, skin rash, sore throat, tingling in the fingers or toes, unusual bleeding or bruising, vomiting, or yellowing of the eyes or skin.

INTERACTIONS

Chlorothiazide diuretic and antihypertensive interacts with several other types of medications:

1. It may decrease the effectiveness of oral anticoagulants, antigout medications, insulin, oral antidiabetic medicines, and methenamine.

2. Fenfluramine can increase the blood-pressure-lowering effects of chlorothiazide, which can be dangerous.

3. Indomethacin can decrease the blood-pressure-lowering effects of chlorothiazide, thereby counteracting the desired effects.

4. Cholestyramine and colestipol decrease the absorption of this medication from the gastrointestinal tract. Chlorothiazide should, therefore, be taken one hour before or four hours after a dose of cholestyramine or colestipol (if you have also been prescribed one of these medications).

5. The side effects of amphotericin B, calcium, cortisone-like steroids (such as cortisone, dexamethasone, hydrocortisone, prednisone, and prednisolone), digoxin, digitalis, lithium, quinidine, sulfonamide antibiotics, and vitamin D may be increased by chlorothiazide.

BE SURE TO TELL YOUR DOCTOR about any medications you are currently taking, especially any of those listed above.

WARNINGS

- Tell your doctor about unusual or allergic reactions you have had to any medications, especially to diuretics or any other sulfa drugs, including oral antidiabetic medications and sulfonamide antibiotics.
- Before you start taking chlorothiazide, tell your doctor if you now have or if you have ever had kidney disease or problems with urination, diabetes mellitus, gout, liver disease, asthma, pancreas disease, or systemic lupus erythematosus.
- Chlorothiazide can cause potassium loss. Signs of potassium loss include dry mouth, thirst, weakness, muscle pain or cramps, nausea, and vomiting. If you experience any of these symptoms, call your doctor. To help avoid potassium loss, take this drug with a glass of fresh or frozen orange or cranberry juice, or eat a banana every day. The use of a salt substitute also helps to prevent potassium loss. Do not change your diet or use a salt substitute, however, before discussing it with your doctor. Too much potassium can also be dangerous. Your doctor may want to have blood tests performed periodically to monitor your potassium levels.
- Limit your intake of alcoholic beverages while taking this medication, in order to prevent dizziness and light-headedness.
- If you have high blood pressure, do not take any over-the-counter (nonprescription) medications for weight control or for cough, cold, allergy, asthma, or sinus problems unless your doctor directs you to do so.
- To prevent dehydration (severe water loss) while taking this medication, check with your doctor if you have any illness that causes severe or continuous nausea, vomiting, or diarrhea.
- This medication can raise blood sugar levels in diabetic patients. Therefore, blood sugar should be carefully monitored by blood or urine tests when this medication is being taken.
- Be sure to tell your doctor if you are pregnant. Although studies in humans have not been conducted, chlorothiazide can cross the placenta and may cause adverse effects in the developing fetus. Also, tell your doctor if you are breast-feeding an infant. Although problems in humans have not

been reported, small amounts of this drug can pass into breast milk, so caution is warranted.

---

chlorpheniramine

BRAND NAMES (Manufacturers)
Aller-chlor* (Rugby)
Chlorate (Major)
Chlor-Niramine* (Whiteworth)
chlorpheniramine maleate (various manufacturers)
Chlorspan-12 (Vortech)
Chlortab (Vortech)
Chlor-Trimeton* (Schering)
Phenetron (Lannett)
Telachlor S.R. (Major)
Teldrin* (Smith Kline Consumer)
Trymegen (Medco Supply)
*Available over-the-counter (without a prescription)

TYPE OF DRUG
Antihistamine

INGREDIENT
chlorpheniramine maleate

DOSAGE FORMS
Tablets (4 mg)
Sustained-release tablets (8 mg and 12 mg)
Sustained-release capsules (8 mg and 12 mg)
Oral syrup (2 mg per 5-ml spoonful, with 7% alcohol)

STORAGE
Chlorpheniramine tablets, capsules, and oral syrup should be stored at room temperature in tightly closed containers.

USES

This medication belongs to a group of drugs known as antihistamines (antihistamines block the action of histamine, a chemical that is released by the body during an allergic reaction). It is, therefore, used to treat or prevent symptoms of allergy.

TREATMENT

To avoid stomach upset, you can take chlorpheniramine with food or with a full glass of milk or water (unless your doctor directs you to do otherwise).

The oral syrup form of chlorpheniramine should be measured carefully with a specially designed 5-ml measuring spoon. An ordinary kitchen teaspoon is not accurate enough.

The sustained-release tablets and capsules should be swallowed whole. Breaking, chewing, or crushing these forms of the medication destroys the sustained-release activity and may increase the side effects.

If you miss a dose of this medication, take the missed dose as soon as possible, unless it is almost time for your next dose. In that case, do not take the missed dose at all; just return to your regular dosing schedule. Do not double the next dose.

SIDE EFFECTS

Minor. Blurred vision; confusion; constipation; diarrhea; difficult or painful urination; dizziness; dry mouth, throat, or nose; headache; irritability; loss of appetite; nausea; restlessness; ringing or buzzing in the ears; stomach upset; or unusual increase in sweating. These side effects should disappear as your body adjusts to the medication.

This medication can cause increased sensitivity to sunlight. It is, therefore, important to avoid prolonged exposure to sunlight and sunlamps. Wear protective clothing, and use an effective sunscreen.

If you are constipated, increase the amount of fiber in your diet (fresh fruits and vegetables, salads, bran, and whole-grain breads), exercise, and drink more water (unless your doctor tells you not to do so).

Chew sugarless gum or suck on ice chips or a piece of hard candy to reduce mouth dryness.

If you feel dizzy or light-headed, sit or lie down for a while; get up from a sitting or lying position slowly, and be careful on stairs.

Major. Tell your doctor about any side effects that are persistent or particularly bothersome. IT IS ESPECIALLY IMPORTANT TO TELL YOUR DOCTOR about change in menstruation, clumsiness, feeling faint, flushing of the face, hallucinations, palpitations, rash, seizures, shortness of breath, sleeping disorders, sore throat or fever, tightness in the chest, unusual bleeding or bruising, or unusual tiredness or weakness.

INTERACTIONS

Chlorpheniramine interacts with other types of medications:

1. Concurrent use of it with other central nervous system depressants (such as alcohol, barbiturates, benzodiazepine tranquilizers, muscle relaxants, narcotics, pain medications, and phenothiazine tranquilizers) or with tricyclic antidepressants can cause extreme drowsiness.

2. Monoamine oxidase (MAO) inhibitors (isocarboxazid, pargyline, phenelzine, tranylcypromine) can increase the side effects of this medication.

3. Chlorpheniramine can also decrease the activity of oral anticoagulants (blood thinners, such as warfarin).

BE SURE TO TELL YOUR DOCTOR about any medications you are currently taking, especially any of those listed above.

WARNINGS

- Tell your doctor about unusual or allergic reactions you have had to any medications, especially to chlorpheniramine or to other antihistamines (such as azatadine, brompheniramine, carbinoxamine, clemastine, cyproheptadine, dexchlorpheniramine, dimenhydrinate, dimethindene, diphenhydramine, diphenylpyraline, doxylamine, hydroxyzine, promethazine, pyrilamine, trimeprazine, tripelennamine, and triprolidine).
- Tell your doctor if you now have or if you have ever had asthma, blood vessel disease, glaucoma, high blood pressure, kidney disease, peptic ulcers, enlarged prostate gland, or thyroid disease.
- Chlorpheniramine can cause drowsiness or dizziness. Your ability to perform tasks that require alertness, such as driving a car or operating potentially dangerous equipment, may be decreased. Appropriate caution should, therefore, be taken.
- Be sure to tell your doctor if you are pregnant. The effects of this medication during pregnancy have not been thoroughly studied in humans. Also, be sure to tell your doctor if

you are breast-feeding an infant. Small amounts of chlorpheniramine pass into breast milk and may cause unusual excitement or irritability in nursing infants.

chlorpheniramine maleate—see chlorpheniramine

---

chlorpromazine

BRAND NAMES (Manufacturers)
chlorpromazine hydrochloride (various manufacturers)
Ormazine (Hauck)
Sonazine (Cord)
Thorazine (Smith Kline & French)
Thorazine Spansules (Smith Kline & French)
Thor-Prom (Major)

TYPE OF DRUG
Phenothiazine tranquilizer

INGREDIENT
chlorpromazine hydrochloride

DOSAGE FORMS
Tablets (10 mg, 25 mg, 50 mg, 100 mg, and 200 mg)
Sustained-release capsules (30 mg, 75 mg, 150 mg, 200 mg, and 300 mg)
Oral concentrate (30 mg per ml and 100 mg per ml)
Oral syrup (10 mg per 5-ml spoonful)
Suppositories (25 mg and 100 mg)

STORAGE
The tablet and capsule forms of this drug should be stored at room temperature in tightly closed, light-resistant containers. The oral concentrate, oral syrup, and suppository forms of this drug should be stored in the refrigerator in tightly closed, light-resistant containers. If the oral concentrate or syrup turns to a slight yellow color, the medicine is still effective and can be used. However, if the oral concentrate or syrup changes color markedly or has particles floating in it, it should not be used; instead, it should be discarded down the sink. Chlorpromazine should never be frozen.

USES

Chlorpromazine is prescribed to treat the symptoms of certain types of mental illness, such as emotional symptoms of psychosis, the manic phase of manic-depressive illness, and severe behavioral problems in children. This medication is thought to relieve the symptoms of mental illness by blocking certain chemicals involved with nerve transmission in the brain.

Chlorpromazine may also be used to treat tetanus, porphyria, uncontrollable hiccups, anxiety before surgery, and nausea and vomiting (this medication works at the vomiting center in the brain to relieve nausea and vomiting).

TREATMENT

In order to avoid stomach irritation, you can take the tablet or capsule forms of this medication with a meal or with a glass of water or milk (unless your doctor directs you to do otherwise).

The sustained-release capsules should be taken whole; do not crush, break, or open them prior to swallowing. Breaking the capsule would release the medication all at once—defeating the purpose of the extended-release capsules.

Measure the oral syrup carefully with a specially designed 5-ml measuring spoon. An ordinary kitchen teaspoon is not accurate enough.

The oral concentrate form of this medication should be measured carefully with the dropper provided, then added to four ounces (one-half cup) or more of water, milk, or a carbonated beverage or to applesauce or pudding immediately prior to administration. Be careful that the serving size is not more than the patient is willing or able to drink or eat; otherwise, the full dose may not be consumed. To prevent possible loss of effectiveness, the medication should not be diluted in tea, coffee, or apple juice.

To use the suppository form of this medication, remove the foil wrapper and moisten the suppository with water (if the suppository is too soft to insert, refrigerate it for half an hour or run cold water over it before removing the wrapper). Lie on your left side with your right knee bent. Push the suppository into the rectum, pointed end first. Lie still for a few minutes. Try to avoid having a bowel movement for at least an hour.

If you miss a dose of this medication, take the missed dose as soon as possible, then return to your regular schedule. If it is almost time for the next dose, however, skip the one you missed and return to your regular schedule. Do not double the dose (unless your doctor directs you to do so).

Antacids and antidiarrheal medicines may decrease the absorption of this medication from the gastrointestinal tract. Therefore, at least one hour should separate doses of one of these medicines and chlorpromazine.

The full effects of this medication for the control of emotional or mental symptoms may not become apparent for two weeks after you start to take it.

SIDE EFFECTS

Minor. Blurred vision, constipation, decreased sweating, diarrhea, dizziness, drooling, drowsiness, dry mouth, fatigue, jitteriness, menstrual irregularities, nasal congestion, restlessness, tremors, vomiting, or weight gain. As your body adjusts to the medication, these side effects should disappear.

This medication can cause increased sensitivity to sunlight. It is, therefore, important to avoid prolonged exposure to sunlight or sunlamps. Wear protective clothing, and use an effective sunscreen.

Chlorpromazine can also cause discoloration of the urine to red, pink, or red-brown. This is a harmless effect.

If you are constipated, increase the amount of fiber in your diet (fresh fruits and vegetables, salads, bran, and whole-grain breads), exercise, and drink more water (unless your doctor directs you to do otherwise).

Chew sugarless gum or suck on ice chips or a piece of hard candy to reduce mouth dryness.

To avoid dizziness or light-headedness when you stand, contract and relax the muscles of your legs for a few moments before rising. Do this by pushing one foot against the floor while raising the other foot slightly, alternating feet so that you are "pumping" your legs in a pedaling motion.

Major. Tell your doctor about any side effects that are persistent or particularly bothersome. IT IS ESPECIALLY IMPORTANT TO TELL YOUR DOCTOR about breast enlargement (in both sexes); chest pain; convulsions; darkened skin; difficulty in swallowing or breathing; fainting; fever; impotence; involuntary movements of the face, mouth, jaw, or tongue; palpitations; rash; sleep disorders; sore throat; uncoordinated movements; unusual bleeding or bruising; visual disturbances; or yellowing of the eyes or skin.

INTERACTIONS

Chlorpromazine interacts with several types of drugs:

1. It can cause extreme drowsiness when combined with alcohol or other central nervous system depressants (such as barbiturates, benzodiazepine tranquilizers, muscle relaxants, narcotics, and pain medications) or with tricyclic antidepressants.

2. Chlorpromazine can decrease the effectiveness of amphetamines, guanethidine, anticonvulsants, and levodopa.

3. The side effects of cyclophosphamide, epinephrine, monoamine oxidase (MAO) inhibitors, phenytoin, and tricyclic antidepressants may be increased by this medication.

4. Chlorpromazine can increase the absorption of propranolol, which can increase the risks of side effects.

5. Lithium may increase the side effects and decrease the effectiveness of this medication.

Before starting to take chlorpromazine, BE SURE TO TELL YOUR DOCTOR about any medications you are currently taking, especially any of those listed above.

WARNINGS

• Tell your doctor about unusual or allergic reactions you have had to any medications, especially to chlorpromazine or any other phenothiazine tranquilizers (such as fluphenazine, mesoridazine, perphenazine, prochlorperazine, promazine, thioridazine, and trifluoperazine) or to loxapine.

• Tell your doctor if you have a history of alcoholism, or if you now have or ever had blood disease, bone marrow disease, brain disease, breast cancer, blockage in the urinary or digestive tract, drug-induced depression, epilepsy, high or low blood pressure, diabetes mellitus, glaucoma, heart or circulatory disease, liver disease, lung disease, Parkinson's disease, peptic ulcers, or an enlarged prostate gland.

• Tell your doctor about any recent exposure to a pesticide or an insecticide. Chlorpromazine may increase the side effects from the exposure.

• To prevent oversedation, avoid drinking alcoholic beverages while taking this medication.

• If this drug makes you dizzy or drowsy, avoid any activity that requires alertness, such as driving a car or operating dangerous equipment. Be careful on stairs, and avoid getting up suddenly from a lying or sitting position.

• Before having surgery or any other medical or dental treatment, be sure to tell your doctor or dentist that you are taking this medication.

• Some of the side effects caused by this drug can be prevented by taking an antiparkinsonism drug. Discuss this with your doctor.

• This medication can decrease sweating and heat release from the body. You should, therefore, avoid becoming overheated by strenuous exercise in hot weather and should avoid taking hot baths, showers, and saunas.

• Do not stop taking this medication suddenly. If the drug is stopped abruptly, you may experience nausea, vomiting, stomach upset, headache, increased heart rate, insomnia, tremors, or a worsening of your condition. Your doctor may want to reduce the dosage gradually.

• If you are planning to have a myelogram or any other procedure in which dye will be injected into your spinal cord, tell your doctor that you are taking this medication.

• Avoid spilling the oral concentrate or oral syrup forms of this medication on your skin or clothing; it may cause redness and irritation of the skin.

• While you are being treated with this medication, do not take any over-the-counter (nonprescription) medication for weight control or for cough, cold, allergy, asthma, or sinus problems without first checking with your doctor. The combination of these medications with chlorpromazine may cause high blood pressure.

• Be sure to tell your doctor if you are pregnant. Small amounts of this medication cross the placenta. Although there are reports of safe use of this drug during pregnancy, there are also reports of liver disease and tremors in newborn infants whose mothers received this medication close to term. Also, tell your doctor if you are breast-feeding an infant. Small amounts of this medication pass into breast milk and may cause unwanted effects in the nursing infant.

chlorpromazine hydrochloride—see chlorpromazine

---

chlorpropamide

BRAND NAMES (Manufacturers)
chlorpropamide (various manufacturers)
Diabinese (Pfizer)

TYPE OF DRUG
Oral antidiabetic

INGREDIENT
chlorpropamide

DOSAGE FORM
Tablets (100 mg and 250 mg)

STORAGE
Store at room temperature in a tightly closed container.

USES

Chlorpropamide is used for the treatment of diabetes mellitus that appears in adulthood and cannot be managed by control of diet alone. This type of diabetes is known as non-insulin-dependent diabetes (sometimes called maturity-onset or Type II diabetes). Chlorpropamide lowers blood sugar by increasing the release of insulin from the pancreas.

TREATMENT

In order for this medication to work correctly, it must be taken as your doctor has directed. It is best to take this medicine at the same time each day in order to maintain a constant blood sugar level. It is important, therefore, to try not to miss any doses of this medication. If you do miss a dose, take it as soon as possible, unless it is almost time for the next dose. In that case, do not take the missed dose at all; just return to your regular dosing schedule. Do not double the next dose. Tell your doctor if you feel any side effects from missing a dose of this drug.

Diabetics who are taking oral antidiabetic medication may need to be switched to insulin if they develop diabetic coma, have a severe infection, are scheduled for major surgery, or become pregnant.

SIDE EFFECTS

Minor. Diarrhea, headache, heartburn, loss of appetite, nausea, stomach discomfort, stomach pain, or vomiting. These side effects usually disappear during treatment, as your body adjusts to the medication.

Chlorpropamide may increase your sensitivity to sunlight. Use caution during exposure to the sun. You may want to wear protective clothing and sunglasses. Use an effective sunscreen, and avoid exposure to sunlamps.

Major. If any side effects are persistent or particularly bothersome, it is important to notify your doctor. IT IS ESPECIALLY IMPORTANT TO TELL YOUR DOCTOR about dark urine, fatigue, itching of the skin, light-colored stools, sore throat and fever, unusual bleeding or bruising, or yellowing of the eyes or skin.

Chlorpropamide can also cause retention of body water, which in turn can lead to drowsiness; muscle cramps; seizures; swelling or puffiness of the face, hands, or ankles; and tiredness or weakness. IT IS IMPORTANT TO TELL YOUR DOCTOR if you notice any of these side effects.

INTERACTIONS

Chlorpropamide interacts with a number of other types of medications:

1. Chloramphenicol, fenfluramine, guanethidine, insulin, miconazole, monoamine oxidase (MAO) inhibitors, oxyphenbutazone, oxytetracycline, phenylbutazone, probenecid, aspirin or other salicylates, sulfinpyrazone, or sulfonamide antibiotics, when combined with chlorpropamide, can lower blood sugar levels—sometimes to dangerously low levels.

2. Thyroid hormones, dextrothyroxine, epinephrine, phenytoin, thiazide diuretics (water pills), or cortisone-like medications (such as dexamethasone, hydrocortisone, and prednisone), when combined with chlorpropamide, can actually increase blood sugar levels—just what you are trying to avoid.

3. Rifampin can decrease the blood levels of chlorpropamide, which can lead to a decrease in its effectiveness.

4. Antidiabetic medications can increase the effects of anticoagulants (blood thinners, such as warfarin), which can lead to bleeding complications.

5. Beta-blocking medications (acebutolol, atenolol, betaxolol, carteolol, esmolol, labetalol, metoprolol, nadolol, penbutolol, pindolol, propranolol, timolol), combined with chlorpropamide, can result in either high or low blood sugar levels. Beta blockers can also mask the symptoms of low blood sugar, which can be dangerous.

6. Avoid drinking alcoholic beverages while taking this medication (unless otherwise directed by your doctor). Some patients who take this medicine suffer nausea, vomiting, dizziness, stomach pain, pounding headache, sweating, or redness of the face and skin when they drink alcohol. Also, large amounts of alcohol can lower blood sugar to dangerously low levels.

BE SURE TO TELL YOUR DOCTOR about any medications you are currently taking, especially any of those listed above.

WARNINGS

- It is important to tell your doctor if you have ever had unusual or allergic reactions to this medicine or to any sulfa medication (sulfonamide antibiotics, acetazolamide, diuretics [water pills], or other oral antidiabetics).
- Tell your doctor if you now have or if you have ever had kidney disease, liver disease, severe infection, or thyroid disease.
- Follow the special diet that your doctor gave you. This is an essential part of controlling your blood sugar and is necessary in order for this medicine to work properly.
- Before having surgery or any other medical or dental treatment, be sure to tell your doctor or dentist that you are taking this medicine.
- Test for sugar in your urine as directed by your doctor. It is a convenient way to determine whether or not your diabetes is being controlled by this medicine.
- Eat or drink something containing sugar right away if you experience any symptoms of low blood sugar (such as anxiety, chills, cold sweats, cool or pale skin, drowsiness, excessive hunger, headache, nausea, nervousness, rapid heartbeat, shakiness, or unusual tiredness or weakness). It is important that your family and friends know the symptoms of low blood sugar and what to do if they observe any of these symptoms in you.

Even if the symptoms of low blood sugar are corrected by eating or drinking sugar, it is important to contact your doctor as soon as possible after experiencing them. The blood-sugar-lowering effects of this medicine can last for hours, and the symptoms may return during this period. Good sources of sugar are orange juice, corn syrup, honey, sugar cubes, and table sugar. You are at greatest risk of developing low blood sugar if you skip or delay meals, exercise more than usual, cannot eat because of nausea or vomiting, or drink large amounts of alcohol.

- Be sure to tell your doctor if you are pregnant. Since extensive studies have not yet been conducted, it is not known whether this medication can cause problems when administered to a pregnant woman. Cautious use is thus warranted. It is also important to tell your doctor if you are breast-feeding an infant. It has been determined that this medicine passes into breast milk. This product is not recommended for use by a woman who is breast-feeding.

---

chlorprothixene

BRAND NAME (Manufacturer)
Taractan (Roche)

TYPE OF DRUG
Antipsychotic

INGREDIENT
chlorprothixene

DOSAGE FORMS
Tablets (10 mg, 25 mg, 50 mg, and 100 mg)
Oral suspension (100 mg as lactate and hydrochloride per 5-ml spoonful)

STORAGE
Store at room temperature in a tightly closed, light-resistant container. This medication should never be frozen.

USES

Chlorprothixene is prescribed to treat the symptoms of certain types of mental illness, such as emotional symptoms of psychosis. This medication is thought to relieve the symptoms of mental illness by blocking certain chemicals involved with nerve transmission in the brain.

TREATMENT

To avoid stomach irritation, you can take the tablet form of this medication with a meal or with a glass of water or milk (unless your doctor directs you to do otherwise).

Measure the oral suspension carefully with a specially designed 5-ml measuring spoon. An ordinary kitchen teaspoon is not accurate enough to ensure that you receive the proper dose of chlorprothixene.

Antacids and antidiarrheal medicines may decrease the absorption of this medication from the gastrointestinal tract. Therefore, at least one hour should separate doses of chlorprothixene and one of these medicines.

If you miss a dose of this medication, take the missed dose as soon as possible and return to your regular schedule. If it is within two hours of your next dose, however, skip the dose you missed and return to your regular schedule. Do not double the dose (unless your doctor directs you to do so).

The full effects of this medication for the control of emotional or mental symptoms may not become apparent for two weeks after you start to take it.

SIDE EFFECTS

Minor. Blurred vision, constipation, decreased sweating, diarrhea, dizziness, drooling, drowsiness, dry mouth, fatigue, jitteriness, menstrual irregularities, nasal congestion, restlessness, tremors, vomiting, or weight gain. As your body adjusts to the medication, these side effects should disappear.

This medication can cause increased sensitivity to sunlight. It is, therefore, important to avoid prolonged exposure to sunlight and sunlamps. Wear protective clothing, and use an effective sunscreen.

Chlorprothixene can also cause discoloration of the urine to red, pink, or red-brown. This is a harmless effect.

If you are constipated, increase the amount of fiber in your diet (fresh fruits and vegetables, salads, bran, and whole-grain breads), exercise, and drink more water (unless your doctor directs you to do otherwise).

Chew sugarless gum or suck on ice chips or a piece of hard candy to reduce mouth dryness.

To avoid dizziness or light-headedness when you stand, contract and relax the muscles of your legs for a few moments before rising. Do this by pushing one foot against the floor while raising the other foot slightly, alternating feet so that you are "pumping" your legs in a pedaling motion.

Major. Tell your doctor about any side effects that are persistent or particularly bothersome. IT IS ESPECIALLY IMPORTANT TO TELL YOUR DOCTOR about breast enlargement (in both sexes); chest pain; convulsions; darkened skin; difficulty in swallowing or breathing; fainting; fever; impotence; involuntary movements of the face, mouth, jaw, or tongue; palpitations; rash; sleep disorders; sore throat; uncoordinated movements; unusual bleeding or bruising; visual disturbances; or yellowing of the eyes or skin.

INTERACTIONS

Chlorprothixene interacts with several other types of medications:

1. It can cause extreme drowsiness when combined with alcohol or other central nervous system depressants (such as barbiturates, benzodiazepine tranquilizers, muscle relaxants, narcotics, and pain medications) or with tricyclic antidepressants.

2. This medication can decrease the effectiveness of amphetamines, guanethidine, anticonvulsants, and levodopa.

3. The side effects of epinephrine, monoamine oxidase (MAO) inhibitors, and tricyclic antidepressants may be increased by this medication.

4. Lithium may increase the side effects and decrease the effectiveness of this medication.

Before starting to take chlorprothixene, BE SURE TO TELL YOUR DOCTOR about any medications you are currently taking, especially any of those listed above.

WARNINGS

- Tell your doctor about unusual or allergic reactions you have had to any medications, especially to chlorprothixene, thiothixene, or any phenothiazine tranquilizer.
- Tell your doctor if you have a history of alcoholism, or if you now have or have ever had blood disease, bone marrow disease, brain disease, breast cancer, blockage in the urinary or digestive tract, drug-induced depression, epilepsy, high or low blood pressure, diabetes mellitus, glaucoma, heart or circulatory disease, liver disease, lung disease, Parkinson's disease, peptic ulcers, or an enlarged prostate gland.
- Avoid drinking alcoholic beverages while taking this medication, in order to prevent oversedation.
- If this medication makes you dizzy or drowsy, do not take part in any activity that requires alertness, such as driving a car or operating potentially dangerous equipment. Be careful on stairs, and avoid getting up suddenly from a lying or sitting position.
- Before having surgery or any other medical or dental treatment, be sure to tell your doctor or dentist that you are taking this medication.
- Some of the side effects caused by this drug can be prevented by taking an antiparkinsonism drug. Discuss this with your doctor.
- Chlorprothixene can decrease sweating and heat release from the body. You should, therefore, avoid becoming overheated by strenuous exercise in hot weather and avoid taking hot baths, showers, and saunas.
- Do not stop taking this medication suddenly. If the drug is stopped abruptly, you may experience nausea, vomiting, stomach upset, headache, increased heart rate, insomnia, tremulousness, or a worsening of your condition. Your doctor may want to reduce the dosage gradually.
- If you are planning to have a myelogram, or any other procedure in which dye will be injected into your spinal cord, tell your doctor that you are taking this medication.
- Avoid spilling the oral suspension form of this medication on your skin or clothing; it can cause redness and irritation of the skin.
- Chlorprothixene tablets contain the color additive FD&C Yellow No. 5 (tartrazine), which can cause allergic-type reactions (fainting, shortness of breath, or rash) in certain susceptible individuals.
- While taking this medication, do not take any over-the-counter (nonprescription) drugs for weight control or for cough, cold, allergy, asthma, or sinus problems without

checking with your doctor. The combination of these medications with chlorprothixene may cause high blood pressure.

• Be sure to tell your doctor if you are pregnant. Small amounts of this medication can cross the placenta. Although there are reports of safe use of this drug during pregnancy, there are also reports of liver disease and tremors in newborn infants whose mothers received this type of medication close to term. Also, tell your doctor if you are breast-feeding an infant. Small amounts of this medication pass into breast milk and may cause unwanted effects in the nursing infant.

Chlorspan-12—see chlorpheniramine

Chlortab—see chlorpheniramine

---

chlorthalidone

BRAND NAMES (Manufacturers)
chlorthalidone (various manufacturers)
Hygroton (Rorer)
Hylidone (Major)
Thalitone (Boehringer Ingelheim)

TYPE OF DRUG
Diuretic and antihypertensive

INGREDIENT
chlorthalidone

DOSAGE FORM
Tablets (25 mg, 50 mg, and 100 mg)

STORAGE
Store at room temperature in a tightly closed container.

USES

Chlorthalidone is prescribed to treat high blood pressure. It is also used to reduce fluid accumulation in the body caused by conditions such as heart failure, cirrhosis of the liver, kidney disease, and the long-term use of some medications. This medication reduces fluid accumulation by increasing the elimination of salt and water through the kidneys.

TREATMENT

To decrease stomach irritation, you can take this medication with a glass of milk or with a meal (unless your doctor directs you to do otherwise). Try to take it at the same time every day. Avoid taking a dose after 6:00 P.M.; otherwise, you may have to get up during the night to urinate.

If you miss a dose of this medication, take the missed dose as soon as possible, unless it is almost time for the next dose. In that case, do not take the missed dose at all; just wait until the next scheduled dose. Do not double the dose.

This medication does not cure high blood pressure, but it will help to control the condition as long as you take it.

SIDE EFFECTS

Minor. Constipation, cramps, diarrhea, dizziness, drowsiness, headache, heartburn, loss of appetite, restlessness, or stomach upset. As your body adjusts to the medication, these side effects should disappear.

This medication can cause increased sensitivity to sunlight. Therefore, avoid prolonged exposure to sunlight and sunlamps. Wear protective clothing, and use an effective sunscreen.

To relieve constipation, increase the amount of fiber in your diet (fresh fruits and vegetables, salads, bran, and whole-grain breads) and exercise (unless your doctor directs you to do otherwise).

To avoid dizziness or light-headedness when you stand, contract and relax the muscles of your legs for a few moments before rising. Do this by pushing one foot against the floor while raising the other foot slightly, alternating feet so that you are "pumping" your legs in a pedaling motion.

Major. Tell your doctor about any side effects that are persistent or particularly bothersome. IT IS ESPECIALLY IMPORTANT TO TELL YOUR DOCTOR about any blurred vision, confusion, difficulty in breathing, dry mouth, excessive thirst, excessive weakness, fever, itching, joint pain, mood changes, muscle pains or spasms, nausea, palpitations, skin rash, sore throat, tingling in the fingers or toes, unusual bleeding or bruising, vomiting, or yellowing of the eyes or skin.

INTERACTIONS

Chlorthalidone interacts with several other types of drugs:

1. It may decrease the effectiveness of oral anticoagulants, antigout medications, insulin, oral antidiabetic medicines, and methenamine.

2. Fenfluramine can increase the blood-pressure-lowering effects of chlorthalidone, which can be dangerous.

3. Indomethacin can decrease the blood-pressure-lowering effects of chlorthalidone, thereby counteracting the desired effects.

4. Cholestyramine and colestipol decrease the absorption of this medication from the gastrointestinal tract. Chlorthalidone should, therefore, be taken one hour before or four hours after a dose of cholestyramine or colestipol (if you have also been prescribed one of these medications).

5. The side effects of amphotericin B, calcium, cortisone-like steroids (such as cortisone, dexamethasone, hydrocortisone, prednisone, prednisolone), digoxin, digitalis, lithium, quinidine, sulfonamide antibiotics, and vitamin D may be increased by chlorthalidone.

BE SURE TO TELL YOUR DOCTOR about any medications you are currently taking, especially any of those listed above.

WARNINGS

• Tell your doctor about unusual or allergic reactions you have had to any drugs, especially to diuretics or any other sulfa drugs, including oral antidiabetics and sulfonamide antibiotics.

• Before you start taking chlorthalidone, tell your doctor if you now have or if you have ever had kidney disease or problems with urination, diabetes mellitus, gout, liver disease, asthma, pancreatic disease, or systemic lupus erythematosus.

• Chlorthalidone can cause potassium loss. Signs of potassium loss include dry mouth, thirst, weakness, muscle pain or cramps, nausea, and vomiting. If you experience any of these symptoms, call your doctor. To help avoid potassium loss, take this drug with a glass of fresh or frozen orange or cranberry juice, or eat a banana every day. The use of a salt substitute also helps to prevent potassium loss. Do not change your diet or use a salt substitute, however, before discussing it with your doctor. Too much potassium can also be dangerous. Your doctor may want to have blood tests performed periodically to monitor your potassium levels.

• Limit your intake of alcoholic beverages while taking this medication, in order to prevent dizziness and light-headedness.

• If you have high blood pressure, do not take any over-the-counter (nonprescription) medications for weight control or for cough, cold, allergy, asthma, or sinus problems unless your doctor directs you to do so.

• To prevent dehydration (severe water loss) while taking this medication, check with your doctor if you have any illness that causes severe or continuous nausea, vomiting, or diarrhea.

• This medication can raise blood sugar levels in diabetic patients. Therefore, blood sugar should be carefully monitored by blood or urine tests when this medication is being taken.

• Be sure to tell your doctor if you are pregnant. Although studies in humans have not been conducted, chlorthalidone can cross the placenta and may cause adverse effects in the developing fetus. Also, tell your doctor if you are breast-feeding an infant. Although problems in humans have not been reported, small amounts of this drug can pass into breast milk, so caution is warranted.

Chlor-Trimeton—see chlorpheniramine

Chlor-Trimeton Decongestant—see pseudoephedrine and chlorpheniramine combination

Chlor-Trimeton Decongestant Repetabs—see pseudoephedrine and chlorpheniramine combination

Chlorzone Forte—see chlorzoxazone and acetaminophen combination

---

chlorzoxazone and acetaminophen combination

BRAND NAMES (Manufacturers)
Blanex (Edwards)
Chlorofon-F (Rugby)
Chlorzone Forte (Schein)
chlorzoxazone and acetaminophen (various manufacturers)
Flexaphen (Trimen)
Lobac (Seatrace)
Mus-Lax (Jones Medical)
Paracet Forte (A.D.I.)
Polyflex (Holloway)

TYPE OF DRUG
Muscle relaxant and analgesic

INGREDIENTS
chlorzoxazone and acetaminophen

DOSAGE FORMS
Tablets (250 mg chlorzoxazone and 300 mg acetaminophen)
Capsules (250 mg chlorzoxazone and 300 mg acetaminophen)

STORAGE
Chlorzoxazone and acetaminophen combination tablets and capsules should be stored at room temperature in a tightly closed container.

USES

Chlorzoxazone and acetaminophen combination is used to relax muscles and to relieve the pain of sprains, strains, and other muscle injuries. Chlorzoxazone acts as a central nervous system (brain and spinal cord) depressant, which blocks reflexes involved in producing and maintaining muscle spasms. It does not act directly on tense muscles.

TREATMENT

This medication should be taken with a full glass of water. In order to avoid stomach irritation, you can also take this medication with food or milk (unless your doctor directs you to do otherwise).

If you miss a dose of this medication, take the missed dose as soon as possible, unless it is within three hours of your next scheduled dose. In that case, do not take the missed dose at all; just return to your regular dosing schedule. Do not double the next dose.

SIDE EFFECTS

Minor. Constipation, diarrhea, dizziness, drowsiness, fatigue, headache, heartburn, light-headedness, nausea, nervousness, overstimulation, stomach cramps, or vomiting. These side effects should disappear as your body adjusts to the medication.

Chlorzoxazone can cause your urine to become orange or reddish-purple in color. This is a harmless effect that will disappear when you stop taking the drug.

If you are constipated, increase the amount of fiber in your diet (fresh fruits and vegetables, salads, bran, and whole-grain breads) and drink more water (unless your doctor directs you to do otherwise).

If you feel dizzy or light-headed, sit or lie down for a while; get up slowly from a sitting or lying position, and be careful on stairs.

Major. Tell your doctor about any side effects that are persistent or particularly bothersome. IT IS ESPECIALLY IMPORTANT TO TELL YOUR DOCTOR about bloody or black, tarry stools; difficulty in urinating; fever; rash; sore throat; severe abdominal pain; unusual bleeding or bruising; unusual weakness; or yellowing of the eyes or skin.

INTERACTIONS

Chlorzoxazone and acetaminophen combination interacts with several other types of medications:

1. Concurrent use of chlorzoxazone with other central nervous system depressants (such as alcohol, antihistamines, barbiturates, benzodiazepine tranquilizers, pain medications, narcotics, phenothiazine tranquilizers, and sleeping medications) or with tricyclic antidepressants can cause extreme drowsiness.

2. Alcohol, barbiturates, and anticonvulsants can increase the liver toxicity of large doses of acetaminophen.

3. Long-term use of large doses of acetaminophen can increase the effects of oral anticoagulants (such as warfarin), which can lead to bleeding complications.

Before starting to take this medication, BE SURE TO TELL YOUR DOCTOR about any medications you are currently taking, especially any of those listed above.

WARNINGS

- Tell your doctor about unusual or allergic reactions you have had to any medications, especially to chlorzoxazone or to acetaminophen.
- Tell your doctor if you now have or if you have ever had blood disorders or heart, kidney, liver, or lung disease.
- If this medication makes you dizzy or drowsy, do not take part in any activity that requires alertness, such as driving a car or operating potentially dangerous equipment.
- This medication should not be taken as a substitute for rest, physical therapy, or other measures recommended by your doctor to treat your condition.
- Because this product contains acetaminophen, additional medications that contain acetaminophen should not be taken without your doctor's approval. Check the labels on over-the-counter (nonprescription) pain, sinus, allergy, asthma, diet, cough, and cold products before you use them to see if they contain acetaminophen.
- Be sure to tell your doctor if you are pregnant. Extensive studies have not been conducted to determine whether chlorzoxazone and acetaminophen combination can be used safely during pregnancy. Since this drug may interfere with fetal development, your doctor should decide if the benefits of its use clearly outweigh the possible risks to the fetus. Also, tell your doctor if you are breast-feeding an infant. Small amounts of acetaminophen pass into breast milk. It is not known whether chlorzoxazone passes into the milk.

Choledyl—see oxtriphylline

Choledyl SA—see oxtriphylline

---

cholestyramine

BRAND NAMES (Manufacturers)
Cholybar (Parke-Davis)
Questran (Bristol Labs)
TYPE OF DRUG
Antihyperlipidemic (lipid-lowering drug)
INGREDIENT
cholestyramine
DOSAGE FORM
Oral powder (4 gm of cholestyramine per 9 gm of powder)
Bar (4 gm of cholestyramine per bar)
STORAGE
Cholestyramine should be stored at room temperature in a tightly closed container.

USES

This medication is used to lower blood cholesterol and to treat itching associated with liver disease. Cholestyramine chemically binds to bile salts in the gastrointestinal tract and prevents the body from producing cholesterol.

TREATMENT

Cholestyramine is usually taken before meals. Each dose should be measured carefully, then placed on the surface of two to six ounces of a beverage (water, milk, fruit juice, or other noncarbonated beverage). The powder should be allowed to sit for one to two minutes without being stirred (to prevent lumpiness). The mixture should then be stirred and completely mixed (the powder does not completely dissolve). After the solution has been drunk, the glass should be refilled with the same beverage and this solution swallowed as well (this assures that the whole dose is taken). The powder can also be mixed with soup, applesauce, or crushed pineapple. You should never take cholestyramine dry; you might accidentally inhale the powder, which could irritate your throat and lungs. For the bar form of the drug, chew thoroughly. As with the powder, this should be followed with plenty of fluids.

If you miss a dose of this medication, take the dose you missed as soon as possible, unless it is almost time for the next dose. In that case, do not take the missed dose at all; just return to your regular dosing schedule. Do not double the next dose.

Cholestyramine does not cure hypercholesterolemia (high blood cholesterol levels), but it will help to control the condition as long as you continue to take it.

SIDE EFFECTS

Minor. Anxiety, belching, constipation, diarrhea, dizziness, drowsiness, fatigue, gas, headache, hiccups, loss of appetite, nausea, stomach pain, vomiting, or weight loss or gain. These side effects should disappear as your body adjusts to the medication.

To relieve constipation, increase the amount of fiber in your diet (fresh fruits and vegetables, salads, bran, and whole-grain breads), exercise, and drink more water (unless your doctor directs you to do otherwise).

If you feel dizzy, sit or lie down for a while; get up slowly from a sitting or reclining position, and be careful on stairs.

Major. Tell your doctor about any side effects that are persistent or particularly bothersome. IT IS ESPECIALLY IMPORTANT TO TELL YOUR DOCTOR about backaches; bloody or black, tarry stools; difficult or painful urination; fluid retention; muscle or joint pains; rash or irritation of the skin, tongue, or rectal area; ringing in the ears; swollen glands; tingling sensations; unusual bleeding or bruising; or unusual weakness.

INTERACTIONS

Cholestyramine interferes with the absorption of a number of other drugs, including phenylbutazone, warfarin, thiazide diuretics (water pills), digoxin, penicillins, tetracycline, phenobarbital, folic acid, iron, thyroid hormones, cephalexin, clindamycin, trimethoprim, and fat-soluble vitamins (A, D, E, and K). The effectiveness of these medications will be decreased by cholestyramine. To avoid this interaction, take the other medications one hour before or four to six hours after a dose of cholestyramine.

Before starting to take this medication, BE SURE TO TELL YOUR DOCTOR about any medications you are currently taking, especially any of those listed above.

WARNINGS

- Tell your doctor about unusual or allergic reactions you have had to any medications, especially to cholestyramine.
- Tell your doctor if you now have or if you have ever had bleeding disorders, biliary obstruction, heart disease, hem-

orrhoids, gallstones or gallbladder disease, kidney disease, malabsorption, stomach ulcers, or an obstructed intestine.

• Cholestyramine should be used only in conjunction with diet, weight reduction, or correction of other conditions that could be causing high blood cholesterol levels.

• This product contains the color additive FD&C Yellow No. 5 (tartrazine), which can cause allergic-type reactions (fainting, rash, shortness of breath) in certain susceptible individuals.

• The color of cholestyramine powder may vary from batch to batch. This does not affect the effectiveness of the drug.

• Be sure to tell your doctor if you are pregnant. Although cholestyramine appears to be safe (because very little is absorbed into the bloodstream), extensive studies in humans during pregnancy have not been conducted. Also, tell your doctor if you are breast-feeding an infant. It is not known whether cholestyramine passes into breast milk. However, cholestyramine can decrease the absorption of some vitamins in the mother, which could result in decreased availability of the vitamins to the nursing infant.

Cholybar—see cholestyramine

Cibalith-S—see lithium

cimetidine

BRAND NAME (Manufacturer)
Tagamet (Smith Kline & French)
TYPE OF DRUG
Gastric acid secretion inhibitor (decreases stomach acid)
INGREDIENT
cimetidine
DOSAGE FORMS
Tablets (200 mg, 300 mg, 400 mg, and 800 mg)
Oral liquid (300 mg per 5-ml spoonful, with 2.8% alcohol)
STORAGE
Cimetidine tablets and oral liquid should be stored at room temperature in tightly closed, light-resistant containers. This medication should never be frozen.

USES

Cimetidine is used to treat duodenal and gastric ulcers. It is also used in the long-term treatment of excessive stomach acid secretion and in the prevention of recurrent ulcers. Cimetidine works by blocking the effects of histamine in the stomach, which reduces stomach acid secretion.

TREATMENT

In order to obtain the maximum effect, cimetidine should be taken with, or shortly after, meals and again at bedtime (unless your doctor directs you to do otherwise).

The tablets should not be crushed or chewed, because cimetidine has a bitter taste and an unpleasant odor.

The oral liquid should be measured carefully with a specially designed 5-ml measuring spoon. An ordinary kitchen teaspoon is not accurate enough.

Antacids can block the absorption of cimetidine. If you are taking antacids as well as cimetidine, at least one hour should separate doses of the two medications.

If you miss a dose of cimetidine, take the missed dose as soon as possible, unless it is almost time for the next dose. In that case, do not take the missed dose at all; just return to your regular dosing schedule. Do not double the next dose.

SIDE EFFECTS

Minor. Diarrhea, dizziness, drowsiness, headache, or muscle pain. These side effects should disappear as your body adjusts to the medication.

If you feel dizzy, sit or lie down for a while; get up slowly from a sitting or reclining position, and be careful on stairs.

Major. Tell your doctor about any side effects that are persistent or particularly bothersome. IT IS ESPECIALLY IMPORTANT TO TELL YOUR DOCTOR about confusion, fever, hair loss, enlarged or painful breasts (in both sexes), hallucinations, impotence, palpitations, rash, sore throat, unusual bleeding or bruising, weakness, or yellowing of the eyes or skin.

INTERACTIONS

Cimetidine interacts with other types of medications:

1. It can decrease the elimination, and thus increase the side effects, of theophylline, aminophylline, oxtriphylline, phenytoin, carbamazepine, beta blockers, benzodiazepine tranquilizers (such as clorazepate, chlordiazepoxide, diazepam, flurazepam, halazepam, and prazepam), tricyclic antidepressants, oral anticoagulants (blood thinners, such as warfarin), lidocaine, verapamil, quinidine, nifedipine, metronidazole, codeine, and morphine.

2. The combination of cimetidine and antineoplastic agents (anticancer drugs) may increase the risk of blood disorders.

3. The absorption of ketoconazole is decreased by cimetidine; at least two hours should separate doses of these two drugs.

4. Cimetidine may decrease the blood levels and effectiveness of digoxin.

BE SURE TO TELL YOUR DOCTOR about any medications you are currently taking, especially any of those listed above.

WARNINGS

• Tell your doctor about any unusual or allergic reactions you have had to medications, especially to cimetidine, famotidine, nizatidine, or ranitidine.

• Tell your doctor if you now have or if you have ever had arthritis, kidney disease, liver disease, or organic brain syndrome.

• Cimetidine can decrease the elimination of alcohol from the body, which can prolong its intoxicating effects.

• Cimetidine should be taken continuously for as long as your doctor prescribes. Stopping therapy early may be a cause of ineffective treatment.

• Cigarette smoking may block the beneficial effects of therapy with cimetidine.

• If this drug makes you dizzy or drowsy, do not take part in any activity that requires alertness, such as driving a car or operating potentially dangerous equipment.

• Be sure to tell your doctor if you are pregnant. Cimetidine appears to be safe during pregnancy; however, extensive testing has not been conducted. Also, tell your doctor if you are breast-feeding an infant. Small amounts of cimetidine pass into breast milk.

Cinobac—see cinoxacin

cinoxacin

BRAND NAME (Manufacturer)
Cinobac (Dista)
TYPE OF DRUG
Antibiotic
INGREDIENT
cinoxacin
DOSAGE FORM
Capsules (250 mg and 500 mg)
STORAGE
Cinoxacin capsules should be stored at room temperature in a tightly closed container.

USES

Cinoxacin is an antibiotic that is used to treat bacterial urinary tract infections. It chemically attaches to the bacteria, preventing their growth and multiplication. It kills susceptible bacteria, but it is not effective against viruses, parasites, or fungi.

TREATMENT

In order to prevent stomach irritation, you can take cinoxacin with food or with a full glass of water or milk (unless your doctor directs you to do otherwise).

Cinoxacin works best when the level of medicine in your urine is kept constant. It is best, therefore, to take the doses at evenly spaced intervals day and night. For example, if you are to take four doses a day, the doses should be spaced six hours apart.

Try not to miss any doses of this medication. If you do miss a dose, take it as soon as you remember. However, if you do not remember to take the missed dose until it is almost time for your next dose, take the missed dose immediately; space the following dose about halfway through the regular interval between doses; then continue with your regular dosing schedule.

It is important to continue to take this medication for the entire time prescribed by your doctor (usually seven to 14 days), even if the symptoms disappear before the end of that period. If you stop taking the drug too soon, resistant bacteria are given a chance to continue growing, and your infection could recur.

SIDE EFFECTS

Minor. Abdominal cramps, diarrhea, dizziness, headache, increased sensitivity of the eyes to light, insomnia, loss of appetite, nausea, nervousness, or rectal itching. These side effects should disappear as your body adjusts to the medication.

To relieve the increased sensitivity of your eyes to light, avoid prolonged exposure to sunlight and bright lights, and wear sunglasses.

Major. Tell your doctor about any side effects that are persistent or particularly bothersome. IT IS ESPECIALLY IMPORTANT TO TELL YOUR DOCTOR about confusion, itching, rapid weight gain (three to five pounds within a week), ringing in the ears, skin rash, tingling sensations, visual disturbances, or yellowing of the eyes or skin. Also, if the symptoms of your infection do not improve within several days, contact your doctor.

INTERACTIONS

Probenecid blocks the excretion of cinoxacin into the urinary tract, decreasing its effectiveness.

BE SURE TO TELL YOUR DOCTOR about any medications you are currently taking, especially probenecid.

WARNINGS

- Tell your doctor about unusual or allergic reactions you have had to any medications, especially to cinoxacin, nalidixic acid, or norfloxacin.
- Tell your doctor if you now have or if you have ever had kidney disease or liver disease.
- If this drug makes you dizzy, do not take part in any activity that requires alertness, such as driving a car or operating potentially dangerous equipment.
- Cinoxacin has been prescribed for your current infection only. Another infection later on, or one that someone else has, may require a different medicine. Do not give your medicine to other people or use it for another infection unless your doctor specifically directs you to do so.
- Be sure to tell your doctor if you are pregnant. Although cinoxacin use appears to be safe during pregnancy, extensive studies in humans have not been conducted. Also, tell your doctor if you are breast-feeding an infant. It is not known whether cinoxacin passes into breast milk.

Cin-Quin—see quinidine

Cipro—see ciprofloxacin

ciprofloxacin

BRAND NAME (Manufacturer)
Cipro (Miles)
TYPE OF DRUG
Antibiotic
INGREDIENT
ciprofloxacin
DOSAGE FORM
Tablets (250 mg, 500 mg, and 750 mg)
STORAGE
Ciprofloxacin tablets should be stored at room temperature in tightly closed containers away from direct light.

USES

Ciprofloxacin is an antibiotic that is used to treat a wide variety of bacterial infections. It chemically attaches to the bacteria and prevents their growth and multiplication. It is not effective against viruses, parasites, or fungi.

TREATMENT

Ciprofloxacin is best taken two hours after a meal with a full glass (8 ounces) of water. You should drink several additional glasses of water every day, unless your doctor directs you to do otherwise. Drinking extra water will help to prevent unwanted effects of ciprofloxacin.

Ciprofloxacin works best when the level of medicine in your bloodstream is kept constant. It is best, therefore, to take the doses at evenly spaced intervals day and night. For example, if you are to take two doses a day, the doses should be spaced 12 hours apart.

It is very important that you do not miss any doses of this medication. If you do miss a dose, take it as soon as you remember. However, if you do not remember to take the missed dose until it is almost time for your next dose, skip the missed dose and go back to your regular dosing schedule. Do not double the next dose.

Ciprofloxacin therapy may be required for four to six weeks or longer. It is important to continue to take this drug for the entire time prescribed, even if the symptoms of infection disappear before the end of that period. If you stop taking the drug too soon, resistant bacteria are given a chance to continue growing, and your infection could recur.

SIDE EFFECTS

Minor. Diarrhea, headache, light-headedness, nausea, stomach irritation, or vomiting. These side effects should disappear as your body adjusts to the medication.

Major. Tell your doctor about any side effects that are persistent or particularly bothersome. IT IS ESPECIALLY IMPORTANT TO TELL YOUR DOCTOR about blood in your urine, change in your vision, confusion, convulsions (seizures), agitation, dizziness, hallucinations, lower back pain, muscle or joint pain, pain or difficulty in urinating, restlessness, skin rash, tremor, unpleasant taste, unusual bleeding or bruising, or yellowing of the eyes or skin. Also, if the symptoms of your infection do not improve in several days, contact your doctor.

INTERACTIONS

Ciprofloxacin interacts with several other drugs:

1. Use of antacids with ciprofloxacin can decrease the absorption of this medicine. Do not take antacids within two hours of taking this medicine.

2. Use of sucralfate with ciprofloxacin can decrease the absorption of ciprofloxacin. Do not take a dose of sucralfate within two hours of a dose of ciprofloxacin unless directed to do so by your doctor.

3. Use of medicine containing theophylline along with ciprofloxacin can lead to increased bloodstream levels of theophylline and therefore to an increased chance of theophylline-related side effects.

4. Regular consumption of large quantities of caffeine-containing products (coffee, tea, or caffeine-containing soft drinks) with ciprofloxacin may lead to exaggerated or prolonged effects of caffeine. Your doctor may wish for you to restrict intake of caffeine during treatment.

5. Use of probenecid with ciprofloxacin can increase the bloodstream levels of ciprofloxacin and thus increase the risk of ciprofloxacin-related side effects.

Before starting to take ciprofloxacin, BE SURE TO TELL YOUR DOCTOR about any other medications you are currently taking, especially any of those listed above.

WARNINGS

- Tell your doctor about unusual or allergic reactions you have had to any medications, especially to ciprofloxacin, enoxacin, norfloxacin, cinoxacin, or nalidixic acid.
- Before starting to take this medication, be sure to tell your doctor if you now have or if you have ever had brain or spinal cord disease, epilepsy, kidney disease, or liver disease.
- To decrease the potential for harmful effects on your kidneys, you should increase your intake of fluids (nonalcoholic) unless your doctor directs you to do otherwise.
- Ciprofloxacin can cause dizziness or light-headedness, so patients taking this medicine should know how they react to this medicine before they operate an automobile or machinery, or engage in activities requiring alertness or coordination.
- This medicine can make your skin more sensitive to the sun. When you first begin taking this drug, avoid too much sun and do not use a sunlamp until you see how your skin responds to short periods of sun exposure. This is especially important if you tend to sunburn easily.
- Ciprofloxacin has been prescribed for your current infection only. Another infection later on, or one that someone else has, may require a different medicine. You should not give your medicine to other people or use it for other infections, unless your doctor specifically directs you to do so.
- Be sure to tell your doctor if you are pregnant. This drug is not recommended for use in pregnant women because it can result in serious adverse effects in the developing fetus. Also, tell your doctor if you are breast-feeding an infant. It is not known whether ciprofloxacin passes into breast milk.

---

clemastine

BRAND NAMES (Manufacturers)

Tavist (Sandoz)
Tavist-1 (Sandoz)

TYPE OF DRUG

Antihistamine

INGREDIENT

clemastine fumarate

DOSAGE FORMS

Tablets (1 mg and 2 mg)
Oral syrup (0.5 mg per 5-ml spoonful, with 5.5% alcohol)

STORAGE

Clemastine tablets and oral syrup should be stored at room temperature in tightly closed containers.

USES

This medication belongs to a group of drugs known as antihistamines (antihistamines block the action of histamine, a chemical that is released by the body during an allergic reaction). It is, therefore, used to treat or prevent symptoms of allergy.

TREATMENT

To avoid stomach upset, you can take clemastine with food or with a full glass of milk or water (unless your doctor directs you to do otherwise).

Each dose of the oral syrup should be measured carefully with a specially designed 5-ml measuring spoon. An ordinary kitchen teaspoon is not accurate enough.

If you miss a dose of this medication, take the missed dose as soon as possible, unless it is almost time for your next dose. In that case, do not take the missed dose at all; just return to your regular dosing schedule. Do not double the next dose.

SIDE EFFECTS

Minor. Blurred vision; confusion; constipation; diarrhea; difficult or painful urination; dizziness; drowsiness; dry mouth, throat, or nose; headache; irritability; loss of appetite; nausea; restlessness; ringing or buzzing in the ears; stomach upset; or unusual increase in sweating. These side effects should disappear as your body adjusts to the medication.

This medication can cause increased sensitivity to sunlight. It is, therefore, important to avoid prolonged exposure to sunlight and sunlamps. Wear protective clothing, and use an effective sunscreen.

If you are constipated, increase the amount of fiber in your diet (fresh fruits and vegetables, salads, bran, and whole-grain breads), exercise, and drink more water (unless your doctor tells you not to do so).

Chew sugarless gum or suck on ice chips or a piece of hard candy to reduce mouth dryness.

If you feel dizzy or light-headed, sit or lie down for a while; get up from a sitting or lying position slowly, and be careful on stairs.

Major. Tell your doctor about any side effects that are persistent or particularly bothersome. IT IS ESPECIALLY IMPORTANT TO TELL YOUR DOCTOR about change in menstruation, clumsiness, feeling faint, flushing of the face, hallucinations, palpitations, rash, seizures, shortness of breath, sleeping disorders, sore throat or fever, tightness in the chest, unusual bleeding or bruising, or unusual tiredness or weakness.

INTERACTIONS

Clemastine interacts with other types of medications:

1. Concurrent use of it with central nervous system depressants (such as alcohol, barbiturates, benzodiazepine tranquilizers, muscle relaxants, narcotics, pain medications, and phenothiazine tranquilizers) or with tricyclic antidepressants can cause extreme drowsiness.

2. Monoamine oxidase (MAO) inhibitors (isocarboxazid, pargyline, phenelzine, tranylcypromine) can increase the side effects of this medication. At least 14 days should separate the use of this drug and the use of an MAO inhibitor.

3. Clemastine can also decrease the activity of oral anticoagulants (blood thinners, such as warfarin).

BE SURE TO TELL YOUR DOCTOR about any medications you are currently taking, especially any of the medications that are listed above.

WARNINGS

- Tell your doctor about unusual or allergic reactions you have had to any medications, especially to clemastine or to other antihistamines (such as astemizole, azatadine, brompheniramine, carbinoxamine, chlorpheniramine, cyproheptadine, dexchlorpheniramine, dimenhydrinate, dimethindene, diphenhydramine, diphenylpyraline, doxylamine, hydroxyzine, phenidamine, promethazine, pyrilamine, terfenadine, trimeprazine, tripelennamine, and triprolidine).
- Tell your doctor if you now have or if you have ever had asthma, blood vessel disease, glaucoma, high blood pressure, kidney disease, peptic ulcers, enlarged prostate gland, or thyroid disease.
- Clemastine can cause drowsiness or dizziness. Your ability to perform tasks that require alertness, such as driving a car or operating potentially dangerous equipment, may be decreased. Appropriate caution should, therefore, be taken.
- Drinking alcoholic beverages can increase the sedative effects of clemastine.
- Be sure to tell your doctor if you are pregnant. The effects of this medication during pregnancy have not been thoroughly studied in humans. Also, tell your doctor if you are breast-feeding an infant. Small amounts of clemastine pass into breast milk and may cause unusual excitement or irritability in nursing infants.

Cleocin—see clindamycin (systemic)

Cleocin Pediatric—see clindamycin (systemic)

Cleocin T—see clindamycin (topical)

---

clindamycin (systemic)

BRAND NAMES (Manufacturers)
Cleocin (Upjohn)
Cleocin Pediatric (Upjohn)
TYPE OF DRUG
Antibiotic
INGREDIENT
clindamycin palmitate hydrochloride
DOSAGE FORMS
Capsules (75 mg and 150 mg)
Oral suspension (75 mg per 5-ml spoonful)
STORAGE
Clindamycin capsules and oral suspension should be stored at room temperature in tightly closed containers. The oral suspension should not be refrigerated or frozen; when chilled, it thickens and becomes difficult to pour. The suspension form of this medication should be discarded after 14 days because it loses potency after that time.

USES

Clindamycin is an antibiotic that is used to treat a wide variety of bacterial infections. It chemically attaches to the bacteria and prevents their growth and multiplication. Clindamycin kills susceptible bacteria, but it is not effective against viruses, parasites, or fungi.

TREATMENT

In order to prevent irritation to your esophagus (swallowing tube) or stomach, you should take clindamycin with food or a full glass of water or milk (unless your doctor directs you to do otherwise).

The suspension form of this medication should be shaken well just before measuring each dose. The contents tend to settle on the bottom of the bottle, so it is necessary to shake the container to distribute the ingredients evenly and equalize the doses. Each dose should then be measured carefully with a specially designed 5-ml measuring spoon. An ordinary kitchen teaspoon is not accurate enough.

Clindamycin works best when the level of medicine in your bloodstream is kept constant. It is best, therefore, to take the doses at evenly spaced intervals day and night. For example, if you are to take four doses a day, the doses should be spaced six hours apart.

Try not to miss any doses of this medication. If you do miss a dose, take it as soon as you remember. However, if you do not remember to take the missed dose until it is almost time for your next dose, take the missed dose immediately; space the following dose about halfway through the regular interval between doses; then continue with your regular dosing schedule.

It is important to continue to take this medication for the entire time prescribed by your doctor (usually seven to 14 days), even if your symptoms of infection disappear before the end of that period. If you stop taking the drug too soon, resistant bacteria are given a chance to continue growing, and your infection could recur.

SIDE EFFECTS

Minor. Diarrhea, loss of appetite, nausea, stomach or throat irritation, or vomiting. These side effects should disappear as your body adjusts to the medication. If the diarrhea becomes prolonged, CONTACT YOUR DOCTOR. Do not take antidiarrheal medicine.

Major. Tell your doctor about any side effects that are persistent or particularly bothersome. IT IS ESPECIALLY IMPORTANT TO TELL YOUR DOCTOR about bloody or pus-containing diarrhea, hives, itching, muscle or joint pain, skin rash, unusual bleeding or bruising, or yellowing of the eyes or skin. Also, if the symptoms of your infection do not improve in several days, contact your doctor. This medication may not be effective for your particular infection.

INTERACTIONS

Clindamycin should not interact with other medications if it is used according to directions.

WARNINGS

- Tell your doctor about unusual or allergic reactions you have had to any medications, especially to clindamycin or lincomycin.
- Before starting to take this medication, be sure to tell your doctor if you now have or if you have ever had colitis, kidney disease, or liver disease.
- Before having surgery or any other medical or dental treatment, be sure to tell your doctor or dentist that you are taking clindamycin.
- The capsule form of this medication contains the color additive FD&C Yellow No. 5 (tartrazine), which can cause allergic-type symptoms (fainting, shortness of breath, rash) in certain susceptible individuals.
- Clindamycin has been prescribed for your current infection only. Another infection later on, or one that someone else has, may require a different medicine. You should not give your medicine to other people or use it for other infections, unless your doctor specifically directs you to do so.
- Be sure to tell your doctor if you are pregnant. Although clindamycin appears to be safe during pregnancy, extensive studies in humans have not been conducted. Also, tell your doctor if you are breast-feeding an infant. Small amounts of clindamycin pass into breast milk.

clindamycin (topical)

BRAND NAME (Manufacturer)
Cleocin T (Upjohn)
TYPE OF DRUG
Antibiotic
INGREDIENT
clindamycin phosphate
DOSAGE FORMS
Topical solution (10 mg per ml)
Topical gel (1%)
Topical lotion (10 mg per ml)
STORAGE
Clindamycin topical solution, gel, or lotion should be stored at room temperature in a tightly closed container. It should be kept away from flames and heat because the solution is flammable (it contains alcohol).

USES

Clindamycin topical solution is used to treat acne vulgaris. It is an antibiotic that is thought to act by suppressing the growth of the bacteria *Propionibacterium acnes*. These bacteria are probably responsible for the formation of the acne sores.

TREATMENT

Before applying topical clindamycin, wash the affected area thoroughly with a mild soap and warm water. Then rinse well and pat dry. To avoid skin irritation from the alcohol, wait at least 30 minutes after washing or shaving before applying this medication.

The solution is packaged in a bottle with an applicator tip that can be used to apply the solution directly to the skin. Press the applicator tip firmly against your skin. The pressure applied determines the amount of medicine released. Use the applicator with a dabbing motion rather than a rolling motion. A thin film of medication should be applied to the entire area of skin affected by acne.

If you miss a dose of this medication, apply it as soon as possible, unless it is almost time for the next dose. In that case, do not apply the missed dose at all; just return to your regular dosing schedule.

Topical clindamycin does not cure acne, but it helps to control the condition as long as you continue to use it.

It is important to continue to apply this medication for the entire time prescribed by your doctor (which may be several months), even if your symptoms disappear in several days. If you stop applying the medication too soon, the bacteria are given a chance to continue growing, and your infection could recur.

If there is no improvement in your condition after six weeks of using this medication, check with your doctor. However, it may take up to 12 weeks before improvement in your acne is readily apparent.

SIDE EFFECTS

Minor. Diarrhea, dry skin, fatigue, headache, nausea, oily skin, or stomach irritation. These side effects should disappear as your body adjusts to the medication.

If diarrhea becomes severe or prolonged, CONTACT YOUR DOCTOR. Do not take any antidiarrheal medicine.

Major. Tell your doctor about any side effects that are per-

sistent or particularly bothersome. IT IS ESPECIALLY IMPORTANT TO TELL YOUR DOCTOR about bloody or pus-containing diarrhea, increased urination, itching, sore throat, or swelling of the face.

INTERACTIONS

If you are using another topical medication as well as clindamycin, it is best to apply them at different times to increase effectiveness and reduce the chance of skin irritation.

Use of abrasive or medicated cleansers, medicated cosmetics, or any topical, alcohol-containing preparations (such as after-shave lotions or perfume) along with topical clindamycin can result in excessive skin dryness and irritation.

WARNINGS

- Tell your doctor about unusual or allergic reactions you have had to any drugs, especially to clindamycin or lincomycin.
- Tell your doctor if you have ever had colitis.
- Because this medication contains alcohol, it can cause skin irritation in sensitive areas. In addition, it has an unpleasant taste if it gets on the mouth or lips. You should avoid getting this medication in your eyes, nose, or mouth, or in the areas surrounding scratches or burns.
- You may continue to use cosmetics while applying this medication (unless otherwise directed by your doctor), but it is best to use only "water-based" cosmetics rather than ones with an oil base.
- Be sure to tell your doctor if you are pregnant. Although topical clindamycin appears to be safe during pregnancy, extensive studies in humans have not been conducted. Also, tell your doctor if you are breast-feeding an infant. It is not known whether topical clindamycin passes into breast milk.

Clindex—see chlordiazepoxide and clidinium combination

Clinoril—see sulindac

Clinoxide—see chlordiazepoxide and clidinium combination

Clipoxide—see chlordiazepoxide and clidinium combination

---

clofibrate

BRAND NAMES (Manufacturers)

Atromid-S (Ayerst)
clofibrate (various manufacturers)

TYPE OF DRUG

Antihyperlipidemic (lipid-lowering drug)

INGREDIENT

clofibrate

DOSAGE FORM

Capsules (500 mg)

STORAGE

Clofibrate should be stored at room temperature in a tightly closed, light-resistant container.

USES

Clofibrate is used to reduce fat (lipid) or cholesterol in the blood in patients with atherosclerosis (hardening of the arteries) and in patients having certain kinds of skin lesions caused by excessive fat levels in the blood. It is not clearly understood how clofibrate works, but it appears to decrease the body's production of cholesterol and fats.

Attempts are usually made to control serum fat levels with diet, exercise, weight loss, or control of diabetes before therapy with this drug is initiated.

TREATMENT

Clofibrate should be taken with food or immediately after a meal (unless your doctor directs you to do otherwise).

If you miss a dose of this medication, take the missed dose as soon as possible, unless it is almost time for the next dose. In that case, do not take the missed dose at all; just return to your regular dosing schedule. Do not double the next dose.

SIDE EFFECTS

Minor. Abdominal cramps, bloating, blurred vision, decreased sexual desire, diarrhea, dizziness, drowsiness, dry and brittle hair, dry skin, fatigue, gas, headache, increased sweating, itching, muscle cramps, nausea, sore mouth, vomiting, weakness, or weight gain. These side effects should disappear as your body adjusts to the medication.

If you feel dizzy, sit or lie down for a while; get up slowly from a sitting or reclining position, and be careful on stairs.

Major. Tell your doctor about any side effects that are persistent or particularly bothersome. IT IS ESPECIALLY IMPORTANT TO TELL YOUR DOCTOR about bloody or black, tarry stools; chest pain; difficult or painful urination; impotence; loss of hair; rash; palpitations; sore joints; tremors; or unusual bleeding or bruising.

INTERACTIONS

Clofibrate interacts with several other types of medications:

1. It can increase the side effects of oral anticoagulants (blood thinners, such as warfarin) and oral antidiabetic agents.
2. Rifampin can decrease the effectiveness of clofibrate.
3. Probenecid and furosemide can increase the side effects of clofibrate.

Before starting to take clofibrate, BE SURE TO TELL YOUR DOCTOR about any medications you are currently taking, especially any of those listed above.

WARNINGS

- Tell your doctor about unusual or allergic reactions you have had to any medications, especially to clofibrate.
- Before starting to take this medication, be sure to tell your doctor if you now have or if you have ever had diabetes mellitus, gallstones, heart disease, kidney disease, liver disease, stomach ulcers, or thyroid disease.
- Do not stop taking this medication without first checking with your doctor. Stopping this medication abruptly may lead to an increase in your blood fat levels. Your doctor may want you to follow a special diet to prevent this from happening.
- Be sure to tell your doctor if you are pregnant. Clofibrate crosses the placenta and can build up in the body of the developing fetus. Because clofibrate has long-term effects on

the body, you should not become pregnant for at least two months after you stop taking this drug. Also, tell your doctor if you are breast-feeding an infant. It is not known whether clofibrate passes into breast milk.

Clomid—see clomiphene

---

clomiphene

BRAND NAMES (Manufacturers)
Clomid (Merrell Dow)
Serophene (Serono)
TYPE OF DRUG
Fertility drug
INGREDIENT
clomiphene
DOSAGE FORM
Tablets (50 mg)
STORAGE
Clomiphene should be stored at room temperature in a tightly closed, light-resistant container.

USES

Clomiphene is used to treat infertility in women. It reverses some types of infertility by stimulating ovulation.

TREATMENT

Clomiphene can be taken either on an empty stomach or with food or milk, as directed by your doctor.

It is very important to follow your dosing schedule carefully. If you have any questions about how to take this medication, BE SURE TO CHECK WITH YOUR DOCTOR.

If you miss a dose of this medication, take the missed dose as soon as possible. If you do not remember until it is time for the next dose, double the dose, then return to your regular dosing schedule. If you miss more than one dose, CHECK WITH YOUR DOCTOR.

SIDE EFFECTS

Minor. Abdominal discomfort, bloating, dizziness, headache, insomnia, nausea, nervousness, or vomiting. These side effects should disappear as your body adjusts to the medication.

If you feel dizzy, sit or lie down for a while; get up slowly from a sitting or reclining position, and be careful on stairs.

Major. Tell your doctor about any side effects that are persistent or particularly bothersome. IT IS ESPECIALLY IMPORTANT TO TELL YOUR DOCTOR about breast tenderness, depression, fatigue, hair loss, hot flashes, pelvic pain, skin rash, or visual disturbances.

INTERACTIONS

Clomiphene should not interact with other medications if it is used according to directions.

WARNINGS

- Tell your doctor about unusual or allergic reactions you have had to any medications, especially to clomiphene.
- Before starting to take clomiphene, tell your doctor if you now have or if you have ever had abnormal vaginal bleeding, clotting problems, tumors or cysts of the uterus or ovaries, liver disease, or mental depression.
- If this drug makes you dizzy, do not take part in any activity that requires alertness, such as driving a car or operating potentially dangerous equipment.
- While taking this medication, it is important to carefully follow your doctor's directions for recording your body temperature and for the timing of sexual intercourse.
- The risk of a multiple pregnancy is increased when clomiphene is used. This medication should not be taken if you are already pregnant. If you should become pregnant during treatment with clomiphene, tell your doctor immediately and, unless directed to do otherwise, discontinue the medication at once. It has been reported to cause birth defects in the offspring of animals that received large doses of clomiphene during pregnancy. Also, tell your doctor if you are breast-feeding an infant. It is not known whether clomiphene passes into breast milk.

---

clonazepam

BRAND NAME (Manufacturer)
Klonopin (Roche)
TYPE OF DRUG
Benzodiazepine anticonvulsant
INGREDIENT
clonazepam
DOSAGE FORM
Tablets (0.5 mg, 1 mg, and 2 mg)
STORAGE
Clonazepam should be stored at room temperature in a tightly closed, light-resistant container.

USES

This medication is used to treat certain seizure disorders. It is unclear exactly how clonazepam works to treat convulsions, but it appears to prevent the spread of seizures to all parts of the brain.

TREATMENT

This medication can be taken either on an empty stomach or with food or milk (as directed by your doctor).

Clonazepam works best when the level of medicine in your bloodstream is kept constant. It is best, therefore, to take the doses at evenly spaced intervals day and night. For example, if you are to take three doses a day, the doses should be spaced eight hours apart.

Try not to miss any doses of this medication. If you do miss a dose and remember within an hour, take the dose immediately. If more than an hour has passed, do not take the missed dose at all; just return to your regular dosing schedule. Do not double the next dose. If you miss two or more doses, CONTACT YOUR DOCTOR.

SIDE EFFECTS

Minor. Constipation, diarrhea, drowsiness, dry mouth, headache, increased appetite, insomnia, loss of appetite, nausea, runny nose, or weight loss or gain. These side effects should disappear as your body adjusts to the medication.

In order to relieve constipation, increase the amount of fiber in your diet (fresh fruits and vegetables, salads, bran, and whole-grain breads), exercise, and drink more water (unless your doctor directs you to do otherwise).

To relieve mouth dryness, chew sugarless gum or suck on ice chips or a piece of hard candy.

Major. Tell your doctor about any side effects that are persistent or particularly bothersome. IT IS ESPECIALLY IMPORTANT TO TELL YOUR DOCTOR about behavioral problems, confusion, depression, fever, fluid retention, hair loss, hallucinations, hysteria, increased or decreased urination, muscle weakness, palpitations, skin rash, slurred speech, sore gums, tremors, unusual bleeding or bruising, unusual body movements, or yellowing of the eyes or skin.

Clonazepam can also produce an increase in salivation, so it should be used cautiously by people who have swallowing difficulties. Contact your doctor if salivation becomes a problem.

INTERACTIONS

Clonazepam interacts with several other types of drugs:

1. Concurrent use of it with other central nervous system depressants (such as alcohol, antihistamines, barbiturates, benzodiazepine tranquilizers, muscle relaxants, narcotics, pain medications, phenothiazine tranquilizers, and sleeping medications) or with tricyclic antidepressants can cause extreme drowsiness.

2. Phenobarbital and phenytoin can decrease the blood levels and effectiveness of clonazepam.

3. Concurrent use of clonazepam and valproic acid can lead to increased seizure activity.

Before starting to take this medication, BE SURE TO TELL YOUR DOCTOR about any medications you are currently taking, especially any of those listed above.

WARNINGS

- Tell your doctor about unusual or allergic reactions you have had to any medications, especially to clonazepam or to other benzodiazepine tranquilizers (such as alprazolam, chlordiazepoxide, clorazepate, diazepam, flurazepam, halazepam, lorazepam, oxazepam, prazepam, temazepam, and triazolam).
- Tell your doctor if you now have or if you have ever had glaucoma, kidney disease, liver disease, or lung disease.
- If this drug makes you dizzy or drowsy, do not take part in any activity that requires alertness, such as driving a car or operating potentially dangerous equipment. Children should be careful while playing.
- Do not stop taking this medication unless you first check with your doctor. If you have been taking this medication for several months or longer, stopping the drug abruptly could lead to a withdrawal reaction and a worsening of your condition. Your doctor may, therefore, want to reduce your dosage of this medication gradually.
- Be sure to tell your doctor if you are pregnant. Although no harmful effects have been reported during pregnancy, extensive studies have not been conducted. The risks and benefits of clonazepam therapy during pregnancy should be discussed with your doctor. Also, tell your doctor if you are breast-feeding an infant. Small amounts of clonazepam pass into breast milk and may cause excessive drowsiness in nursing infants.

clonidine

BRAND NAMES (Manufacturers)
Catapres (Boehringer Ingelheim)
Catapres-TTS (Boehringer Ingelheim)
clonidine hydrochloride (various manufacturers)

TYPE OF DRUG
Antihypertensive

INGREDIENT
clonidine hydrochloride

DOSAGE FORMS
Tablets (0.1 mg, 0.2 mg, and 0.3 mg)
Transdermal patch (2.5 mg, 5 mg, and 7.5 mg per patch; release rate of clonidine is 0.1 mg, 0.2 mg, and 0.3 mg per 24 hours)

STORAGE
Clonidine tablets should be stored at room temperature in a tightly closed container. Do not remove a patch from its packaging until just before you apply it.

USES

This medication works on the central nervous system (brain and spinal cord) to prevent the release of chemicals responsible for maintaining high blood pressure.

TREATMENT

To avoid stomach irritation, you can take clonidine tablets with food or with a full glass of milk or water. In order to become accustomed to taking this medication, try to take it at the same time(s) every day.

Clonidine transdermal patches come with detailed patient instructions that should be carefully followed. Apply the patch to a hairless area of unbroken skin on the upper arm or chest. If the patch becomes loose before it is time to remove it (after seven days), apply adhesive tape over the patch to ensure good adhesion. To avoid skin irritation, apply each new patch to a different site after removing the old one.

If you miss a dose of clonidine tablets, take the missed dose as soon as possible, unless it is almost time for your next dose. In that case, do not take the missed dose at all; just return to your regular dosing schedule. Do not double the next dose. If you miss more than two doses of this medication, contact your doctor.

If you forget to remove the clonidine transdermal patch after seven days, remove the old patch as soon as you remember. Apply a new patch immediately to a different site.

Clonidine does not cure high blood pressure, but it will help control the condition as long as it is taken.

SIDE EFFECTS

Minor. Anxiety, constipation, decreased sexual desire, dizziness, drowsiness, dry eyes, dry mouth, fatigue, headache, insomnia, jaw pain, loss of appetite, nasal congestion, nausea, nervousness, or vomiting. These side effects should disappear as your body adjusts to the medication.

The patches can also cause burning, inflammation, itching, rash, or increased or decreased pigmentation of the skin at the site of application. TELL YOUR DOCTOR if the skin reactions persist or become bothersome.

To prevent constipation, increase the amount of fiber in your diet (fresh fruits and vegetables, salads, bran, and whole-grain breads), unless your doctor tells you not to.

To relieve mouth dryness, suck on ice chips or a piece of hard candy or chew sugarless gum.

"Artificial tears" eye drops may help relieve eye dryness.

To avoid dizziness or light-headedness when you stand, contract and relax the muscles of your legs for a few moments before rising. Do this by pushing one foot against the floor while raising the other foot slightly, alternating feet so that you are "pumping" your legs in a pedaling motion.

Major. Tell your doctor about any side effects that are persistent or particularly bothersome. IT IS ESPECIALLY IMPORTANT TO TELL YOUR DOCTOR about chest pain; cold fingertips or toes; depression; difficulty in breathing; difficulty in urinating; enlarged, painful breasts (in both sexes); hair loss; hives; impotence; itching; nightmares; rash; swelling of the hands or feet; weight gain; or yellowing of the eyes or skin.

INTERACTIONS

Clonidine interacts with several other types of medications:

1. Concurrent use of clonidine with other central nervous system depressants (such as alcohol, antihistamines, barbiturates, benzodiazepine tranquilizers, muscle relaxants, narcotics, pain medications, phenothiazine tranquilizers, and sleeping medications) or with tricyclic antidepressants can cause extreme drowsiness.

2. Tolazoline and tricyclic antidepressants may block the blood-pressure-lowering effects of clonidine.

Before you start to take this medication, BE SURE TO TELL YOUR DOCTOR about any medications you are currently taking, especially any of those listed above.

WARNINGS

- Tell your doctor about any unusual or allergic reactions you have had to medications, especially to clonidine.
- Tell your doctor if you have ever had heart disease, kidney disease, depression, Raynaud's disease, or a heart attack or stroke.
- Before having surgery or any other medical or dental treatment, tell your doctor or dentist you are taking this drug.
- Do not take any over-the-counter (nonprescription) medication for weight control or for allergy, asthma, sinus, cough, or cold problems unless you first check with your doctor.
- If this drug makes you dizzy or drowsy, do not take part in any activity that requires alertness, such as driving a car or operating potentially dangerous equipment.
- Tolerance to this medication develops occasionally; consult your doctor if you feel that the drug is becoming less effective.
- Do not stop taking this medication without first consulting your doctor. If therapy with this drug is stopped abruptly, you may experience nervousness, agitation, headache, and a rise in blood pressure. Your doctor may, therefore, want to reduce your dosage of the drug gradually or start you on another medication.
- Make sure you have enough medication on hand to last through weekends, vacations, and holidays.
- Drinking alcoholic beverages, standing for prolonged periods, exercising, and hot weather can each increase the blood-pressure-lowering effects of clonidine and can cause fainting or dizziness.
- Be sure to tell your doctor if you are pregnant. Although clonidine appears to be safe in animals, extensive studies in humans during pregnancy have not been conducted. Also, tell your doctor if you are breast-feeding an infant. Small amounts of clonidine pass into breast milk.

clonidine hydrochloride—see clonidine

---

clorazepate

BRAND NAMES (Manufacturers)
clorazepate (various manufacturers)
Tranxene-SD (Abbott)
Tranxene T-Tabs (Abbott)

TYPE OF DRUG
Benzodiazepine sedative/hypnotic

INGREDIENT
clorazepate

DOSAGE FORMS
Capsules (3.75 mg, 7.5 mg, and 15 mg)
Tablets (3.75 mg, 7.5 mg, 11.25 mg, 15 mg, and 22.5 mg)

STORAGE
This medication should be stored at room temperature in tightly closed, light-resistant containers.

USES

Clorazepate is prescribed to treat the symptoms of anxiety and sometimes to treat seizures and alcohol withdrawal symptoms. It is not clear exactly how this medicine works, but it may relieve anxiety by acting as a depressant of the central nervous system. Clorazepate is currently used by many people to relieve nervousness. It is effective for this purpose for short periods, but it is important to try to remove the cause of the anxiety as well.

TREATMENT

This medication should be taken exactly as directed by your doctor. It can be taken with food or a full glass of water if stomach upset occurs. Do not take this medication with a dose of antacids, since they may retard its absorption.

If you are taking this medication regularly and you miss a dose, take the missed dose immediately if you remember within an hour. If more than an hour has passed, skip the dose you missed and wait for the next scheduled dose. Do not double the next dose.

SIDE EFFECTS

Minor. Bitter taste in the mouth, constipation, depression, diarrhea, dizziness, drowsiness (after a night's sleep), dry mouth, excessive salivation, fatigue, flushing, headache, heartburn, loss of appetite, nausea, nervousness, sweating, or vomiting. As your body adjusts to the medicine, these side effects should disappear.

To relieve constipation, increase the amount of fiber in your diet (fresh fruits and vegetables, salads, bran, and whole-grain breads), exercise, and drink more water (unless your doctor directs you to do otherwise).

Dry mouth can be relieved by chewing sugarless gum or by sucking on ice chips.

If you feel dizzy, sit or lie down for a while; get up slowly from a sitting or reclining position, and be careful on stairs.

Major. Tell your doctor about any side effects that are per-

sistent or particularly bothersome. IT IS ESPECIALLY IMPORTANT TO TELL YOUR DOCTOR about blurred or double vision, chest pain, difficulty in urinating, fainting, falling, fever, joint pain, hallucinations, mouth sores, nightmares, palpitations, rash, severe depression, shortness of breath, slurred speech, sore throat, uncoordinated movements, unusual excitement, unusual tiredness, or yellowing of the eyes or skin.

INTERACTIONS

Clorazepate interacts with several other types of drugs:

1. To prevent oversedation, this drug should not be taken with alcohol or other sedative drugs, central nervous system depressants (such as antihistamines, barbiturates, muscle relaxants, pain medicines, narcotics, medicines for seizures, and phenothiazine tranquilizers), or with antidepressants.

2. This medication may decrease the effectiveness of carbamazepine, levodopa, and oral anticoagulants (blood thinners) and may increase the effects of phenytoin.

3. Disulfiram, oral contraceptives (birth control pills), isoniazid, and cimetidine can increase the blood levels of clorazepate, which can lead to increased sedation.

4. Concurrent use of rifampin may decrease the effectiveness of clorazepate.

BE SURE TO TELL YOUR DOCTOR about any medications you are currently taking, especially any of those listed above.

WARNINGS

• Tell your doctor about unusual or allergic reactions you have had to any medications, especially to clorazepate or other benzodiazepine tranquilizers (such as alprazolam, chlordiazepoxide, diazepam, flurazepam, halazepam, lorazepam, oxazepam, prazepam, temazepam, and triazolam).

• Tell your doctor if you now have or if you have ever had liver disease, kidney disease, epilepsy, lung disease, myasthenia gravis, porphyria, depression, or mental illness.

• This medicine can cause drowsiness. Avoid tasks that require alertness, such as driving a car or using potentially dangerous equipment.

• This medication has the potential for abuse and must be used with caution. Tolerance may develop quickly; do not increase the dosage without first consulting your doctor. It is also important not to stop taking this drug suddenly if you have been taking it in large amounts or if you have used it for several weeks. Your doctor may want to reduce the dosage gradually.

• This is a safe drug when used properly. When it is combined with other sedative drugs or alcohol, however, serious side effects may develop.

• Be sure to tell your doctor if you are pregnant. This medicine may increase the chance of birth defects if it is taken during the first three months of pregnancy. In addition, too much use of this medicine during the last six months of pregnancy may cause the baby to become dependent on it. This may result in withdrawal symptoms in the newborn. Also, use of this medicine during the last weeks of pregnancy may cause excessive drowsiness, slowed heartbeat, and breathing difficulties in the newborn. Tell your doctor if you are breast-feeding an infant. This medicine can pass into the breast milk and cause excessive drowsiness, slowed heartbeat, and breathing difficulties in the nursing infant.

clotrimazole (topical)

BRAND NAMES (Manufacturers)
Lotrimin (Schering)
Mycelex (Miles)

TYPE OF DRUG
Antifungal

INGREDIENT
clotrimazole

DOSAGE FORMS
Topical cream (1%)
Topical solution (1%)
Topical lotion (1%)

STORAGE
Store at room temperature in tightly closed containers. This medication should never be frozen.

USES

This medication is used to treat superficial fungal infections of the skin. Clotrimazole is an antifungal agent that is active against a broad range of fungi and yeasts. It acts by preventing the growth and multiplication of these organisms.

TREATMENT

Apply this medication in the morning and evening, unless your doctor directs you to do otherwise. Before applying clotrimazole, you should wash your hands. Then (unless otherwise directed) cleanse the affected area with soap and water. Pat the skin with a clean towel until it is almost dry. Gently massage a small amount of the cream, solution, or lotion over the entire area that is affected and the skin immediately surrounding this area. Do not bandage or cover the infection after applying the medication unless your doctor instructs you to do so. Wash your hands again after use.

Improvement in your condition may not become apparent for as much as a week after you begin treatment with this drug. However, you should be sure to complete the full course of therapy. If you stop using this drug too soon, resistant fungi are given a chance to continue growing, and the infection could recur. If your condition has not improved after four weeks of treatment with this medication, however, CONTACT YOUR DOCTOR. Clotrimazole may not be effective against the organism that is causing your infection.

If you miss a dose of this medication, apply the missed dose as soon as possible. If you do not remember until it is almost time for the next dose, however, do not apply the missed dose at all; just return to your regular dosing schedule. Do not use a double dose of the medication at the next application.

SIDE EFFECTS

Minor. You may experience some burning, itching, stinging, or redness when this drug is applied to the skin. These side effects should disappear as your body adjusts to the drug.

Major. Tell your doctor about any side effects that are persistent or particularly bothersome. IT IS ESPECIALLY IMPORTANT TO TELL YOUR DOCTOR about blistering, irritation, peeling of the skin, or swelling.

INTERACTIONS

Clotrimazole should not interact with other medications as long as it is used according to directions.

WARNINGS

• Tell your doctor about any unusual or allergic reactions you have had to medications, especially to clotrimazole.
• This medication has been prescribed for your current infection only. Another infection may require a different medication. Therefore, you should not give your medicine to other people or use it for other infections, unless your doctor specifically directs you to do so.
• Clotrimazole should not be used in or around the eyes.
• In order to avoid reinfection, keep the affected area clean and dry, wear freshly laundered clothing, and try to avoid wearing tight-fitting clothing.
• Be sure to tell your doctor if you are pregnant. Small amounts of clotrimazole may be absorbed through the skin. It should, therefore, be used cautiously, especially during the first three months of pregnancy. Also, tell your doctor if you are breast-feeding an infant. It is not known whether clotrimazole passes into breast milk.

---

clotrimazole (vaginal)

BRAND NAMES (Manufacturers)
Gyne-Lotrimin*(Schering)
Mycelex-G (Miles)
*Available without a prescription in 1% cream or 100 mg tablet.

TYPE OF DRUG
Antifungal

INGREDIENT
clotrimazole

DOSAGE FORMS
Vaginal cream (1%)
Vaginal tablets (100 mg and 500 mg)

STORAGE
Store at room temperature in a tightly closed container. This medication should never be frozen.

USES

This medication is used to treat fungal infections of the vagina. Clotrimazole is an antifungal agent that prevents the growth and multiplication of a wide range of fungi and yeast, including *Candida*.

TREATMENT

Clotrimazole vaginal cream and tablets are packaged with detailed directions for use. Follow these instructions carefully. An applicator will probably be provided for inserting the cream into the vagina. Use this medication at bedtime, unless otherwise directed by your doctor.

You should wash the area carefully prior to inserting the cream or tablet into the vagina.

If you begin to menstruate while being treated with clotrimazole, continue your regular dosing schedule.

If you miss a dose of this medication, insert the missed dose as soon as possible. However, if you do not remember until the following day, do not insert the missed dose at all; just return to your regular dosing schedule. Do not use a double dose of the medication at the next application.

It is important to continue to insert this medication for the entire time prescribed by your doctor—even if the symptoms disappear before the end of that period. If you stop using the drug too soon, resistant fungus is given a chance to continue growing, and your infection could recur.

SIDE EFFECTS

Minor. You may experience vaginal burning, itching, or irritation when this drug is inserted. This sensation should disappear as your body adjusts to the medication. Your sexual partner may also experience some burning or irritation.

Do not treat any side effects that occur in the area of the infection unless you first consult your doctor.

Major. Tell your doctor about any side effects that are persistent or particularly bothersome. IT IS ESPECIALLY IMPORTANT TO TELL YOUR DOCTOR about abdominal cramps, blistering, bloating, excessive irritation, painful urination, or peeling of the skin.

INTERACTIONS

Clotrimazole should not interact with other medications if it is used according to directions.

WARNINGS

• Tell your doctor about unusual or allergic reactions you have had to any medications, especially to clotrimazole.
• Tell your doctor if you have had other vaginal infections, especially if they have been resistant to treatment.
• To prevent reinfection, avoid sexual intercourse or ask your partner to use a condom until treatment is completed.
• There may be some vaginal drainage while using this medication; therefore, you may want to use a sanitary napkin or panty liner to prevent the staining of clothing. However, the use of tampons is not recommended since they may soak up too much of the medicine.
• Wear cotton panties rather than those made of nylon or other nonporous materials while being treated for a vaginal fungus infection. Also, in order to prevent reinfection, always wear freshly laundered underclothes.
• If there is no improvement in your condition, or if irritation in the area continues after several days of treatment, CONTACT YOUR DOCTOR. This medication may be causing an allergic reaction, or it may not be effective against the organism causing your infection.
• This medication has been prescribed for your current infection only. Another infection that develops later on, or one that someone else has, may require a different medication. Therefore, you should not give your medication to other women or use it for other infections unless your doctor specifically directs you to do so.
• Tell your doctor if you are pregnant. Clotrimazole appears to be safe during pregnancy. However, extensive studies have not been conducted. In addition, your doctor may want to change the instructions on how you are to use this drug if you are pregnant. Also, tell your doctor if you are breast-feeding. It is not known whether this drug passes into breast milk.

---

cloxacillin

BRAND NAMES (Manufacturers)
cloxacillin sodium (various manufacturers)

Cloxapen (Beecham)
Tegopen (Bristol)

TYPE OF DRUG
Penicillin antibiotic

INGREDIENT
cloxacillin

DOSAGE FORMS
Capsules (250 mg and 500 mg)
Oral solution (125 mg per 5-ml spoonful)

STORAGE
Cloxacillin capsules should be stored at room temperature in a tightly closed container. The oral solution should be stored in the refrigerator in a tightly closed container. Any unused portion of the solution should be discarded after 14 days because the drug loses its potency after that time. This medication should never be frozen.

USES

Cloxacillin is used to treat a wide variety of bacterial infections, especially those caused by *Staphylococcus* bacteria. It acts by severely injuring the cell walls of the infecting bacteria, thereby preventing them from growing and multiplying. Cloxacillin kills susceptible bacteria, but it is not effective against viruses, parasites, or fungi.

TREATMENT

Cloxacillin should be taken on an empty stomach or with a glass of water one hour before or two hours after a meal. This medication should never be taken with fruit juices or carbonated beverages because the acidity of these drinks destroys the drug in the stomach.

The oral solution should be measured carefully with a specially designed 5-ml measuring spoon. An ordinary kitchen teaspoon is not accurate enough.

Cloxacillin works best when the level of medicine in your bloodstream is kept constant. Therefore, take the doses at evenly spaced intervals day and night. For example, if you are taking four doses a day, the doses should be spaced six hours apart.

If you miss a dose of this medication, take the missed dose immediately. However, if you do not remember to take the missed dose until it is almost time for your next dose, take it; space the following dose about halfway through the regular interval between doses; then return to your regular schedule. Try not to skip any doses.

It is important to continue to take this medication for the entire time prescribed by your doctor (usually seven to 14 days), even if the symptoms of the infection disappear before the end of that period. If you stop taking the drug too soon, resistant bacteria are given the chance to continue growing, and the infection could recur.

SIDE EFFECTS

Minor. Diarrhea, heartburn, nausea, or vomiting. These side effects should disappear as your body adjusts to the medication.

Major. Tell your doctor about any side effects that are persistent or particularly bothersome. IT IS ESPECIALLY IMPORTANT TO TELL YOUR DOCTOR about bloating, chills, cough, darkened tongue, difficulty in breathing, fever, irritation of the mouth, muscle aches, rash, rectal or vaginal itching, severe diarrhea, or sore throat. Also, if your symptoms of infection seem to be getting worse rather than improving, you should contact your physician.

INTERACTIONS

Cloxacillin interacts with several other types of medications:

1. Probenecid can increase the blood concentrations and side effects of this medication.

2. Cloxacillin may decrease the effectiveness of birth control pills, and pregnancy could result. You should, therefore, use a different or additional form of birth control while taking this drug. Discuss this with your doctor.

BE SURE TO TELL YOUR DOCTOR about any medications you are currently taking, especially any listed above.

WARNINGS

• Tell your doctor about unusual or allergic reactions you have had to any medications, especially to cloxacillin or penicillins, cephalosporin antibiotics, penicillamine, or griseofulvin.

• Tell your doctor if you now have or if you have ever had kidney disease, asthma, or allergies.

• This medication has been prescribed for your current infection only. Another infection that develops later on, or one that someone else has, may require a different medicine. You should not give your medicine to other people to use or use your medication for other infections, unless your doctor specifically directs you to do so.

• Diabetics taking cloxacillin should know that this drug can cause a false-positive sugar reaction with a Clinitest urine glucose test. To avoid this problem, switch to Clinistix or Tes-Tape in order to test your urine for sugar.

• Be sure to tell your doctor if you are pregnant. Although cloxacillin appears to be safe during pregnancy, extensive studies in humans have not been conducted. Also, tell your doctor if you are breast-feeding an infant. Small amounts of this medication pass into breast milk and may temporarily alter the bacterial balance in the intestinal tract of the nursing infant, resulting in diarrhea.

cloxacillin sodium—see cloxacillin

Cloxapen—see cloxacillin

---

clozapine

BRAND NAME (Manufacturer)
Clozaril (Sandoz)

TYPE OF DRUG
Antipsychotic

INGREDIENT
clozapine

DOSAGE FORM
Tablets (25 mg and 100 mg)

STORAGE
Clozapine tablets should be stored at room temperature in the unit-dose packages provided by the manufacturer.

USES

Clozapine is prescribed for the treatment of schizophrenia in patients who have not been helped by or could not tolerate other medications. It is available only through the Clozaril Patient Management Program, which your doctor will arrange for you. This program provides a week's supply of the drug at the time your blood is drawn for testing. Clozapine is not available from your pharmacy or drugstore.

TREATMENT

To avoid stomach irritation, you can take this medication with a meal or a glass of water or milk (unless your doctor directs you to do otherwise).

If you miss a dose of this medication, take the missed dose as soon as possible, then return to your regular dosing schedule. If it is almost time for the next dose, however, skip the one you missed and return to your regular schedule. Do not double the next dose (unless your doctor directs you to do so).

The full effects of this medication for the control of emotional or mental symptoms may not become apparent for two weeks after you start to take it.

SIDE EFFECTS

Minor. Abdominal discomfort, constipation, dizziness, drowsiness, dry mouth, headache, heartburn, increased saliva production, light-headedness, nausea, vomiting, or weight gain. As your body adjusts to the medication, these side effects should disappear.

If you are constipated, increase the amount of fiber in your diet (fresh fruits and vegetables, salads, bran, and whole-grain breads), exercise, and drink more water (unless your doctor directs you to do otherwise).

Chew sugarless gum or suck on ice chips or a piece of hard candy to reduce mouth dryness.

To avoid dizziness or light-headedness when you stand, contract and relax the muscles of your legs for a few moments before rising. Do this by pushing one foot against the floor while raising the other foot slightly, alternating feet so that you are "pumping" your legs in a pedaling motion.

Major. Tell your doctor about any side effects that are persistent or particularly bothersome. IT IS ESPECIALLY IMPORTANT TO TELL YOUR DOCTOR about anxiety, blurred vision, chest pain, chills, confusion, convulsions, difficulty in urinating, fainting, fever, increased sweating, loss of bladder control, mouth sores, muscle stiffness, nightmares, rapid heart rate, rash, restlessness, severe headache, sore throat, tremor, trouble sleeping, or unusual bleeding or bruising.

INTERACTIONS

Clozapine antipsychotic medication interacts with several other types of medications:

1. It can cause extreme drowsiness when combined with alcohol or other central nervous system (brain and spinal cord) depressants, such as barbiturates, benzodiazepine tranquilizers, muscle relaxants, phenothiazine tranquilizers, narcotics, and pain medications, or with tricyclic antidepressants.

2. Lithium may increase the side effects of this drug.

3. The effect of clozapine on blood cells may be increased by other drugs, such as antineoplastics (cancer medicine), antithyroid drugs, azathioprine, chloramphenicol, colchicine, flucytosine, interferon, and zidovudine.

4. The side effects of digoxin, phenytoin, and warfarin may be increased by this medication.

Before starting to take clozapine, BE SURE TO TELL YOUR DOCTOR about any medications you are currently taking, especially any of those listed above.

WARNINGS

- Tell your doctor about unusual or allergic reactions you have had to any medications, especially to clozapine.
- Tell your doctor if you have a history of alcoholism or if you now have or have ever had blood disease, depression, enlarged prostate, gastrointestinal problems, glaucoma, heart or circulatory disease, liver disease, or seizures.
- To avoid oversedation, avoid drinking alcoholic beverages while taking this medication.
- If this drug makes you dizzy or drowsy, do not take part in any activity that requires alertness, such as driving a car or operating potentially dangerous equipment. Be careful on stairs, and avoid getting up suddenly from a lying or sitting position.
- Do not stop taking this medication suddenly. Your doctor may want to gradually reduce the amount you are taking before stopping the drug.
- It is very important that you have your blood tested weekly and that your doctor check your progress regularly. You can only receive the drug after your blood is drawn. The results of your blood tests will assist your doctor in making safe dosage adjustments for you.
- Be sure to tell your doctor if you are pregnant. Although clozapine appears to be safe in animals, extensive studies in humans have not been conducted. Also, tell your doctor if you are breast-feeding an infant. Small amounts of this medication pass into breast milk and may cause unwanted effects in the nursing infant.

Clozaril—see clozapine

---

codeine

BRAND NAMES (Manufacturers)
Codeine Phosphate (various manufacturers)
Codeine Sulfate (various manufacturers)
TYPE OF DRUG
Analgesic and cough suppressant
INGREDIENT
codeine
DOSAGE FORM
Tablets (15 mg, 30 mg, and 60 mg)
STORAGE
Codeine tablets should be stored at room temperature in a tightly closed, light-resistant container.

USES

Codeine is a narcotic analgesic that acts directly on the central nervous system (brain and spinal cord). It is used to relieve mild to moderate pain or to suppress coughing.

TREATMENT

In order to avoid stomach upset, you can take codeine with food or milk.

This drug works best if you take it at the onset of pain, rather than waiting until the pain becomes intense.

If you are taking this medication on a regular schedule and you miss a dose, take the missed dose as soon as possible, unless it is almost time for your next dose. In that case, do not take the missed dose at all; just return to your regular dosing schedule. Do not double the next dose.

SIDE EFFECTS

Minor. Constipation, dizziness, drowsiness, dry mouth, false sense of well-being, flushing, light-headedness, loss of appetite, nausea, painful or difficult urination, or sweating. These side effects should disappear as your body adjusts to the medication.

If you are constipated, increase the amount of fiber in your diet (fresh fruits and vegetables, salads, bran, and whole-grain breads), exercise, and drink more water (unless your doctor directs you to do otherwise).

Chew sugarless gum or suck on ice chips or a piece of hard candy to reduce mouth dryness.

If you feel dizzy, light-headed, or nauseated, sit or lie down for a while; get up from a sitting or lying position slowly, and be careful on stairs.

Major. Tell your doctor about any side effects that are persistent or particularly bothersome. IT IS ESPECIALLY IMPORTANT TO TELL YOUR DOCTOR about anxiety, breathing difficulties, excitation, fatigue, palpitations, rash, restlessness, sore throat and fever, tremors, or weakness.

INTERACTIONS

Codeine interacts with several other types of medications:

1. Concurrent use of this medication with other central nervous system depressants (such as alcohol, antihistamines, barbiturates, benzodiazepine tranquilizers, muscle relaxants, and phenothiazine tranquilizers) or with tricyclic antidepressants can cause extreme drowsiness.

2. A monoamine oxidase (MAO) inhibitor taken within 14 days of this medication can lead to unpredictable and severe side effects.

3. Cimetidine, combined with this medication, can cause confusion, disorientation, and shortness of breath.

BE SURE TO TELL YOUR DOCTOR about any medications you are currently taking, especially any listed above.

WARNINGS

- Tell your doctor about unusual or allergic reactions you have had to medications, especially to codeine or to any other narcotic analgesics (such as hydrocodone, hydromorphone, meperidine, methadone, morphine, oxycodone, and propoxyphene).
- Tell your doctor if you now have or if you have ever had acute abdominal conditions, asthma, brain disease, colitis, epilepsy, gallstones or gallbladder disease, head injuries, heart disease, kidney disease, liver disease, lung disease, mental illness, emotional disorders, prostate disease, thyroid disease, or urethral stricture.
- If this drug makes you dizzy or drowsy, do not take part in any activity that requires alertness, such as driving a car or operating potentially dangerous equipment.
- Before having surgery or other medical or dental treatment, tell your doctor or dentist you are taking this drug.
- Because this product contains codeine, it has the potential for abuse and must be used with caution. Usually, it should not be taken on a regular schedule for longer than ten days (unless your doctor directs you to do so). Tolerance develops quickly; do not increase the dosage or stop taking the drug abruptly unless you first consult your doctor. If you have been taking large amounts of this medication for long periods, you may experience a withdrawal reaction (muscle aches, diarrhea, gooseflesh, runny nose, nausea, vomiting, shivering, trembling, stomach cramps, sleep disorders, irritability, weakness, excessive yawning, or sweating) when you stop taking it. Your doctor may, therefore, want to reduce the dosage gradually.
- Be sure to tell your doctor if you are pregnant. The effects of this medication during the early stages of pregnancy have not been thoroughly studied in humans. However, codeine, used regularly in large doses during the later stages of pregnancy, can result in addiction of the fetus, leading to withdrawal symptoms (irritability, excessive crying, tremors, fever, vomiting, diarrhea, sneezing, or excessive yawning) at birth. Also, tell your doctor if you are breast-feeding an infant. Small amounts of this medication may pass into breast milk and cause excessive drowsiness in the nursing infant.

---

codeine and guaifenesin combination

BRAND NAMES (Manufacturers)

Cheracol (Upjohn)
Guiatuss A.C. (various manufacturers)
Guiatussin with Codeine (Rugby)
Mytussin AC (PBI)
Nortussin with Codeine (Vortech)
Robitussin A-C (Robins)
Tolu-Sed (Scherer)

TYPE OF DRUG

Cough suppressant and expectorant combination

INGREDIENTS

codeine and guaifenesin

DOSAGE FORM

Oral syrup (10 mg codeine and 100 mg guaifenesin per 5-ml spoonful, with 3.5%, 4.75%, or 10% alcohol)

STORAGE

Codeine and guaifenesin combination should be stored at room temperature in a tightly closed container.

USES

This medication is used to relieve coughs due to colds or infections or inflammation of the upper respiratory tract. Guaifenesin is an expectorant, which loosens bronchial secretions. Codeine is a narcotic cough suppressant, which acts on the cough center in the brain.

TREATMENT

You can take codeine and guaifenesin combination syrup either on an empty stomach or, to avoid stomach irritation, with food or milk (as directed by your doctor).

Each dose should be measured carefully with a specially designed 5-ml measuring spoon. An ordinary kitchen teaspoon is not accurate enough.

To help loosen the mucus in the bronchi, you should drink a glass of water after each dose.

If you miss a dose of this medication, take the missed one as soon as possible, unless it is almost time for the next dose. In that case, do not take the missed dose at all; just return to your regular dosing schedule. Do not double the next dose.

SIDE EFFECTS

Minor. Constipation, dizziness, drowsiness, nausea, restlessness, stomach upset, vomiting, or weakness. These side effects should disappear as your body adjusts to the medication.

If you feel dizzy, sit or lie down for a while; get up slowly from a sitting or reclining position, and be careful on stairs.

To relieve constipation, increase the amount of fiber in your diet (fresh fruits and vegetables, salads, bran, and whole-grain breads), exercise, and drink more water (unless your doctor directs you to do otherwise).

Major. Tell your doctor about any side effects that are persistent or particularly bothersome. IT IS ESPECIALLY IMPORTANT TO TELL YOUR DOCTOR about blurred vision; cold, clammy skin; confusion; difficulty in breathing; or fainting.

INTERACTIONS

Codeine and guaifenesin combination can interact with several other types of medications:

1. Concurrent use with other central nervous system depressants (such as alcohol, barbiturates, benzodiazepine tranquilizers, muscle relaxants, other narcotics, pain medications, phenothiazine tranquilizers, and sleeping medications) or with tricyclic antidepressants can lead to extreme drowsiness.

2. Use of a monoamine oxidase (MAO) inhibitor within 14 days of use of codeine and guaifenesin combination can lead to serious side effects.

3. Cimetidine combined with this medication can cause confusion, disorientation, and shortness of breath.

Before starting codeine and guaifenesin combination, BE SURE TO TELL YOUR DOCTOR about any medications you are currently taking, especially any of those listed above.

WARNINGS

- Tell your doctor about unusual or allergic reactions you have had to any medications, especially to guaifenesin or codeine, or to other narcotics (such as hydrocodone, hydromorphone, meperidine, methadone, opium, oxycodone, propoxyphene, and pentazocine).
- Before starting to take this medication, be sure to tell your doctor if you now have or if you have ever had asthma, brain disease, enlarged prostate gland, gallstones or gallbladder disease, gastrointestinal diseases, heart disease, kidney disease, liver disease, lung disease, mental disorders, or thyroid disease.
- If this drug makes you dizzy or drowsy, do not take part in activities that require alertness, such as driving a car or operating potentially dangerous equipment.
- While you are taking this medication, drink at least eight glasses of water a day (to help loosen bronchial secretions).
- Because this product contains codeine, it has the potential for abuse and must be used with caution. Tolerance may develop quickly; you should not use it in higher doses or for longer periods than recommended by your doctor. If you have been taking it for longer than several weeks, do not stop taking it until you first check with your doctor. Stopping the drug abruptly can lead to a withdrawal reaction (body aches, diarrhea, gooseflesh, vomiting, restlessness, runny nose, sneezing, sweating, trembling, or excessive yawning). Your doctor may, therefore, want to reduce your dosage gradually.
- Be sure to tell your doctor if you are pregnant. Large amounts of codeine taken during pregnancy can lead to addiction in the developing fetus, resulting in withdrawal reactions in the newborn infant. Also, tell your doctor if you are breast-feeding an infant. Codeine may pass into breast milk and can cause extreme drowsiness in the nursing infant.

---

codeine and iodinated glycerol combination

BRAND NAMES (Manufacturers)

Iophen-C (various manufacturers)
Oridol C (LuChem)
Tussi-Organidin (Wallace)
Tussi-R-Gen (Goldline)

TYPE OF DRUG

Cough suppressant and expectorant combination

INGREDIENTS

codeine and iodinated glycerol

DOSAGE FORM

Oral liquid (10 mg codeine and 30 mg iodinated glycerol per 5-ml spoonful)

STORAGE

Codeine and iodinated glycerol combination should be stored at room temperature in a tightly closed container. Avoid exposure of this medication to high temperatures.

USES

This drug is used to relieve coughs due to colds or infection or inflammation of the upper respiratory tract. Iodinated glycerol is an expectorant, which loosens bronchial secretions. Codeine is a narcotic cough suppressant, which acts on the cough center in the brain.

TREATMENT

You can take codeine and iodinated glycerol combination on an empty stomach or, to avoid stomach irritation, with food or milk (as directed by your doctor).

Each dose should be measured carefully with a specially designed 5-ml measuring spoon. An ordinary kitchen teaspoon is not accurate enough.

To help loosen the mucus in the bronchi, you should drink a glass of water after each dose.

If you miss a dose of this medication, take the missed one as soon as possible, unless it is almost time for the next dose. In that case, do not take the missed dose at all; just return to your regular dosing schedule. Do not double the next dose.

SIDE EFFECTS

Minor. Constipation, dizziness, drowsiness, nausea, restlessness, stomach upset, vomiting, or weakness. These side effects should disappear as your body adjusts to the medication.

If you feel dizzy, sit or lie down for a while; get up slowly from a sitting or reclining position, and be careful on stairs.

To relieve constipation, increase the amount of fiber in your diet (fresh fruits and vegetables, salads, bran, and whole-grain breads), exercise, and drink more water (unless your doctor directs you to do otherwise).

Major. Tell your doctor about any side effects that are persistent or particularly bothersome. IT IS ESPECIALLY IMPORTANT TO TELL YOUR DOCTOR about blurred vision; cold, clammy skin; confusion; difficulty in breathing; fainting; skin rash; or swollen lymph nodes.

INTERACTIONS

This drug can interact with other types of drugs:

1. Concurrent use with other central nervous system depressants (such as alcohol, barbiturates, benzodiazepine tranquilizers, muscle relaxants, other narcotics, pain medications, phenothiazine tranquilizers, and sleeping medications) or with tricyclic antidepressants can lead to extreme drowsiness.

2. Use of a monoamine oxidase (MAO) inhibitor within 14 days of use of codeine and iodinated glycerol combination can lead to serious side effects.

3. The iodine component of iodinated glycerol can increase the side effects of lithium on the thyroid gland. It can also increase the effects of antithyroid medications.

4. Cimetidine combined with this medication can cause confusion, disorientation, and shortness of breath.

Before starting codeine and iodinated glycerol combination, BE SURE TO TELL YOUR DOCTOR about any medications you are currently taking, especially any of those listed above.

WARNINGS

• Tell your doctor about unusual or allergic reactions you have had to any medications, especially to codeine, or to other narcotics (such as hydrocodone, hydromorphone, meperidine, methadone, opium, oxycodone, propoxyphene, and pentazocine), or to iodinated glycerol, iodine, or iodine-containing dyes.

• Before starting to take this medication, be sure to tell your doctor if you now have or if you have ever had acne, asthma, brain disease, cystic fibrosis, gallstones or gallbladder disease, gastrointestinal diseases, heart disease, kidney disease, liver disease, lung disease, mental disorders, enlarged prostate gland, or thyroid disease.

• If this drug makes you dizzy or drowsy, do not take part in activities that require alertness, such as driving a car or operating potentially dangerous equipment.

• While you are taking this medication, drink at least eight glasses of water a day (to help loosen bronchial secretions).

• Because this product contains codeine, it has the potential for abuse and must be used with caution. Tolerance may develop quickly; you should not use it in higher doses, or for longer periods, than recommended by your doctor. If you have been taking it for longer than several weeks, do not stop taking it until you first check with your doctor. Stopping the drug abruptly can lead to a withdrawal reaction (body aches, diarrhea, gooseflesh, vomiting, restlessness, runny nose, sneezing, sweating, trembling, or excessive yawning). Your doctor may, therefore, want to reduce your dosage gradually.

• Be sure to tell your doctor if you are pregnant. This medication should not be taken during pregnancy. Large amounts of codeine taken during pregnancy can lead to addiction in the developing fetus, resulting in withdrawal reactions in the newborn infant. Iodinated glycerol can cause goiter (an enlarged thyroid gland) in the developing fetus. Also, tell your doctor if you are breast-feeding an infant. Both codeine and iodinated glycerol can pass into the breast milk and cause side effects in the nursing infant.

Codeine Phosphate—see codeine

Codeine Sulfate—see codeine

Codimal-L.A.—see pseudoephedrine and chlorpheniramine combination

Codoxy—see aspirin and oxycodone combination

Cogentin—see benztropine

Co-Gesic—see acetaminophen and hydrocodone combination

---

colchicine

BRAND NAMES (Manufacturers)
colchicine (various manufacturers)
Colchicine (Abbott)
TYPE OF DRUG
Antigout
INGREDIENT
colchicine
DOSAGE FORM
Tablets (0.5 mg, 0.54 mg, 0.6 mg, 0.65 mg)
STORAGE
Colchicine should be stored at room temperature in a tightly closed, light-resistant container.

USES

Colchicine is used to relieve the symptoms of a gout attack and to prevent further attacks. Colchicine prevents the movement of uric acid crystals, which is responsible for the pain in the joints that occurs during an attack of gout.

TREATMENT

Colchicine can be taken on an empty stomach or with food or a full glass of water or milk (as directed by your doctor).

If you are taking colchicine to control a gout attack, it is important that you understand how to take it and when it should be stopped. CHECK WITH YOUR DOCTOR.

If you miss a dose of this medication, take the missed dose as soon as possible, unless it is almost time for the next dose. In that case, do not take the missed dose at all; just return to your regular dosing schedule. Do not double the next dose.

SIDE EFFECTS

Minor. Abdominal pain, diarrhea, nausea, or vomiting. These side effects should disappear as your body adjusts to the medication.

Major. Tell your doctor about any side effects that are persistent or particularly bothersome. IT IS ESPECIALLY IMPORTANT TO TELL YOUR DOCTOR about difficult or painful urination, fever, loss of hair, muscle pain, persistent diarrhea, skin rash, sore throat, tingling in the hands or feet, or unusual bleeding or bruising.

INTERACTIONS

Colchicine interacts with several other types of medications:

1. It can decrease absorption of vitamin B_{12}.

2. The action of colchicine can be blocked by vitamin C and can be enhanced by sodium bicarbonate or ammonium chloride.

3. Colchicine can increase the drowsiness caused by central nervous system depressants.

BE SURE TO TELL YOUR DOCTOR about any medications you are currently taking, especially any of those listed above.

WARNINGS

- Tell your doctor about unusual or allergic reactions you have had to any medications, especially to colchicine.
- Tell your doctor if you now have or if you have ever had blood disorders, gastrointestinal disorders, heart disease, kidney disease, or liver disease.
- Large amounts of alcohol can increase the blood levels of uric acid, which can decrease the effectiveness of colchicine. Alcohol ingestion should, therefore, be limited while you are taking this medication.
- Colchicine is not an analgesic (pain reliever) and does not relieve pain other than that of gout.
- Be sure to tell your doctor if you are pregnant. Colchicine is not recommended for use during pregnancy because it has been reported to cause birth defects in both animals and humans. Also, tell your doctor if you are breast-feeding an infant. It is not known whether colchicine passes into breast milk.

Colchicine—see colchicine

Colestid—see colestipol

---

colestipol

BRAND NAME (Manufacturer)
Colestid (Upjohn)

TYPE OF DRUG
Antihyperlipidemic (lipid-lowering drug)

INGREDIENT
colestipol

DOSAGE FORM
Oral granules (5 g per level 5-ml measuring spoon)

STORAGE
Colestipol should be stored at room temperature in a tightly closed container.

USES

This medication is used to lower blood cholesterol levels. It chemically binds to bile salts in the gastrointestinal tract and prevents the body from producing cholesterol.

TREATMENT

Colestipol is usually taken before meals. Each dose should be measured carefully with a specially designed 5-ml measuring spoon. An ordinary kitchen teaspoon is not accurate enough. The dose should then be added to at least three ounces of fluid (water, milk, fruit juice, or other carbonated or noncarbonated beverage). The mixture should be stirred and completely mixed (the granules do not completely dissolve). After the solution has been drunk, the glass should be refilled with the same beverage and this solution swallowed as well. This ensures that the whole dose is taken. The granules can also be mixed with soup, applesauce, or crushed pineapple. You should never take colestipol dry; you might accidentally inhale the granules, which could irritate your throat and lungs.

If you miss a dose of this medication, take the missed dose as soon as possible, unless it is almost time for the next dose. In that case, do not take the missed dose at all; just return to your regular dosing schedule. Do not double the next dose.

Colestipol does not cure hypercholesterolemia (high blood cholesterol levels), but it will help to control the condition as long as you continue to take it.

SIDE EFFECTS

Minor. Anxiety, belching, constipation, diarrhea, dizziness, drowsiness, fatigue, gas, headache, hiccups, loss of appetite, nausea, stomach pain, vomiting, or weight loss or gain. These side effects should disappear as your body adjusts to the medication.

To relieve constipation, increase the amount of fiber in your diet (fresh fruits and vegetables, salads, bran, and whole-grain breads), exercise, and drink more water (unless your doctor directs otherwise). A stool softener may also be helpful; ask your pharmacist to recommend one.

If you feel dizzy, sit or lie down for a while; get up slowly from a sitting or reclining position, and be careful on stairs.

Major. Tell your doctor about any side effects that are persistent or particularly bothersome. IT IS ESPECIALLY IMPORTANT TO TELL YOUR DOCTOR about backaches; bleeding gums; bloating; bloody or black, tarry stools; difficult or painful urination; muscle or joint pains; rash or irritation of the skin, tongue, or rectal area; ringing in the ears; swollen glands; tingling sensations; unusual bleeding or bruising; or unusual weakness.

INTERACTIONS

Colestipol interferes with the absorption of a number of other drugs, including phenylbutazone, warfarin, thiazide diuretics (water pills), digoxin, penicillins, tetracycline, phenobarbital, folic acid, iron, thyroid hormones, oral vancomycin, adrenocorticosteroids, and the fat-soluble vitamins (vitamins A, D, E, and K). The effectiveness of these medications will be decreased by colestipol. To avoid this interaction, take the other medications one hour before or four to six hours after a dose of colestipol.

BE SURE TO TELL YOUR DOCTOR about any medications you are currently taking, especially any of those listed above.

WARNINGS

- Tell your doctor if you have ever had unusual or allergic reactions to any type of drug, especially to colestipol.

• Before starting to take this drug, be sure to tell your doctor if you now have or if you have ever had bleeding disorders, biliary obstruction, heart disease, hemorrhoids, gallstones or gallbladder disease, kidney disease, malabsorptive disorders, stomach ulcers, or an obstructed intestine.
• Colestipol should be used only in conjunction with a carefully regulated diet, weight reduction, or correction of other conditions that could be causing high blood cholesterol levels.
• Be sure to tell your doctor if you are pregnant. Although colestipol appears to be safe (because none is absorbed into the bloodstream), extensive studies in humans during pregnancy have not been conducted. Also, be sure to tell your doctor if you are breast-feeding an infant. This medication can decrease absorption of some vitamins in the mother, which could result in decreased availability of the vitamins to the nursing infant.

Compazine—see prochlorperazine

Compazine Spansules—see prochlorperazine

Compoz—see diphenhydramine

Condrin-LA—see phenylpropanolamine and chlorpheniramine combination

Conex D.A.—see phenylpropanolamine and chlorpheniramine combination

conjugated estrogens—see estrogens, conjugated

Constant-T—see theophylline

Contac 12-Hour—see phenylpropanolamine and chlorpheniramine combination

Co-Pyronil 2—see pseudoephedrine and chlorpheniramine combination

Coracin—see hydrocortisone, polymyxin B, neomycin, and bacitracin combination (ophthalmic)

Cordran—see flurandrenolide (topical)

Cordran SP—see flurandrenolide (topical)

Corgard—see nadolol

Corque—see hydrocortisone and iodochlorhydroxyquin combination (topical)

Cortaid—see hydrocortisone (topical)

Cortatrigen Modified Ear Drops—see hydrocortisone, polymyxin B, and neomycin combination (otic)

Cort-Dome—see hydrocortisone (topical)

Cortef—see hydrocortisone (systemic)

Cortef Feminine Itch—see hydrocortisone (topical)

Cortin—see hydrocortisone and iodochlorhydroxyquin combination (topical)

cortisone (systemic)

BRAND NAMES (Manufacturers)
cortisone acetate (various manufacturers)
Cortone Acetate (Merck Sharp & Dohme)

TYPE OF DRUG
Adrenocorticosteroid hormone

INGREDIENT
cortisone

DOSAGE FORM
Tablets (5 mg, 10 mg, and 25 mg)

STORAGE
Cortisone tablets should be stored at room temperature in a tightly closed container.

USES

Your adrenal glands naturally produce certain cortisone-like chemicals. These chemicals are involved in various regulatory processes in the body (such as those involving fluid balance, temperature, and reaction to inflammation). Cortisone belongs to a group of drugs known as adrenocorticosteroids (or cortisone-like medications). It is used to treat a variety of disorders, including hormonal disorders; asthma; blood diseases; certain cancers; eye disorders; gastrointestinal disturbances, such as ulcerative colitis; respiratory diseases; and inflammations such as arthritis, dermatitis, and poison ivy. How this drug acts to relieve these disorders is not completely understood.

TREATMENT

In order to prevent stomach irritation, you can take cortisone with food or with milk.

If you are taking only one dose of this medication each day, try to take it before 9:00 A.M. This will mimic the body's normal production of this type of chemical.

It is important to try not to miss any doses of cortisone. However, if you do miss a dose of this medication, follow these guidelines:

1. If you are taking it more than once a day, take the missed dose as soon as possible and return to your regular schedule. If it is already time for the next dose, double the dose.
2. If you are taking this medication once a day, take the dose you missed as soon as possible, unless you don't remember until the next day. In that case, do not take the missed dose at all; just follow your regular dosing schedule. Do not double the next dose.
3. If you are taking this drug every other day, take it as soon as you remember. If you missed the scheduled time by a whole day, take it when you remember, then skip a day before you take the next dose. Do not double the dose.

If you miss more than one dose of cortisone, CONTACT YOUR DOCTOR.

SIDE EFFECTS

Minor. Dizziness, false sense of well-being, fatigue, increased appetite, increased sweating, indigestion, menstrual irregularities, muscle weakness, nausea, reddening of the skin on the face, restlessness, sleep disorders, thinning of the skin, or weight gain. These side effects should disappear as your body adjusts to the medication.

To help avoid potassium loss while using this drug, you can take your dose with a glass of fresh or frozen orange juice, or eat a banana each day. The use of a salt substitute also helps to prevent potassium loss. Do not change your diet or take a salt substitute, however, before discussing it with your doctor.

Major. Tell your doctor about any side effects that are persistent or particularly bothersome. IT IS ESPECIALLY IMPORTANT TO TELL YOUR DOCTOR about abdominal enlargement; acne or other skin problems; back or rib pain; bloody or black, tarry stools; blurred vision; convulsions; depression; eye pain; fever; glaucoma; growth impairment (in children); headaches; impaired healing of wounds; increased thirst and urination; mood changes; muscle wasting; nightmares; rapid weight gain (three to five pounds within a week); rash; severe abdominal pain; shortness of breath; sore throat; unusual bleeding or bruising; or unusual weakness.

INTERACTIONS

Cortisone interacts with several other types of medications:

1. Alcohol, aspirin, and anti-inflammatory medications (such as diflunisal, ibuprofen, indomethacin, ketoprofen, mefenamic acid, meclofenamate, naproxen, piroxicam, sulindac, and tolmetin) aggravate the stomach problems that may occur with use of this medication.

2. The dosage of oral anticoagulants (blood thinners, such as warfarin) and oral antidiabetic drugs or insulin may need to be altered when this medication is started or stopped.

3. The loss of potassium caused by cortisone can lead to serious side effects in individuals taking digoxin. Thiazide diuretics (water pills) and furosemide can increase the potassium loss caused by cortisone.

4. Phenobarbital, phenytoin, rifampin, and ephedrine can increase the elimination of cortisone from the body, thereby decreasing its effectiveness.

5. Oral contraceptives (birth control pills) and estrogen-containing drugs may decrease the elimination of this drug from the body, which can lead to an increase in side effects.

6. Cortisone can increase elimination of aspirin and isoniazid from the body, decreasing their effectiveness.

7. Cholestyramine and colestipol can chemically bind this medication in the stomach and gastrointestinal tract, preventing its absorption.

BE SURE TO TELL YOUR DOCTOR about any medications you are currently taking, especially any listed above.

WARNINGS

- Tell your doctor about unusual or allergic reactions you have had to any medications, especially to cortisone or other adrenocorticosteroids (such as betamethasone, dexamethasone, hydrocortisone, methylprednisolone, paramethasone, prednisolone, prednisone, or triamcinolone).
- Tell your doctor if you now have or if you have ever had bone disease, diabetes mellitus, emotional instability, glaucoma, fungal infections, heart disease, high blood pressure, high cholesterol levels, myasthenia gravis, peptic ulcers, osteoporosis, thyroid disease, tuberculosis, ulcerative colitis, kidney disease, or liver disease.
- If you are using this medication for longer than a week, you may need to receive higher dosages if you are subjected to stress, such as serious infections, injury, or surgery. Discuss this with your doctor.
- If you have been taking this drug for more than a week, do not stop taking it suddenly. If it is stopped suddenly, you may experience abdominal or back pain, dizziness, extreme weakness, fainting, fever, muscle or joint pain, nausea, vomiting, or shortness of breath. Your doctor may, therefore, want to reduce the dosage gradually. Never increase the dose or take the drug for longer than the prescribed time unless you first consult your doctor.
- While you are taking this drug, you should not be vaccinated or immunized. This medication decreases the effectiveness of vaccines and can lead to infection if a live-virus vaccine is administered.
- Before having surgery or any other medical or dental treatment, be sure to tell your doctor or dentist that you are taking this medication.
- If you are taking this medication for prolonged periods of time, you should wear or carry an identification card or notice indicating that you are taking an adrenocorticosteroid drug.
- Because this drug can cause glaucoma and cataracts with long-term use, your doctor may want you to have your eyes examined by an ophthalmologist periodically during treatment.
- This medication can raise blood sugar levels in diabetic patients. Blood sugar should, therefore, be monitored carefully with blood or urine tests when this medication is being taken.
- Be sure to tell your doctor if you are pregnant. This drug crosses the placenta. Although studies in humans have not been conducted, birth defects have been observed in the offspring of animals that were given large doses of this type of drug during pregnancy. Also, tell your doctor if you are breast-feeding an infant. Small amounts of this drug pass into breast milk and can cause growth suppression or a decrease in natural adrenocorticosteroid production in the nursing infant.

cortisone acetate—see cortisone (systemic)

Cortisporin Ophthalmic—see hydrocortisone, polymyxin B, neomycin, and bacitracin combination (ophthalmic)

Cortisporin Otic—see hydrocortisone, polymyxin B, and neomycin combination (otic)

Cortizone-5—see hydrocortisone (topical)

Cortone Acetate—see cortisone (systemic)

Cortril—see hydrocortisone (topical)

Corzide—see nadolol and bendroflumethiazide

Cotazym-S—see pancrelipase

Cotrim—see sulfamethoxazole and trimethoprim combination

Cotrim DS—see sulfamethoxazole and trimethoprim combination

Cotrim Pediatric—see sulfamethoxazole and trimethoprim combination

Coumadin—see warfarin

cromolyn sodium (inhalation)

BRAND NAME (Manufacturer)
Intal (Fisons)
TYPE OF DRUG
Antiallergic (antiasthmatic)
INGREDIENT
cromolyn
DOSAGE FORMS
Capsules (20 mg): for inhalation only
Solution (20 mg per 2-ml ampule): for inhalation only
Aerosol spray 8.1 g and 14.2 g (800 mcg per spray): for inhalation only
STORAGE
Cromolyn sodium capsules and solution should be kept at room temperature in tightly closed, light-resistant storage containers. The container of the aerosol form is pressurized; it should, therefore, never be punctured or broken. It should also be stored away from heat and direct sunlight.

USES

This medication is used to prevent asthma attacks. It is not effective in relieving asthma symptoms once an attack has begun. It works by preventing release of the body chemicals responsible for the symptoms of asthma or allergy.

TREATMENT

Cromolyn sodium capsules are for inhalation only—they should NOT be swallowed. The medication is not effective if swallowed. This medication comes packaged with instructions for use of the capsules with the Spinhaler device. It is very important that you completely understand how to use this device.

The Spinhaler should be cleaned at least once a week. Take the Spinhaler apart and rinse it in clear, warm water. Do not use soap. Allow the inhaler to air-dry before you use it again. If properly cared for, the inhaler should last about six months.

The solution form of this medication should be used only with a power-operated nebulizer equipped with a face mask. It should never be used with a hand-held nebulizer.

The aerosol form of this medication comes packaged with instructions for use. Read the instructions carefully; if you have any questions, check with your doctor or pharmacist. The aerosol can should be shaken well just before each dose is sprayed. The contents tend to settle on the bottom of the container, so it should be shaken to disperse the medication and equalize the doses. The 14.2 g container provides about 200 measured sprays, and the 8.1 g container provides about 112 measured sprays.

Cromolyn sodium is most effective when therapy is started before contact with allergens (the suspected offending agents causing your allergy), so if you expect to be exposed to something to which you know you are allergic, it is a good idea to start taking your medication first.

This medication works best when the level of medicine in your bloodstream is kept constant. It is best, therefore, to take the doses at evenly spaced intervals day and night. For example, if you are to take four doses a day, the doses should be spaced six hours apart.

If you are using another inhaler to open up the lungs (a bronchodilator), it should be used 20 to 30 minutes before using cromolyn sodium. This allows the cromolyn sodium to penetrate more deeply into the lungs.

The full benefits of this medication may not become apparent for up to four weeks after you start to take it.

If you miss a dose of this medication and remember within an hour or so, take the missed dose immediately. If more than an hour has passed, however, do not take the missed dose at all; just return to your regular dosing schedule. Do not double the next dose of this medication.

SIDE EFFECTS

Minor. Cough, dizziness, drowsiness, headache, increased urination, nasal congestion, nasal itching, nausea, sneezing, stomach irritation, or tearing. These side effects should disappear as your body adjusts to the medication.

If you feel dizzy, sit or lie down for a while; get up slowly from a sitting or reclining position, and be careful on stairs.

This medication can cause mouth dryness, throat irritation, and hoarseness. Gargling and rinsing your mouth after each dose helps to prevent these effects.

Major. Tell your doctor about any side effects that are persistent or particularly bothersome. IT IS ESPECIALLY IMPORTANT TO TELL YOUR DOCTOR about itching, joint swelling or pain, nosebleeds, nose burning, painful or increased urination, rash, swelling of the face or eyes, swollen glands, or wheezing.

INTERACTIONS

Cromolyn sodium should not interact with other medications if it is used according to directions.

WARNINGS

- Tell your doctor about unusual or allergic reactions you have had to any drugs, especially to cromolyn sodium.
- Patients who are allergic to lactose, milk, or milk products may be allergic to the capsule form of this drug.
- Before starting to take this medication, tell your doctor if you now have or if you have ever had kidney or liver disease.
- Do not stop taking this medication unless you first check with your doctor. Stopping the drug abruptly may lead to a worsening of your condition.
- Be sure to tell your doctor if you are pregnant. Extensive safety studies in humans have not been conducted. Also, tell your doctor if you are breast-feeding an infant. It is not known whether cromolyn sodium passes into breast milk.

cromolyn sodium (nasal)

BRAND NAME (Manufacturer)
Nasalcrom (Fisons)

TYPE OF DRUG
Antiallergic
INGREDIENT
cromolyn
DOSAGE FORM
Nasal solution (each spray delivers 5.2 mg)
STORAGE
Cromolyn sodium should be stored at room temperature in its original container.

USES

Cromolyn sodium nasal solution is used to prevent and treat allergic rhinitis (inflammation of the nasal passages resulting from allergies). Cromolyn sodium works by preventing the release of the body chemicals responsible for inflammation and swelling.

TREATMENT

This medication is for use within the nose only. The nasal passages should be cleared before administering the spray. You should inhale through the nose as you spray the solution. The container provides about 100 measured sprays.

This medication is most effective when therapy is started before contact with allergens (the suspected offending agents causing your allergy), so if you expect to be exposed to something to which you know you are allergic, it is a good idea to start taking your medication first.

This medication works best when the level of medicine in your bloodstream is kept constant. It is best, therefore, to take the doses at evenly spaced intervals day and night. For example, if you are to take four doses a day, the doses should be spaced six hours apart.

Maximum benefits of this medication may not become apparent for up to four weeks after starting therapy.

If you miss a dose of this medication, take the missed dose as soon as possible, unless it is almost time for the next dose. In that case, do not take the missed dose at all; just return to your regular dosing schedule. Do not double the next dose.

SIDE EFFECTS

Minor. Bad taste in the mouth, headaches, irritation or stinging, nasal burning, postnasal drip, or sneezing. These side effects should disappear as your body adjusts to the medication.

Major. Tell your doctor about any side effects that are persistent or particularly bothersome. IT IS ESPECIALLY IMPORTANT TO TELL YOUR DOCTOR about nosebleeds or skin rash.

INTERACTIONS

Cromolyn sodium should not interact with other medications if it is used according to directions.

WARNINGS

- Tell your doctor about unusual or allergic reactions you have had to any medication, especially to cromolyn sodium.
- Before starting to take this medication, be sure to tell your doctor if you now have or if you have ever had kidney or liver disease.
- Do not stop taking this medication unless you first check with your doctor, even if the symptoms of your disorder disappear. Stopping the drug abruptly can lead to a worsening of your condition. Cromolyn sodium should be continued as long as you have contact with the substance causing your allergic symptoms.
- Be sure to tell your doctor if you are pregnant. Extensive safety studies in humans have not been conducted. Also, tell your doctor if you are breast-feeding an infant. It is not known whether cromolyn sodium passes into breast milk.

Crystodigin—see digitoxin

Cuprimine—see penicillamine

Curretab—see medroxyprogesterone

Cyclan—see cyclandelate

---

cyclandelate

BRAND NAMES (Manufacturers)
Cyclan (Major)
cyclandelate (various manufacturers)
Cyclospasmol (Wyeth)
TYPE OF DRUG
Vasodilator
INGREDIENT
cyclandelate
DOSAGE FORMS
Tablets (200 mg and 400 mg)
Capsules (200 mg and 400 mg)
STORAGE
Cyclandelate should be stored at room temperature in a tightly closed container.

USES

Cyclandelate is used to treat vascular (blood vessel) disease in the legs or brain. It acts directly on the muscle tissue of the blood vessels to increase the blood supply to various parts of the body.

TREATMENT

You can take cyclandelate on an empty stomach (unless your doctor gives you different instructions). However, if the drug causes stomach irritation, you may take it with food, milk, or antacids.

If you miss a dose of this medication, take the missed dose as soon as possible, unless it is almost time for the next dose. In that case, do not take the missed dose at all; just return to your regular dosing schedule. Do not double the next dose of this medication.

SIDE EFFECTS

Minor. Dizziness, drowsiness, flushing, headache, heartburn, stomach distress, or sweating. These side effects should disappear as your body adjusts to the medication.

If you feel dizzy, sit or lie down for a while; get up slowly from a sitting or reclining position, and be careful on stairs.

Major. Tell your doctor about any side effects that are persistent or particularly bothersome. IT IS ESPECIALLY IMPORTANT TO TELL YOUR DOCTOR about palpitations, skin rash, tingling in the hands or feet, or weakness.

INTERACTIONS

Cyclandelate does not interact with other medications if it is used according to directions.

WARNINGS

- Tell your doctor about unusual or allergic reactions you have had to any medications, especially to cyclandelate.
- Before starting to take this medication, tell your doctor if you have ever had angina, bleeding disorders, glaucoma, or a heart attack.
- A government panel has recently reviewed the effectiveness of this medication in the treatment of leg cramps and hardening of the arteries and in the prevention of stroke. This drug may not be as effective as was once thought. Discuss this with your doctor.
- Before taking any over-the-counter (nonprescription) cough, cold, allergy, asthma, sinus, or diet medication, check with your doctor or pharmacist. Some of these products can decrease the effectiveness of cyclandelate.
- If this drug makes you dizzy or drowsy, do not take part in any activity that requires alertness, such as driving a car or operating potentially dangerous equipment.
- The beneficial effects of this medication may be decreased by the nicotine in cigarettes. Try to stop smoking.
- To prevent dizziness and fainting while taking this medication, avoid getting overheated by exercising strenuously in hot weather or by taking hot baths, showers, and saunas.
- Be sure to tell your doctor if you are pregnant. Although cyclandelate appears to be safe during pregnancy, extensive studies in humans have not been conducted, and cautious use is warranted. Also, tell your doctor if you are breast-feeding an infant. It is not known whether cyclandelate passes into breast milk.

---

cyclobenzaprine

BRAND NAMES (Manufacturers)
cyclobenzaprine (various manufacturers)
Flexeril (Merck Sharp & Dohme)
TYPE OF DRUG
Muscle relaxant
INGREDIENT
cyclobenzaprine
DOSAGE FORM
Tablets (10 mg)
STORAGE
Cyclobenzaprine tablets should be stored at room temperature in a tightly closed container.

USES

Cyclobenzaprine is prescribed to relieve muscle pain and stiffness caused by injuries such as sprains or strains. It is not clear how this drug works, but it is thought to act as a central nervous system (brain and spinal cord) depressant that blocks reflexes involved in producing and maintaining muscle spasms. It does not act directly on tense muscles.

TREATMENT

In order to avoid stomach irritation, you can take cyclobenzaprine with food or with a full glass of water or milk.

If you miss a dose of this medication and remember within an hour, take the missed dose; then return to your regular dosing schedule. If more than an hour has passed, do not take the missed dose at all; just return to your dosing schedule. Do not double the next dose.

SIDE EFFECTS

Minor. Abdominal pain, black tongue, blurred vision, constipation, diarrhea, dizziness, drowsiness, dry mouth, fatigue, indigestion, insomnia, loss of appetite, muscle pain, nausea, nervousness, sweating, unpleasant taste in the mouth, vomiting, or weakness. These side effects should disappear as your body adjusts to the medication.

If you are constipated, increase the amount of fiber in your diet (fresh fruits and vegetables, salads, bran, and whole-grain breads) and drink more water (unless your doctor directs you to do otherwise).

If you feel dizzy or light-headed, sit or lie down for a while; get up slowly from a sitting or reclining position, and be careful on stairs.

To relieve mouth dryness, chew sugarless gum, or suck on ice chips or hard candy.

Major. Tell your doctor about any side effects that are persistent or particularly bothersome. IT IS ESPECIALLY IMPORTANT TO TELL YOUR DOCTOR about confusion, depression, difficulty in urinating, disorientation, hallucinations, headache, itching, numbness in the fingers or toes, palpitations, rash, swelling of the face or tongue, tremors, or yellowing of your skin or eyes.

INTERACTIONS

Cyclobenzaprine interacts with several other types of drugs:

1. Concurrent use of cyclobenzaprine with other central nervous system depressants (such as alcohol, antihistamines, barbiturates, antianxiety medications, narcotics, pain medications, tranquilizers, and sleeping medications) or with tricyclic antidepressants can cause extreme drowsiness.

2. Cyclobenzaprine can block the blood-pressure-lowering effects of clonidine and guanethidine.

3. Use of this drug within 14 days of a monoamine oxidase (MAO) inhibitor (tranylcypromine, phenelzine, isocarboxazid, pargyline) can lead to severe reactions and high blood pressure.

Before starting to take this medication, BE SURE TO TELL YOUR DOCTOR about any medications you are currently taking, especially any of those listed above.

WARNINGS

- Tell your doctor about unusual or allergic reactions you have had to medications, especially to cyclobenzaprine or to tricyclic antidepressants (such as amitriptyline, amoxapine, desipramine, doxepin, imipramine, nortriptyline, protriptyline, and trimipramine).
- Tell your doctor if you have ever had blood clots, epilepsy, heart disease, a heart attack, narrow-angle glaucoma, thyroid disease, or urinary retention.
- Use of cyclobenzaprine for periods longer than two to three weeks is not recommended because there is no evidence of benefit with prolonged use and because muscle spasm caused by sprain or strain is generally of short duration.
- This medication should not be taken as a substitute for

rest, physical therapy, or other measures recommended by your doctor to treat your condition.

• If this medication makes you dizzy or drowsy or blurs your vision, do not take part in any activity that requires alertness, such as driving a car or operating potentially dangerous equipment.

• If you have been taking large doses of this medication for prolonged periods, you may experience nausea, headache, or fatigue when you stop taking it, until your body adjusts to the absence of the drug.

• Be sure to tell your doctor if you are pregnant. Although cyclobenzaprine appears to be safe during pregnancy, extensive studies in humans have not been conducted. Also, tell your doctor if you are breast-feeding an infant. It is not known whether cyclobenzaprine passes into breast milk.

---

cyclophosphamide

BRAND NAME (Manufacturer)
Cytoxan (Bristol Myers USP)
TYPE OF DRUG
Antineoplastic (anticancer drug)
INGREDIENT
cyclophosphamide
DOSAGE FORM
Tablets (25 mg and 50 mg)
STORAGE
Cyclophosphamide should be stored at room temperature in a tightly closed container.

USES

Cyclophosphamide belongs to a group of drugs known as alkylating agents or nitrogen mustards. It is used to treat a variety of cancers. Cyclophosphamide works by binding to the rapidly growing cancer cells, preventing their multiplication and growth. This drug has also been used as an immunosuppressant to treat severe rheumatoid arthritis.

TREATMENT

In order to obtain maximum benefit, you should take cyclophosphamide on an empty stomach. However, if stomach upset occurs, you can take it with food or milk (unless your doctor directs you to do otherwise).

The timing of the doses of this anticancer medication is important. Be sure you completely understand your doctor's instructions on how and when this medication should be taken. Try not to miss any doses.

If you miss a dose of this medication, do not take the missed dose at all; just return to your regular dosing schedule. Do not double the next dose.

SIDE EFFECTS

Minor. Diarrhea, loss of appetite, nausea, or vomiting. These side effects may disappear as your body adjusts to the medication. However, it is important to continue taking this medication despite the nausea and vomiting that may occur. Cyclophosphamide also causes hair loss, which is reversible when the medication is stopped.

Major. Tell your doctor about any side effects that are persistent or particularly bothersome. IT IS ESPECIALLY IMPORTANT TO TELL YOUR DOCTOR about blood in the urine, chills, cough, darkening of the skin or fingernails, difficult or painful urination, fever, menstrual irregularities, mouth sores, sore throat, unusual bleeding or bruising, or yellowing of the eyes or skin.

INTERACTIONS

This drug interacts with several other types of drugs:

1. It can decrease the absorption of digoxin from the gastrointestinal tract.

2. Phenobarbital can increase the side effects of cyclophosphamide.

3. Concurrent use of allopurinol, chloramphenicol, chlorpromazine, or thiazide diuretics (water pills) with cyclophosphamide can lead to bone marrow suppression.

4. It can increase the effect of warfarin (blood thinner).

Before starting to take this medication, BE SURE TO TELL YOUR DOCTOR about any medications you are currently taking, especially any of those listed above.

WARNINGS

• Tell your doctor about unusual or allergic reactions you have had to any medications, especially to cyclophosphamide.

• Before starting to take this medication, be sure to tell your doctor if you have ever had blood disorders, chronic or recurrent infections, gout, kidney disease, or liver disease.

• Before having surgery or any other medical or dental treatment, be sure to tell your doctor or dentist that you are taking this medication.

• Cyclophosphamide tablets contain the color additive FD&C Yellow No. 5 (tartrazine), which can cause allergic-type reactions (fainting, shortness of breath, rash) in certain susceptible individuals.

• You should not receive any immunizations or vaccinations while taking this medication. Cyclophosphamide decreases the effectiveness of the vaccine and may result in an infection if a live-virus vaccine is administered.

• It is important to drink plenty of fluids (three quarts each day) while taking this medication. If the drug is allowed to concentrate in the bladder, it can cause bloody urine and can damage the kidneys or bladder.

• This medication can lower your platelet count, which can decrease your body's ability to form blood clots. You should, therefore, be especially careful while brushing your teeth, flossing, or using toothpicks, razors, or fingernail scissors. Try to avoid falls and other injuries.

• This drug can decrease fertility in both men and women.

• Be sure to tell your doctor if you are pregnant. Birth defects have been reported in both animals and humans whose mothers received cyclophosphamide during pregnancy. The risks should be discussed with your doctor. Also, tell your doctor if you are breast-feeding an infant. Since the drug passes into breast milk, a woman should stop breast-feeding before starting cyclophosphamide therapy.

Women of childbearing potential who are not already pregnant when treatment with cyclophosphamide is begun need to use some sort of birth control to prevent pregnancy from occurring. However, oral contraceptives (birth control pills) may not be recommended by your doctor since they may interfere with this medication. Consult with your physician about alternative methods of birth control.

Cyclospasmol—see cyclandelate

---

cyclosporine

BRAND NAME (Manufacturer)
Sandimmune (Sandoz)
TYPE OF DRUG
Immunosuppressant
INGREDIENT
cyclosporine
DOSAGE FORM
Oral solution (100 mg per ml, with 12.5% alcohol)
STORAGE
Cyclosporine oral solution should be stored in the original container at room temperature. This medication should never be refrigerated or frozen. Once the container has been opened, the contents should be used within two months.

USES

Cyclosporine is used to prevent organ rejection after kidney, liver, and heart transplants. It is not clearly understood how cyclosporine works, but it appears to prevent the body's rejection of foreign tissue.

TREATMENT

To make it more palatable, the solution should be diluted with milk, chocolate milk, or orange juice (preferably at room temperature). The dose should be measured carefully with the dropper provided and placed in one of the fluids listed above. Use a glass container (cyclosporine chemically binds to wax-lined and plastic surfaces). Stir well and drink at once—do not allow the mixture to stand before drinking. Refill the glass with the same beverage and drink this solution to ensure that the whole dose is taken. The dropper should be wiped with a clean towel after use and stored in its container. If the dropper needs to be cleaned, make sure it is completely dry before using it again.

It is important not to miss any doses of this medication. If you do miss a dose, take the missed dose as soon as possible, unless it is almost time for the next dose. In that case, do not take the missed dose at all; just return to your regular dosing schedule. Do not double the next dose.

SIDE EFFECTS

Minor. Abdominal discomfort, diarrhea, flushing, headache, hiccups, leg cramps, loss of appetite, nausea, or vomiting. These side effects should disappear as your body adjusts to the medication.

Major. Tell your doctor about any side effects that are persistent or particularly bothersome. IT IS ESPECIALLY IMPORTANT TO TELL YOUR DOCTOR about acne; bleeding, tender, or enlarged gums; convulsions; difficult or painful urination; enlarged and painful breasts (in both sexes); fever; hair growth; hearing loss; muscle pain; rapid weight gain (three to five pounds within a week); sore throat; tingling of the hands or feet; tremors; unusual bleeding or bruising; or yellowing of the eyes or skin.

INTERACTIONS

Cyclosporine interacts with several other types of drugs:

1. Carbamazepine, isoniazid, rifampin, phenytoin, phenobarbital, and trimethoprim/sulfamethoxazole can decrease the blood levels of cyclosporine, decreasing its effectiveness.
2. Cimetidine, diltiazem, erythromycin, ketoconazole, oral contraceptives, danazol, and amphotericin B can increase the blood levels of cyclosporine, which can lead to an increase in side effects.
3. It is important to tell your doctor if you are currently taking corticosteroids, verapamil, or nonsteroidal anti-inflammatory drugs.

BE SURE TO TELL YOUR DOCTOR about any medications you are currently taking, especially any listed above.

WARNINGS

- Tell your doctor about unusual or allergic reactions you have had to any medications, especially to cyclosporine or to polyoxyethylated castor oil.
- Before starting to take this medication, be sure to tell your doctor if you now have or if you have ever had hypertension (high blood pressure) or gastrointestinal disorders.
- Repeated laboratory tests are necessary while you are taking cyclosporine to ensure that you are receiving the correct dosage and to avoid liver and kidney damage.
- Certain cancers have occurred in patients receiving cyclosporine and other immunosuppressant drugs after transplantation. No causal effect has been established, however.
- Do not stop taking this medication without first consulting your doctor. If the drug is stopped abruptly, organ rejection may occur. Your doctor may, therefore, want to reduce your dosage gradually or start you on another drug if treatment with this drug is to be discontinued.
- Be sure to tell your doctor if you are pregnant. Although extensive studies in humans have not been conducted, cyclosporine has caused fetal damage when administered to animals. Also, tell your doctor if you are breast-feeding, because cyclosporine passes into breast milk.

Cycrin—see medroxyprogesterone

Cylert—see pemoline

---

cyproheptadine

BRAND NAMES (Manufacturers)
cyproheptadine hydrochloride (various manufacturers)
Periactin (Merck Sharp & Dohme)
TYPE OF DRUG
Antihistamine
INGREDIENT
cyproheptadine
DOSAGE FORMS
Tablets (4 mg)
Oral syrup (2 mg per 5-ml spoonful, with 5% alcohol)
STORAGE
Store at room temperature in a tightly closed container. Freezing of the oral syrup should be avoided.

USES

This medication belongs to a group of drugs known as antihistamines (antihistamines block the action of histamine, a chemical that is released by the body during an allergic reaction). It is, therefore, used to treat or prevent symptoms of allergy.

TREATMENT

To avoid stomach upset, you can take cyproheptadine with food or with a full glass of milk or water (unless your doctor directs you to do otherwise).

The oral syrup should be measured carefully with a specially designed 5-ml measuring spoon. An ordinary kitchen teaspoon is not accurate enough.

If you miss a dose of this medication, take the missed dose as soon as possible, unless it is almost time for your next dose. If it is almost time for the next dose, do not take the missed dose at all; just return to your regular dosing schedule. Do not double the next dose.

SIDE EFFECTS

Minor. Blurred vision; confusion; constipation; diarrhea; difficult or painful urination; dizziness; dry mouth, throat, or nose; headache; increased or decreased appetite; irritability; nausea; restlessness; ringing or buzzing in the ears; stomach upset; or unusual increase in sweating. These side effects should disappear as your body adjusts to the medication.

This medication can cause increased sensitivity to sunlight. It is, therefore, important to avoid prolonged exposure to sunlight and sunlamps. Wear protective clothing and use an effective sunscreen.

If you are constipated, increase the amount of fiber in your diet (fresh fruits and vegetables, salads, bran, and whole-grain breads), exercise, and drink more water (unless your doctor directs you not to do so).

Chew sugarless gum or suck on ice chips or a piece of hard candy to reduce mouth dryness.

If you feel dizzy or light-headed, sit or lie down for a while; get up from a sitting or lying position slowly, and be careful on stairs.

Major. Tell your doctor about any side effects that are persistent or particularly bothersome. IT IS ESPECIALLY IMPORTANT TO TELL YOUR DOCTOR about change in menstruation, clumsiness, feeling faint, flushing of the face, hallucinations, palpitations, rash, seizures, shortness of breath, sleeping disorders, sore throat or fever, tightness in the chest, unusual bleeding or bruising, unusual tiredness or weakness, or yellowing of the eyes or skin.

INTERACTIONS

This drug interacts with several other types of drugs:

1. Concurrent use of this medication with other central nervous system depressants (such as alcohol, barbiturates, benzodiazepine tranquilizers, muscle relaxants, narcotics, pain medications, and phenothiazine tranquilizers) or with tricyclic antidepressants can cause extreme drowsiness.

2. Monoamine oxidase (MAO) inhibitors (such as isocarboxazid, pargyline, phenelzine, and tranylcypromine) can increase the side effects of this medication.

BE SURE TO TELL YOUR DOCTOR about any medications you are currently taking, especially any listed above.

WARNINGS

- Tell your doctor about unusual or allergic reactions you have had to any medications, especially to cyproheptadine or to other antihistamines (such as azatadine, astemizole, brompheniramine, carbinoxamine, chlorpheniramine, clemastine, cyproheptadine, dimenhydrinate, dimethindene, diphenhydramine, diphenylpyraline, doxylamine, hydroxyzine, phenidamine, promethazine, pyrilamine, terfenadine, trimeprazine, tripelennamine, and triprolidine).
- Tell your doctor if you now have or if you have ever had asthma, blood vessel disease, glaucoma, high blood pressure, kidney disease, peptic ulcers, enlarged prostate gland, or thyroid disease.
- Cyproheptadine can cause drowsiness or dizziness. Your ability to perform tasks that require alertness, such as driving a car or operating potentially dangerous equipment, may be decreased. Appropriate caution should, therefore, be taken.
- Be sure to tell your doctor if you are pregnant. The effects of this medication during pregnancy have not been thoroughly studied in humans. Also, tell your doctor if you are breast-feeding an infant. Small amounts of cyproheptadine pass into breast milk and may cause unusual excitement or irritability in nursing infants. The drug may also inhibit lactation.

cyproheptadine hydrochloride—see cyproheptadine

Cyronine—see liothyronine

Cytomel—see liothyronine

Cytotec—see misoprostal

Cytoxan—see cyclophosphamide

Dallergy-D—see pseudoephedrine and chlorpheniramine combination

Dalmane—see flurazepam

D-Amp—see ampicillin

Dantrium—see dantrolene

---

dantrolene

BRAND NAME (Manufacturer)
Dantrium (Norwich-Eaton)
TYPE OF DRUG
Muscle relaxant
INGREDIENT
dantrolene
DOSAGE FORM
Capsules (25 mg, 50 mg, and 100 mg)
STORAGE
Dantrolene should be stored at room temperature in a tightly closed container.

USES

This medication is used to relieve the spasticity caused by spinal cord injury, stroke, cerebral palsy, or multiple sclerosis. It works directly on muscles to prevent contraction. Dantrolene is also used prior to anesthesia to prevent malignant hyperthermia in patients known or suspected to be at risk for developing this complication.

TREATMENT

You can take dantrolene either on an empty stomach or with food or milk (as directed by your doctor). If you are unable to swallow the capsule, you can open it and mix the contents with fruit juice or another nonalcoholic beverage. Stir gently to mix the powder with the liquid before drinking. You should then take the dose immediately after mixing. Rinse the glass with a little more liquid and drink that as well to make sure that you have taken all of the medicine.

If you miss a dose and remember within an hour, take the missed dose immediately. If more than an hour has passed, do not take the missed dose; just return to your regular dosing schedule. Do not double the next dose.

SIDE EFFECTS

Minor. Abnormal hair growth, alteration of taste, constipation, diarrhea, dizziness, drowsiness, excessive tearing, fatigue, headache, insomnia, loss of appetite, or stomach upset. These side effects should disappear as your body adjusts to the medication.

This medication can increase your sensitivity to sunlight. You should, therefore, try to avoid prolonged exposure to sunlight and sunlamps. Wear protective clothing, and use an effective sunscreen.

To relieve constipation, increase the amount of fiber in your diet (fresh fruits and vegetables, salads, bran, and whole-grain breads), exercise, and drink more water (unless your doctor directs you to do otherwise).

If you feel dizzy, sit or lie down for a while; get up slowly from a sitting or reclining position, and be careful on stairs.

Major. Tell your doctor about any side effects that are persistent or particularly bothersome. IT IS ESPECIALLY IMPORTANT TO TELL YOUR DOCTOR about backaches; bloody or black, tarry stools; blurred vision; chills; confusion; convulsions; depression; difficult or painful urination; difficulty in breathing; difficulty in swallowing; feeling of suffocation; fever; increased urination; muscle pain; nervousness; palpitations; skin rash; speech disturbances; unusual weakness; or yellowing of the eyes or skin.

INTERACTIONS

Dantrolene interacts with several other types of drugs:

1. Concurrent use of dantrolene with central nervous system depressants (such as alcohol, antihistamines, barbiturates, benzodiazepine tranquilizers, muscle relaxants, narcotics, pain medications, phenothiazine tranquilizers, and sleeping medications) or with tricyclic antidepressants can lead to extreme drowsiness.

2. Concurrent use of dantrolene and estrogen by women over 35 years of age can increase their risk of liver damage.

BE SURE TO TELL YOUR DOCTOR about any medications you are currently taking, especially any listed above.

WARNINGS

- Tell your doctor about unusual or allergic reactions you have had to any medications, especially to dantrolene.
- Before starting to take this medication, be sure to tell your doctor if you now have or if you have ever had heart disease, liver disease, or lung disease.
- Repeated laboratory tests are necessary while you are taking dantrolene to monitor changes that may indicate liver damage.
- If this drug makes you dizzy or drowsy or blurs your vision, do not take part in any activity that requires alertness, such as driving a car or operating potentially dangerous equipment.
- Be sure to tell your doctor if you are pregnant. Although extensive studies in humans have not been conducted, animal studies involving large doses of dantrolene have demonstrated adverse effects on the fetus. Also, tell your doctor if you are breast-feeding. This drug is not recommended for nursing women.

Dapex—see phentermine

Darvocet-N 50—see acetaminophen and propoxyphene combination

Darvocet-N 100—see acetaminophen and propoxyphene combination

Darvon—see propoxyphene

Darvon Compound-65—see aspirin, caffeine, and propoxyphene combination

Darvon-N—see propoxyphene

Dazamide—see acetazolamide

Decadron—see dexamethasone (systemic)

Deconamine—see pseudoephedrine and chlorpheniramine combination

Deconamine SR—see pseudoephedrine and chlorpheniramine combination

Decongestabs—see phenylpropanolamine, phenylephrine, chlorpheniramine, and phenyltoloxamine combination

Dehist—see phenylpropanolamine and chlorpheniramine combination

Delacort—see hydrocortisone (topical)

Delaxin—see methocarbamol

Delta-Cortef—see prednisolone (systemic)

Deltasone—see prednisone (systemic)

Demazin—see phenylpropanolamine and chlorpheniramine combination

Demerol—see meperidine

Demulen—see oral contraceptives

Depakene—see valproic acid

Depakote—see valproic acid

Depen Titratable Tablets—see penicillamine

Deponit—see nitroglycerin (topical)

Dermacort—see hydrocortisone (topical)

DermiCort—see hydrocortisone (topical)

Dermolate Anti-Itch—see hydrocortisone (topical)

Dermolate Scalp-Itch—see hydrocortisone (topical)

Dermtex HC—see hydrocortisone (topical)

---

desipramine

BRAND NAMES (Manufacturers)
Norpramin (Merrell Dow)
Pertofrane (Rorer)
TYPE OF DRUG
Tricyclic antidepressant
INGREDIENT
desipramine
DOSAGE FORMS
Capsules (25 mg and 50 mg)
Tablets (10 mg, 25 mg, 50 mg, 75 mg, 100 mg, and 150 mg)
STORAGE
Desipramine capsules and tablets should be stored at room temperature in tightly closed containers.

USES

Desipramine is used to relieve the symptoms of mental depression. This medication belongs to a group of drugs referred to as the tricyclic antidepressants. These medicines are thought to relieve depression by increasing the concentration of certain chemicals necessary for nerve transmission in the brain.

TREATMENT

This medication should be taken exactly as your doctor prescribes. You can take it with food to lessen the chance of stomach irritation, unless your doctor tells you to do otherwise.

If you miss a dose of this medication, take the missed dose as soon as possible, then return to your regular dosing schedule. If, however, the dose you missed was a once-a-day bedtime dose, do not take that dose in the morning; check with your doctor instead. If the dose is taken in the morning, it may cause some unwanted side effects. Never double the dose.

The effects of therapy with this medication may not become apparent for several weeks.

SIDE EFFECTS

Minor. Agitation, anxiety, blurred vision, confusion, constipation, cramps, diarrhea, dizziness, drowsiness, dry mouth, fatigue, heartburn, insomnia, loss of appetite, nausea, peculiar tastes in the mouth, restlessness, sweating, vomiting, weakness, or weight gain or loss. As your body adjusts to the medication, these side effects should disappear.

This medication may increase your sensitivity to sunlight. You should, therefore, avoid prolonged exposure to sunlight and sunlamps. Wear protective clothing and sunscreen.

Dry mouth can be relieved by chewing sugarless gum or by sucking on ice chips or a piece of hard candy.

To relieve constipation, increase the amount of fiber in your diet (fresh fruits and vegetables, salads, bran, and whole-grain breads), exercise, and drink more water (unless your doctor directs you to do otherwise).

To avoid dizziness or light-headedness when you stand, contract and relax the muscles of your legs for a few moments before rising. Do this by pushing one foot against the floor while raising the other foot slightly, alternating feet so that you are "pumping" your legs in a pedaling motion.

Major. Tell your doctor about any side effects that are persistent or particularly bothersome. IT IS ESPECIALLY IMPORTANT TO TELL YOUR DOCTOR about chest pain, convulsions, difficulty in urinating, enlarged or painful breasts (in both sexes), fainting, fever, fluid retention, hair loss, hallucinations, headaches, impotence, mood changes, mouth sores, nervousness, nightmares, nosebleeds, numbness in the fingers or toes, palpitations, ringing in the ears, seizures, skin rash, sleep disorders, sore throat, tremors, uncoordinated movements or balance problems, unusual bleeding or bruising, or yellowing of the eyes or skin.

INTERACTIONS

Desipramine interacts with several other types of drugs:

1. Extreme drowsiness can occur when this medicine is taken with central nervous system depressants (such as alcohol, antihistamines, barbiturates, benzodiazepine tranquilizers, muscle relaxants, narcotics, pain medications, phenothiazine tranquilizers, and sleeping medications) or with other antidepressants.

2. Desipramine may decrease the effectiveness of antiseizure medications.

3. It may block the blood-pressure-lowering effects of clonidine and guanethidine.

4. Cimetidine can decrease the elimination of desipramine from the body, increasing the possibility of side effects.

5. Birth control pills or estrogen-containing drugs can increase the side effects and reduce the effectiveness of the tricyclic antidepressants (including desipramine).

6. Tricyclic antidepressants may increase the side effects of thyroid medication and of over-the-counter (nonprescription) cough, cold, allergy, asthma, sinus, and diet drugs.

7. The concurrent use of tricyclic antidepressants and monoamine oxidase (MAO) inhibitors should be avoided, because the combination may result in fever, convulsions, or high blood pressure. At least 14 days should separate the use of this drug and the use of an MAO inhibitor.

BE SURE TO TELL YOUR DOCTOR about any medications you are currently taking, especially any listed above.

WARNINGS

- Tell your doctor if you have had unusual or allergic reactions to medications, especially to desipramine or any of the other tricyclic antidepressants (such as amitriptyline, imipramine, doxepin, trimipramine, amoxapine, protriptyline, maprotiline, and nortriptyline).

• Tell your doctor if you have a history of alcoholism or if you have ever had asthma, high blood pressure, liver disease, kidney disease, heart disease, a heart attack, circulatory disease, stomach problems, intestinal problems, difficulty in urinating, enlarged prostate gland, epilepsy, seizures, glaucoma, thyroid disease, mental illness, or electroshock therapy.
• If this drug makes you dizzy or drowsy, do not take part in any activity that requires alertness, such as driving a car or operating potentially dangerous equipment.
• Before having surgery or other medical or dental treatment, tell your doctor or dentist about this drug.
• Do not stop taking this drug suddenly. Abruptly stopping it can cause nausea, headache, stomach upset, fatigue, or a worsening of your condition. Your doctor may want to reduce the dosage gradually.
• The effects of this medication may last as long as seven days after you have stopped taking it, so continue to observe all precautions during that period.
• The tablet form of this medication contains the color additive FD&C Yellow No. 5 (tartrazine), which can cause allergic-type symptoms (fainting, shortness of breath, rash) in certain susceptible individuals.
• Be sure to tell your doctor if you are pregnant. Problems in humans have not been reported; however, studies in animals have shown that this medication can cause side effects in the fetus when given to the mother in large doses during pregnancy. Also, tell your doctor if you are breast-feeding an infant. Small amounts of this drug can pass into breast milk, which may cause unwanted effects, such as irritability or sleeping problems, in the nursing infant.

Desoxyn—see methamphetamine

Desoxyn Gradumets—see methamphetamine

Desyrel—see trazodone

Desyrel Dividose—see trazodone

Detuss—see phenylpropanolamine and caramiphen combination

Dexacidin—see dexamethasone, neomycin, and polymyxin B combination (ophthalmic)

Dexameth—see dexamethasone

dexamethasone (systemic)

BRAND NAMES (Manufacturers)
Decadron (Merck Sharp & Dohme)
Dexameth (Major)
dexamethasone (various manufacturers)
Dexone (Reid-Rowell)
Hexadrol (Organon)
TYPE OF DRUG
Adrenocorticosteroid hormone
INGREDIENT
dexamethasone
DOSAGE FORMS
Tablets (0.25 mg, 0.5 mg, 0.75 mg, 1 mg, 1.5 mg, 2 mg, 4 mg, and 6 mg)
Oral elixir (0.5 mg per 5-ml spoonful, with 5% alcohol)
Oral solution (0.5 mg per 5-ml spoonful)
Oral concentrate (0.5 mg per 0.5 ml, with 30% alcohol)
STORAGE
Dexamethasone should be stored at room temperature in a tightly closed container.

USES

Your adrenal glands naturally produce certain cortisone-like chemicals. These chemicals are involved in various regulatory processes in the body (such as those involving fluid balance, temperature, and reaction to inflammation). Dexamethasone belongs to a group of drugs known as adrenocorticosteroids (or cortisone-like medications). It is used to treat a variety of disorders, including endocrine and rheumatic disorders; asthma; blood diseases; certain cancers; eye disorders; gastrointestinal disturbances, such as ulcerative colitis; respiratory diseases; and inflammations such as arthritis, dermatitis, and poison ivy. How this drug acts to relieve these disorders is not completely understood.

TREATMENT

In order to prevent stomach irritation, you can take dexamethasone with food or milk.

If you are taking only one dose of this medication each day, try to take it before 9:00 A.M. This will mimic the body's normal production of this type of chemical.

The oral elixir and solution forms of this medication should be measured carefully with a specially designed 5-ml measuring spoon. An ordinary kitchen teaspoon is not accurate enough.

The oral concentrate may be diluted in juice, other liquids, or semi-solid foods like applesauce.

It is important to try not to miss any doses of dexamethasone. However, if you do miss a dose of this medication, follow these guidelines:

1. If you are taking this medication more than once a day, take the missed dose as soon as possible and return to your regular schedule. If it is already time for the next dose of medication, double the dose.
2. If you are taking this medication once a day, take the dose you missed as soon as possible, unless you don't remember until the next day. In that case, do not take the missed dose at all, just follow your regular dosing schedule. Do not double the next dose.
3. If you are taking this drug every other day, take it as soon as you remember. If you missed the scheduled time by a whole day, take it when you remember, then skip a day before you take the next dose. Do not double the dose.

If you miss more than one dose of dexamethasone, CONTACT YOUR DOCTOR.

SIDE EFFECTS

Minor. Dizziness, false sense of well-being, fatigue, increased appetite, increased sweating, indigestion, leg cramps, menstrual irregularities, muscle weakness, nausea, reddening of the skin on the face, restlessness, sleep disorders, thinning of the skin, or weight gain. These side effects should disappear as your body adjusts to the medication.

To help avoid potassium loss while using this drug, you can take your dose with a glass of fresh or frozen orange juice, or eat a banana each day. The use of a salt substitute also helps to prevent potassium loss. Check with your doctor before changing your diet or using a salt substitute.

Major. Tell your doctor about any side effects that are persistent or particularly bothersome. IT IS ESPECIALLY IMPORTANT TO TELL YOUR DOCTOR about abdominal enlargement or pain; acne or other skin problems; back or rib pain; bloody or black, tarry stools; blurred vision; convulsions; eye pain; fever and sore throat; growth impairment (in children); headaches; impaired healing of wounds; increased thirst and urination; mental depression; mood changes; muscle wasting; nightmares; peptic ulcers; rapid weight gain (three to five pounds within a week); rash; shortness of breath; unusual bleeding or bruising; or unusual weakness.

INTERACTIONS

This drug interacts with several other types of drugs:

1. Alcohol, aspirin, and anti-inflammatory medications (such as diclofenac, diflunisal, fenoprofen, flurbiprofen, ibuprofen, indomethacin, ketoprofen, mefenamic acid, meclofenamate, naproxen, piroxicam, sulindac, and tolmetin) aggravate the stomach problems that may occur with use of this medication.

2. The dosage of oral anticoagulants (blood thinners, such as warfarin), oral antidiabetic drugs, or insulin may need to be altered when this medication is started or stopped.

3. The loss of potassium caused by this medication can lead to serious side effects in individuals taking digoxin.

4. Thiazide diuretics (water pills) can increase the potassium loss caused by dexamethasone.

5. Phenobarbital, phenytoin, rifampin, and ephedrine can increase the elimination of dexamethasone from the body, thereby decreasing its effectiveness.

6. Oral contraceptives (birth control pills) and estrogen-containing drugs may decrease the elimination of this drug from the body, which can lead to an increase in side effects.

7. Dexamethasone can increase the elimination of aspirin and isoniazid from the body, thereby decreasing the effectiveness of these two medications.

8. Cholestyramine and colestipol can chemically bind this medication in the stomach and gastrointestinal tract, preventing its absorption.

BE SURE TO TELL YOUR DOCTOR about any medications you are currently taking, especially any of those listed above.

WARNINGS

• Tell your doctor about unusual or allergic reactions you have had to any medications, especially to dexamethasone or other adrenocorticosteroids (such as alcometasone, amcinonide, betamethasone, clobetasol, clocortolone, cortisone, desonide, desoximetasone, diflorasone, flumethasone, fluocinolone, fluocinonide, fluorometholone, flurandrenolide, halcinonide, hydrocortisone, methylprednisolone, paramethasone, prednisolone, prednisone, and triamcinolone).

• Tell your doctor if you now have or if you have ever had bone disease, diabetes mellitus, emotional instability, glaucoma, fungal infections, heart disease, high blood pressure, high cholesterol levels, myasthenia gravis, peptic ulcers, osteoporosis, thyroid disease, tuberculosis, ulcerative colitis, kidney disease, or liver disease.

• If you are using this medication for longer than a week, you may need to receive higher doses if you are subjected to stress, such as serious infections, injury, or surgery. Discuss this with your doctor.

• If you have been taking this drug for more than one or two weeks, do not stop taking it suddenly. If it is stopped abruptly, you may experience abdominal or back pain, dizziness, extreme weakness, fainting, fever, muscle or joint pain, nausea, vomiting, or shortness of breath. Your doctor may, therefore, want to reduce the dosage gradually. Never increase the dosage or take the drug for longer than the prescribed time, unless you first consult your doctor.

• While you are taking this drug, you should not be vaccinated or immunized. This medication decreases the effectiveness of vaccines and can lead to infection if a live-virus vaccine is administered.

• Before having surgery or other medical or dental treatment, tell your doctor or dentist you are taking this drug.

• Because this drug can cause glaucoma and cataracts with long-term use, your doctor may want to have your eyes examined by an ophthalmologist periodically during treatment.

• If you are taking this medication for prolonged periods, you should wear or carry an identification card or notice stating that you are taking an adrenocorticosteroid.

• This drug can raise blood sugar levels in diabetic patients. Blood sugar should, therefore, be monitored carefully with blood or urine tests when this drug is being taken.

• Be sure to tell your doctor if you are pregnant. This drug crosses the placenta and may cause adverse effects in the fetus. Birth defects have been observed in the offspring of animals that were given large doses of this type of drug during pregnancy. Also, tell your doctor if you are breast-feeding an infant. Small amounts of this drug pass into breast milk and may cause growth suppression or a decrease in natural adrenocorticosteroid production in the nursing infant.

---

dexamethasone, neomycin, and polymyxin B combination (ophthalmic)

BRAND NAMES (Manufacturers)

AK-Trol (Akorn)
Dexacidin (Iolab Pharm)
Dexasporin (various manufacturers)
Maxitrol (Alcon)

TYPE OF DRUG

Ophthalmic adrenocorticosteroid and antibiotic

INGREDIENTS

dexamethasone, neomycin, and polymyxin B

DOSAGE FORMS

Ophthalmic suspension (0.1% dexamethasone, 3.5 mg neomycin, and 10,000 units polymyxin B per ml)
Ophthalmic ointment (0.1% dexamethasone, 3.5 mg neomycin, and 10,000 units polymyxin B per gram)

STORAGE

The ophthalmic suspension and ointment should be stored at room temperature (never frozen) in tightly closed containers. If the suspension or ointment changes color, don't use the medication. A change in color indicates a loss of effectiveness.

USES

This medication is used for the short-term treatment of bacterial infections and inflammation of the eyes.

Your adrenal glands naturally produce certain cortisone-like chemicals. These chemicals are involved in various regulatory processes in the body (such as those involving fluid balance, temperature, and reaction to inflammation). Dexamethasone belongs to a group of drugs known as adrenocorticosteroids (or cortisone-like medications). It is used to relieve inflammation (redness, swelling, itching, and discomfort). How it does so is not completely understood.

Neomycin and polymyxin B are antibiotics, which act to prevent the growth and multiplication of infecting bacteria.

TREATMENT

Wash your hands with soap and water before using this medication. If you are using the suspension, shake the bottle well before measuring out the drops. The contents tend to settle on the bottom of the bottle, so it is necessary to shake the container to distribute the ingredients evenly and to equalize the doses.

In order to prevent contamination of the medicine, be careful not to touch the tube portion of the dropper, and do not let the dropper touch the eye.

Note that the bottle of the eye drops is not completely full. This is to allow control of the number of drops used.

To apply the drops, tilt your head back and pull down the lower eyelid with one hand to make a pouch below the eyeball. Drop the medicine into the pouch and slowly close your eyes. Do not blink. Place one finger at the corner of the eye next to your nose, applying slight pressure (this is done to prevent loss of medication through the duct that drains fluid from the surface of the eye into the nose and throat), and keep your eyes closed for a minute or two. If you think that the medicine did not get into your eye, repeat the process once. If you are using more than one type of eye drops, wait at least five minutes between doses of the two drugs.

Follow the same general procedure for applying the ointment. Tilt your head back, pull down the lower eyelid, and squeeze the prescribed amount of ointment in a line along the pouch below the eyeball. Close your eyes, and place your finger at the corner of the eye near the nose for a minute or two. Do not rub your eyes. Wipe off excess ointment and the tip of the tube with clean tissues.

Since applying the medication is somewhat difficult to do, you may want someone else to apply it for you.

If you miss a dose of this drug, insert the drops or apply the ointment as soon as possible, unless it is almost time for the next application. In that case, do not use the missed dose at all; just return to your regular dosing schedule.

Your doctor may advise you to reduce the number of times you are applying this medication when the inflammation and infection begin to improve. Continue to take this medication for the entire time prescribed by your doctor, even if the symptoms of infection disappear before then. If you stop applying the drug too soon, bacteria are given a chance to continue growing, and the infection could recur.

SIDE EFFECTS

Minor. Blurred vision, burning, or stinging. These side effects should disappear as your body adjusts to the drug.

Major. Tell your doctor about any side effects that are persistent or particularly bothersome. IT IS ESPECIALLY IMPORTANT TO TELL YOUR DOCTOR about disturbed or reduced vision; eye pain, itching, or swelling; headache; rash; or severe irritation.

INTERACTIONS

This medication should not interact with any other medications as long as it is used according to directions.

WARNINGS

- Tell your doctor about any reactions you have had to medications, especially to dexamethasone or other adrenocorticosteroids (such as alcometasone, amcinonide, betamethasone, clobetasol, clocortolone, cortisone, desonide, desoximetasone, diflorasone, flumethasone, fluocinolone, fluorometholone, flurandrenolide, halcinonide, hydrocortisone, methylprednisolone, prednisolone, prednisone, and triamcinolone), to polymyxin B, to neomycin, or to any related antibiotic (amikacin, gentamicin, kanamycin, netilmicin, paromomycin, streptomycin, tobramycin).
- Tell your doctor if you have ever had fungal or viral infections of the eye, inner ear disease, kidney disease, or myasthenia gravis.
- If there is no change in your condition two or three days after starting to take this drug, contact your doctor. The drug may not be effective for your particular infection.
- Do not use this medication for longer than ten consecutive days unless your doctor directs you to do so. Prolonged use of this drug may result in glaucoma, secondary infection, cataracts, or eye damage. If you need to take this medication for several weeks, your doctor may want you to have an eye examination by an ophthalmologist.
- This medication has been prescribed for your current infection only. A subsequent infection, or one that someone else has, may require a different medicine. You should not give your medicine to other people or use it to treat other infections, unless your doctor specifically directs you to do so.
- Do not apply makeup to the affected eye.
- Be sure to tell your doctor if you are pregnant. When large amounts of dexamethasone are applied for prolonged periods, some of it is absorbed into the bloodstream. It may cross the placenta. Birth defects have been observed in the offspring of animals that were given large oral doses of this drug during pregnancy. Also, tell your doctor if you are breast-feeding an infant. If absorbed through the eye, small amounts of dexamethasone can pass into breast milk and may cause growth suppression or a decrease in natural adrenocorticosteroid production in the nursing infant.

Dexasporin—see dexamethasone, neomycin, and polymyxin B combination (ophthalmic)

dexbrompheniramine and pseudoephedrine—see pseudoephedrine and dexbrompheniramine combination

Dexchlor—see dexchlorpheniramine

dexchlorpheniramine

BRAND NAMES (Manufacturers)
Dexchlor (Henry Schein)
dexchlorpheniramine (various manufacturers)
Poladex T.D. (Major)
Polaramine (Schering)
Polaramine Repetabs (Schering)
Polargen (Goldline)
TYPE OF DRUG
Antihistamine
INGREDIENT
dexchlorpheniramine
DOSAGE FORMS
Tablets (2 mg)
Repeat-action tablets (4 mg and 6 mg)
Oral syrup (2 mg per 5-ml spoonful, with 6% alcohol)
STORAGE
Dexchlorpheniramine tablets and oral syrup should be stored in tightly closed containers. This medication should be stored at room temperature.

USES

This medication belongs to a group of drugs known as antihistamines (antihistamines block the action of histamine, a chemical that is released by the body during an allergic reaction). It is, therefore, used to treat or prevent symptoms of allergy.

TREATMENT

To avoid stomach upset, you can take dexchlorpheniramine with food or with a full glass of milk or water (unless your doctor directs you to do otherwise).

The syrup form of this medication should be measured carefully with a specially designed 5-ml measuring spoon. An ordinary kitchen teaspoon is not accurate enough to ensure that you receive the proper dose.

The repeat-action tablet form of this medication should be swallowed whole. Breaking, chewing, or crushing these tablets destroys their sustained-release activity and may increase the side effects.

If you miss a dose of this medication, take the missed dose as soon as possible, unless it is almost time for your next dose. In that case, do not take the missed dose at all; just return to your regular dosing schedule. Do not double the next dose.

SIDE EFFECTS

Minor. Blurred vision; confusion; constipation; diarrhea; difficult or painful urination; dizziness; dry mouth, throat, or nose; headache; irritability; loss of appetite; nausea; rash; restlessness; ringing or buzzing in the ears; stomach upset; or unusual increase in sweating. These side effects should disappear as your body adjusts to the medication.

This medication can cause increased sensitivity to sunlight. It is, therefore, important to avoid prolonged exposure to sunlight and sunlamps. Wear protective clothing, and use an effective sunscreen.

If you are constipated, increase the amount of fiber in your diet (fresh fruits and vegetables, salads, bran, and whole-grain breads), exercise, and drink more water (unless your doctor directs you to do otherwise).

If you experience mouth or throat dryness, you may wish to chew sugarless gum or suck on ice chips or a piece of hard candy to minimize these side effects.

If you feel dizzy or light-headed, sit or lie down for a while; get up from a sitting or lying position slowly, and be careful on stairs.

Major. Tell your doctor about any side effects that are persistent or particularly bothersome. IT IS ESPECIALLY IMPORTANT TO TELL YOUR DOCTOR about changes in menstruation, clumsiness, feeling faint, flushing of the face, hallucinations, seizures, shortness of breath, sleeping disorders, sore throat or fever, palpitations, tightness in the chest, unusual bleeding or bruising, or unusual tiredness or weakness.

INTERACTIONS

Dexchlorpheniramine interacts with several other types of medications:

1. Concurrent use of it with central nervous system depressants (such as alcohol, barbiturates, benzodiazepine tranquilizers, muscle relaxants, narcotics, pain medications, and phenothiazine tranquilizers) or with tricyclic antidepressants can cause extreme drowsiness.

2. Monoamine oxidase (MAO) inhibitors (such as isocarboxazid, pargyline, phenelzine, and tranylcypromine) can increase the side effects of this medication. At least 14 days should separate the use of this drug and the use of an MAO inhibitor.

BE SURE TO TELL YOUR DOCTOR about any medications you are currently taking, especially any of those listed above.

WARNINGS

• Tell your doctor about unusual or allergic reactions you have had to any medications, especially to dexchlorpheniramine or other antihistamines (such as astemizole, azatadine, brompheniramine, carbinoxamine, chlorpheniramine, clemastine, cyproheptadine, dimenhydrinate, dimethindene, diphenhydramine, diphenylpyraline, doxylamine, hydroxyzine, phenidamine, promethazine, pyrilamine, terfenadine, trimeprazine, tripelennamine, and triprolidine).

• Tell your doctor if you now have or if you have ever had asthma, blood vessel disease, glaucoma, high blood pressure, kidney disease, peptic ulcers, enlarged prostate gland, or thyroid disease.

• Dexchlorpheniramine can cause drowsiness or dizziness. Your ability to perform tasks that require alertness, such as driving a car or operating potentially dangerous equipment, may be decreased. Appropriate caution should, therefore, be taken.

• Be sure to tell your doctor if you are pregnant. The effects of this medication during pregnancy have not been thoroughly studied in humans. It is recommended that use of this drug be avoided during the last three months of pregnancy. Also, tell your doctor if you are breast-feeding an infant. Small amounts of dexchlorpheniramine pass into breast milk and may cause unusual excitement or irritability in nursing infants.

Dexedrine—see dextroamphetamine

Dexedrine Spansules—see dextroamphetamine

Dexone—see dexamethasone (systemic)

---

dextroamphetamine

BRAND NAMES (Manufacturers)
Dexedrine (Smith Kline & French)
Dexedrine Spansules (Smith Kline & French)
dextroamphetamine sulfate (various manufacturers)
Oxydess II (Vortech)
Spancap No. 1 (Vortech)

TYPE OF DRUG
Amphetamine

INGREDIENT
dextroamphetamine

DOSAGE FORMS
Tablets (5 mg, 10 mg, and 15 mg)
Capsules (15 mg)
Sustained-release capsules (5 mg, 10 mg, and 15 mg)
Oral elixir (5 mg per 5-ml spoonful, with 10% alcohol)

STORAGE
Dextroamphetamine tablets, capsules, and oral elixir should be stored at room temperature in tightly closed containers.

USES

This medication is a central nervous system stimulant that increases mental alertness and decreases fatigue. It is used to treat narcolepsy (problems in staying awake) and abnormal behavioral syndrome in children (hyperkinetic syndrome or attention deficit disorder). The way this medication acts to control abnormal behavioral syndrome in children is not clearly understood.

Dextroamphetamine is also used as an appetite suppressant during the first few weeks of dieting (while you are trying to establish new eating habits). It is thought to relieve hunger by altering nerve impulses to the appetite control center in the brain. Its effectiveness as an appetite suppressant lasts only for short periods (three to 12 weeks), however.

TREATMENT

In order to avoid stomach upset, you can take dextroamphetamine with food or with a full glass of milk or water (unless your doctor directs you to do otherwise).

If this medication is being used to treat narcolepsy or abnormal behavioral syndrome in children, the first dose each day should be taken soon after awakening. Subsequent doses should be spaced at four- to six-hour intervals.

If this medication has been prescribed as a diet aid, it should be taken one hour before each meal.

The oral elixir form of this medication should be measured carefully with a specially designed 5-ml measuring spoon. An ordinary kitchen teaspoon is not accurate enough.

The sustained-release form of this medication should be swallowed whole. Breaking, chewing, or crushing these capsules destroys their sustained-release activity and may increase the side effects.

In order to avoid difficulty in falling asleep, the last dose of this medication each day should be taken four to six hours before bedtime (tablets and capsules) or ten to 14 hours before bedtime (sustained-release capsules).

If you miss a dose of this medication, take the missed dose as soon as possible, unless it is almost time for your next dose. In that case, do not take the missed dose at all; just return to your regular dosing schedule. Do not double the next dose.

SIDE EFFECTS

Minor. Abdominal cramps, constipation, diarrhea, dizziness, dry mouth, false sense of well-being, insomnia, loss of appetite, irritability, nausea, overstimulation, restlessness, unpleasant taste in the mouth, or vomiting. These side effects should disappear as your body adjusts to the drug.

To prevent constipation, increase the amount of fiber in your diet (fresh fruits and vegetables, bran, salads, and whole-grain cereals and breads), exercise, and drink more water (unless your doctor directs you to do otherwise).

Dry mouth can be relieved by sucking on ice chips or a piece of hard candy or by chewing sugarless gum.

If you feel dizzy, sit or lie down for a while; get up from a sitting or lying position slowly, and be careful on stairs.

Major. Tell your doctor about any side effects that are persistent or particularly bothersome. IT IS ESPECIALLY IMPORTANT TO TELL YOUR DOCTOR about blurred vision, confusion, fatigue, headaches, impotence, mental depression, nosebleeds, palpitations, rash, sweating, tightness in the chest, tremors, or uncoordinated movements.

INTERACTIONS

Dextroamphetamine interacts with several other types of medications:

1. Use of dextroamphetamine within 14 days of use of a monoamine oxidase (MAO) inhibitor (such as isocarboxazid, pargyline, phenelzine, tranylcypromine) can result in high blood pressure and other side effects.

2. Barbiturate medications, certain tranquilizers (especially chlorpromazine), and tricyclic antidepressants can reverse the effect of this medication.

3. Amphetamines can decrease the blood-pressure-lowering effects of antihypertensive medications (especially guanethidine) and may alter dosage requirements for insulin and oral antidiabetic medication in diabetic patients.

4. The side effects of other central nervous system stimulants (such as caffeine, nonprescription appetite suppressants, and cough, sinus, allergy, asthma, or cold preparations) may be increased by dextroamphetamine.

5. Acetazolamide and sodium bicarbonate can decrease the elimination of the amphetamines from the body, thereby prolonging their duration of action.

BE SURE TO TELL YOUR DOCTOR about any medications you are currently taking, especially any listed above.

WARNINGS

- Tell your doctor about unusual or allergic reactions you have had to any medications, especially to dextroamphetamine or other central nervous system stimulants (such as albuterol, amphetamine, ephedrine, epinephrine, isoproterenol, metaproterenol, norepinephrine, phenylephrine, phenylpropanolamine, pseudoephedrine, and terbutaline).

• Tell your doctor if you have a history of drug abuse or if you have ever had problems with agitation, diabetes mellitus, glaucoma, heart or blood vessel disease, high blood pressure, or thyroid disease.
• Dextroamphetamine can mask the symptoms of extreme fatigue and can cause dizziness. Your ability to perform tasks that require alertness, such as driving a car or operating potentially dangerous equipment, may be decreased. Appropriate caution should, therefore, be taken.
• Before surgery or other medical or dental treatment, tell your doctor or dentist you are taking this drug.
• Dextroamphetamine is related to amphetamine and may be habit-forming when taken for long periods of time (both physical and psychological dependence can occur). Therefore, you should not increase the dosage of this medication or take it for longer than 12 weeks unless you first consult your doctor. It is also important that you not stop taking this medication abruptly; fatigue, sleep disorders, mental depression, nausea, vomiting, stomach cramps, or pain could occur. Your doctor may, therefore, want to decrease the dosage gradually in order to prevent these side effects.
• Some of these products contain the color additive FD&C Yellow No. 5 (tartrazine), which can cause allergic-type reactions (difficulty in breathing, fainting, rash, wheezing) in certain susceptible individuals.
• Be sure to tell your doctor if you are pregnant. Although side effects in humans have not been thoroughly studied, some of the amphetamines have caused heart, brain, and biliary tract abnormalities in the fetuses of animals that received large doses of these drugs during pregnancy. Also, tell your doctor if you are breast-feeding an infant. Small amounts of this drug pass into breast milk.

dextroamphetamine sulfate—see dextroamphetamine

---

dextromethorphan and iodinated glycerol combination

BRAND NAMES (Manufacturers)
Iophen DM (various manufacturers)
Oridol DM (LuChem)
Torganic-DM (Major)
Tusside (Ortega)
Tussi-Organidin DM (Wallace)
Tussi-R-Gen DM (Goldline)
TYPE OF DRUG
Cough suppressant and expectorant combination
INGREDIENTS
dextromethorphan and iodinated glycerol
DOSAGE FORM
Oral liquid (10 mg dextromethorphan and 30 mg iodinated glycerol per 5-ml spoonful)
STORAGE
This medicine should be stored at room temperature in a tightly closed container. Avoid exposure of this medication to high temperatures during storage.

USES
Dextromethorphan and iodinated glycerol combination is used to relieve coughs due to colds or infections or inflammation of the upper respiratory tract. Iodinated glycerol is an expectorant, which loosens bronchial secretions. Dextromethorphan is a cough suppressant, which acts on the cough center in the brain.

TREATMENT
You can take dextromethorphan and iodinated glycerol combination either on an empty stomach or, to avoid stomach irritation, with food or milk (as directed by your doctor).

Each dose should be measured carefully with a specially designed 5-ml measuring spoon. An ordinary kitchen teaspoon is not accurate enough.

To help loosen the mucus in the bronchi, you should drink a glass of water after each dose.

If you miss a dose of this medication, take the missed dose as soon as possible, unless it is almost time for the next dose. In that case, do not take the missed dose at all; just return to your regular dosing schedule. Do not double the next dose.

SIDE EFFECTS
Minor. Drowsiness or stomach upset. These side effects should disappear as your body adjusts to this medication.
Major. Tell your doctor about any side effects that are persistent or particularly bothersome. IT IS ESPECIALLY IMPORTANT TO TELL YOUR DOCTOR about extreme weakness, skin rash, or swollen lymph nodes.

INTERACTIONS
This medicine can interact with other types of drugs:
1. Concurrent use with other central nervous system depressants (such as alcohol, barbiturates, benzodiazepine tranquilizers, muscle relaxants, narcotics, pain medications, phenothiazine tranquilizers, and sleeping medications) or with tricyclic antidepressants can lead to extreme drowsiness.
2. The iodine component of iodinated glycerol can increase the side effects of lithium on the thyroid gland. It can also increase the effects of antithyroid medications.

Before starting dextromethorphan and iodinated glycerol combination, BE SURE TO TELL YOUR DOCTOR about any medications you are currently taking, especially any of those listed above.

WARNINGS
• Tell your doctor about unusual or allergic reactions you have had to any medications, especially to dextromethorphan or to iodinated glycerol or iodine.
• Before starting to take this medication, be sure to tell your doctor if you now have or if you have ever had acne, cystic fibrosis, heart disease, or thyroid disease.
• If this drug makes you dizzy or drowsy, do not take part in activities that require alertness, such as driving a car or operating potentially dangerous equipment.
• While you are taking this medication, drink at least eight glasses of water a day (to help loosen bronchial secretions).
• Be sure to tell your doctor if you are pregnant. This medication should not be taken during pregnancy. Iodinated glycerol can cause goiter (an enlarged thyroid gland) in the developing fetus. Also, tell your doctor if you are breast-feeding an infant. Iodinated glycerol can pass into breast milk and cause side effects in the nursing infant.

DiaBeta—see glyburide

Diabinese—see chlorpropamide

Diachlor—see chlorothiazide

Diamine T.D.—see brompheniramine

Diamox—see acetazolamide

Diamox Sequels—see acetazolamide

Diaqua—see hydrochlorothiazide

---

diazepam

BRAND NAMES (Manufacturers)
diazepam (various manufacturers)
Diazepam Intensol (Roxene)
Valium (Roche)
Valrelease (Roche)
Vazepam (Major)

TYPE OF DRUG
Sedative/hypnotic

INGREDIENT
diazepam

DOSAGE FORMS
Oral solution (5 mg per 5 ml spoonful)
Oral intensol solution (5 mg per ml)
Tablets (2 mg, 5 mg, and 10 mg)
Sustained-release capsules (15 mg)

STORAGE
This medication should be stored at room temperature in a tightly closed, light-resistant container.

USES

Diazepam is prescribed to treat symptoms of anxiety and sometimes to treat muscle spasms, convulsions, seizures, or alcohol withdrawal. It is not clear exactly how this medicine works, but it may relieve anxiety by acting as a depressant of the central nervous system (brain and spinal cord). Diazepam is currently used by many people to relieve nervousness. It is effective for this purpose for short periods, but it is important to try to remove the cause of the anxiety as well.

TREATMENT

The oral intensol solution should be mixed with a nonalcoholic liquid or semi-solid food such as water, juice, soda or soda-like beverages, applesauce, or pudding. Use only the calibrated dropper provided. Stir the liquid or food gently for a few seconds after adding the oral intensol solution. The entire amount of the mixture should be consumed immediately. Do not store prepared mixtures for future use. The tablet or capsule form of this medication should be taken exactly as directed by your doctor. It can be taken with food or a full glass of water if stomach upset occurs. Do not take this medication with a dose of antacids, since they may retard its absorption.

If you are taking this medication regularly and you miss a dose and remember within an hour, take the missed dose immediately. If more than an hour has passed, skip the dose you missed and wait for the next scheduled dose. Do not double the next dose.

SIDE EFFECTS

Minor. Bitter taste in the mouth, constipation, depression, diarrhea, dizziness, drowsiness (after a night's sleep), dry mouth, excessive salivation, fatigue, flushing, headache, heartburn, loss of appetite, nausea, nervousness, sweating, or vomiting. These side effects should disappear as your body adjusts to the medication.

To relieve constipation, increase the amount of fiber in your diet (fresh fruits and vegetables, salads, bran, and whole-grain breads), exercise, and drink more water (unless your doctor directs you to do otherwise).

Dry mouth can be relieved by chewing sugarless gum or by sucking on ice chips.

If you feel dizzy, sit or lie down for a while; get up slowly from a sitting or reclining position, and be careful on stairs.

Major. Tell your doctor about any side effects that are persistent or particularly bothersome. IT IS ESPECIALLY IMPORTANT TO TELL YOUR DOCTOR about blurred or double vision, chest pain, difficulty in urinating, fainting, falling, fever, joint pain, hallucinations, mouth sores, nightmares, palpitations, rash, severe depression, shortness of breath, slurred speech, sore throat, uncoordinated movements, unusual excitement, unusual tiredness, or yellowing of the eyes or skin.

INTERACTIONS

This medication interacts with several other types of medications:

1. To prevent oversedation, this drug should not be taken with alcohol, other sedative drugs, or central nervous system depressants (such as antihistamines, barbiturates, muscle relaxants, pain medicines, narcotics, medicines for seizures, and tranquilizers), or with antidepressants.

2. This medication may decrease the effectiveness of carbamazepine, levodopa, and oral anticoagulants (blood thinners) and may increase the effects of phenytoin.

3. Disulfiram, oral contraceptives (birth control pills), isoniazid, fluoxetine, valproic acid, propranolol, metoprolol, and cimetidine can increase the blood levels of diazepam, which can lead to toxic effects.

4. Concurrent use of rifampin may decrease the effectiveness of diazepam.

BE SURE TO TELL YOUR DOCTOR about any medications you are currently taking, especially any of those listed above.

WARNINGS

- Tell your doctor about unusual or allergic reactions you have had to any medications, especially to diazepam or other benzodiazepine tranquilizers (such as alprazolam, flurazepam, halazepam, lorazepam, oxazepam, prazepam, temazepam, and triazolam).
- Tell your doctor if you now have or if you have ever had liver disease, kidney disease, epilepsy, lung disease, myasthenia gravis, porphyria, mental depression, or mental illness.
- This medicine can cause drowsiness. Avoid tasks that require alertness, such as driving a car or operating potentially dangerous machinery.
- This medication has the potential for abuse and must be used with caution. Tolerance may develop quickly; do not increase your dosage of the drug without first consulting your doctor. It is also important not to stop taking this drug

suddenly if you have been taking it in large amounts or if you have used it for several weeks. Your doctor may want to reduce your dosage gradually.

• This is a safe drug when used properly. When it is combined with other sedative drugs or alcohol, however, serious side effects can develop.

• Be sure to tell your doctor if you are pregnant. This medicine may increase the chance of birth defects if it is taken during the first three months of pregnancy. In addition, too much use of this medicine during the last six months of pregnancy may cause the baby to become dependent on it, resulting in withdrawal side effects in the newborn. Also, use of this medicine during the last weeks of pregnancy may cause excessive drowsiness, slowed heartbeat, and breathing difficulties in the infant. Tell your doctor if you are breastfeeding an infant. This medicine can pass into breast milk and cause excessive drowsiness, slowed heartbeat, and breathing difficulties in nursing infants.

Diazepam Intensol—see diazepam

Di-Azo—see phenazopyridine

---

diclofenac

BRAND NAME (Manufacturer)
Voltaren (Ciba-Geigy)
TYPE OF DRUG
Nonsteroidal anti-inflammatory analgesic
INGREDIENT
diclofenac
DOSAGE FORM
Enteric-coated tablets (25 mg, 50 mg, 75 mg)
STORAGE
This medication should be stored in a tightly closed container at room temperature away from heat and direct sunlight.

USES

Diclofenac is used to treat the inflammation (pain, swelling, and stiffness) of arthritis and ankylosing spondylitis. Diclofenac has been shown to block the production of certain body chemicals, called prostaglandins, that may trigger pain. However, it is not yet fully understood how it works.

TREATMENT

You should take this medication on an empty stomach 30 to 60 minutes before meals or two hours after meals, so that it gets into your bloodstream quickly. To decrease stomach irritation, your doctor may want you to take this medication with food or antacids.

Do not break, crush, or chew the tablets before swallowing. They should be swallowed whole to lessen side effects.

It may take two weeks before you feel the full effects of this medication. Diclofenac does not cure arthritis or ankylosing spondylitis, but it will help to control the condition as long as you continue to take it.

It is important that you take diclofenac on schedule and do not miss any doses. If you do miss a dose, take it as soon as possible, unless it is almost time for your next dose. In that case, do not take the missed dose at all; just return to your regular dosing schedule. Do not double the next dose.

SIDE EFFECTS

Minor. Abdominal cramps, constipation, diarrhea, dizziness, headache, indigestion, or nausea. As your body adjusts to the drug, these side effects should disappear.

To relieve constipation, increase the amount of fiber in your diet (fresh fruits and vegetables, salads, bran, and whole-grain breads), exercise, and drink more water (unless your doctor directs you to do otherwise).

If you become dizzy, sit or lie down; get up slowly from a sitting or reclining position, and be careful on stairs.

Major. Tell your doctor about any side effects that are persistent or particularly bothersome. IT IS ESPECIALLY IMPORTANT TO TELL YOUR DOCTOR about bloody or black, tarry stools; blurred vision; confusion; difficult or painful urination; palpitations; a problem with hearing, or ringing or buzzing in your ears; skin rash, hives, or itching; stomach pain; swelling of the feet or hands; tightness in the chest; unexplained sore throat and fever; soreness of the tongue or mouth; unusual fatigue or weakness; unusual weight gain; wheezing or difficulty in breathing; or yellowing of the eyes or skin.

INTERACTIONS

Diclofenac interacts with several other types of medications:

1. Anticoagulants (blood thinners such as warfarin) can lead to an increase in bleeding complications.

2. Aspirin, other salicylates, and other anti-inflammatory medications can increase stomach irritation. Aspirin may also decrease the effectiveness of diclofenac. Therefore, aspirin should not be used concurrently with diclofenac.

3. Diclofenac can decrease the elimination of digoxin, methotrexate, and lithium from the body, which can lead to serious side effects.

4. The activity of diuretics (water pills) and drugs to lower blood pressure (propranolol, metoprolol) may be inhibited by diclofenac.

5. Diclofenac may alter a diabetic patient's response to insulin, oral hypoglycemic agents, or antiseizure medication (phenytoin).

Before starting to take diclofenac, BE SURE TO TELL YOUR DOCTOR about any medications you are taking, especially any of those listed above.

WARNINGS

• Before you start to take this medication, it is important to tell your doctor if you have ever had unusual or allergic reactions to diclofenac or to any of the other chemically related drugs (aspirin, other salicylates, diflunisal, fenoprofen, flurbiprofen, indomethacin, ketoprofen, meclofenamate, mefenamic acid, naproxen, oxyphenbutazone, phenylbutazone, piroxicam, sulindac, or tolmetin).

• Tell your doctor if you now have or if you have ever had asthma, bleeding problems, colitis, stomach ulcers or other stomach problems, epilepsy, heart disease, high blood pressure, kidney disease, liver disease, mental illness, or Parkinson's disease.

• If diclofenac makes you dizzy or drowsy, do not take part in any activity that requires alertness, such as driving a car or operating potentially dangerous machinery.

• Because this drug can prolong your bleeding time, it is important to tell your doctor or dentist that you are taking this drug before having surgery or any other medical or dental treatment.
• Stomach problems are more likely to occur if you take aspirin regularly or drink alcohol while being treated with this medication. These should, therefore, be avoided (unless your doctor directs you to do otherwise).
• Be sure to tell your doctor if you are pregnant or planning to become pregnant. This medication can cause unwanted effects on the heart or blood flow of the fetus. Studies in animals have also shown that this medicine, if taken late in pregnancy, may increase the length of pregnancy, prolong labor, or cause other problems during delivery. Also tell your doctor if you are breast-feeding an infant. Small amounts of diclofenac can pass into breast milk.

Dicloxacil—see dicloxacillin

---

dicloxacillin

BRAND NAMES (Manufacturers)
Dicloxacil (Goldline)
dicloxacillin sodium (various manufacturers)
Dycill (Beecham)
Dynapen (Bristol)
Pathocil (Wyeth)
TYPE OF DRUG
Penicillin antibiotic
INGREDIENT
dicloxacillin
DOSAGE FORMS
Capsules (125 mg, 250 mg, and 500 mg)
Oral suspension (62.5 mg per 5-ml spoonful)
STORAGE
Dicloxacillin capsules should be stored at room temperature in a tightly closed container. The oral suspension should be stored in the refrigerator in a tightly closed container. Any unused portion of the suspension should be discarded after 14 days because the drug loses its potency after that time. This medication should never be frozen.

USES

Dicloxacillin is used to treat a wide variety of bacterial infections, especially those caused by *Staphylococcus* bacteria. It acts by severely injuring the cell membranes of the infecting bacteria, thereby preventing them from growing and multiplying. Dicloxacillin kills susceptible bacteria, but it is not effective against viruses, parasites, or fungi.

TREATMENT

Dicloxacillin should be taken on an empty stomach or with a glass of water, one hour before or two hours after a meal. This medication should never be taken with fruit juices or carbonated beverages, because the acidity of these drinks destroys the drug in the stomach.

The suspension form of this medication should be shaken well just before measuring each dose. The contents tend to settle at the bottom of the bottle, so it is necessary to shake the container to distribute the ingredients evenly and equalize the doses. Each dose should then be measured carefully with a specially designed 5-ml measuring spoon. An ordinary kitchen teaspoon is not accurate enough.

Dicloxacillin works best when the level of medicine in your bloodstream is kept constant. It is best, therefore, to take the doses at evenly spaced intervals day and night. For example, if you are taking four doses a day, the doses should be spaced six hours apart.

If you miss a dose of this medication, take the missed dose immediately. However, if you do not remember to take the missed dose until it is almost time for your next dose, take it; space the following dose about halfway through the regular interval between doses; then return to your regular schedule. Try not to skip any doses.

It is important for you to continue to take this medication for the entire time prescribed by your doctor (usually seven to 14 days), even if the symptoms of your infection disappear before the end of that period. If you stop taking the drug too soon, bacteria are given a chance to continue growing, and the infection could recur.

SIDE EFFECTS

Minor. Diarrhea, heartburn, nausea, or vomiting. These side effects should disappear as you adjust to the drug.
Major. Tell your doctor about any side effects that are persistent or particularly bothersome. IT IS ESPECIALLY IMPORTANT TO TELL YOUR DOCTOR about bloating, chills, cough, darkened tongue, difficulty in breathing, fever, irritation of the mouth, muscle aches, rash, rectal or vaginal itching, severe diarrhea, or sore throat. In addition, if the symptoms of your infection seem to be getting worse rather than improving, you should contact your doctor.

INTERACTIONS

Dicloxacillin interacts with other types of medications:
1. Probenecid can increase the blood concentrations and side effects of this medication.
2. Dicloxacillin may decrease the effectiveness of oral contraceptives (birth control pills), and pregnancy could result. You should, therefore, use a different or additional form of birth control while taking this medication. Discuss this with your doctor.

BE SURE TO TELL YOUR DOCTOR about any medications you are currently taking, especially any of those listed above.

WARNINGS

• Tell your doctor about unusual or allergic reactions you have had to any medications, especially to dicloxacillin or penicillins, or to cephalosporin antibiotics, penicillamine, or griseofulvin.
• Tell your doctor if you now have or if you have ever had kidney disease, asthma, or allergies.
• This medication has been prescribed for your current infection only. Another infection later on, or one that someone else has, may require a different medicine. You should not give your medicine to other people or use it for other infections, unless your doctor specifically directs you to do so.
• Diabetics taking dicloxacillin should know that this drug can cause interference with a Clinitest urine glucose test. To avoid this problem while taking dicloxacillin, you should switch to Clinistix or Tes-Tape to test your urine for sugar.

• Be sure to tell your doctor if you are pregnant. Although dicloxacillin appears to be safe during pregnancy, extensive studies in humans have not been conducted. Also, tell your doctor if you are breast-feeding an infant. Small amounts of this medication pass into breast milk and may temporarily alter the bacterial balance in the intestinal tract of the nursing infant, resulting in diarrhea.

dicloxacillin sodium—see dicloxacillin

---

dicyclomine

BRAND NAMES (Manufacturers)
Bentyl (Lakeside Pharmaceutical)
Byclomine (Major)
dicyclomine hydrochloride (various manufacturers)
Di-Spaz (Vortech)
TYPE OF DRUG
Antispasmodic
INGREDIENT
dicyclomine
DOSAGE FORMS
Tablets (20 mg)
Capsules (10 mg and 20 mg)
Oral liquid (10 mg per 5-ml spoonful)
STORAGE
Dicyclomine tablets, capsules, and oral liquid should be stored at room temperature in tightly closed containers. This medication should never be frozen.

USES

Dicyclomine is used to treat gastrointestinal tract disorders and irritable bowel syndrome. Dicyclomine acts directly on the muscles of the gastrointestinal tract to decrease tone and slow their activity.

TREATMENT

Dicyclomine can be taken before or after meals. Consult your doctor for specific recommendations.

Antacids and antidiarrheal medicines may prevent absorption of this drug; therefore, at least one hour should separate doses of dicyclomine and one of these medications.

Measure the liquid form of dicyclomine carefully with a specially designed 5-ml measuring spoon. An ordinary kitchen teaspoon is not accurate enough. You can then dilute the oral liquid in other liquids to mask its taste.

If you miss a dose of this medication, do not take the missed dose at all; just return to your regular dosing schedule. Do not double the next dose.

SIDE EFFECTS

Minor. Bloating; blurred vision; confusion; constipation; dizziness; drowsiness; dry mouth, throat, and nose; headache; increased sensitivity to light; insomnia; loss of taste; nausea; nervousness; decreased sweating; vomiting; or weakness. These side effects should disappear as your body adjusts to the medication.

If you are constipated, increase the amount of fiber in your diet (fresh fruits and vegetables, salads, bran, and whole-grain breads), exercise, and drink more water (unless your doctor directs you to do otherwise).

Chew sugarless gum or suck on ice chips or a piece of hard candy to reduce mouth dryness.

Wear sunglasses if your eyes become sensitive to light.

To avoid dizziness or light-headedness when you stand, contract and relax the muscles of your legs for a few moments before rising. Do this by pushing one foot against the floor while raising the other foot slightly, alternating feet so that you are "pumping" your legs in a pedaling motion.

Major. Tell your doctor about any side effects that are persistent or particularly bothersome. IT IS ESPECIALLY IMPORTANT TO TELL YOUR DOCTOR about difficulty in urinating, fever, hallucinations, impotence, palpitations, rash, short-term memory loss, or sore throat.

INTERACTIONS

Dicyclomine interacts with several other types of drugs:

1. It can cause extreme drowsiness when combined with central nervous system depressants (such as alcohol, antihistamines, barbiturates, benzodiazepine tranquilizers, muscle relaxants, narcotics, pain medications, and phenothiazine tranquilizers) or with tricyclic antidepressants.

2. Amantadine, antihistamines, haloperidol, monoamine oxidase (MAO) inhibitors, phenothiazine tranquilizers, procainamide, quinidine, and tricyclic antidepressants can increase the side effects of dicyclomine.

Before starting to take this medication, BE SURE TO TELL YOUR DOCTOR about any medications you are currently taking, especially any of those listed above.

WARNINGS

• Tell your doctor about unusual or allergic reactions you have had to any medications, especially to dicyclomine.

• Tell your doctor if you have ever had glaucoma; heart disease; hiatal hernia; high blood pressure; kidney, liver, or thyroid disease; myasthenia gravis; obstructed bladder; obstructed intestine; enlarged prostate gland; ulcerative colitis; or internal bleeding.

• If this medication makes you dizzy or drowsy or blurs your vision, do not take part in any activity that requires alertness, such as driving a car or operating potentially dangerous equipment. Be careful on stairs, and avoid getting up from a lying or sitting position suddenly.

• This drug can decrease sweating and heat release from the body. Avoid taking hot baths, showers, or saunas, and avoid getting overheated by exercising in hot weather.

• Before having surgery or other medical or dental treatment, tell your doctor or dentist you are taking this drug.

• Tell your doctor if you are pregnant. Although this drug appears to be safe during pregnancy, extensive studies in humans have not been conducted. Also, tell your doctor if you are breast-feeding an infant. Small amounts of dicyclomine pass into breast milk.

dicyclomine hydrochloride—see dicyclomine

---

diethylpropion

BRAND NAMES (Manufacturers)
diethylpropion hydrochloride (various manufacturers)
Tenuate (Lakeside Pharmaceutical)
Tenuate Dospan (Lakeside Pharmaceutical)

Tepanil (Riker)
Tepanil Ten-Tab (Riker)

TYPE OF DRUG
Anorectic

INGREDIENT
diethylpropion

DOSAGE FORMS
Tablets (25 mg)
Sustained-release tablets (75 mg)

STORAGE
Diethylpropion tablets should be stored at room temperature in tightly closed, light-resistant containers.

USES

Diethylpropion is used as an appetite suppressant during the first few weeks of dieting to help establish new eating habits. This medication is thought to relieve hunger by altering nerve impulses to the appetite control center in the brain. Its effectiveness lasts only for short periods (three to 12 weeks), however.

TREATMENT

You can take diethylpropion with a full glass of water one hour before meals (unless your doctor directs you to do otherwise).

In order to avoid difficulty in falling asleep, the last dose of this medication each day should be taken four to six hours before bedtime (regular tablets) or ten to 14 hours before bedtime (sustained-release tablets).

The sustained-release form of this medication should be swallowed whole. Breaking, chewing, or crushing these tablets destroys their sustained-release activity and may increase the side effects.

If you miss a dose, take the missed dose as soon as possible, unless it is almost time for your next dose. In that case, do not take the missed dose; just return to your regular dosing schedule. Do not double the next dose.

SIDE EFFECTS

Minor. Blurred vision, constipation, diarrhea, dizziness, dry mouth, euphoria, fatigue, insomnia, irritability, nausea, nervousness, restlessness, stomach pain, sweating, tremors, unpleasant taste in the mouth, or vomiting. These side effects should disappear as your body adjusts to the medication.

Dry mouth can be relieved by sucking on ice chips or a piece of hard candy or by chewing sugarless gum.

In order to prevent constipation, increase the amount of fiber in your diet (fresh fruits and vegetables, salads, bran, and whole-grain breads), exercise, and drink more water (unless your doctor directs you to do otherwise).

Major. Tell your doctor about any side effects that are persistent or particularly bothersome. IT IS ESPECIALLY IMPORTANT TO TELL YOUR DOCTOR about changes in sexual desire, chest pain, difficulty in urinating, enlarged breasts (in both sexes), fever, hair loss, headaches, impotence, menstrual irregularities, mental depression, mood changes, mouth sores, muscle pains, nosebleeds, palpitations, rash, or sore throat.

INTERACTIONS

Diethylpropion interacts with several other types of drugs:

1. Use of diethylpropion within 14 days of use of a monoamine oxidase (MAO) inhibitor (such as isocarboxazid, pargyline, phenelzine, tranylcypromine) can result in high blood pressure and other side effects.

2. Barbiturate medications and phenothiazine tranquilizers (especially chlorpromazine) can antagonize (act against) the appetite suppressant activity of this medication, decreasing its effectiveness.

3. Diethylpropion can decrease the blood-pressure-lowering effects of antihypertensive medications (especially guanethidine) and may alter insulin and oral antidiabetic medication dosage requirements in diabetic patients.

4. The side effects of other central nervous system stimulants (such as caffeine and nonprescription appetite suppressants and cough, allergy, asthma, sinus, and cold preparations) may be increased by this medication.

BE SURE TO TELL YOUR DOCTOR about any medications you are currently taking, especially any listed above.

WARNINGS

- Tell your doctor about unusual or allergic reactions you have had to any medications, especially to diethylpropion or other appetite suppressants (including benzphetamine, phendimetrazine, phenmetrazine, fenfluramine, mazindol, and phentermine), or to epinephrine, norepinephrine, ephedrine, amphetamine, dextroamphetamine, phenylephrine, phenylpropanolamine, pseudoephedrine, albuterol, metaproterenol, or terbutaline.
- Tell your doctor if you have a history of drug abuse, or if you have ever had angina, diabetes mellitus, emotional disturbances, glaucoma, heart or cardiovascular disease, high blood pressure, thyroid disease, or epilepsy.
- Diethylpropion can mask the symptoms of extreme fatigue and can cause dizziness or light-headedness. Your ability to perform tasks that require alertness, such as driving a car or operating potentially dangerous equipment, may be decreased. Appropriate caution should, therefore, be taken.
- Before surgery or other medical or dental treatment, tell your doctor or dentist you are taking this drug.
- Diethylpropion is related to amphetamine and may be habit-forming when taken for long periods (both physical and psychological dependence can occur). Therefore, you should not increase the dosage of this drug or take it for longer than 12 weeks unless you first consult your doctor. It is also important that you not stop taking this drug abruptly if you have been taking large doses for a long time. Fatigue, sleep disorders, mental depression, nausea or vomiting, or stomach cramps or pain could occur. Your doctor may want to decrease your dosage gradually.
- Be sure to tell your doctor if you are pregnant. Although side effects in humans have not been thoroughly studied, some of the appetite suppressants have been shown to cause side effects in the fetuses of animals that received large doses during pregnancy. Also, tell your doctor if you are breast-feeding an infant. It is not known whether this medication passes into breast milk.

diethylpropion hydrochloride—see diethylpropion

---

diflunisal

BRAND NAME (Manufacturer)
Dolobid (Merck Sharp & Dohme)

TYPE OF DRUG
Nonsteroidal anti-inflammatory analgesic
INGREDIENT
diflunisal
DOSAGE FORM
Tablets (250 mg and 500 mg)
STORAGE
This medication should be stored in a closed container at room temperature, away from heat and direct sunlight.

USES

Diflunisal is used to treat the inflammation (pain, swelling, and stiffness) of osteoarthritis and muscle or skeletal injury. Diflunisal has been shown to block the production of certain body chemicals, called prostaglandins, that may trigger pain. However, it is not yet fully understood how diflunisal works.

TREATMENT

You should take this drug immediately after meals or with food in order to reduce stomach irritation. Do not break, crush, or chew the tablets before swallowing—they should be swallowed whole to lessen side effects and to maintain their benefits for a full 12 hours. Ask your doctor if you can take diflunisal with an antacid.

If you are taking diflunisal to relieve osteoarthritis, you must take it regularly, as directed by your doctor. It may take several days before you feel the full benefits of this medication. Diflunisal does not cure osteoarthritis, but it will help to control the condition as long as you continue to take the medication.

It is important to take diflunisal on schedule and not to miss any doses. If you do miss a dose of this medication, take the missed dose as soon as possible, unless more than six hours has passed. In that case, do not take the missed dose at all; just return to your regular dosing schedule. Do not double the next dose.

SIDE EFFECTS

Minor. Bloating, constipation, diarrhea, difficulty in sleeping, dizziness, drowsiness, headache, heartburn, indigestion, light-headedness, loss of appetite, nausea, nervousness, unusual sweating, or vomiting. As your body adjusts to the drug, these side effects should disappear.

To relieve constipation, increase the amount of fiber in your diet (fresh fruits and vegetables, salads, bran, and whole-grain breads), exercise, and drink more water (unless your doctor directs you to do otherwise).

If you become dizzy, sit or lie down for a while; get up slowly from a sitting or reclining position, and be careful on stairs.

Major. Tell your doctor about any side effects that are persistent or particularly bothersome. IT IS ESPECIALLY IMPORTANT TO TELL YOUR DOCTOR about bloody or black, tarry stools; blurred vision; confusion; depression; difficult or painful urination; difficulty in breathing; palpitations; ringing or buzzing in the ears or difficulty in hearing; skin rash, hives, or itching; stomach pain; swelling of the feet; tightness in the chest; unexplained sore throat and fever; unusual bleeding or bruising; unusual fatigue or weakness; unusual weight gain; wheezing; or yellowing of the eyes or skin.

INTERACTIONS

Diflunisal interacts with several other types of medications:
1. Anticoagulants (blood thinners, such as warfarin), in combination with diflunisal, can lead to an increase in bleeding complications.
2. Aspirin, salicylates, or other anti-inflammatory medications may cause increased stomach irritation.
3. Antacids can lower blood diflunisal concentrations, decreasing its effectiveness.
4. Diflunisal can increase the blood concentrations and side effects of acetaminophen.
5. Diflunisal can increase or decrease some effects of hydrochlorothiazide and furosemide.

BE SURE TO TELL YOUR DOCTOR about any medications you are currently taking, especially any of those listed above.

WARNINGS

- Before you take this medication, it is important to tell your doctor if you have ever had unusual or allergic reactions to diflunisal or any chemically related drug (including aspirin or other salicylates, diclofenac, fenoprofen, flurbiprofen, ibuprofen, indomethacin, ketoprofen, meclofenamate, mefenamic acid, naproxen, oxyphenbutazone, phenylbutazone, piroxicam, sulindac, or tolmetin).
- Tell your doctor if you now have or if you have ever had bleeding problems, colitis, stomach ulcers or other stomach problems, epilepsy, heart disease, high blood pressure, asthma, kidney disease, liver disease, mental illness, or Parkinson's disease.
- If this drug makes you dizzy or drowsy, do not take part in any activity that requires alertness, such as driving a car or operating potentially dangerous equipment.
- Because diflunisal can prolong your bleeding time, it is important to tell your doctor or dentist that you are taking this drug before having surgery or any other medical or dental treatment.
- Stomach problems are more likely to occur if you take aspirin regularly or drink alcohol while being treated with this medication. These should, therefore, be avoided (unless your doctor directs you to do otherwise).
- Be sure to tell your doctor if you are pregnant. Although studies in humans have not been conducted, unwanted side effects (defects in the spine and ribs) have been reported in the offspring of animals that received diflunisal during pregnancy. If taken during the last three months of pregnancy, this drug can cause heart problems in the fetus; it can also prolong labor. Also, tell your doctor if you are breast-feeding an infant. Because diflunisal can pass into breast milk, breast-feeding while taking this drug is not recommended.

---

digitoxin

BRAND NAMES (Manufacturers)
Crystodigin (Lilly)
digitoxin (various manufacturers)
TYPE OF DRUG
Cardiac glycoside
INGREDIENT
digitoxin

DOSAGE FORM
Tablets (0.05 mg, 0.1 mg, 0.15 mg, and 0.2 mg)
STORAGE
Store at room temperature in a tightly closed container.

USES

Digitoxin belongs to a group of drugs known as digitalis glycosides. It is used to treat heart arrhythmias and congestive heart failure. Digitoxin improves the strength and efficiency of the heart and controls the heart rhythm.

TREATMENT

In order to avoid stomach irritation, you can take digitoxin with food or with a full glass of water or milk (unless your doctor directs you to do otherwise).

In order to become accustomed to taking this medication, try to take it at the same time each day.

If you miss a dose of this medication, take the missed dose as soon as possible, unless it is almost time for the next dose. In that case, do not take the missed dose at all; just return to your regular dosing schedule. Do not double the next dose. If you miss two or more doses, check with your doctor.

Digitoxin does not cure heart failure, but it will help to control the condition as long as you continue to take it.

SIDE EFFECTS

Minor. Drowsiness, headache, loss of appetite, nausea, stomach upset, or vomiting. These side effects should disappear as your body adjusts to the medication.
Major. Tell your doctor about any side effects that are persistent or particularly bothersome. IT IS ESPECIALLY IMPORTANT TO TELL YOUR DOCTOR about bad dreams, blurred vision, breast enlargement (in both sexes), confusion, depression, disorientation, hallucinations, muscle weakness, palpitations, or tingling sensations.

INTERACTIONS

Digitoxin interacts with several other types of medications:
1. Barbiturates, phenytoin, aminoglutethimide, levodopa, penicillamine, oral antidiabetic medications, phenylbutazone, and rifampin can decrease the blood levels and effectiveness of digitoxin.
2. The absorption of digitoxin from the gastrointestinal tract is reduced when it is taken with colestipol, cholestyramine, metoclopramide, antacids, neomycin, antineoplastic (anticancer) drugs, or sulfasalazine.
3. Tetracycline can increase the absorption of digitoxin from the gastrointestinal tract, which can increase the risk of side effects.
4. Spironolactone can unpredictably increase or decrease the side effects of digitoxin.
5. Concurrent use of quinidine, procainamide, hydroxychloroquine, calcium, reserpine, ephedrine, or beta blockers (acebutolol, atenolol, betaxolol, carteolol, esmolol, labetalol, metoprolol, nadolol, penbutolol, pindolol, propranolol, timolol) with digitoxin can lead to additive effects on the heart.
6. The dosage of digitoxin may require adjustment if therapy with thyroid hormones, methimazole, or propylthiouracil is started.
7. Concurrent use of digitoxin and quinidine, quinine, erythromycin, amiodarone, benzodiazepine tranquilizers, diltiazem, nifedipine, or verapamil can increase the blood levels and the side effects of digitoxin.

Before starting to take digitoxin, BE SURE TO TELL YOUR DOCTOR about any medications you are currently taking, especially any of those listed above.

WARNINGS

- Tell your doctor about unusual or allergic reactions you have had to medications, especially to digitoxin or any other digitalis glycoside.
- Before starting to take this medication, be sure to tell your doctor if you now have or if you have ever had blood electrolyte disorders (too much or too little calcium, magnesium, or potassium), heart disease, kidney disease, lung disease, liver disease, or thyroid disease.
- Before having surgery or any other medical or dental treatment, be sure to tell your doctor or dentist that you are taking this medication.
- Check with your doctor or pharmacist before taking any over-the-counter (nonprescription) allergy, asthma, cough, cold, diet, or sinus product. Some of these products can increase the side effects of digitoxin.
- Do not stop taking this medication unless you first check with your doctor. Stopping abruptly may lead to a worsening of your condition.
- While you are taking digitoxin, your doctor may want you to check your pulse every day. If your pulse is slower than your doctor has told you it should be or if the rhythm is irregular, CONTACT YOUR DOCTOR IMMEDIATELY.
- Be sure to tell your doctor if you are pregnant. Although digitoxin appears to be safe during pregnancy, extensive studies in humans have not been conducted. In addition, the dosage of digitoxin required to control your disorder may change during pregnancy. Also, tell your doctor if you are breast-feeding an infant. It is not known if digitoxin passes into breast milk.

---

digoxin

BRAND NAMES (Manufacturers)
digoxin (various manufacturers)
Lanoxicaps (Burroughs Wellcome)
Lanoxin (Burroughs Wellcome)
TYPE OF DRUG
Cardiac glycoside
INGREDIENT
digoxin
DOSAGE FORMS
Tablets (0.125 mg, 0.25 mg, and 0.5 mg)
Capsules (0.05 mg, 0.1 mg, and 0.2 mg)
Pediatric elixir (0.05 mg per ml, with 10% alcohol)
STORAGE
Digoxin tablets, capsules, and pediatric elixir should be stored at room temperature in tightly closed, light-resistant containers. This medication should never be frozen.

USES

Digoxin is used to strengthen the heartbeat and improve heart rhythm. It works directly on the muscle of the heart to improve contraction.

TREATMENT

In order to avoid stomach irritation, you can take digoxin with a full glass of water or with food. Try to take it at the same time every day.

Measure the dose of the pediatric elixir carefully with the dropper provided. An ordinary kitchen teaspoon is not accurate enough.

Antacids decrease the absorption of digoxin from the gastrointestinal tract. Therefore, if you are taking both digoxin and an antacid, the dose of digoxin should be taken one hour before or two hours after a dose of antacids.

Try not to miss any doses of this medication. If you do miss a dose, take the missed dose as soon as possible, unless it is almost time for the next dose. In that case, do not take the missed dose at all; just return to your regular dosing schedule. Do not double the next dose. If you miss more than two doses of digoxin, contact your doctor.

Digoxin does not cure congestive heart failure, but it will help to control the condition as long as you continue to take the medication.

SIDE EFFECTS

Minor. Apathy, diarrhea, drowsiness, headache, muscle weakness, or tiredness. These side effects should disappear as your body adjusts to the medication.

Major. Tell your doctor about any side effects that are persistent or particularly bothersome. IT IS ESPECIALLY IMPORTANT TO TELL YOUR DOCTOR about disorientation, enlarged and painful breasts (in both sexes), hallucinations, loss of appetite, mental depression, nausea, palpitations, severe abdominal pain, slowed heart rate, visual disturbances (such as blurred or yellow vision), or vomiting.

INTERACTIONS

Digoxin interacts with several other types of medications (interactions may vary depending upon the dosage form of digoxin being used):

1. Penicillamine, antiseizure medications, rifampin, aminoglutethimide, and levodopa can decrease the blood levels and, therefore, the effectiveness of digoxin.

2. Erythromycin, amiodarone, captopril, benzodiazepine tranquilizers, flecainide, tetracycline, hydroxychloroquine, verapamil, nifedipine, diltiazem, quinidine, quinine, and spironolactone can increase the blood levels of digoxin, which can lead to an increase in side effects.

3. Thyroid hormone, propylthiouracil, and methimazole can change the dosage requirements of digoxin.

4. Antacids, kaolin-pectin, sulfasalazine, aminosalicylic acid, metoclopramide, antineoplastic agents (anticancer drugs), neomycin, colestipol, and cholestyramine can decrease the absorption of digoxin from the gastrointestinal tract, decreasing its effectiveness.

5. Calcium, tolbutamide, and reserpine can increase the side effects of digoxin.

6. Diuretics (water pills) and adrenocorticosteroids (cortisone-like medications) can cause hypokalemia (low potassium blood levels), which can increase the side effects of digoxin.

BE SURE TO TELL YOUR DOCTOR about any medications you are currently taking, especially any of those listed above.

WARNINGS

- Tell your doctor about unusual or allergic reactions you have had to any medications, especially to digoxin, digitoxin, or gitalin.
- Tell your doctor if you now have or if you have ever had kidney disease, lung disease, thyroid disease, hypokalemia (low blood levels of potassium), or hypercalcemia (high blood levels of calcium).
- The pharmacologic activity of the different brands of this drug varies widely—the tablets dissolve in the stomach and bowel at different rates and to varying degrees. Because of this variability, it is important not to change brands of the drug without consulting your doctor.
- Meals high in bran fiber may reduce the absorption of digoxin from the gastrointestinal tract. Avoid these types of meals when taking your dose of medication.
- Your doctor may want you to take your pulse daily while you are using digoxin. Contact your doctor if your pulse becomes slower than what your doctor tells you is normal, or if it drops below 50 beats per minute.
- Before having surgery or any other medical or dental treatment, be sure to tell your doctor or dentist that you are taking this medication.
- Before taking any over-the-counter (nonprescription) asthma, allergy, cough, cold, sinus, or diet product, be sure to check with your doctor or pharmacist. Some of these drugs can increase the side effects of digoxin.
- Be sure to tell your doctor if you are pregnant. Although this drug appears to be safe during pregnancy, extensive studies in humans have not been conducted. In addition, the dosage of digoxin required to control your symptoms may change during pregnancy. Also, tell your doctor if you are breast-feeding an infant. Small amounts of digoxin pass into breast milk.

---

dihydrotachysterol

BRAND NAMES (Manufacturers)

dihydrotachysterol or DHT (Roxane)
Hytakerol (Winthrop)

TYPE OF DRUG

Vitamin D analog

INGREDIENT

dihydrotachysterol

DOSAGE FORMS

Tablets (0.125 mg, 0.2 mg, and 0.4 mg)
Capsules (0.125 mg)
Oral solution (0.2 mg per ml, with 4% alcohol)
Oral concentrate (0.2 mg per ml, with 20% alcohol)

STORAGE

Dihydrotachysterol tablets, capsules, oral solution, and oral concentrate should be stored at room temperature in tightly closed, light-resistant containers. This medication should never be frozen.

USES

Vitamin D is essential to many body systems (including muscle and heart function). Dihydrotachysterol is a vitamin D analog—it raises blood calcium levels. This medication is used to treat tetany and hypoparathyroidism, conditions characterized by low blood calcium levels.

TREATMENT

You can take dihydrotachysterol either on an empty stomach or with food or milk (as directed by your doctor).

Each dose of the oral solution form of this medication should be measured carefully with the dropper provided. The solution can then be swallowed directly or mixed with fruit juice, cereal, or other foods.

If you miss a dose of this medication, take the missed dose as soon as possible, unless it is almost time for the next dose. In that case, do not take the missed dose; just return to your regular dosing schedule. Do not double the dose.

SIDE EFFECTS

Minor. None, at the dosages normally prescribed.

Major. The side effects associated with dihydrotachysterol therapy are usually the result of too much medication (vitamin D intoxication). Tell your doctor about any side effects that are persistent or particularly bothersome. IT IS ESPECIALLY IMPORTANT TO TELL YOUR DOCTOR about blurred vision, bone pain, constipation, dry mouth, headache, increased thirst, increased urination, irritability, loss of appetite, mental disorders, metallic taste in the mouth, muscle pain, nausea, palpitations, runny nose, vomiting, weakness, or weight loss.

INTERACTIONS

This drug interacts with several other drugs.

1. If you are being treated for hypoparathyroidism, concurrent use of dihydrotachysterol and thiazide diuretics (water pills) can lead to hypercalcemia (high blood calcium levels).

2. The effects of this medication may be increased or decreased by digoxin, antacids, verapamil, or cholestyramine.

BE SURE TO TELL YOUR DOCTOR about any medications you are currently taking, especially any listed above.

WARNINGS

- Tell your doctor about unusual or allergic reactions you have had to any medications, especially to dihydrotachysterol, calcitriol, calcifediol, ergocalciferol, or vitamin D.
- Before starting to take this medication, be sure to tell your doctor if you now have or if you have ever had heart or blood vessel disease, hypercalcemia, hyperphosphatemia, vitamin D intoxication, or sarcoidosis.
- Before taking any over-the-counter (nonprescription) products that contain calcium, phosphates, magnesium, or vitamin D, check with your doctor. These ingredients can increase the side effects of dihydrotachysterol.
- Dihydrotachysterol is more expensive than vitamin D products, but it is often prescribed instead of vitamin D because it is faster-acting and does not persist in the body once therapy is stopped.
- Be sure to tell your doctor if you are pregnant. Although dihydrotachysterol has not been studied during pregnancy in humans, birth defects have been reported in the offspring of animals that received large doses of this medication during pregnancy. Also, tell your doctor if you are breastfeeding an infant. It is not known if this drug passes into breast milk.

Dilantin—see phenytoin

Dilantin Infatab—see phenytoin

Dilantin Kapseal—see phenytoin

Dilatrate-SR—see isosorbide dinitrate

Dilaudid—see hydromorphone

---

diltiazem

BRAND NAMES (Manufacturers)

Cardizem (Marion)
Cardizem SR (Marion)

TYPE OF DRUG

Antianginal and antihypertensive

INGREDIENT

diltiazem

DOSAGE FORMS

Tablets (30 mg, 60 mg, 90 mg, and 120 mg)
Sustained-release capsules (60 mg, 90 mg, 120 mg)

STORAGE

Diltiazem should be stored at room temperature in a tightly closed container.

USES

This medication is used to prevent the symptoms of angina (chest pain). It belongs to a group of drugs known as calcium channel blockers. It is unclear exactly how it does so, but diltiazem dilates the blood vessels of the heart and increases the amount of oxygen that reaches the heart muscle. This drug is also prescribed to lower blood pressure in patients with hypertension.

TREATMENT

If stomach irritation occurs, diltiazem can be taken either on an empty stomach or with meals, as directed by your doctor. The sustained-release capsules should be swallowed whole; chewing, crushing, or crumbling them destroys their controlled-release activity and possibly increases the side effects.

In order to become accustomed to taking this medication, try to take it at the same times each day.

Diltiazem does not relieve chest pain once it has begun; this medication is used to prevent angina attacks.

If you miss a dose of this medication, take the missed dose as soon as possible, unless it is within four hours of the next scheduled dose. In that case, do not take the missed dose at all; just return to your regular dosing schedule. Do not double the next dose.

This medication does not cure angina, but it will help to control the condition as long as you continue to take it.

SIDE EFFECTS

Minor. Constipation, diarrhea, dizziness, drowsiness, headache, insomnia, light-headedness, nausea, nervousness, stomach upset, or vomiting. These side effects should disappear as your body adjusts to the medication.

This drug can increase your sensitivity to sunlight. Therefore, avoid prolonged exposure to sunlight and sunlamps. Wear protective clothing and sunglasses, and use an effective sunscreen.

If you feel dizzy or light-headed, sit or lie down for a while; get up slowly from a sitting or reclining position, and be careful on stairs.

To relieve constipation, increase the amount of fiber in your diet (fresh fruits and vegetables, salads, bran, and whole-grain breads), exercise, and drink more water (unless your doctor directs you to do otherwise).

Major. Tell your doctor about any side effects that are persistent or particularly bothersome. IT IS ESPECIALLY IMPORTANT TO TELL YOUR DOCTOR about confusion, depression, fainting, fatigue, flushing, fluid retention, hallucinations, palpitations, skin rash, tingling in the fingers or toes, unusual weakness, or yellowing of the eyes or skin.

INTERACTIONS

Diltiazem can interact with several other types of medications:

1. Diltiazem should be used cautiously with beta blockers (acebutolol, atenolol, betaxolol, carteolol, esmolol, labetalol, metoprolol, nadolol, penbutolol, propranolol, pindolol, timolol), digitoxin, digoxin, or disopyramide. Side effects on the heart may be increased by the concurrent use of these medications.

2. Cimetidine can decrease the elimination of diltiazem from the body, which can increase the risk of side effects.

3. Diltiazem can increase the blood concentrations of cyclosporine, which can increase the risk of side effects.

BE SURE TO TELL YOUR DOCTOR about any medications you are currently taking, especially any listed above.

WARNINGS

- Tell your doctor about unusual or allergic reactions you have had to any medications, especially to diltiazem.
- Before starting to take this medication, be sure to tell your doctor if you now have or if you have ever had bradycardia (slow heartbeat), heart block, heart failure, kidney disease, liver disease, low blood pressure, or sick sinus syndrome.
- If this drug makes you dizzy or drowsy, avoid taking part in any activity that requires alertness, such as driving a car or operating potentially dangerous equipment.
- To prevent fainting while taking this drug, avoid drinking large amounts of alcohol. Also, avoid prolonged standing and strenuous exercise in hot weather.
- Be sure to tell your doctor if you are pregnant. Extensive studies in pregnant women have not been conducted, but birth defects have been reported in the offspring of animals that received large doses of diltiazem during pregnancy. It is also known that diltiazem passes into breast milk. If you are breast-feeding an infant while being treated with this medication, tell your doctor. Unless directed to do otherwise, breast-feeding is not recommended at this time.

Dimetane—see brompheniramine

Dimetane Extentabs—see brompheniramine

Dimetapp Extentabs—see phenylpropanolamine, phenylephrine, and brompheniramine combination

Diphenatol—see diphenoxylate and atropine combination

Diphen Cough Syrup—see diphenhydramine

---

diphenhydramine

BRAND NAMES (Manufacturers)

AllerMax (Pfeiffer)
Belix* (Halsey)
Benadryl* (Parke-Davis)
Benadryl Kapseals (Parke-Davis)
Benylin Cough Syrup* (Parke-Davis)
Bydramine Cough Syrup* (Major)
Compoz* (Jeffrey Martin)
Diphen Cough Syrup* (My-K Lab)
diphenhydramine hydrochloride (various manufacturers)
Dormarex 2* (Republic)
Hydramine* (Goldline)
Nervine Night-time Sleep Aid* (Miles)
Nordryl (Vortech)
Nytol (Block)
Sleep-Eze 3* (Whitehall)
Sominex 2* (Beecham)
Tusstat (Century)
Twilite* (Pfeiffer)
Unisom Nighttime Sleep Aid*(Leeming)
*Available over-the-counter (without a prescription)

TYPE OF DRUG

Antihistamine and sedative/hypnotic

INGREDIENT

diphenhydramine

DOSAGE FORMS

Tablets (50 mg)
Capsules (25 mg and 50 mg)
Elixir (12.5 mg per 5-ml spoonful, with 14% alcohol)
Oral syrup (12.5 mg per 5-ml spoonful, with 5% alcohol)

STORAGE

Store at room temperature in a tightly closed container.

USES

This medication has multiple uses. It belongs to a group of drugs known as antihistamines (antihistamines block the action of histamine, a chemical that is released by the body during an allergic reaction). It is, therefore, used to treat or prevent symptoms of allergy.

Diphenhydramine is also used to treat motion sickness and Parkinson's disease, and it is used as a nighttime sleeping aid and nonnarcotic cough suppressant.

TREATMENT

To avoid stomach upset, you can take diphenhydramine with food or with a full glass of milk or water (unless your doctor directs you to do otherwise).

The elixir and oral syrup forms of this medication should be measured carefully with a specially designed 5-ml measuring spoon. An ordinary teaspoon is not accurate enough.

If you miss a dose of this medication, take the missed dose as soon as possible, unless it is almost time for your next dose. In that case, do not take the missed dose at all; just return to your regular dosing schedule. Do not double the next dose.

SIDE EFFECTS

Minor. Blurred vision; confusion; constipation; diarrhea; dizziness; dry mouth, throat, or nose; headache; irritability; loss of appetite; nausea; restlessness; stomach upset; or unusual increase in sweating. These side effects should disappear as your body adjusts to the medication.

This medication can cause increased sensitivity to sunlight. It is, therefore, important to avoid prolonged exposure to sunlight and sunlamps. Wear protective clothing, and use an effective sunscreen.

If you are constipated, increase the amount of fiber in your diet (fresh fruits and vegetables, salads, bran, and whole-grain breads), exercise, and drink more water (unless your doctor tells you not to do so).

To reduce mouth dryness, chew sugarless gum or suck on ice chips or a piece of hard candy.

If you feel dizzy or light-headed, sit or lie down for a while; get up slowly from a sitting or reclining position, and be careful on stairs.

Major. Tell your doctor about any side effects that are persistent or particularly bothersome. IT IS ESPECIALLY IMPORTANT TO TELL YOUR DOCTOR about changes in menstruation, clumsiness, difficult or painful urination, feeling faint, flushing of the face, hallucinations, palpitations, ringing or buzzing in the ears, rash, seizures, shortness of breath, sleeping disorders, sore throat or fever, tightness in the chest, unusual bleeding or bruising, or unusual tiredness or weakness.

INTERACTIONS

Diphenhydramine interacts with several types of drugs:

1. Concurrent use of it with other central nervous system depressants (such as alcohol, barbiturates, benzodiazepine tranquilizers, muscle relaxants, narcotics, pain medications, and phenothiazine tranquilizers) or with tricyclic antidepressants can cause extreme drowsiness.

2. Monoamine oxidase (MAO) inhibitors (isocarboxazid, pargyline, phenelzine, tranylcypromine) can increase the side effects of this medication. At least 14 days should separate the use of this drug and the use of an MAO inhibitor.

3. Diphenhydramine can also decrease the activity of oral anticoagulants (blood thinners, such as warfarin).

BE SURE TO TELL YOUR DOCTOR about any medications you are currently taking, especially any of those listed above.

WARNINGS

- Tell your doctor about unusual or allergic reactions you have had to any medications, especially to diphenhydramine or to any other antihistamine (such as astemizole, azatadine, brompheniramine, carbinoxamine, chlorpheniramine, clemastine, cyproheptadine, dexchlorpheniramine, dimenhydrinate, dimethindene, diphenylpyraline, doxylamine, hydroxyzine, phenidamine, promethazine, pyrilamine, terfenadine, trimeprazine, tripelennamine, and triprolidine).
- Tell your doctor if you now have or if you have ever had asthma, blood vessel disease, glaucoma, high blood pressure, kidney disease, peptic ulcers, enlarged prostate gland, or thyroid disease.
- Diphenhydramine can cause drowsiness or dizziness. Your ability to perform tasks that require alertness, such as driving a car or operating potentially dangerous equipment, may be decreased. Appropriate caution should, therefore, be taken.
- Be sure to tell your doctor if you are pregnant. The effects of this medication during pregnancy have not been thoroughly studied in humans. Also, tell your doctor if you are breast-feeding an infant. Small amounts of diphenhydramine pass into breast milk and may cause unusual excitement or irritability in nursing infants.

diphenhydramine hydrochloride—see diphenhydramine

---

diphenoxylate and atropine combination

BRAND NAMES (Manufacturers)

Diphenatol (Rugby)
diphenoxylate hydrochloride with atropine sulfate (various manufacturers)
Lofene (Lannett)
Logen (Goldline)
Lomanate (Barre)
Lomotil (Searle)
Lonox (Geneva Generics)
Lo-Trol (Vangard)
Low-Quel (Halsey)
Nor-Mil (Vortech)

TYPE OF DRUG

Antidiarrheal (antispasmodic and anticholinergic)

INGREDIENTS

diphenoxylate and atropine

DOSAGE FORMS

Tablets (2.5 mg diphenoxylate and 0.025 mg atropine)
Oral liquid (2.5 mg diphenoxylate and 0.025 mg atropine per 5-ml spoonful, with 15% alcohol)

STORAGE

Diphenoxylate and atropine combination tablets and oral liquid should be stored at room temperature in tightly closed, light-resistant containers. Neither form of this medication should be frozen.

USES

Diphenoxylate and atropine combination is used to treat severe diarrhea. Diphenoxylate is related to the narcotic analgesics and acts by slowing the movement of the gastrointestinal tract. Small amounts of atropine are added to this medication to prevent abuse of the narcotic diphenoxylate.

TREATMENT

In order to avoid stomach upset, you can take this medication with food or with a full glass of water or milk.

The oral liquid form of this medication should be measured carefully using a specially designed 5-ml measuring spoon. An ordinary kitchen teaspoon is not accurate enough.

If you miss a dose of this medication, do not take the missed dose at all; just return to your regular dosing schedule. Do not double the next dose.

SIDE EFFECTS

Minor. Blurred vision, constipation, dizziness, drowsiness, dry mouth, flushing, headache, loss of appetite, nervousness, sweating, or swollen gums. These side effects should disappear as your body adjusts to the medication.

If you become constipated, exercise and drink more water (unless your doctor directs you to do otherwise).

To relieve mouth dryness, chew sugarless gum or suck on ice chips or a piece of hard candy.

If you feel dizzy or light-headed, sit or lie down for a while; get up slowly from a sitting or reclining position, and be careful on stairs.

Major. Tell your doctor about any side effects that are persistent or particularly bothersome. IT IS ESPECIALLY IMPORTANT TO TELL YOUR DOCTOR about abdominal pain, bloating, breathing difficulties, depression, difficult or painful urination, false sense of well-being, fever, hives, itching, numbness in the fingers or toes, palpitations, rash, severe nausea, vomiting, or weakness.

INTERACTIONS

This medication interacts with several other types of medications:

1. Concurrent use of this medication with central nervous system depressants (such as alcohol, antihistamines, barbiturates, benzodiazepine tranquilizers, muscle relaxants, narcotics, pain medications, and phenothiazine tranquilizers) or with tricyclic antidepressants can cause extreme drowsiness.

2. A monoamine oxidase (MAO) inhibitor (tranylcypromine, phenelzine, isocarboxazid, pargyline) taken within 14 days of this medication can lead to unpredictable and severe side effects.

3. The side effects of the atropine component of this medication may be increased by amantadine, haloperidol, phenothiazine tranquilizers, procainamide, and quinidine.

BE SURE TO TELL YOUR DOCTOR about any medications you are currently taking, especially any of those listed above.

WARNINGS

- Tell your doctor about unusual or allergic reactions you have had to medications, especially to diphenoxylate or to atropine.
- Tell your doctor if you now have or if you have ever had drug-induced diarrhea, gallstones or gallbladder disease, glaucoma, heart disease, hiatal hernia, high blood pressure, kidney disease, liver disease, lung disease, myasthenia gravis, enlarged prostate gland, thyroid disease, or ulcerative colitis.
- If this drug makes you dizzy or drowsy, do not take part in any activity that requires alertness, such as driving a car or operating potentially dangerous equipment.
- Before having surgery or any other medical or dental treatment, be sure to tell your doctor or dentist that you are taking this medication.
- Because this product contains diphenoxylate, it has the potential for abuse and must be used with caution. Tolerance develops quickly; do not increase the dosage or stop taking the drug unless you first consult your doctor. If you have been taking large amounts of this medication for long periods and then stop abruptly, you may experience a withdrawal reaction (muscle aches, diarrhea, gooseflesh, runny nose, nausea, vomiting, shivering, trembling, stomach cramps, sleep disorders, irritability, weakness, excessive yawning, or sweating). Your doctor may, therefore, want to reduce the dosage gradually.
- Check with your doctor if your diarrhea does not subside within two to three days. Unless your doctor prescribes otherwise, do not take this drug for more than five days.
- While taking this medication, drink lots of fluids to replace those lost with the diarrhea.
- Be sure to tell your doctor if you are pregnant. Although this medication has been shown to be safe in animals, its effects in humans during pregnancy have not been thoroughly studied. Also, tell your doctor if you are breast-feeding an infant. Small amounts of this medication may pass into breast milk and cause excessive drowsiness in nursing infants.

diphenoxylate hydrochloride with atropine sulfate—see diphenoxylate and atropine combination

Diphenylan—see phenytoin

Diprolene—see betamethasone dipropionate (topical)

Diprosone—see betamethasone dipropionate (topical)

---

dipyridamole

BRAND NAMES (Manufacturers)
dipyridamole (various manufacturers)
Persantine (Boehringer Ingelheim)
Pyridamole (Major)

TYPE OF DRUG
Antianginal

INGREDIENT
dipyridamole

DOSAGE FORM
Tablets (25 mg, 50 mg, and 75 mg)

STORAGE
Store at room temperature in a tightly closed container.

USES

Dipyridamole is used to prevent chronic chest pain (angina) due to heart disease. It relieves chest pain by dilating the blood vessels of the heart and providing more oxygen to the heart muscle. Dipyridamole is also used to prevent blood clot formation, especially in patients who have artificial heart valves.

TREATMENT

You should take this medication on an empty stomach with a full glass of water one hour before or two hours after a meal. If this drug upsets your stomach, check with your doctor to see if you can take it with food.

The full benefits of this medication may not become apparent for up to two to three months.

If you miss a dose of this medication, take the missed dose as soon as possible, unless it is within four hours of your next scheduled dose. In that case, do not take the missed dose at all; just return to your regular dosing schedule. Do not double the next dose.

SIDE EFFECTS

Minor. Dizziness, fatigue, flushing, headache, nausea, stomach cramps, or weakness. These side effects should disappear as your body adjusts to the medication.

To avoid dizziness or light-headedness when you stand, contract and relax the muscles of your legs for a few moments before rising. Do this by pushing one foot against the floor while raising the other foot slightly, alternating feet so that you are "pumping" your legs in a pedaling motion.

Major. Tell your doctor about any side effects that are persistent or particularly bothersome. IT IS ESPECIALLY IMPORTANT TO TELL YOUR DOCTOR about fainting, skin rash, or a worsening of your chest pain.

INTERACTIONS

Dipyridamole should not interact with other medications if it is used according to directions.

WARNINGS

- Tell your doctor about unusual or allergic reactions you have had to any medications, especially to dipyridamole.
- Tell your doctor if you have ever had low blood pressure.
- The effectiveness of dipyridamole in controlling chronic angina is controversial. This drug is more frequently prescribed to prevent blood clot formation, although use of dipyridamole for this purpose has not yet been approved by the Food and Drug Administration (FDA).
- This drug does not stop chest pain from angina that has already begun. It is used only to prevent such pain from occurring.
- If this drug makes you dizzy, do not take part in any activity that requires alertness, such as driving a car or operating potentially dangerous equipment.
- Before having any surgery or other medical or dental treatment, be sure to tell your doctor or dentist that you are taking this medication.
- Be sure to tell your doctor if you are pregnant. Although this drug appears to be safe, extensive studies in humans during pregnancy have not been conducted. Also, tell your doctor if you are breast-feeding an infant. Small amounts of dipyridamole pass into breast milk.

Disophrol—see pseudoephedrine and dexbrompheniramine combination

Disophrol Chronotabs—see pseudoephedrine and dexbrompheniramine combination

---

disopyramide

BRAND NAMES (Manufacturers)

Napamide (Major)
Norpace (Searle)
Norpace CR (Searle)

TYPE OF DRUG

Antiarrhythmic

INGREDIENT

disopyramide

DOSAGE FORMS

Capsules (100 mg and 150 mg)
Sustained-release capsules (100 mg and 150 mg)

STORAGE

Disopyramide capsules should be stored at room temperature in tightly closed containers.

USES

Disopyramide is used for the treatment of heart arrhythmias. It corrects irregular heartbeats and helps to achieve a more normal rhythm.

TREATMENT

Disopyramide can be taken with or without food. Check with your doctor for a recommendation.

Try to take disopyramide at the same time(s) each day. This medication works best if the amount of the drug in your bloodstream is kept at a constant level. It is best, therefore, to take this medication at evenly spaced intervals day and night. For example, if you are to take it three times per day, the doses should be spaced eight hours apart.

Try not to miss any doses of this medication. If you do miss a dose and remember within two hours, take the missed dose as soon as possible. If more than two hours have passed, do not take the missed dose; just wait for your next scheduled dose. Do not double the dose.

SIDE EFFECTS

Minor. Abdominal pain; aches and pain; blurred vision; constipation; decreased sweating; diarrhea; dizziness; dry mouth, eyes, and throat; fatigue; gas; headache; impotence; loss of appetite; nausea; nervousness; or vomiting. These side effects should disappear as you adjust to the drug.

To relieve constipation, increase the amount of fiber in your diet (fresh fruits and vegetables, salads, bran, and whole-grain breads), exercise, and drink more water (unless your doctor directs you to do otherwise).

If you feel dizzy or light-headed, sit or lie down for a while; get up slowly from a sitting or reclining position, and be careful on stairs.

To relieve mouth dryness, suck on ice chips or a piece of hard candy or chew sugarless gum.

"Artificial tears" eye drops may help to relieve eye dryness.

Major. Tell your doctor about any side effects that are persistent or particularly bothersome. IT IS ESPECIALLY IMPORTANT TO TELL YOUR DOCTOR about chest pain; depression; difficult or painful urination; enlarged, painful breasts (in both sexes); fainting; fever; muscle pain; muscle weakness; numbness or tingling sensations; palpitations; rash; shortness of breath; sore throat; swelling of the feet or ankles; weight gain; or yellowing of the eyes or skin.

INTERACTIONS

Disopyramide interacts with several other types of medications:

1. Phenytoin, rifampin, barbiturates, and glutethimide can decrease its effectiveness.

2. The combination of alcohol and disopyramide can lead

to dizziness and hypoglycemia (low blood sugar levels). You should, therefore, avoid drinking alcoholic beverages while you are taking this medication.

3. The concurrent use of disopyramide and beta blockers (acebutolol, atenolol, betaxolol, carteolol, esmolol, labetalol, metoprolol, nadolol, penbutolol, pindolol, propranolol, timolol) can have additive negative effects on the heart.

4. Disopyramide may interact with verapamil.

Before starting to take disopyramide, BE SURE TO TELL YOUR DOCTOR about any medications you are currently taking, especially any of those listed above.

WARNINGS

• Tell your doctor about unusual or allergic reactions you have had to any medications, especially to disopyramide.

• Tell your doctor if you now have or if you have ever had glaucoma, hypoglycemia (low blood sugar levels), hypokalemia (low blood potassium levels), kidney disease, liver disease, myasthenia gravis, urinary retention, or an enlarged prostate gland.

• If this drug makes you dizzy or drowsy or blurs your vision, do not take part in any activity that requires alertness, such as driving a car or operating potentially dangerous equipment.

• This medication can decrease sweating and heat release from the body. You should, therefore, avoid getting overheated by strenuous exercise in hot weather and should avoid taking hot baths, showers, and saunas.

• Before having surgery or any other medical or dental treatment, be sure to tell your doctor or dentist that you are taking this medication.

• Disopyramide can cause hypoglycemia. Signs of hypoglycemia include anxiety, chills, pale skin, headache, hunger, nausea, nervousness, shakiness, sweating, and weakness. If you experience this reaction, eat or drink something containing sugar, and CONTACT YOUR DOCTOR.

• Be sure to tell your doctor if you are pregnant. The effects of this medication during pregnancy have not been thoroughly studied in humans. It is known that disopyramide passes into breast milk. If you are breast-feeding an infant while being treated with this medication, tell your doctor. Unless directed to do otherwise, breast-feeding is not recommended during treatment with this medication.

Di-Spaz—see dicyclomine

---

disulfiram

BRAND NAMES (Manufacturers)
Antabuse (Wyeth-Ayerst)
disulfiram (various manufacturers)

TYPE OF DRUG
Antialcoholic

INGREDIENT
disulfiram

DOSAGE FORM
Tablets (250 mg and 500 mg)

STORAGE
Disulfiram should be stored at room temperature in a tightly closed, light-resistant container.

USES

Disulfiram is used as an aid to treat alcoholics who are strongly motivated to remain sober. Disulfiram blocks the breakdown of alcohol by the body, leading to an accumulation of the chemical acetaldehyde in the bloodstream. Buildup of acetaldehyde in the body can lead to a severe and very unpleasant reaction after alcohol consumption. Alcohol must, therefore, be avoided to prevent this reaction.

TREATMENT

Disulfiram can be taken either on an empty stomach or with food or milk (as directed by your doctor). The tablets can also be crushed and mixed with beverages (nonalcoholic).

If you miss a dose of this medication, take the missed dose as soon as possible, unless it is almost time for the next dose. In that case, do not take the missed dose at all; just return to your regular dosing schedule. Do not double the next dose.

SIDE EFFECTS

Minor. Drowsiness, fatigue, headache, metallic or garlic-like aftertaste, and restlessness. These side effects should disappear as your body adjusts to the medication.

Major. Tell your doctor about any side effects that are persistent or particularly bothersome. IT IS ESPECIALLY IMPORTANT TO TELL YOUR DOCTOR about blurred vision, impotence, joint pain, mental disorders, skin rash, tingling sensations, or yellowing of the eyes or skin.

INTERACTIONS

Disulfiram interacts with several other types of medications:

1. It can increase the blood levels and side effects of diazepam, chlordiazepoxide, phenytoin, and oral anticoagulants (blood thinners, such as warfarin).

2. Concurrent use of disulfiram with isoniazid, antidepressants, metronidazole, or marijuana can lead to severe reactions.

BE SURE TO TELL YOUR DOCTOR about any medications you are currently taking, especially any of those listed above. Also, be sure to tell your doctor if you use marijuana.

WARNINGS

• Tell your doctor about unusual or allergic reactions you have had to any medications, especially to disulfiram, rubber, pesticides, or fungicides.

• Before starting to take this medication, be sure to tell your doctor if you have ever had brain damage, dermatitis, diabetes mellitus, epilepsy, heart disease, kidney disease, liver disease, mental disorders, or thyroid disease.

• It is important not to drink or to use any alcohol-containing preparations, medications, or foods (including beer, elixirs, tonics, wine, liquor, vinegar, sauces, after-shave lotions, liniments, or colognes) while taking this medication. Be sure to check the labels on any over-the-counter (nonprescription) products for their alcohol content, especially cough syrups, mouthwashes, and gargles.

• It is important that you understand the serious nature of the disulfiram-alcohol reaction. If you take disulfiram within 12 hours after ingesting alcohol or drink alcohol within two weeks after your last dose of disulfiram, you may experience blurred vision, chest pain, confusion, dizziness, fainting, flushing, headache, nausea, pounding heartbeat, sweating, vomiting, or weakness. The reaction usually occurs within five to ten minutes of drinking alcohol and can last from half an hour to two hours, depending on the dose of disulfiram and the quantity of alcohol ingested.

- If this drug makes you drowsy, do not take part in any activity that requires alertness, such as driving a car or operating potentially dangerous machinery.
- Be sure to tell your doctor if you are pregnant. Birth defects have been reported in both animals and humans whose mothers received disulfiram during pregnancy. It must also be kept in mind that alcohol, even in small amounts, can cause a variety of birth defects when ingested during pregnancy. Discuss the risks with your doctor. Also, tell your doctor if you are breast-feeding an infant. It is not known if disulfiram passes into breast milk.

Ditropan—see oxybutynin

Diulo—see metolazone

Diurese—see trichlormethiazide

Diurigen—see chlorothiazide

Diuril—see chlorothiazide

Dizmiss—see meclizine

Dolacet—see acetaminophen and hydrocodone combination

Dolene—see propoxyphene

Dolene AP-65—see acetaminophen and propoxyphene combination

Dolene Compound-65—see aspirin, caffeine, and propoxyphene combination

Dolobid—see diflunisal

Dolophine—see methadone

Donnamor—see atropine, scopolamine, hyoscyamine, and phenobarbital combination

Donna-Sed—see atropine, scopolamine, hyoscyamine, and phenobarbital combination

Donnatal—see atropine, scopolamine, hyoscyamine, and phenobarbital combination

Dopar—see levodopa

Dorcol Children's Liquid Cold Formula—see pseudoephedrine and chlorpheniramine combination

Dormarex 2—see diphenhydramine

Doryx—see doxycycline

Doxaphene Compound—see aspirin, caffeine, and propoxyphene combination

doxepin

BRAND NAMES (Manufacturers)
Adapin (Pennwalt)
doxepin (various manufacturers)
Sinequan (Fisons)

TYPE OF DRUG
Tricyclic antidepressant

INGREDIENT
doxepin

DOSAGE FORMS
Capsules (10 mg, 25 mg, 50 mg, 75 mg, 100 mg, and 150 mg)
Oral concentrate (10 mg per ml)

STORAGE
Doxepin capsules and oral concentrate should be stored at room temperature in tightly closed containers. This medication should never be frozen.

USES

Doxepin is used to relieve the symptoms of mental depression. This medication belongs to a group of drugs referred to as the tricyclic antidepressants. These medicines are thought to relieve depression by increasing the concentration of certain chemicals necessary for nerve transmission in the brain.

TREATMENT

This medication should be taken exactly as your doctor prescribes. You can take it with food to lessen the chance of stomach irritation (unless your doctor tells you to do otherwise).

Each dose of the oral concentrate should be diluted in at least four ounces (half a glass) of water, milk, or fruit juice just prior to administration. Measure the correct amount carefully with the dropper provided. DO NOT mix the medication with grape juice or with carbonated beverages, since they may decrease the medicine's effectiveness.

If you miss a dose of this medication, take the missed dose as soon as possible, then return to your regular dosing schedule. If, however, the dose you missed was a once-a-day bedtime dose, do not take that dose in the morning; check with your doctor instead. If the dose is taken in the morning, it may cause some unwanted side effects. Never double the dose.

The antidepressant effects of therapy with this medication may not become apparent for two or three weeks.

SIDE EFFECTS

Minor. Blurred vision, constipation, cramps, diarrhea, dizziness, drowsiness, dry mouth, fatigue, indigestion, insomnia, loss of appetite, nausea, peculiar tastes in the mouth, restlessness, sweating, vomiting, weakness, or weight gain or loss. As your body adjusts to the medication, these side effects should disappear.

This drug may cause increased sensitivity to sunlight. Therefore, avoid prolonged exposure to sunlight and sunlamps. Wear protective clothing, and use an effective sunscreen.

Dry mouth can be relieved by chewing sugarless gum or by sucking on ice chips or a piece of hard candy.

To relieve constipation, increase the amount of fiber in your diet (fresh fruits and vegetables, salads, bran, and

whole-grain breads), exercise, and drink more water (unless your doctor directs you to do otherwise).

To avoid dizziness or light-headedness when you stand, contract and relax the muscles of your legs for a few moments before rising. Do this by pushing one foot against the floor while raising the other foot slightly, alternating feet so that you are "pumping" your legs in a pedaling motion.

Major. Tell your doctor about any side effects that are persistent or particularly bothersome. IT IS ESPECIALLY IMPORTANT TO TELL YOUR DOCTOR about agitation, anxiety, chest pain, confusion, convulsions, difficulty in urinating, enlarged or painful breasts (in both sexes), fainting, fever, fluid retention, hair loss, hallucinations, headaches, impotence, mood changes, mouth sores, nervousness, nightmares, numbness in the fingers or toes, palpitations, ringing in the ears, seizures, skin rash, sleep disorders, sore throat, a tendency to bleed or bruise, tremors, uncoordinated movements or balance problems, or yellowing of the eyes or skin.

INTERACTIONS

Doxepin interacts with a number of other types of medications:

1. Extreme drowsiness can occur when this medicine is taken with central nervous system depressants (such as alcohol, antihistamines, barbiturates, benzodiazepine tranquilizers, muscle relaxants, narcotics, pain medications, phenothiazine tranquilizers, and sleeping medications) or with other antidepressants.

2. Doxepin may decrease the effectiveness of antiseizure medications and may block the blood-pressure-lowering effects of clonidine and guanethidine.

3. Oral contraceptives (birth control pills) and estrogen-containing drugs can increase the side effects and reduce the effectiveness of the tricyclic antidepressants (including doxepin).

4. Cimetidine can decrease the elimination of doxepin from the body, increasing the possibility of side effects.

5. Tricyclic antidepressants may increase the side effects of thyroid medications and over-the-counter (nonprescription) cough, cold, allergy, asthma, sinus, and diet medications.

6. The concurrent use of tricyclic antidepressants and monoamine oxidase (MAO) inhibitors should be avoided, because the combination may result in fever, convulsions, or high blood pressure. At least 14 days should separate the use of this drug and the use of an MAO inhibitor.

BE SURE TO TELL YOUR DOCTOR about any medications you are currently taking, especially any listed above.

WARNINGS

- Tell your doctor if you have had unusual or allergic reactions to any medications, especially to doxepin or any of the other tricyclic antidepressants (amitriptyline, imipramine, trimipramine, amoxapine, protriptyline, desipramine, maprotiline, nortriptyline).
- Tell your doctor if you have a history of alcoholism or if you have ever had asthma, high blood pressure, liver or kidney disease, heart disease, a heart attack, circulatory disease, stomach problems, intestinal problems, difficulty in urinating, enlarged prostate gland, epilepsy, glaucoma, thyroid disease, mental illness, or electroshock therapy.
- If this drug makes you dizzy or drowsy, do not take part in any activity that requires alertness, such as driving a car or operating potentially dangerous equipment.
- Before having surgery or any other medical or dental treatment, be sure to tell your doctor or dentist that you are taking this medication.
- Do not stop taking this drug suddenly. Abruptly stopping it can cause nausea, headache, stomach upset, fatigue, or a worsening of your condition. Your doctor may want to reduce the dosage gradually.
- The effects of this medication may last as long as seven days after you have stopped taking it, so continue to observe all precautions during that period.
- Be sure to tell your doctor if you are pregnant. The effects of this drug during pregnancy have not been thoroughly studied in humans. Studies in animals have shown that this medication can cause side effects to the fetus if given to the mother in large doses during pregnancy. Also, tell your doctor if you are breast-feeding an infant. Small amounts of this drug can pass into breast milk and may cause unwanted effects in the nursing infant.

Doxy-Caps—see doxycycline

Doxychel Hyclate—see doxycycline

---

doxycycline

BRAND NAMES (Manufacturers)

AK-Ramycin (Akorn)
AK-Ratabs (Akorn)
Doryx (Parke-Davis)
Doxy-Caps (Edwards)
Doxychel Hyclate (Rachelle)
doxycycline (various manufacturers)
Doxy-Lemmon (Lemmon)
Vibramycin Hyclate (Pfizer)
Vibra Tabs (Pfizer)
Vivox (Squibb)

TYPE OF DRUG

Tetracycline antibiotic

INGREDIENT

doxycycline

DOSAGE FORMS

Tablets (50 mg and 100 mg)
Capsules (50 mg and 100 mg)
Capsules, coated pellets (100 mg)
Oral suspension (25 mg per 5-ml spoonful)
Oral syrup (50 mg per 5-ml spoonful)

STORAGE

Doxycycline tablets, capsules, oral suspension, and oral syrup should be stored at room temperature in tightly closed, light-resistant containers. Any unused portion of the suspension should be discarded after 14 days because the drug loses its potency after that period. This medication should never be frozen.

USES

Doxycycline is used to treat a wide variety of bacterial infections and to prevent or treat traveler's diarrhea. It acts by inhibiting the growth of bacteria.

Doxycycline kills susceptible bacteria, but it is not effective against viruses or fungi.

TREATMENT

To avoid stomach upset, you can take this medication with food (unless your doctor directs you to do otherwise).

The suspension should be shaken well just before measuring each dose. The contents tend to settle on the bottom of the bottle, so it is necessary to shake the container to distribute the ingredients evenly and equalize the doses. Each dose of the oral suspension or oral syrup should be measured carefully with a specially designed 5-ml measuring spoon. An ordinary kitchen teaspoon is not accurate enough.

Do not mix the oral syrup form of this drug with other substances unless so directed by your doctor.

Doxycycline works best when the level of medicine in your bloodstream is kept constant. It is best, therefore, to take the doses at evenly spaced intervals day and night. For example, if you are to take two doses a day, the doses should be spaced 12 hours apart.

If you miss a dose of this medication, take the missed dose immediately. However, if you do not remember to take the missed dose until it is almost time for your next dose, take it; space the following dose about halfway through the regular interval between doses; then return to your regular dosing schedule. Try not to skip any doses.

Take this drug for the entire time prescribed, even if the symptoms disappear before the end of that period. If you stop taking the drug too soon, resistant bacteria can continue to grow, and the infection could recur.

SIDE EFFECTS

Minor. Diarrhea, discoloration of the nails, dizziness, loss of appetite, nausea, stomach cramps and upset, or vomiting. These side effects should disappear as your body adjusts to the medication.

Doxycycline can increase your sensitivity to sunlight. You should, therefore, try to avoid prolonged exposure to sunlight and sunlamps. Wear protective clothing and sunglasses, and use an effective sunscreen.

Major. Tell your doctor about any side effects that are persistent or particularly bothersome. IT IS ESPECIALLY IMPORTANT TO TELL YOUR DOCTOR about darkened tongue, difficulty in breathing, joint pain, mouth irritation, rash, rectal or vaginal itching, sore throat and fever, unusual bleeding or bruising, or yellowing of the eyes or skin. Also, if your symptoms of infection seem to be getting worse rather than improving, you should contact your doctor.

INTERACTIONS

Doxycycline interacts with other types of medications:

1. It can increase the absorption of digoxin, which may lead to digoxin toxicity.

2. The gastrointestinal side effects (nausea, vomiting, stomach upset) of theophylline may be increased by doxycycline.

3. The dosage of oral anticoagulants (blood thinners, such as warfarin) may need to be adjusted when this medication is started.

4. Doxycycline may decrease the effectiveness of oral contraceptives (birth control pills), and pregnancy could result. You should, therefore, use a different or additional form of birth control while taking doxycycline. Discuss this with your doctor.

5. Barbiturates, carbamazepine, phenytoin, and antacids can lower the blood levels of doxycycline, decreasing its effectiveness.

6. Iron can bind to doxycycline in the gastrointestinal tract, which can decrease its absorption and, therefore, its effectiveness.

BE SURE TO TELL YOUR DOCTOR about any medications you are currently taking, especially any of those listed above.

WARNINGS

- Tell your doctor about unusual or allergic reactions you have had to any medications, especially to doxycycline, oxytetracycline, tetracycline, or minocycline.
- Tell your doctor if you now have or if you have ever had kidney or liver disease.
- Doxycycline can affect tests for syphilis; tell your doctor you are taking this medication if you are also being treated for this disease.
- Make sure that your prescription for this medication is marked with the drug's expiration date. The drug should be discarded after the expiration date. If doxycycline is used after it has expired, serious side effects (especially to the kidneys) could result.
- This medication has been prescribed for your current infection only. Another infection later on, or one that someone else has, may require a different medicine. You should not give your medicine to other people or use it for other infections, unless your doctor specifically directs you to do so.
- Be sure to tell your doctor if you are pregnant or if you are breast-feeding an infant. Doxycycline should not be used during pregnancy and breast-feeding. Doxycycline crosses the placenta and passes into breast milk. This drug can cause permanent discoloration of the teeth and can inhibit tooth and bone growth if used during their development. Also, this drug should not be used by children less than eight years old.

Doxy-Lemmon—see doxycycline

Drisdol—see ergocalciferol (vitamin D)

Drixoral—see pseudoephedrine and dexbrompheniramine combination

Drize—see phenylpropanolamine and chlorpheniramine combination

Drotic—see hydrocortisone, polymyxin B, and neomycin combination (otic)

Duotrate—see pentaerythritol tetranitrate

Duradyne DHC—see acetaminophen and hydrocodone combination

Duralex—see pseudoephedrine and chlorpheniramine combination

Duraquin—see quinidine

Dura-Vent—see phenylpropanolamine and guaifenesin combination

Dura-Vent/A—see phenylpropanolamine and chlorpheniramine combination

Duricef—see cefadroxil

Durrax—see hydroxyzine

Duvoid—see bethanechol

Dyazide—see triamterene and hydrochlorothiazide combination

Dycill—see dicloxacillin

Dymelor—see acetohexamide

Dynapen—see dicloxacillin

Dyrenium—see triamterene

Dyrexan-OD—see phendimetrazine

Earocol—see antipyrine, benzocaine, oxyquinoline, and glycerin combination

Easprin—see aspirin

Ecotrin—see aspirin

Edecrin—see ethacrynic acid

E.E.S.—see erythromycin

E.E.S. 400—see erythromycin

Elavil—see amitriptyline

Eldepryl—see selegiline

Elixicon—see theophylline

Elixomin—see theophylline

Elixophyllin—see theophylline

Empirin—see aspirin

Empirin with Codeine—see aspirin and codeine combination

E-Mycin—see erythromycin

E-Mycin E—see erythromycin

---

enalapril

BRAND NAME (Manufacturer)
Vasotec (Merck Sharp & Dohme)
TYPE OF DRUG
Antihypertensive
INGREDIENT
enalapril
DOSAGE FORM
Tablets (2.5 mg, 5 mg, 10 mg, and 20 mg)
STORAGE
Enalapril should be stored at room temperature in a tightly closed container.

USES

Enalapril is used to treat high blood pressure. It is a vasodilator (it widens the blood vessels) that acts by blocking the production of chemicals that may be responsible for constricting or narrowing the blood vessels.

TREATMENT

Enalapril can be taken either on an empty stomach or with food if it causes stomach irritation. To become accustomed to taking this medication, try to take it at the same time(s) every day.

It may be several weeks before you notice the full effects of this medication.

If you miss a dose of enalapril, take the missed dose as soon as possible, unless it is almost time for the next dose. In that case, do not take the missed dose at all; just wait until the next scheduled dose. Do not double the dose.

Enalapril does not cure high blood pressure, but it will help to control the condition as long as you continue to take the medication.

SIDE EFFECTS

Minor. Abdominal pain, cough, diarrhea, dizziness, drowsiness, fatigue, headache, heartburn, insomnia, nausea, nervousness, sweating, or vomiting. These side effects should disappear as your body adjusts to the medication.

To avoid dizziness when you stand, contract and relax the muscles of your legs for a few moments before rising. Do this by alternately pushing one foot against the floor while lifting the other foot slightly, so that you are "pumping" your legs in a pedaling motion.

Major. Tell your doctor about any side effects that are persistent or particularly bothersome. IT IS ESPECIALLY IMPORTANT TO TELL YOUR DOCTOR about chest pain; difficulty in breathing; fainting; fever; itching; lightheadedness (especially during the first few days); muscle cramps; palpitations; rash; sore throat; swelling of the face, eyes, lips, or tongue; tingling in the fingers or toes; or yellowing of the eyes or skin.

INTERACTIONS

Enalapril interacts with several other types of medications:

1. Diuretics (water pills) and other antihypertensive medications can cause an excessive drop in blood pressure when combined with enalapril (especially with the first dose).

2. The combination of enalapril with spironolactone, triamterene, amiloride, potassium supplements, or salt substitutes can lead to hyperkalemia (dangerously high levels of potassium in the bloodstream).

Before starting to take enalapril, BE SURE TO TELL YOUR DOCTOR about any medications you are currently taking, especially any of those listed above.

WARNINGS

- Tell your doctor about unusual or allergic reactions you have had to any medications, especially to enalapril.
- Tell your doctor if you now have or if you have ever had blood disorders, heart failure, renal disease, or systemic lupus erythematosus.

• Excessive perspiration, dehydration, or prolonged vomiting or diarrhea can lead to an excessive drop in blood pressure while you are taking this medication. Contact your doctor if you have any of these symptoms.
• Before having surgery or other medical or dental treatment, tell your doctor or dentist you are taking this drug.
• If this drug makes you dizzy or drowsy, do not take part in any activity that requires alertness, such as driving a car or operating potentially dangerous equipment.
• If you have high blood pressure, do not take any over-the-counter (nonprescription) medication for weight control or for asthma, sinus, cough, cold, or allergy problems unless you first check with your doctor.
• Be sure to tell your doctor if you are pregnant. Although enalapril appears to be safe in animals, studies in pregnant women have not been conducted. Also, tell your doctor if you are breast-feeding an infant. It is not yet known if enalapril passes into human breast milk.

Endep—see amitriptyline

Enduron—see methyclothiazide

Enovid-E—see oral contraceptives

Entex L.A.—see phenylpropanolamine and guaifenesin combination

Epifrin—see epinephrine (ophthalmic)

Epinal—see epinephrine (ophthalmic)

epinephrine (ophthalmic)

BRAND NAMES (Manufacturers)
Epifrin (Allergan)
Epinal (Alcon)
Epitrate (Ayerst)
Eppy/N (Barnes-Hind)
Glaucon (Alcon)

TYPE OF DRUG
Antiglaucoma ophthalmic solution

INGREDIENT
epinephrine (adrenaline)

DOSAGE FORM
Ophthalmic solution (0.1%, 0.25%, 0.5%, 1%, and 2%)

STORAGE
Store at room temperature in a tightly closed, light-resistant container. This medication should never be frozen. The solution should be discarded if it turns brown or cloudy because this indicates deterioration and loss of potency.

USES

Epinephrine (ophthalmic) is used to treat glaucoma. It lowers the pressure in the eye by decreasing the production of aqueous humor (a particular fluid in the eye) and increasing its drainage.

TREATMENT

Wash your hands with soap and water before applying this medication. In order to avoid contamination of the eye drops, be careful not to touch the tube portion of the dropper or let it touch your eye; and DO NOT wipe off or rinse the dropper after each use.

To apply the eye drops, tilt your head back and pull down your lower eyelid with one hand to make a pouch below the eye. Drop the prescribed amount of medicine into this pouch and slowly close your eyes. Try not to blink. Keep your eyes closed, and place one finger at the corner of the eye next to your nose for a minute or two, applying slight pressure (this is done to prevent loss of the medication through the duct that drains fluid from the surface of the eye into the nose and throat). Then wipe away any excess with a clean tissue. Since the drops are somewhat difficult to apply, you may want to have someone else apply them for you.

If more than one type of eye drop has been prescribed for you, wait at least five minutes after applying epinephrine before using the other eye medication (to give the epinephrine time to work). However, if you are also using an eye drop that constricts your pupils, check with your doctor to see which drug should be applied first.

If you miss a dose of epinephrine, apply the missed dose as soon as possible, unless it is almost time for the next dose. In that case, do not apply the missed dose at all; just return to your regular dosing schedule. Do not double the next dose.

SIDE EFFECTS

Minor. Headache or transitory stinging on initial application. These side effects should disappear as your body adjusts to the medication.
Major. Tell your doctor about any side effects that are persistent or particularly bothersome. IT IS ESPECIALLY IMPORTANT TO TELL YOUR DOCTOR about blurred vision, eye pain, fainting, palpitations, sweating, or trembling.

INTERACTIONS

Epinephrine interacts with several other types of medications:
1. Concurrent use of epinephrine and monoamine oxidase (MAO) inhibitors or tricyclic antidepressants can lead to serious side effects. At least 21 days should, therefore, separate doses of epinephrine and either of these types of medications.
2. Digoxin can increase the side effects of epinephrine.

BE SURE TO TELL YOUR DOCTOR about any medications you are currently taking, especially any listed above.

WARNINGS

• Tell your doctor about unusual or allergic reactions you have had to any medications, especially to epinephrine.
• Tell your doctor if you are allergic to sulfites.
• Before starting to take this medication, be sure to tell your doctor if you now have or if you have ever had diabetes mellitus, heart or blood vessel disease, high blood pressure, a stroke, or thyroid disease.
• If this medication blurs your vision, try to avoid activities that require visual acuity, such as driving a car or operating potentially dangerous equipment.
• Epinephrine can cause discoloration of soft contact lenses. If you currently wear soft contact lenses, you should discuss with your doctor whether your medication or your contact lenses should be changed.
• Be sure to tell your doctor if you are pregnant. Although

epinephrine (ophthalmic) appears to be safe during pregnancy, studies in humans have not been conducted. Also, tell your doctor if you are breast-feeding an infant. It is not known whether epinephrine passes into breast milk.

Epitol—see carbamazepine

Epitrate—see epinephrine (ophthalmic)

E.P. Mycin—see oxytetracycline

Eppy/N—see epinephrine (ophthalmic)

Epromate—see meprobamate and aspirin combination

Equagesic—see meprobamate and aspirin combination

Equanil—see meprobamate

Equazine M—see meprobamate and aspirin combination

Eramycin—see erythromycin

Ercatab—see ergotamine and caffeine combination

Ergo Caff—see ergotamine and caffeine combination

---

ergocalciferol (vitamin D)

BRAND NAMES (Manufacturers)
Calciferol (Kremers-Urban)
Drisdol (Winthrop)
vitamin D (various manufacturers)
TYPE OF DRUG
Vitamin
INGREDIENT
ergocalciferol
DOSAGE FORMS
Tablets (50,000 units)
Capsules (50,000 units)
Oral liquid (8,000 units per ml)*
*The oral liquid is available without a prescription.
STORAGE
Store at room temperature in a tightly closed, light-resistant container. This medication should never be frozen.

USES

Ergocalciferol is used to treat rickets, hypophosphatemia (low blood levels of phosphate), and hypoparathyroidism (underactive parathyroid gland). This medication is converted by the liver and kidney to the active form of vitamin D—a vitamin essential to many body systems (including bone and tooth structure, regulation of blood calcium levels, and heart and muscle contraction).

TREATMENT

Ergocalciferol can be taken either on an empty stomach or with food or milk (as directed by your doctor).

Each dose of the oral liquid form of this medication should be measured carefully with the dropper provided. The liquid can then be taken directly or mixed with fruit juice, cereal, or other foods.

If you miss a dose of this medication, take the missed dose as soon as possible, unless it is almost time for the next dose. In that case, do not take the missed dose at all; just return to your regular dosing schedule. Do not double the next dose.

SIDE EFFECTS

Minor. None, at the dosages normally prescribed.
Major. The side effects associated with ergocalciferol therapy are usually the result of too much medication (vitamin D intoxication). Tell your doctor about any side effects that are persistent or particularly bothersome. IT IS ESPECIALLY IMPORTANT TO TELL YOUR DOCTOR about blurred vision, bone pain, constipation, dry mouth, headache, increased thirst, increased urination, irritability, loss of appetite, metallic taste in the mouth, mental disorders, muscle pain, nausea, palpitations, runny nose, vomiting, weakness, or weight loss.

INTERACTIONS

Cholestyramine, colestipol, and mineral oil can decrease the absorption of ergocalciferol from the gastrointestinal tract, decreasing its effectiveness.

BE SURE TO TELL YOUR DOCTOR about any medications you are currently taking, especially any of those listed above.

WARNINGS

- Tell your doctor about unusual or allergic reactions you have had to any medications, especially to ergocalciferol (vitamin D), calcitriol, calcifediol, or dihydrotachysterol.
- Before starting to take this medication, be sure to tell your doctor if you now have or if you have ever had heart or blood vessel disease, hypercalcemia (high blood levels of calcium), hyperphosphatemia (high blood levels of phosphate), vitamin D intoxication, or sarcoidosis.
- Before taking any over-the-counter (nonprescription) products that contain calcium, phosphates, magnesium, or vitamin D, check with your doctor. These ingredients can increase the side effects of ergocalciferol.
- Some forms of this medication contain the color additive FD&C Yellow No. 5 (tartrazine), which can cause allergic-type symptoms (fainting, shortness of breath, rash) in certain susceptible individuals.
- Be sure to tell your doctor if you are pregnant. Although the effects of this medication have not been thoroughly studied during human pregnancy, animal studies have shown that this medication can cause side effects to the fetus if given to the mother in large doses during pregnancy. Also, tell your doctor if you are breast-feeding an infant. It is not known if this medication passes into breast milk.

---

ergoloid mesylates

BRAND NAMES (Manufacturers)
ergoloid mesylates (various manufacturers)
Gerimal (Rugby)
Hydergine (Sandoz)
Niloric (Ascher)

TYPE OF DRUG
Vasodilator
INGREDIENTS
ergoloid mesylates
DOSAGE FORMS
Capsules, liquid (1 mg)
Oral tablets (0.5 mg and 1 mg)
Sublingual tablets (0.5 mg and 1 mg)
Oral liquid (1 mg per ml, with 30% alcohol)
STORAGE
Ergoloid mesylates capsules, tablets, and oral liquid should be stored at room temperature in tightly closed, light-resistant containers. Never freeze this medication.

USES
This medication is used to reduce the symptoms associated with senility. It is not clear how ergoloid mesylates work, but it is thought that they act by dilating (widening) the blood vessels, thus increasing blood flow to the brain.

TREATMENT
In order to avoid stomach irritation, you can take the capsules, tablets, or oral liquid with food or milk. Be sure to measure the dose of the liquid form of this medication carefully with the dropper provided.

The sublingual form of this medication must be placed under the tongue and allowed to dissolve completely. Try not to swallow for as long as possible, because the drug is more completely absorbed through the lining of the mouth than it is from the stomach. Do not drink any liquid, eat, or smoke for at least ten minutes after placing the tablet under the tongue.

If you miss a dose of this medication, take the missed dose as soon as possible, unless it is almost time for the next dose. In that case, do not take the missed dose at all; just return to your regular dosing schedule. Do not double the next dose.

It may take three or four weeks for the effects of this medication to become apparent.

SIDE EFFECTS
Minor. Blurred vision, dizziness, drowsiness, flushing, headache, irritation under the tongue (with the sublingual form only), light-headedness, loss of appetite, nasal congestion, nausea, stomach cramps, or vomiting. These side effects should disappear as your body adjusts to the medication.

If you feel dizzy or light-headed, sit or lie down for a while; get up slowly from a sitting or reclining position, and be careful on stairs.

Major. Tell your doctor about any side effects that are persistent or particularly bothersome. IT IS ESPECIALLY IMPORTANT TO TELL YOUR DOCTOR about a slowed heart rate.

INTERACTIONS
Ergoloid mesylates should not interact with other medications if they are used according to directions.

WARNINGS
- Tell your doctor about unusual or allergic reactions you have had to any medications, especially to ergoloid mesylates or ergot alkaloids (such as ergonovine, ergotamine, or bromocriptine).
- Before starting to take this medication, be sure to tell your doctor if you now have or if you have ever had liver disease, low blood pressure, porphyria, severe mental illness, or a slowed heart rate.
- Ergoloid mesylates may lessen your ability to adjust to the cold. Therefore, since you may experience increased sensitivity, do not expose your body to very cold temperatures for prolonged periods.
- Your doctor may want you to take your pulse daily while you are using this medication. Contact your doctor if your pulse becomes slower than normal or if it drops below 50 beats per minute.
- If this drug makes you dizzy or drowsy or blurs your vision, do not take part in any activity that requires alertness, such as driving a car or operating potentially dangerous equipment.
- Some of these products contain the color additive FD&C Yellow No. 5 (tartrazine), which can cause allergic-type reactions (rash, shortness of breath, fainting) in certain susceptible individuals.

Ergomar—see ergotamine

---

ergonovine

BRAND NAMES (Manufacturers)
ergonovine maleate (various manufacturers)
Ergotrate Maleate (Lilly)
TYPE OF DRUG
Uterine stimulant
INGREDIENT
ergonovine
DOSAGE FORM
Tablets (0.2 mg)
STORAGE
Ergonovine should be stored at room temperature in a tightly closed container.

USES
Ergonovine is used to prevent or treat postpartum (immediately after delivery) or postabortion uterine bleeding. This medication is usually administered for only a short period of time (usually 48 hours). It acts directly on the uterus to cause contractions and to constrict blood vessels.

TREATMENT
Ergonovine tablets can be taken either on an empty stomach or with food or milk (as directed by your doctor). For more rapid effect, the tablet can also be placed under the tongue to dissolve.

If you miss a dose of this medication, do not take the missed dose at all; just return to your regular dosing schedule. Do not double the next dose.

SIDE EFFECTS
Minor. Diarrhea, headache, nausea, or vomiting. These side effects should disappear as your body adjusts to the medication.

Major. Tell your doctor about any side effects that are persistent or particularly bothersome. IT IS ESPECIALLY IMPOR-

TANT TO TELL YOUR DOCTOR about chest pain, confusion, convulsions, excitement, hallucinations, hives, itching, numbness or coldness of the fingers or toes, ringing in the ears, shortness of breath, skin rash, or tingling sensations—even if these side effects appear or continue after you stop taking ergonovine.

INTERACTIONS

Ergonovine should not interact with other medications if it is used according to directions.

WARNINGS

• Tell your doctor about unusual or allergic reactions you have had to medications, especially to ergonovine or to any other ergot alkaloid (bromocriptine, ergotamine, ergoloid mesylates).

• Before starting to take this medication, tell your doctor if you now have or if you have ever had hypocalcemia, heart disease, high blood pressure, kidney or liver disease, or peripheral vascular disease (poor circulation).

• Be sure to tell your doctor if you are breast-feeding an infant. Ergonovine can pass into breast milk and may cause side effects in the nursing infant. It can also decrease milk production.

ergonovine maleate—see ergonovine

Ergostat—see ergotamine

---

ergotamine

BRAND NAMES (Manufacturers)
Ergomar (Fisons)
Ergostat (Parke-Davis)
Medihaler Ergotamine (Riker)
Wigrettes (Organon)
TYPE OF DRUG
Antimigraine (vasoconstrictor)
INGREDIENT
ergotamine
DOSAGE FORMS
Sublingual tablets (2 mg)
Aerosol (0.36 mg per spray)
STORAGE
This medication should be stored at room temperature in tightly closed, light-resistant containers.

The container of the aerosol is pressurized; it should, therefore, never be punctured or broken. It should also be stored away from heat and direct sunlight.

USES

This medication is used to treat migraine and cluster headaches. These headaches are thought to be caused by an increase in the diameter of the blood vessels in the head, which results in increased blood flow, increased pressure, and pain. Ergotamine is a vasoconstrictor; it acts by constricting (narrowing) the blood vessels.

TREATMENT

It is best to take this medication as soon as you notice your migraine headache symptoms. If you wait until the headache becomes severe, the drug takes longer to work and may not be as effective.

After you take either of these forms of ergotamine, you should try to lie down in a quiet, dark room for at least two hours (in order to help the medication work). The drug usually takes effect in 30 to 60 minutes.

It is very important that you understand how often you can repeat a dose of this medication during an attack (usually every 30 to 60 minutes for the sublingual tablets, and every five minutes for the aerosol spray) and the maximum amount of medication you can take per day (usually three sublingual tablets or six inhalations). Five is generally the maximum number of sublingual tablets and 15 is about the maximum number of inhalations that can be taken in any one-week period. CHECK WITH YOUR DOCTOR if you have any questions.

The sublingual tablets should be placed under your tongue. DO NOT swallow these tablets—they are more efficiently absorbed through the lining of the mouth than from the gastrointestinal tract. Try not to eat, drink, chew, or smoke while the tablet is dissolving.

The aerosol form of this medication comes packaged with instructions for use. Read the directions carefully; if you have any questions, check with your doctor or pharmacist. The aerosol can should be shaken well just before each dose is sprayed. The contents tend to settle on the bottom of the container, so it should be shaken to disperse the medication and equalize the doses. The container provides about 300 measured sprays.

If you are on prolonged treatment with this drug and you miss a dose, take it as soon as you remember. Wait four hours to take the next dose. It is very important that you consult your doctor before you discontinue using this drug. Your doctor may want to reduce your dosage gradually.

SIDE EFFECTS

Minor. Diarrhea, dizziness, headache, nausea, vomiting, or sensation of cold hands and feet with MILD numbness or tingling. These side effects should disappear as your body adjusts to the medication.

The aerosol form of ergotamine can cause hoarseness or throat irritation. Gargling or rinsing your mouth out with water after taking the dose may help prevent this side effect.

Major. Tell your doctor about any side effects that are persistent or particularly bothersome. IT IS ESPECIALLY IMPORTANT TO TELL YOUR DOCTOR about chest pain; coldness, numbness, pain, tingling, or dark discoloration of the fingers or toes; confusion; fluid retention; itching; localized swelling; muscle pain; severe abdominal pain and swelling; or unusual weakness.

INTERACTIONS

Ergotamine interacts with several other types of medications:

1. Ergotamine interacts with amphetamines, ephedrine, epinephrine (adrenaline), pseudoephedrine, erythromycin, and troleandomycin. Such combinations can lead to increases in blood pressure or increased risk of adverse reaction to ergotamine.

2. Do not drink alcoholic beverages while you are taking this medication. Since alcohol dilates (widens) the blood vessels (which are already dilated during migraine headaches), drinking will only make your headache worse.

3. Ergotamine interacts with marijuana to produce cold sensations in the arms and legs or even persistent chill.
4. Nicotine and cocaine decrease the effectiveness of ergotamine and, therefore, make the headache worse.
5. The caffeine in tea, coffee, and cola drinks also interacts with this medication. It may actually help to relieve your headache.

BE SURE TO TELL YOUR DOCTOR about any medications or substances you are currently taking or using, especially any of those listed above.

WARNINGS

- Tell your doctor about unusual or allergic reactions you have had to any medications, especially to ergotamine or other ergot alkaloids (such as ergonovine or bromocriptine).
- Before starting to take this medication, be sure to tell your doctor if you now have or if you have ever had heart or blood vessel disease, high blood pressure, infections, kidney disease, liver disease, or thyroid disease.
- Avoid any foods to which you are allergic—they may make your headache worse.
- If this drug makes you dizzy or drowsy, do not take part in any activity that requires alertness, such as driving a car or operating potentially dangerous equipment.
- Try to avoid exposure to cold. Since this drug acts by constricting blood vessels throughout the body, your fingers and toes may become especially sensitive to the cold.
- This medication should not be taken for longer periods or in higher doses than recommended by your doctor. Extended use of this drug can lead to serious side effects. In addition, tolerance can develop—higher doses would be required to obtain the same beneficial effects (at the same time increasing the risk of side effects).
- Be sure to tell your doctor if you are pregnant. Ergotamine can cause contractions of the uterus, which can harm the developing fetus. This drug should not be used during pregnancy. Also, tell your doctor if you are breast-feeding an infant. Ergotamine passes into breast milk and may cause vomiting, diarrhea, or convulsions in the nursing infant.

MONEY-SAVING TIP

Save the inhaler piece from the aerosol container. Refill units, which are less expensive, are available.

---

ergotamine and caffeine combination

BRAND NAMES (Manufacturers)
Cafergot (Sandoz)
Cafetrate (Schein)
Ercatab (Parmed)
Ergo Caff (Rugby)
Wigraine (Organon)

TYPE OF DRUG
Antimigraine (vasoconstrictor)

INGREDIENTS
ergotamine and caffeine

DOSAGE FORMS
Tablets (1 mg ergotamine, 100 mg caffeine)
Suppositories (2 mg ergotamine, 100 mg caffeine)

STORAGE
Ergotamine and caffeine combination tablets should be stored at room temperature in tightly closed, light-resistant containers. They should also be stored away from heat and direct sunlight.

The suppository form of this medication should be stored in the refrigerator (never frozen) in a tightly closed container.

USES

This medication is used to treat migraine and cluster headaches. These headaches are thought to be caused by an increase in the diameter of the blood vessels in the head, which results in increased blood flow, increased pressure, and pain. Ergotamine is a vasoconstrictor: it acts by constricting (narrowing) the blood vessels. Caffeine helps in both the absorption of the drug from the gastrointestinal tract and in constricting blood vessels.

TREATMENT

It is best to take this medication as soon as you notice your migraine headache symptoms. If you wait until the headache becomes severe, the drug takes longer to work and may not be as effective.

After you take either of these forms of ergotamine and caffeine combination, you should try to lie down in a quiet, dark room for at least two hours (in order to help the medication work). The drug usually takes effect within 30 to 60 minutes.

It is very important that you understand how often you can repeat a dose of this medication during an attack (usually every 30 to 60 minutes) and the maximum number of tablets you can take per day (usually six tablets). Ten is generally the maximum number of tablets that can be taken in any one-week period. CHECK WITH YOUR DOCTOR if you have any questions.

The tablets should be swallowed with liquid. Take one tablet when you first notice your migraine headache symptoms. If necessary, take a second dose 30 to 60 minutes later to relieve your headache.

To use the suppository form of this medication, first unwrap it and moisten it slightly with water (if the suppository is too soft to insert, run cold water over it or refrigerate it for 30 minutes before you unwrap it). Lie down on your left side, with your right knee bent. Push the suppository well into the rectum with your finger. Try to avoid having a bowel movement for at least an hour to give the medication time to be absorbed. Insert one suppository when you first notice your migraine symptoms. If necessary, insert a second suppository one hour later for full relief of your migraine headache.

If you are on prolonged treatment with this drug and you miss a dose, take it as soon as you remember. Wait four hours to take the next dose. It is very important that you consult your doctor before you discontinue using this drug. Your doctor may want to reduce your dosage gradually.

SIDE EFFECTS

Minor. Diarrhea, dizziness, headache, nausea, nervousness or jitters, vomiting, or sensation of cold hands and feet with MILD numbness or tingling. These side effects should disappear as your body adjusts to the medication.

Major. Tell your doctor about any side effects that are persistent or particularly bothersome. IT IS ESPECIALLY IM-

PORTANT TO TELL YOUR DOCTOR about chest pain; coldness, numbness, pain, tingling, or dark discoloration of the fingers or toes; confusion; fluid retention; itching; localized swelling; muscle pain; severe abdominal pain and swelling; severe nausea or vomiting; or unusual weakness.

INTERACTIONS

Ergotamine and caffeine combination interacts with several other types of medications:

1. Ergotamine interacts with amphetamines, ephedrine, epinephrine (adrenaline), pseudoephedrine, erythromycin, and troleandomycin. Such combinations can lead to increases in blood pressure or increased risk of adverse reaction to ergotamine.

2. Do not drink alcoholic beverages while you are taking this medication. Since alcohol dilates (widens) the blood vessels, drinking will only make your headache worse.

3. Ergotamine interacts with marijuana to produce cold sensations in the arms and legs or even persistent chill.

4. Tobacco (nicotine) and cocaine decrease the effectiveness of ergotamine and, therefore, make the headache worse.

5. The caffeine in tea, coffee, and cola drinks also interacts with this medication.

BE SURE TO TELL YOUR DOCTOR about any medications or substances you are currently taking or using, especially any of those listed above.

WARNINGS

• Tell your doctor about unusual or allergic reactions you have had to medications, especially to ergotamine, caffeine, or any ergot alkaloid (ergonovine, ergoloid mesylates, bromocriptine).

• Before starting to take this medication, be sure to tell your doctor if you now have or if you have ever had heart or blood vessel disease, high blood pressure, infections, kidney disease, liver disease, or thyroid disease.

• Avoid any foods to which you are allergic—they may make your headache worse.

• If this drug makes you dizzy or drowsy, do not take part in any activity that requires alertness, such as driving a car or operating potentially dangerous equipment.

• Try to avoid exposure to cold. Since this drug acts by constricting blood vessels throughout the body (not just in the head), your fingers and toes may become especially sensitive to the cold.

• Elderly patients are more sensitive to the effects of ergotamine. Consult your doctor if the side effects become bothersome.

• This medication should not be taken for longer periods or in higher doses than recommended by your doctor. Extended use of this drug can lead to serious side effects. In addition, tolerance can develop—higher doses would be required to obtain the same beneficial effects (at the same time increasing the risk of side effects).

• Be sure to tell your doctor if you are pregnant. This medication can cause contractions of the uterus, which can harm the developing fetus. This drug should not be used during pregnancy. Also, tell your doctor if you are breast-feeding an infant. Ergotamine and caffeine combination passes into breast milk and may cause vomiting, diarrhea, irritability, or convulsions in the nursing infant.

Ergotrate Maleate—see ergonovine

Eridium—see phenazopyridine

Eryc—see erythromycin

Erypar—see erythromycin

EryPed—see erythromycin

Ery-Tab—see erythromycin

Erythrocin Stearate Filmtabs—see erythromycin

---

erythromycin

BRAND NAMES (Manufacturers)

E.E.S. (Abbott)
E.E.S. 400 (Abbott)
E-Mycin (Upjohn)
E-Mycin E (Upjohn)
Eramycin (Wesley)
Eryc (Parke-Davis)
Erypar (Parke-Davis)
EryPed (Abbott)
Ery-Tab (Abbott)
Erythrocin Stearate Filmtabs (Abbott)
Erythromycin Base (Abbott)
Ilosone (Dista)
Ilosone Pulvules (Dista)
Ilotycin (Dista)
PCE Dispertab (Abbott)
Pediamycin (Ross)
Robimycin (Robins)
Wyamycin E (Wyeth)
Wyamycin S (Wyeth)

TYPE OF DRUG

Antibiotic

INGREDIENT

erythromycin

DOSAGE FORMS

Tablets (250 mg, 333 mg, and 500 mg)
Chewable tablets (125 mg, 200 mg, and 250 mg)
Enteric-coated tablets (250 mg, 333 mg, and 500 mg)
Film-coated tablets (250 mg, 400 mg, and 500 mg)
Polymer-coated tablets (333 mg)
Capsules (125 mg and 250 mg)
Oral drops (100 mg per ml)
Oral suspension (125 mg, 200 mg, 250 mg, and 400 mg per 5-ml spoonful)

STORAGE

Erythromycin tablets and capsules should be stored at room temperature in tightly closed, light-resistant containers. Erythromycin oral drops and oral suspension should be stored in the refrigerator in tightly closed, light-resistant containers. Any unused portion of the liquid forms should be discarded after 14 days because the drug loses its potency after that time. Erythromycin ethylsuccinate liquid does not need to be refrigerated; however, refrigeration helps to preserve the taste. This medication should never be frozen.

USES

Erythromycin is used to treat a wide variety of bacterial infections, including infections of the middle ear and the respiratory tract. It is also used to treat infections in persons who are allergic to penicillin. It acts by preventing the bacteria from manufacturing protein, which prevents their growth. It is not effective against viruses, parasites, or fungi.

TREATMENT

In order to prevent stomach upset, erythromycin coated tablets and erythromycin estolate or ethylsuccinate can be taken with food or milk. Other erythromycin products should be taken with a full glass of water, preferably on an empty stomach, one hour before or two hours after a meal.

The liquid forms should be taken undiluted.

Each dose of the oral drops should be measured carefully with the dropper provided.

The oral suspension form of this medication should be shaken well just before measuring each dose. The contents tend to settle on the bottom of the bottle, so it is necessary to shake the container to distribute the ingredients evenly and equalize the doses. Each dose should then be measured carefully with a specially designed 5-ml measuring spoon. An ordinary kitchen teaspoon is not accurate enough.

In order to prevent gastrointestinal side effects, the coated tablets and capsules should be swallowed whole; do not break, chew, or crush these products.

Erythromycin works best when the level of medicine in your bloodstream is kept constant. It is best, therefore, to take the doses at evenly spaced intervals day and night. For example, if you are to take four doses a day, the doses should be spaced six hours apart.

If you miss a dose of this medication, take the missed dose immediately. However, if you do not remember to take the missed dose until it is almost time for your next dose, take it; space the following dose about halfway through the regular interval between doses; then return to your regular schedule. Try not to skip any doses.

It is important to continue to take this medication for the entire time prescribed by your doctor (usually seven to 14 days), even if the symptoms disappear before the end of that period. If you stop taking this drug too soon, resistant bacteria are given a chance to continue growing, and the infection could recur.

SIDE EFFECTS

Minor. Abdominal cramps, black tongue, cough, diarrhea, fatigue, irritation of the mouth, loss of appetite, nausea, or vomiting. These side effects should disappear as your body adjusts to the medication.

Major. Tell your doctor about any side effects that are persistent or particularly bothersome. IT IS ESPECIALLY IMPORTANT TO TELL YOUR DOCTOR about fever, hearing loss, hives, rash, rectal or vaginal itching, or yellowing of the eyes or skin. Also, if your symptoms of infection seem to be getting worse rather than improving, you should contact your doctor.

INTERACTIONS

1. Erythromycin can decrease the elimination of aminophylline, oxtriphylline, theophylline, digoxin, oral anticoagulants (blood thinners, such as warfarin), and carbamazepine from the body, which can lead to serious side effects.

2. Therapy with erythromycin may increase the effects of methylprednisolone.

BE SURE TO TELL YOUR DOCTOR about any medications you are currently taking, especially any listed above.

WARNINGS

- Tell your doctor about unusual or allergic reactions you have had to any medications, especially to erythromycin.
- Tell your doctor if you have ever had liver disease.
- This medication has been prescribed for your current infection only. Another infection later on, or one that someone else has, may require a different medicine. You should not give your medicine to other people or use it for other infections, unless your doctor specifically directs you to do so.
- Before having surgery or any other medical or dental treatment, be sure to tell your doctor or dentist that you are taking erythromycin.
- Not all erythromycin products are chemically equivalent. However, they all produce the same therapeutic effect. Discuss with your doctor or pharmacist which forms of erythromycin are appropriate for you, and then choose the least expensive product among those recommended.
- Some of these products contain the color additive FD&C Yellow No. 5 (tartrazine), which can cause allergic-type reactions (difficulty in breathing, rash, fainting) in certain susceptible individuals.
- Be sure to tell your doctor if you are pregnant. Although erythromycin appears to be safe during pregnancy, extensive studies in humans have not been conducted. Also, tell your doctor if you are breast-feeding an infant. Small amounts of this medication pass into breast milk and may temporarily alter the bacterial balance in the intestinal tract of the nursing infant, resulting in diarrhea.

---

erythromycin and sulfisoxazole combination

BRAND NAME (Manufacturer)
Pediazole (Ross)

TYPE OF DRUG
Antibiotic

INGREDIENTS
erythromycin and sulfisoxazole

DOSAGE FORM
Oral suspension (200 mg erythromycin and 600 mg sulfisoxazole per 5-ml spoonful)

STORAGE
Store in the refrigerator (never frozen) in a tightly closed container. Any unused portion of the suspension should be discarded after the expiration date (usually after 14 days) because the drug loses its potency after that time.

USES

Erythromycin and sulfisoxazole combination is used to treat acute otitis media (middle ear infection) in children. Erythromycin acts by preventing the bacteria from manufacturing protein, thereby preventing their growth. Sulfisoxazole also acts by preventing production of nutrients that are required for growth of the infecting bacteria. Erythromycin and sulfisoxazole combination kills a wide range of susceptible bacteria, but it is not effective against viruses, parasites, or fungi.

TREATMENT

In order to avoid stomach upset, you can take this medication either with food or with a full glass of water or milk. You can also take it on an empty stomach.

The oral suspension should be shaken well just before measuring each dose. The contents tend to settle on the bottom of the bottle, so it is necessary to shake the container to distribute the ingredients evenly and equalize the doses. Each dose should then be measured carefully with a specially designed 5-ml measuring spoon. An ordinary kitchen teaspoon is not accurate enough.

This medication works best when the level of medicine in the bloodstream is kept constant. It is best, therefore, to take the doses at evenly spaced intervals day and night. For example, if you are to take four doses a day, the doses should be spaced six hours apart.

If you miss a dose of this medication, take the missed dose immediately. However, if you do not remember to take the missed dose until it is almost time for your next dose, take it; space the following dose about halfway through the regular interval between doses; then return to your regular schedule. Try not to skip any doses.

It is important to continue to take this medication for the entire time prescribed by your doctor (usually seven to 14 days), even if the symptoms disappear before the end of that period. If you stop taking the drug too soon, resistant bacteria are given a chance to continue growing, and the infection could recur.

SIDE EFFECTS

Minor. Diarrhea, dizziness, headache, loss of appetite, nausea, sleep disorders, sore mouth or tongue, or vomiting. These side effects should disappear as your body adjusts to the medication.

This medication can cause increased sensitivity to sunlight. It is, therefore, important to avoid prolonged exposure to sunlight and sunlamps. Wear protective clothing and sunglasses, and use an effective sunscreen. However, sunscreens containing para-aminobenzoic acid (PABA) interfere with the antibacterial activity of sulfisoxazole and should not be used.

If you feel dizzy, sit or lie down for a while; get up slowly from a sitting or reclining position, and be careful on stairs.

Major. Tell your doctor about any side effects that are persistent or particularly bothersome. IT IS ESPECIALLY IMPORTANT TO TELL YOUR DOCTOR about aching, or joint and muscle pain; convulsions; difficult or painful urination; difficulty in swallowing; hallucinations; mental depression; loss of hearing; redness, blistering, or peeling of the skin; itching; rash; sore throat and fever; uncoordinated movements; unusual bleeding or bruising; unusual tiredness; or yellowing of the eyes or skin. Also, if the symptoms of infection seem to be getting worse, contact your doctor.

INTERACTIONS

This medication interacts with several other types of drugs:

1. Erythromycin can decrease the elimination of aminophylline, oxtriphylline, theophylline, digoxin, oral anticoagulants (blood thinners, such as warfarin), and carbamazepine from the body, which can lead to serious side effects.

2. Sulfisoxazole can increase the active blood levels of oral anticoagulants (blood thinners, such as warfarin), oral antidiabetic agents, methotrexate, oxyphenbutazone, phenylbutazone, and phenytoin, which can lead to serious side effects.

3. Methenamine can increase the side effects to the kidneys caused by sulfisoxazole.

4. Probenecid and sulfinpyrazone can increase the blood levels of sulfisoxazole.

5. Erythromycin may increase the effects of methylprednisolone.

Before starting to take this medication, BE SURE TO TELL YOUR DOCTOR about any medications you are currently taking, especially any of those listed above.

WARNINGS

- Tell your doctor about unusual or allergic reactions you have had to any medications, especially to erythromycin, sulfisoxazole, any other sulfa medication (sulfonamide antibiotics, diuretics, dapsone, sulfoxone, oral antidiabetic medicines) or acetazolamide.
- Tell your doctor if you now have or if you have ever had glucose-6-phosphate dehydrogenase (G6PD) deficiency, kidney disease, liver disease, or porphyria.
- This medication has been prescribed for your current infection only. Another infection later on, or one that someone else has, may require a different medicine. You should not give your medicine to other people or use it for other infections, unless your doctor specifically directs you to do so.
- Be sure to tell your doctor if you are pregnant. Small amounts of erythromycin and sulfisoxazole cross the placenta. Although these antibiotics appear to be safe during pregnancy, extensive studies in humans have not been conducted. Also, tell your doctor if you are breast-feeding an infant. Small amounts of this drug pass into breast milk and may temporarily alter the bacterial balance in the intestinal tract of the infant, resulting in diarrhea. This drug should not be used in an infant less than two months of age in order to avoid side effects involving the liver.

Erythromycin Base—see erythromycin

Esidrix—see hydrochlorothiazide

Eskalith—see lithium

Eskalith CR—see lithium

Estinyl—see ethinyl estradiol

Estraderm—see estradiol (topical)

---

estradiol (topical)

BRAND NAME (Manufacturer)

Estraderm (Ciba)

TYPE OF DRUG
Estrogen
INGREDIENT
estradiol
DOSAGE FORM
Transdermal patch (delivers 0.05 mg or 0.1 mg per 24 hours)
STORAGE
Estradiol transdermal patches should be stored at room temperature in their original packages.

USES

Estradiol is a synthetic estrogen that is used to treat menopausal symptoms or other conditions associated with estrogen deficiency.

TREATMENT

Your prescription of estradiol will come with patient instructions. It is important that you follow the directions carefully.

Wash and dry your hands before and after applying the patch. Apply the patch to a clean, dry, hairless area of the skin on the trunk of the body or on the abdomen. Do not apply to the breasts. Avoid applying the patch over a cut or to any area of the body where tight clothes might rub against the patch and loosen it. Apply the patch immediately after opening the packet and removing the protective liner. Press the patch firmly to the skin with the palm of your hand for about ten seconds. Make sure there is good contact of the patch to the skin, especially around the edges. Rotate the application sites on the skin, waiting at least one week before applying to the same site.

If the patch becomes loose or falls off, the same one can be reapplied. If necessary, however, a new patch can be applied. In either case, continue with your original treatment schedule.

If you miss an application of this medication, apply a new patch as soon as possible unless it is almost time for the next application. In that case, return to your regular schedule. Do not apply a double dose.

SIDE EFFECTS

Minor. Acne, abdominal cramping, abnormal vaginal bleeding, bloating, breast tenderness, change in sexual desire, darkening of the skin, diarrhea, dizziness, fluid retention, frequent or painful urination, hair loss, headache, nausea, nervousness, skin irritation at patch site, vomiting, or weight gain. These side effects should disappear as your body adjusts to the drug.

If you feel dizzy, sit or lie down for a while; get up slowly from a sitting or reclining position, and be careful on stairs.

Eating a full breakfast or having a midmorning snack may help to relieve the nausea and vomiting.

This medication can increase your sensitivity to sunlight. You should, therefore, try to avoid prolonged exposure to sunlight and sunlamps. Wear protective clothing and sunglasses, and use an effective sunscreen.

Major. Tell your doctor about any side effects that are persistent or particularly bothersome. IT IS ESPECIALLY IMPORTANT TO TELL YOUR DOCTOR about blurred vision, chest pain, convulsions, depression, itching, loss of coordination, pain or inflammation of the calves or thighs, shortness of breath, skin rash, slurred speech, or yellowing of the eyes or skin.

INTERACTIONS

Estradiol interacts with several other types of medications:

1. It can decrease the effectiveness of oral anticoagulants (blood thinners, such as warfarin).

2. Carbamazepine, phenobarbital, phenytoin, primidone, and rifampin can reduce the effectiveness of estradiol.

3. Estradiol can increase the side effects and decrease the effectiveness of tricyclic antidepressants.

BE SURE TO TELL YOUR DOCTOR about any medications you are currently taking, especially any listed above.

WARNINGS

- Tell your doctor about unusual or allergic reactions you have had to any medications, especially to estradiol, other estrogens, or oral contraceptives.
- Tell your doctor if you now have or if you have ever had asthma, blood clot disorders, breast disease, depression, diabetes mellitus, epilepsy, endometriosis, gallstones or gallbladder disease, heart disease, high blood pressure, kidney disease, liver disease, migraine headaches, porphyria, or uterine tumors.
- Estrogens may cause a change in glucose tolerance in diabetic patients. Be sure to tell your doctor if you notice any abnormalities in your urine or blood glucose levels.
- Estrogens can change your blood's clotting ability, so be especially careful to avoid injuries.
- Although it is not known if estrogens can increase the risk of breast cancer, it is important that you examine your breasts regularly for lumps or discharge.
- If you notice tenderness, swelling, or bleeding of your gums, consult your doctor or dentist.
- Your doctor may schedule regular office visits to be sure your medication is working properly.
- Before having surgery or any other medical or dental treatment, be sure to tell your doctor or dentist that you are taking this medication.
- A package insert titled "Information for the Patient" should be dispensed with your prescription. It is important that you understand the possible risks and benefits of this medication. If you have any questions, check with your doctor or pharmacist.
- Cigarette smoking can greatly increase the risk of developing heart or blood vessel disorders while taking this medication. The risks increase with the amount of smoking and the age of the smoker.
- Be sure to tell your doctor if you are pregnant. If you suspect you are pregnant, discontinue use of the medication immediately. Estrogens have been shown to cause birth defects in the offspring of women who received these medications during pregnancy. Also, tell your doctor if you are breast-feeding an infant. Small amounts of estrogen pass into breast milk. Estradiol can also decrease milk production.

---

estrogens, conjugated

BRAND NAMES (Manufacturers)
conjugated estrogens (various manufacturers)
Premarin (Ayerst)
TYPE OF DRUG
Estrogen

INGREDIENTS
conjugated estrogens
DOSAGE FORM
Tablets (0.3 mg, 0.625 mg, 0.9 mg, 1.25 mg, and 2.5 mg)
STORAGE
These tablets should be stored at room temperature in a tightly closed container.

USES

Conjugated estrogens are a group of estrogen-like products obtained from natural sources (the urine of pregnant mares). They are used to treat menopausal symptoms, prostatic cancer, uterine bleeding, and some cases of breast cancer. They can also be used in replacement therapy for women who do not produce enough estrogen of their own.

TREATMENT

In order to avoid stomach irritation, you can take conjugated estrogens with food or immediately after a meal.

Follow your doctor's instructions carefully when you take this medication. Often, conjugated estrogens are prescribed to be taken for three-week periods, with one week off (in order to reduce potential side effects).

If you miss a scheduled dose of this medication, take the missed dose as soon as possible, unless it is almost time for the next dose. In that case, do not take the missed dose at all; just return to your regular dosing schedule. Do not double the next dose.

SIDE EFFECTS

Minor. Acne, bloating, change in sexual desire, depression, diarrhea, dizziness, headache, loss of appetite, nausea, or vomiting. These side effects should disappear as your body adjusts to the medication.

This medication can increase your sensitivity to sunlight. You should, therefore, try to avoid prolonged exposure to sunlight and sunlamps. Wear protective clothing and sunglasses, and use an effective sunscreen.

If you feel dizzy or light-headed, sit or lie down for a while; get up slowly from a sitting or reclining position, and be careful on stairs.

Major. Tell your doctor about side effects that are persistent or particularly bothersome. IT IS ESPECIALLY IMPORTANT TO TELL YOUR DOCTOR about changes in menstrual patterns; chest pain; difficulty in breathing; eye pain; loss of coordination; lumps in the breast; painful urination; pain in the calves; skin color changes; slurred speech; sudden, severe headache; swelling of the feet or ankles; vision changes; weight gain or loss; or yellowing of eyes or skin.

INTERACTIONS

Conjugated estrogens interact with several other drugs:

1. Estrogens can decrease the effectiveness of oral anticoagulants (blood thinners, such as warfarin).

2. Carbamazepine, ampicillin, phenobarbital, phenytoin, primidone, and rifampin can increase the elimination of estrogen from the body, thus decreasing its effectiveness.

3. Estrogens can increase the side effects, and decrease the effectiveness, of the tricyclic antidepressants.

Before starting to take conjugated estrogens, BE SURE TO TELL YOUR DOCTOR about any medications you are currently taking, especially any of those listed above.

WARNINGS

- Tell your doctor about unusual or allergic reactions you have had to any medications, especially to conjugated estrogens, to oral contraceptives (birth control pills), or to any other estrogen product.
- Before starting to take this drug, tell your doctor if you have ever had asthma, blood clot disorders, breast cancer, diabetes mellitus, endometriosis, epilepsy, gallbladder disease, heart disease, high blood pressure, hypercalcemia, kidney disease, liver disease, migraines, porphyria, uterine fibroid tumors, vaginal bleeding, or depression.
- Studies have shown that estrogens increase the risk of certain types of cancer. Ask your pharmacist for the brochure "Information for the Patient." It is important that you understand the possible risks and benefits of this medication. If you have any questions, check with your doctor or pharmacist.
- Although it is not known if estrogens can increase the risk of breast cancer, it is important that you examine your breasts regularly for lumps or discharge.
- If you notice tenderness, swelling, or bleeding of your gums, consult your doctor or dentist.
- Estrogens can cause a change in glucose tolerance in diabetic patients. If you are diabetic, be sure to tell your doctor if you notice any abnormalities in your urine or blood glucose levels.
- Do not change your brand of medication without the consent of your doctor. If your refill does not look the same, consult your doctor or pharmacist.
- Cigarette smoking increases the risk of serious side effects from estrogens. The risk increases with both age and the amount of smoking.
- If this medication makes you dizzy or light-headed, do not take part in any activity that requires alertness, such as driving a car or operating potentially dangerous equipment.
- Estrogens can change your blood's clotting ability, so be especially careful to avoid injuries.
- Before having surgery or any other medical or dental treatment, be sure to tell your doctor or dentist that you are taking this medication.
- Be sure to tell your doctor if you are pregnant. If you suspect you are pregnant, discontinue use of this medication immediately. Several studies have shown that estrogens taken during pregnancy can cause birth defects. Also, tell your doctor if you are breast-feeding an infant. Estrogens pass into breast milk.

---

ethacrynic acid

BRAND NAME (Manufacturer)
Edecrin (Merck Sharp & Dohme)
TYPE OF DRUG
Diuretic and antihypertensive
INGREDIENT
ethacrynic acid
DOSAGE FORM
Tablets (25 mg and 50 mg)
STORAGE
Ethacrynic acid should be stored at room temperature in a tightly closed, light-resistant container.

USES

Ethacrynic acid is prescribed to treat high blood pressure. It is also used to reduce fluid accumulation in the body caused by conditions such as heart failure, cirrhosis of the liver, kidney disease, and the long-term use of some medications. This medication reduces fluid accumulation by increasing the elimination of salt and water through the kidneys.

TREATMENT

To decrease stomach irritation, you can take ethacrynic acid with a glass of milk or with a meal (unless your doctor directs you to do otherwise). Try to take it at the same time every day. Avoid taking a dose after 6:00 P.M.; otherwise, you may have to get up during the night to urinate.

If you miss a dose of this medication, take the missed dose as soon as possible, unless it is almost time for the next dose. In that case, do not take the missed dose at all; just return to your regular dosing schedule. Do not double the next dose.

This medication does not cure high blood pressure, but it will help to control the condition as long as you take it.

SIDE EFFECTS

Minor. Blurred vision, constipation, cramping, diarrhea, dizziness, headache, loss of appetite, sore mouth, or stomach upset. As your body adjusts to the medication, these side effects should disappear.

This medication will cause an increase in the amount of urine or in the frequency of urination when you first begin to take it. It may also cause you to have an unusual feeling of tiredness. These effects should lessen after several days.

This medication can also cause increased sensitivity to sunlight. It is, therefore, important to avoid prolonged exposure to sunlight and sunlamps. Wear protective clothing, and use an effective sunscreen.

To relieve constipation, increase the amount of fiber in your diet (fresh fruits and vegetables, salads, bran, and whole-grain breads) and exercise more (unless your doctor directs you to do otherwise).

To avoid dizziness or light-headedness when you stand, contract and relax the muscles of your legs for a few moments before rising. Do this by pushing one foot against the floor while raising the other foot slightly, alternating feet so that you are "pumping" your legs in a pedaling motion.

Major. Tell your doctor about any side effects that are persistent or particularly bothersome. IT IS ESPECIALLY IMPORTANT TO TELL YOUR DOCTOR about black, tarry stools; confusion; difficulty in breathing; dry mouth; fainting; increased thirst; itching; joint pains; loss of appetite; mood changes; muscle cramps; nausea; palpitations; rash; ringing in the ears; sore throat; severe abdominal pain; tingling in the fingers and toes; unusual bleeding or bruising; vomiting; watery diarrhea; weakness; or yellowing of the eyes or skin.

INTERACTIONS

Ethacrynic acid interacts with several other types of drugs:

1. It can increase the side effects of alcohol, barbiturates, narcotics, cephalosporin antibiotics, chloral hydrate, cortisone and cortisone-like steroids (such as dexamethasone, hydrocortisone, prednisone, and prednisolone), digoxin, digitalis, lithium, amphotericin B, heparin, and warfarin.

2. Probenecid and indomethacin may decrease the effectiveness of this medicine.

3. The effectiveness of antigout medications, insulin, and oral antidiabetic medications may be decreased by ethacrynic acid.

Before taking ethacrynic acid, BE SURE TO TELL YOUR DOCTOR about any medications you are currently taking, especially any of those listed above.

WARNINGS

- Tell your doctor about unusual or allergic reactions you have had to any medications, especially to ethacrynic acid or other diuretics.
- Before you start taking this medication, tell your doctor if you now have or if you have ever had kidney disease, problems with urination, or liver disease.
- This drug can cause potassium loss. Signs of potassium loss include dry mouth, thirst, weakness, muscle pain or cramps, nausea, and vomiting. If you experience any of these symptoms, call your doctor. Your doctor may have blood tests performed periodically to monitor your potassium levels. To help avoid potassium loss, take this drug with a glass of fresh or frozen orange or cranberry juice, or eat a banana every day. The use of a salt substitute also helps to prevent potassium loss. Do not change your diet or use a salt substitute, however, before discussing it with your doctor. Too much potassium can also be dangerous.
- To prevent severe water loss (dehydration) while taking this medication, check with your doctor if you have any illness that causes severe or continuous nausea, vomiting, or diarrhea.
- Before having any kind of surgery or other medical or dental treatment, be sure to tell your doctor or dentist that you are taking ethacrynic acid.
- To prevent dizziness, light-headedness, and fainting, get up from a sitting or lying position slowly, avoid standing for long periods of time, and avoid strenuous exercise and prolonged exposure to hot weather.
- While taking this medication, limit your intake of alcoholic beverages in order to prevent dizziness or light-headedness.
- If you have high blood pressure, do not take any over-the-counter (nonprescription) medication for weight control or for allergy, asthma, cough, cold, or sinus problems unless you first check with your doctor.
- The elderly may be more sensitive to the effects of this medication.
- Be sure to tell your doctor if you are pregnant. This drug crosses the placenta. Although studies in humans have not been conducted, adverse effects have been observed in the fetuses of animals that received large doses of this drug during pregnancy. Also, tell your doctor if you are breast-feeding an infant. Small amounts of this drug pass into breast milk.

---

ethinyl estradiol

BRAND NAMES (Manufacturers)

Estinyl (Schering)
Feminone (Upjohn)

TYPE OF DRUG
Estrogen
INGREDIENT
ethinyl estradiol
DOSAGE FORM
Tablets (0.02 mg, 0.05 mg, and 0.5 mg)
STORAGE
Ethinyl estradiol should be stored at room temperature in a tightly closed container.

USES

Ethinyl estradiol is a synthetic estrogen that is used to treat menopausal symptoms, certain types of breast cancer, and prostate cancer.

TREATMENT

In order to avoid stomach irritation, you can take ethinyl estradiol with food or with a full glass of milk or water (unless your doctor directs you to do otherwise).

If you miss a dose of this medication, take the missed dose as soon as possible, unless it is almost time for the next dose. In that case, do not take the missed dose at all; just return to your regular dosing schedule. Do not double the next dose.

SIDE EFFECTS

Minor. Abdominal cramping, abnormal vaginal bleeding, acne, bloating, breast tenderness, darkening of the skin, diarrhea, dizziness, fluid retention, frequent or painful urination, headache, nausea, nervousness, vomiting, or weight gain. These side effects should disappear as your body adjusts to the medication.

This medication can increase your sensitivity to sunlight. You should, therefore, try to avoid prolonged exposure to sunlight and sunlamps. Wear protective clothing and sunglasses, and use an effective sunscreen.

If you feel dizzy, sit or lie down for a while; get up slowly from a sitting or reclining position, and be careful on stairs.

Eating a full breakfast or having a midmorning snack may help to relieve the nausea and vomiting.

Major. Tell your doctor about any side effects that are persistent or particularly bothersome. IT IS ESPECIALLY IMPORTANT TO TELL YOUR DOCTOR about blurred vision, chest pain, convulsions, depression, hair loss, itching, pain or inflammation of the calves or thighs, shortness of breath, skin rash, or yellowing of the eyes or skin.

INTERACTIONS

Ethinyl estradiol interacts with other types of medications:

1. It can decrease the effectiveness of oral anticoagulants (blood thinners, such as warfarin).

2. Carbamazepine, phenobarbital, phenytoin, primidone, and rifampin can reduce the effectiveness of ethinyl estradiol.

3. Ethinyl estradiol can increase the side effects and decrease the effectiveness of tricyclic antidepressants.

BE SURE TO TELL YOUR DOCTOR about any medications you are currently taking, especially any listed above.

WARNINGS

- Tell your doctor about unusual or allergic reactions you have had to any medications, especially to ethinyl estradiol or other estrogens or to oral contraceptives (birth control pills).
- Tell your doctor if you now have or if you have ever had asthma, blood clot disorders, breast disease, depression, diabetes mellitus, epilepsy, endometriosis, gallstones or gallbladder disease, heart disease, high blood pressure, kidney disease, liver disease, migraine headaches, porphyria, or uterine tumors.
- Some of these products contain the color additive FD&C Yellow No. 5 (tartrazine), which can cause allergic-type reactions (shortness of breath, fainting, rash) in certain susceptible individuals.
- Estrogens can change your blood's clotting ability, so be especially careful to avoid injuries.
- Estrogens can cause a change in glucose tolerance in diabetic patients. Be sure to tell your doctor if you notice any abnormalities in your urine or blood glucose levels.
- Before having surgery or any other medical or dental treatment, be sure to tell your doctor or dentist that you are taking this medication.
- A package insert titled "Information for the Patient" should be dispensed with your prescription. It is important that you understand the possible risks and benefits of this medication. If you have any questions, check with your doctor or pharmacist.
- Although it is not known if estrogens increase the risk of breast cancer, it is important that you examine your breasts regularly for lumps or discharge.
- Cigarette smoking can greatly increase the risk of developing heart or blood vessel disorders while taking this medication. The risks increase with the amount of smoking and the age of the smoker.
- Be sure to tell your doctor if you are pregnant. If you suspect you are pregnant, discontinue use of this medication immediately. Estrogens have been shown to cause birth defects in the offspring of women who received these medications during pregnancy. Also, tell your doctor if you are breast-feeding an infant. Small amounts of estrogen pass into breast milk. Ethinyl estradiol can also decrease milk production.

Ethon—see methyclothiazide

---

ethosuximide

BRAND NAME (Manufacturer)
Zarontin (Parke-Davis)
TYPE OF DRUG
Anticonvulsant
INGREDIENT
ethosuximide
DOSAGE FORMS
Capsules (250 mg)
Oral syrup (250 mg per 5-ml spoonful)
STORAGE
Ethosuximide capsules and oral syrup should be stored at room temperature in tightly closed, light-resistant containers. This medication should never be frozen. Discard any outdated medication.

USES

This medication is used to treat absence (petit mal) seizures. Although it is not exactly clear how it does so, ethosuximide seems to prevent seizure activity by decreasing the activity of certain chemicals (nerve transmitters) in the brain.

TREATMENT

In order to avoid stomach irritation, you can take ethosuximide with food or with a full glass of water or milk (unless your doctor directs you to do otherwise).

Each dose of the oral syrup form of this medication should be measured carefully with a specially designed 5-ml measuring spoon. An ordinary kitchen teaspoon is not accurate enough.

Ethosuximide works best when the level of medicine in your bloodstream is kept constant. It is best, therefore, to take the doses at evenly spaced intervals day and night. For example, if you are to take three doses a day, the doses should be spaced eight hours apart.

It is important to try not to miss any doses of this medication. If you do miss a dose, and remember within four hours, take the missed dose immediately and then return to your normal schedule. If more than four hours have passed, do not take the missed dose at all; just return to your regular dosing schedule. Do not double the next dose.

SIDE EFFECTS

Minor. Constipation, diarrhea, dizziness, drowsiness, headache, hiccups, loss of appetite, nausea, stomach upset, or weight loss. These side effects should disappear as your body adjusts to the medication.

To relieve constipation, increase the amount of fiber in your diet (fresh fruits and vegetables, salads, bran, and whole-grain breads), exercise, and drink more water (unless your doctor directs you to do otherwise).

If you feel dizzy, sit or lie down for a while; get up slowly from a sitting or reclining position, and be careful on stairs.

Major. Tell your doctor about any side effects that are persistent or particularly bothersome. IT IS ESPECIALLY IMPORTANT TO TELL YOUR DOCTOR about blurred vision, confusion, depression, difficult or painful urination, false sense of well-being, fatigue, irritability, joint pains, loss of coordination, mental disorders, mood changes, nervousness, skin rash, swelling of the eyes or tongue, unusual bleeding or bruising, or vaginal bleeding.

INTERACTIONS

This drug can interact with several other types of drugs:

1. Tricyclic antidepressants, haloperidol, thiothixene, phenothiazine tranquilizers, and alcohol can increase the risk of seizures. Dosage adjustments of ethosuximide may be necessary when any of these medications are started.

2. Isoniazid can increase the side effects of ethosuximide.

BE SURE TO TELL YOUR DOCTOR about any medications you are currently taking, especially any listed above.

WARNINGS

- Tell your doctor about unusual or allergic reactions you have had to any medications, especially to ethosuximide, methsuximide, or phensuximide.
- Tell your doctor if you now have or if you have ever had blood disorders, kidney disease, or liver disease.
- If this drug makes you dizzy or drowsy, do not take part in any activity that requires alertness, such as driving a car or operating potentially dangerous equipment. Children should be careful while playing.
- Before having surgery or any other medical or dental treatment, be sure to tell your doctor or dentist that you are taking ethosuximide.
- Do not stop taking this medication unless you first check with your doctor. Stopping the drug abruptly may lead to a worsening of your condition. Your doctor may want to reduce your dosage gradually or start you on another drug when treatment with ethosuximide is discontinued.
- Your doctor may schedule regular office visits, especially during the first few months of therapy, to be sure the drug is working properly.
- Be sure to tell your doctor if you are pregnant. Birth defects have been reported more often in infants whose mothers have seizure disorders. It is unclear if the increased risk of birth defects is associated with the disorder or with the anticonvulsant medications, such as ethosuximide, that are used to treat the condition. The risks and benefits of treatment should be discussed with your doctor. Also, tell your doctor if you are breast-feeding an infant. Ethosuximide passes into breast milk.

Etrafon—see perphenazine and amitriptyline combination

Eutonyl Filmtabs—see pargyline

Exna—see benzthiazide

---

famotidine

BRAND NAME (Manufacturer)

Pepcid (Merck Sharp & Dohme)

TYPE OF DRUG

Gastric acid secretion inhibitor (decreases stomach acid)

INGREDIENT

famotidine

DOSAGE FORMS

Tablets (20 mg and 40 mg)

Oral suspension (40 mg per 5-ml spoonful)

STORAGE

Famotidine should be stored at room temperature (never frozen) in a tightly closed container. Avoid exposure of this medication to high temperatures during storage.

USES

Famotidine is used to treat active duodenal ulcers. It is also used in the long-term treatment of excessive stomach acid secretion (Zollinger-Ellison syndrome) and in the prevention of recurrent ulcers. Famotidine reduces stomach acid secretion by blocking the effects of histamine in the stomach.

TREATMENT

If you are taking a single daily dose of famotidine, it is best to take the dose at bedtime in order to obtain the maximum benefits from it. Antacids will not affect the activity of famotidine. Check with your doctor to see if you should be taking antacids as part of your ulcer treatment.

The oral liquid should be measured carefully with a specially designed 5-ml measuring spoon. An ordinary kitchen teaspoon is not accurate enough to ensure that the proper dose will be taken.

If you miss a dose of famotidine, take the missed dose as soon as possible, unless it is almost time for the next dose. In that case, do not take the missed dose at all; just return to your regular dosing schedule. Do not double the next dose.

SIDE EFFECTS

Minor. Abdominal pain, acne, change in taste, constipation, diarrhea, dizziness, dry mouth, dry skin, fatigue, flushing, headache, insomnia, loss of appetite, nausea, or vomiting. These side effects should disappear as your body adjusts to this drug.

If you are constipated, exercise and drink more water (unless your doctor tells you not to do so).

To reduce mouth dryness, chew sugarless gum or suck on ice chips or hard candy.

If you feel dizzy or light-headed, sit or lie down for a while; get up slowly from a sitting or reclining position, and be careful on stairs.

Major. Tell your doctor about any side effects that are persistent or particularly bothersome. IT IS ESPECIALLY IMPORTANT TO TELL YOUR DOCTOR about anxiety, confusion, depression, fever, hair loss, hallucinations, itching, muscle or joint pain, palpitations, ringing in the ear, seizures, shortness of breath, tingling in the fingers or toes, or yellowing of the eyes or skin.

INTERACTIONS

No drug interactions with famotidine have yet been confirmed. It is still very important, however, to tell your doctor about all of the medications you are taking before starting famotidine.

WARNINGS

- Tell your doctor about any unusual or allergic reactions you have had to any medications, especially to famotidine or to the other gastric acid secretion inhibitors (cimetidine and ranitidine).
- Before starting famotidine, tell your doctor if you now have or if you have ever had kidney disease.
- Famotidine should be taken continuously for as long as your doctor prescribes. Stopping therapy early may be a cause of ineffective treatment.
- Cigarette smoking may interfere with the beneficial effects of famotidine.
- Aspirin, foods known to cause stomach upset, and certain drinks (such as those containing caffeine) may worsen your stomach irritation.
- If this drug makes you dizzy or drowsy, do not take part in any activity that requires alertness, such as driving a car or operating potentially dangerous equipment.
- Be sure to tell your doctor if you are pregnant. Studies in pregnant women have not been conducted. Also, tell your doctor if you are breast-feeding an infant. Small amounts of famotidine pass into animal milk; studies on human milk have not been done.

Fastin—see phentermine

Fedahist—see pseudoephedrine and chlorpheniramine combination

Feldene—see piroxicam

Feminone—see ethinyl estradiol

---

fenfluramine

BRAND NAME (Manufacturer)
Pondimin (Robins)
TYPE OF DRUG
Anorectic
INGREDIENT
fenfluramine
DOSAGE FORM
Tablets (20 mg)
STORAGE
Fenfluramine should be stored at room temperature in a tightly closed, light-resistant container.

USES

Fenfluramine is used as an appetite suppressant during the first few weeks of dieting to help establish new eating habits. This medication is thought to relieve hunger by altering nerve impulses to the appetite control center in the brain. Its effectiveness lasts only for short periods (three to 12 weeks), however.

TREATMENT

You can take fenfluramine with a full glass of water, one hour before meals (unless your doctor directs you to do otherwise).

If you miss a dose of this medication, take the missed dose as soon as possible, unless it is almost time for your next dose. In that case, do not take the missed dose at all; just return to your regular dosing schedule. Do not double the next dose.

SIDE EFFECTS

Minor. Blurred vision, constipation, diarrhea, dizziness, dry mouth, euphoria, fatigue, frequent urination, headache, insomnia, irritability, nausea, nervousness, restlessness, stomach pain, sweating, unpleasant taste in the mouth, or vomiting. These side effects should disappear as your body adjusts to the medication.

Dry mouth can be relieved by sucking on ice chips or a piece of hard candy or by chewing sugarless gum.

In order to prevent constipation, increase the amount of fiber in your diet (fresh fruits and vegetables, salads, bran, and whole-grain breads), exercise, and drink more water (unless your doctor tells you not to do so).

Major. Tell your doctor about any side effects that are persistent or particularly bothersome. IT IS ESPECIALLY IMPORTANT TO TELL YOUR DOCTOR about changes in sexual desire, chest pain, difficulty in urinating, enlarged breasts (in both sexes), fever, hair loss, headaches, impotence, increased blood pressure, menstrual irregularities, mental depression, mood changes, mouth sores, muscle pains, nosebleeds, palpitations, rash, sore throat, or tremors.

INTERACTIONS

Fenfluramine anorectic medication interacts with several other types of medications:

1. Concurrent use of it with central nervous system depres-

sants (such as alcohol, antihistamines, barbiturates, muscle relaxants, narcotics, pain medications, and phenothiazine tranquilizers) or with tricyclic antidepressants can cause extreme drowsiness.

2. Fenfluramine may alter insulin and oral antidiabetic medication dosage requirements in diabetic patients.

3. The blood-pressure-lowering effects of antihypertensive medications, especially guanethidine, reserpine, methyldopa, and diuretics (water pills), may be increased by this medication.

4. Use of fenfluramine within 14 days of a monoamine oxidase (MAO) inhibitor (isocarboxazid, pargyline, phenelzine, tranylcypromine) can result in high blood pressure and other side effects.

BE SURE TO TELL YOUR DOCTOR about any medications you are currently taking, especially any of those listed above.

WARNINGS

- Tell your doctor about unusual or allergic reactions you have had to any medications, especially to fenfluramine or other appetite suppressants (such as benzphetamine, phendimetrazine, diethylpropion, phenmetrazine, mazindol, and phentermine), or to epinephrine, norepinephrine, ephedrine, amphetamines, dextroamphetamine, phenylephrine, phenylpropanolamine, pseudoephedrine, albuterol, metaproterenol, or terbutaline.
- Tell your doctor if you have a history of drug abuse or alcoholism or if you have ever had angina, diabetes mellitus, emotional disturbances, glaucoma, heart or cardiovascular disease, high blood pressure, thyroid disease, epilepsy, or mental depression.
- Fenfluramine can mask the symptoms of extreme fatigue and can cause dizziness or light-headedness. Your ability to perform tasks that require alertness, such as driving a car or operating potentially dangerous equipment, may be decreased during therapy with this medication. Appropriate caution should, therefore, be taken.
- Before having surgery or any other medical or dental treatment, be sure to tell your doctor or dentist that you are taking this medication.
- Fenfluramine is related to amphetamine and may be habit-forming when taken for long periods of time (both physical and psychological dependence can occur). You should, therefore, not increase the dosage of this medication or take it for longer than 12 weeks, unless you first consult your doctor. It is also important that you not stop taking this medication abruptly. Fatigue, sleep disorders, mental depression, nausea, vomiting, stomach cramps, or pain could occur. Your doctor may want to decrease your dosage gradually in order to prevent these side effects.
- Fenfluramine can alter blood sugar levels in diabetic patients. Therefore, if you are diabetic and starting to take this medication, you should carefully monitor your blood or urine glucose levels for the first several days.
- Be sure to tell your doctor if you are pregnant. Although side effects in humans have not been studied, some of the appetite suppressants have been shown to cause side effects in the fetuses of animals that received large doses during pregnancy. Also, tell your doctor if you are breast-feeding an infant. It is not known whether this medication passes into breast milk.

fenoprofen

BRAND NAMES (Manufacturers)

fenoprofen (various manufacturers)
Nalfon (Dista)
Nalfon 200 (Dista)

TYPE OF DRUG

Nonsteroidal anti-inflammatory analgesic

INGREDIENT

fenoprofen

DOSAGE FORMS

Capsules (200 mg, 300 mg, and 600 mg)
Tablets (600 mg)

STORAGE

This medication should be stored in tightly closed containers at room temperature away from heat and direct sunlight.

USES

Fenoprofen is used to treat the inflammation (pain, swelling, and stiffness) of certain types of arthritis, gout, bursitis, and tendinitis. Fenoprofen has been shown to block the production of certain body chemicals, called prostaglandins, that trigger pain. However, it is not yet fully understood how fenoprofen works.

TREATMENT

You should take this medication on an empty stomach 30 to 60 minutes before meals or two hours after meals, so that it gets into your bloodstream quickly. Since fenoprofen can cause stomach irritation, however, your doctor may want you to take this medicine with food or antacids.

If you are taking fenoprofen to relieve arthritis, you must take it regularly as directed by your doctor. It may take up to three weeks before you feel its full benefits. This medication does not cure arthritis, but it will help to control the condition as long as you continue to take it.

It is important to take fenoprofen on schedule and not to miss any doses. If you do miss a dose, take the missed dose as soon as possible, unless it is almost time for your next dose. In that case, do not take the missed dose at all; just return to your regular dosing schedule. Do not double the next dose.

SIDE EFFECTS

Minor. Bloating, constipation, diarrhea, difficulty in sleeping, dizziness, drowsiness, headache, heartburn, indigestion, light-headedness, loss of appetite, nausea, nervousness, soreness of the mouth, unusual sweating, or vomiting. As your body adjusts to the drug, these side effects should disappear.

To relieve constipation, increase the amount of fiber in your diet (fresh fruits and vegetables, salads, bran, and whole-grain breads), exercise, and drink more water (unless your doctor directs you to do otherwise).

If you become dizzy, sit or lie down for a while; get up slowly from a sitting or reclining position, and be careful on stairs.

Major. If any side effects are persistent or particularly bothersome, you should report them to your doctor. IT IS ESPECIALLY IMPORTANT TO TELL YOUR DOCTOR about bloody or black, tarry stools; blurred vision; confusion; depression; difficult or painful urination; difficulty in breathing; hearing difficulties; palpitations; ringing or buzzing in the ears; skin rash, hives, or itching; stomach pain; swelling of the feet; tightness in the chest; unexplained sore throat and fever; unusual bleeding or bruising; unusual fatigue or weakness; unusual weight gain; or yellowing of the eyes or skin.

INTERACTIONS

Fenoprofen interacts with several types of medications:

1. Anticoagulants (blood thinners, such as warfarin) can lead to an increase in bleeding complications.
2. Aspirin, salicylates, and other anti-inflammatory medications can lead to an increase in stomach irritation caused by fenoprofen.
3. Fenoprofen levels may be affected by concurrent use of phenobarbital.
4. Probenecid may increase blood levels of fenoprofen, which may increase the risk of side effects.
5. The action of beta blockers may be decreased by this drug.

BE SURE TO TELL YOUR DOCTOR about any medications you are currently taking, especially any of those listed above.

WARNINGS

- Tell your doctor if you have ever had unusual or allergic reactions to medications, especially to fenoprofen or any chemically related drug (such as aspirin or other salicylates, diclofenac, diflunisal, flurbiprofen, indomethacin, ibuprofen, ketoprofen, meclofenamate, mefenamic acid, naproxen, oxyphenbutazone, piroxicam, sulindac, or tolmetin).
- Tell your doctor if you have ever had bleeding problems, colitis, stomach ulcers or other stomach problems, epilepsy, heart disease, high blood pressure, asthma, kidney disease, liver disease, mental illness, or Parkinson's disease.
- If this drug makes you dizzy or drowsy, do not take part in any activity that requires alertness, such as driving a car or operating potentially dangerous equipment.
- Before having surgery or other medical or dental treatment, tell your doctor or dentist about this drug.
- Stomach problems are more likely to occur if you take aspirin regularly or drink alcohol while being treated with this medication. These should, therefore, be avoided (unless your doctor directs you to do otherwise).
- Be sure to tell your doctor if you are pregnant. Although studies in humans have not been conducted, unwanted heart side effects have been reported in the offspring of animals that received fenoprofen during pregnancy. Also, tell your doctor if you are breast-feeding an infant. Small amounts of this medication can pass into breast milk.

Festal II—see pancrelipase

Fiorgen PF—see aspirin, caffeine, and butalbital combination

Fiorinal—see aspirin, caffeine, and butalbital combination

Fiorinal with Codeine—see aspirin, caffeine, butalbital, and codeine combination

Flagyl—see metronidazole

Flexaphen—see chlorzoxazone and acetaminophen combination

Flexeril—see cyclobenzaprine

Florvite—see vitamins, multiple, with fluoride

---

flunisolide (nasal)

BRAND NAME (Manufacturer)
Nasalide (Syntex)
TYPE OF DRUG
Nasal adrenocorticosteroid hormone
INGREDIENT
flunisolide
DOSAGE FORM
Nasal solution (25 mcg flunisolide per ml)
STORAGE
Flunisolide nasal solution should be stored at room temperature in a tightly closed container. Opened containers of this medication should be discarded after three months.

USES

Flunisolide nasal solution is used to relieve symptoms of rhinitis (inflammation of the nasal passages). How this drug acts to relieve these symptoms is not completely understood. Your adrenal glands naturally produce certain cortisone-like chemicals. These chemicals are involved in various regulatory processes in the body (such as those involving fluid balance, temperature, and reaction to inflammation). Flunisolide belongs to a group of drugs known as adrenocorticosteroids (or cortisone-like medications).

TREATMENT

Just before applying flunisolide nasal solution, clear your nasal passages of all secretions. Then carefully follow the patient instructions, which you should receive when your prescription is dispensed. The instructions will explain how to properly apply this medication. To avoid the risk of side effects, measure the dose carefully. Do not increase the dose of flunisolide or increase the number of applications per day without first checking with your doctor.

If your doctor recommends that you use a nasal decongestant to clear your nasal passages, use the decongestant just before you apply flunisolide.

Relief from the symptoms of inflammation may not become apparent for up to three weeks after starting flunisolide. This drug does not cure the cause of inflammation, but it may help relieve the symptoms as long as you continue to use it. Therefore, its effectiveness depends on regular use while the condition is present. Your doctor may then recommend that you gradually decrease the number of daily doses as your condition improves.

If there is no improvement in your condition within three weeks after starting flunisolide, check with your doctor. He or she may want you to stop the medication. Try not to miss any doses of this medication.

If you do miss a dose, apply the dose as soon as possible, unless it is almost time for the next dose. In that case, do not apply the missed dose; just return to your regular dosing schedule. Do not double the next dose.

SIDE EFFECTS

Minor. Drying of nasal passages, headache, loss of smell or taste, nasal congestion, nasal irritation, nausea, nosebleeds, sneezing, sore throat, vomiting, or watery eyes. These side effects should disappear as your body adjusts to this medication. A mild, temporary burning or stinging sensation may occur after this medication is applied.

Major. Tell your doctor about any side effects that are persistent or particularly bothersome. IT IS ESPECIALLY IMPORTANT TO TELL YOUR DOCTOR about persistent burning or stinging after application.

INTERACTIONS

This medication should not interact with any other medications as long as it is used according to directions.

WARNINGS

- Tell your doctor about unusual or allergic reactions you have had to any medications, especially to flunisolide or other adrenocorticosteroids (such as amcinonide, beclomethasone, betamethasone, clocortolone, cortisone, desonide, desoximetasone, dexamethasone, diflorasone, flumethasone, fluocinolone, fluocinonide, fluorometholone, flurandrenolide, halcinonide, hydrocortisone, methylprednisolone, paramethasone, prednisolone, prednisone, and triamcinolone).
- Before starting flunisolide, tell your doctor if you now have or if you have ever had chicken pox, diabetes mellitus, or tuberculosis.
- Flunisolide can slow the healing of wounds. Therefore, tell your doctor about recent nasal surgery or injury, recurrent nosebleeds, or nasal ulcers.
- Be sure to tell your doctor if you are pregnant. Studies in humans have not been conducted; however, birth defects have been observed in the offspring of animals that were given large oral doses of this drug during pregnancy. Also, tell your doctor if you are breast-feeding an infant. Small amounts of adrenocorticosteroids do pass into breast milk and may cause growth suppression or a decrease in natural adrenocorticosteroid production in the nursing infant.

---

fluocinolone (topical)

BRAND NAMES (Manufacturers)
fluocinolone acetonide (various manufacturers)
Fluonid (Herbert)
Flurosyn (Rugby)
Synalar (Syntex)
Synalar-HP (Syntex)
Synemol (Syntex)

TYPE OF DRUG
Adrenocorticosteroid hormone

INGREDIENT
fluocinolone

DOSAGE FORMS
Cream (0.01%, 0.025%, and 0.2%)
Ointment (0.025%)
Solution (0.01%)

STORAGE
Store at room temperature in a tightly closed container. This medication should never be frozen.

USES

Your adrenal glands naturally produce certain cortisone-like chemicals. These chemicals are involved in various regulatory processes in the body (such as those involving fluid balance, temperature, and reaction to inflammation). Fluocinolone belongs to a group of drugs known as adrenocorticosteroids (or cortisone-like medications). It is used to relieve the skin inflammation (redness, swelling, itching, and discomfort) associated with conditions such as dermatitis, eczema, and poison ivy. How this drug works is not completely understood.

TREATMENT

Before applying this medication, wash your hands. Then, unless your doctor gives you different instructions, gently wash the area of the skin where the medication is to be applied. With a clean towel, pat the area almost dry; it should be slightly damp when you put the medicine on.

Apply a small amount of fluocinolone to the affected area in a thin layer. Do not bandage the area unless your doctor tells you to do so. If you are to apply an occlusive dressing (like kitchen plastic wrap), ask for instructions. Wash your hands again after application.

If you miss a dose of this medication, apply the missed dose as soon as possible, unless it is almost time for the next application. In that case, do not apply the missed dose at all; just return to your regular schedule. Do not put twice as much of the medication on your skin at the next application.

SIDE EFFECTS

Minor. Acne, burning, itching, rash, or skin dryness.

If the affected area is extremely dry or scaling, the skin may be moistened before applying the medication by soaking in water or by applying water with a clean cloth. The ointment form is probably better for dry skin.

A mild, temporary stinging sensation may occur after this medication is applied. If this persists, contact your doctor.

Major. Tell your doctor about any side effects that are persistent or particularly bothersome. IT IS ESPECIALLY IMPORTANT TO TELL YOUR DOCTOR about blistering, increased hair growth, irritation of the affected area, loss of skin color, secondary infection in the area being treated, or thinning of the skin with easy bruising.

INTERACTIONS

This medication should not interact with other medications as long as it is used according to directions.

WARNINGS

- Tell your doctor about unusual or allergic reactions you have had to any medications, especially to fluocinolone or any other adrenocorticosteroid (such as amcinonide, beclomethasone, betamethasone, clocortolone, cortisone, desonide, desoximetasone, dexamethasone, diflorasone, flumethasone, fluocinonide, fluorometholone, flurandrenolide, halcinonide, hydrocortisone, methylprednisolone, paramethasone, prednisolone, prednisone, and triamcinolone).
- Tell your doctor if you now have or if you have ever had blood vessel disease, chicken pox, diabetes mellitus, fungal infection, peptic ulcers, shingles, tuberculosis, tuberculosis of the skin, vaccinia, or any other type of infection, especially at the site currently being treated.

• If irritation develops while using this drug, immediately discontinue its use and notify your doctor.
• This product is not for use in the eyes, nose, or mouth; contact may result in side effects.
• Do not use this product with an occlusive wrap unless your doctor directs you to do so. Systemic absorption of this drug is increased if large areas of the body are treated, particularly if occlusive bandages are used. If it is necessary for you to use this drug under a wrap, follow your doctor's instructions exactly; do not leave the wrap in place longer than specified.
• If you are using fluocinolone on a child's diaper area, do not put tight-fitting diapers or plastic pants on the child. This could lead to increased systemic absorption of the drug and a possible increase in side effects.
• Be sure to tell your doctor if you are pregnant. If large amounts of this drug are applied for prolonged periods, some of it will be absorbed and may cross the placenta. Although studies in humans have not been conducted, birth defects have been observed in the offspring of animals that were given large oral doses of this type of drug during pregnancy. Also, tell your doctor if you are breast-feeding an infant. If absorbed through the skin, small amounts of this medication pass into breast milk and may cause growth suppression or a decrease in natural adrenocorticosteroid hormone production in the nursing infant.

fluocinolone acetonide—see fluocinolone (topical)

---

fluocinonide (topical)

BRAND NAMES (Manufacturers)
fluocinonide (various manufacturers)
Lidex (Syntex)
Lidex-E (Syntex)
TYPE OF DRUG
Adrenocorticosteroid hormone
INGREDIENT
fluocinonide
DOSAGE FORMS
Ointment (0.05%)
Cream (0.05%)
Gel (0.05%)
Solution (0.05%, with 35% alcohol)
STORAGE
Fluocinonide ointment, cream, gel, and solution should be stored at room temperature in tightly closed containers. This medication should never be frozen.

USES

Your adrenal glands naturally produce certain cortisone-like chemicals. These chemicals are involved in various regulatory processes in the body (such as those involving fluid balance, temperature, and reaction to inflammation). Fluocinonide belongs to a group of drugs known as adrenocorticosteroids (or cortisone-like medications). It is used to relieve the skin inflammation (redness, swelling, itching, and discomfort) associated with conditions such as dermatitis, eczema, and poison ivy. How this drug works is not completely understood.

TREATMENT

Before applying this medication, wash your hands. Then, unless your doctor gives you different instructions, gently wash the area of the skin where the medication is to be applied. With a clean towel, pat the area almost dry; it should be slightly damp when you put the medicine on.

Apply a small amount of fluocinonide to the affected area in a thin layer. Do not bandage the area unless your doctor tells you to do so. If you are to apply an occlusive dressing (like kitchen plastic wrap), be sure you understand the instructions. Wash your hands again after application.

If you miss a dose of this medication, apply the missed dose as soon as possible, unless it is almost time for the next application. In that case, do not apply the missed dose at all; just return to your regular schedule. Do not put twice as much of the medication on your skin at the next application.

SIDE EFFECTS

Minor. Acne, burning sensation, itching, rash, or skin dryness.

If the affected area is extremely dry or scaling, the skin may be moistened before applying the medication by soaking in water or by applying water with a clean cloth. The ointment form is probably better for dry skin.

A mild, temporary stinging sensation may occur after this medication is applied. If this persists, contact your doctor.

Major. Tell your doctor about any side effects that are persistent or particularly bothersome. IT IS ESPECIALLY IMPORTANT TO TELL YOUR DOCTOR about blistering, increased hair growth, irritation of the affected area, loss of skin color, secondary infection in the area being treated, or thinning of the skin with easy bruising.

INTERACTIONS

This medication should not interact with any other medications as long as it is used according to directions.

WARNINGS

• Tell your doctor about unusual or allergic reactions you have had to any medications, especially to fluocinonide or any other adrenocorticosteroid (such as amcinonide, betamethasone, clocortolone, cortisone, desonide, desoximetasone, dexamethasone, diflorasone, flumethasone, fluocinolone, fluorometholone, flurandrenolide, halcinonide, hydrocortisone, methylprednisolone, paramethasone, prednisolone, prednisone, and triamcinolone).
• Tell your doctor if you now have or if you have ever had blood vessel disease, chicken pox, diabetes mellitus, fungal infection, peptic ulcers, shingles, tuberculosis, tuberculosis of the skin, vaccinia, or any other type of infection, especially at the site currently being treated.
• If irritation develops while using this drug, immediately discontinue its use and notify your doctor.
• This product is not for use in the eyes, nose, or mouth; contact may result in side effects.
• Do not use this product with an occlusive wrap unless your doctor directs you to do so. Systemic absorption of this drug is increased if large areas of the body are treated, particularly if occlusive bandages are used. If it is necessary for you to use this drug under a wrap, follow your doctor's instructions exactly; do not leave the wrap in place longer than specified.

• If you are using fluocinonide on a child's diaper area, do not put tight-fitting diapers or plastic pants on the child. This may lead to increased systemic absorption of the drug and a possible increase in side effects.
• Be sure to tell your doctor if you are pregnant. If large amounts of this drug are applied for prolonged periods, some of it will be absorbed and may cross the placenta. Although studies in humans have not been conducted, birth defects have been observed in the offspring of animals that were given large oral doses of this type of drug during pregnancy. Also, tell your doctor if you are breast-feeding an infant. If absorbed through the skin, small amounts of fluocinonide pass into breast milk and may cause growth suppression or a decrease in natural adrenocorticosteroid hormone production in the nursing infant.

Fluonid—see fluocinolone (topical)

---

fluoxetine

BRAND NAME (Manufacturer)
Prozac (Dista)
TYPE OF DRUG
Cyclic antidepressant
INGREDIENT
fluoxetine
DOSAGE FORM
Capsules (20 mg)
STORAGE
Store at room temperature in a tightly closed container. Do not store in the bathroom. Heat or moisture can cause this medicine to break down.

USES

Fluoxetine is used to treat the symptoms of mental depression. It relieves depression by increasing the concentration of certain chemicals necessary for nerve transmission in the brain.

TREATMENT

This medication should be taken exactly as prescribed by your doctor. In order to avoid stomach irritation, you can take fluoxetine with food or with a full glass of water (unless your doctor directs you to do otherwise).

The effects of therapy with this medication may not become apparent for one to three weeks.

If you miss a dose of this medicine, it is not necessary to make up the missed dose. Skip that dose and continue at the next scheduled time. You should never take a double dose to make up for one you missed.

SIDE EFFECTS

Minor. Agitation, change in vision, changes in taste, constipation, decreased appetite, decreased mental concentration, decreased sex drive, diarrhea, dizziness, drowsiness, dry mouth, fast heartbeat, flushing, frequent urination, headache, increased sweating, nausea, stomach cramps, stuffy nose, vomiting, or weight gain or loss.

Dry mouth can be relieved by chewing sugarless gum or sucking on hard candy.

To relieve constipation, increase the amount of fiber in your diet (fresh fruits and vegetables, salads, bran, and whole-grain breads), exercise, and drink more water (unless your doctor directs you to do otherwise).

To avoid dizziness when you stand, contract and relax the muscles of your legs for a few moments before rising.

Major. Tell your doctor about any side effects that are persistent or particularly bothersome. IT IS ESPECIALLY IMPORTANT TO TELL YOUR DOCTOR about anxiety, chills or fever, convulsions (seizures), enlarged lymph glands (swelling under jaw or in armpits or groin area), difficulty in breathing, joint or muscle pain, skin rash or hives, or swelling of the feet or lower legs.

INTERACTIONS

Fluoxetine interacts with a number of other types of drugs:

1. Extreme drowsiness can occur when this medicine is taken with central nervous system depressants (such as alcohol, antihistamines, barbiturates, benzodiazepine tranquilizers, muscle relaxants, narcotics, pain medications, phenothiazine tranquilizers, and sleeping medications) or with other antidepressants.

2. Fluoxetine may increase the effects of anticoagulants (blood thinners) such as warfarin, and certain heart medications (such as digitoxin).

3. Serious side effects may occur if a monoamine oxidase (MAO) inhibitor (such as furazolidone, isocarboxazid, pargyline, phenelzine, procarbazine, or tranylcypromine) is taken with fluoxetine. At least 14 days should separate the use of fluoxetine and the use of an MAO inhibitor.

4. Fluoxetine can increase agitation, restlessness, and stomach irritation when taken along with tryptophan.

Before starting to take fluoxetine, BE SURE TO TELL YOUR DOCTOR about any medications you are currently taking, especially any of those listed above.

WARNINGS

• Tell your doctor immediately if you develop a skin rash or hives while taking this medication, or if you have ever had an allergic reaction to fluoxetine.
• Tell your doctor if you have a history of allergy to any substance, such as foods, sulfites or other preservatives, or dyes.
• Before starting to take this medication, be sure to tell your doctor if you have a history of alcoholism or if you have ever had a heart attack, asthma, circulatory disease, difficulty in urinating, electroshock therapy, enlarged prostate gland, epilepsy, glaucoma, high blood pressure, intestinal problems, liver or kidney disease, mental illness, stomach problems, or thyroid disease.
• If this drug makes you dizzy or drowsy, do not take part in any activity that requires alertness, such as driving a car or operating potentially dangerous equipment.
• Do not stop taking this drug suddenly. Abruptly stopping it can cause nausea, headache, stomach upset, or a worsening of your condition. Your doctor may want to reduce the dosage gradually.
• The elderly may be at increased risk for side effects. Use this drug cautiously, and report any mental status changes to your doctor immediately.
• The effects of this medication may persist for as long as five weeks after you stop taking it, so continue to observe all precautions during that period.

• Be sure to tell your doctor if you are pregnant. Although birth defects have not been documented in animal studies, it is not known if fluoxetine is safe during human pregnancy. It is also not known if fluoxetine passes into breast milk, so be sure to tell your doctor if you are breast-feeding an infant.

---

fluphenazine

BRAND NAMES (Manufacturers)
Permitil (Schering)
Prolixin (Princeton)
TYPE OF DRUG
Phenothiazine tranquilizer
INGREDIENT
fluphenazine
DOSAGE FORMS
Tablets (1 mg, 2.5 mg, 5 mg, and 10 mg)
Oral concentrate (5 mg per ml, with 1% alcohol)
Oral elixir (2.5 mg per 5-ml spoonful, with 14% alcohol)
STORAGE
The tablet form should be stored at room temperature in a tightly closed, light-resistant container. The oral concentrate and the elixir forms should be stored in the refrigerator in tightly closed, light-resistant containers. If the concentrate or elixir turns slightly yellow, the medicine is still effective and can be used. However, if it changes color markedly or has particles floating in it, it should not be used; discard it down the sink. This drug should never be frozen.

USES

Fluphenazine is prescribed to treat the symptoms of certain types of mental illness, such as emotional symptoms of psychosis, the manic phase of manic-depressive illness, and severe behavioral problems in children and adults. This medication is thought to relieve the symptoms of mental illness by blocking certain chemicals involved with nerve transmission in the brain.

TREATMENT

To avoid stomach irritation, you can take the tablet or elixir form of this medication with a meal or with a glass of water or milk (unless your doctor directs you to do otherwise).

Measure the oral elixir carefully with a specially designed 5-ml measuring spoon. An ordinary kitchen teaspoon is not accurate enough.

The oral concentrate form of this medication should be measured carefully with the dropper provided, then added to four ounces (1/2 cup) or more of water, milk, or a cola-free, caffeine-free carbonated beverage or to applesauce or pudding immediately prior to administration. To prevent possible loss of effectiveness, the medication should not be diluted in tea, coffee, or apple juice.

Antacids and antidiarrheal medicines may decrease the absorption of this medication from the gastrointestinal tract. Therefore, at least one hour should separate doses of one of these medicines and fluphenazine.

The full effects of this medication for the control of emotional or mental symptoms may not become apparent until two weeks after you start to take it.

If you miss a dose of this medication, take the missed dose as soon as possible and return to your regular dosing schedule. If it is almost time for the next dose, however, skip the one you missed and return to your regular schedule. Do not double the dose (unless your doctor directs you to do so).

SIDE EFFECTS

Minor. Blurred vision, constipation, decreased sweating, diarrhea, dizziness, drooling, drowsiness, dry mouth, fatigue, jitteriness, menstrual irregularities, nasal congestion, restlessness, vomiting, or weight gain. As your body adjusts to the medication, these side effects should disappear.

Fluphenazine can also cause discoloration of the urine to red, pink, or red-brown. This is a harmless effect.

This drug can cause increased sensitivity to sunlight. Therefore, avoid prolonged exposure to sunlight and sunlamps. Wear protective clothing, and use an effective sunscreen.

If you are constipated, increase the amount of fiber in your diet (fresh fruits and vegetables, salads, bran, and whole-grain breads) and drink more water (unless your doctor directs you to do otherwise).

Chew sugarless gum or suck on ice chips or a piece of hard candy to reduce mouth dryness.

To avoid dizziness or light-headedness when you stand, contract and relax the muscles of your legs for a few moments before rising. Do this by pushing one foot against the floor while raising the other foot slightly, alternating feet so that you are "pumping" your legs in a pedaling motion.

Major. Tell your doctor about any side effects that are persistent or particularly bothersome. IT IS ESPECIALLY IMPORTANT TO TELL YOUR DOCTOR about breast enlargement (in both sexes); chest pain; convulsions; darkened skin; difficulty in swallowing or breathing; fainting; fever; impotence; involuntary movements of the face, mouth, jaw, tongue, or limbs; palpitations; rash; sleep disorders; sore throat; tremors; uncoordinated movements; unusual bleeding or bruising; visual disturbances; or yellowing of the eyes or skin. Also, tell your doctor if your original symptoms worsen or change.

INTERACTIONS

Fluphenazine interacts with several other types of medications:

1. It can cause extreme drowsiness when combined with alcohol or other central nervous system depressants (such as barbiturates, benzodiazepine tranquilizers, muscle relaxants, narcotics, and pain medications) or with tricyclic antidepressants.

2. Fluphenazine can decrease the effectiveness of amphetamines, guanethidine, anticonvulsants, and levodopa.

3. The side effects of epinephrine, monoamine oxidase (MAO) inhibitors, propranolol, phenytoin, and tricyclic antidepressants may be increased by this medication. At least 14 days should separate the use of this drug and the use of an MAO inhibitor.

4. Lithium may increase the side effects, and decrease the effectiveness, of this medication.

Before starting to take fluphenazine, BE SURE TO TELL YOUR DOCTOR about any medications you are currently taking, especially any of those listed above.

WARNINGS

• Tell your doctor about unusual or allergic reactions you have had to medications, especially to fluphenazine or any other phenothiazine tranquilizers (such as chlorpromazine, mesoridazine, perphenazine, prochlorperazine, promazine, thioridazine, trifluoperazine, and triflupromazine) or to loxapine.

- Tell your doctor if you have a history of alcoholism or if you now have or have ever had any blood disease, bone marrow disease, brain disease, breast cancer, blockage of the urinary or digestive tract, drug-induced depression, epilepsy, high or low blood pressure, diabetes mellitus, glaucoma, heart or circulatory disease, liver disease, lung disease, Parkinson's disease, peptic ulcers, or an enlarged prostate gland.
- Tell your doctor about any recent exposure to a pesticide or an insecticide. Fluphenazine may increase the side effects from the exposure.
- To prevent oversedation, avoid drinking alcoholic beverages while taking this medication.
- If this drug makes you dizzy or drowsy, do not take part in any activity that requires alertness, such as driving a car or operating potentially dangerous equipment. Be careful on stairs, and avoid getting up suddenly from a lying or sitting position.
- Prior to having surgery or any other medical or dental treatment, be sure to tell your doctor or dentist that you are taking this medication.
- Some of the side effects caused by this drug can be prevented by taking an antiparkinsonism drug. Discuss this with your doctor.
- This medication can decrease sweating and heat release from the body. You should, therefore, avoid getting overheated by strenuous exercise in hot weather and should avoid hot baths, showers, and saunas.
- Do not stop taking this medication suddenly. If the drug is stopped abruptly, you may experience nausea, vomiting, stomach upset, headache, increased heart rate, insomnia, tremors, or a worsening of your condition. Your doctor may want to reduce the dosage gradually.
- If you are planning to have a myelogram, or any other procedure in which dye will be injected into your spinal cord, tell your doctor that you are taking this medication.
- Avoid spilling the oral concentrate or elixir form of this medication on your skin or clothing; it may cause redness and irritation of the skin.
- While taking this medication, do not take any over-the-counter (nonprescription) medication for weight control or for cough, cold, allergy, asthma, or sinus problems without first checking with your doctor. The combination of these medications may cause high blood pressure.
- Some of these products contain the color additive FD&C Yellow No. 5 (tartrazine), which can cause allergic-type reactions (shortness of breath, rash, fainting) in certain susceptible individuals.
- A potentially permament movement disorder called tardive dyskinesia may develop with the use of these medications. It is important to discuss this with your doctor and to report any unusual or uncontrolled movements.
- The elderly may be at greater risk for adverse effects when using this drug.
- Be sure to tell your doctor if you are pregnant. Small amounts of this medication cross the placenta. Although there are reports of safe use of this drug during pregnancy, there are also reports of liver disease and tremors in newborn infants whose mothers received this type of medication close to term. Also, tell your doctor if you are breast-feeding an infant. Small amounts of this medication pass into breast milk and may cause unwanted effects in the nursing infant.

---

flurandrenolide (topical)

BRAND NAMES (Manufacturers)
Cordran (Dista)
Cordran SP (Dista)
flurandrenolide (various manufacturers)

TYPE OF DRUG
Adrenocorticosteroid hormone

INGREDIENT
flurandrenolide

DOSAGE FORMS
Ointment (0.025% and 0.05%)
Cream (0.025% and 0.05%)
Lotion (0.05%)
Tape (4 mcg per square centimeter of tape)

STORAGE
Flurandrenolide ointment, cream, lotion, and tape should be stored at room temperature in tightly closed containers. This medication should never be frozen.

USES

Your adrenal glands naturally produce certain cortisone-like chemicals. These chemicals are involved in various regulatory processes in the body (such as those involving fluid balance, temperature, and reaction to inflammation). Flurandrenolide belongs to a group of drugs known as adrenocorticosteroids (or cortisone-like medications). It is used to relieve the skin inflammation (redness, swelling, itching, and discomfort) associated with conditions such as dermatitis, eczema, and poison ivy. How this drug acts to relieve these disorders is not completely understood.

TREATMENT

Before applying this medication, wash your hands. Then, unless your doctor gives you different instructions, gently wash the area of the skin where the medication is to be applied. With a clean towel, pat the area almost dry; it should be slightly damp when you put the medicine on.

If you are using the lotion form of this medication, shake the bottle well before pouring out the medicine. The contents tend to settle on the bottom of the bottle, so it is necessary to shake the container to distribute the ingredients evenly and equalize the doses. Apply a small amount of the medication to the affected area in a thin layer. Do not bandage the area unless your doctor tells you to do so. If you are to apply an occlusive dressing (like kitchen plastic wrap), be sure you understand the instructions.

When using the tape form of this medication, dry the skin thoroughly before applying the tape. Remove the tape from the package and cut a piece slightly larger than the area to be covered. Round off the corners. Pull the white paper from the transparent tape (be careful that the tape does not stick to itself). Press the tape into place, keeping the skin smooth. If ends of the tape loosen, they may be trimmed off and replaced with fresh tape. The tape should be cut, never torn.

If you miss a dose of this medication, apply the dose as soon as possible, unless it is almost time for the next application. In that case, do not apply the missed dose; just return to your regular schedule. Do not put twice as much of the medication on your skin at the next application.

SIDE EFFECTS

Minor. Acne, burning sensation, itching, rash, or skin dryness.

If the affected area is extremely dry or scaling, the skin may be moistened before applying the medication by soaking in water or by applying water with a clean cloth. The ointment form is probably better for dry skin.

A mild, temporary stinging sensation may occur after this medication is applied. If this persists, contact your doctor.

Major. Tell your doctor about any side effects that are persistent or particularly bothersome. IT IS ESPECIALLY IMPORTANT TO TELL YOUR DOCTOR about blistering, increased hair growth, irritation of the affected area, loss of skin color, secondary infection in the area being treated, or thinning of the skin with easy bruising.

INTERACTIONS

This medication does not interact with any other medications as long as it is used according to directions.

WARNINGS

- Tell your doctor about unusual or allergic reactions you have had to medications, especially to flurandrenolide or any other adrenocorticosteroid (such as amcinonide, betamethasone, clocortolone, cortisone, desonide, desoximetasone, dexamethasone, diflorasone, flumethasone, fluocinolone, fluocinonide, fluorometholone, halcinonide, hydrocortisone, methylprednisolone, paramethasone, prednisolone, prednisone, and triamcinolone).
- Tell your doctor if you now have or if you have ever had blood vessel disease, chicken pox, diabetes mellitus, fungal infection, peptic ulcers, shingles, tuberculosis, tuberculosis of the skin, vaccinia, or any other type of infection, especially at the site currently being treated.
- If irritation develops while using this drug, immediately discontinue its use and notify your doctor.
- This product is not for use in the eyes or mucous membranes; contact may result in side effects.
- Do not use this product with an occlusive wrap unless your doctor directs you to do so. Systemic absorption of this drug is increased if extensive areas of the body are treated, particularly if occlusive bandages are used. If it is necessary for you to use this drug under a wrap, follow your doctor's instructions exactly; do not leave the wrap in place longer than specified.
- If you are using this medication on a child's diaper area, do not put tight-fitting diapers or plastic pants on the child. This could lead to increased systemic absorption of the drug and a possible increase in side effects.
- Be sure to tell your doctor if you are pregnant. If large amounts of this drug are applied for prolonged periods, some of it will be absorbed and may cross the placenta. Although studies in humans have not been conducted, birth defects have been observed in the offspring of animals that were given large oral doses of this type of drug during pregnancy. Also, tell your doctor if you are breast-feeding an infant. If absorbed through the skin, small amounts of flurandrenolide pass into breast milk and may cause decreased growth or a decrease in natural adrenocorticosteroid hormone production in the nursing infant.

---

flurazepam

BRAND NAMES (Manufacturers)
Dalmane (Roche)
flurazepam (various manufacturers)

TYPE OF DRUG
Benzodiazepine sedative/hypnotic

INGREDIENT
flurazepam

DOSAGE FORM
Capsules (15 mg and 30 mg)

STORAGE
This medication should be stored at room temperature in a tightly closed, light-resistant container.

USES

Flurazepam is prescribed to treat insomnia (including problems in falling asleep, waking during the night, and early morning wakefulness). It is not clear exactly how this medicine works, but it may relieve insomnia by acting as a depressant of the central nervous system (brain and spinal cord).

TREATMENT

Flurazepam should be taken ten to 15 minutes before bedtime. It can be taken with food or a full glass of water if stomach upset occurs. Do not take this medication with antacids, since they may slow its absorption from the gastrointestinal tract.

Your sleeping problem may improve the first night you take this medication, but it may take two or three nights before the effectiveness of flurazepam is noticed.

SIDE EFFECTS

Minor. Bitter taste in the mouth, constipation, depression, diarrhea, dizziness, daytime drowsiness, dry mouth, excessive salivation, fatigue, flushing, headache, heartburn, loss of appetite, nausea, nervousness, sweating, or vomiting. As your body adjusts to the medicine, these side effects should disappear.

To relieve constipation, increase the amount of fiber in your diet (fresh fruits and vegetables, salads, bran, and whole-grain breads), exercise more, and drink more water (unless your doctor directs you to do otherwise).

Dry mouth can be relieved by chewing sugarless gum or by sucking on ice chips.

If you feel dizzy while taking this medication, sit or lie down for a while; get up slowly from a sitting or reclining position, and be careful on stairs.

Major. Tell your doctor about any side effects that are persistent or particularly bothersome. IT IS ESPECIALLY IMPORTANT TO TELL YOUR DOCTOR about blurred or double vision, chest pain, fainting, falling, fever, hallucinations, joint pain, nightmares, palpitations, rash, severe depression, shortness of breath, slurred speech, sore throat, uncoordinated movements, unusual excitement, unusual tiredness, or yellowing of the eyes or skin.

INTERACTIONS

Flurazepam interacts with several other types of drugs:

1. To prevent oversedation, this drug should not be taken with alcohol, other sedative drugs, or central nervous system depressants (such as antihistamines, barbiturates, muscle relaxants, pain medicines, narcotics, medicines for seizures, phenothiazine tranquilizers) or with antidepressants.
2. This medication may decrease the effectiveness of carbamazepine, levodopa, and oral anticoagulants (blood thinners) and may decrease the effects of phenytoin.
3. Disulfiram, oral contraceptives (birth control pills), isoniazid, and cimetidine can increase the blood levels of flurazepam, which can lead to increased side effects.
4. Concurrent use of rifampin may decrease the effectiveness of flurazepam.

BE SURE TO TELL YOUR DOCTOR about any medications you are currently taking, especially any listed above.

WARNINGS

- Tell your doctor about any unusual or allergic reactions you have had to any medications, especially to flurazepam or other benzodiazepine tranquilizers (such as alprazolam, chlordiazepoxide, clorazepate, diazepam, halazepam, lorazepam, oxazepam, prazepam, temazepam, and triazolam).
- Tell your doctor if you now have or if you have ever had liver disease, kidney disease, epilepsy, lung disease, myasthenia gravis, porphyria, mental depression, or mental illness.
- Flurazepam can cause drowsiness. Avoid tasks that require alertness, such as driving a car or using potentially dangerous equipment.
- This medication has the potential for abuse and must be used with caution. Tolerance may develop quickly; do not increase the dosage of the drug without first consulting your doctor. It is also important not to stop taking this drug suddenly if you have been taking it in large amounts or if you have used it for several weeks. Your doctor may want to reduce the dosage gradually.
- This is a safe drug when used properly. When it is combined with other sedative drugs or with alcohol, however, serious side effects may develop.
- The elderly may be at increased risk for side effects, especially daytime drowsiness or confusion. Report any changes in mental status to your doctor immediately.
- Be sure to tell your doctor if you are pregnant. This type of medicine may increase the chance of birth defects if it is taken during the first three months of pregnancy. In addition, too much use of this medicine during the last six months of pregnancy may result in addiction of the fetus—leading to withdrawal side effects at birth. Also, use of this medicine during the last weeks of pregnancy may cause excessive drowsiness, slowed heartbeat, and breathing difficulties in the newborn. Tell your doctor if you are breast-feeding an infant. This medicine can pass into breast milk and cause excessive drowsiness, slowed heartbeat, and breathing difficulties in nursing infants.

---

flurbiprofen

BRAND NAME (Manufacturer)
Ansaid (Upjohn)

TYPE OF DRUG
Nonsteroidal anti-inflammatory analgesic

INGREDIENT
flurbiprofen

DOSAGE FORM
Tablets (50 mg, 100 mg)

STORAGE
This medication should be stored in a tightly closed container at room temperature away from heat and direct light.

USES

Flurbiprofen is used to treat the inflammation (pain, swelling, and stiffness) of arthritis and osteoarthritis. Flurbiprofen has been shown to block the production of certain body chemicals, called prostaglandins, that may trigger pain. However, it is not yet fully understood how flurbiprofen works.

TREATMENT

You should take this medication on an empty stomach 30 to 60 minutes before meals or two hours after meals, so that it gets into your bloodstream quickly. However, to decrease stomach irritation, your doctor may want you to take this medication with food or antacids.

It may take up to two weeks before you feel the full effects of this medication. Flurbiprofen does not cure arthritis or osteoarthritis, but it will help to control the condition as long as you continue to take it.

It is important to take flurbiprofen on schedule and not to miss any doses. If you do miss a dose, take it as soon as possible, unless it is almost time for your next dose. In that case, do not take the missed dose at all; just return to your regular dosing schedule. Do not double the next dose.

SIDE EFFECTS

Minor. Indigestion, diarrhea, abdominal pain, nausea, constipation, headache, or dizziness. As your body adjusts to the drug, these side effects should disappear.

To relieve constipation, increase the amount of fiber in your diet (fresh fruits and vegetables, salads, bran, and whole-grain breads), exercise, and drink more water (unless your doctor directs you to do otherwise).

If you become dizzy, sit or lie down for a while; get up slowly from a sitting or reclining position, and be careful on stairs.

Major. Tell your doctor about any side effects that are persistent or particularly bothersome. IT IS ESPECIALLY IMPORTANT TO TELL YOUR DOCTOR about bloody or black, tarry stools; blurred vision; confusion; difficult or painful urination; palpitations; a problem with hearing, or ringing or buzzing in your ears; skin rash, hives, or itching; stomach pain; swelling of the feet or hands; chest tightness; unexplained sore throat and fever; unusual bleeding or bruising; unusual weight gain; wheezing or difficulty in breathing; or yellowing of the eyes or skin.

INTERACTIONS

Flurbiprofen interacts with several other types of medications:

1. Anticoagulants (blood thinners, such as warfarin) can lead to an increase in bleeding complications.
2. Aspirin, other salicylates, and other anti-inflammatory

medications can increase stomach irritation. Aspirin may also decrease the effectiveness of flurbiprofen; therefore, it should not be used concurrently with flurbiprofen.
3. Flurbiprofen may block the blood-pressure-lowering effects of beta-blocking drugs such as propranolol.
4. The activity of diuretics (water pills) may be inhibited by flurbiprofen.
5. Flurbiprofen may alter a diabetic patient's response to insulin or oral hypoglycemic agents.

Before starting to take flurbiprofen, BE SURE TO TELL YOUR DOCTOR about any medications you are currently taking, especially any of those listed above.

WARNINGS

- Before taking this medication, tell your doctor if you have ever had unusual or allergic reactions to flurbiprofen or to any of the other chemically related drugs (aspirin, other salicylates, diclofenac, diflunisal, fenoprofen, ibuprofen, indomethacin, ketoprofen, meclofenamate, mefenamic acid, naproxen, oxyphenbutazone, phenylbutazone, piroxicam, sulindac, or tolmetin).
- Tell your doctor if you now have or if you have ever had asthma, bleeding problems, epilepsy, heart disease, high blood pressure, kidney disease, liver disease, mental illness, or Parkinson's disease.
- If flurbiprofen makes you dizzy or drowsy, do not take part in any activity that requires alertness, such as driving a car or operating potentially dangerous machinery.
- Because this drug can prolong your bleeding time, it is important to tell your doctor or dentist that you are taking this drug before having surgery or any other medical or dental treatment.
- Stomach problems are more likely to occur if you take aspirin regularly or drink alcohol while being treated with this medication. These should, therefore, be avoided (unless your doctor directs you to do otherwise).
- The elderly may be at increased risk for side effects.
- Be sure to tell your doctor if you are pregnant or if you are planning to become pregnant. This medication can cause unwanted effects on the heart or blood flow of the fetus. Studies in animals have also shown that this medication, if taken late in pregnancy, may increase the length of pregnancy, prolong labor, or cause other problems during delivery. Also tell your doctor if you are breast-feeding an infant. Small amounts of flurbiprofen can pass into breast milk.

Flurosyn—see fluocinolone (topical)

Flutex—see triamcinolone (topical)

FoilleCort—see hydrocortisone (topical)

Fulvicin P/G—see griseofulvin

Fulvicin U/F—see griseofulvin

Fumide—see furosemide

Furadantin—see nitrofurantoin

Furalan—see nitrofurantoin

Furan—see nitrofurantoin

Furanite—see nitrofurantoin

---

furosemide

BRAND NAMES (Manufacturers)
Fumide (Everett)
furosemide (various manufacturers)
Lasix (Hoechst-Roussel)
Luramide (Major)
TYPE OF DRUG
Diuretic and antihypertensive
INGREDIENT
furosemide
DOSAGE FORMS
Tablets (20 mg, 40 mg, and 80 mg)
Oral solution (10 mg per ml, and 40 mg per ml, with 0.02% or 11.57% alcohol)
STORAGE
Furosemide tablets and oral solution should be stored at room temperature in a tightly closed, light-resistant container. This medication should never be frozen.

USES

Furosemide is prescribed to treat high blood pressure. It is also used to reduce fluid accumulation in the body caused by conditions such as heart failure, cirrhosis of the liver, kidney disease, and the long-term use of some medications. Furosemide reduces fluid accumulation by increasing the elimination of salt and water through the kidneys.

TREATMENT

To decrease stomach irritation, you can take furosemide with a glass of milk or with a meal (unless your doctor directs you to do otherwise). Try to take it at the same time every day. Avoid taking a dose after 6:00 P.M.; otherwise, you may have to get up during the night to urinate.

Each dose of the oral solution should be carefully measured with a specially designed measuring spoon. An ordinary kitchen teaspoon is not accurate enough.

This medication does not cure high blood pressure, but it will help to control the condition as long as you continue to take it.

If you miss a dose of this medication, take the missed dose as soon as possible, unless it is almost time for the next dose. In that case, do not take the missed dose at all; just wait until the next scheduled dose. Do not double the dose.

SIDE EFFECTS

Minor. Blurred vision, constipation, cramping, diarrhea, dizziness, headache, sore mouth, or stomach upset. As your body adjusts to the medication, these side effects should disappear.

This medication will cause an increase in the amount of urine or in your frequency of urination when you first begin to take it. It may also cause you to have an unusual feeling of tiredness. These effects should subside after several days.

Furosemide can cause increased sensitivity to sunlight. Avoid prolonged exposure to sunlight and sunlamps. Wear protective clothing, and use an effective sunscreen.

To relieve constipation, increase the amount of fiber in your diet (fresh fruits and vegetables, salads, bran, and

whole-grain breads) and exercise more (unless your doctor directs you to do otherwise).

To avoid dizziness and light-headedness when you stand, contract and relax the muscles of your legs for a few moments before rising. Do this by pushing one foot against the floor while raising the other foot slightly, alternating feet so that you are "pumping" your legs in a pedaling motion.

Major. Tell your doctor about any side effects that are persistent or particularly bothersome. IT IS ESPECIALLY IMPORTANT TO TELL YOUR DOCTOR about confusion, difficulty in breathing, dry mouth, fainting, increased thirst, itching, joint pains, loss of appetite, mood changes, muscle cramps, nausea, palpitations, rash, ringing in the ears, severe abdominal pain, sore throat, tingling in the fingers or toes, unusual bleeding or bruising, vomiting, weakness, or yellowing of the eyes or skin.

INTERACTIONS

Furosemide interacts with several other types of drugs:

1. It can increase the side effects of alcohol, chloral hydrate, digoxin, digitalis, lithium, aspirin, and theophylline.

2. The effectiveness of antigout medications, insulin, and oral antidiabetic medications may be decreased by furosemide.

3. Phenytoin can decrease the absorption and effectiveness of furosemide.

4. Indomethacin can decrease the diuretic effects of furosemide.

Before taking furosemide, BE SURE TO TELL YOUR DOCTOR about any medications you are currently taking, especially any of those listed above.

WARNINGS

- Tell your doctor about unusual or allergic reactions you have had to any medications, especially to diuretics or to any other sulfa drugs including oral antidiabetic medicines or sulfonamide antibiotics.
- Tell your doctor if you have ever had kidney disease or problems with urination, diabetes mellitus, gout, liver disease, asthma, pancreatic disease, or systemic lupus erythematosus.
- Furosemide can cause potassium loss. Signs of potassium loss include dry mouth, thirst, weakness, muscle pain or cramps, nausea, and vomiting. If you experience any of these symptoms, call your doctor. Your doctor may want to have blood tests performed periodically in order to monitor your blood potassium levels. To help avoid potassium loss, take this medication with a glass of fresh or frozen orange juice or cranberry juice, or eat a banana every day. The use of a salt substitute also helps to prevent potassium loss. Do not change your diet, however, before discussing it with your doctor. Too much potassium may also be dangerous.
- Before having surgery or any other medical or dental treatment, be sure to tell your doctor or dentist that you are taking furosemide.
- To avoid dizziness, light-headedness, or fainting, get up from a sitting or lying position slowly, and avoid standing for long periods of time. You should also avoid strenuous exercise and prolonged exposure to hot weather.
- Furosemide oral solution contains the color additive FD&C Yellow No. 5 (tartrazine), which may cause allergic symptoms (shortness of breath, rash, fainting) in certain susceptible individuals.
- While taking this drug, limit your intake of alcohol in order to prevent dizziness and light-headedness.
- If you have high blood pressure, do not take any over-the-counter (nonprescription) medication for weight control or for cough, cold, asthma, allergy, or sinus problems unless you first check with your doctor.
- To prevent severe water loss (dehydration) while taking this medication, check with your doctor if you have any illness that causes severe nausea, vomiting, or diarrhea.
- This medication can raise blood sugar levels in diabetic patients. Blood sugar should be monitored carefully with blood or urine tests when this medication is started.
- Be sure to tell your doctor if you are pregnant. This drug crosses the placenta. Although studies in humans have not been conducted, adverse effects have been observed in the fetuses of animals that received large doses of this drug during pregnancy. Also, tell your doctor if you are breast-feeding an infant. Small amounts of furosemide pass into breast milk.

Gamazole—see sulfonamide antibiotics (oral)

Gantanol—see sulfonamide antibiotics (oral)

Gantanol DS—see sulfonamide antibiotics (oral)

Gantrisin—see sulfonamide antibiotics (oral)

---

gemfibrozil

BRAND NAME (Manufacturer)
Lopid (Parke-Davis)
TYPE OF DRUG
Antihyperlipidemic (lipid-lowering drug)
INGREDIENT
gemfibrozil
DOSAGE FORMS
Tablets (600 mg)
Capsules (300 mg)
STORAGE
Store at room temperature in a tightly closed container.

USES

Gemfibrozil is used to treat hyperlipidemia (high blood fat levels). It may be prescribed in conjunction with other lipid-lowering measures such as diet, weight reduction, exercise, and control of blood sugar level. It is not clear how gemfibrozil lowers blood lipid levels, but it is thought to decrease the body's production of certain fats.

TREATMENT

In order to maximize its effectiveness, gemfibrozil should be taken 30 minutes before meals.

If you miss a dose of this medication, take the missed dose as soon as possible, unless it is almost time for the next dose. In that case, do not take the missed dose; just return to your regular dosing schedule. Do not double the next dose.

SIDE EFFECTS

Minor. Constipation, diarrhea, dizziness, dry mouth, gas, headache, insomnia, loss of appetite, nausea, or stomach upset. These side effects should disappear as your body adjusts to the medication.

To relieve constipation, increase the amount of fiber in your diet (fresh fruits and vegetables, salads, bran, and whole-grain breads), exercise, and drink more water (unless your doctor directs you to do otherwise).

If you feel dizzy, sit or lie down for a while; get up slowly from a sitting or reclining position, and be careful on stairs.

To help relieve mouth dryness, chew sugarless gum or suck on ice chips.

Major. Tell your doctor about any side effects that are persistent or particularly bothersome. IT IS ESPECIALLY IMPORTANT TO TELL YOUR DOCTOR about back pain, blurred vision, fatigue, muscle cramps, rash, ringing in the ears, swollen or painful joints, tingling sensations, or yellowing of the eyes or skin.

INTERACTIONS

Gemfibrozil can increase the effects of oral anticoagulants (blood thinners, such as warfarin), which can lead to bleeding complications.

BE SURE TO TELL YOUR DOCTOR about any drugs you are taking, especially oral anticoagulants.

WARNINGS

- Tell your doctor about unusual or allergic reactions you have had to any medications, especially to gemfibrozil.
- Before starting this drug, tell your doctor if you now have or if you have ever had biliary disorders, gallstones or gallbladder disease, kidney disease, or liver disease.
- If this drug makes you dizzy or blurs your vision, avoid activities that require alertness, such as driving a car.
- Do not stop taking this medication unless you first check with your doctor. Stopping the drug abruptly may lead to a rapid increase in blood lipid (fat) and cholesterol levels. Your doctor may, therefore, want to start you on a special diet or another medication when gemfibrozil is discontinued.
- Gemfibrozil may affect blood glucose levels. Glucose levels should be closely monitored.
- Be sure to tell your doctor if you are pregnant. Although gemfibrozil appears to be safe during pregnancy, extensive studies in humans have not been conducted. Also, tell your doctor if you are breast-feeding an infant. It is not known whether gemfibrozil passes into breast milk.

Genagesic—see acetaminophen and propoxyphene combination

Genamin—see phenylpropanolamine and chlorpheniramine combination

Gencold—see phenylpropanolamine and chlorpheniramine combination

Genpril—see ibuprofen

Geocillin—see carbenicillin

Geridium—see phenazopyridine

Gerimal—see ergoloid mesylates

Glaucon—see epinephrine (ophthalmic)

glipizide

BRAND NAME (Manufacturer)
Glucotrol (Roerig)
TYPE OF DRUG
Oral antidiabetic
INGREDIENT
glipizide
DOSAGE FORM
Tablets (5 mg and 10 mg)
STORAGE
This medication should be stored at room temperature in a tightly closed container.

USES

Glipizide is usually used for the treatment of the type of diabetes mellitus (sugar diabetes) that appears in adulthood and cannot be managed by control of diet alone. This type of diabetes is known as non-insulin-dependent diabetes (sometimes called maturity-onset or Type II diabetes). Glipizide lowers blood sugar levels by increasing the release of insulin from the pancreas. It may also increase the effectiveness of insulin.

TREATMENT

Take this drug on an empty stomach 30 minutes before a meal (unless your doctor directs you to do otherwise).

It is important to try not to miss any doses of this medication. If you do miss a dose, take it as soon as possible, unless it is almost time for the next dose. In that case, do not take the missed dose at all; just return to your regular dosing schedule. Do not double the next dose. Tell your doctor if you feel any side effects from missing a dose of this drug.

Diabetics who are taking oral antidiabetic medication may need to be switched to insulin if they develop diabetic coma, have a severe infection, are scheduled for major surgery, or become pregnant. Sometimes your doctor may prescribe insulin while you are taking an oral antidiabetic agent.

SIDE EFFECTS

Minor. Diarrhea, headache, heartburn, loss of appetite, nausea, stomach pain, stomach discomfort, or vomiting. These side effects usually disappear during treatment as your body adjusts to the medicine.

Glipizide may increase your sensitivity to sunlight. It is, therefore, important to use caution during exposure to the sun. Use an effective sunscreen and avoid exposure to sunlamps.

Major. If any side effects are persistent or particularly bothersome, it is important to notify your doctor. IT IS ESPECIALLY IMPORTANT TO TELL YOUR DOCTOR about continuous thirst, dark urine, fatigue, frequent urination, itching of the skin, light-colored stools, rash, sore throat and fever, unusual bleeding or bruising, or yellowing of the eyes or skin.

INTERACTIONS

Glipizide interacts with several other types of medications:

1. The combination of glipizide and chloramphenicol, cimetidine, ranitidine, fenfluramine, guanethidine, insulin, monoamine oxidase (MAO) inhibitors, oxyphenbutazone, oxytetracycline, phenylbutazone, probenecid, aspirin or other aspirin-like drugs such as ibuprofen or other nonsteroidal anti-inflammatory analgesics, or sulfonamide antibiotics can lower blood sugar levels—sometimes to dangerously low levels.

2. The combination of glipizide and thyroid hormones, dextrothyroxine, epinephrine, phenytoin, thiazide diuretics (water pills), or cortisone-like medications (such as dexamethasone, hydrocortisone, and prednisone) can actually increase blood sugar levels—just what you are trying to avoid.

3. Rifampin can decrease the blood concentration of glipizide, which can lead to a decrease in its effectiveness.

4. Antidiabetic medications can increase the effects of the blood thinner warfarin, which can lead to bleeding complications.

5. The combination of glipizide and beta-blocking medications (acebutolol, atenolol, betaxolol, carteolol, esmolol, labetalol, metoprolol, nadolol, penbutolol, pindolol, propranolol, or timolol) can result in either high or low blood sugar levels. Beta blockers can also mask the symptoms of low blood sugar, which can be dangerous.

BE SURE TO TELL YOUR DOCTOR about any medications you are currently taking, especially any listed above.

WARNINGS

- It is important to tell your doctor if you have ever had any unusual or allergic reaction to this medicine or to any other sulfa medication, including sulfonamide antibiotics, diuretics (water pills), or other oral antidiabetics.
- It is also important to tell your doctor if you now have or if you have ever had kidney disease, liver disease, severe infection, or thyroid disease.
- Avoid drinking alcoholic beverages while taking this medication (unless otherwise directed by your doctor). Some patients who take this medicine suffer nausea, vomiting, dizziness, stomach pain, pounding headache, sweating, or redness of the face and skin when they drink alcohol. Also, large amounts of alcohol can lower blood sugar to dangerously low levels.
- Follow the special diet that your doctor gave you. This is an important part of controlling your blood sugar and is necessary in order for this medicine to work properly.
- Before having surgery or any other medical or dental treatment, be sure to tell your doctor or dentist that you are taking this medicine.
- Test for sugar in your urine or blood as directed by your doctor. It is a convenient way to determine whether your diabetes is being controlled by this medicine. Urine tests only indicate possible elevated blood sugar. They do not indicate low blood sugar.
- Eat or drink something containing sugar right away if you experience any symptoms of low blood sugar (such as anxiety, chills, cold sweats, cool or pale skin, drowsiness, excessive hunger, headache, nausea, nervousness, rapid heartbeat, shakiness, or unusual tiredness or weakness). It is also important that your family and friends know the symptoms of low blood sugar and what to do if they observe any of these symptoms in you.

Even if the symptoms of low blood sugar are corrected by eating or drinking sugar-containing products, it is important to contact your doctor as soon as possible after experiencing them. The blood-sugar-lowering effects of this medicine can last for hours, and the symptoms may return during this period. Good sources of sugar are orange juice, corn syrup, honey, sugar cubes, and table sugar. You are at greatest risk of developing low blood sugar if you skip or delay meals, exercise more than usual, cannot eat because of nausea or vomiting, or drink large amounts of alcohol.

- The elderly may have a heightened response to this drug. It is important to monitor your symptoms and blood sugar level carefully.
- Be sure to tell your doctor if you are pregnant. Glipizide appears to be safe in animals; however, studies have not been conducted in humans. Also, tell your doctor if you are breast-feeding an infant. Small amounts of glipizide pass into breast milk.

Glucotrol—see glipizide

---

glutethimide

BRAND NAME (Manufacturer)
glutethimide (various manufacturers)
TYPE OF DRUG
Sedative/hypnotic
INGREDIENT
glutethimide
DOSAGE FORMS
Tablets (250 mg and 500 mg)
Capsules (500 mg)
STORAGE
Store at room temperature in a tightly closed container.

USES

This medication is used for short-term treatment of insomnia. It is not clearly understood how glutethimide works to produce sleep, but it is a central nervous system depressant (a drug that slows the activity of the brain and spinal cord). This drug loses its effectiveness in producing and maintaining sleep after three to seven days of continuous treatment.

TREATMENT

You can take glutethimide tablets or capsules either on an empty stomach or, to avoid stomach irritation, with food or milk (unless your doctor directs you to do otherwise). The dose should be taken 15 to 30 minutes before bedtime.

SIDE EFFECTS

Minor. Drowsiness during the daytime, dizziness, a "hangover" feeling, headache, nausea, or vomiting. These side effects should disappear as your body adjusts to the medication.

If you feel dizzy, sit or lie down for a while; change positions slowly, and be careful on stairs.

Major. Tell your doctor about any side effects that are persistent or particularly bothersome. IT IS ESPECIALLY IMPORTANT TO TELL YOUR DOCTOR about blurred vision, clumsiness, confusion, convulsions, difficulty in breathing, fever, hallucinations, muscle cramps, nightmares, skin rash, slurred speech, sore throat, trembling, unusual bleeding or bruising, or unusual weakness.

INTERACTIONS

Glutethimide interacts with other types of medications:

1. Concurrent use of it with other central nervous system depressants (such as alcohol, antihistamines, barbiturates, benzodiazepine tranquilizers, muscle relaxants, narcotics, pain medications, phenothiazine tranquilizers, and other sleeping medications) or with tricyclic antidepressants can lead to extreme drowsiness and can be dangerous.

2. Glutethimide can decrease the blood levels and effectiveness of oral anticoagulants (blood thinners, such as warfarin).

BE SURE TO TELL YOUR DOCTOR about any medications you are currently taking, especially any listed above.

WARNINGS

- Tell your doctor about unusual or allergic reactions you have had to any medications, especially to glutethimide.
- Before starting to take this medication, be sure to tell your doctor if you now have or if you have ever had glaucoma, heart arrhythmias, kidney disease, severe pain, peptic ulcers, enlarged prostate gland, porphyria, or blockage of the intestines or urinary tract.
- If this medication makes you drowsy or dizzy or blurs your vision, do not take part in any activity that requires alertness, such as driving a car or operating potentially dangerous machinery.
- This medication has the potential for abuse. Therefore, it should not be used in higher doses or for longer periods than recommended by your doctor. If you have been taking glutethimide for longer than several weeks, check with your doctor before discontinuing it. Stopping abruptly can lead to a withdrawal reaction. Your doctor may want to reduce the dosage gradually to prevent this reaction.
- The elderly may be more sensitive to the effects of glutethimide and may therefore be at increased risk of experiencing side effects.
- Be sure to tell your doctor if you are pregnant. Extensive studies in pregnant women using glutethimide have not been conducted. However, it is known that large amounts of the drug taken during the last three months of pregnancy can cause the baby to become dependent on the medication, leading to withdrawal side effects at birth. Also, tell your doctor if you are breast-feeding an infant. Small amounts of glutethimide pass into breast milk and can cause extreme drowsiness in the nursing infant.

---

glyburide

BRAND NAMES (Manufacturers)
DiaBeta (Hoechst-Roussel)
Micronase (Upjohn)

TYPE OF DRUG
Oral antidiabetic

INGREDIENT
glyburide

DOSAGE FORM
Tablets (1.25 mg, 2.5 mg, and 5 mg)

STORAGE
This medication should be stored at room temperature in a tightly closed container.

USES

Glyburide is usually used for the treatment of the type of diabetes mellitus (sugar diabetes) that appears in adulthood and cannot be managed by control of diet alone. This type of diabetes is known as non-insulin-dependent diabetes (sometimes called maturity-onset or Type II diabetes). Glyburide lowers blood sugar levels by increasing the release of insulin from the pancreas. It may also increase the effectiveness of insulin.

TREATMENT

In order for glyburide to work correctly, it must be taken as directed by your doctor. To maintain a constant blood sugar level, it is best to take this medication at the same time(s) each day. It is, therefore, important to try not to miss any doses of this medication. If you do miss a dose, take it as soon as possible, unless it is almost time for the next dose. In that case, do not take the missed dose at all; just return to your regular dosing schedule. Do not double the next dose. Tell your doctor if you feel any side effects from missing a dose of this drug.

Diabetics who are taking oral antidiabetic medication may need to be switched to insulin if they develop diabetic coma, have a severe infection, are scheduled for major surgery, or become pregnant. Sometimes your doctor may prescribe insulin while you are taking an oral antidiabetic agent.

SIDE EFFECTS

Minor. Diarrhea, headache, heartburn, loss of appetite, nausea, vomiting, stomach pain, or stomach discomfort. These side effects usually disappear during treatment, as your body adjusts to the medicine.

Glyburide may increase your sensitivity to sunlight. It is, therefore, important to use caution during exposure to the sun. You may want to wear protective clothing and sunglasses. Use an effective sunscreen, and avoid exposure to sun lamps.

Major. If any side effects are persistent or particularly bothersome, it is important to notify your doctor. IT IS ESPECIALLY IMPORTANT TO TELL YOUR DOCTOR about continuous thirst, dark urine, fatigue, frequent urination, itching of the skin, light-colored stools, rash, sore throat and fever, unusual bleeding or bruising, or yellowing of the eyes or skin.

INTERACTIONS

Glyburide interacts with several other types of medications:

1. The combination of glyburide and chloramphenicol, cimetidine, ranitidine, fenfluramine, guanethidine, insulin, monoamine oxidase (MAO) inhibitors, oxyphenbutazone, oxytetracycline, phenylbutazone, probenecid, aspirin or other aspirin-like drugs such as ibuprofen or other nonsteroidal anti-inflammatory analgesics, or sulfonamide antibiotics can lower blood sugar levels—sometimes to dangerously low levels.

2. The combination of glyburide and thyroid hormones, dextrothyroxine, epinephrine, phenytoin, thiazide diuretics (water pills), or cortisone-like medications (such as dexamethasone, hydrocortisone, and prednisone) can actually increase blood sugar levels—just what you are trying to avoid.

3. Rifampin can decrease the blood concentration of glyburide, which can lead to a decrease in its effectiveness.
4. Antidiabetic medications can increase the effects of the blood thinner warfarin, which can lead to bleeding complications.
5. The combination of glyburide and beta-blocking medications (acebutolol, atenolol, betaxolol, carteolol, esmolol, labetalol, metoprolol, nadolol, penbutolol, pindolol, propranolol, timolol) can result in either high or low blood sugar levels. Beta blockers can also mask the symptoms of low blood sugar, which can be dangerous.

BE SURE TO TELL YOUR DOCTOR about any medications you are currently taking, especially any of those listed above.

WARNINGS

- It is important to tell your doctor if you have ever had unusual or allergic reactions to medications, especially to glyburide or to any other sulfa medication, including sulfonamide antibiotics, diuretics (water pills), or other oral antidiabetics.
- Tell your doctor if you now have or if you have ever had kidney disease, liver disease, severe infection, or thyroid disease.
- Follow the special diet that your doctor gave you. This is an important part of controlling your blood sugar and is necessary in order for this medicine to work properly.
- Avoid drinking alcoholic beverages while taking this medication (unless otherwise directed by your doctor). Some patients who take this medicine suffer nausea, vomiting, dizziness, stomach pain, pounding headache, sweating, and redness of the face and skin when they drink alcohol. Also, large amounts of alcohol can lower blood sugar to dangerously low levels.
- Before having surgery or any other medical or dental treatment, be sure to tell your doctor or dentist that you are taking this medication.
- Test for sugar in your urine or blood as directed by your doctor. It is a convenient way to determine whether your diabetes is being controlled by this medicine. Urine tests may only indicate elevated blood sugar. They do not indicate low blood sugar.
- Eat or drink something containing sugar right away if you experience any symptoms of low blood sugar (such as anxiety, chills, cold sweats, cool or pale skin, drowsiness, excessive hunger, headache, nausea, nervousness, rapid heartbeat, shakiness, or unusual tiredness or weakness). It is also important that your family and friends know the symptoms of low blood sugar and what to do if they observe any of these symptoms in you.

Even if the symptoms of low blood sugar are corrected by eating or drinking sugar-containing products, it is important to contact your doctor as soon as possible after experiencing them. The blood-sugar-lowering effects of this medicine can last for hours, and the symptoms may return during this period. Good sources of sugar are orange juice, corn syrup, honey, sugar cubes, and table sugar. You are at greatest risk of developing low blood sugar if you skip or delay meals, exercise more than usual, cannot eat because of nausea or vomiting, or drink large amounts of alcohol.

- DiaBeta brand glyburide contains the color additive FD&C Yellow No. 5 (tartrazine), which may cause allergic-type reactions (shortness of breath, rash, fainting) in certain susceptible individuals.
- The elderly may have a heightened response to this drug. It is important to monitor your symptoms and blood sugar level carefully.
- Be sure to tell your doctor if you are pregnant. Glyburide appears to be safe in animals; however, studies have not been conducted in humans. It is also important to tell your doctor if you are breast-feeding an infant. Small amounts of glyburide may pass into breast milk.

Glyceryl-T—see theophylline and guaifenesin combination

Grifulvin V—see griseofulvin

Grisactin—see griseofulvin

Grisactin Ultra—see griseofulvin

---

griseofulvin

BRAND NAMES (Manufacturers)
Fulvicin P/G (Schering)
Fulvicin U/F (Schering)
Grifulvin V (Ortho)
Grisactin (Ayerst)
Grisactin Ultra (Ayerst)
griseofulvin (various manufacturers)
Gris-PEG (Herbert)

TYPE OF DRUG
Antifungal

INGREDIENT
griseofulvin

DOSAGE FORMS
Tablets (125 mg, 165 mg, 250 mg, 330 mg, and 500 mg)
Capsules (125 mg and 250 mg)
Oral suspension (125 mg per 5-ml spoonful)

STORAGE
Griseofulvin tablets, capsules, and oral suspension should be stored at room temperature in tightly closed containers. This medication should never be frozen.

USES

This medication is used to treat certain fungal infections of the skin and nails. Griseofulvin prevents the multiplication of susceptible fungi. It also enters the cells of skin, hair, and nails and protects them from fungal invasion.

TREATMENT

In order to avoid stomach irritation, you can take griseofulvin with food or milk.

The oral suspension form of this medication should be shaken well just before measuring each dose. The contents tend to settle on the bottom of the bottle, so it is necessary to shake the container to distribute the ingredients evenly and equalize the doses. Each dose should then be measured carefully with a specially designed 5-ml measuring spoon. An ordinary kitchen teaspoon is not accurate enough for measuring your dose of this medication.

If you miss a dose of this medication, take the missed dose as soon as possible, unless it is almost time for the next dose. In that case, do not take the missed dose at all; just return to your regular dosing schedule. Do not double the next dose.

It is important to continue to take this medication for the entire time prescribed by your doctor (perhaps six months or more), even if the symptoms disappear before the end of that period. If you stop taking this drug too soon, resistant fungi are given a chance to continue growing, and your infection could recur.

SIDE EFFECTS

Minor. Diarrhea, dizziness, fatigue, headache, insomnia, nausea, stomach upset, or vomiting. These side effects should disappear as your body adjusts to the medication.

This medication can increase your sensitivity to sunlight. You should, therefore, avoid prolonged exposure to sunlight and sunlamps. Wear protective clothing and sunglasses, and use an effective sunscreen.

If you feel dizzy, sit or lie down for a while; get up slowly from a sitting or reclining position, and be careful on stairs.

Major. Tell your doctor about any side effects that are persistent or particularly bothersome. IT IS ESPECIALLY IMPORTANT TO TELL YOUR DOCTOR about confusion; itching; skin rash; sore throat; swelling of lips, tongue, or eyelids; tingling of the hands or feet; or whitish tongue.

INTERACTIONS

Griseofulvin interacts with several other types of medications:

1. It can increase the effects of alcohol, resulting in flushing and an increased heart rate.

2. Barbiturates such as phenobarbital can decrease the effectiveness of griseofulvin.

3. Griseofulvin can decrease the effectiveness of oral contraceptives (birth control pills) and oral anticoagulants (blood thinners, such as warfarin).

Before starting to take griseofulvin, BE SURE TO TELL YOUR DOCTOR about any medications you are currently taking, especially any of those listed above.

WARNINGS

- Tell your doctor about unusual or allergic reactions you have had to any medications, especially to griseofulvin, penicillins, cephalosporin antibiotics, or penicillamine.
- Before starting to take griseofulvin, be sure to tell your doctor if you now have or if you have ever had liver disease, porphyria, or systemic lupus erythematosus.
- If this drug makes you dizzy, do not take part in any activity that requires alertness, such as driving a car or operating potentially dangerous machinery.
- Observe good hygiene to control the source of infection and to prevent reinfection.
- Concurrent use of an appropriate topical antifungal medication may be necessary to help clear the infection.
- Be sure to tell your doctor if you are pregnant. Extensive studies in pregnant women have not been conducted, but birth defects have been reported in the offspring of animals that received large doses of griseofulvin during pregnancy. Also, tell your doctor if you are breast-feeding an infant. It is not known whether griseofulvin passes into breast milk.

Gris-PEG—see griseofulvin

guanabenz

BRAND NAME (Manufacturer)
Wytensin (Wyeth)

TYPE OF DRUG
Antihypertensive

INGREDIENT
guanabenz

DOSAGE FORM
Tablets (4 mg and 8 mg)

STORAGE
Guanabenz should be stored at room temperature in a tightly closed, light-resistant container.

USES

This medication is used to control high blood pressure. It works by decreasing the release of chemicals in the brain that are responsible for increasing blood pressure.

TREATMENT

Guanabenz can be taken either on an empty stomach or, to avoid stomach irritation, with food or milk (as directed by your doctor).

Try to take the doses at the same times each day, so that you become accustomed to taking this medication. Your doctor may want you to take the last dose of the day at bedtime, in order to control blood pressure at night and to reduce daytime drowsiness.

If you miss a dose of this medication, take the missed dose as soon as possible, unless it is almost time for your next dose. In that case, do not take the missed dose at all; just return to your regular dosing schedule. Do not double the next dose. If you miss more than two consecutive doses, contact your doctor as soon as possible.

Guanabenz does not cure high blood pressure but will help control the condition as long as you continue to take it.

SIDE EFFECTS

Minor. Constipation, diarrhea, dizziness, drowsiness, dry mouth, headache, nasal congestion, nausea, sleep disturbances, stomach upset, taste disorders, vomiting, or weakness. These should disappear as you adjust to the drug.

To relieve constipation, increase the amount of fiber in your diet (fresh fruits and vegetables, salads, bran, and whole-grain breads), exercise, and drink more water (unless your doctor directs you to do otherwise).

If you feel dizzy or light-headed, sit or lie down for a while; get up slowly, and be careful on stairs.

To help relieve mouth dryness, chew sugarless gum or suck on ice chips or a piece of hard candy.

Major. Tell your doctor about any side effects that are persistent or particularly bothersome. IT IS ESPECIALLY IMPORTANT TO TELL YOUR DOCTOR about anxiety, blurred vision, chest pain, depression, disturbances in sexual function, drowsiness or sedation, enlarged or painful breasts (in both sexes), increased urination, itching, loss of coordination, muscle aches, palpitations, rapid weight gain (three to five pounds within a week), shortness of breath, or skin rash.

INTERACTIONS

Concurrent use of guanabenz with central nervous system depressants (such as alcohol, antihistamines, barbiturates, benzodiazepine tranquilizers, muscle relaxants, narcotics, pain medications, phenothiazine tranquilizers, and sleeping medications) or with tricyclic antidepressants can lead to extreme drowsiness.

BE SURE TO TELL YOUR DOCTOR about any medications you are currently taking, especially any of those listed above.

WARNINGS

- Tell your doctor about unusual or allergic reactions you have had to any medications, especially to guanabenz.
- Before starting to take this medication, be sure to tell your doctor if you now have or if you have ever had heart or blood vessel disease, kidney disease, or liver disease.
- If this medication makes you dizzy or drowsy or blurs your vision, avoid taking part in activities that require alertness, such as driving a car or operating potentially dangerous machinery.
- Before having surgery or any other medical or dental treatment, be sure to tell your doctor or dentist that you are taking this medication.
- Do not stop taking guanabenz unless you first check with your doctor. If this drug is stopped abruptly, you may experience nervousness, agitation, headache, and a rise in blood pressure. Your doctor may, therefore, want to decrease your dosage gradually or start you on another drug when this medication is stopped.
- Check with your doctor or pharmacist before taking any over-the-counter (nonprescription) asthma, allergy, cough, cold, diet, or sinus preparations. Some of these products can reduce the effectiveness of guanabenz.
- Be sure to tell your doctor if you are pregnant. Although guanabenz appears to be safe during pregnancy, extensive studies in humans have not been conducted. Studies on birth defects in animals have produced conflicting results. Also, tell your doctor if you are breast-feeding an infant. It is not known whether guanabenz passes into breast milk.

---

guanadrel

BRAND NAME (Manufacturer)
Hylorel (Pennwalt)

TYPE OF DRUG
Antihypertensive

INGREDIENT
guanadrel

DOSAGE FORM
Tablets (10 mg and 25 mg)

STORAGE
Guanadrel tablets should be stored at room temperature in a tightly closed container.

USES

Guanadrel is used to control high blood pressure. It works by blocking the action of the body chemicals responsible for increasing blood pressure.

TREATMENT

Guanadrel can be taken either on an empty stomach or, to avoid stomach irritation, with food or milk (as directed by your doctor). Try to take your doses at the same times each day in order to become accustomed to taking this medication.

If you miss a dose of this medication, take the missed dose as soon as possible, unless it is almost time for your next dose. In that case, do not take the missed dose at all; just return to your regular dosing schedule. Do not double the next dose.

This medication does not cure high blood pressure, but it will help to control the condition as long as you continue to take it.

SIDE EFFECTS

Minor. Constipation, diarrhea, dizziness, drowsiness, dry throat or mouth, fatigue, gas, headache, loss of appetite, nausea, sleep disorders, stomach upset, or weight gain or loss. These side effects should disappear as your body adjusts to the medication.

To relieve constipation, increase the amount of fiber in your diet (fresh fruits and vegetables, salads, bran, and whole-grain breads), exercise, and drink more water (unless your doctor directs you to do otherwise).

If you feel dizzy, sit or lie down for a while; change positions slowly, and be careful on stairs.

To help relieve mouth dryness, chew sugarless gum or suck on ice chips or a piece of hard candy.

Major. Tell your doctor about any side effects that are persistent or particularly bothersome. IT IS ESPECIALLY IMPORTANT TO TELL YOUR DOCTOR about backache, blurred vision, chest pain, confusion, coughing, depression, fainting, impotence, increased urination, joint pain, leg cramps, mental disorders, mouth sores, palpitations, rapid weight gain (three to five pounds within a week), shortness of breath, or tingling sensations.

INTERACTIONS

Guanadrel interacts with several other types of medications:

1. Concurrent use of guanadrel and alcohol can lead to fainting or extreme drowsiness.

2. Amphetamines, diet preparations, ephedrine, methylphenidate, phenothiazine tranquilizers, phenylpropanolamine, and tricyclic antidepressants can decrease the beneficial effects of guanadrel.

3. Concurrent use of guanadrel with monoamine oxidase (MAO) inhibitors can lead to serious side effects. At least 14 days should separate doses of these two types of medications.

BE SURE TO TELL YOUR DOCTOR about any of the medications you are currently taking, especially any of those listed above.

WARNINGS

- Tell your doctor about unusual or allergic reactions you have had to any medications, especially to guanadrel.
- Before starting to take this medication, be sure to tell your doctor if you now have or if you have ever had asthma, fevers, heart or blood vessel disease, peptic ulcers, pheochromocytoma, or a slowed heartbeat.
- If this drug makes you dizzy or drowsy or blurs your vision, avoid taking part in activities that require alertness, such as driving a car or operating potentially dangerous machinery.

• Before having surgery or any other medical or dental treatment, be sure to tell your doctor or dentist that you are taking this medication.
• Check with your doctor or pharmacist before taking any over-the-counter (nonprescription) asthma, allergy, cough, cold, diet, or sinus preparation. Some of these products can decrease the effectiveness of guanadrel.
• To prevent feeling faint while you are taking guanadrel, you should avoid drinking alcoholic beverages. You should also avoid standing for prolonged periods, exercising excessively, and taking hot showers and saunas.
• This medication can cause a rapid decrease in blood pressure when you change positions or stand up. To avoid this, always stand up slowly.
• Be sure to tell your doctor if you are pregnant. Although guanadrel appears to be safe during pregnancy, extensive studies in humans have not been conducted. Also, tell your doctor if you are breast-feeding an infant. It is not known whether guanadrel passes into breast milk.

---

guanethidine

BRAND NAMES (Manufacturers)
guanethidine (various manufacturers)
Ismelin (Ciba)
TYPE OF DRUG
Antihypertensive
INGREDIENT
guanethidine
DOSAGE FORM
Tablets (10 mg and 25 mg)
STORAGE
Guanethidine should be stored at room temperature in a tightly closed container.

USES

Guanethidine is used to control high blood pressure. It works by blocking the action of the chemicals responsible for increasing blood pressure.

TREATMENT

Guanethidine can be taken either on an empty stomach or, to avoid stomach irritation, with food or milk (as directed by your doctor). Try to take your doses at the same times each day to become accustomed to taking this medication.

If you miss a dose of this medication, take the missed dose as soon as possible, unless it is almost time for the next dose. In that case, do not take the missed dose at all; just return to your regular dosing schedule. Do not double the next dose.

This medication does not cure high blood pressure, but it will help to control the condition as long as you continue to take it.

SIDE EFFECTS

Minor. Diarrhea, dizziness, dry mouth, fatigue, nasal congestion, nausea, vomiting, weakness, or weight gain. These side effects should disappear as your body adjusts to the medication.

If you feel dizzy, sit or lie down for a while; change positions slowly, and be careful on stairs.

To help relieve mouth dryness, chew sugarless gum or suck on ice chips or a piece of hard candy.

Major. Tell your doctor about any side effects that are persistent or particularly bothersome. IT IS ESPECIALLY IMPORTANT TO TELL YOUR DOCTOR about blurred vision, chest pain, decreased sexual ability, depression, drooping eyelids, hair loss, increased urination, itching, muscle pain or tremors, rapid weight gain (three to five pounds within a week), skin rash, shortness of breath, or swollen or tender glands.

INTERACTIONS

Guanethidine interacts with several other types of drugs:

1. Concurrent use of guanethidine and alcohol can lead to fainting or extreme drowsiness.
2. Amphetamines, appetite suppressants, ephedrine, haloperidol, methylphenidate, phenothiazine tranquilizers, chlorprothixene, thiothixine, phenylpropanolamine, and tricyclic antidepressants can decrease the beneficial effects of guanethidine.
3. Minoxidil, methotrimeprazine, narcotics, fenfluramine, and reserpine can increase guanethidine's blood-pressure-lowering effects, which can be dangerous.
4. The dosage of oral antidiabetic medications may need to be adjusted when guanethidine is being taken.
5. Concurrent use of guanethidine with monoamine oxidase (MAO) inhibitors can lead to serious side effects. At least 14 days should the use of this drug and the use of an MAO inhibitor.

BE SURE TO TELL YOUR DOCTOR about any medications you are currently taking, especially any listed above.

WARNINGS

• Tell your doctor about unusual or allergic reactions you have had to any medications, especially to guanethidine.
• Before starting to take this medication, be sure to tell your doctor if you now have or if you have ever had asthma, diabetes mellitus, fever, heart or blood vessel disease, kidney disease, liver disease, peptic ulcers, pheochromocytoma, or a slowed heart rate.
• If this medication makes you dizzy or drowsy, avoid taking part in activities that require alertness, such as driving a car or operating potentially dangerous machinery.
• To prevent fainting while you are taking guanethidine, you should avoid drinking alcoholic beverages. You should also avoid standing for prolonged periods, excercising excessively, and taking hot showers and saunas.
• Before having surgery or any other medical or dental treatment, be sure to tell your doctor or dentist that you are taking this medication.
• Check with your doctor or pharmacist before taking any over-the-counter (nonprescription) asthma, allergy, cough, cold, diet, or sinus preparation. Some of these products can reduce the effectiveness of guanethidine.
• Be sure to tell your doctor if you are pregnant. Although guanethidine appears to be safe during pregnancy, extensive studies in humans have not been conducted. Also, tell your doctor if you are breast-feeding an infant. It is not known whether guanethidine passes into breast milk.

Guiatuss A.C.—see codeine and guaifenesin combination

Guiatussin with Codeine—see codeine and guaifenesin combination

Guipax—see phenylpropanolamine and guaifenesin combination

Gulfasin—see sulfonamide antibiotics (oral)

G-well—see lindane

Gynecort—see hydrocortisone (topical)

Gyne-Lotrimin—see clotrimazole (vaginal)

---

halazepam

BRAND NAME (Manufacturer)
Paxipam (Schering)
TYPE OF DRUG
Benzodiazepine sedative/hypnotic/antianxiety
INGREDIENT
halazepam
DOSAGE FORM
Tablets (20 mg and 40 mg)
STORAGE
This medication should be stored at room temperature in a tightly closed, light-resistant container.

USES

Halazepam is prescribed to treat symptoms of anxiety. It is not clear exactly how this medicine works, but it may relieve anxiety by acting as a depressant of the central nervous system. Halazepam is used by many people to relieve nervousness. It is effective for this purpose for short periods, but it is important to try to remove the cause of the anxiety as well.

TREATMENT

This medication should be taken exactly as directed by your doctor. It can be taken with food or a full glass of water if stomach upset occurs. Do not take this medication with antacids, since they may retard its absorption from the gastrointestinal tract.

If you are taking this medication regularly and you miss a dose, take the missed dose immediately if you remember within an hour. If more than an hour has passed, skip the dose you missed and wait for the next scheduled dose. Do not double the dose.

SIDE EFFECTS

Minor. Bitter taste, constipation, diarrhea, dizziness, drowsiness (after a night's sleep), dry mouth, excessive salivation, fatigue, flushing, headache, heartburn, loss of appetite, nausea, nervousness, sweating, or vomiting. As you adjust to the medicine, these effects should disappear.

To relieve constipation, increase the amount of fiber in your diet (fresh fruits and vegetables, salads, bran, and whole-grain breads), exercise, and drink more water (unless your doctor directs you to do otherwise).

Dry mouth can be relieved by chewing sugarless gum or by sucking on ice chips.

If you feel dizzy, sit or lie down for a while; get up slowly from a sitting or reclining position, and be careful on stairs.

Major. Tell your doctor about any side effects that are persistent or particularly bothersome. IT IS ESPECIALLY IMPORTANT TO TELL YOUR DOCTOR about blurred or double vision, chest pain, depression, difficulty in urinating, fainting, falling, fever, joint pain, hallucinations, mouth sores, nightmares, palpitations, rash, shortness of breath, slurred speech, sore throat, uncoordinated movements, unusual excitement, unusual tiredness, or yellowing of the eyes or skin.

INTERACTIONS

Halazepam interacts with several other types of drugs:

1. To prevent oversedation, halazepam should not be taken with alcohol, other sedative drugs, central nervous system depressants (such as antihistamines, barbiturates, muscle relaxants, pain medicines, narcotics, medicines for seizures, and phenothiazine tranquilizers), or antidepressants unless otherwise directed by your doctor.

2. This medication may decrease the effectiveness of carbamazepine, levodopa, and oral anticoagulants and may increase the effects of phenytoin.

3. Disulfiram, oral contraceptives (birth control pills), isoniazid, and cimetidine can increase the blood levels of halazepam, which can lead to toxic effects.

4. Concurrent use of rifampin may decrease the effectiveness of halazepam.

BE SURE TO TELL YOUR DOCTOR about any medications you are currently taking, especially any of those listed above.

WARNINGS

- Tell your doctor about unusual or allergic reactions you have had to any medications, especially to halazepam or any other benzodiazepine tranquilizers (such as alprazolam, chlordiazepoxide, clorazepate, diazepam, flurazepam, lorazepam, oxazepam, prazepam, temazepam, and triazolam).
- Tell your doctor if you now have or if you have ever had liver or kidney disease, epilepsy, lung disease, myasthenia gravis, porphyria, mental depression, or mental illness.
- This medicine can cause drowsiness. You should, therefore, avoid tasks that require alertness, such as driving a car or using potentially dangerous machinery.
- This medication has the potential for abuse and must be used with caution. Tolerance may develop quickly; do not increase the dosage without first consulting your doctor. It is also important not to stop taking this drug suddenly if you have been taking it in large amounts or if you have used it for several weeks. Your doctor may want to reduce the dosage gradually.
- The combination of this medication with other sedative drugs or alcohol can result in serious side effects.
- The elderly may have a heightened response to this drug.
- This type of medication may actually have the opposite effect on some individuals (it may cause an increase in anxiety or agitation). Report any such changes in mental status to your physician immediately.
- Be sure to tell your doctor if you are pregnant. This type of medicine may increase the chance of birth defects if it is taken during the first three months of pregnancy. In addition,

too much use of this medicine during the last six months of pregnancy may result in addiction of the fetus, leading to withdrawal side effects in the newborn. Also, use of this medicine during the last weeks of pregnancy may cause excessive drowsiness, slowed heartbeat, and breathing difficulties in the infant. Tell your doctor if you are breast-feeding an infant. This medicine can pass into breast milk and cause excessive drowsiness, slowed heartbeat, and breathing difficulties in nursing infants.

---

halcinonide (topical)

BRAND NAMES (Manufacturers)
Halog (Princeton)
Halog-E (Princeton)
TYPE OF DRUG
Adrenocorticosteroid hormone
INGREDIENT
halcinonide
DOSAGE FORMS
Ointment (0.1%)
Cream (0.025% and 0.1%)
Solution (0.1%)
STORAGE
Halcinonide ointment, cream, and solution should be stored at room temperature in tightly closed containers. This medication should never be frozen.

USES

Your adrenal glands naturally produce certain cortisone-like chemicals. These chemicals are involved in various regulatory processes in the body (such as those involving fluid balance, temperature, and reaction to inflammation). Halcinonide belongs to a group of drugs known as adrenocorticosteroids (or cortisone-like medications). It is used to relieve the skin inflammation (redness, swelling, itching, and discomfort) associated with conditions such as dermatitis, eczema, and poison ivy. How this drug acts to relieve inflammation is not completely understood.

TREATMENT

Before applying this medication, wash your hands. Then, unless your doctor gives you different instructions, gently wash the area of the skin where the medication is to be applied. With a clean towel, pat the area almost dry; it should be slightly damp when you put the medicine on.

Apply a small amount of the medication to the affected area in a thin layer. Do not bandage the area unless your doctor tells you to do so. If you are to apply an occlusive dressing (like kitchen plastic wrap), be sure you understand the instructions. Wash your hands again after application.

If you miss a dose of this medication, apply the dose as soon as possible, unless it is almost time for the next application. In that case, do not apply the missed dose at all; just return to your regular schedule. Do not put twice as much of the medication on your skin at the next application.

SIDE EFFECTS

Minor. Acne, burning sensation, itching, rash, or skin dryness. If the affected area is extremely dry or scaling, the skin may be moistened before applying the medication by soaking in water or by applying water with a clean cloth. The ointment form is probably better for dry skin.

A mild, temporary stinging sensation may occur after this medication is applied. If this persists, contact your doctor.
Major. Tell your doctor about any side effects that are persistent or particularly bothersome. IT IS ESPECIALLY IMPORTANT TO TELL YOUR DOCTOR about blistering, increased hair growth, irritation of the affected area, loss of skin color, secondary infection in the area being treated, or thinning of the skin with easy bruising.

INTERACTIONS

This medication should not interact with any other medications as long as it is used according to directions.

WARNINGS

- Tell your doctor about unusual or allergic reactions you have had to any medications, especially to halcinonide or any other adrenocorticosteroids (such as amcinonide, betamethasone, cortisone, desonide, desoximetasone, dexamethasone, flumethasone, fluocinolone, fluocinonide, fluorometholone, flurandrenolide, hydrocortisone, methylprednisolone, paramethasone, prednisolone, prednisone, and triamcinolone).
- Tell your doctor if you now have or if you have ever had blood vessel disease, chicken pox, diabetes mellitus, fungal infection, peptic ulcers, shingles, tuberculosis, tuberculosis of the skin, vaccinia, or any other type of infection, especially at the site currently being treated.
- If irritation develops while using this drug, immediately discontinue its use and notify your doctor.
- This product is not for use in the eyes, nose, or mouth; contact may result in side effects.
- Do not use this product with an occlusive wrap unless your doctor directs you to do so. Systemic absorption of this drug is increased if extensive areas of the body are treated, particularly if occlusive bandages are used. If it is necessary for you to use this drug under a wrap, follow your doctor's instructions exactly; do not leave the wrap in place longer than specified.
- If you are using this medication on a child's diaper area, do not put tight-fitting diapers or plastic pants on the child. This may lead to increased systemic absorption of the drug and a possible increase in side effects.
- Be sure to tell your doctor if you are pregnant. If large amounts of this drug are applied for prolonged periods, some of it will be absorbed and may cross the placenta. Studies in humans have not been conducted; however, birth defects have been observed in the offspring of animals that were given large oral doses of this type of drug during pregnancy. Also, tell your doctor if you are breast-feeding an infant. If absorbed through the skin, small amounts of halcinonide pass into breast milk and may cause growth suppression or a decrease in natural adrenocorticosteroid hormone production in the nursing infant.

Halcion—see triazolam

Haldol—see haloperidol

Halog—see halcinonide (topical)

Halog-E—see halcinonide (topical)

---

haloperidol

BRAND NAMES (Manufacturers)
Haldol (McNeil)
haloperidol (various manufacturers)
TYPE OF DRUG
Antipsychotic
INGREDIENT
haloperidol
DOSAGE FORMS
Tablets (0.5 mg, 1 mg, 2 mg, 5 mg, 10 mg, and 20 mg)
Oral concentrate (2 mg per ml)
STORAGE
Haloperidol tablets and oral concentrate should be stored at room temperature in a tightly closed, light-resistant container. This medication should never be frozen.

USES

Haloperidol is prescribed to treat the symptoms of certain types of mental illness, such as the emotional symptoms of psychosis, the manic phase of manic-depressive illness, Tourette's syndrome, and severe behavioral problems in children. This drug is thought to relieve symptoms of mental illness by blocking certain chemicals involved with nerve transmission in the brain.

TREATMENT

To avoid stomach irritation, you can take haloperidol tablets with a meal or with a glass of water or milk (unless your doctor directs you to do otherwise).

The oral concentrate form of this medication should be measured carefully with the dropper provided, then added to four ounces (1/2 cup) or more of water, milk, or a cola-free, caffeine-free carbonated beverage or to applesauce or pudding immediately prior to administration. To prevent possible loss of effectiveness, haloperidol should not be diluted with tea, coffee, caffeine-containing beverages, or apple juice.

If you miss a dose of this medication and remember within six hours, take the missed dose as soon as possible; then return to your regular schedule. If more than six hours have passed, however, skip the missed dose and return to your regular dosing schedule. Do not double the next dose unless your doctor directs you to do so.

The full effects of haloperidol may not become apparent for two weeks after you start to take it.

SIDE EFFECTS

Minor. Blurred vision, constipation, decreased or increased sweating, diarrhea, dizziness, drooling, drowsiness, dry mouth, fatigue, headache, heartburn, jitteriness, loss of appetite, menstrual irregularities, nausea, restlessness, sleep disorders, vomiting, or weakness. As your body adjusts to the medication, these side effects should disappear.

This medication can cause increased sensitivity to sunlight. It is, therefore, important to avoid prolonged exposure to sunlight and sunlamps. Wear protective clothing, and use an effective sunscreen.

If you are constipated, increase the amount of fiber in your diet (fresh fruits and vegetables, salads, bran, and whole-grain breads), exercise, and drink more water (unless your doctor directs you to do otherwise).

To reduce mouth dryness, chew sugarless gum or suck on ice chips or a piece of hard candy.

To avoid dizziness or light-headedness when you stand, contract and relax the muscles of your legs for a few moments before rising. Do this by pushing one foot against the floor while raising the other foot slightly, alternating feet so that you are "pumping" your legs in a pedaling motion.

Major. Tell your doctor about any side effects that are persistent or particularly bothersome. IT IS ESPECIALLY IMPORTANT TO TELL YOUR DOCTOR about aching joints and muscles; breast enlargement (in both sexes); chest pain; confusion; convulsions; difficulty in breathing or swallowing; difficulty in urinating; fainting; fever; fluid retention; hair loss; hallucinations; impotence; involuntary movements of the mouth, face, neck, tongue, or limbs; mouth sores; palpitations; skin darkening; skin rash; sore throat; tremors; unusual bleeding or bruising; visual disturbances; or yellowing of the eyes or skin.

INTERACTIONS

Haloperidol interacts with several other types of medications:

1. It can cause extreme drowsiness when combined with alcohol or other central nervous system depressants (such as antihistamines, barbiturates, benzodiazepine tranquilizers, muscle relaxants, narcotics, and pain medications) or with tricyclic antidepressants.

2. This medication can decrease the effectiveness of guanethidine and anticonvulsants (antiseizure medications).

3. The blood-pressure-lowering effects of antihypertensive medications may be dangerously increased by haloperidol.

4. Haloperidol may increase the side effects of epinephrine, lithium, and methyldopa.

5. It is important to note that tea or coffee can reduce the gastrointestinal absorption of haloperidol, decreasing its effectiveness. Therefore, haloperidol should not be taken within an hour of drinking tea or coffee (before or after).

Before starting to take haloperidol, BE SURE TO TELL YOUR DOCTOR about any medications you are currently taking, especially any of those listed above.

WARNINGS

- Tell your doctor about unusual or allergic reactions you have had to any medications, especially to haloperidol or to any other medicines used to treat mental illness.
- Tell your doctor if you now have or if you have ever had any blood disorders, blockage of the urinary tract, drug-induced depression, enlarged prostate gland, epilepsy, glaucoma, heart or circulatory disease, kidney disease, liver disease, lung disease, mental depression, Parkinson's disease, peptic ulcers, or thyroid disease.
- Avoid drinking alcoholic beverages while taking this medication in order to prevent oversedation.
- If this medication makes you dizzy or drowsy, do not take part in any activity that requires alertness, such as driving a car or operating potentially dangerous machinery. Be careful on stairs, and avoid getting up suddenly from a lying or sitting position.

• Prior to having surgery or any other medical or dental treatment, be sure to tell your doctor or dentist that you are taking this medication.
• Some of the side effects caused by this drug can be prevented by taking an antiparkinsonism drug. Discuss this with your doctor.
• This medication can decrease sweating and heat release from the body. You should, therefore, avoid getting overheated by strenuous exercise in hot weather and should avoid taking hot baths, showers, and saunas.
• Do not stop taking this medication suddenly. If the drug is stopped abruptly, you may experience nausea, vomiting, stomach upset, headache, increased heart rate, insomnia, tremors, or a worsening of your condition. Your doctor may want to reduce the dosage gradually.
• The elderly may be at increased risk for side effects. Watch closely for side effects or other changes, especially in mental status, and report them to your doctor.
• If you are planning to have a myelogram, or any other procedure in which dye is injected into the spinal cord, tell your doctor that you are taking this medication.
• Avoid spilling the oral concentrate form of this medication on your skin or clothing; it can cause redness and irritation of the skin.
• While taking haloperidol, do not take any over-the-counter (nonprescription) medication for weight control or for cough, cold, allergy, asthma, or sinus problems unless you first check with your doctor. The combination of these medications may cause high blood pressure.
• Haloperidol has the potential to cause a permanent movement disorder called tardive dyskinesia. It is important to discuss this with your doctor and to report any unusual or uncontrolled body movements.
• Be sure to tell your doctor if you are pregnant. A few cases of limb malformations have occurred in infants whose mothers had received haloperidol in combination with several other drugs during the first three months of pregnancy. Whether haloperidol was the cause is still not known. Also, tell your doctor if you are breast-feeding an infant. Small amounts of haloperidol pass into breast milk.

Haltran—see ibuprofen

HC-Form—see hydrocortisone and iodochlorhydroxyquin combination (topical)

HC-Jel—see hydrocortisone (topical)

Hemorrhoidal HC—see hydrocortisone, benzyl benzoate, bismuth resorcin compound, bismuth subgallate, zinc oxide, and Peruvian balsam combination (topical)

Hexadrol—see dexamethasone (systemic)

H-H-R—see hydralazine, hydrochlorothiazide, and reserpine combination

Hi-Cor—see hydrocortisone (topical)

Hiprex—see methenamine

Hismanal—see astemizole

Histabid Duracaps—see phenylpropanolamine and chlorpheniramine combination

Histalet—see pseudoephedrine and chlorpheniramine combination

Histamic—see phenylpropanolamine, phenylephrine, chlorpheniramine, and phenyltoloxamine combination

H_2Cort—see hydrocortisone (topical)

Humulin L—see insulin

Humulin N—see insulin

Humulin R—see insulin

Hydergine—see ergoloid mesylates

---

hydralazine

BRAND NAMES (Manufacturers)
Alazine (Major)
Apresoline (Ciba)
hydralazine hydrochloride (various manufacturers)
TYPE OF DRUG
Antihypertensive
INGREDIENT
hydralazine
DOSAGE FORM
Tablets (10 mg, 25 mg, 50 mg, and 100 mg)
STORAGE
Hydralazine tablets should be stored at room temperature in a tightly closed, light-resistant container.

USES

This medication is used to treat high blood pressure or heart failure. Hydralazine is a vasodilator that directly relaxes the muscle of the blood vessels and allows the blood to flow at a lower force, which causes a lowering of blood pressure.

TREATMENT

In order to avoid stomach irritation while you are taking this medication, you can take your dose of hydralazine with food or with a glass of water or milk. To become accustomed to taking this medication, try to take it at the same time(s) each day. It may take up to two weeks before the full effects of this medication are observed.

Try not to miss any doses of this medication. If you do miss a dose, take the missed dose as soon as possible, unless it is almost time for the next dose. In that case, do not take the missed dose at all; just return to your regular dosing schedule. Do not double the next dose.

Hydralazine does not cure high blood pressure, but it will help to control the condition as long as you continue to take the medication.

SIDE EFFECTS

Minor. Constipation, diarrhea, dizziness, drowsiness, flushing, headache, light-headedness, loss of appetite, muscle

(continued on page 209)

Tablet/Capsule Identification Guide

On the following pages, you will find color photos of hundreds of the most commonly prescribed drugs in tablet and capsule form. These photos will help you identify your prescription medications and will enable you to make certain that the prescription your doctor wrote refers to the same medication you received from your pharmacist. If you note any discrepancy, call your pharmacist immediately.

HOW TO USE THIS SECTION

Prescription drugs are displayed in alphabetical order by brand name. Included are one or more dosage forms of the particular medication. The generic name is listed below the brand name of each prescription medication. A generic name is generally a shortened form of the chemical name of the drug or, in the case of a combination medication, a list of its active ingredients. This is the name under which you will be able to read more about your medication in the Drug Profiles section of this book. For example, if you have been prescribed the antibiotic Amoxil, you will find a detailed discussion of this medication under its generic name, amoxicillin. If you have been prescribed Darvon Compound-65, you will find your medication discussed in detail within the "aspirin, caffeine, and propoxyphene combination" profile.

For drugs that have only one active ingredient, the amount of that ingredient is listed. For example, in the sample photo for Amoxil shown below, the quantity of amoxicillin in the capsule is indicated. Some medications however, are, composed of more than one active ingredient. For such medications, the quantities of each ingredient are listed in the order in which they appear in the generic name. For example, Darvon Compound-65 contains 389 mg of aspirin, 32.4 mg of caffeine, and 65 mg of propoxyphene. Note that the number 65 appears in the drug's brand name, thus indicating the drug's narcotic content. Other combination drugs containing a narcotic often use the terms No. 1, No. 2, No. 3, or No.4 to designate the narcotic content. (This is described in more detail within the appropriate drug profiles.)

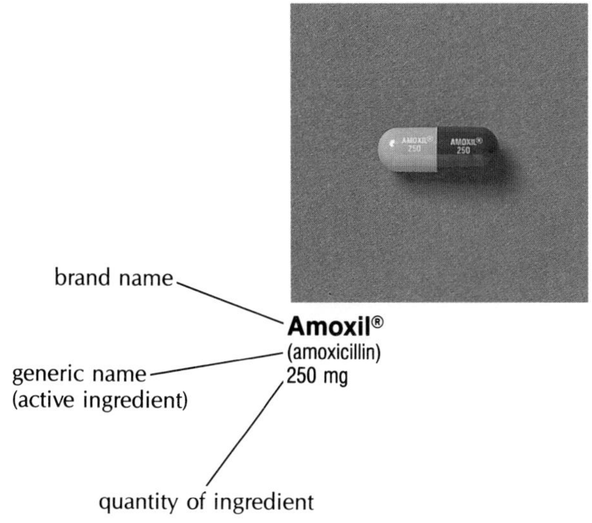

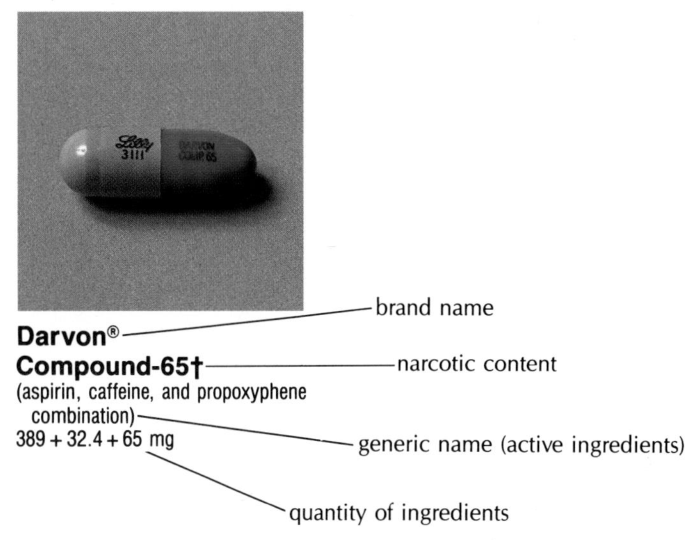

†Drug contains multiple ingredients; ingredients and quantities are listed respectively.

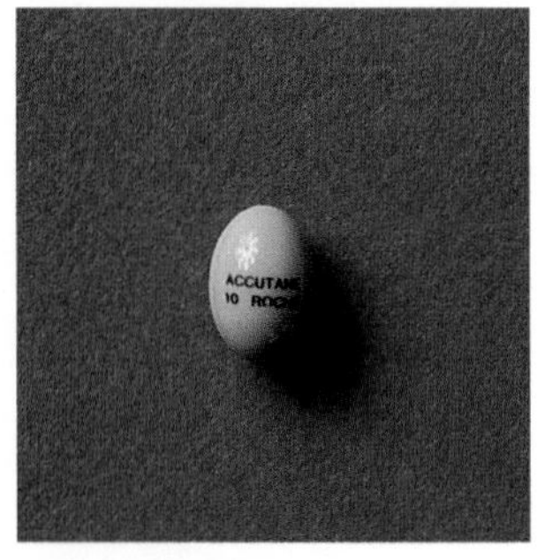

Accutane®
(isotretinoin)
10 mg

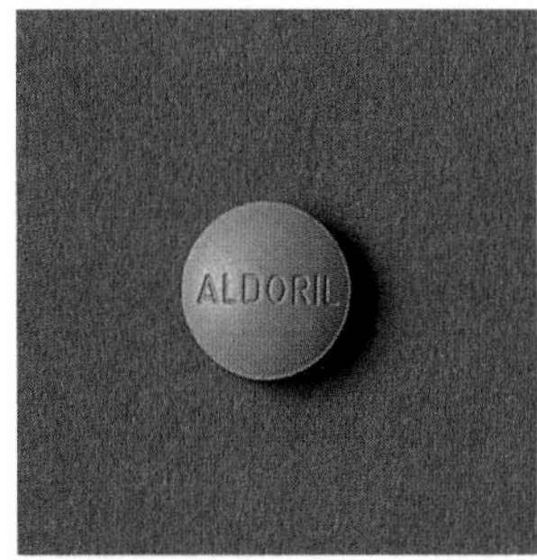

Aldoril®†
(methyldopa and
hydrochlorothiazide combination)
250 + 15 mg

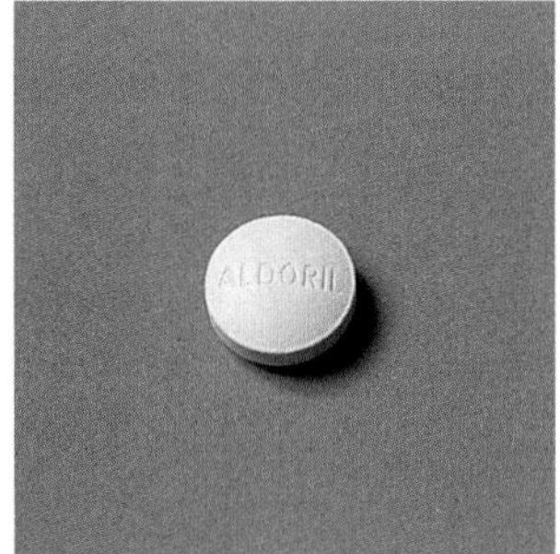

Aldoril®†
(methyldopa and
hydrochlorothiazide combination)
250 + 25 mg

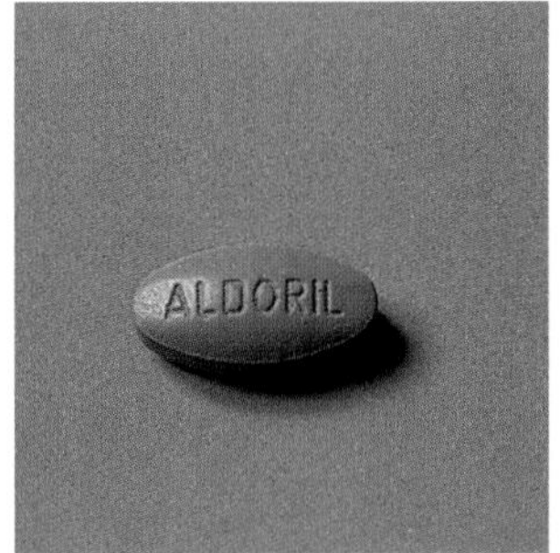

Aldoril®†
(methyldopa and
hydrochlorothiazide combination)
500 + 30 mg

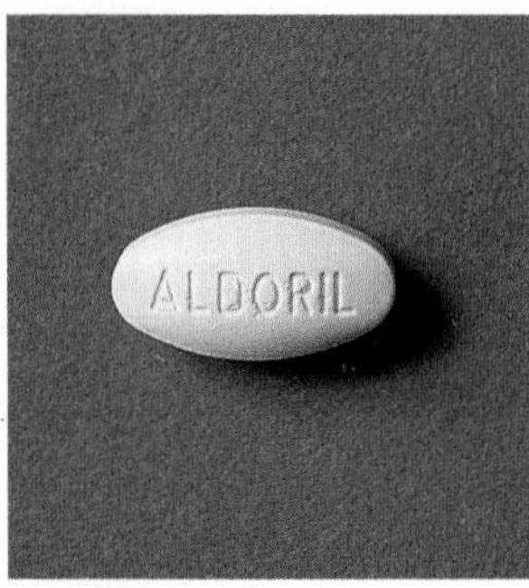

Aldoril®†
(methyldopa and
hydrochlorothiazide combination)
500 + 50 mg

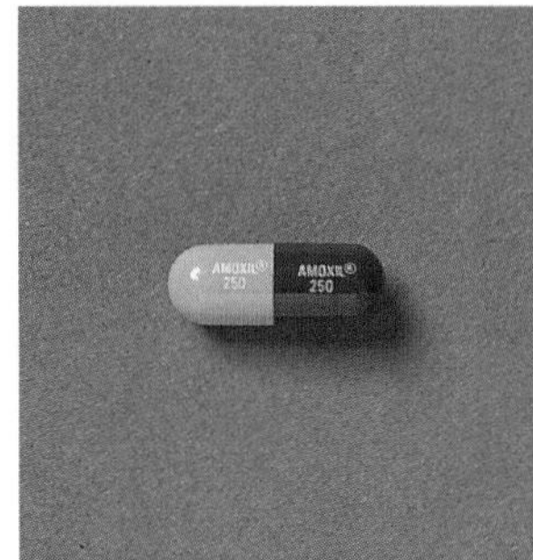

Amoxil®
(amoxicillin)
250 mg

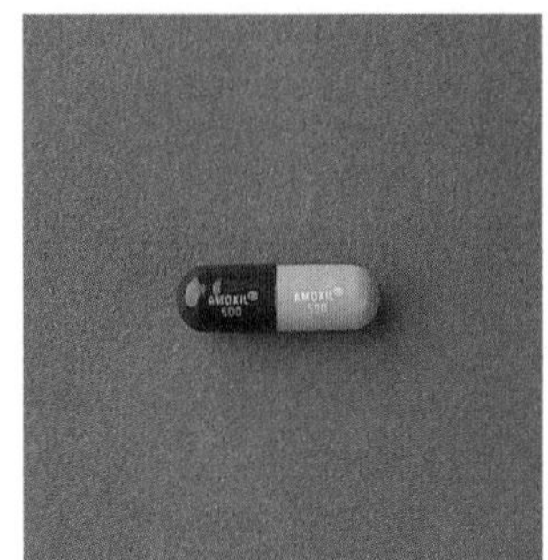

Amoxil®
(amoxicillin)
500 mg

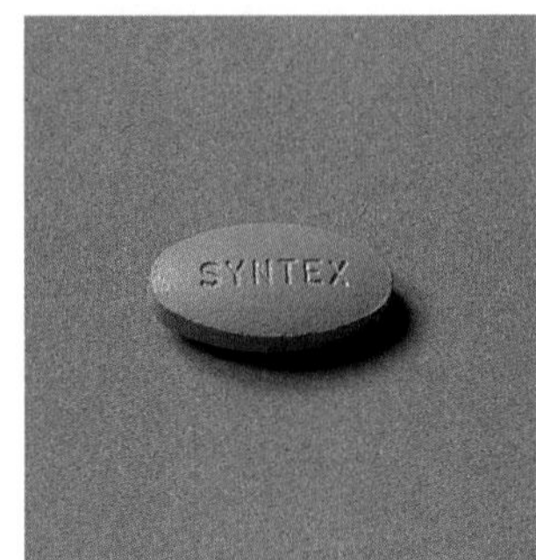

Anaprox®
(naproxen sodium)
275 mg

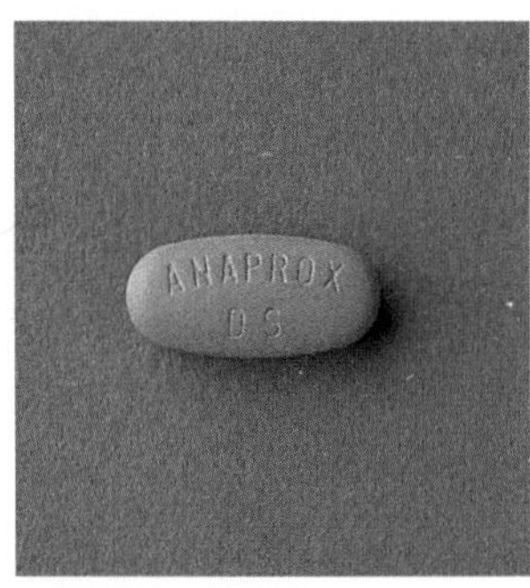

Anaprox® DS
(naproxen sodium)
550 mg

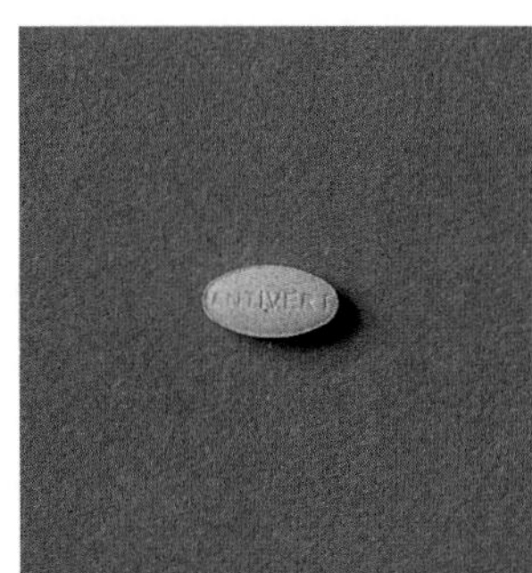

Antivert®
(meclizine)
12.5 mg

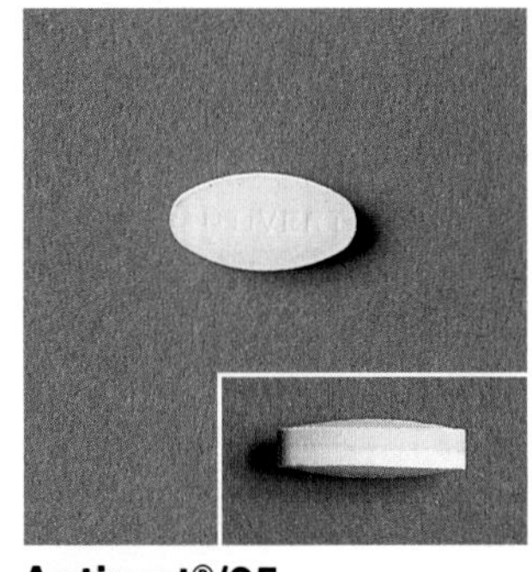

Antivert®/25
(meclizine)
25 mg

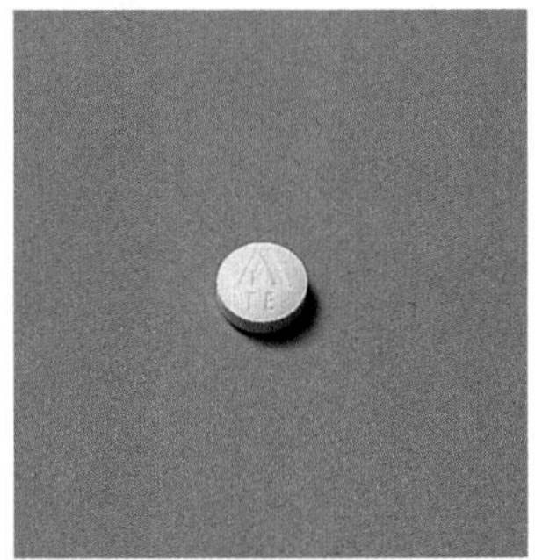

Armour® Thyroid
(thyroid hormone)
65 mg

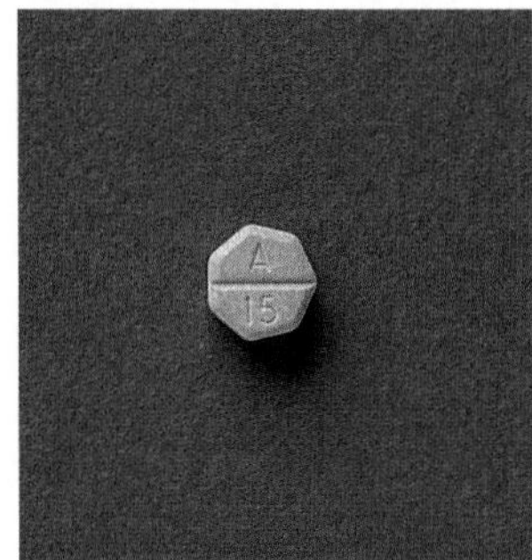

Asendin®
(amoxapine)
50 mg

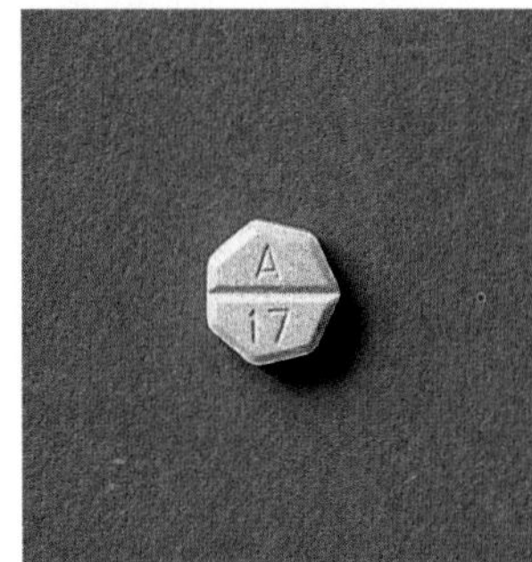

Asendin®
(amoxapine)
100 mg

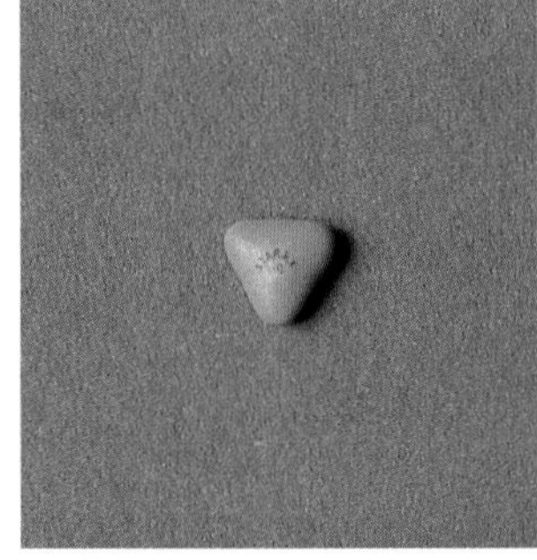

Atarax®
(hydroxyzine)
10 mg

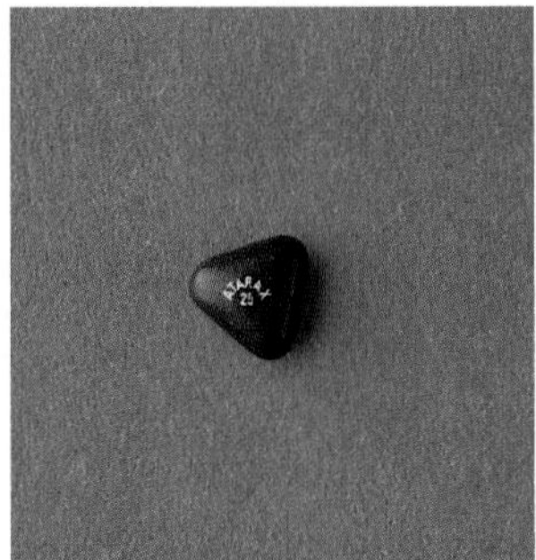

Atarax®
(hydroxyzine)
25 mg

†Drug contains multiple ingredients; ingredients and quantities are listed respectively.

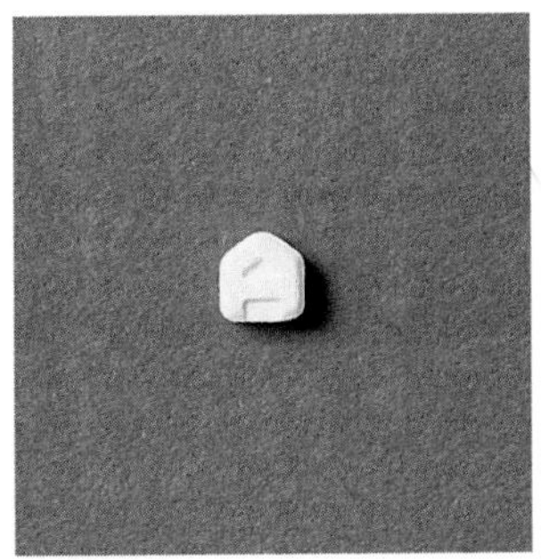

Ativan®
(lorazepam)
0.5 mg

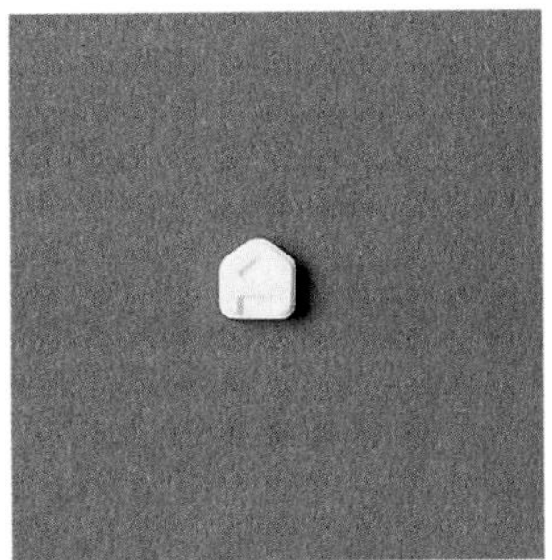

Ativan®
(lorazepam)
1 mg

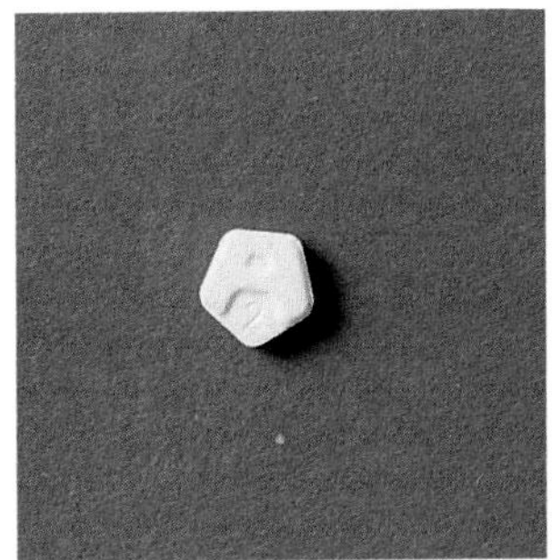

Ativan®
(lorazepam)
2 mg

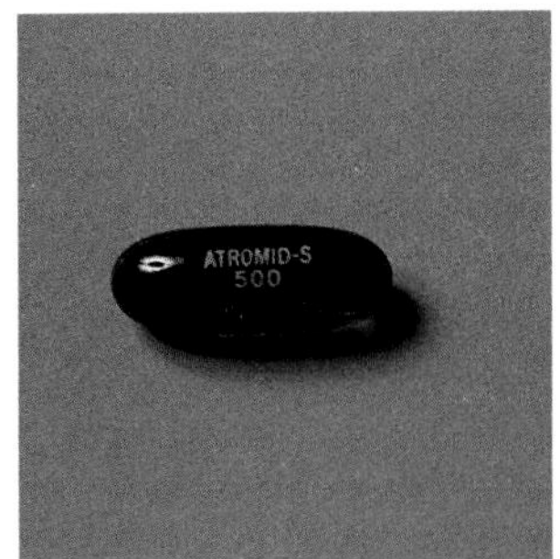

Atromid-S®
(clofibrate)
500 mg

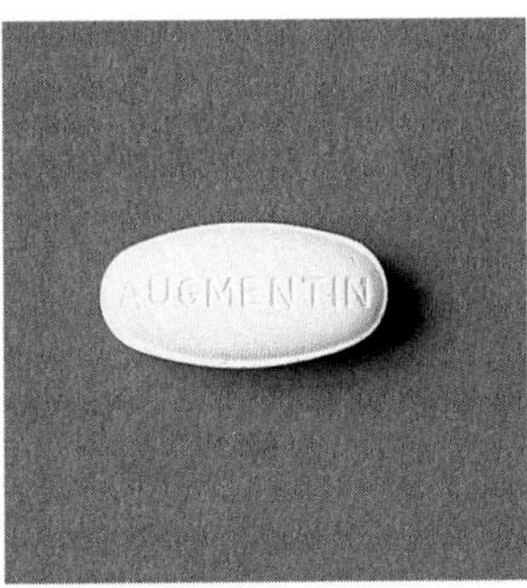

Augmentin®†
(amoxicillin and clavulanic acid combination)
500 + 125 mg

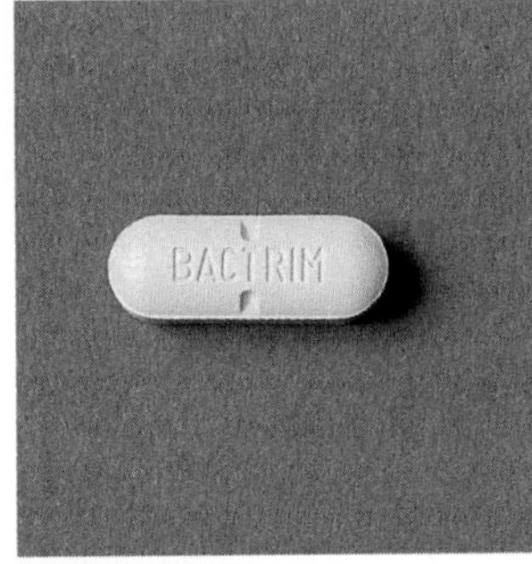

Bactrim™†
(sulfamethoxazole and trimethoprim combination)
400 + 80 mg

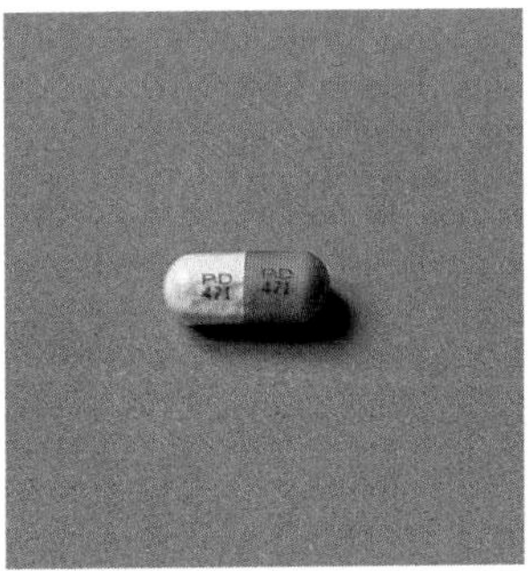

Benadryl®
(diphenhydramine)
25 mg

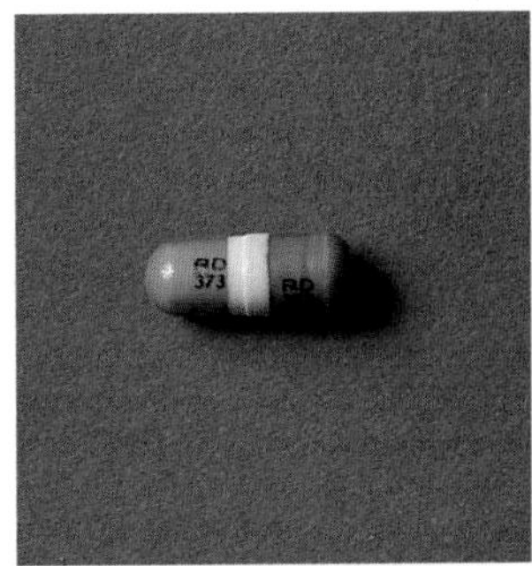

Benadryl® Kapseals®
(diphenhydramine)
50 mg

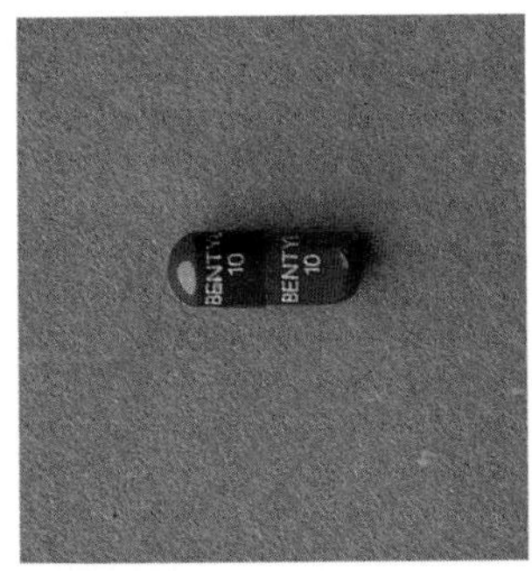

Bentyl®
(dicyclomine)
10 mg

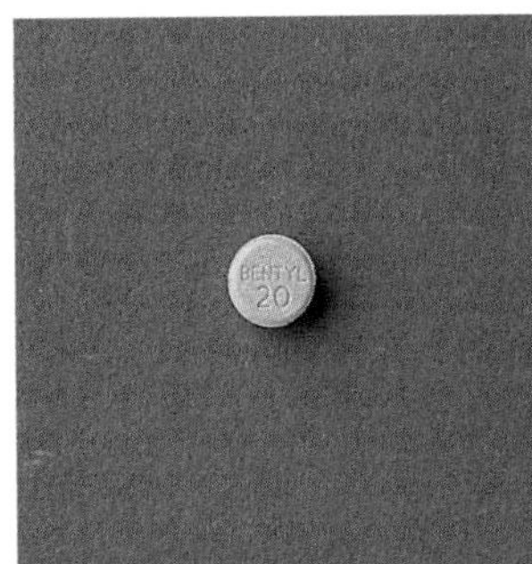

Bentyl®
(dicyclomine)
20 mg

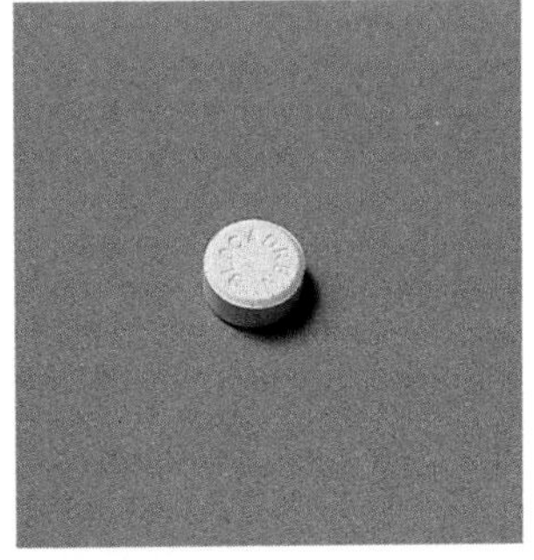

Blocadren®
(timolol)
10 mg

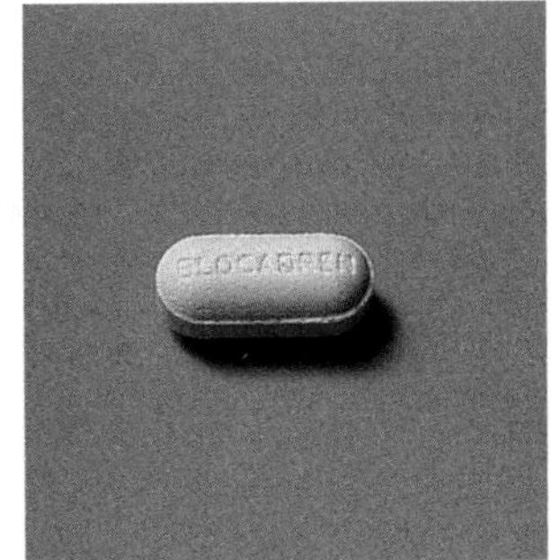

Blocadren®
(timolol)
20 mg

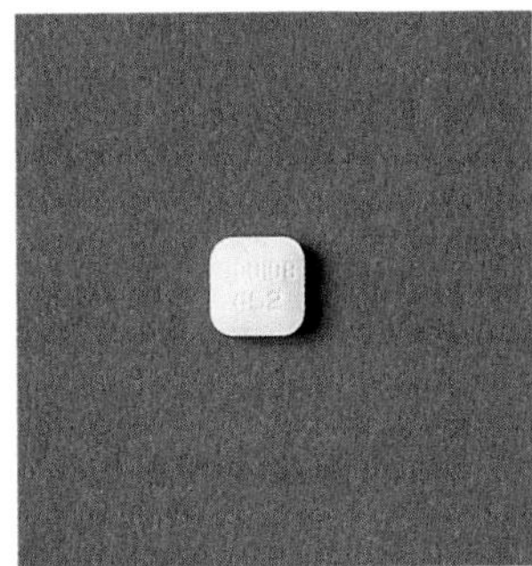

Capoten®
(captopril)
25 mg

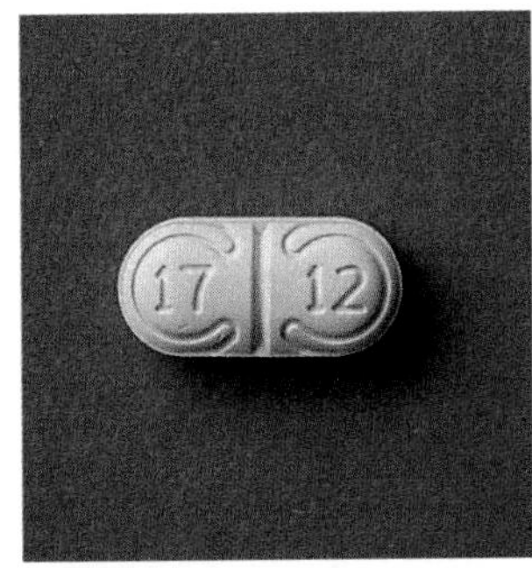

Carafate®
(sucralfate)
1 g

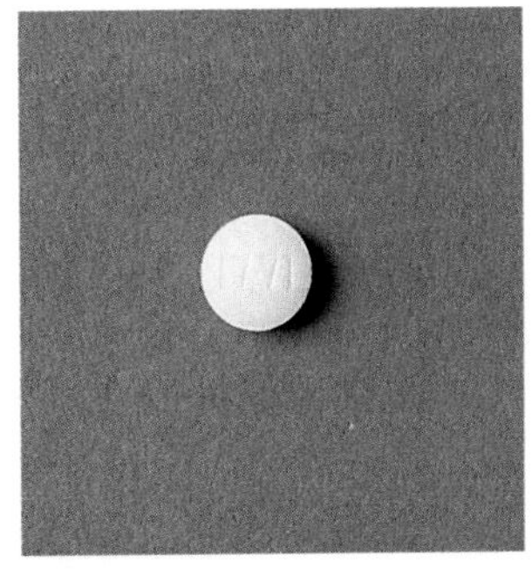

Cardizem®
(diltiazem)
30 mg

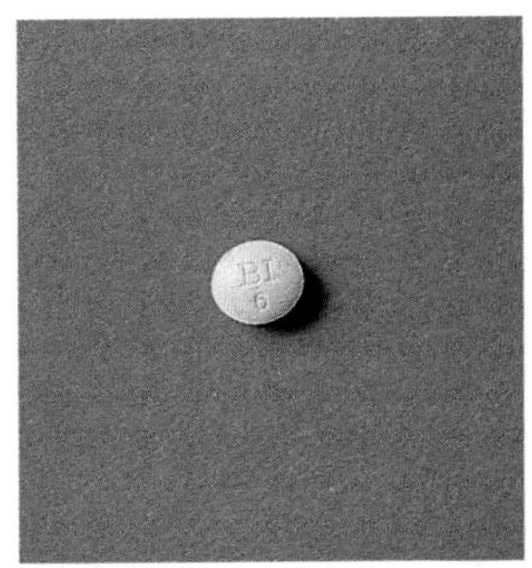

Catapres®
(clonidine)
0.1 mg

†Drug contains multiple ingredients; ingredients and quantities are listed respectively.

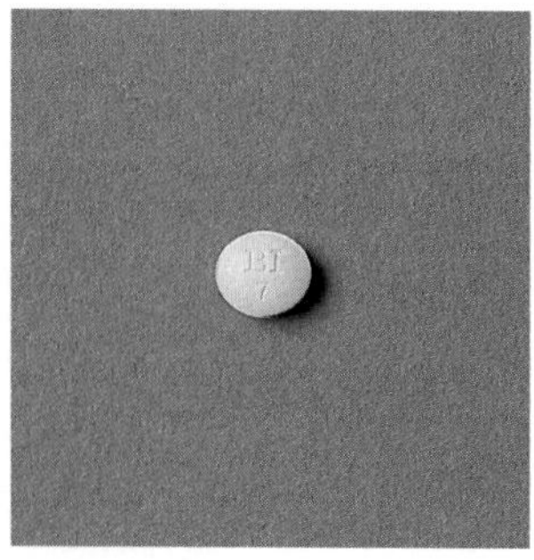

Catapres®
(clonidine)
0.2 mg

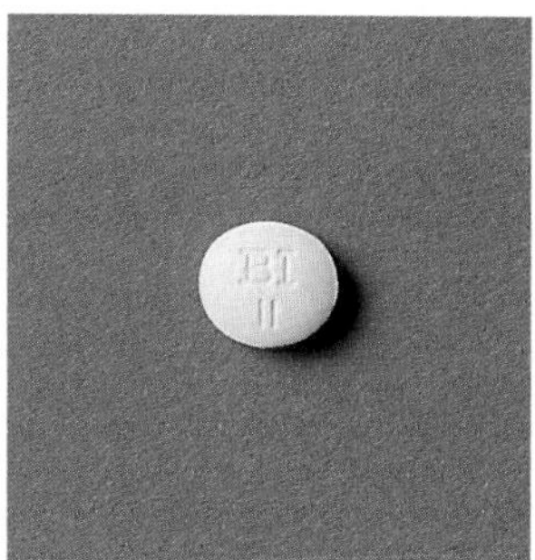

Catapres®
(clonidine)
0.3 mg

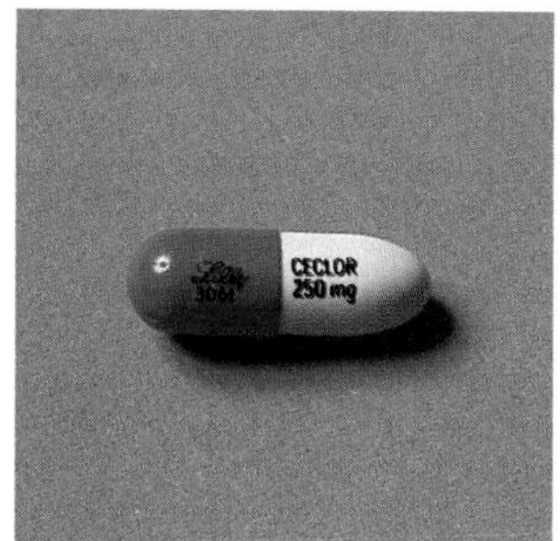

Ceclor®
(cefaclor)
250 mg

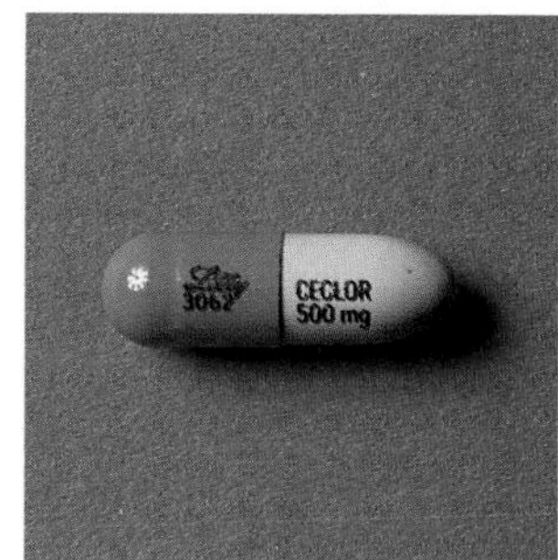

Ceclor®
(cefaclor)
500 mg

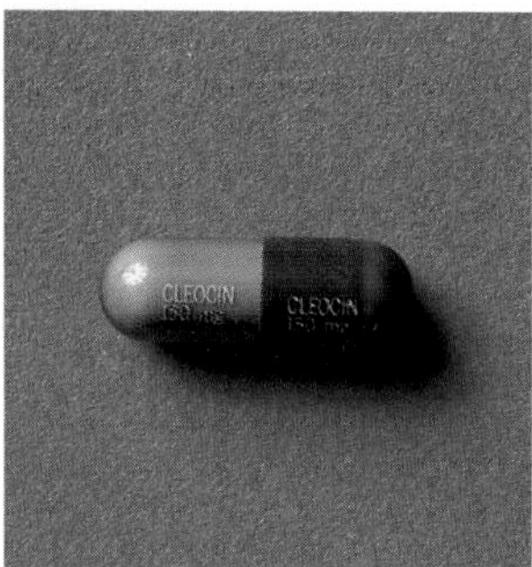

Cleocin HCl®
(clindamycin)
150 mg

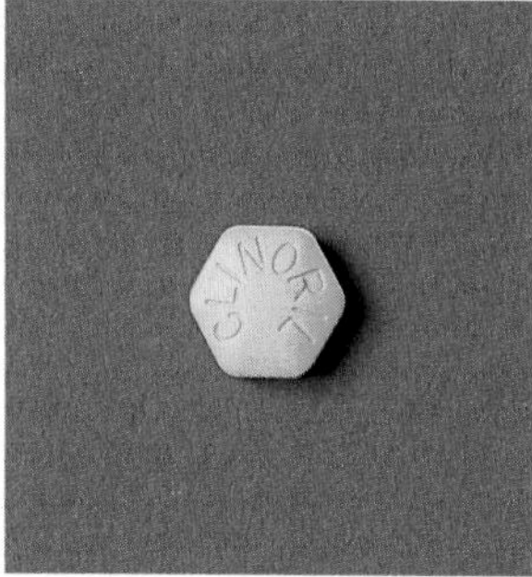

Clinoril®
(sulindac)
150 mg

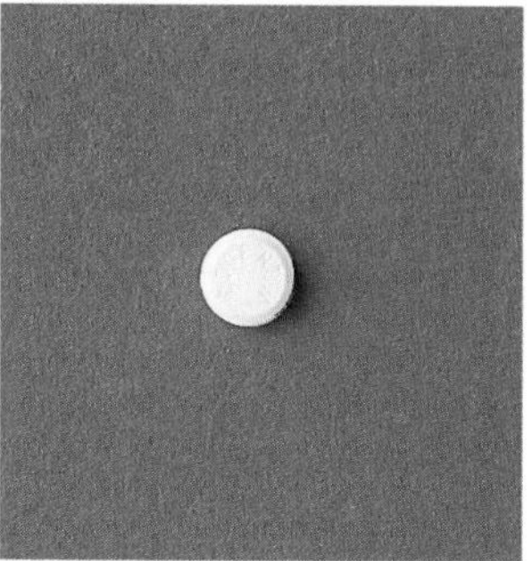

Cogentin®
(benztropine)
0.5 mg

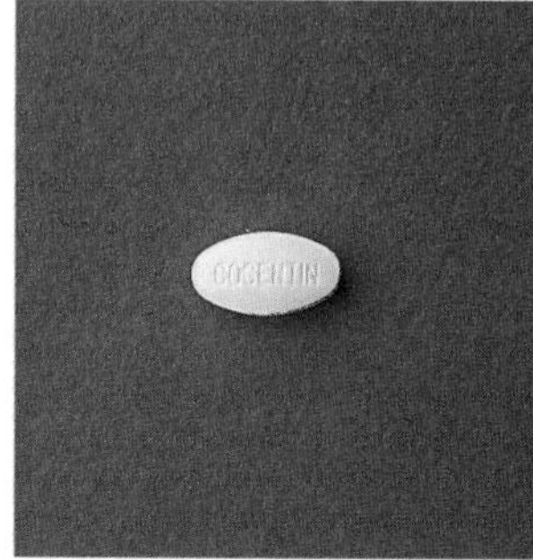

Cogentin®
(benztropine)
1 mg

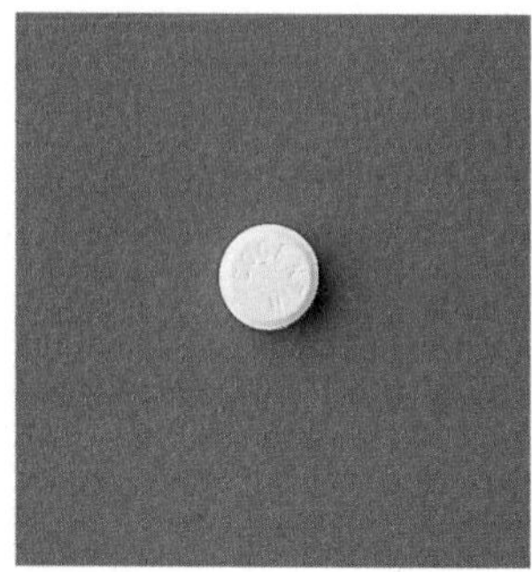

Cogentin®
(benztropine)
2 mg

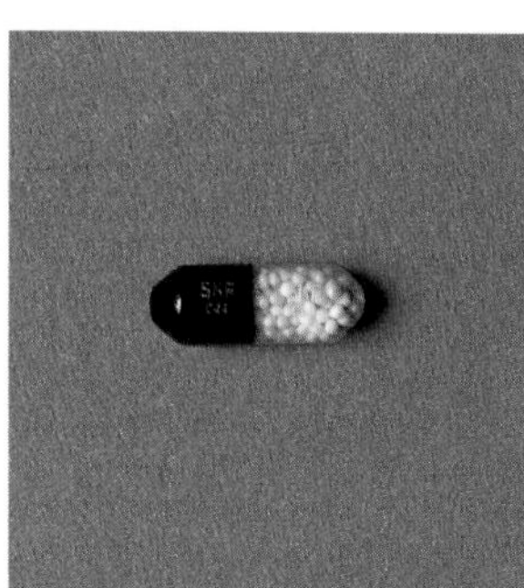

Compazine® Spansule®
(prochlorperazine)
10 mg

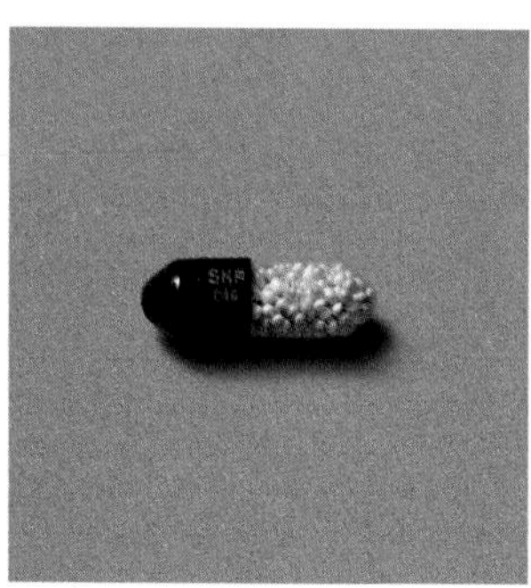

Compazine® Spansule®
(prochlorperazine)
15 mg

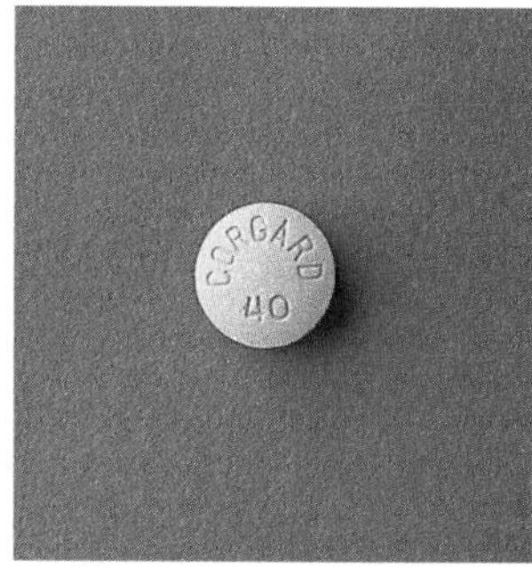

Corgard®
(nadolol)
40 mg

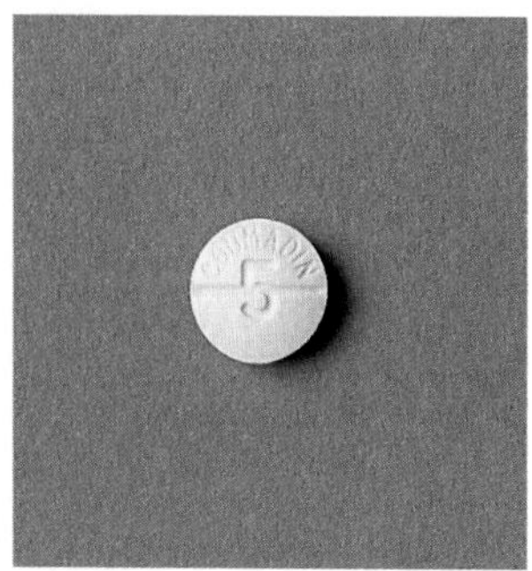

Coumadin®
(warfarin)
5 mg

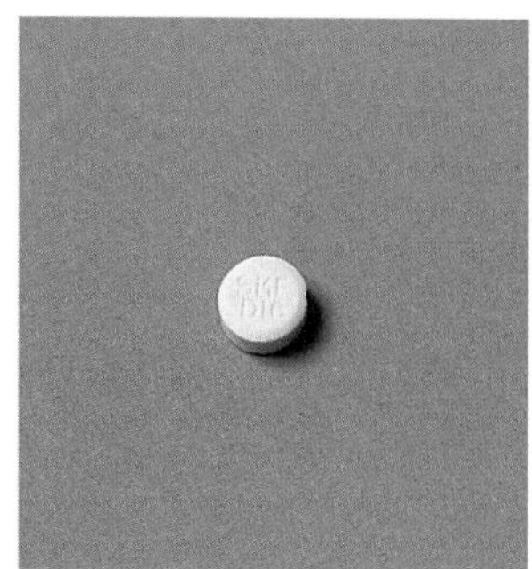

Cytomel®
(liothyronine)
25 mcg

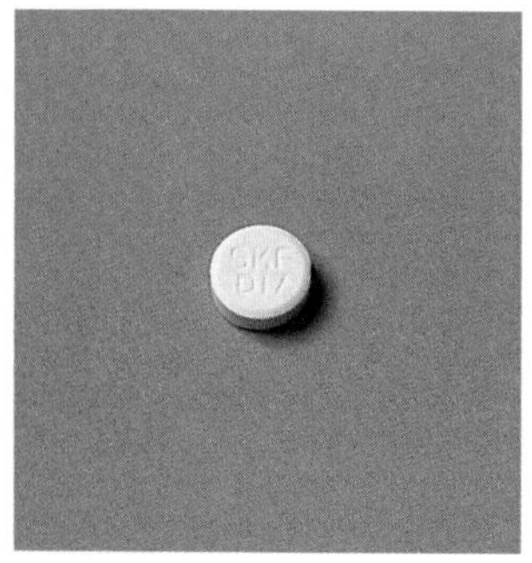

Cytomel®
(liothyronine)
50 mcg

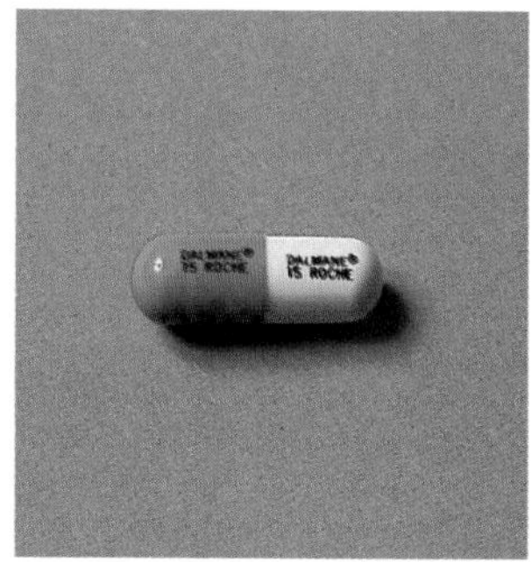

Dalmane®
(flurazepam)
15 mg

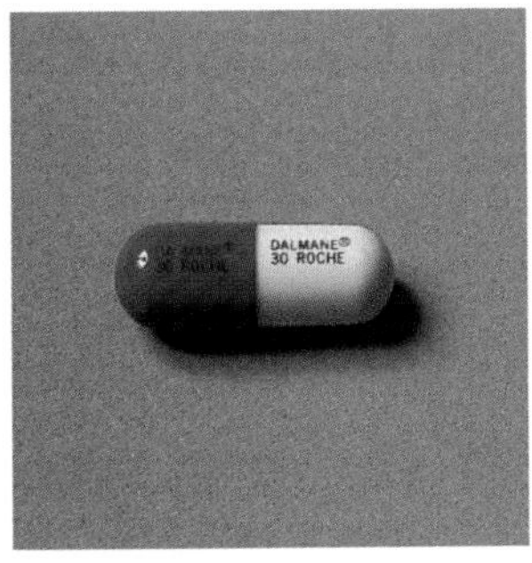

Dalmane®
(flurazepam)
30 mg

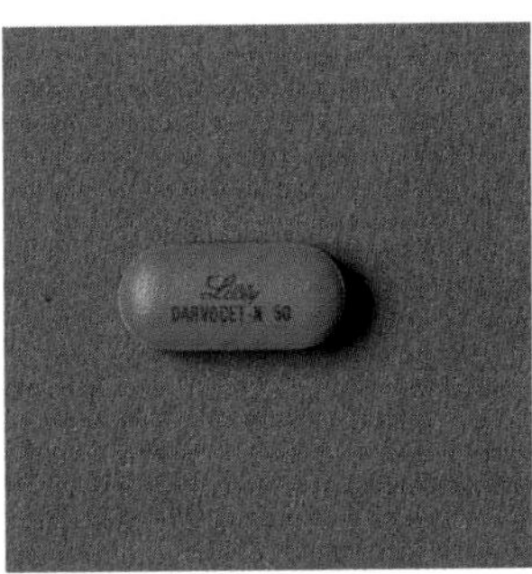

Darvocet-N® 50†
(acetaminophen and propoxyphene combination)
325 + 50 mg

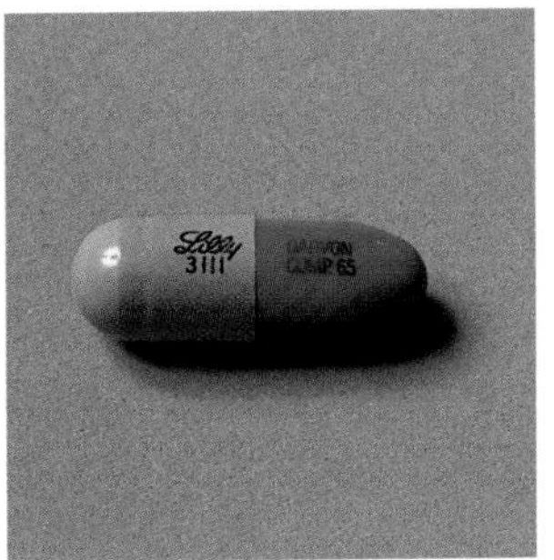

Darvon® Compound-65†
(aspirin, caffeine, and propoxyphene combination)
389 + 32.4 + 65 mg

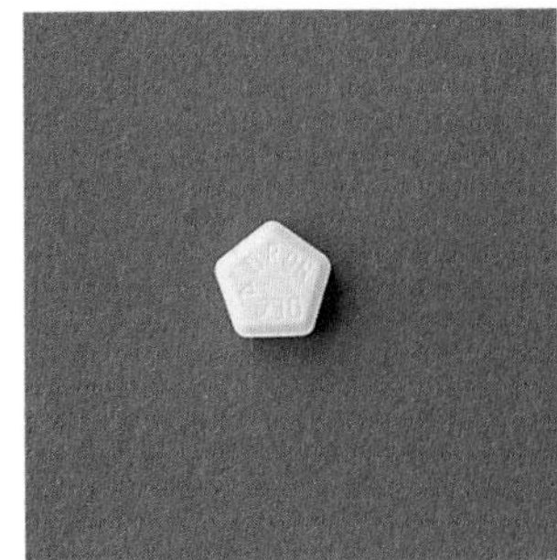

Decadron®
(dexamethasone)
0.5 mg

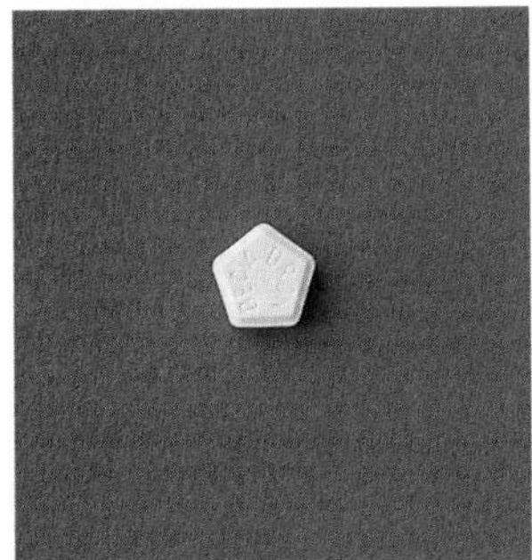

Decadron®
(dexamethasone)
0.75 mg

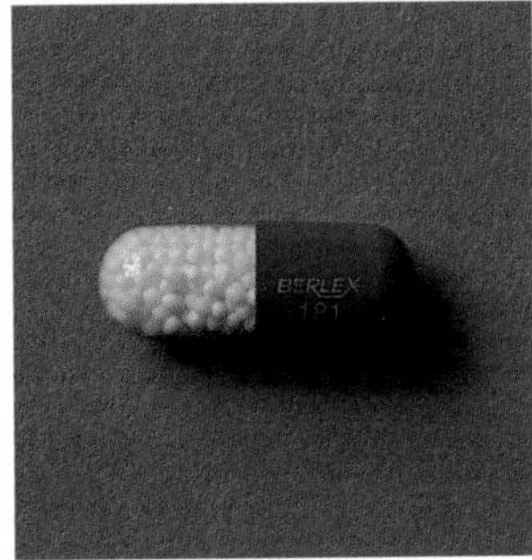

Deconamine® SR†
(pseudoephedrine and chlorpheniramine combination)
120 + 8 mg

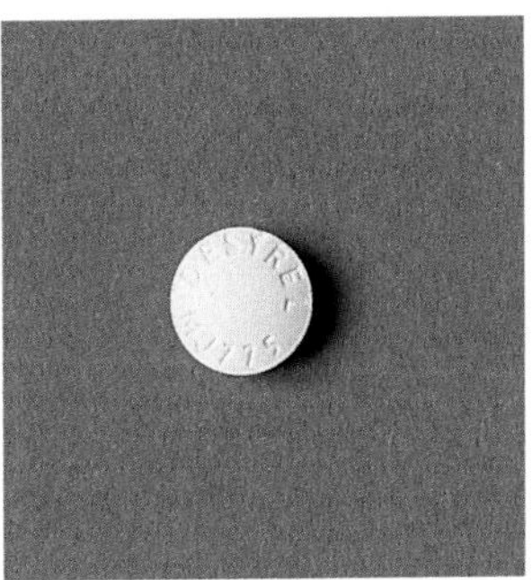

Desyrel®
(trazodone)
50 mg

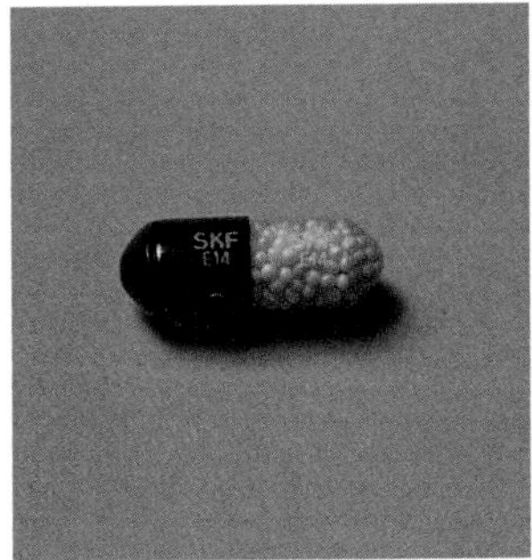

Dexedrine® Spansule®
(dextroamphetamine)
15 mg

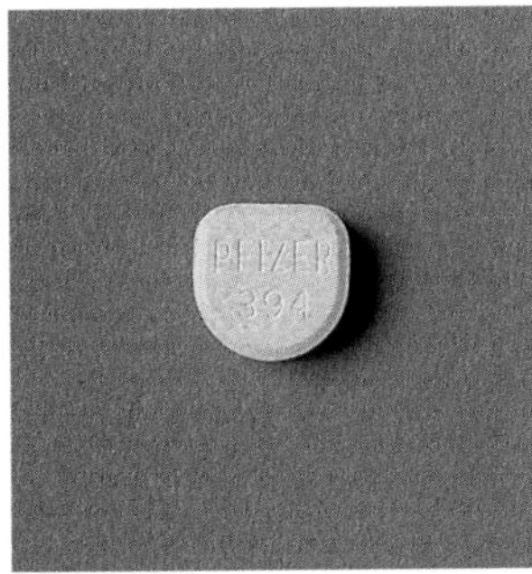

Diabinese®
(chlorpropamide)
250 mg

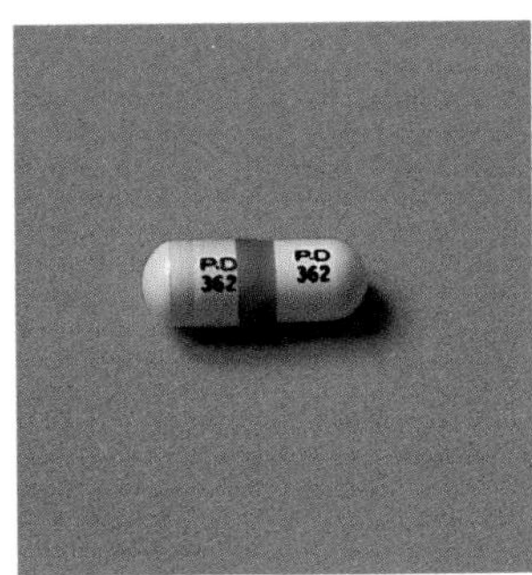

Dilantin® Kapseals®
(phenytoin)
100 mg

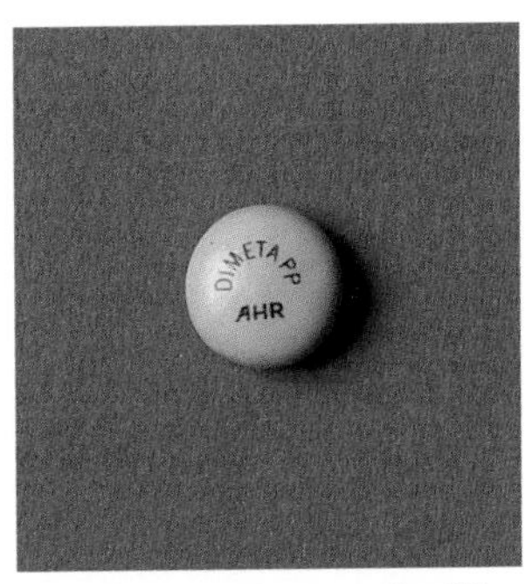

Dimetapp Extentabs®†
(phenylpropanolamine and brompheniramine combination)
75 + 12 mg

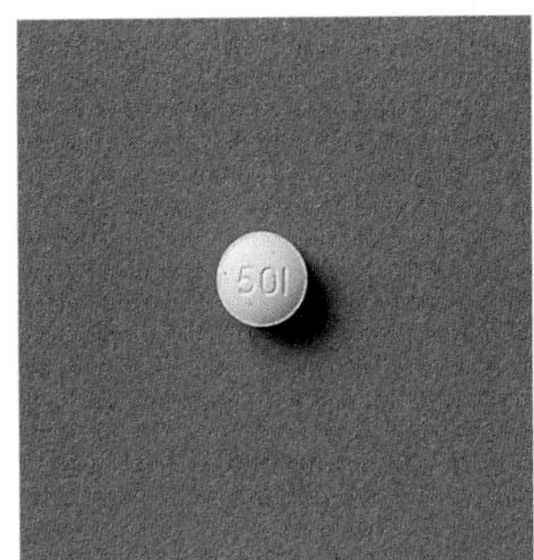

Diulo®
(metolazone)
2.5 mg

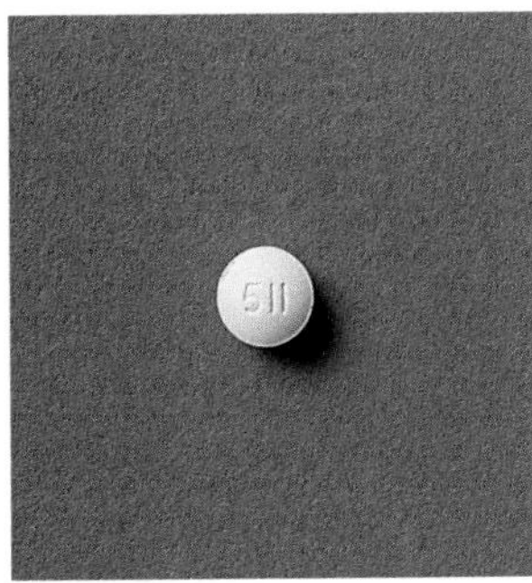

Diulo®
(metolazone)
5 mg

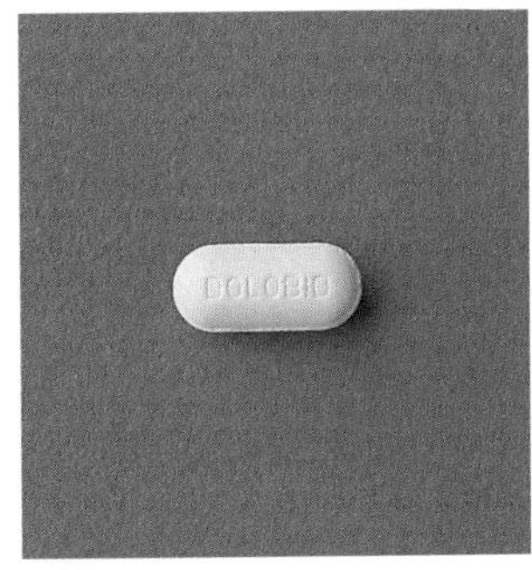

Dolobid®
(diflunisal)
250 mg

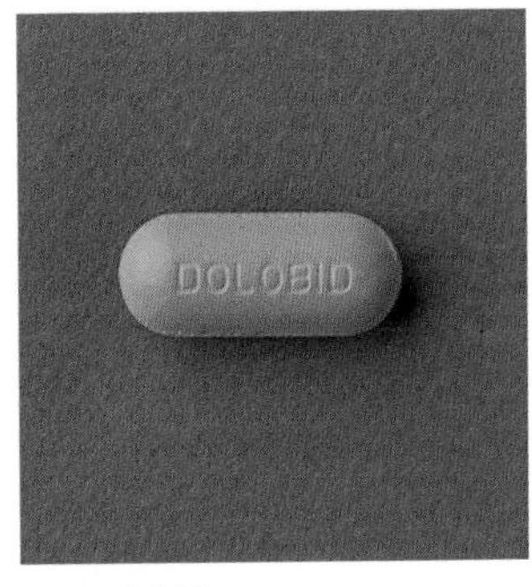

Dolobid®
(diflunisal)
500 mg

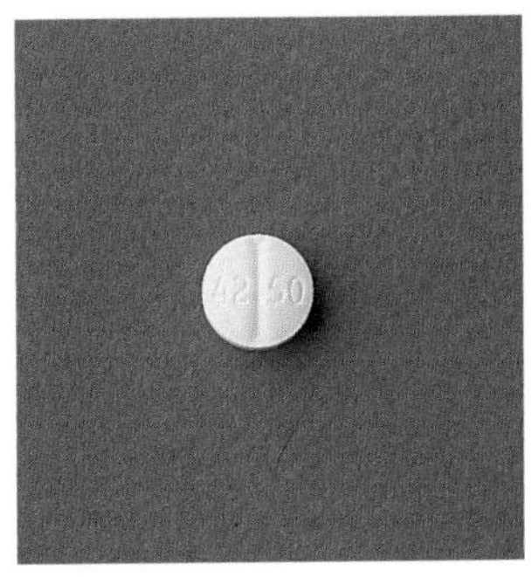

Donnatal®†
(atropine, scopolamine, hyoscyamine, and phenobarbital combination)
0.0194 + 0.0065 + 0.1037 + 16.2

†Drug contains multiple ingredients; ingredients and quantities are listed respectively.

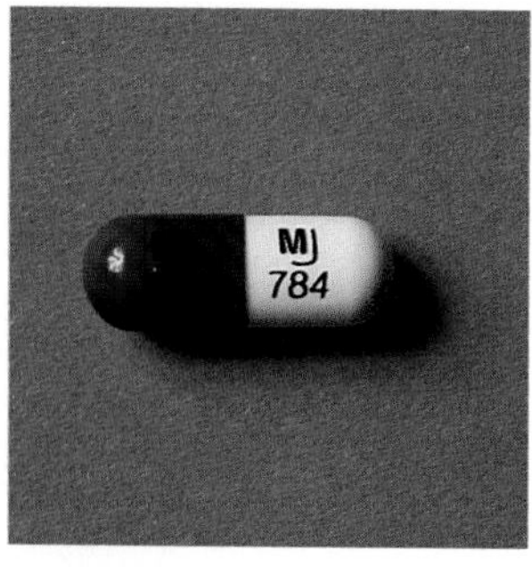

Duricef®
(cefadroxil)
500 mg

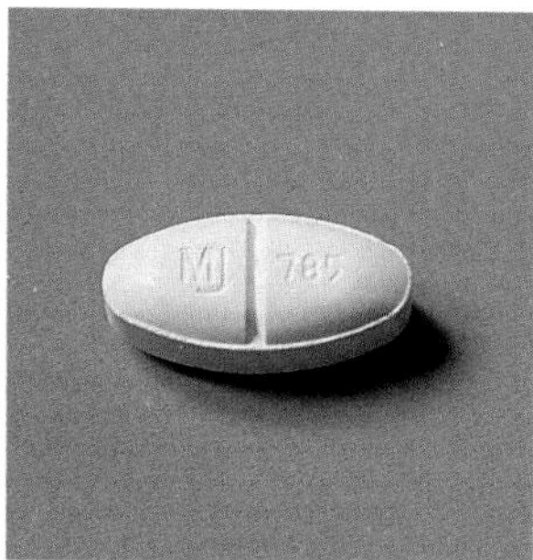

Duricef®
(cefadroxil)
1 g

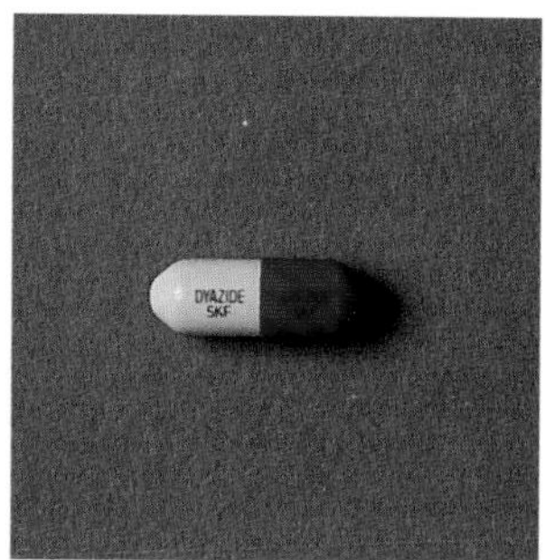

Dyazide®†
(triamterene and hydrochlorothiazide combination)
50 + 25 mg

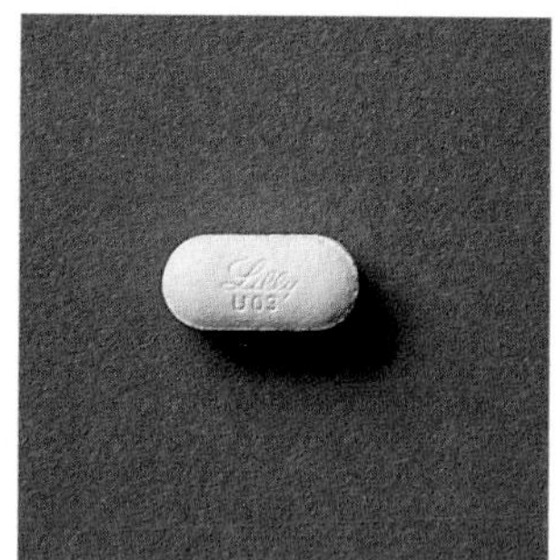

Dymelor®
(acetohexamide)
250 mg

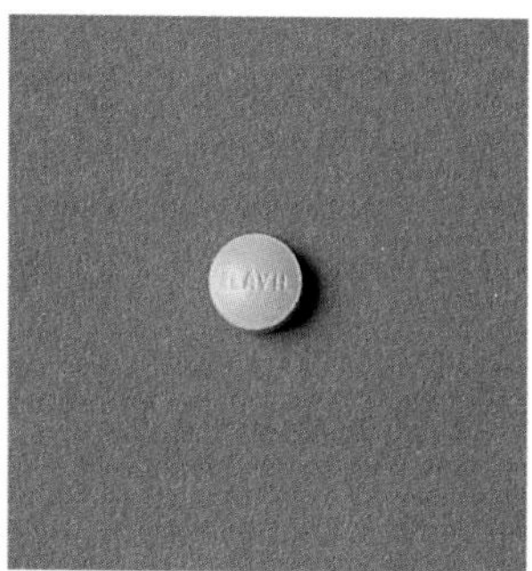

Elavil®
(amitriptyline)
10 mg

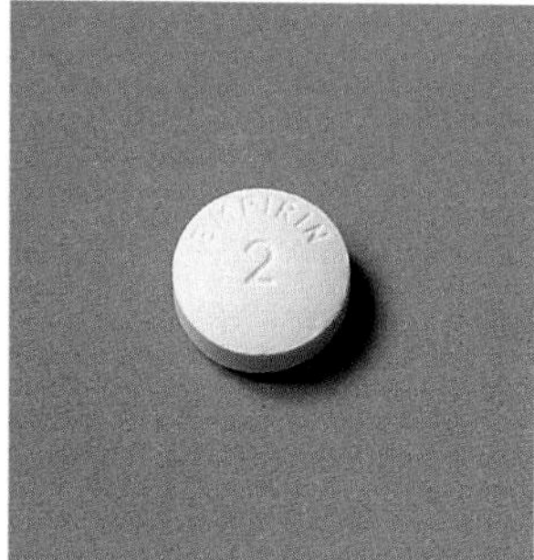

Empirin® with Codeine No. 2†
(aspirin and codeine combination)
325 + 15 mg

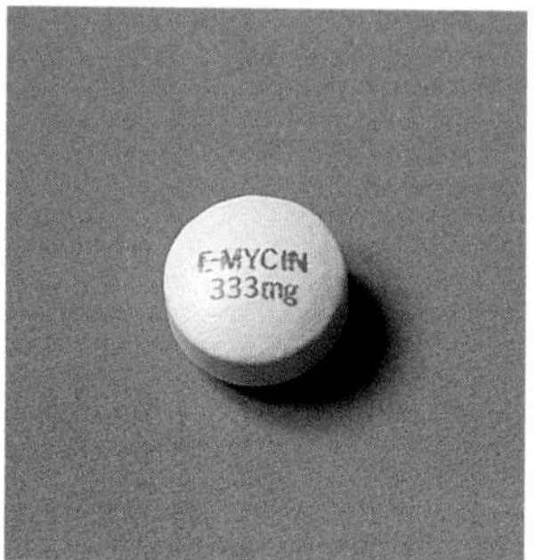

E-Mycin®
(erythromycin)
333 mg

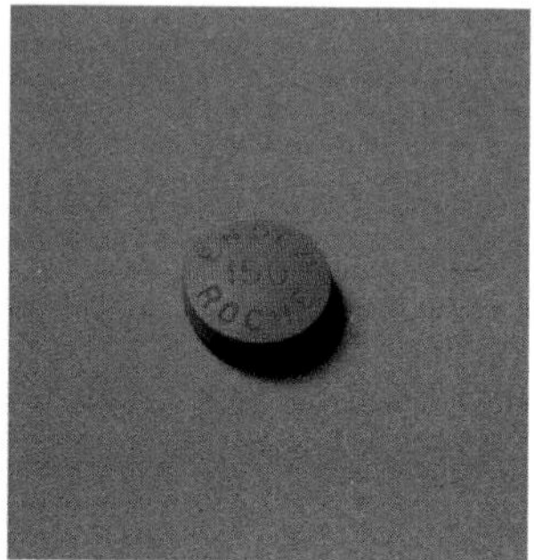

Endep®
(amitriptyline)
150 mg

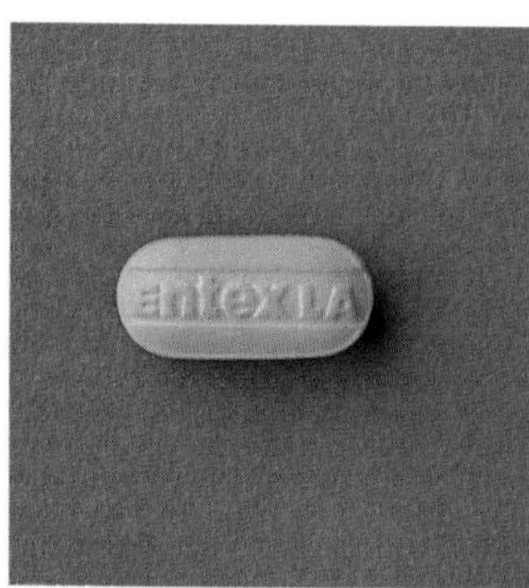

Entex® LA†
(phenylpropanolamine and guaifenesin combination)
75 + 400 mg

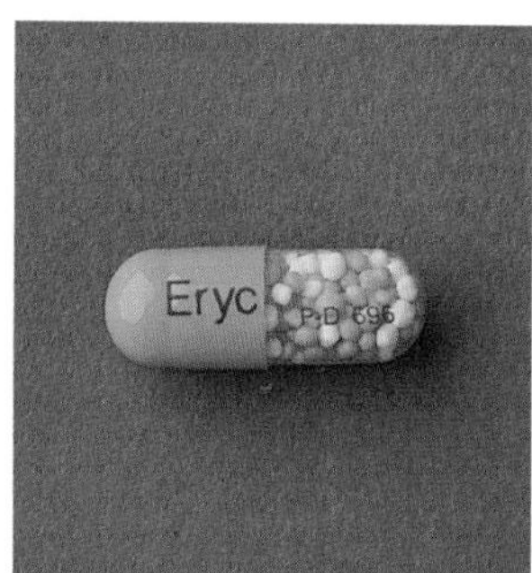

Eryc®
(erythromycin)
250 mg

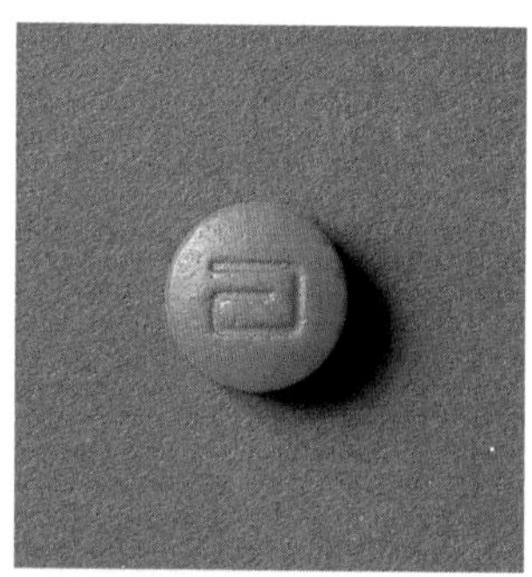

Erythrocin® Stearate Filmtab®
(erythromycin)
250 mg

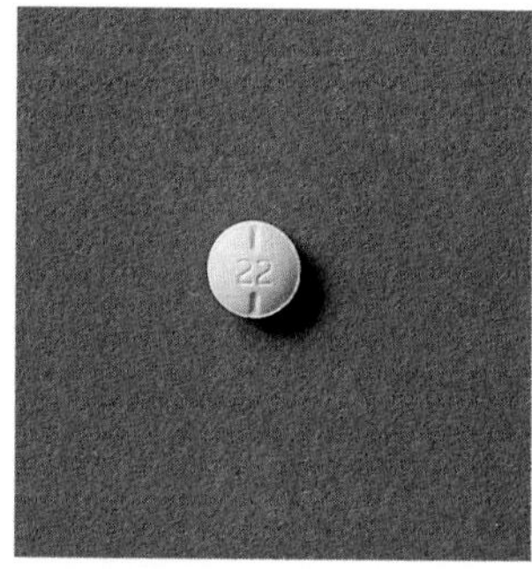

Esidrix®
(hydrochlorothiazide)
25 mg

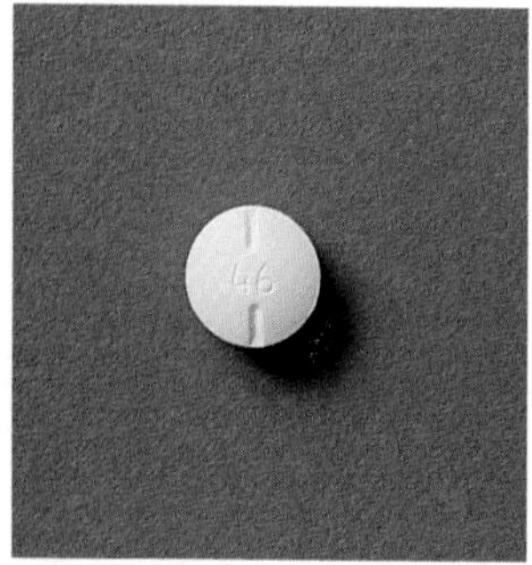

Esidrix®
(hydrochlorothiazide)
50 mg

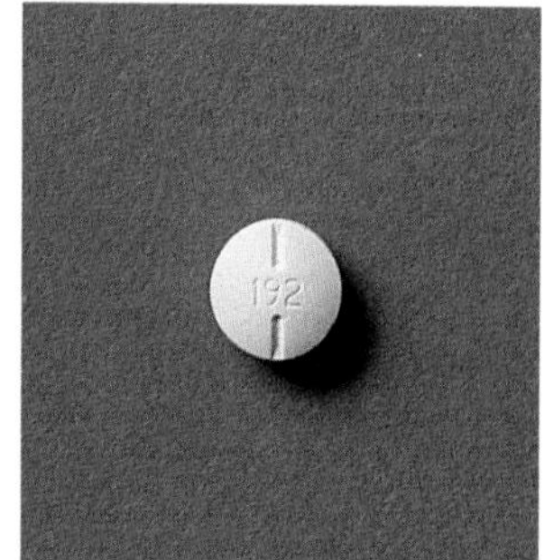

Esidrix®
(hydrochlorothiazide)
100 mg

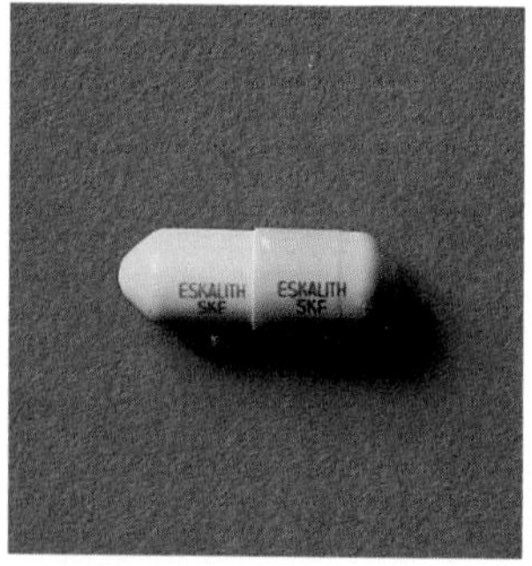

Eskalith®
(lithium)
300 mg

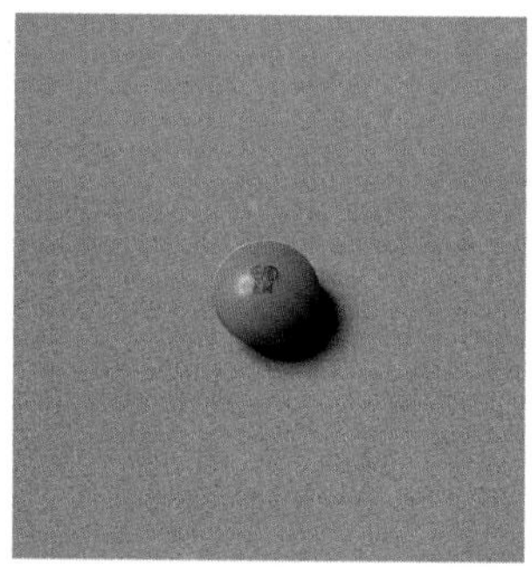

Estinyl®
(ethinyl estradiol)
0.05 mg

†Drug contains multiple ingredients; ingredients and quantities are listed respectively.

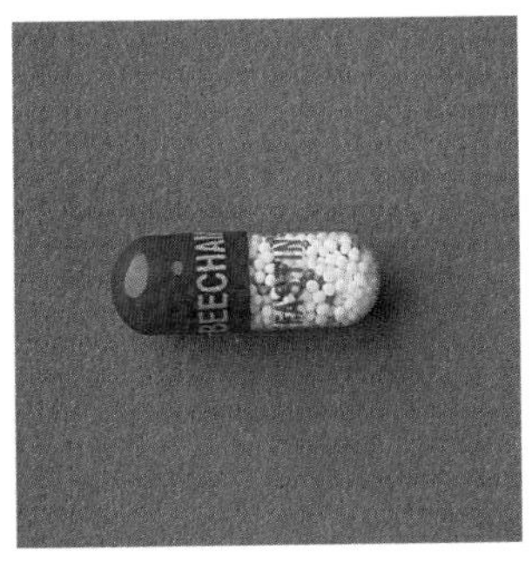

Fastin®
(phentermine)
30 mg

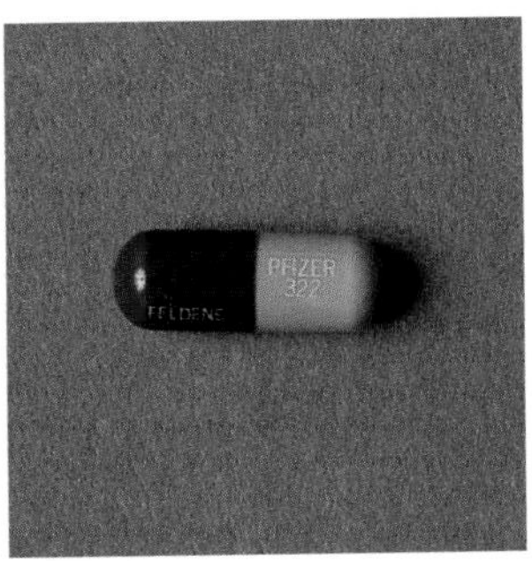

Feldene®
(piroxicam)
10 mg

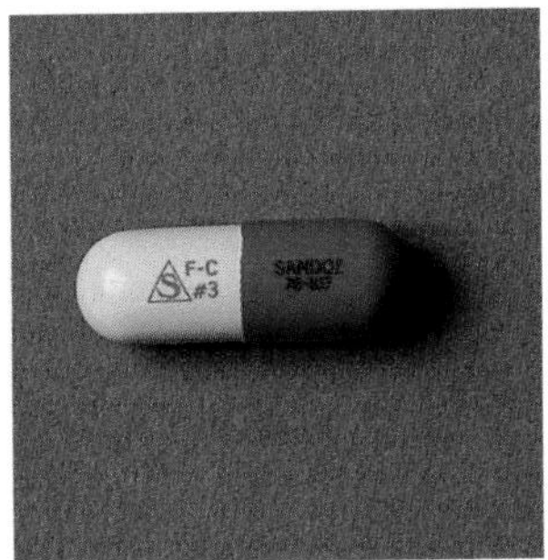

Fiorinal® with Codeine No. 3† (aspirin, caffeine, butalbital, and codeine combination)
325 + 40 + 50 + 30 mg

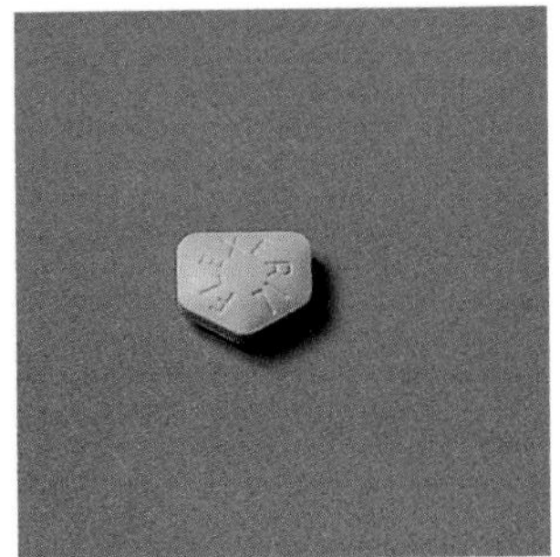

Flexeril®
(cyclobenzaprine)
10 mg

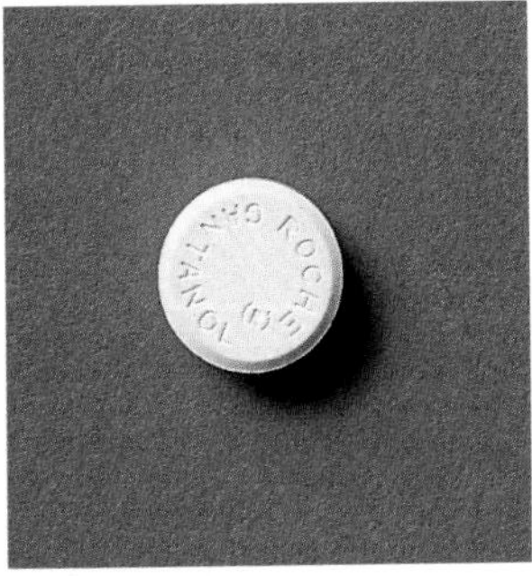

Gantanol®
(sulfamethoxazole)
500 mg

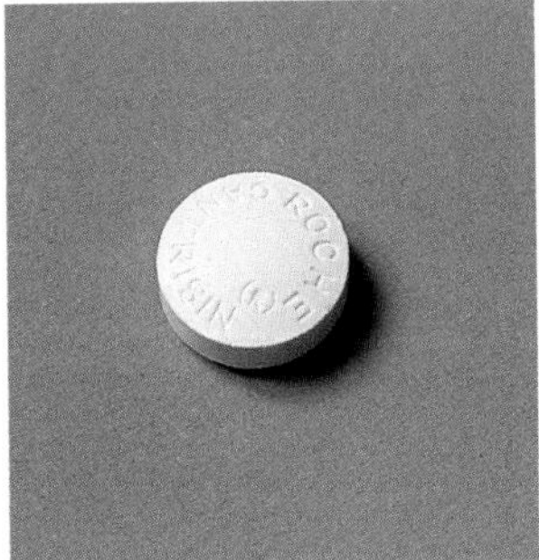

Gantrisin®
(sulfisoxazole)
500 mg

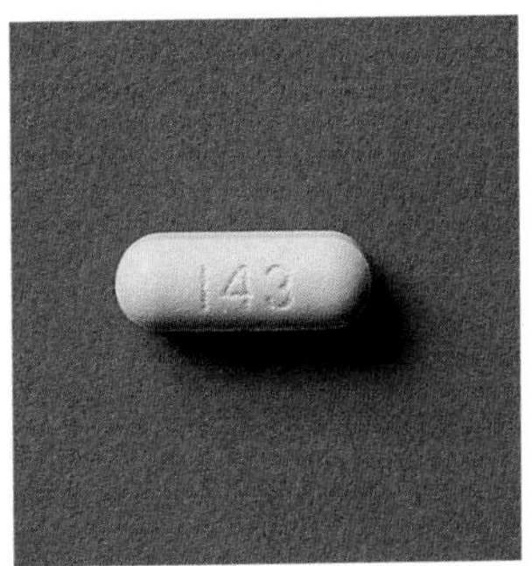

Geocillin®
(carbenicillin)
382 mg

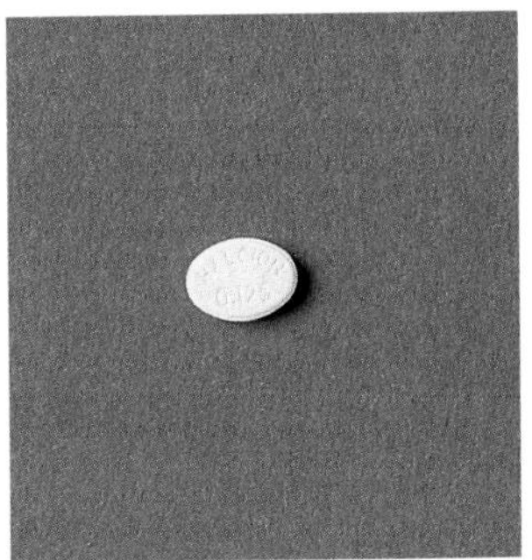

Halcion®
(triazolam)
0.125 mg

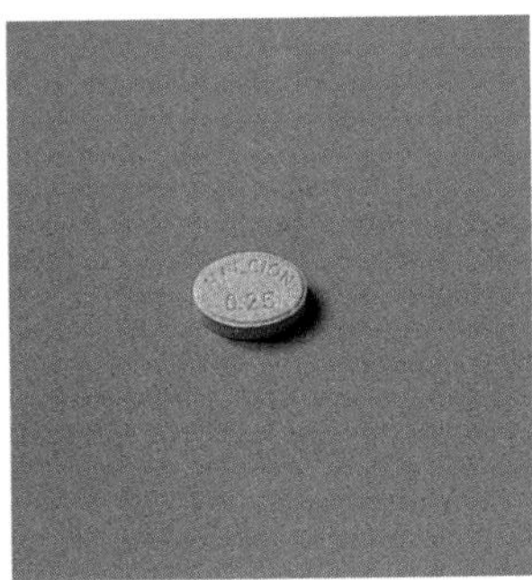

Halcion®
(triazolam)
0.25 mg

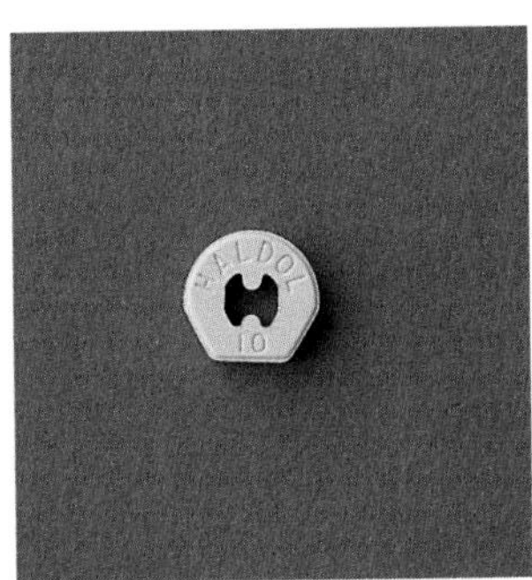

Haldol®
(haloperidol)
10 mg

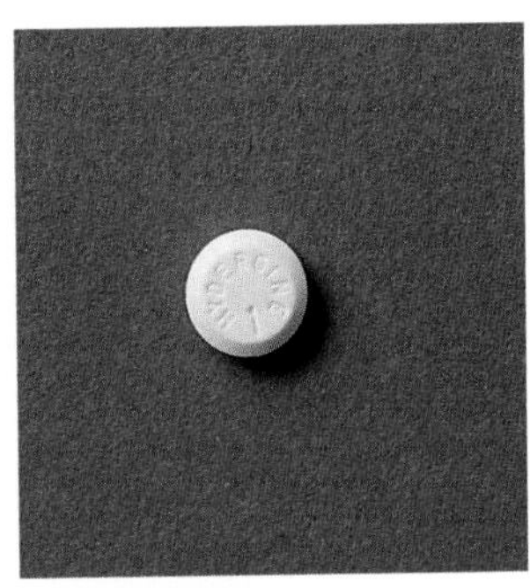

Hydergine®
(ergoloid mesylates)
1 mg

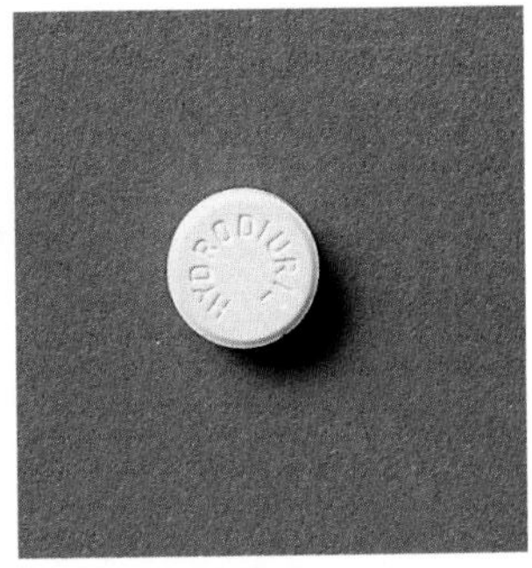

HydroDIURIL®
(hydrochlorothiazide)
100 mg

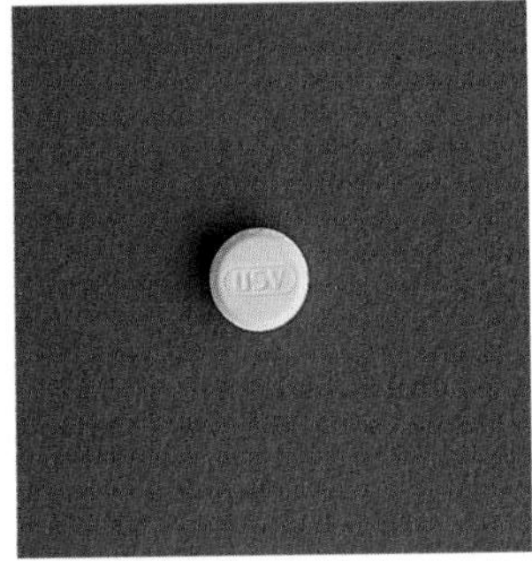

Hygroton®
(chlorthalidone)
100 mg

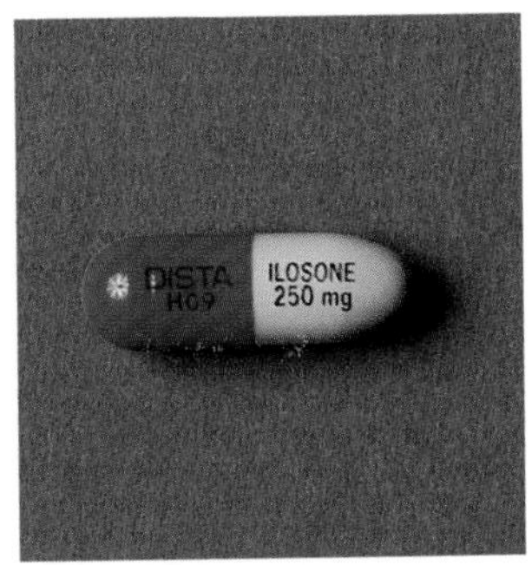

Ilosone® Pulvules
(erythromycin)
250 mg

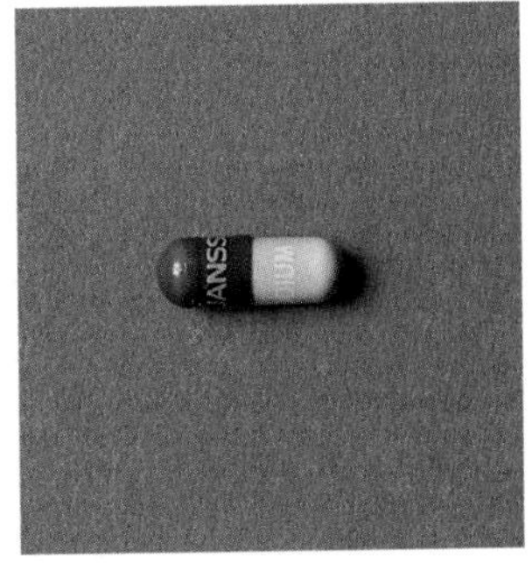

Imodium®
(loperamide)
2 mg

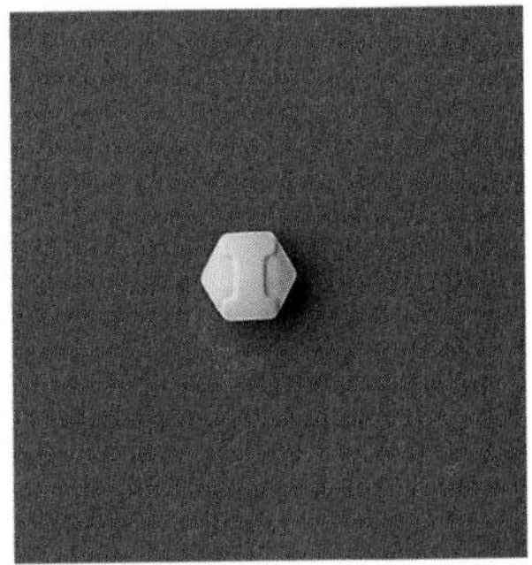

Inderal®
(propranolol)
10 mg

†Drug contains multiple ingredients; ingredients and quantities are listed respectively.

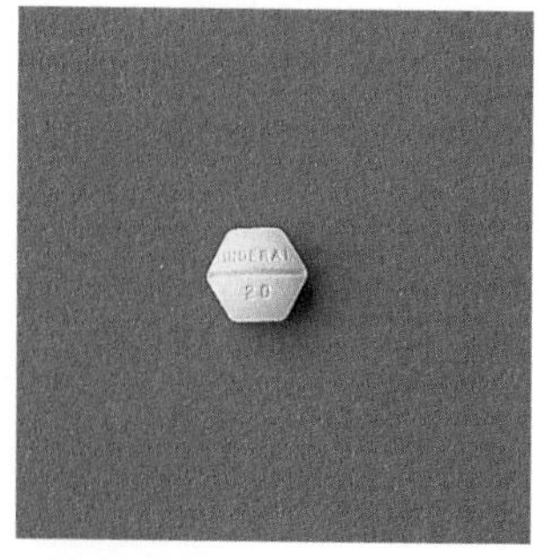

Inderal®
(propranolol)
20 mg

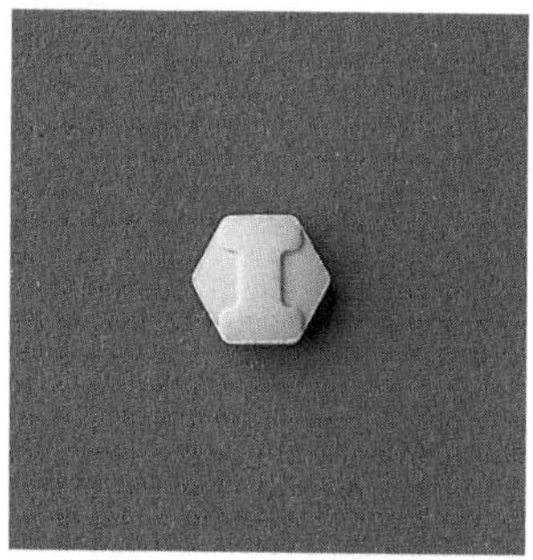

Inderal®
(propranolol)
40 mg

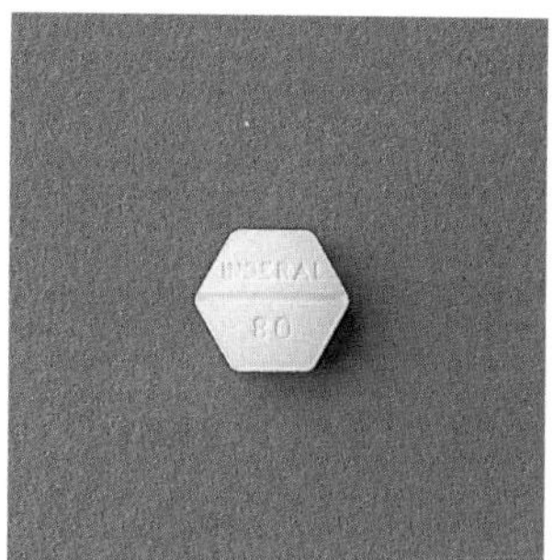

Inderal®
(propranolol)
80 mg

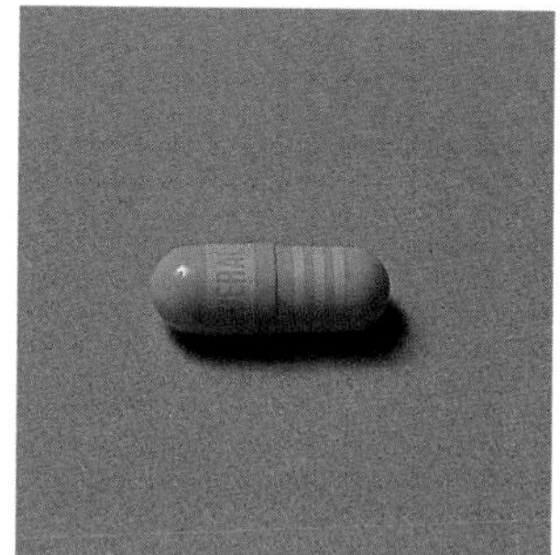

Inderal® LA
(propranolol)
80 mg

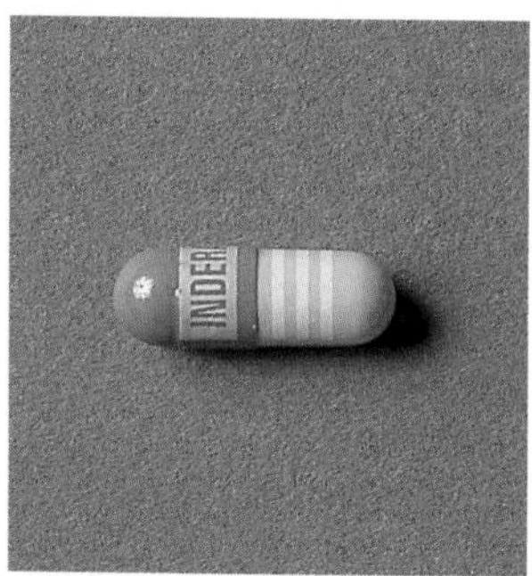

Inderal® LA
(propranolol)
120 mg

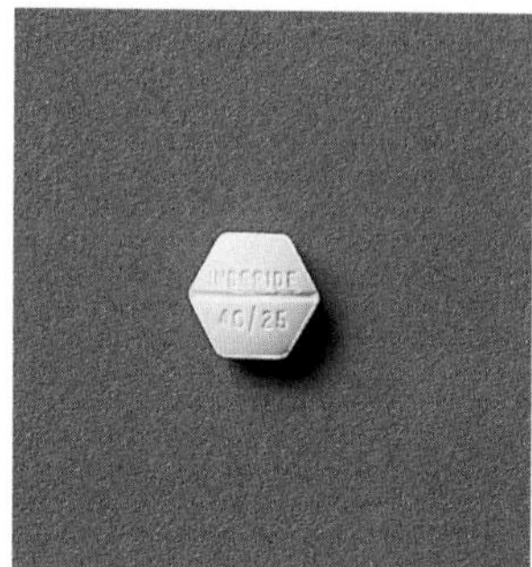

Inderide®†
(propranolol and hydrochlorothiazide combination)
40 + 25 mg

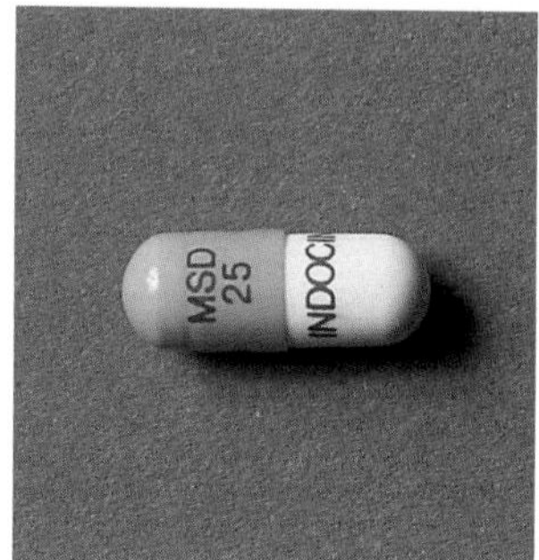

Indocin®
(indomethacin)
25 mg

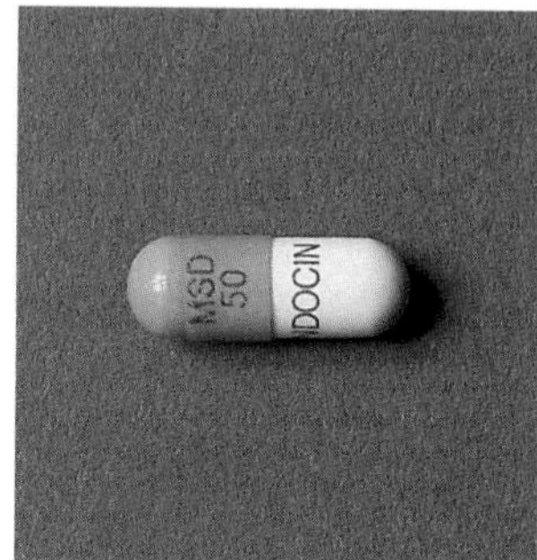

Indocin®
(indomethacin)
50 mg

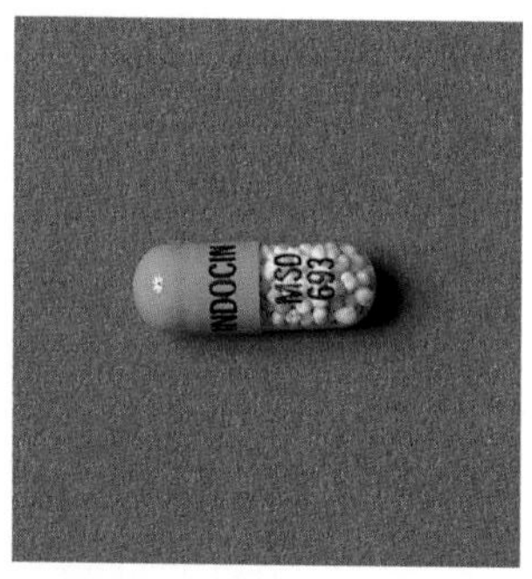

Indocin® SR
(indomethacin)
75 mg

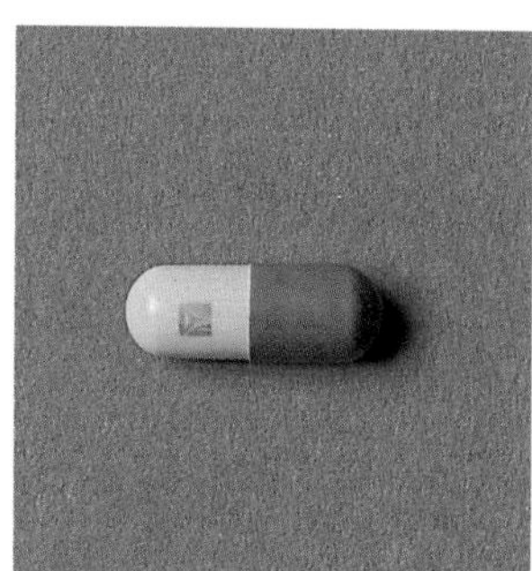

Ionamin®
(phentermine)
15 mg

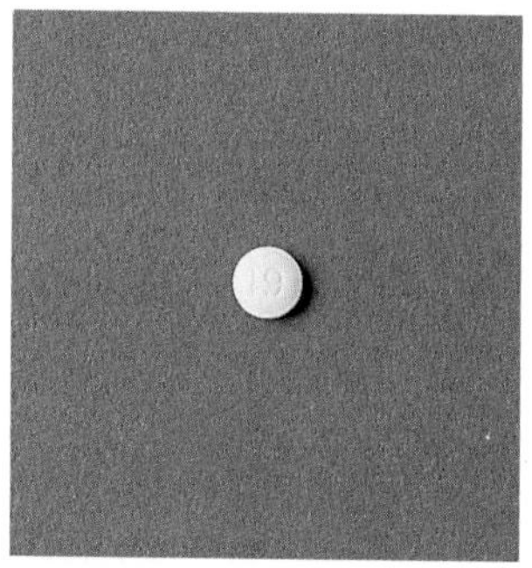

Isordil®
(isosorbide dinitrate)
5 mg

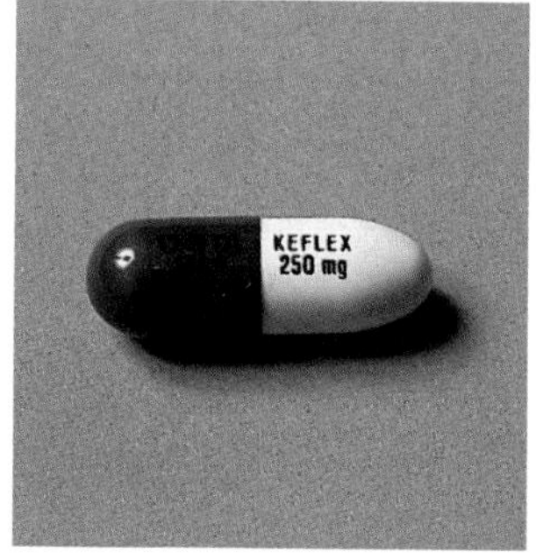

Keflex®
(cephalexin)
250 mg

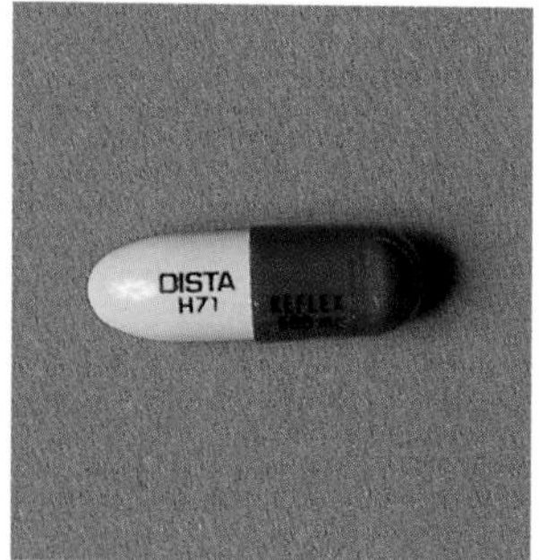

Keflex®
(cephalexin)
500 mg

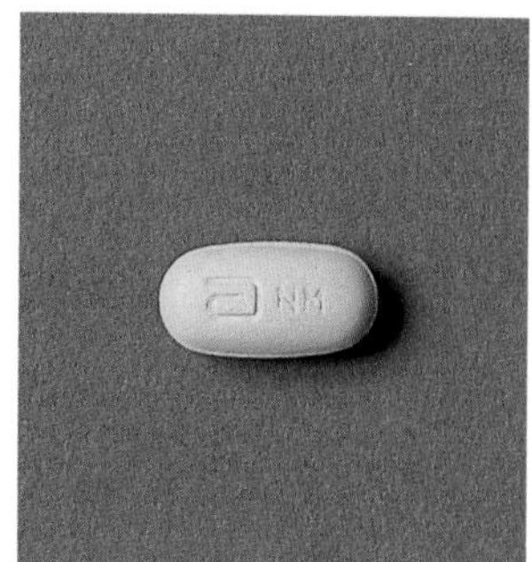

K-Tab®
(potassium chloride)
750 mg

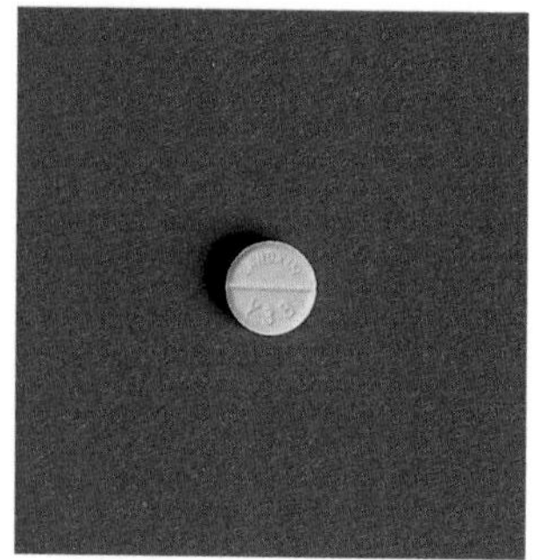

Lanoxin®
(digoxin)
0.125 mg

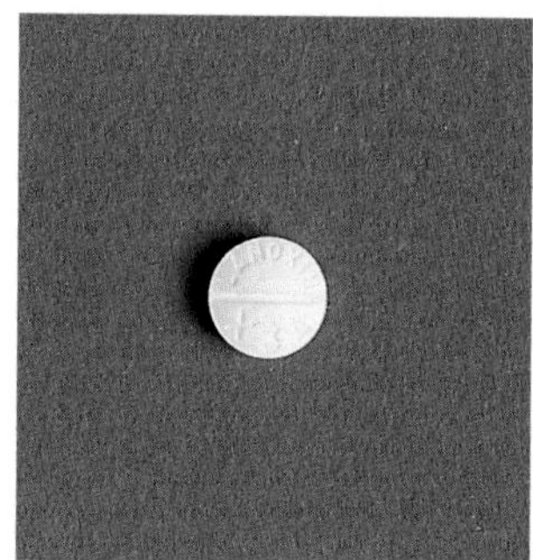

Lanoxin®
(digoxin)
0.25 mg

†Drug contains multiple ingredients; ingredients and quantities are listed respectively.

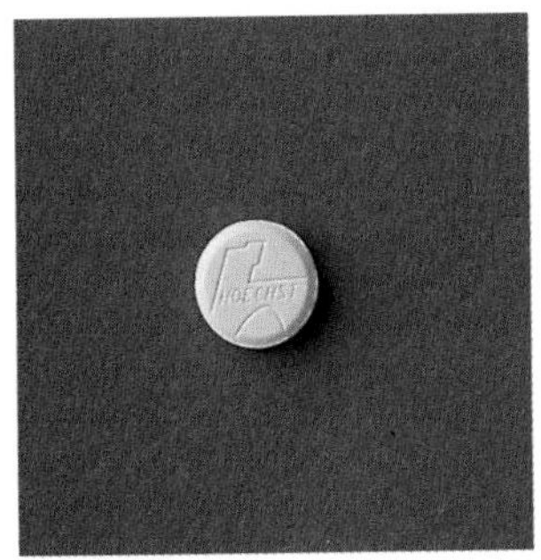

Lasix®
(furosemide)
40 mg

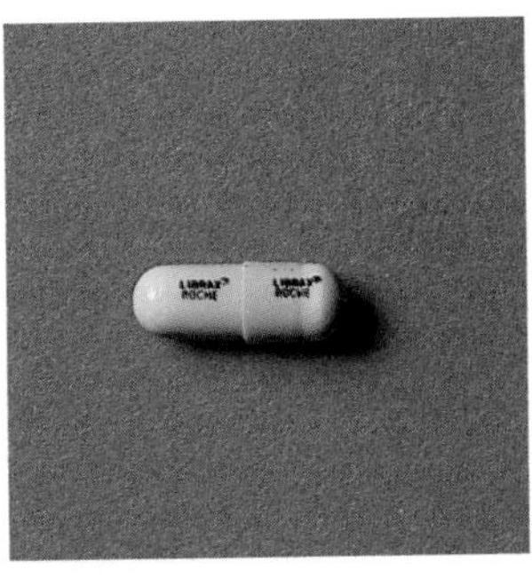

Librax®†
(chlordiazepoxide and clidinium combination)
5 + 2.5 mg

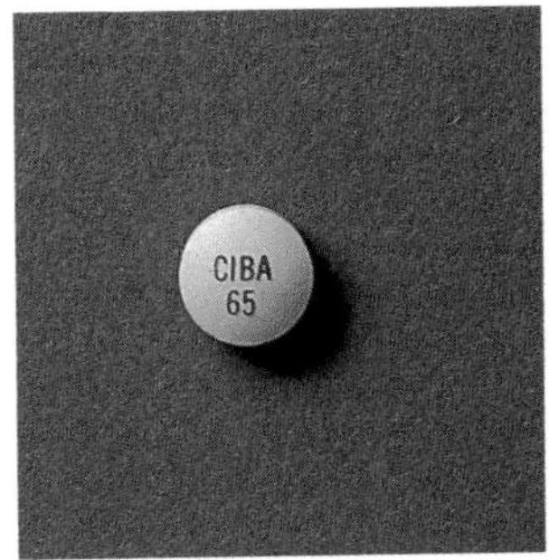

Lithobid®
(lithium)
300 mg

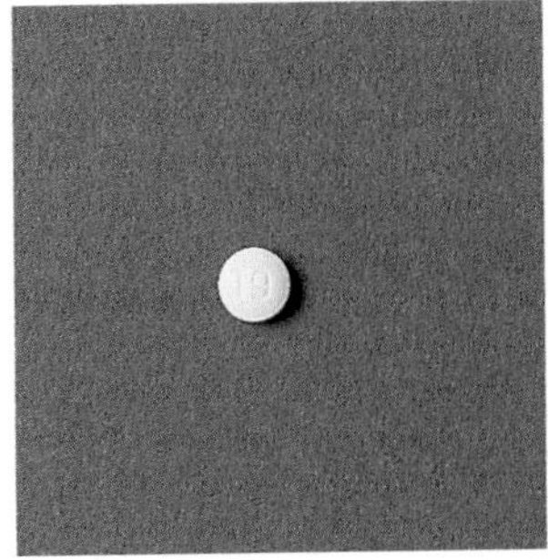

Lomotil®†
(diphenoxylate and atropine combination)
2.5 + 0.025 mg

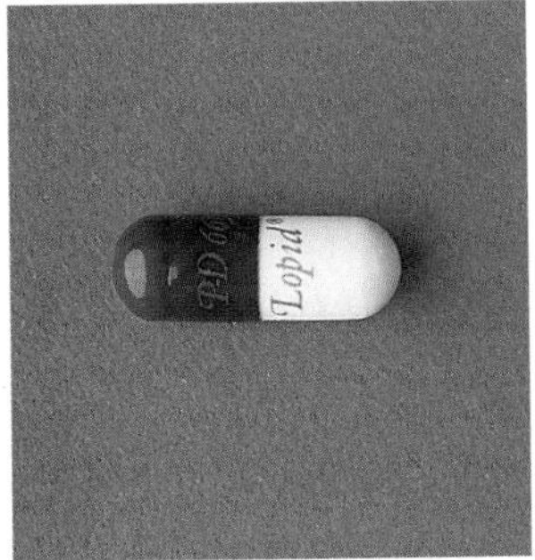

Lopid®
(gemfibrozil)
300 mg

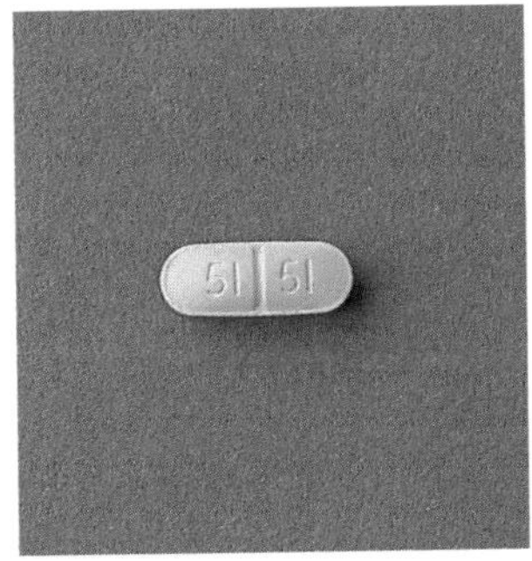

Lopressor®
(metoprolol)
50 mg

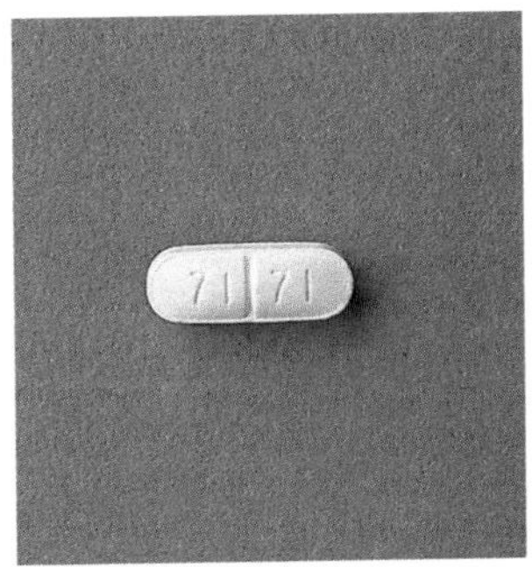

Lopressor®
(metoprolol)
100 mg

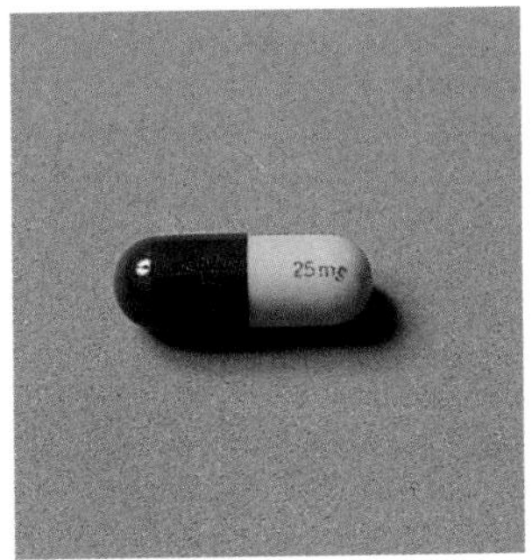

Loxitane®
(loxapine)
25 mg

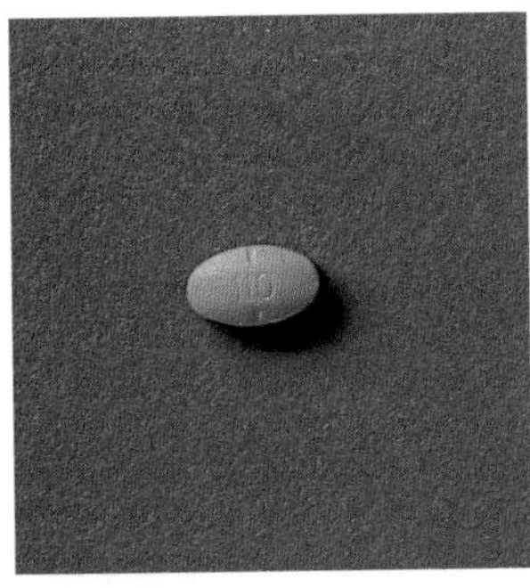

Ludiomil®
(maprotiline)
25 mg

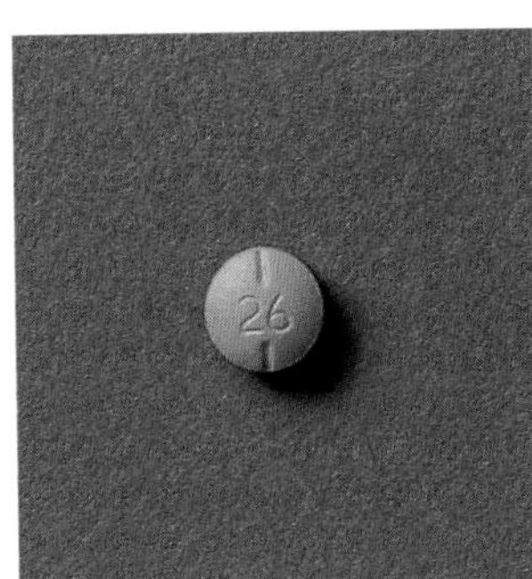

Ludiomil®
(maprotiline)
50 mg

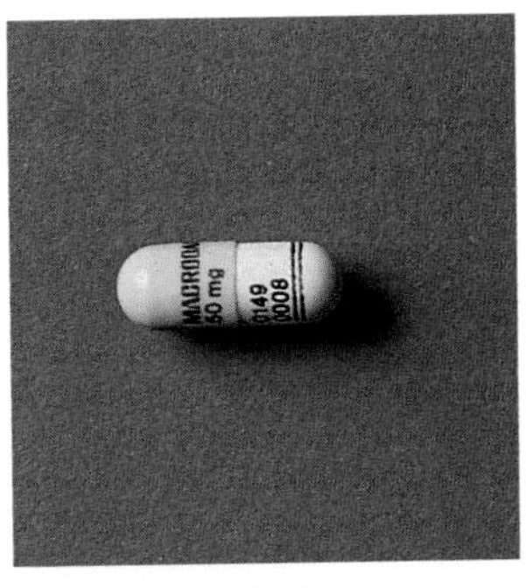

Macrodantin®
(nitrofurantoin)
50 mg

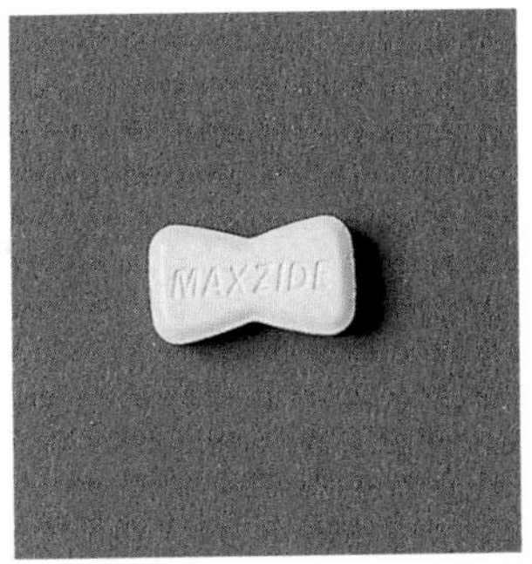

Maxzide®†
(triamterene and hydrochlorothiazide combination)
75 + 50 mg

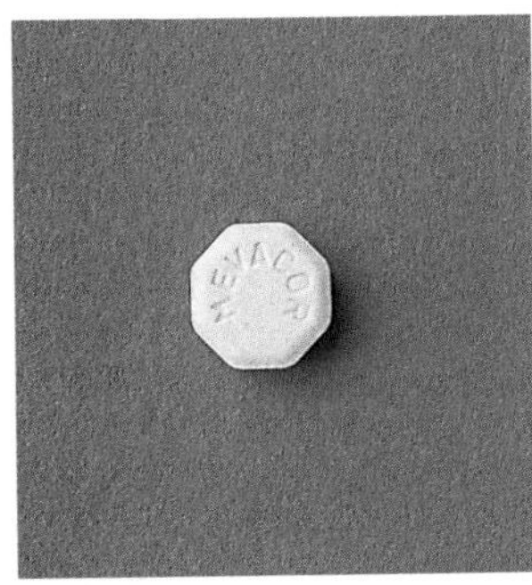

Mevacor®
(lovastatin)
20 mg

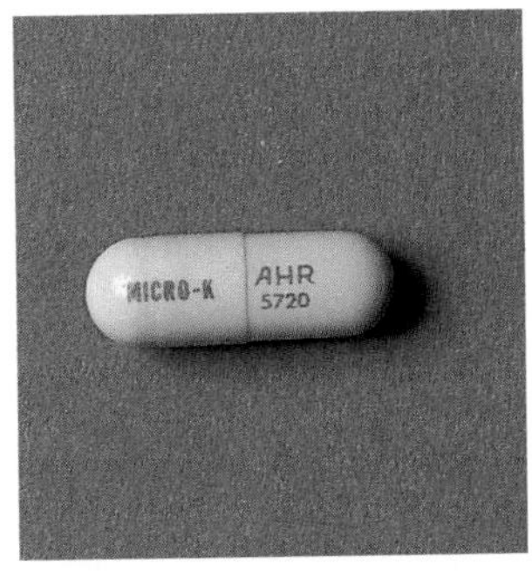

Micro-K Extencaps®
(potassium chloride)
600 mg (8 mEq)

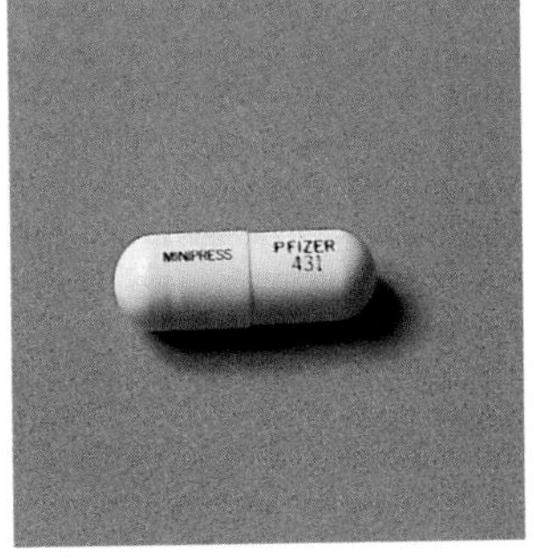

Minipress®
(prazosin)
1 mg

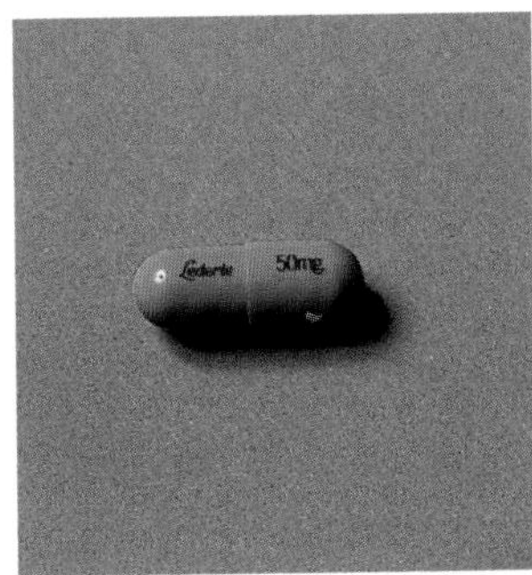

Minocin®
(minocycline)
50 mg

†*Drug contains multiple ingredients; ingredients and quantities are listed respectively.*

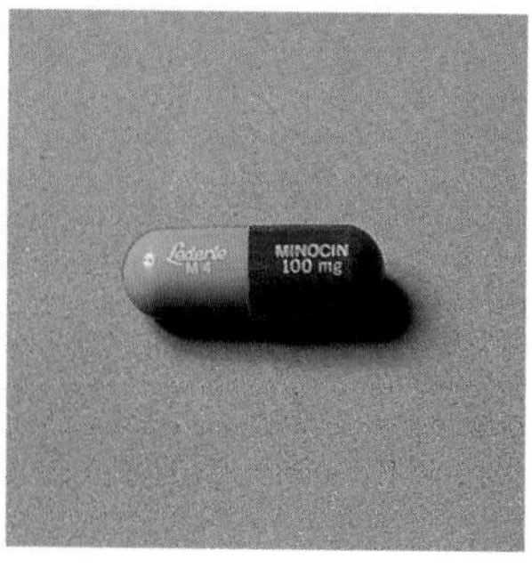

Minocin®
(minocycline)
100 mg

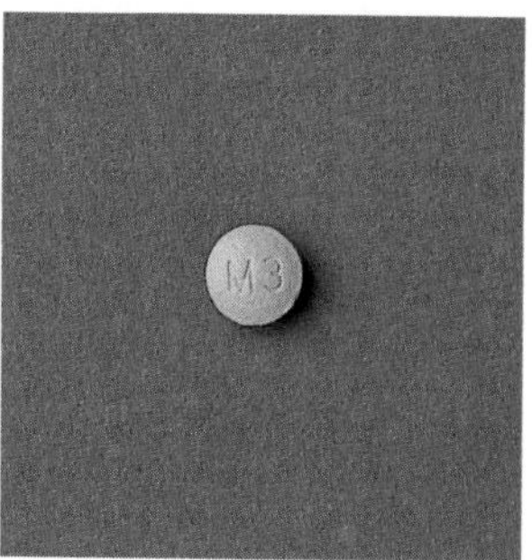

Minocin®
(minocycline)
50 mg

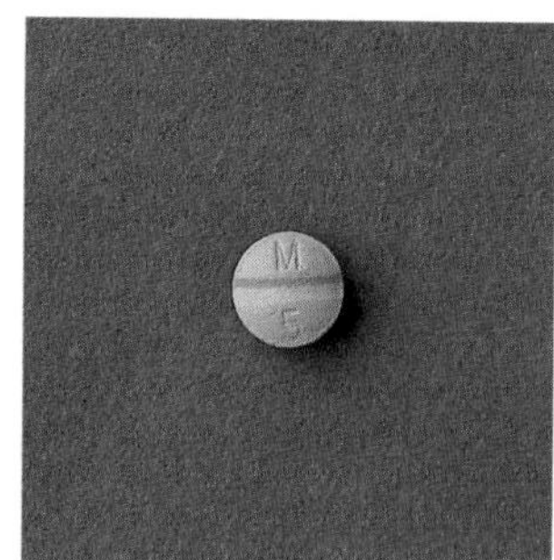

Minocin®
(minocycline)
100 mg

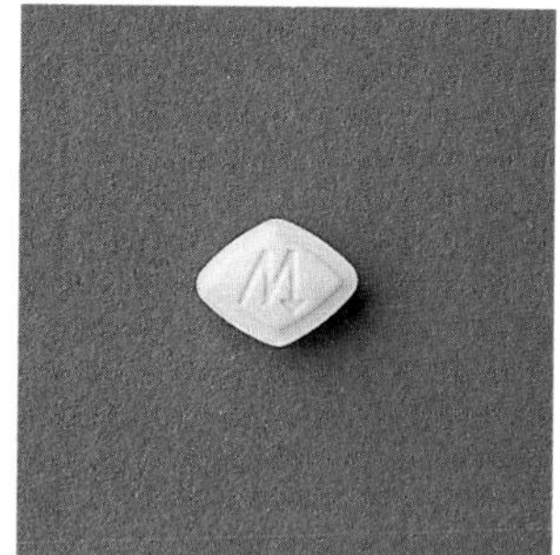

Moduretic®†
(amiloride and hydrochlorothiazide combination)
5 + 50 mg

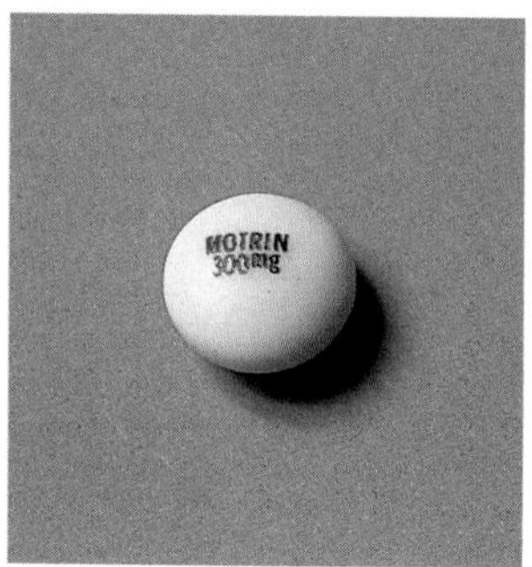

Motrin®
(ibuprofen)
300 mg

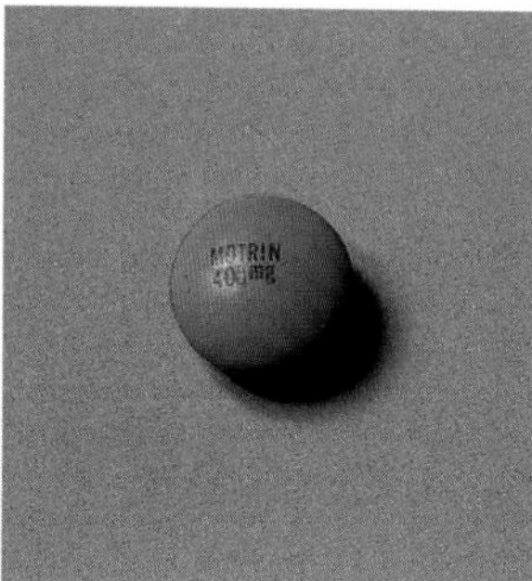

Motrin®
(ibuprofen)
400 mg

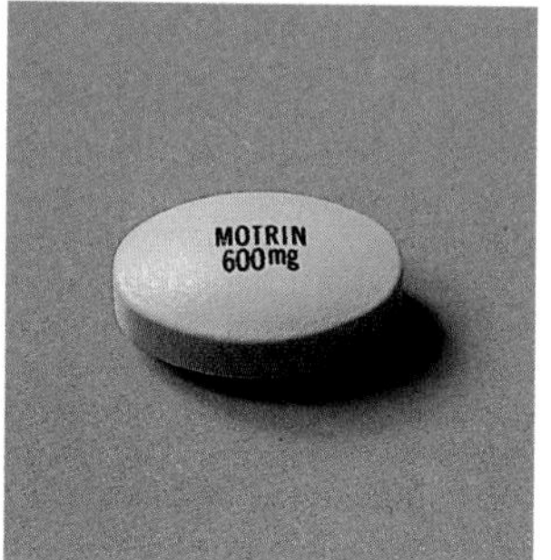

Motrin®
(ibuprofen)
600 mg

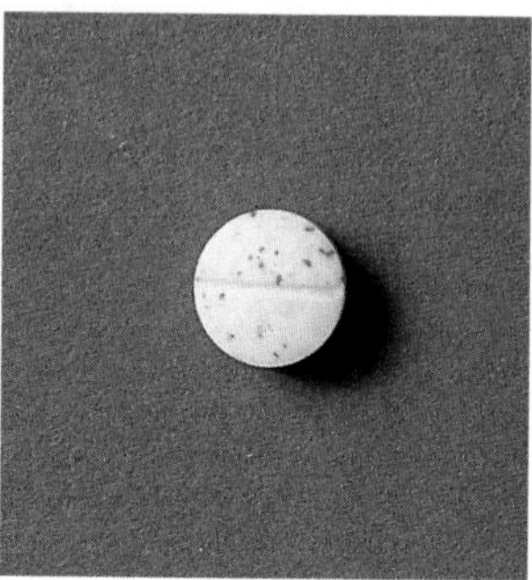

Naldecon®†
(phenylpropanolamine, phenylephrine, chlorpheniramine, and phenyltoloxamine combination)
40 + 10 + 5 + 15 mg

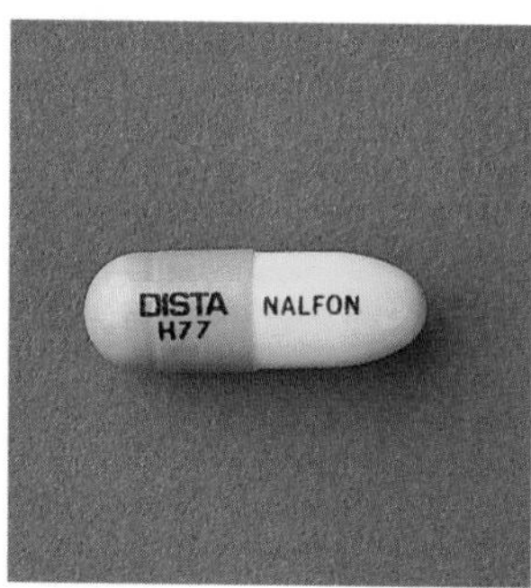

Nalfon®
(fenoprofen)
300 mg

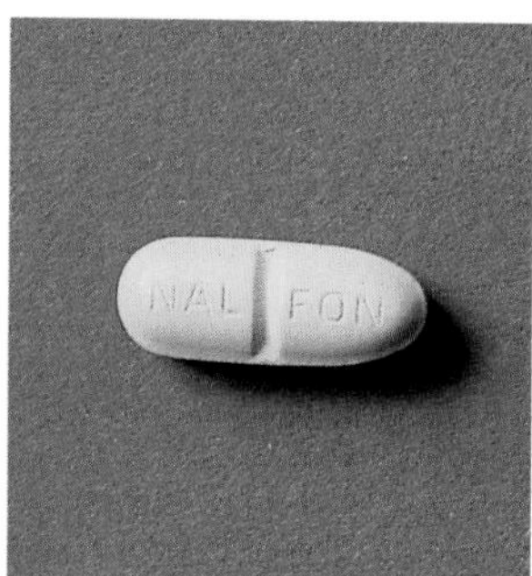

Nalfon®
(fenoprofen)
600 mg

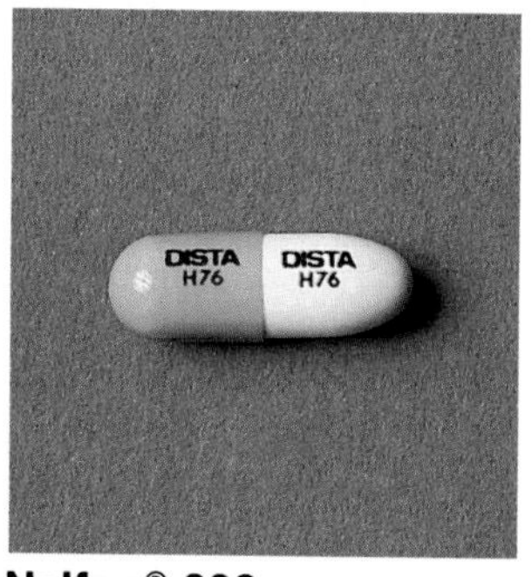

Nalfon® 200
(fenoprofen)
200 mg

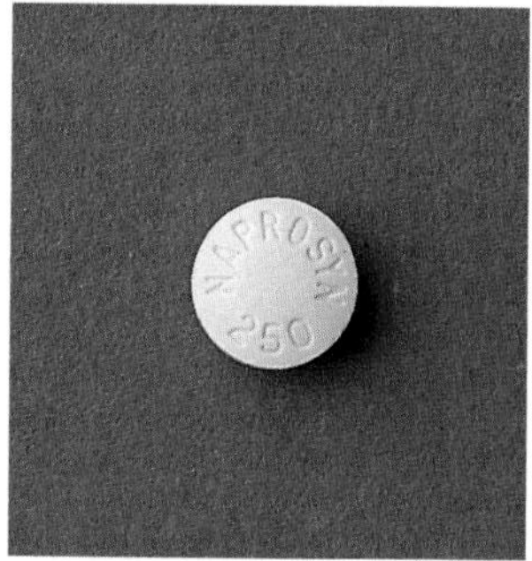

Naprosyn®
(naproxen)
250 mg

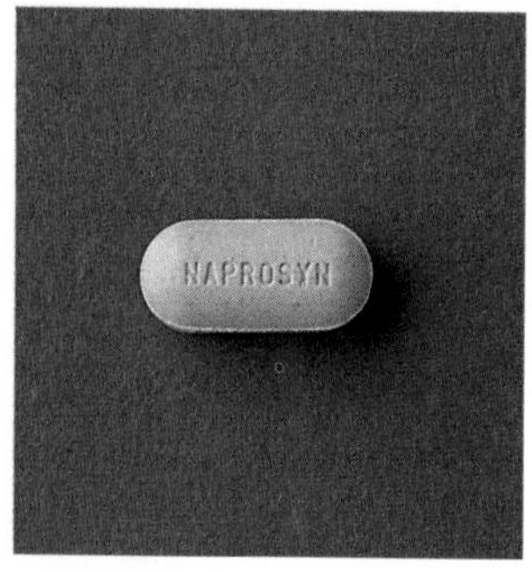

Naprosyn®
(naproxen)
375 mg

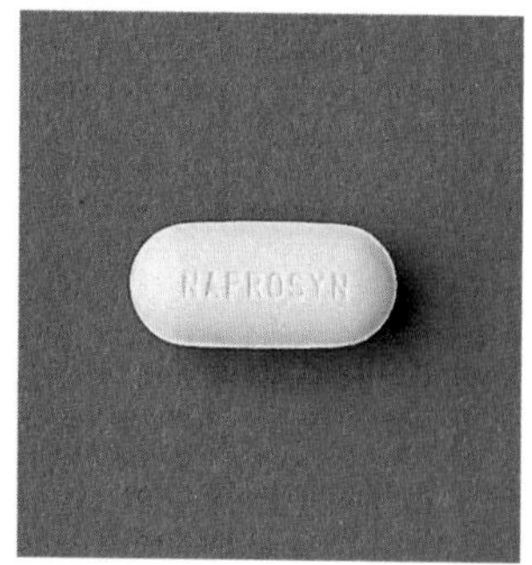

Naprosyn®
(naproxen)
500 mg

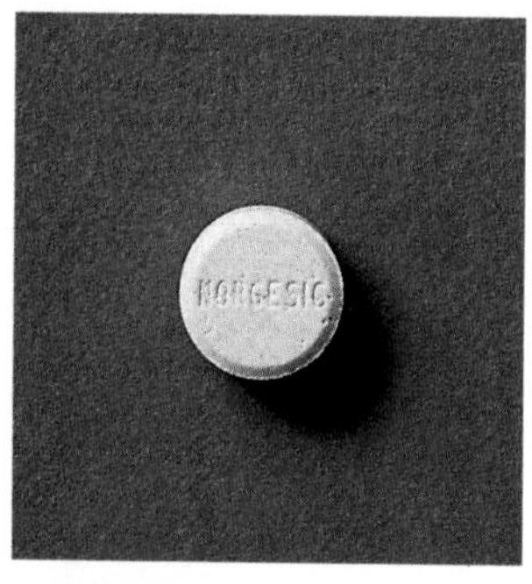

Norgesic®†
(orphenadrine, aspirin, and caffeine combination)
25 + 385 + 30 mg

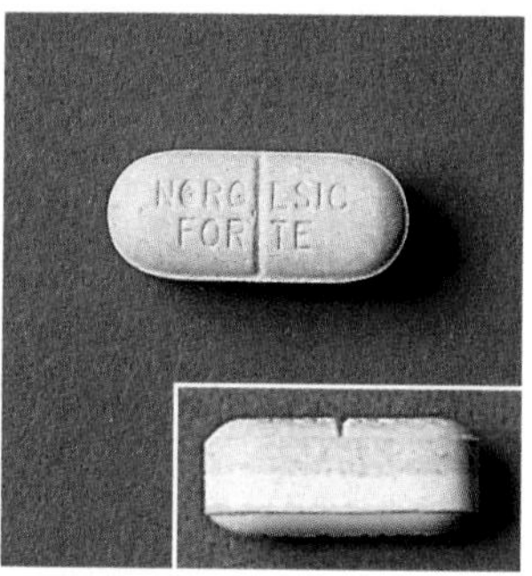

Norgesic® Forte†
(orphenadrine, aspirin, and caffeine combination)
50 + 770 + 60 mg

†Drug contains multiple ingredients; ingredients and quantities are listed respectively.

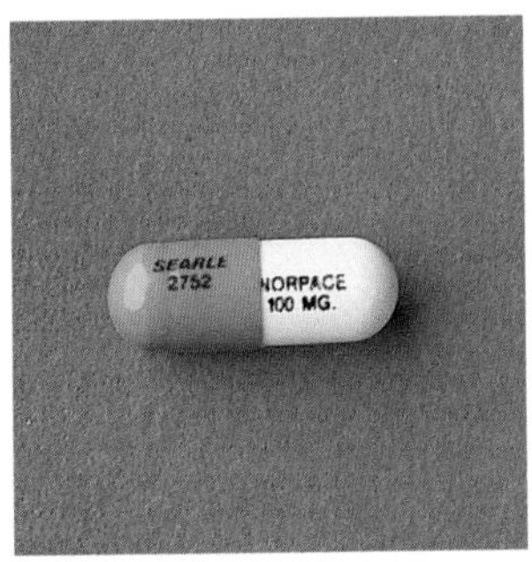

Norpace®
(disopyramide)
100 mg

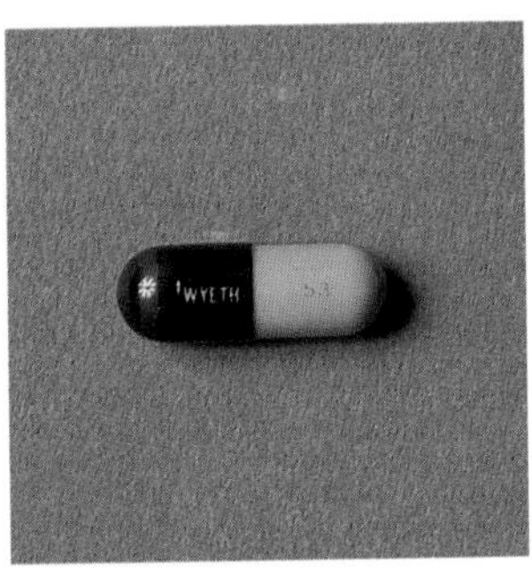

Omnipen®
(ampicillin)
250 mg

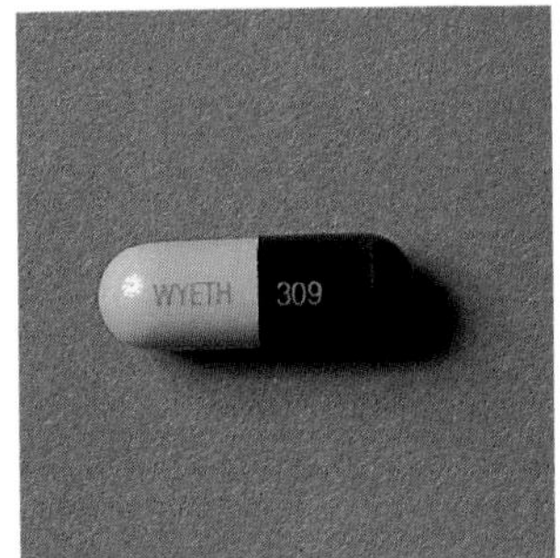

Omnipen®
(ampicillin)
500 mg

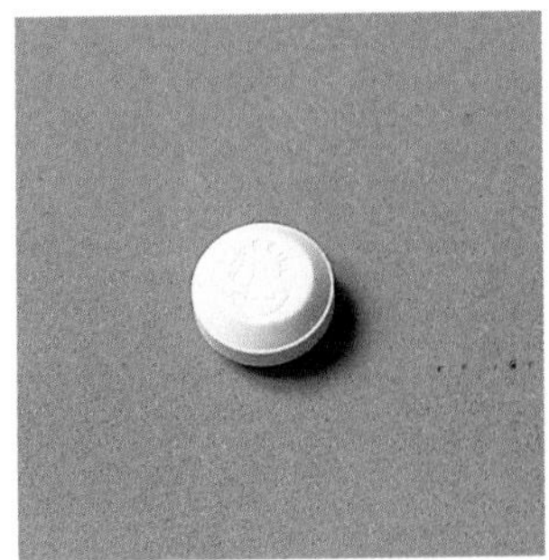

Optimine®
(azatadine)
1 mg

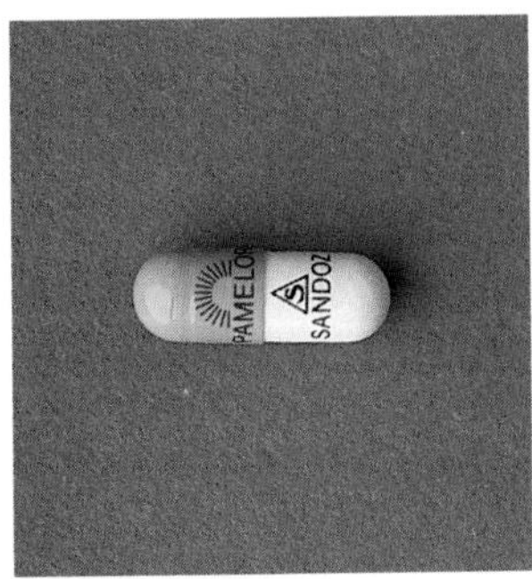

Pamelor®
(nortriptyline)
25 mg

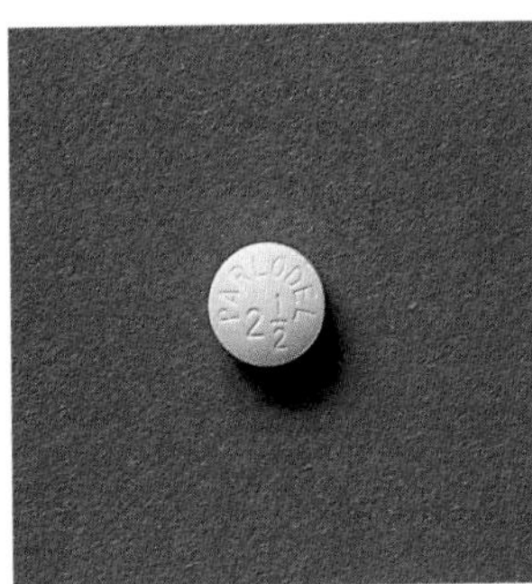

Parlodel® SnapTabs™
(bromocriptine)
2.5 mg

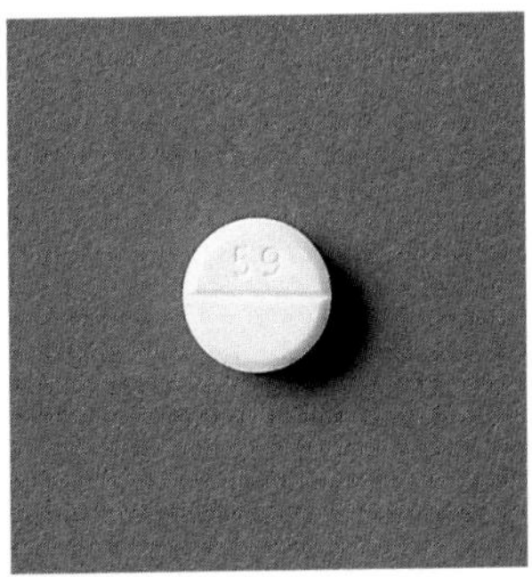

Pen-Vee® K
(penicillin VK)
250 mg

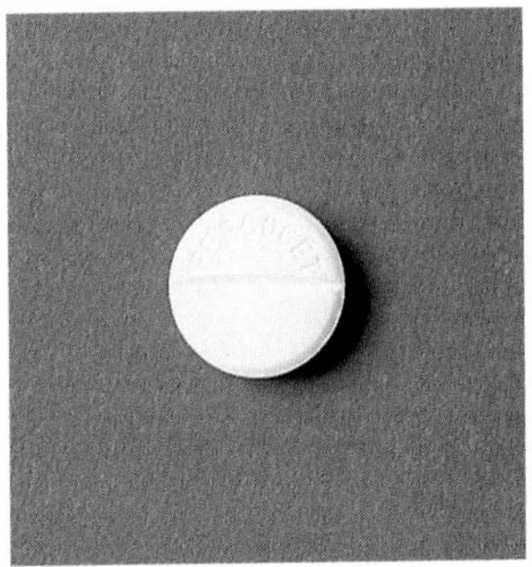

Percocet®†
(acetaminophen and oxycodone combination)
325 + 5 mg

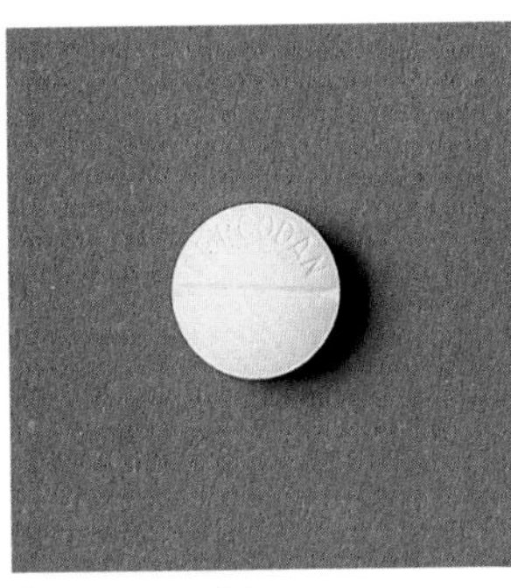

Percodan®†
(aspirin, oxycodone hydrochloride, and oxycodone terephthalate combination) 325 + 4.5 + 0.38 mg

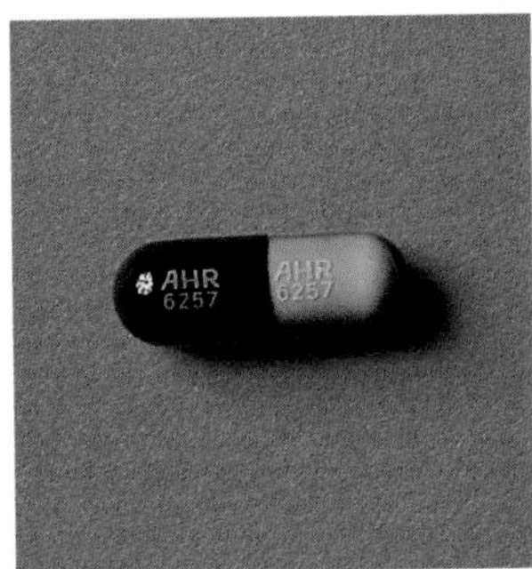

Phenaphen® with Codeine No. 3†
(acetaminophen and codeine combination) 325 + 30 mg

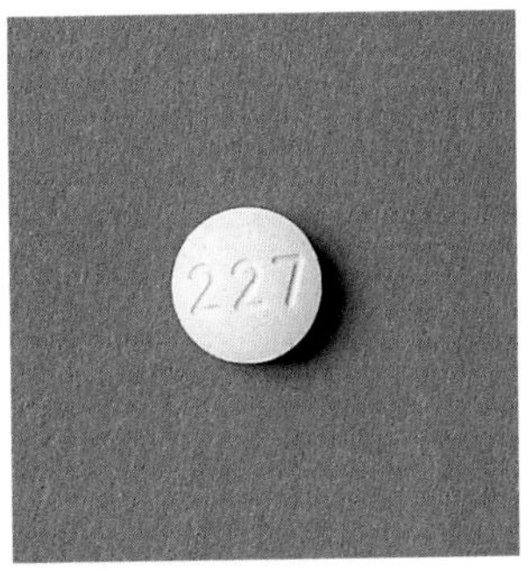

Phenergan®†
(promethazine)
50 mg

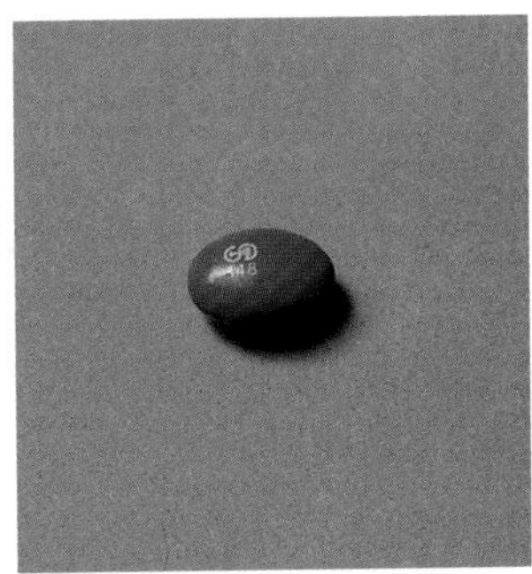

Polaramine® Repetabs®
(dexchlorpheniramine)
6 mg

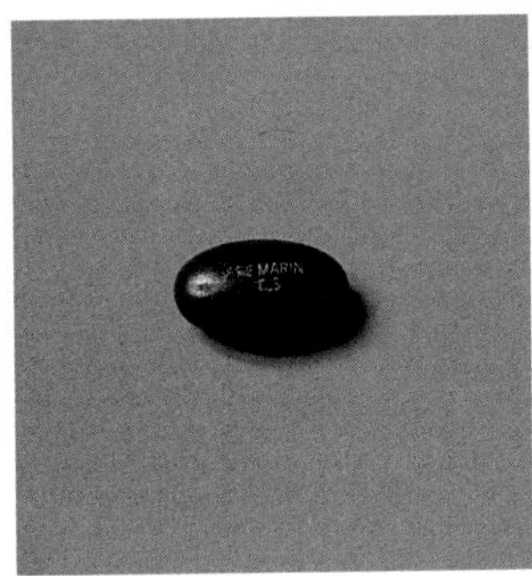

Premarin®
(estrogens, conjugated)
0.3 mg

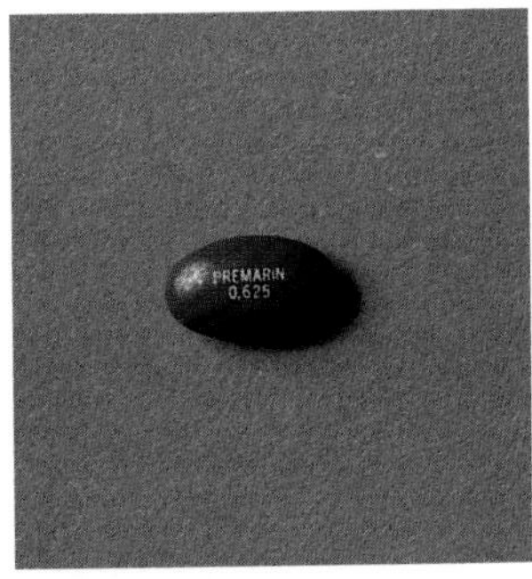

Premarin®
(estrogens, conjugated)
0.625

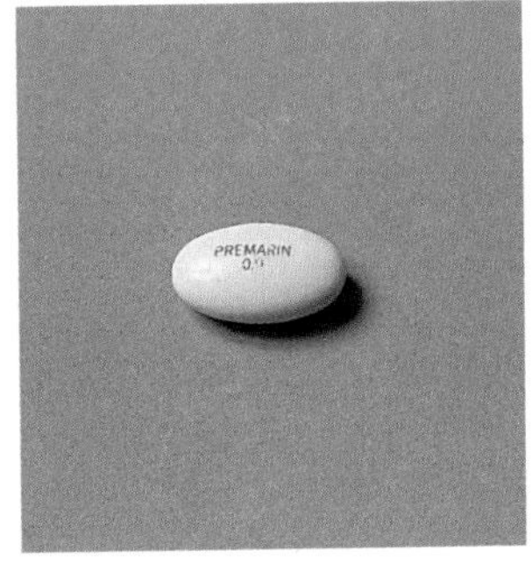

Premarin®
(estrogens, conjugated)
0.9 mg

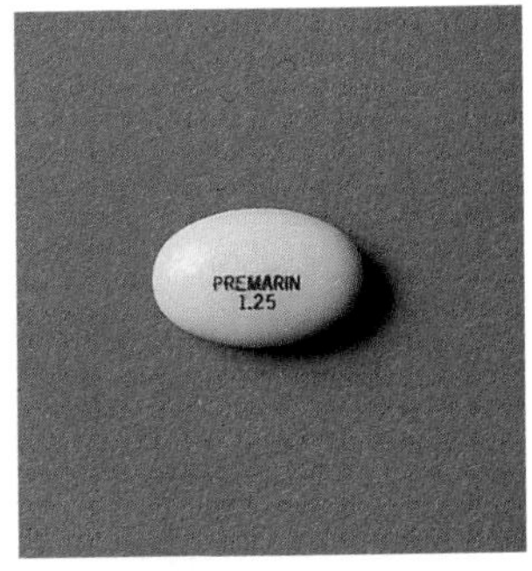

Premarin®
(estrogens, conjugated)
1.25 mg

†*Drug contains multiple ingredients; ingredients and quantities are listed respectively.*

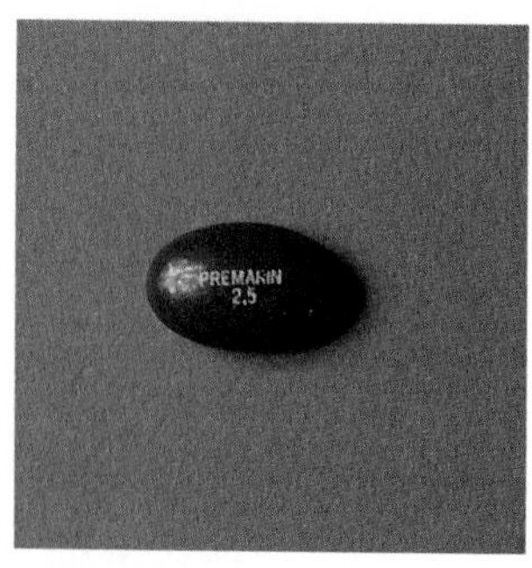

Premarin®
(estrogens, conjugated)
2.5 mg

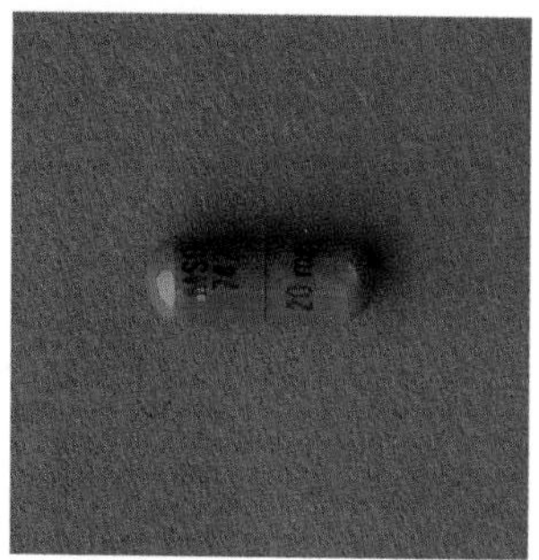

Prilosec™
(omeprazole)
20 mg

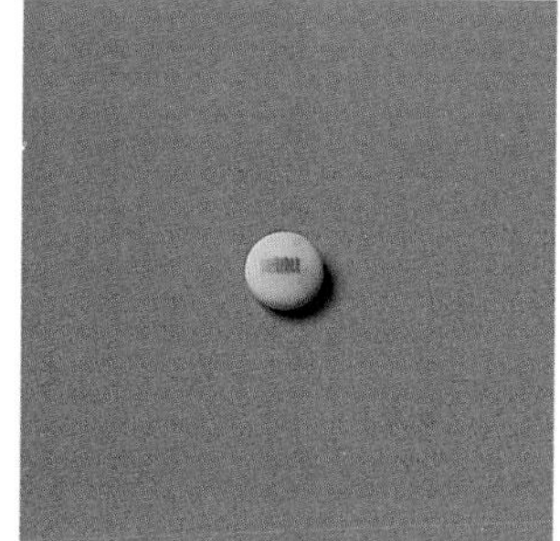

Pro-Banthine®
(propantheline)
15 mg

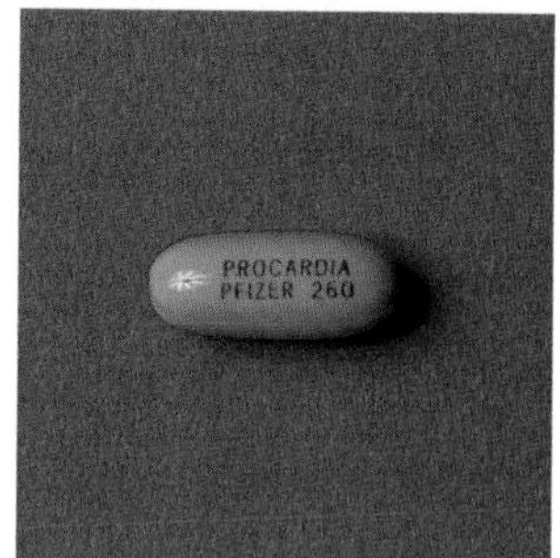

Procardia®
(nifedipine)
10 mg

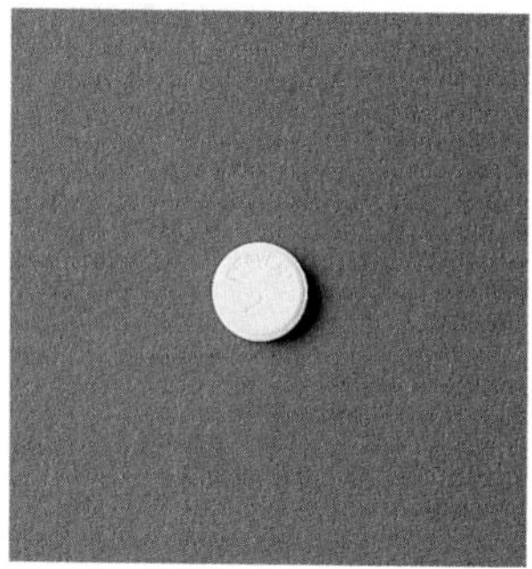

Proventil®
(albuterol)
2 mg

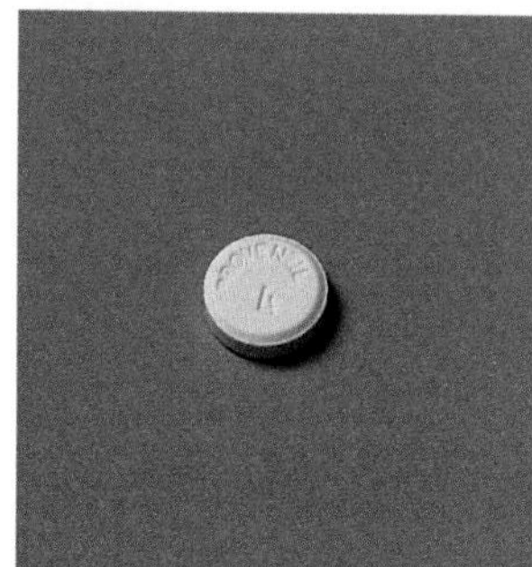

Proventil®
(albuterol)
4 mg

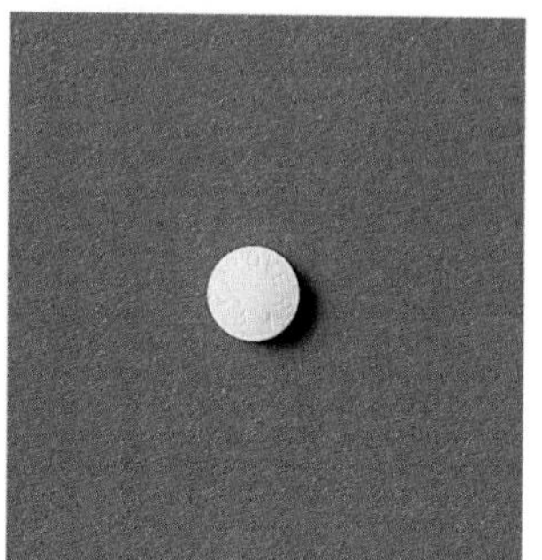

Provera®
(medroxyprogesterone)
2.5 mg

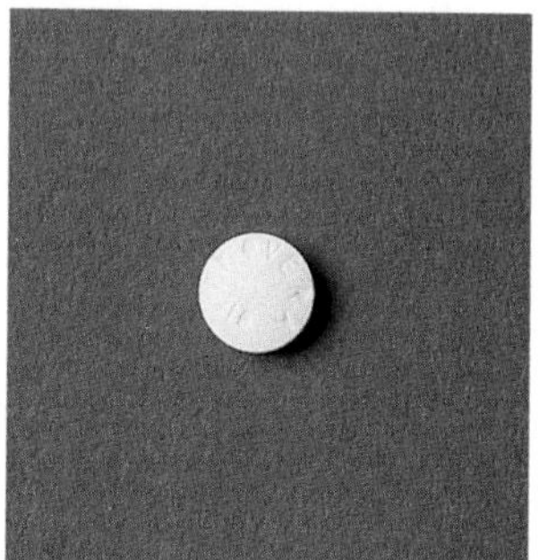

Provera®
(medroxyprogesterone)
10 mg

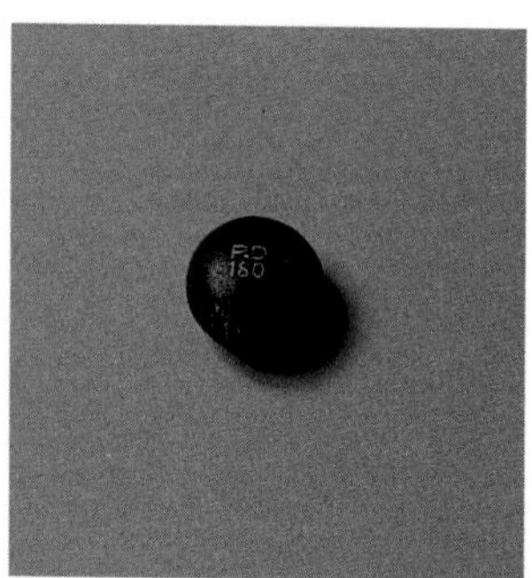

Pyridium®
(phenazopyridine)
100 mg

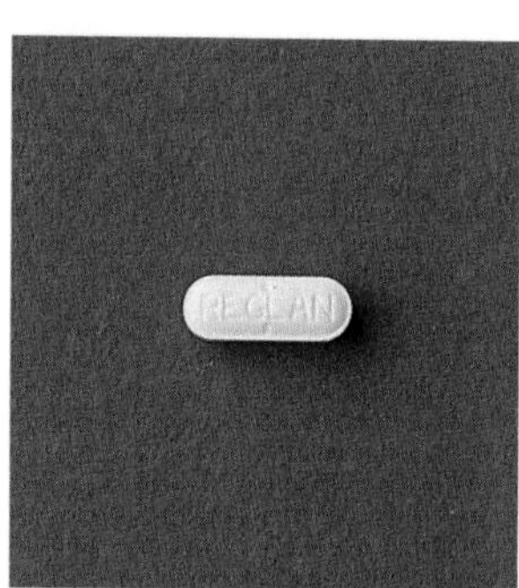

Reglan®
(metoclopramide)
10 mg

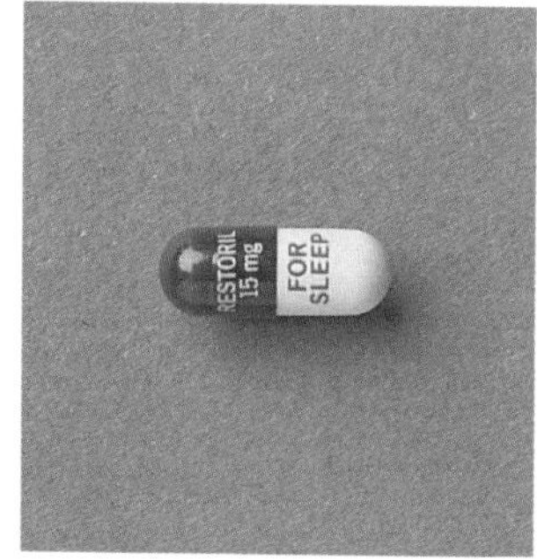

Restoril®
(temazepam)
15 mg

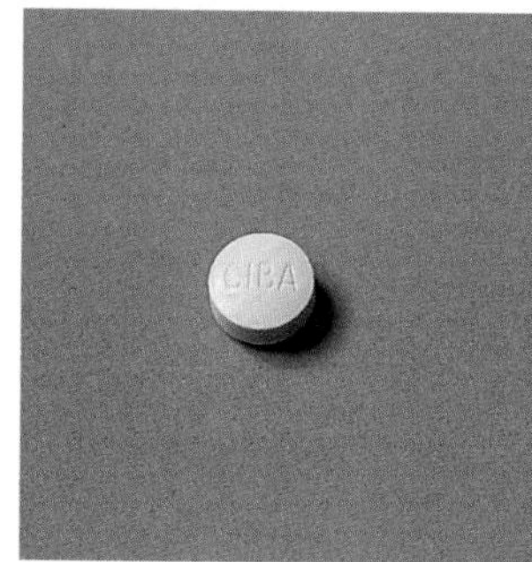

Ritalin®
(methylphenidate)
5 mg

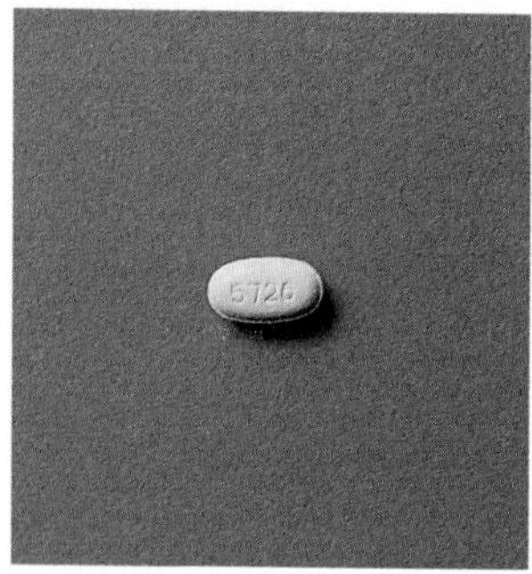

Rondec®†
(pseudoephedrine and carbinoxamine combination)
60 + 4 mg

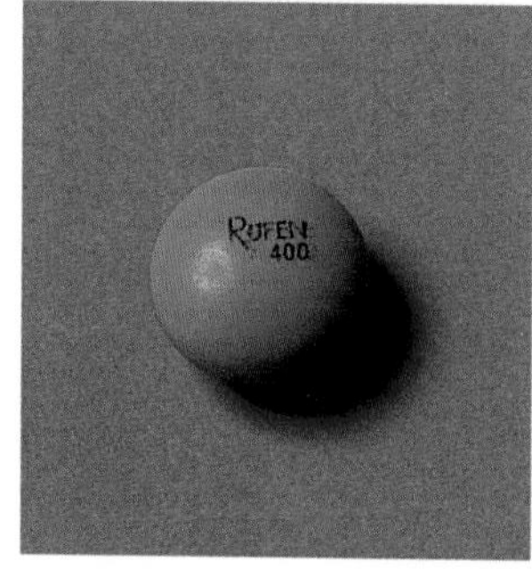

Rufen®
(ibuprofen)
400 mg

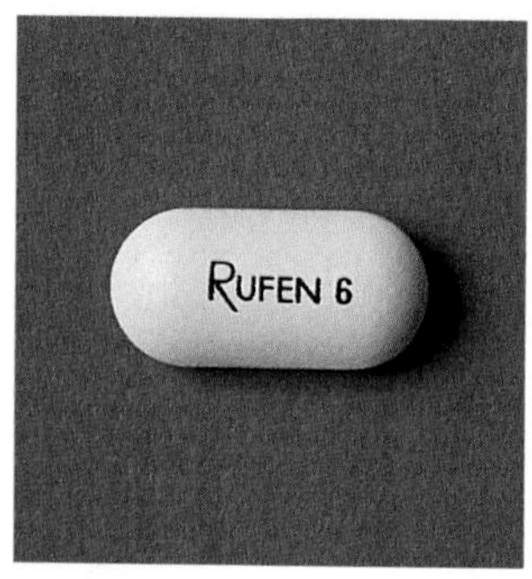

Rufen®
(ibuprofen)
600 mg

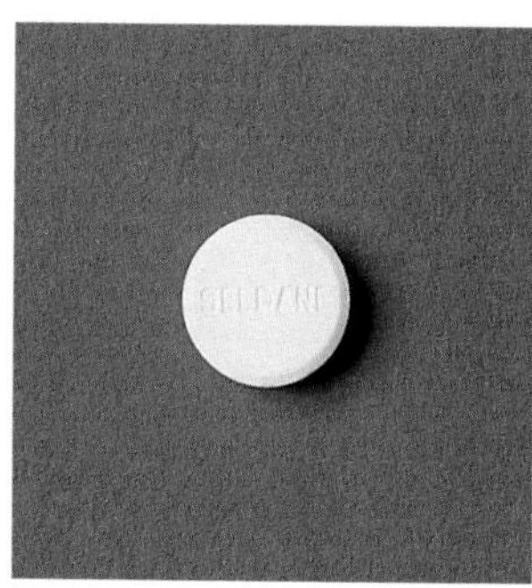

Seldane®
(terfenadine)
60 mg

†*Drug contains multiple ingredients; ingredients and quantities are listed respectively.*

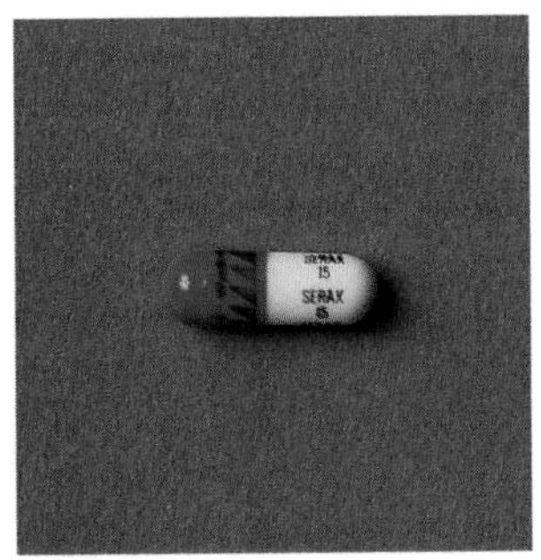

Serax®
(oxazepam)
15 mg

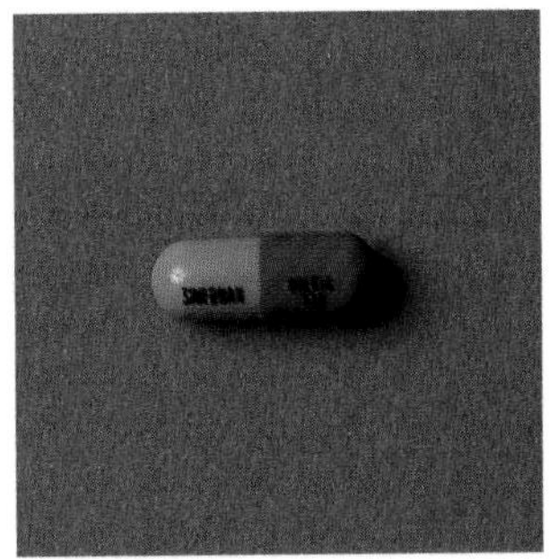

Sinequan®
(doxepin)
10 mg

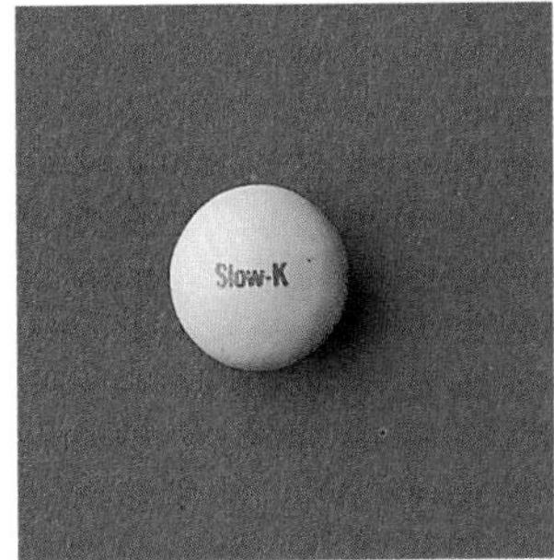

Slow-K®
(potassium chloride)
600 mg (8 mEq)

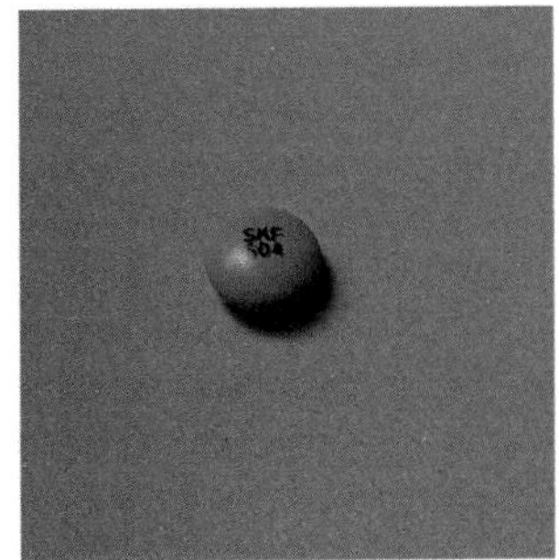

Stelazine®
(trifluoperazine)
2 mg

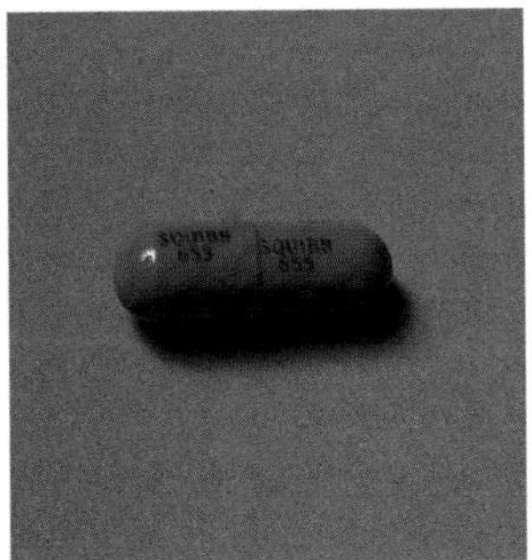

Sumycin®
(tetracycline)
250 mg

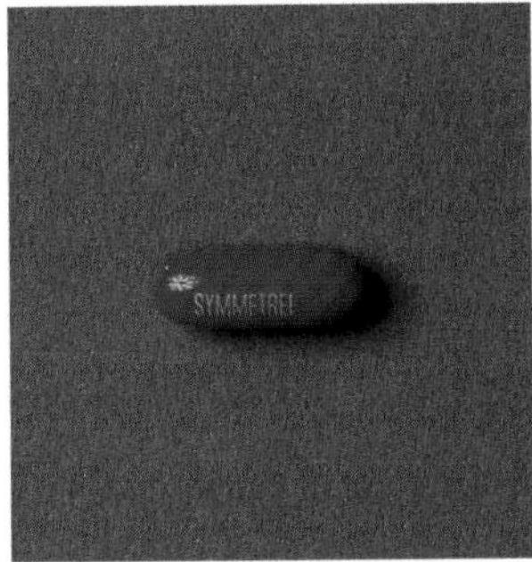

Symmetrel®
(amantadine)
100 mg

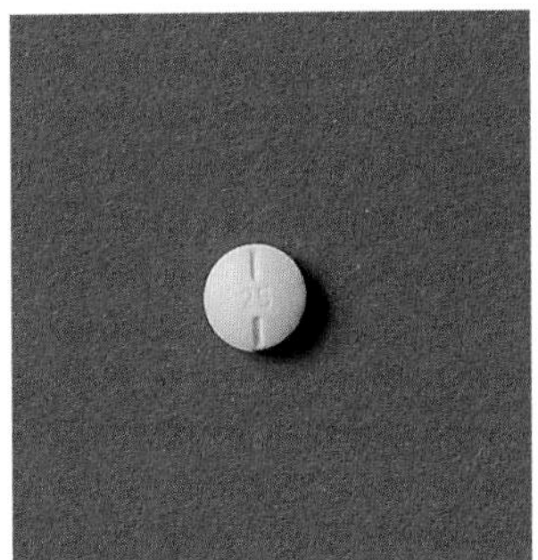

Synthroid®
(levothyroxine)
0.025 mg

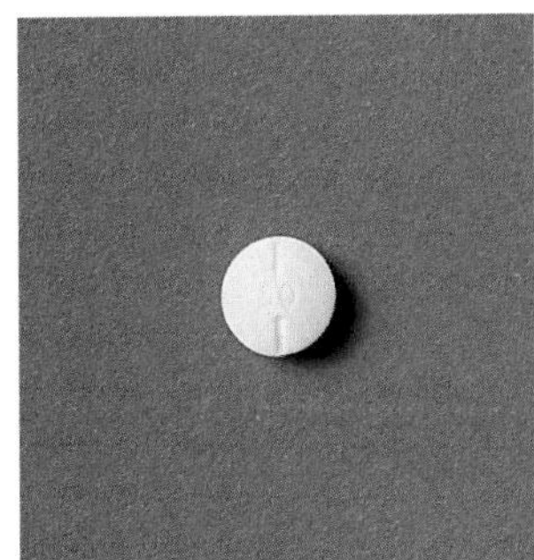

Synthroid®
(levothyroxine)
0.05 mg

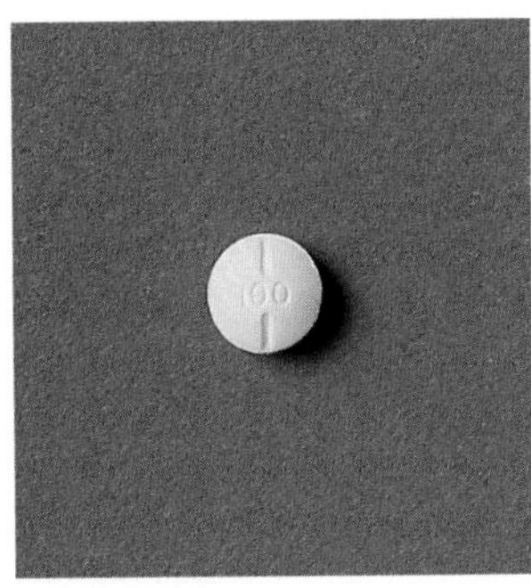

Synthroid®
(levothyroxine)
0.1 mg

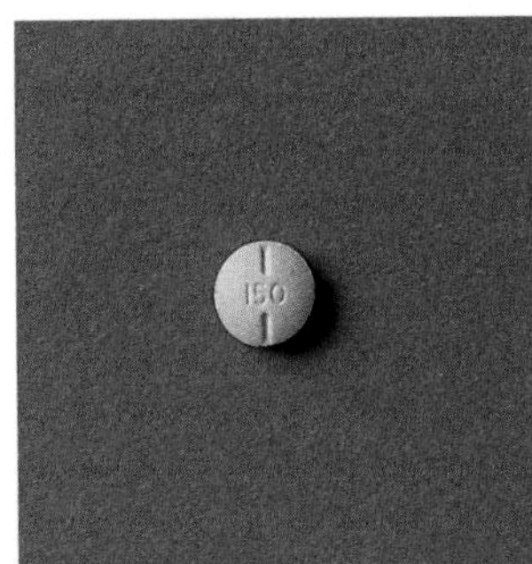

Synthroid®
(levothyroxine)
0.15

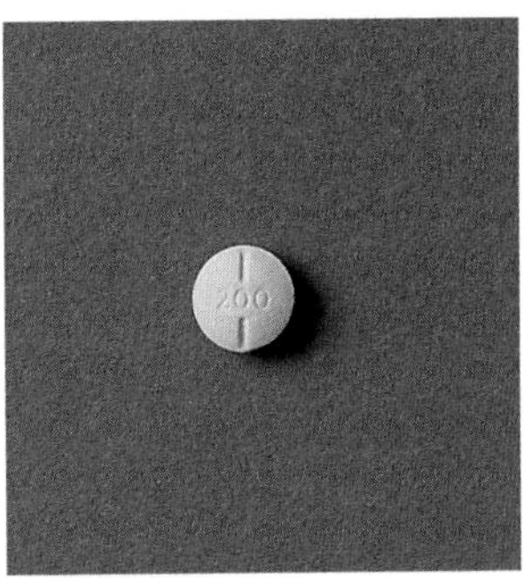

Synthroid®
(levothyroxine)
0.2 mg

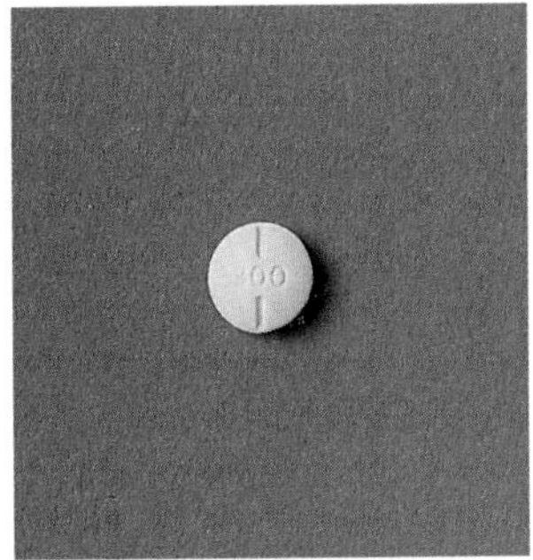

Synthroid®
(levothyroxine)
0.3 mg

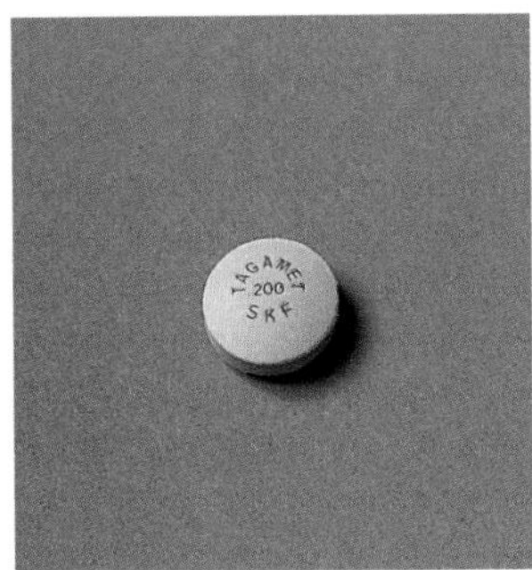

Tagamet®
(cimetidine)
200 mg

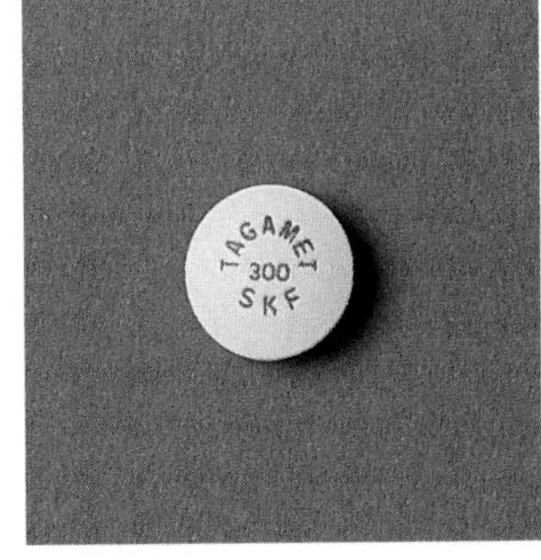

Tagamet®
(cimetidine)
300 mg

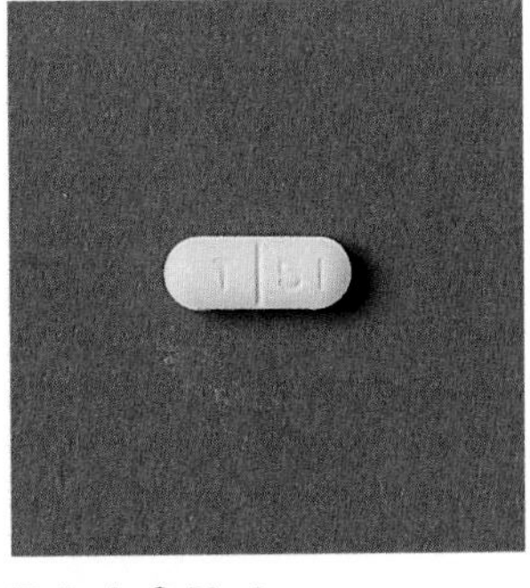

Talwin® Nx†
(pentazocine and naloxone combination)
50 + 0.5 mg

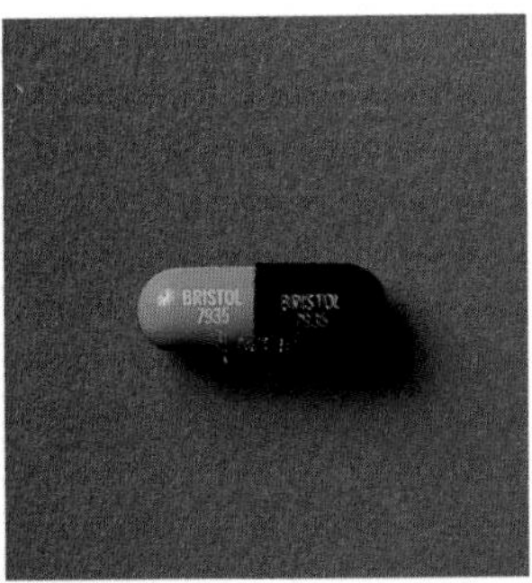

Tegopen®
(cloxacillin)
250 mg

†Drug contains multiple ingredients; ingredients and quantities are listed respectively.

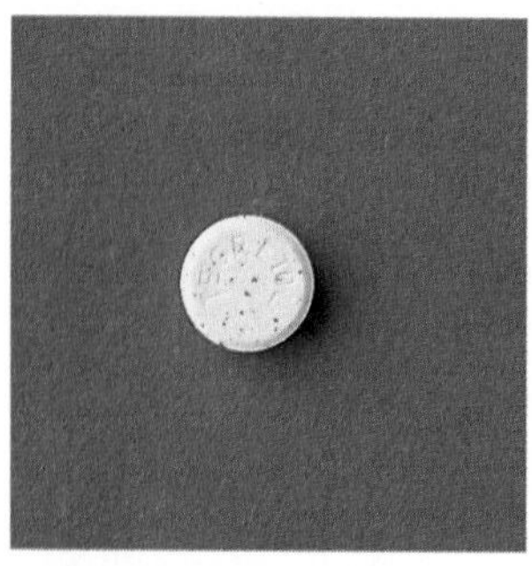

Tegretol® Chewable
(carbamazepine)
100 mg

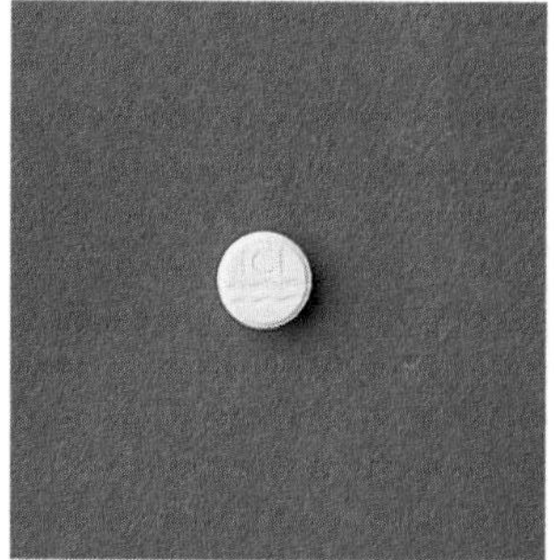

Tenormin®
(atenolol)
50 mg

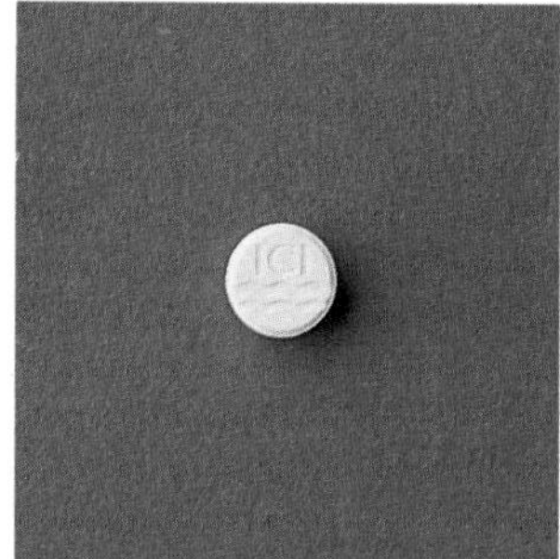

Tenormin®
(atenolol)
100 mg

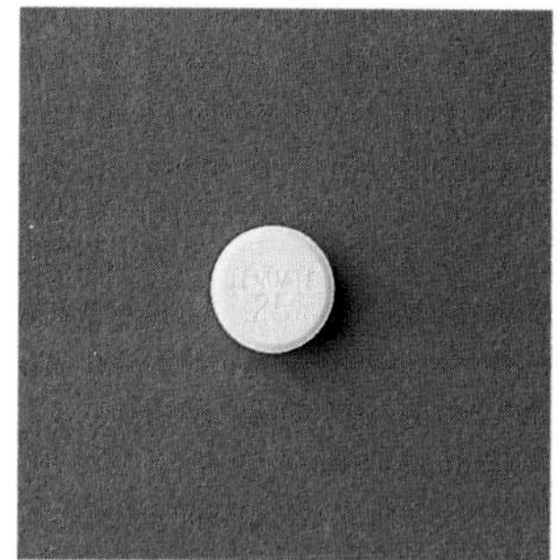

Tenuate®
(diethylpropion)
25 mg

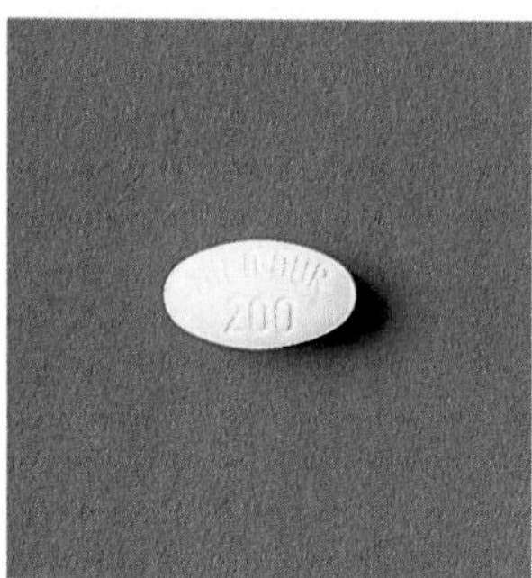

Theo-Dur®
(theophylline)
200 mg

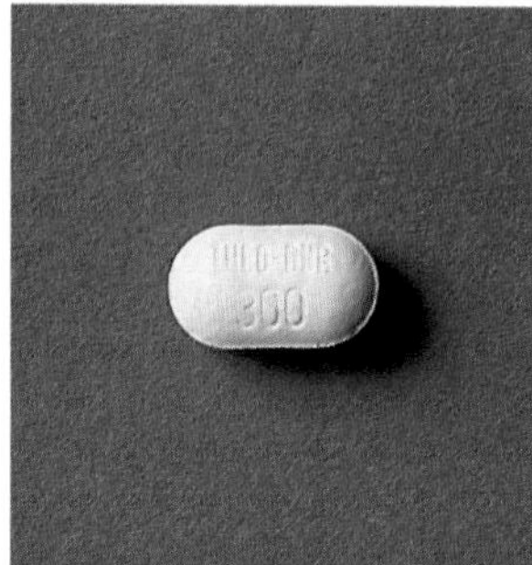

Theo-Dur®
(theophylline)
300 mg

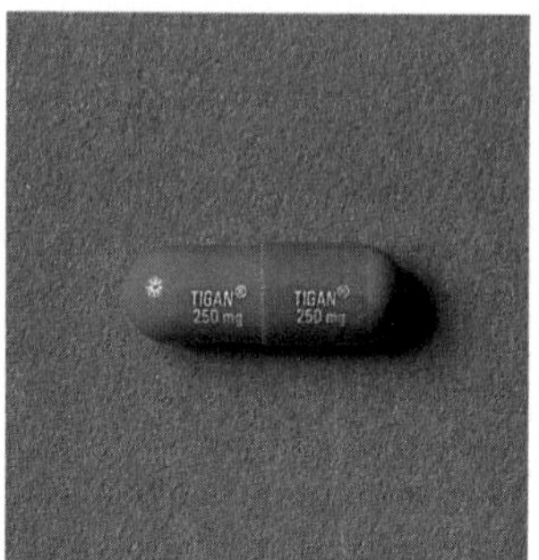

Tigan®
(trimethobenzamide)
250 mg

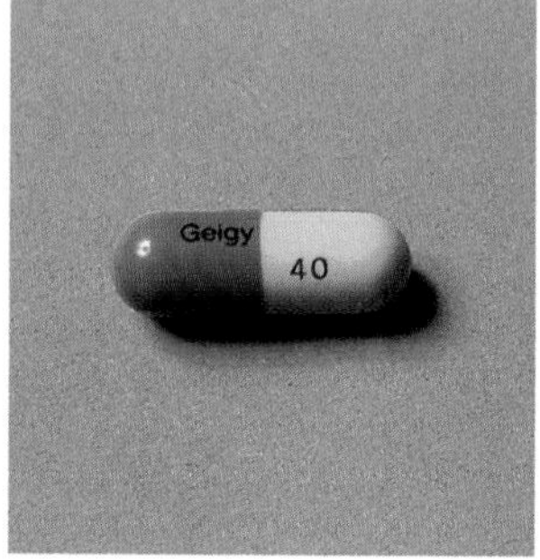

Tofranil-PM®
(imipramine)
100 mg

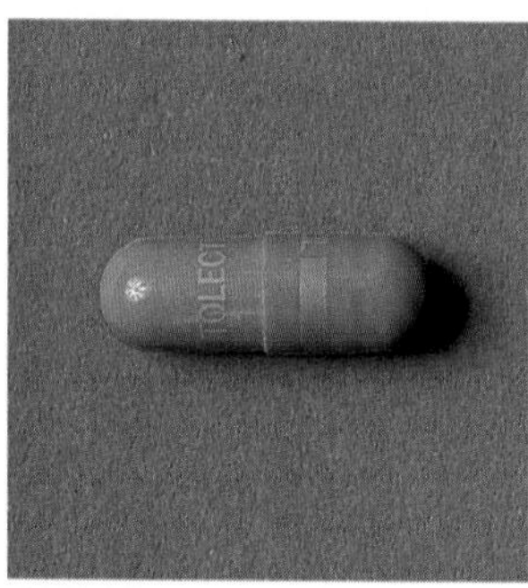

Tolectin® DS
(tolmetin)
400 mg

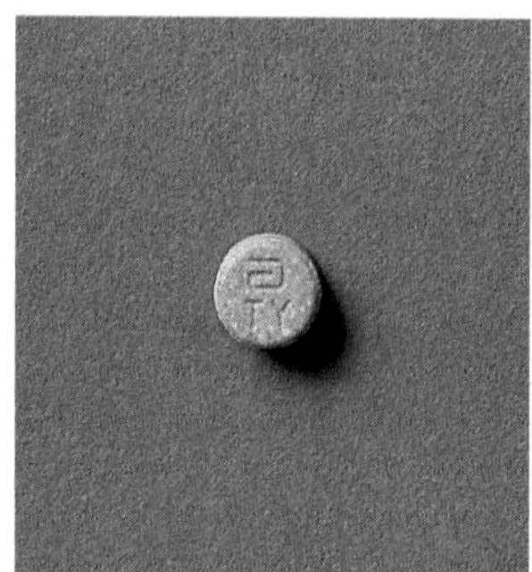

Tranxene®-SD
(clorazepate)
22.5 mg

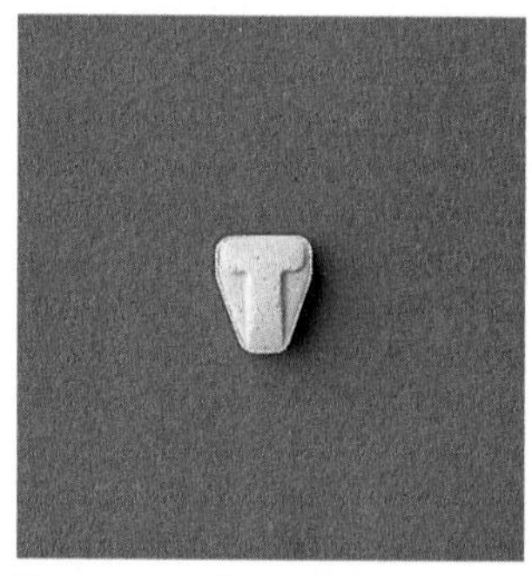

Tranxene® T-Tab™
(clorazepate)
3.75

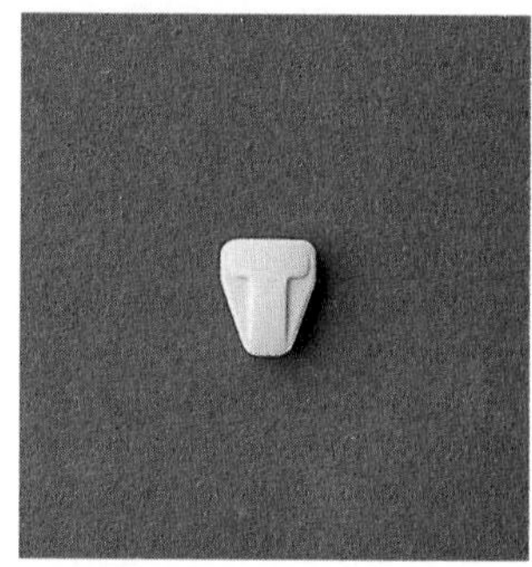

Tranxene® T-Tab™
(clorazepate)
7.5 mg

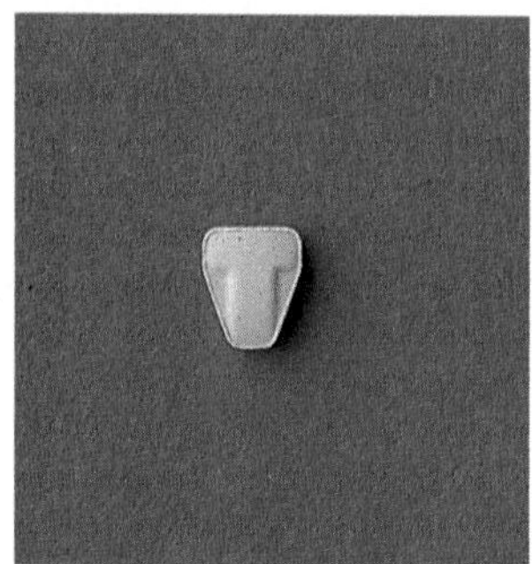

Tranxene® T-Tab™
(clorazepate)
15 mg

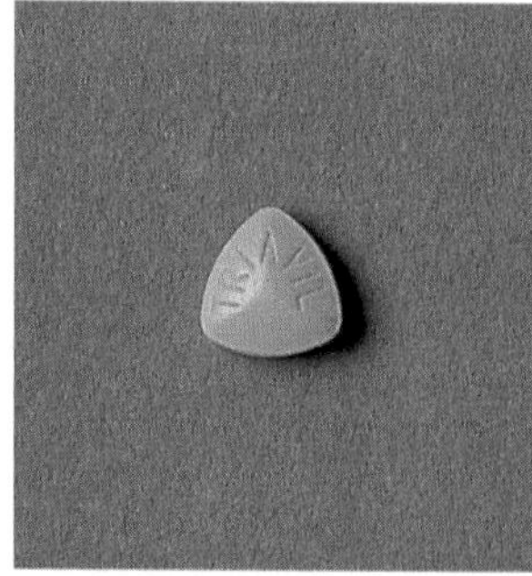

Triavil®†
(perphenazine and amitriptyline combination)
2 + 10 mg

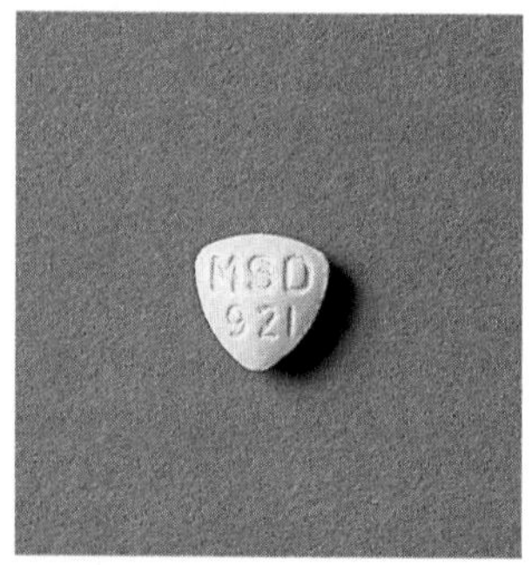

Triavil®†
(perphenazine and amitriptyline combination)
2 + 25 mg

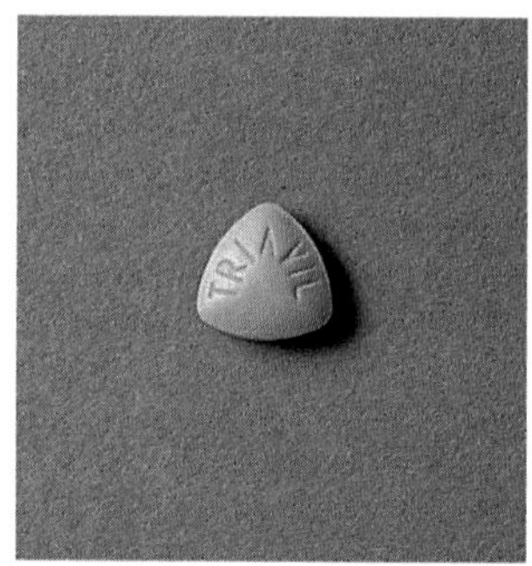

Triavil®†
(perphenazine and amitriptyline combination)
4 + 10 mg

†Drug contains multiple ingredients; ingredients and quantities are listed respectively.

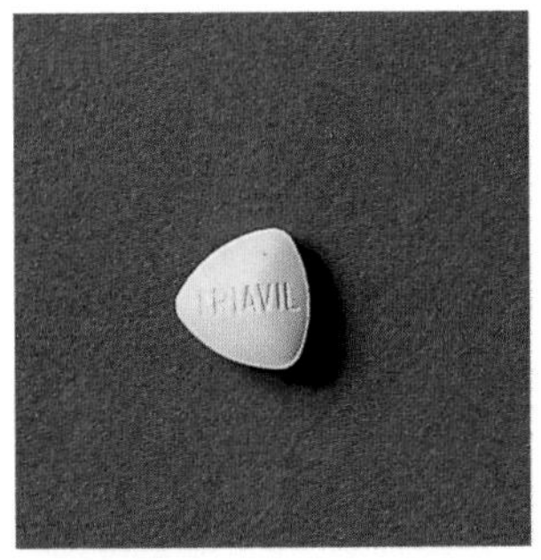

Triavil®†
(perphenazine and amitriptyline combination)
4 + 25 mg

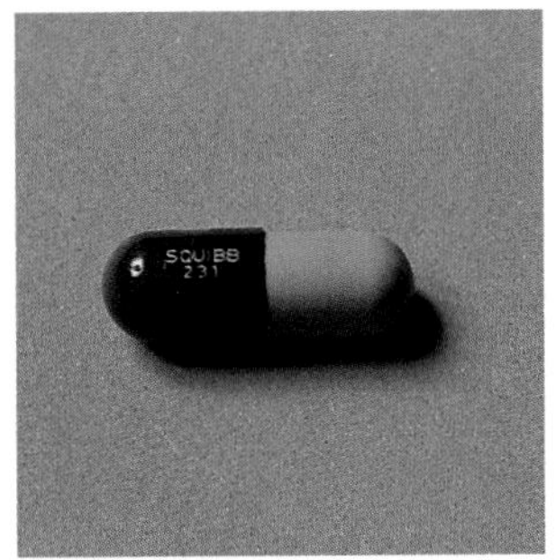

Trimox®
(amoxicillin)
500 mg

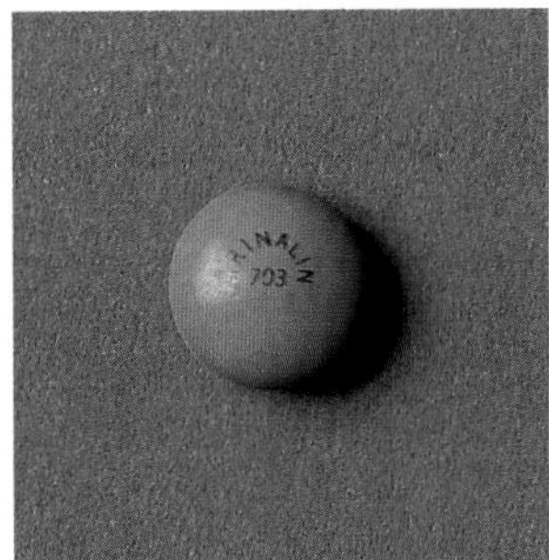

Trinalin® Repetabs®†
(pseudoephedrine and azatadine combination)
120 + 1 mg

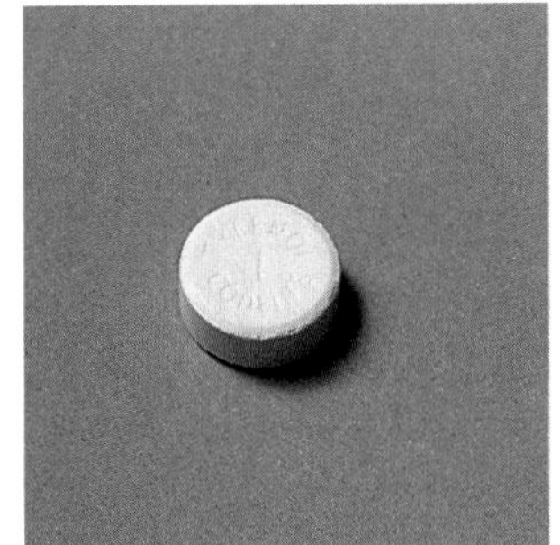

Tylenol® No. 1†
(acetaminophen and codeine combination)
300 + 7.5 mg

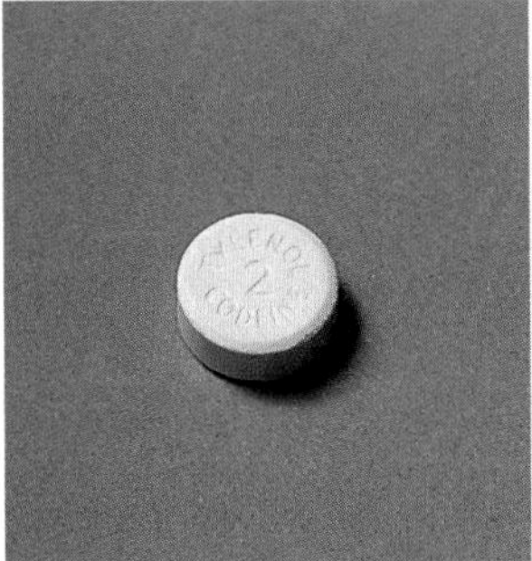

Tylenol® No. 2†
(acetaminophen and codeine combination)
300 + 15 mg

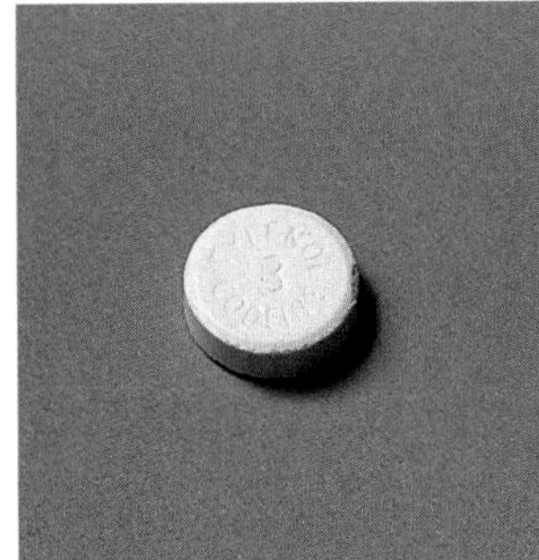

Tylenol® No. 3†
(acetaminophen and codeine combination)
300 + 30 mg

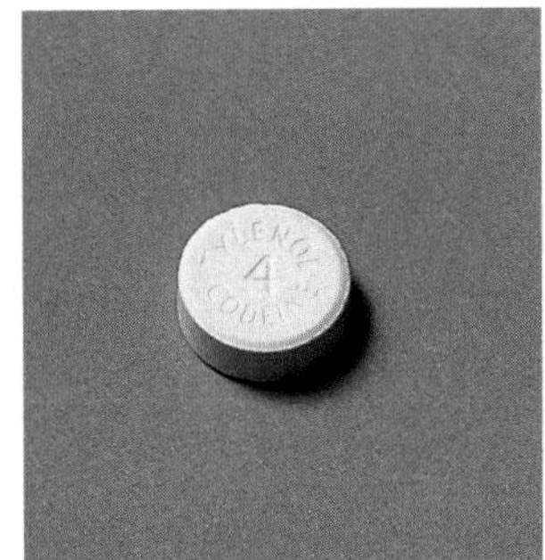

Tylenol® No. 4†
(acetaminophen and codeine combination)
300 + 60 mg

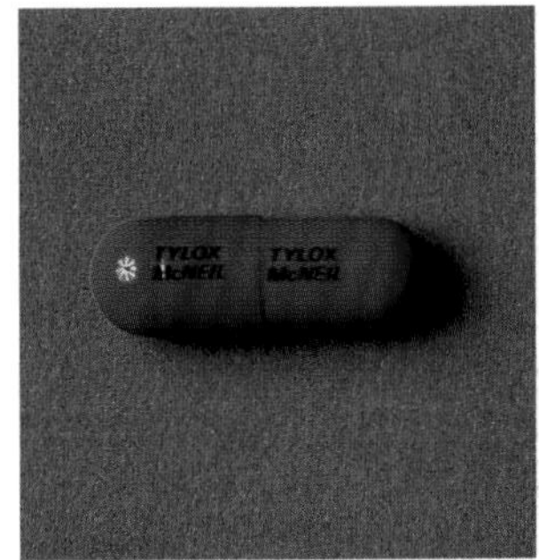

Tylox®†
(acetaminophen and oxycodone combination)
500 + 5 mg

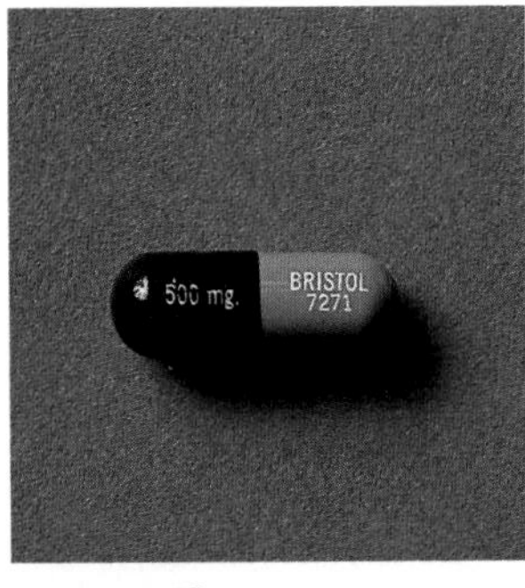

Ultracef®
(cefadroxil)
500 mg

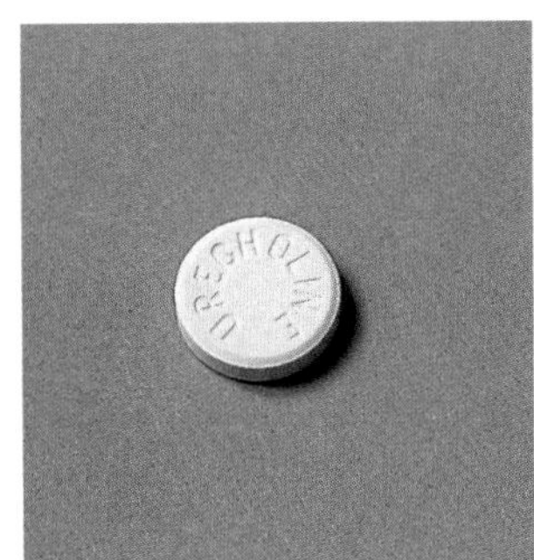

Urecholine®
(bethanechol)
10 mg

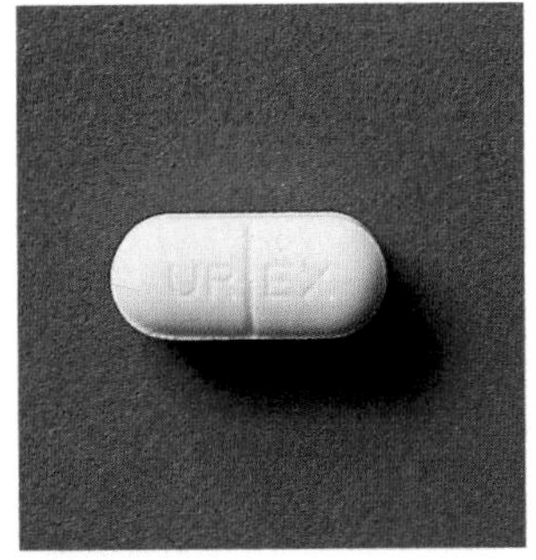

Urex®
(methenamine)
1,000 mg

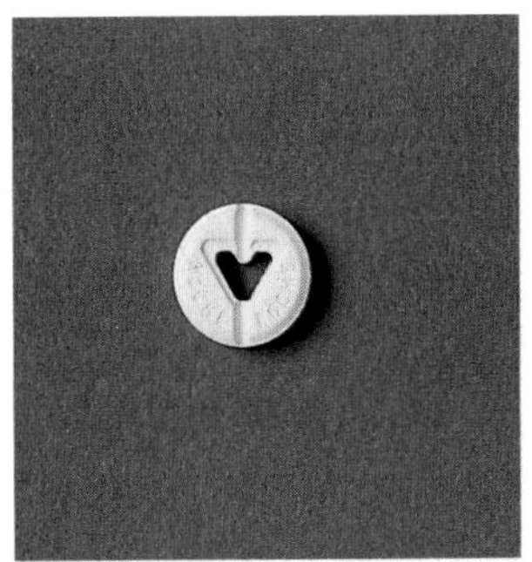

Valium®
(diazepam)
5 mg

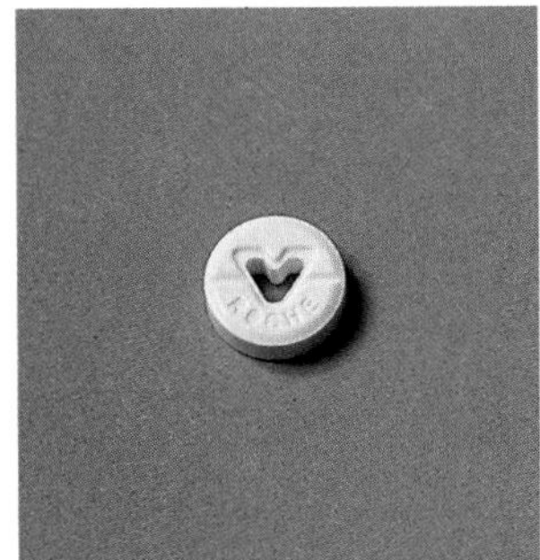

Valium®
(diazepam)
10 mg

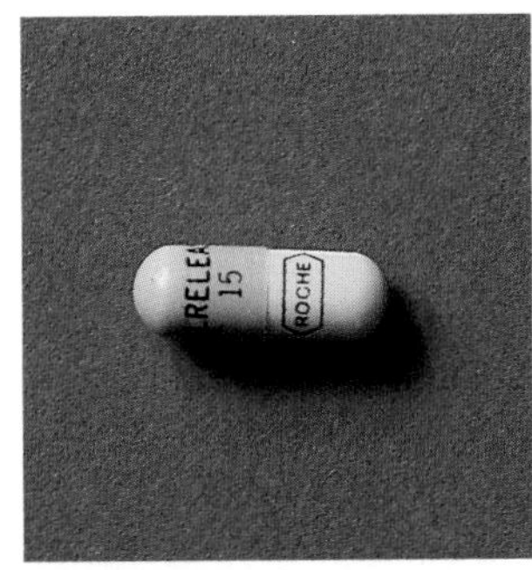

Valrelease®
(diazepam)
15 mg

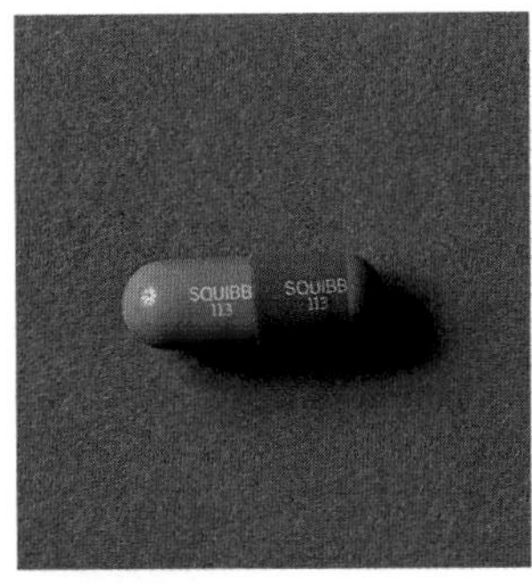

Velosef®
(cephradine)
250 mg

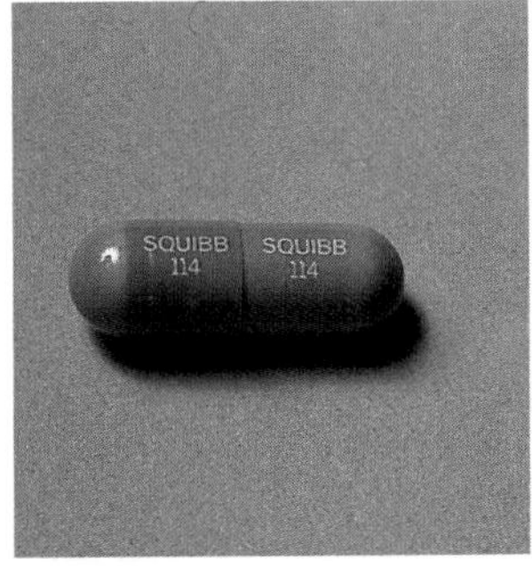

Velosef®
(cephradine)
500 mg

†Drug contains multiple ingredients; ingredients and quantities are listed respectively.

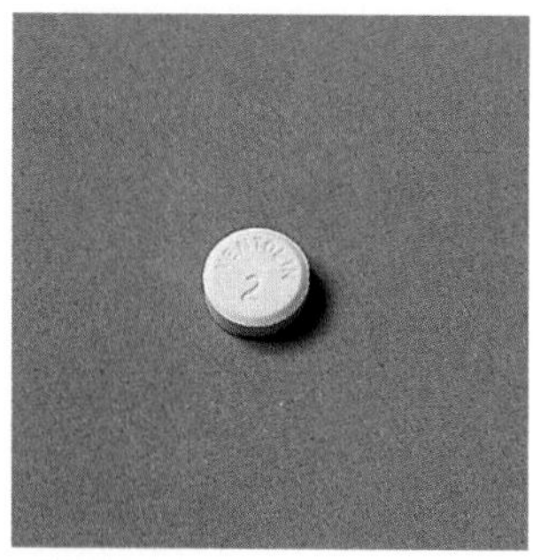

Ventolin®
(albuterol)
2 mg

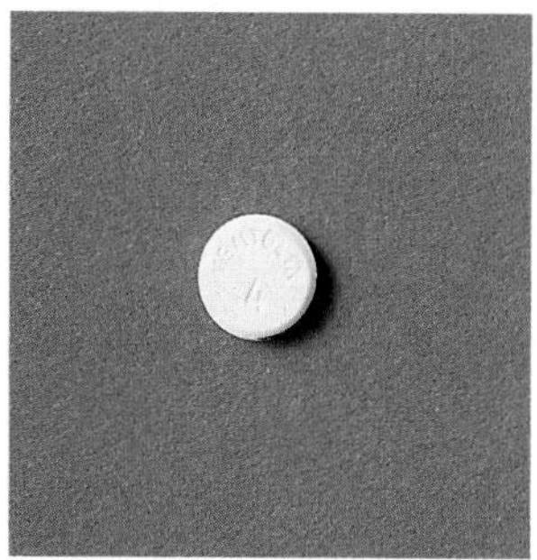

Ventolin®
(albuterol)
4 mg

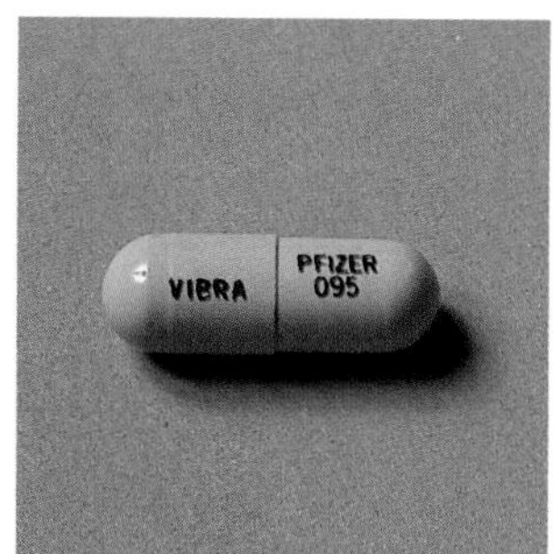

Vibramycin® Hyclate
(doxycycline)
100 mg

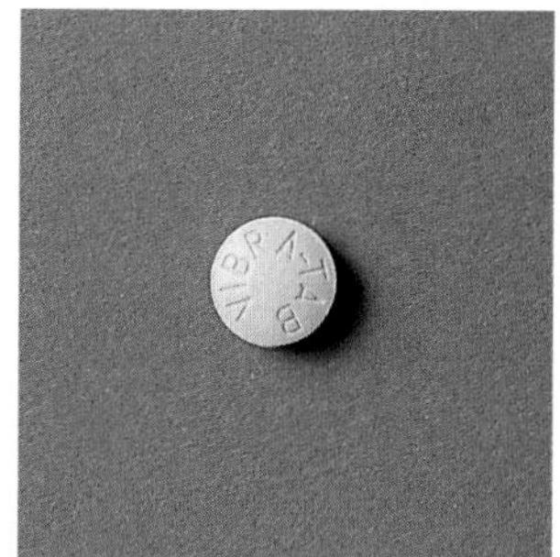

Vibra-Tabs®
(doxycycline)
100 mg

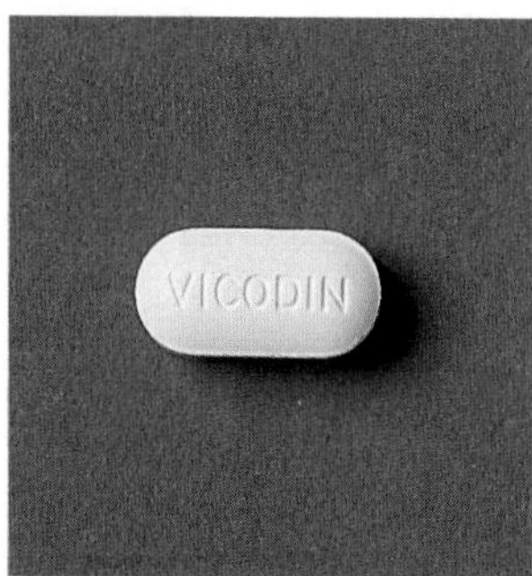

Vicodin®†
(acetaminophen and hydrocodone combination)
500 + 5 mg

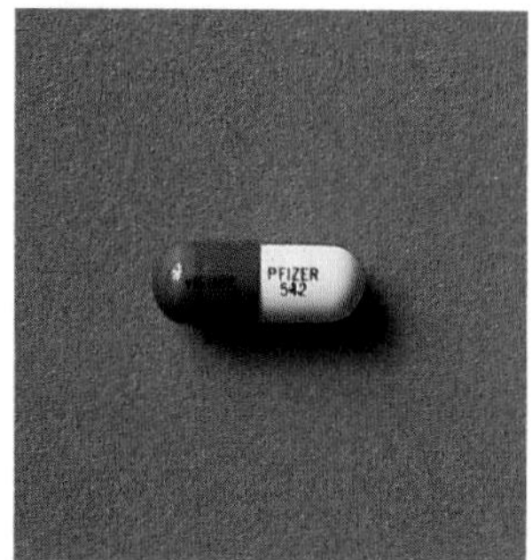

Vistaril®
(hydroxyzine)
50 mg

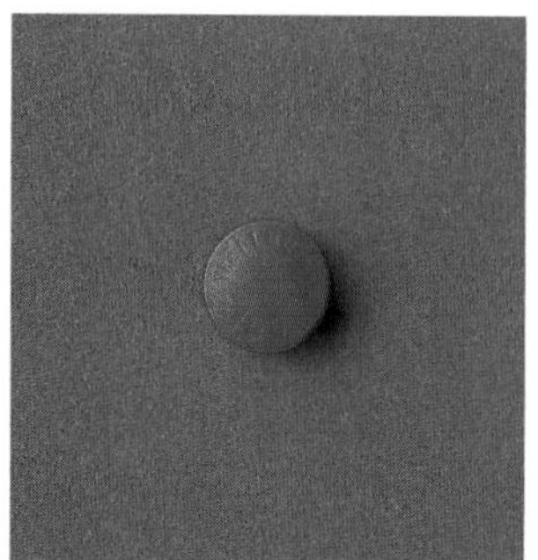

Wellbutrin®
(bupropion)
100 mg

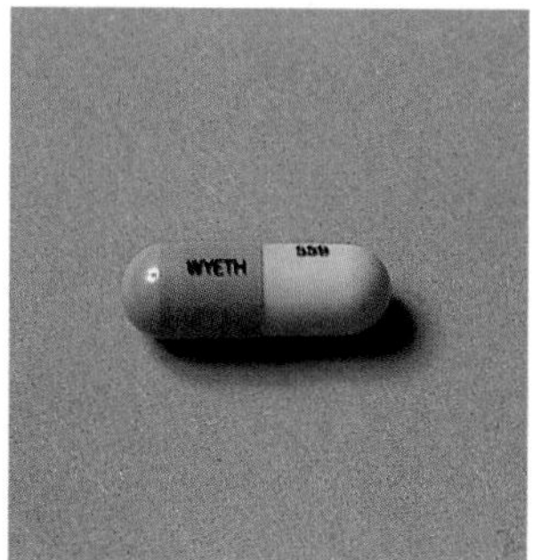

Wymox®
(amoxicillin)
250 mg

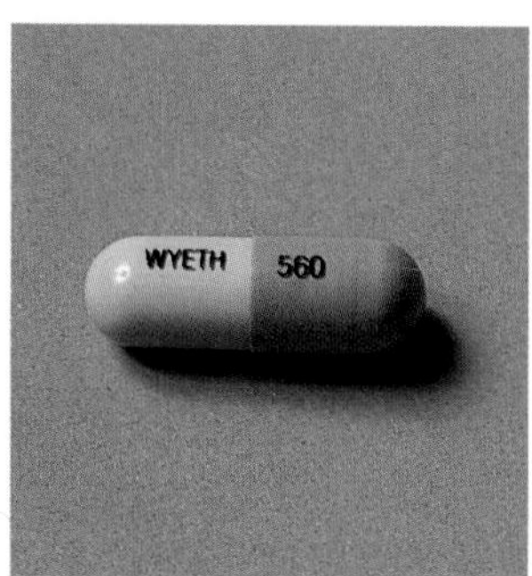

Wymox®
(amoxicillin)
500 mg

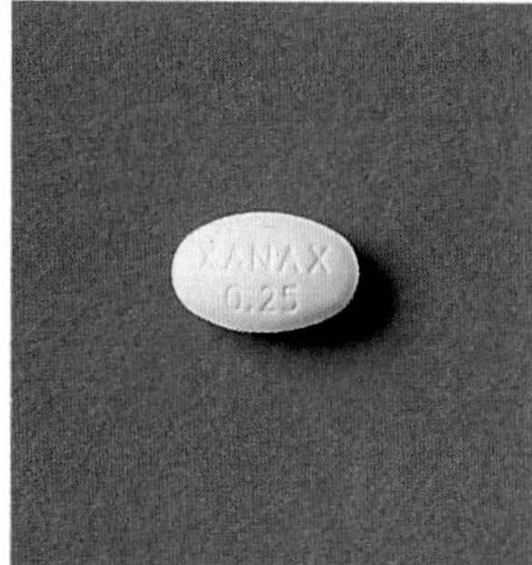

Xanax®
(alprazolam)
0.25 mg

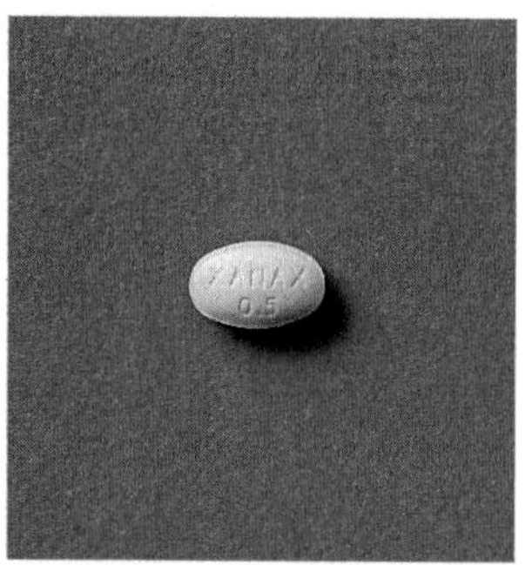

Xanax®
(alprazolam)
0.5 mg

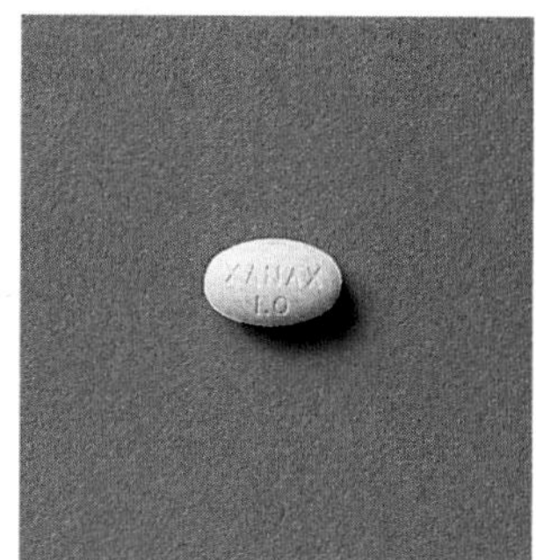

Xanax®
(alprazolam)
1 mg

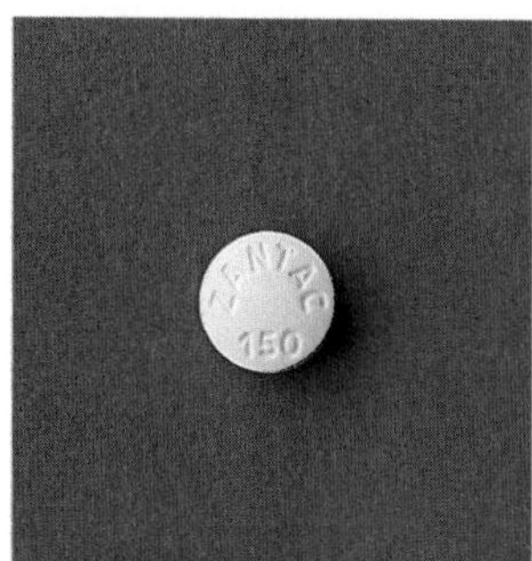

Zantac® 150 Tablets
(ranitidine)
150 mg

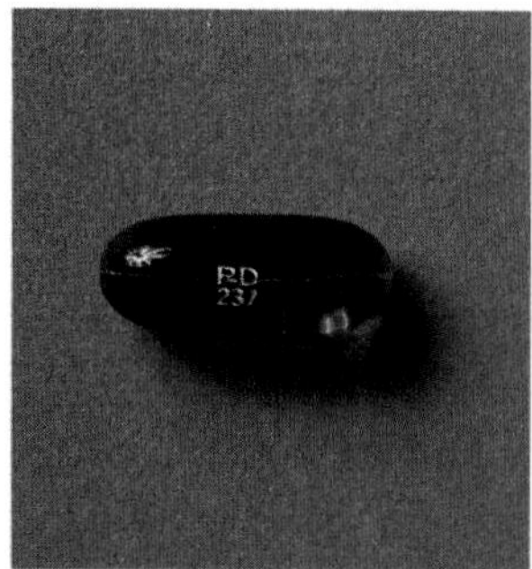

Zarontin® Capsules
(ethosuximide)
250 mg

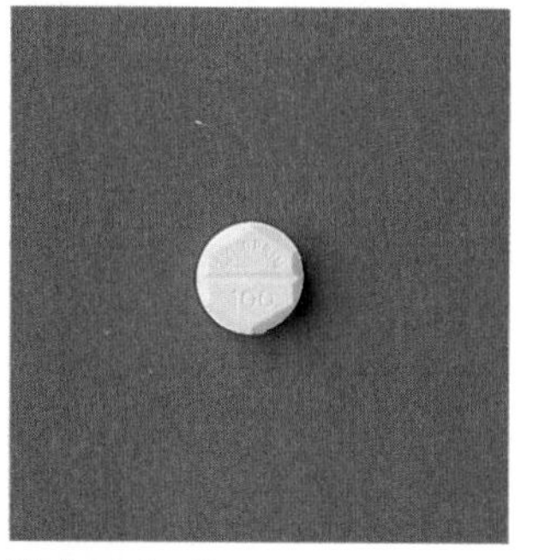

Zyloprim®
(allopurinol)
100 mg

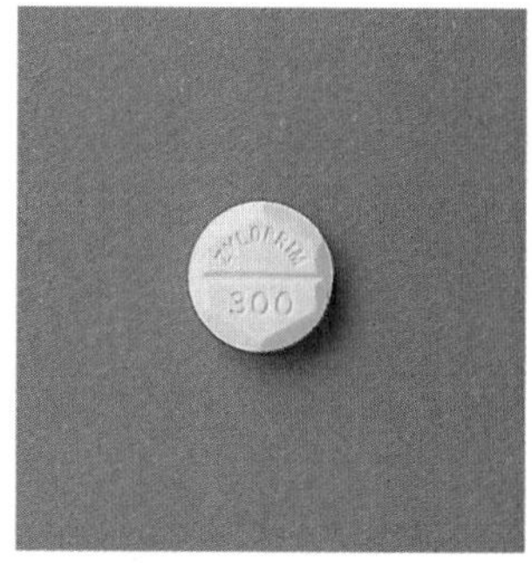

Zyloprim®
(allopurinol)
300 mg

†Drug contains multiple ingredients; ingredients and quantities are listed respectively.

cramps, nasal congestion, nausea, or vomiting. These minor side effects should disappear as your body adjusts to therapy with this medication.

To relieve constipation, increase the amount of fiber in your diet (fresh fruits and vegetables, salads, bran, and whole-grain breads), exercise, and drink more water (unless your doctor directs you to do otherwise).

If you feel dizzy or light-headed, sit or lie down for a while; get up slowly from a sitting or reclining position, and be careful on stairs. To avoid dizziness or light-headedness when you stand, contract and relax the muscles of your legs for a few moments before rising. Do this by pushing one foot against the floor while raising the other foot slightly, alternating feet so that you are "pumping" your legs in a pedaling motion.

Major. Tell your doctor about any side effects that are persistent or particularly bothersome. IT IS ESPECIALLY IMPORTANT TO TELL YOUR DOCTOR about anxiety, chest pain, confusion, cramping, depression, difficulty in urinating, fever, itching, numbness or tingling in the fingers or toes, palpitations, rapid weight gain (three to five pounds within a week), rash, shortness of breath, sore throat, tenderness in the joints and muscles, tiredness, unusual bleeding or bruising, or yellowing of the eyes or skin.

INTERACTIONS

Hydralazine interacts with several other types of drugs:

1. The combination of alcohol and hydralazine can lead to dizziness and fainting. You should, therefore, avoid drinking alcoholic beverages while taking this medication.

2. Used within 14 days of a monoamine oxidase (MAO) inhibitor, hydralazine can cause severe reactions.

Before you start to take hydralazine, BE SURE TO TELL YOUR DOCTOR about any medications you are currently taking, especially an MAO inhibitor.

WARNINGS

- Tell your doctor about any unusual or allergic reactions you have had to any medications, especially to hydralazine.
- Tell your doctor if you have ever had angina, heart disease, stroke, a heart attack, or kidney disease.
- To avoid dizziness or fainting, try not to stand for long periods of time, and avoid drinking alcohol. You should also try not to get overheated (avoid exercising strenuously in hot weather and avoid taking hot baths, showers, and saunas).
- If this drug makes you dizzy or drowsy, avoid taking part in any activities that require alertness, such as driving a car or operating potentially dangerous machinery.
- Before having surgery or any other medical or dental treatment, be sure to tell your doctor or dentist that you are taking this medication.
- Do not take any over-the-counter (nonprescription) allergy, asthma, sinus, cough, cold, or diet products unless you first consult your doctor or pharmacist. The combination of these medications with hydralazine may cause an increase in blood pressure.
- Some hydralazine formulations contain the color additive FD&C Yellow No. 5 (tartrazine), which can cause allergic-type reactions (rash, shortness of breath, fainting) in certain susceptible individuals.
- Do not stop taking this medication until you check with your doctor. If this drug is stopped abruptly, you could experience a sudden rise in blood pressure and other complications. Your doctor may, therefore, want to decrease your dosage gradually.
- Be sure to tell your doctor if you are pregnant. Although studies in humans have not been conducted, hydralazine crosses the placenta, and studies have shown that it causes birth defects in the offspring of animals that received large doses of it during pregnancy. Also, tell your doctor if you are breast-feeding an infant. It is not known whether hydralazine passes into breast milk.

hydralazine hydrochloride—see hydralazine

---

hydralazine, hydrochlorothiazide, and reserpine combination

BRAND NAMES (Manufacturers)

Cam-ap-es (Camall)
Cherapas (Kay)
H-H-R (Geneva Generics)
Ser-A-Gen (Goldline)
Seralazide (Lannett)
Ser-Ap-Es (Ciba)
Serpazide (Major)
Tri-Hydroserpine (Rugby)
Unipres (Reid-Rowell)

TYPE OF DRUG

Antihypertensive

INGREDIENTS

hydralazine, hydrochlorothiazide, and reserpine

DOSAGE FORM

Tablets (25 mg hydralazine, 15 mg hydrochlorothiazide, and 0.1 mg reserpine)

STORAGE

These tablets should be stored at room temperature in a tightly closed, light-resistant container.

USES

Hydralazine, hydrochlorothiazide, and reserpine combination is used to treat high blood pressure. Hydralazine is a vasodilator; it relaxes the muscles of the blood vessels, resulting in a lowering of blood pressure. Hydrochlorothiazide is a diuretic (water pill), which reduces body fluid accumulation by increasing the elimination of salt and water through the kidneys. Reserpine acts by depleting the body of certain chemicals that are responsible for maintaining high blood pressure.

TREATMENT

In order to avoid stomach irritation, you can take hydralazine, hydrochlorothiazide, and reserpine combination with food or with a full glass of water or milk. To become accustomed to taking this medication, try to take it at the same time(s) each day. Avoid taking a dose after 6:00 P.M.

This medication does not cure high blood pressure, but it will help to control the condition as long as you continue to take it.

If you miss a dose of this medication, take the missed dose as soon as possible, unless it is almost time for the next dose. In that case, do not take the missed dose at all; just wait until the next scheduled dose. Do not double the dose.

The effects of therapy with this medication may not become apparent for two weeks.

SIDE EFFECTS

Minor. Abdominal pain, constipation, decrease in sexual desire, diarrhea, dizziness, flushing, loss of appetite, nasal congestion, or weight gain. These side effects should disappear as your body adjusts to the medication.

This medication can cause an increase in sensitivity to sunlight. It is, therefore, important to avoid prolonged exposure to sunlight and sunlamps. Wear protective clothing and sunglasses, and use an effective sunscreen.

To relieve constipation, increase the amount of fiber in your diet (fresh fruits and vegetables, salads, bran, and whole-grain breads) and exercise more (unless your doctor directs you to do otherwise).

To relieve mouth dryness, chew sugarless gum or suck on ice chips or a piece of hard candy.

If you feel dizzy or light-headed, sit or lie down for a while; get up slowly from a sitting or reclining position, and be careful on stairs. To avoid dizziness or light-headedness when you stand, contract and relax the muscles of your legs for a few moments before rising. Do this by pushing one foot against the floor while raising the other foot slightly, alternating feet so that you are "pumping" your legs in a pedaling motion.

Major. Tell your doctor about any side effects that are persistent or particularly bothersome. IT IS ESPECIALLY IMPORTANT TO TELL YOUR DOCTOR about anxiety; blurred vision; breast enlargement (in both sexes); chest pain; depression; difficulty in urinating; drowsiness; dry mouth; fainting; fatigue; fever; headaches; hearing loss; impotence; itching; joint pain; mood changes; muscle pain or spasms; nausea; nervousness; nightmares; palpitations; rapid weight gain (three to five pounds within a week); rash; shortness of breath; sore throat; swelling of the feet, ankles, or lower legs; thirst; tingling in the fingers or toes; tremors; unusual bleeding or bruising; vomiting; weakness; or yellowing of the eyes or skin.

INTERACTIONS

This medication interacts with several other types of drugs:

1. Concurrent use of it with central nervous system depressants (such as alcohol, antihistamines, barbiturates, benzodiazepine tranquilizers, muscle relaxants, narcotics, pain medications, phenothiazine tranquilizers, and sleeping medications) or with tricyclic antidepressants can cause extreme drowsiness.

2. The use of a monoamine oxidase (MAO) inhibitor within 14 days of this medication can lead to a severe reaction.

3. Reserpine combined with tricyclic antidepressants can lead to a severe drop in blood pressure (which can be dangerous). Reserpine can also decrease the effectiveness of levodopa and increase side effects (to the heart) of digoxin and quinidine.

4. Hydrochlorothiazide can decrease the effectiveness of warfarin, antigout medications, insulin, oral antidiabetic medicines, and methenamine.

5. Fenfluramine may increase the blood-pressure-lowering effects of hydrochlorothiazide (which can be dangerous).

6. Indomethacin may decrease the blood-pressure-lowering effects of hydrochlorothiazide, thereby counteracting the desired effects.

7. This medication should be taken one hour before or four hours after a dose of cholestyramine or colestipol (if you have also been prescribed one of these medications) because these medications can decrease the absorption of hydrochlorothiazide from the gastrointestinal tract.

8. Hydrochlorothiazide may increase the side effects of amphotericin B, calcium, adrenocorticosteroids (cortisone-like drugs), digitalis, digoxin, lithium, quinidine, sulfonamide antibiotics, and vitamin D.

BE SURE TO TELL YOUR DOCTOR about any medications you are currently taking, especially any listed above.

WARNINGS

- Tell your doctor about unusual or allergic reactions you have had to any medications, especially to hydralazine, reserpine, or hydrochlorothiazide, or to any other sulfa drugs (other diuretics, oral antidiabetic medicines, or sulfonamide antibiotics).
- Before starting to take this medication, be sure to tell your doctor if you have ever had anuria (decreased urination), blood disorders, chest pain, diabetes mellitus, epilepsy, electroshock therapy, kidney disease, heart disease, liver disease, depression, gallstones or gallbladder disease, Parkinson's disease, peptic ulcers, stroke, systemic lupus erythematosus, or ulcerative colitis.
- Some of these products contain the color additive FD&C Yellow No. 5 (tartrazine), which can cause allergic-type reactions (rash, shortness of breath, fainting) in certain susceptible individuals.
- A doctor does not usually prescribe this drug or other "fixed-dose" products as the first choice in the treatment of high blood pressure. Generally, the patient first receives each ingredient singly. If the response is adequate to the fixed dose contained in this product, it can then be substituted. An advantage of a combination product is increased convenience.
- This drug can cause potassium loss. Signs of potassium loss include dry mouth, thirst, weakness, muscle pain or cramps, nausea, and vomiting. If you experience any of these symptoms, CONTACT YOUR DOCTOR. To help prevent this problem, your doctor may want to have blood tests performed periodically to monitor your potassium levels. To help avoid potassium loss, take this product with a glass of fresh or frozen orange or cranberry juice, or eat a banana every day. The use of a salt substitute also helps to prevent potassium loss. Do not change your diet or use a salt substitute, however, until you discuss it with your doctor. Too much potassium can also be dangerous.
- To prevent severe water loss (dehydration) while taking this medication, check with your doctor if you have any illness that causes severe or continuous nausea, vomiting, or diarrhea.
- Hydrochlorothiazide can raise blood sugar levels in diabetic patients. Blood sugar should, therefore, be monitored carefully (using blood or urine tests) when this medication is being taken.
- In order to prevent dizziness or fainting while taking this medication, try not to stand for long periods of time. You

should also avoid drinking excessive amounts of alcohol, and avoid becoming overheated by exercising strenuously in hot weather or by taking hot baths, showers, and saunas.

• If this drug makes you dizzy or drowsy, avoid taking part in any activity that requires alertness, such as driving a car or operating potentially dangerous machinery.

• Before having surgery or other medical or dental treatment, tell your doctor or dentist you are taking this drug.

• Before taking any over-the-counter (nonprescription) allergy, asthma, sinus, cough, cold, or diet product, check with your doctor or pharmacist. Some of these products can cause an increase in blood pressure.

• Do not stop taking this medication until you first check with your doctor. If this drug is stopped abruptly, you may experience a sudden rise in blood pressure. Your doctor may, therefore, want to decrease your dosage gradually.

• The elderly may be at increased risk for side effects, especially depression, confusion, or other mental changes. Report any such changes to your doctor.

• Be sure to tell your doctor if you are pregnant. Birth defects have been observed in the offspring of animals that received large doses of reserpine and hydralazine during pregnancy. Studies of this drug in humans during pregnancy have not been conducted. Also, tell your doctor if you are breast-feeding an infant. Small amounts of this drug pass into breast milk and can cause side effects in nursing infants.

Hydramine—see diphenhydramine

Hydrex—see benzthiazide

---

hydrochlorothiazide

BRAND NAMES (Manufacturers)
Diaqua (Hauck)
Esidrix (Ciba)
hydrochlorothiazide (various manufacturers)
Hydro-Clor (Vortech)
HydroDIURIL (Merck Sharp & Dohme)
Hydromal (Hauck)
Hydro-T (Major)
Hydro-Z 50 (Mayrand)
Hydrozide-50 (T.E. Williams)
Mictrin (EconoMed)
Oretic (Abbott)
Thiuretic (Warner-Chilcott)

TYPE OF DRUG
Diuretic and antihypertensive

INGREDIENT
hydrochlorothiazide

DOSAGE FORMS
Tablets (25 mg, 50 mg, and 100 mg)
Oral solution (50 mg per 5-ml spoonful)
Intensol oral solution (100 mg per ml)

STORAGE
This medication should be stored at room temperature in a tightly closed container.

USES

Hydrochlorothiazide is prescribed to treat high blood pressure (hypertension). It is also used to reduce fluid accumulation in the body caused by conditions such as heart failure, cirrhosis of the liver, kidney disease, and the long-term use of some medications. This medication reduces body fluid accumulation by increasing the elimination of salt and water through the kidneys.

TREATMENT

To decrease stomach irritation, you can take this medication with a glass of milk or with a meal (unless your doctor directs you to do otherwise). Each dose of the oral solution should be measured carefully with the dropper provided (Intensol solution) or a specially designed 5-ml measuring spoon. An ordinary kitchen teaspoon is not accurate enough. Try to take it at the same time every day. Avoid taking a dose after 6:00 P.M.

If you miss a dose of this medication, take the missed dose as soon as possible, unless it is almost time for the next dose. In that case, do not take the missed dose at all; just wait until the next scheduled dose. Do not double the dose.

This medication does not cure high blood pressure, but it will help to control the condition as long as you continue to take it.

SIDE EFFECTS

Minor. Constipation, cramps, diarrhea, dizziness, drowsiness, headache, heartburn, loss of appetite, restlessness, or upset stomach. As your body adjusts to the medication, these side effects should disappear.

This drug can cause increased sensitivity to sunlight. Therefore, avoid prolonged exposure to sunlight and sunlamps. Wear protective clothing, and use an effective sunscreen.

To relieve constipation, increase the amount of fiber in your diet (fresh fruits and vegetables, salads, bran, and whole-grain breads) and exercise more (unless your doctor directs you to do otherwise).

To avoid dizziness or light-headedness when you stand, contract and relax the muscles of your legs for a few moments before rising. Do this by pushing one foot against the floor while raising the other foot slightly, alternating feet so that you are "pumping" your legs in a pedaling motion.

Major. Tell your doctor about any side effects that are persistent or particularly bothersome. IT IS ESPECIALLY IMPORTANT TO TELL YOUR DOCTOR about blurred vision, confusion, difficulty in breathing, dry mouth, excessive thirst, excessive weakness, fever, itching, joint pain, mood changes, muscle pain or spasms, nausea, palpitations, skin rash, sore throat, thirst, tingling in the fingers or toes, vomiting, or yellowing of the eyes or skin.

INTERACTIONS

Hydrochlorothiazide interacts with several other types of medications:

1. It can decrease the effectiveness of oral anticoagulants, antigout medications, insulin, oral antidiabetic medicines, and methenamine.

2. Fenfluramine can increase the blood-pressure-lowering effects of hydrochlorothiazide (which can be dangerous).

3. Indomethacin can decrease the blood-pressure-lowering effects of hydrochlorothiazide, thereby counteracting the desired effects.

4. Cholestyramine and colestipol decrease the absorption of this medication from the gastrointestinal tract. Hydro-

chlorothiazide should, therefore, be taken one hour before or four hours after a dose of cholestyramine or colestipol (if you have also been prescribed one of these medications).
5. Hydrochlorothiazide may increase the side effects of amphotericin B, calcium, cortisone and cortisone-like steroids (such as dexamethasone, hydrocortisone, prednisone, or prednisolone), digoxin, digitalis, lithium, quinidine, sulfonamide antibiotics, and vitamin D.

BE SURE TO TELL YOUR DOCTOR about any medications you are currently taking, especially any of those listed above.

WARNINGS

- Tell your doctor about unusual or allergic reactions you have had to any medications, especially to hydrochlorothiazide or other sulfa drugs, including other diuretics, oral antidiabetic medications, and sulfonamide antibiotics.
- Tell your doctor if you now have or if you have ever had kidney disease or problems with urination, diabetes mellitus, gout, liver disease, asthma, pancreatic disease, or systemic lupus erythematosus.
- Hydrochlorothiazide can cause potassium loss. Signs of potassium loss include dry mouth, thirst, weakness, muscle pain or cramps, nausea, and vomiting. If you experience any of these symptoms, call your doctor. To help avoid potassium loss, take this drug with a glass of fresh or frozen orange or cranberry juice, or eat a banana every day. The use of a salt substitute also helps to prevent potassium loss. Do not change your diet or use a salt substitute, however, before discussing it with your doctor. Too much potassium can also be dangerous. Your doctor may want you to have blood tests performed periodically in order to monitor your potassium levels while you are taking this drug.
- Limit your intake of alcoholic beverages while taking this medication, in order to prevent dizziness and lightheadedness.
- Becoming overheated can be hazardous while you are taking this medication. Avoid strenuous exercise in hot weather and do not take hot baths, showers, or saunas.
- If you have high blood pressure, do not take any over-the-counter (nonprescription) medications for weight control or for allergy, asthma, cough, cold, or sinus problems unless your doctor directs you to do so.
- To prevent dehydration (severe water loss) while taking this medication, check with your doctor if you have any illness that causes severe or continuous nausea, vomiting, or diarrhea.
- This medication can raise blood sugar levels in diabetic patients. Therefore, blood sugar should be carefully monitored by blood or urine tests when this medication is being taken.
- Before having surgery or any other medical or dental treatment, be sure to tell your doctor or dentist that you are taking this medication.
- Be sure to tell your doctor if you are pregnant. Hydrochlorothiazide can cross the placenta and may cause adverse effects on the developing fetus. Also, tell your doctor if you are breast-feeding an infant. Although problems in humans have not been reported, small amounts of this drug can pass into breast milk, so caution is warranted.

Hydro-Clor—see hydrochlorothiazide

hydrocortisone (systemic)

BRAND NAMES (Manufacturers)
Cortef (Upjohn)
hydrocortisone (various manufacturers)
Hydrocortone (Merck Sharp & Dohme)
TYPE OF DRUG
Adrenocorticosteroid hormone
INGREDIENT
hydrocortisone (cortisol)
DOSAGE FORMS
Tablets (5 mg, 10 mg, and 20 mg)
Oral suspension (10 mg per 5-ml spoonful)
STORAGE
Store at room temperature in a tightly closed container.

USES

Your adrenal glands naturally produce certain cortisone-like chemicals. These chemicals are involved in various regulatory processes in the body (such as those involving fluid balance, temperature, and reaction to inflammation). Hydrocortisone belongs to a group of drugs known as adrenocorticosteroids (or cortisone-like medications). It is used to treat a variety of disorders, including endocrine (hormonal) and rheumatic disorders; asthma; blood diseases; certain cancers; eye disorders; gastrointestinal disturbances, such as ulcerative colitis; respiratory diseases; and inflammations such as arthritis, dermatitis, poison ivy, and other allergic conditions. How this drug acts to relieve these disorders is not completely understood.

TREATMENT

In order to prevent stomach irritation, you can take hydrocortisone with food or milk.

If you are taking only one dose of this medication each day, try to take it before 9:00 A.M. This will mimic the body's normal production of this type of chemical.

The oral suspension form of this medication should be shaken well just before measuring each dose. The contents tend to settle on the bottom of the bottle, so it is necessary to shake the container to distribute the ingredients evenly and equalize the doses. Each dose should then be measured carefully with a specially designed 5-ml measuring spoon. An ordinary kitchen teaspoon is not accurate enough.

It is important to try not to miss any doses of hydrocortisone. However, if you do miss a dose of this medication, follow these guidelines:
1. If you are taking it more than once a day, take the missed dose as soon as possible, then return to your regular schedule. If it is already time for the next dose, double the dose.
2. If you are taking this medication once a day, take the dose you missed as soon as possible, unless you don't remember until the next day. In that case, do not take the missed dose at all; just follow your regular schedule. Do not double the next dose.
3. If you are taking this drug every other day, take the missed dose as soon as you remember. If you missed the scheduled dose by a whole day, take it when you remember and then skip a day before you take the next dose. Do not double the dose.

If you miss more than one dose of hydrocortisone, CONTACT YOUR DOCTOR.

SIDE EFFECTS

Minor. Dizziness, false sense of well-being, increased appetite, increased sweating, indigestion, menstrual irregularities, nausea, reddening and swelling of the skin on the face, restlessness, sleep disorders, or weight gain. These side effects should disappear as your body adjusts to the medication.

To help avoid potassium loss while using this drug, take your dose with a glass of fresh or frozen orange juice, or eat a banana each day. The use of a salt substitute also helps to prevent potassium loss. Check with your doctor before changing your diet or using a salt substitute.

Major. Tell your doctor about any side effects that are persistent or particularly bothersome. IT IS ESPECIALLY IMPORTANT TO TELL YOUR DOCTOR about abdominal (area around and above the waist) enlargement; acne or other skin problems; back or rib pain; bloody or black, tarry stools; blurred vision; convulsions; eye pain; fever and sore throat; growth impairment (in children); headaches; slow healing of wounds; increased thirst and urination; mental depression; mood changes; muscle wasting; muscle weakness; nightmares; rapid weight gain (three to five pounds within a week); rash; red lines across the abdomen; severe abdominal pain; shortness of breath; thinning of the skin; unusual bleeding or bruising; or unusual weakness.

INTERACTIONS

The systemic form of hydrocortisone adrenocorticosteroid hormone interacts with several other types of medications:

1. Alcohol, aspirin, and anti-inflammatory medications (such as diclofenac, diflunisal, flurbiprofen, ibuprofen, indomethacin, ketoprofen, mefenamic acid, meclofenamate, naproxen, piroxicam, sulindac, and tolmetin) aggravate the stomach problems that are common with use of this medication.

2. The dosage of oral anticoagulants (blood thinners, such as warfarin), oral antidiabetic drugs, or insulin may need to be adjusted when this medication is started or stopped.

3. The loss of potassium caused by hydrocortisone can lead to serious side effects in individuals taking digoxin. Also, thiazide diuretics (water pills) can increase the potassium loss caused by hydrocortisone.

4. Phenobarbital, phenytoin, rifampin, and ephedrine can increase the elimination of hydrocortisone from the body, thereby decreasing its effectiveness.

5. Oral contraceptives (birth control pills) and estrogen-containing drugs may decrease the elimination of this drug from the body, which can lead to an increase in side effects.

6. Hydrocortisone can increase the elimination of aspirin and isoniazid from the body, thereby decreasing the effectiveness of these two medications.

7. Cholestyramine and colestipol can chemically bind this medication in the stomach and gastrointestinal tract, preventing its absorption and decreasing its effectiveness.

BE SURE TO TELL YOUR DOCTOR about any medications you are currently taking, especially any of those listed above.

WARNINGS

- Tell your doctor about unusual or allergic reactions you have had to any medications, especially to hydrocortisone or other adrenocorticosteroids (such as betamethasone, cortisone, dexamethasone, fluocinolone, methylprednisolone, prednisolone, prednisone, and triamcinolone).
- Tell your doctor if you now have or if you have ever had bone disease, diabetes mellitus, emotional instability, glaucoma, fungal infections, heart disease, high blood pressure, high cholesterol levels, myasthenia gravis, peptic ulcers, osteoporosis, thyroid disease, tuberculosis, ulcerative colitis, kidney disease, or liver disease.
- If you are using this medication for longer than a week, you may need to receive higher dosages if you are subjected to stress, such as serious infections, injury, or surgery. Discuss this with your doctor.
- If you have been taking this drug for more than a week, do not stop taking it suddenly. If it is stopped suddenly, you may experience abdominal or back pain, dizziness, fainting, fever, muscle or joint pain, nausea, vomiting, shortness of breath, or extreme weakness. Your doctor may, therefore, want to reduce the dosage gradually. Never increase the dosage or take the drug for longer than the prescribed time, unless you first consult your doctor.
- While you are taking this drug, you should not be vaccinated or immunized. This medication decreases the effectiveness of vaccines and can lead to overwhelming infection if a live-virus vaccine is administered.
- Before having surgery or any other medical or dental treatment, be sure to tell your doctor or dentist that you are taking this medication.
- Because this drug can cause glaucoma and cataracts with long-term use, your doctor may want you to have your eyes examined by an ophthalmologist periodically during treatment.
- If you are taking this medication for prolonged periods, you should wear or carry an identification card or notice stating that you are taking an adrenocorticosteroid.
- This medication can raise blood sugar levels in diabetic patients. Blood sugar levels should, therefore, be monitored carefully with blood or urine tests when this medication is being taken.
- Be sure to tell your doctor if you are pregnant. This drug crosses the placenta. Although studies in humans have not been conducted, birth defects have been observed in the offspring of animals that were given large doses of this drug during pregnancy. Also, tell your doctor if you are breast-feeding an infant. Small amounts of this drug pass into breast milk and may cause growth suppression or a decrease in natural adrenocorticosteroid hormone production in the nursing infant.

---

hydrocortisone (topical)

BRAND NAMES (Manufacturers)

Acticort 100 (Baker/Cummins)
Aeroseb-HC (Herbert)
Ala-Cort (Del-Ray)
Ala-Scalp (Del-Ray)
Bactine Hydrocortisone* (Miles)
Caladryl Hydrocortisone* (Parke-Davis)
CaldeCort Anti-Itch* (Pharmacraft)
CaldeCort Light with Aloe* (Pharmacraft)
Cetacort (Owen)

Cortaid* (Upjohn)
Cort-Dome (Miles)
Cortef Feminine Itch* (Upjohn)
Cortizone-5* (Thompson)
Cortril* (Pfipharmecs)
Cortril (Pfizer)
Delacort* (Mericon)
Dermacort (Reid-Rowell)
DermiCort* (Republic Drug)
Dermolate Anti-Itch* (Schering)
Dermolate Scalp-Itch* (Schering)
Dermtex HC* (Pfeiffer)
FoilleCort* (Blistex)
Gynecort (Combe)
HC-Jel (Recsei)
Hi-Cor (C & M Pharmaceuticals)
H_2 Cort* (Vangard)
hydrocortisone acetate (various manufacturers)
Hydrocortone Acetate (Merck Sharp & Dohme)
Hydro-Tex (Syosset)
Hydro-Tex* (Syosset)
Hytone (Dermik)
Hytone* (Dermik)
LactiCare-HC (Stiefel)
Lanacort* (Combe)
Locoid (Owen)
My Cort (Scrip)
Nutracort (Owen)
Penecort (Herbert Labs)
Pharma-Cort* (Purepac)
Racet SE* (Lemmon)
Rhulicort* (Lederle)
Sensacort* (Plough)
Synacort (Syntex)
Texacort (GenDerm)
Westcort (Westwood)
*Available over-the-counter (without a prescription) in concentrations of 0.5% or less.

TYPE OF DRUG
Adrenocorticosteroid hormone

INGREDIENT
hydrocortisone

DOSAGE FORMS
Cream (0.1%, 0.2%, 0.25%, 0.5%, 1%, and 2.5%)
Ointment (0.1%, 0.2%, 0.5%, 1%, and 2.5%)
Lotion (0.25%, 0.5%, 1%, 2%, and 2.5%)
Gel (1%)
Pump spray (0.5%)
Aerosol (0.5%)

STORAGE
Hydrocortisone cream, ointment, lotion, gel, pump spray, and aerosol should be stored at room temperature in tightly closed containers. This medication should never be frozen.

The aerosol form of this medication is packaged under pressure. It should not be stored near heat or an open flame or in direct sunlight, and the container should never be punctured.

USES
Your adrenal glands naturally produce certain cortisone-like chemicals. These chemicals are involved in various regulatory processes in the body (such as those involving fluid balance, temperature, and reaction to inflammation). Hydrocortisone belongs to a group of drugs known as adrenocorticosteroids (or cortisone-like medications). It is used to relieve the skin inflammation (redness, swelling, itching, and discomfort) associated with conditions such as dermatitis, eczema, and poison ivy. How this drug acts to relieve inflammation is not completely understood.

TREATMENT
Before applying this medication, wash your hands. Then, unless your doctor gives you different instructions, gently wash the area of the skin where the medication is to be applied. With a clean towel, pat the area almost dry; it should be slightly damp when you put the medicine on.

Apply a small amount of the medication to the affected area in a thin layer. Do not bandage the area unless your doctor tells you to do so. If you are to apply an occlusive dressing (like kitchen plastic wrap), be sure you understand the instructions. Wash your hands again after application.

If you are using the aerosol form, shake the can in order to disperse the medication evenly. Hold the can upright six to eight inches from the area to be sprayed, and spray the area for one to three seconds. DO NOT SMOKE while you are using the aerosol; the contents are under pressure and may explode when exposed to heat or flames.

If you miss a dose of this medication, apply the dose as soon as possible, unless it is almost time for the next application. In that case, do not apply the missed dose at all; just return to your regular dosing schedule. Do not put twice as much of the medication on your skin at the next application.

SIDE EFFECTS
Minor. Acne, burning sensation, itching, skin dryness, or rash.

If the affected area is extremely dry or scaling, the skin may be moistened before applying the medication by soaking in water or by applying water with a clean cloth. The ointment form is probably better for dry skin.

A mild, temporary stinging sensation may occur after this medication is applied. If this persists, contact your doctor.

Major. Tell your doctor about any side effects that are persistent or particularly bothersome. IT IS ESPECIALLY IMPORTANT TO TELL YOUR DOCTOR about blistering, increased hair growth, irritation of the affected area, loss of skin color, secondary infection in the area being treated, or thinning of the skin with easy bruising.

INTERACTIONS
This medication should not interact with other medications as long as it is used according to the directions given to you by your doctor or pharmacist.

WARNINGS
• Tell your doctor about unusual or allergic reactions you have had to any medications, especially to hydrocortisone or other adrenocorticosteroids (such as amcinonide, betamethasone, clocortolone, cortisone, desonide, desoximetasone, dexamethasone, diflorasone, flumethasone, fluocinolone, fluocinonide, flurandrenolide, halcinonide, methylprednisolone, paramethasone, prednisolone, prednisone, and triamcinolone).

• Tell your doctor if you now have or if you have ever had blood vessel disease, chicken pox, diabetes mellitus, fungal infections, peptic ulcers, shingles, tuberculosis, tuberculosis of the skin, vaccinia, or any other type of infection, especially at the site currently being treated.
• If any irritation develops while using hydrocortisone, immediately discontinue its use and notify your doctor.
• This product is not for use in the eyes, nose, or mouth; contact may result in side effects.
• Do not use this product with an occlusive wrap unless your doctor directs you to do so. Systemic absorption of hydrocortisone is increased if large areas of the body are treated, particularly if occlusive bandages are used. If it is necessary for you to use this drug under a wrap, follow your doctor's instructions exactly; do not leave the wrap in place longer than specified.
• If you are using this medication on a child's diaper area, do not put tight-fitting diapers or plastic pants on the child. This may lead to increased systemic absorption of the drug and a possible increase in side effects.
• In order to avoid freezing skin tissue when using the aerosol or pump spray form of hydrocortisone, make sure that you do not spray for more than three seconds; and hold the container at least six inches away from the skin.
• When using the aerosol or pump spray form of this medication on the face, cover your eyes, and do not inhale the spray (in order to avoid side effects).
• Be sure to tell your doctor if you are pregnant. If large amounts of this drug are applied for prolonged periods, some of it will be absorbed and may cross the placenta. Although studies in humans have not been conducted, birth defects have been observed in the offspring of animals that were given large oral doses of this drug during pregnancy. Also, tell your doctor if you are breast-feeding an infant. If absorbed through the skin, small amounts of hydrocortisone pass into breast milk and may cause growth suppression or a decrease in natural adrenocorticosteroid hormone production in the nursing infant.

hydrocortisone acetate—see hydrocortisone (topical)

---

hydrocortisone and iodochlorhydroxyquin combination (topical)

BRAND NAMES (Manufacturers)
Ala-Quin (Del-Ray)
Caquin (Forest)
Corque (Geneva Generics)
Cortin (C & M)
HC-Form (Recsei)
hydrocortisone with iodochlorhydroxyquin (various manufacturers)
Hysone (Mallard)
Lanvisone (Lannett)
Pedi-Cort V (Pedinol)
Racet (Lemmon)
Viodo HC (NMC Labs)
Vioform-Hydrocortisone (Ciba)
Vytone (Dermik)

TYPE OF DRUG
Adrenocorticosteroid hormone and anti-infective

INGREDIENTS
hydrocortisone and iodochlorhydroxyquin

DOSAGE FORMS
Cream (0.5% hydrocortisone with 1% or 3% iodochlorhydroxyquin; 1% hydrocortisone with 1% or 3% iodochlorhydroxyquin)
Ointment (1% hydrocortisone with 3% iodochlorhydroxyquin)
Lotion (0.5% or 1% hydrocortisone with 3% iodochlorhydroxyquin)
Jelly (1% hydrocortisone with 3% iodochlorhydroxyquin)

STORAGE
Hydrocortisone and iodochlorhydroxyquin combination cream, ointment, lotion, and jelly should be stored at room temperature in tightly closed, light-resistant containers. This medication should never be frozen.

USES

Your adrenal glands naturally produce certain cortisone-like chemicals. These chemicals are involved in various regulatory processes in the body (such as those involving fluid balance, temperature, and reactions to inflammation). Hydrocortisone belongs to a group of drugs known as adrenocorticosteroids (or cortisone-like medications). It is used to relieve the skin inflammation (redness, swelling, itching, and discomfort) associated with conditions such as dermatitis and eczema. How this drug acts to relieve inflammation is not completely understood. Iodochlorhydroxyquin is an antibiotic that acts to prevent the growth and multiplication of the infecting bacteria or fungi.

TREATMENT

Before applying this medication, wash your hands. Then, unless your doctor gives you different instructions, gently wash the area of the skin where the medication is to be applied. With a clean towel, pat the area almost dry; it should be slightly damp when you put the medication on.

If you are using the lotion form of this medication, shake the bottle well before pouring out a dose of medication. The contents tend to settle on the bottom of the bottle, so it is necessary to shake the container to distribute the ingredients evenly and equalize the doses.

Apply a small amount of the cream, ointment, lotion, or jelly to the affected area in a thin layer. Do not bandage the area unless your doctor tells you to do so. If you are to apply an occlusive dressing (like kitchen plastic wrap), be sure you understand the instructions. Wash your hands again after application.

If you miss a dose of this medication, apply the dose as soon as possible, unless it is almost time for the next application. In that case, do not apply the missed dose at all; just return to your regular schedule. Do not put twice as much of the medication on your skin at the next application.

It is important to continue to take the medication for the entire time prescribed by your doctor, even if the symptoms of infection disappear before the end of that period. If you stop applying the drug too soon, resistant bacteria are given a chance to continue growing, and the infection could recur.

SIDE EFFECTS

Minor. Acne, burning sensation, skin dryness, itching, or rash. These side effects should disappear as your body adjusts to the medication.

If the affected area is extremely dry or scaling, the skin may be moistened before applying the medication by soaking in water or by applying water with a clean cloth. The ointment form is probably better for dry skin.

A mild, temporary stinging sensation may occur after this medication is applied. If this persists, contact your doctor.

Major. Tell your doctor about any side effects that are persistent or particularly bothersome. IT IS ESPECIALLY IMPORTANT TO TELL YOUR DOCTOR about blistering, increased hair growth, irritation of the affected area, loss of skin color, secondary infection at the affected site, or thinning of the skin with easy bruising.

INTERACTIONS

This medication should not interact with other medications as long as it is used according to directions.

WARNINGS

- Tell your doctor about unusual or allergic reactions you have had to medications, especially to hydrocortisone or any other adrenocorticosteroid (such as amcinonide, betamethasone, clocortolone, cortisone, desonide, desoximetasone, dexamethasone, diflorasone, flumethasone, fluocinolone, fluocinonide, fluorometholone, flurandrenolide, halcinonide, methylprednisolone, prednisolone, prednisone, and triamcinolone), to iodochlorhydroxyquin, or to iodine.
- Tell your doctor if you now have or if you have ever had tuberculosis or viral or fungal infections of the skin.
- This product may affect the results of thyroid function tests. If you are scheduled to have such a test, be sure your doctor knows that you are using this medication.
- If additional irritation develops while using this drug, immediately discontinue its use and notify your doctor.
- This product is not for use in the eyes or mucous membranes; contact may result in side effects.
- Do not use this product with an occlusive wrap unless your doctor directs you to do so. Systemic absorption of this drug is increased if extensive areas of the body are treated, particularly if occlusive bandages are used. If it is necessary for you to use this drug under a wrap, follow your doctor's instructions exactly; do not leave the wrap in place longer than specified.
- If you are using this medication on a child's diaper area, do not put tight-fitting diapers or plastic pants on the child. This may lead to increased systemic absorption of the drug and a possible increase in side effects.
- This medication has been prescribed for your current infection only. Another infection later on, or one that someone else has, may require a different medicine. You should not give your medicine to other people or use it for other infections, unless your doctor specifically directs you to do so.
- Be sure to tell your doctor if you are pregnant. If large amounts of this drug are applied for prolonged periods, some of it will be absorbed and may cross the placenta. Studies in humans have not been conducted, but birth defects have been observed in the offspring of animals that were given large oral doses of hydrocortisone during pregnancy. Also, tell your doctor if you are breast-feeding an infant. If absorbed through the skin, small amounts of hydrocortisone pass into breast milk and may cause growth suppression or a decrease in natural adrenocorticosteroid hormone production in the nursing infant.

---

hydrocortisone, benzyl benzoate, bismuth resorcin compound, bismuth subgallate, zinc oxide, and Peruvian balsam combination (topical)

BRAND NAMES (Manufacturers)

Anucort (G & W)
Anumed HC (Major)
Anusol HC (Parke-Davis)
Hemorrhoidal HC (various manufacturers)
Rectacort (Century)

TYPE OF DRUG

Adrenocorticosteroid-containing hemorrhoidal and anorectal product

INGREDIENTS

hydrocortisone, benzyl benzoate, bismuth resorcin compound, bismuth subgallate, zinc oxide, and Peruvian balsam

DOSAGE FORMS

Rectal cream (0.5% hydrocortisone, 1.2% benzyl benzoate, 1.75% bismuth resorcin compound, 2.25% bismuth subgallate, 11% zinc oxide, and 1.8% Peruvian balsam)

Rectal suppositories (10 mg hydrocortisone, 1.2% benzyl benzoate, 1.75% bismuth resorcin compound, 2.25% bismuth subgallate, 11% zinc oxide, and 1.8% Peruvian balsam per suppository)

STORAGE

The rectal cream should be stored at room temperature (never frozen) in a tightly closed container. The rectal suppositories should be stored in a cool, dry place or in the refrigerator.

USES

This combination medication is used to relieve the pain, itching, and discomfort arising from hemorrhoids and irritated anorectal tissues.

Your adrenal glands naturally produce certain cortisone-like chemicals. These chemicals are involved in various regulatory processes in the body (such as those involving fluid balance, temperature, and reaction to inflammation). Hydrocortisone belongs to a group of drugs known as adrenocorticosteroids (or cortisone-like drugs). Hydrocortisone is used to relieve inflammation (redness, swelling, itching, and discomfort). Zinc oxide is an astringent that causes shrinking and provides relief of irritation. The other ingredients provide a drying and softening effect.

TREATMENT

Wash your hands before applying this medication. To apply the rectal cream, first wash and dry the rectal area and then gently rub in a small amount of the cream. If you must insert the cream inside the rectum, attach the applicator tip to the opened tube. It may be helpful to lubricate the applicator with a small amount of petroleum jelly to ease insertion. Insert the applicator tip into the rectum and squeeze the tube. Remove the applicator from the tube and wash it with hot water and soap; then thoroughly dry it before storing. Be sure to put the top back on the tube. Wash your hands again after application.

To insert the suppository, unwrap the suppository and moisten it slightly with water (if the suppository is too soft to insert, run cold water over it or refrigerate it for up to 30 minutes before you unwrap it). Lie down on your left side with your right knee bent. Push the suppository well into the rectum with your finger. Try not to have a bowel movement for at least an hour. Wash your hands again after application.

If you miss a dose of this medication, apply the cream or insert the suppository as soon as possible, unless it is almost time for the next application. In that case, do not use the missed dose at all; just wait until the next scheduled dose.

SIDE EFFECTS

Minor. Burning sensation upon application. The burning should disappear as your body adjusts to the medication.

Major. Tell your doctor about any side effects that are persistent or particularly bothersome. IT IS ESPECIALLY IMPORTANT TO TELL YOUR DOCTOR about any additional inflammation or infection at the site of application, as well as rectal pain, bleeding, leakage, itching, or blistering.

INTERACTIONS

This medication should not interact with any other medications as long as it is used according to the directions given to you by the doctor or pharmacist.

WARNINGS

- Tell your doctor about unusual or allergic reactions you have had to medications, especially to benzyl benzoate, bismuth resorcin compound, bismuth subgallate, Peruvian balsam, or to hydrocortisone or any other adrenocorticosteroid (such as amcinonide, betamethasone, clocortolone, cortisone, desonide, desoximetasone, dexamethasone, diflorasone, flumethasone, fluocinolone, fluocinonide, fluorometholone, flurandrenolide, halcinonide, methylprednisolone, paramethasone, prednisolone, prednisone, and triamcinolone).
- If additional irritation develops while using this drug, immediately discontinue its use and notify your doctor.
- You should not use this medication for more than seven consecutive days unless your doctor specifically directs you to do so.
- If this drug stains your clothing, the stain may be removed by washing with laundry detergent.
- Wearing a sanitary napkin may help to protect clothing and to keep the medication in the area.
- Be sure to tell your doctor if you are pregnant. If large amounts of hydrocortisone are applied for prolonged periods, some of it will be absorbed and may cross the placenta. Studies in humans have not been conducted, but birth defects have been observed in the offspring of animals that were given large oral doses of hydrocortisone during pregnancy. Also, tell your doctor if you are breast-feeding an infant. If absorbed through the skin, small amounts of hydrocortisone pass into breast milk and may cause growth suppression or a decrease in natural adrenocorticosteroid hormone production in the nursing infant.

---

hydrocortisone, polymyxin B, and neomycin combination (otic)

BRAND NAMES (Manufacturers)
AK-Spore H.C. Otic (Akorn)
Cortatrigen Modified Ear Drops (Goldline)
Cortisporin Otic (Burroughs Wellcome)
Drotic (Ascher)
Ortega-Otic M (Ortega)
Otocort (Lemmon)
Otomycin-Hpn Otic (Misemer)
Otoreid-HC (Reid-Rowell)

TYPE OF DRUG
Otic adrenocorticosteroid and antibiotic

INGREDIENTS
hydrocortisone, polymyxin B, and neomycin

DOSAGE FORMS
Otic solution (1% hydrocortisone, 10,000 units polymyxin B, and 5 mg neomycin per ml)
Otic suspension (1% hydrocortisone, 10,000 units polymyxin B, and 5 mg neomycin per ml)

STORAGE
The medication should be stored at room temperature (never frozen) in tightly closed, light-resistant containers.

USES

This medication is used to treat superficial bacterial infections of the outer ear. Your adrenal glands naturally produce certain cortisone-like chemicals. These chemicals are involved in various regulatory processes in the body (such as those involving fluid balance, temperature, and reaction to inflammation). Hydrocortisone belongs to a group of drugs known as adrenocorticosteroids (or cortisone-like medications). It is used to relieve inflammation (redness, swelling, itching, pain). Polymyxin B and neomycin are antibiotics, which act to prevent the growth and multiplication of the infecting bacteria.

TREATMENT

For accuracy, and in order to avoid contamination, another person should insert the ear drops if possible.

To warm the drops before administration, roll the bottle back and forth between your hands. DO NOT place the bottle in boiling water; high temperatures destroy the medication.

Before administration, the suspension form of this medication should be shaken well. The contents tend to settle on the bottom of the bottle, so it is necessary to shake the container to distribute the ingredients evenly and equalize the doses.

To administer the ear drops, tilt the head to one side with the affected ear turned upward. Grasp the earlobe and gently pull it upward and back to straighten the ear canal. (If administering ear drops to a child, gently pull the earlobe downward and back.) Fill the dropper and place the prescribed number of drops into the ear. Be careful not to touch the dropper to the ear canal, since the dropper can easily become contaminated. Keep the ear tilted upward for about five minutes. Your doctor may want you to put a piece of cotton soaked with the medication into your ear to keep the medicine from leaking out. To avoid contamination, DO NOT wash or wipe the dropper after you use it.

If you miss a dose, insert the drops as soon as possible, unless it is almost time for the next dose. In that case, don't use the missed dose at all; just return to your regular dosing schedule.

It is important to continue to take this medication for the entire time prescribed by your doctor, even if the symptoms of infection disappear before the end of that period. If you stop using the drug too soon, resistant bacteria are given a chance to continue growing, and the infection could recur.

SIDE EFFECTS

Minor. Burning sensation upon application. The burning should disappear as your body adjusts to the medication.

Major. Tell your doctor about any side effects that are persistent or particularly bothersome. IT IS ESPECIALLY IMPORTANT TO TELL YOUR DOCTOR about itching, rash, redness, or swelling at the site of application.

INTERACTIONS

This medication should not interact with any other medications as long as it is used according to directions.

WARNINGS

- Tell your doctor about unusual or allergic reactions you have had to medications, especially to hydrocortisone or any other adrenocorticosteroids (such as amcinonide, betamethasone, clocortolone, cortisone, desonide, desoximetasone, dexamethasone, diflorasone, flumethasone, fluocinolone, fluocinonide, fluorometholone, flurandrenolide, halcinonide, methylprednisolone, prednisolone, prednisone, and triamcinolone), to polymyxin B, or to neomycin or any related antibiotic (such as amikacin, colistimethate, colistin, gentamicin, kanamycin, netilmicin, paromycin, streptomycin, tobramycin, or viomycin).
- Tell your doctor if you now have or if you have ever had viral or fungal infections of the ear, a punctured eardrum, myasthenia gravis, or kidney disease.
- Do not use this medication for longer than ten consecutive days, unless your doctor directs you to do so. If there is no change in your condition within two or three days after starting to take this medication, contact your doctor. The medication may not be effective for the type of infection you have.
- This medication has been prescribed for your current infection only. Another infection later on, or one that someone else has, may require a different medicine. You should not give your medicine to other people or use it for other infections, unless your doctor specifically directs you to do so.
- Be sure to tell your doctor if you are pregnant. If large amounts of hydrocortisone are applied for prolonged periods, some of it will be absorbed and may cross the placenta. Studies in humans have not been conducted, but birth defects have been observed in the offspring of animals that were given large oral doses of hydrocortisone during pregnancy. Also, tell your doctor if you are breast-feeding an infant. If absorbed through the skin, small amounts of the drug pass into breast milk and may cause growth suppression or a decrease in natural adrenocorticosteroid hormone production in the infant.

---

hydrocortisone, polymyxin B, neomycin, and bacitracin combination (ophthalmic)

BRAND NAMES (Manufacturers)

Coracin (Hauck)
Cortisporin Ophthalmic (Burroughs Wellcome)
Triple Antibiotic (various manufacturers)
Triple-Gen (Goldline)

TYPE OF DRUG

Ophthalmic adrenocorticosteroid and antibiotic

INGREDIENTS

hydrocortisone, polymyxin B, neomycin, and bacitracin (ointment only)

DOSAGE FORMS

Ophthalmic drops (1% hydrocortisone; 10,000 units polymyxin B; 0.5% neomycin; and 0.001% thimerosal per ml)
Ophthalmic ointment (1% hydrocortisone; 10,000 units polymyxin B; 0.5% neomycin; 400 units bacitracin; and 0.001% thimerosal per gram of ointment)

STORAGE

This medication should be stored at room temperature (never frozen) in tightly closed containers. If the drops or ointment change color, do not use the medication. A change in color signifies a loss of effectiveness.

USES

This medication is used for the short-term treatment of bacterial infections of the eyes.

Your adrenal glands naturally produce certain cortisone-like chemicals. These chemicals are involved in various regulatory processes in the body (such as those involving fluid balance, temperature, and reaction to inflammation). Hydrocortisone belongs to a group of drugs known as adrenocorticosteroids (or cortisone-like medications). It is used to relieve inflammation (redness, swelling, itching, and discomfort). How it does so is not completely understood.

Polymyxin B, neomycin, and bacitracin are antibiotics, which act to prevent the growth and multiplication of infecting bacteria. Thimerosal is a preservative.

TREATMENT

Wash your hands with soap and water before using this medication. If you are using the drops, shake the bottle well before measuring out the drops. The contents tend to settle on the bottom of the bottle, so it is necessary to shake the container to distribute the ingredients evenly and equalize the doses.

To prevent contamination of the medicine, do not touch the tube portion of the dropper or let it touch the eye.

Note that the bottle of the eye drops is not completely full. This is to allow control of the number of drops used.

To apply the drops, tilt your head back and pull down the lower eyelid with one hand to make a pouch below the eye. Drop the prescribed amount of medicine into the pouch and slowly close your eyes. Try not to blink. Keep your eyes closed, and place one finger at the corner of the eye next to your nose for a minute or two, applying a slight pressure (this is done to prevent loss of medication through the duct that drains fluid from the surface of the eye into the nose and throat). Then wipe away any excess with a clean tissue. If you don't think the medicine got into your eye, repeat the process once. If you are using more than one type of eye drop, wait at least five minutes between doses of the two types of medication.

Follow the same general procedure for applying the ointment. Tilt your head back, pull down the lower eyelid, and squeeze the ointment in a line along the pouch below the eye. Close your eyes, and place your finger at the corner of the eye near the nose for a minute or two. Do not rub your eyes. Wipe off excess ointment and the tip of the tube with clean tissues.

Since applying the medication is somewhat difficult to do, you may want someone else to apply it for you.

If you miss a dose of this medication, insert the drops or apply the ointment as soon as possible, unless it is almost time for the next application. In that case, do not use the missed dose at all; just wait until the next scheduled dose.

It is important to continue to take this medication for the entire time prescribed by your doctor, even if the symptoms of infection disappear before the end of that period. If you stop applying the drug too soon, resistant bacteria are given a chance to continue growing, and the infection could recur.

SIDE EFFECTS

Minor. Blurred vision, burning, or stinging. These side effects should disappear as your body adjusts to the medication.

Major. Tell your doctor about any side effects that are persistent or particularly bothersome. IT IS ESPECIALLY IMPORTANT TO TELL YOUR DOCTOR about disturbed or reduced vision; eye pain, itching, or swelling; headache; rash; continued burning; or severe irritation.

INTERACTIONS

This medication should not interact with other medications as long as it is used according to the directions given to you by your doctor or pharmacist.

WARNINGS

- Tell your doctor about unusual or allergic reactions you have had to any medications, especially to hydrocortisone or other adrenocorticosteroids (such as amcinonide, betamethasone, clocortolone, cortisone, desonide, desoximetasone, dexamethasone, diflorasone, flumethasone, fluocinolone, fluorometholone, flurandrenolide, halcinonide, methylprednisolone, prednisolone, prednisone, and triamcinolone) or to polymyxin B, neomycin, bacitracin, or any related antibiotic (amikacin, colistimethate, colistin, gentamicin, kanamycin, neomycin, netilmicin, paromycin, streptomycin, tobramycin, or viomycin), or to thimerosal or other mercury compounds.
- Tell your doctor if you now have or if you have ever had fungal or viral infections of the eye, cataracts, glaucoma, inner ear disease, kidney disease, or myasthenia gravis.
- Tell your doctor if you wear contact lenses. Your doctor may suggest that you wear eyeglasses until the infection is gone.
- If there is no change in your condition two or three days after starting to take this medication, contact your doctor. The medication may not be effective for your particular infection.
- Do not use this medication for longer than ten consecutive days, unless your doctor directs you to do so. Prolonged use of this drug may result in glaucoma, secondary infection, cataracts, or eye damage. If you need to take this medication for as long as six weeks, your doctor may want you to have an eye examination by an ophthalmologist.
- This medication has been prescribed for your current infection only. Another infection later on, or one that a family member or friend has, may require a different medicine. You should not give your medicine to other people or use it for other infections, unless your doctor specifically directs you to do so.
- In order to allow your eye infection to clear, you should not apply makeup to the affected eye during treatment with this medication.
- Be sure to tell your doctor if you are pregnant. When large amounts of hydrocortisone are applied for prolonged periods, some of it is absorbed into the bloodstream. It may cross the placenta. Studies in humans have not been conducted, but birth defects have been observed in the offspring of animals that were given large oral doses of hydrocortisone during pregnancy. Also, tell your doctor if you are breastfeeding. If absorbed through the skin, small amounts of hydrocortisone pass into breast milk and may cause growth suppression or a decrease in natural adrenocorticosteroid hormone production in the nursing infant.

Hydrocortone—see hydrocortisone (systemic)

Hydrocortone Acetate—see hydrocortisone (topical)

HydroDIURIL—see hydrochlorothiazide

Hydrogesic—see acetaminophen and hydrocodone combination

Hydromal—see hydrochlorothiazide

---

hydromorphone

BRAND NAMES (Manufacturers)
Dilaudid (Knoll)
hydromorphone hydrochloride (Roxane)

TYPE OF DRUG
Analgesic

INGREDIENT
hydromorphone

DOSAGE FORMS
Tablets (1 mg, 2 mg, 3 mg, and 4 mg)
Suppositories (3 mg)

STORAGE

Hydromorphone tablets should be stored at room temperature in a tightly closed, light-resistant container. The suppositories should be stored in the refrigerator.

USES

Hydromorphone is a narcotic analgesic that acts directly on the central nervous system (brain and spinal cord). It is used to relieve moderate to severe pain.

TREATMENT

In order to avoid stomach upset, you can take hydromorphone tablets with food or milk.

To use the suppository, remove the foil wrapper and moisten the suppository with water (if the suppository is too soft to insert, refrigerate it for half an hour or run cold water over it before removing the wrapper). Lie on your left side with your right knee bent. Push the suppository into the rectum, pointed end first. Lie still for a few minutes. Try to avoid having a bowel movement for at least an hour.

Hydromorphone works most effectively if you take it at the onset of pain, rather than waiting until the pain becomes intense.

If you are taking this medication on a regular schedule and you miss a dose, take the missed dose as soon as possible, unless it is almost time for your next dose. In that case, do not take the missed dose at all; just return to your regular dosing schedule. Do not double the next dose.

SIDE EFFECTS

Minor. Constipation, dizziness, drowsiness, dry mouth, false sense of well-being, flushing, light-headedness, loss of appetite, nausea, or sweating. These side effects should disappear as your body adjusts to the medication.

If you are constipated, increase the amount of fiber in your diet (fresh fruits and vegetables, salads, bran, and whole-grain breads), exercise, and drink more water (unless your doctor directs you to do otherwise).

Chew sugarless gum or suck on ice chips or a piece of hard candy to reduce mouth dryness.

If you feel dizzy or light-headed, sit or lie down for a while; get up from a sitting or lying position slowly, and be careful on stairs.

Major. Tell your doctor about any side effects that are persistent or particularly bothersome. IT IS ESPECIALLY IMPORTANT TO TELL YOUR DOCTOR about anxiety, confusion, continued constipation, difficult or painful urination, difficulty in breathing, excitation, fatigue, rash, restlessness, sore throat and fever, tremors, or weakness.

INTERACTIONS

Hydromorphone interacts with several other types of drugs:

1. Concurrent use of it with other central nervous system depressants (such as alcohol, antihistamines, barbiturates, benzodiazepine tranquilizers, muscle relaxants, and phenothiazine tranquilizers) or with tricyclic antidepressants can cause extreme drowsiness.

2. A monoamine oxidase (MAO) inhibitor taken within 14 days of this medication can lead to unpredictable and severe side effects.

Before starting to take hydromorphone, BE SURE TO TELL YOUR DOCTOR about any medications you are currently taking, especially any of those listed above.

WARNINGS

- Tell your doctor about unusual or allergic reactions you have had to any medications, especially to hydromorphone or to any other narcotic analgesics (such as codeine, hydrocodone, meperidine, methadone, morphine, oxycodone, and propoxyphene).
- Tell your doctor if you now have or if you have ever had acute abdominal conditions, asthma, brain disease, colitis, epilepsy, gallstones or gallbladder disease, head injuries, heart disease, kidney disease, liver disease, lung disease, mental illness, emotional disorders, prostate disease, thyroid disease, or urethral stricture.
- If this drug makes you dizzy or drowsy, do not take part in any activity that requires alertness, such as driving a car or operating potentially dangerous machinery.
- Before having surgery or any other medical or dental treatment, be sure to tell your doctor or dentist that you are taking this medication.
- Hydromorphone has the potential for abuse and must be used with caution. Usually, you should not take it on a regular schedule for longer than ten days (unless your doctor directs you to do so). Tolerance develops quickly; do not increase the dosage or stop taking the drug abruptly, unless you first consult your doctor. If you have been taking large amounts of this medication for long periods, you may experience a withdrawal reaction (muscle aches, diarrhea, gooseflesh, runny nose, nausea, vomiting, shivering, trembling, stomach cramps, sleep disorders, irritability, weakness, excessive yawning, or sweating). Your doctor may, therefore, want to reduce the dosage gradually.
- Some of these products contain the color additive FD&C Yellow No. 5 (tartrazine), which can cause allergic-type reactions (rash, fainting, difficulty in breathing) in certain susceptible individuals.
- The elderly may be more sensitive to side effects, especially constipation, mental effects, or breathing problems. Report any such effects to your doctor.
- Be sure to tell your doctor if you are pregnant. The effects of this medication during the early stages of pregnancy have not been thoroughly studied in humans. However, hydromorphone used regularly in large doses during the later stages of pregnancy can result in addiction of the fetus, leading to withdrawal symptoms (irritability, excessive crying, tremors, fever, vomiting, diarrhea, sneezing, or excessive yawning) at birth. Also, tell your doctor if you are breast-feeding an infant. Small amounts of this medication may pass into breast milk and cause excessive drowsiness in the nursing infant.

hydromorphone hydrochloride—see hydromorphone

Hydro-T—see hydrochlorothiazide

Hydro-Tex—see hydrocortisone (topical)

---

hydroxyzine

BRAND NAMES (Manufacturers)

Anxanil (EconoMed)
Atarax (Roerig)
Durrax (Dermik)

hydroxyzine hydrochloride (various manufacturers)
hydroxyzine pamoate (various manufacturers)
Vamate (Major)
Vistaril (Pfizer)

TYPE OF DRUG
Antihistamine and sedative/hypnotic

INGREDIENT
hydroxyzine

DOSAGE FORMS
Tablets (10 mg, 25 mg, 50 mg, and 100 mg)
Capsules (25 mg, 50 mg, and 100 mg)
Oral syrup (10 mg per 5-ml spoonful, with 0.5% alcohol)
Oral suspension (25 mg per 5-ml spoonful)

STORAGE
Hydroxyzine tablets, capsules, oral syrup, and oral suspension should be stored at room temperature (never frozen) in tightly closed, light-resistant containers.

USES

Hydroxyzine belongs to a group of drugs known as antihistamines (antihistamines block the action of histamine, which is a chemical that is released by the body during an allergic reaction). This medication is, therefore, used to treat or prevent symptoms of allergy. Hydroxyzine is also used as a sleeping aid and can be used to relieve the symptoms of anxiety and tension.

TREATMENT

To avoid stomach upset, you can take hydroxyzine with food or with a full glass of milk or water (unless your doctor directs you to do otherwise).

The oral suspension form of this medication should be shaken well just before measuring each dose. The contents tend to settle on the bottom of the bottle, so it is necessary to shake the container to distribute the ingredients evenly and equalize the doses. Each dose of the oral syrup or oral suspension should be measured carefully with a specially designed 5-ml measuring spoon. An ordinary kitchen teaspoon is not accurate enough.

If you miss a dose of this medication, take the missed dose as soon as possible, unless it is almost time for your next dose. In that case, don't take the missed dose at all; just return to your regular dosing schedule. Do not double the next dose.

SIDE EFFECTS

Minor. Drowsiness or dry mouth. These side effects should disappear as your body adjusts to the medication.

Dry mouth can be relieved by chewing sugarless gum or by sucking on ice chips or a piece of hard candy.

Major. Tell your doctor about any side effects that are persistent or particularly bothersome. IT IS ESPECIALLY IMPORTANT TO TELL YOUR DOCTOR about convulsions, feeling faint, irritability, mental confusion, rash, or trembling or shakiness.

INTERACTIONS

Hydroxyzine can interact with other types of drugs: Concurrent use of it with other central nervous system depressants (such as alcohol, barbiturates, benzodiazepine tranquilizers, muscle relaxants, narcotics, pain medications, and phenothiazine tranquilizers) or with tricyclic antidepressants can cause extreme drowsiness.

BE SURE TO TELL YOUR DOCTOR about any medications you are currently taking, especially any listed above.

WARNINGS

- Tell your doctor about allergic or unusual reactions you have had to medications, especially to hydroxyzine or to any other antihistamines (such as azatadine, brompheniramine, carbinoxamine, chlorpheniramine, clemastine, cyproheptadine, dexchlorpheniramine, dimenhydrinate, dimethindene, diphenhydramine, diphenylpyraline, doxylamine, promethazine, pyrilamine, trimeprazine, tripelennamine, and triprolidine).
- Hydroxyzine can cause drowsiness or dizziness. Your ability to perform tasks that require alertness, such as driving a car or operating potentially dangerous machinery, may be decreased. Appropriate caution should, therefore, be taken.
- Elderly patients may be more sensitive to side effects, especially drowsiness, confusion, and irritability. Report any such effects to your doctor.
- Be sure to tell your doctor if you are pregnant. The effects of this medication during pregnancy have not been thoroughly studied in humans. Also, tell your doctor if you are breast-feeding an infant. Small amounts of hydroxyzine pass into breast milk and may cause unusual excitement or irritability in nursing infants.

hydroxyzine hydrochloride—see hydroxyzine

hydroxyzine pamoate—see hydroxyzine

Hydro-Z 50—see hydrochlorothiazide

Hydrozide-50—see hydrochlorothiazide

Hygroton—see chlorthalidone

Hylidone—see chlorthalidone

Hylorel—see guanadrel

Hyosophen—see atropine, scopolamine, hyoscyamine, and phenobarbital combination

Hy-Phen—see acetaminophen and hydrocodone combination

Hysone—see hydrocortisone and iodochlorhydroxyquin combination (topical)

Hytakerol—see dihydrotachysterol

Hytone—see hydrocortisone (topical)

Ibuprin—see ibuprofen

---

ibuprofen

BRAND NAMES (Manufacturers)
Aches-N-Pain* (Lederle)
Advil* (Whitehall)
Genpril* (Goldline)

Haltran* (Upjohn)
Ibuprin* (Thompson Medical)
ibuprofen (various manufacturers)
Ifen (Everett)
Medipren* (McNeil)
Midol 200* (Glenbrook)
Motrin (Upjohn)
Motrin IB*
Nuprin* (Bristol-Myers)
Pamprin-IB* (Chettem)
Rufen (Boots)
Trendar* (Whitehall)
*Available over-the-counter (without a prescription) as 200-mg tablets.

TYPE OF DRUG

Nonsteroidal anti-inflammatory analgesic

INGREDIENT

ibuprofen

DOSAGE FORM

Tablets (200 mg, 300 mg, 400 mg, 600 mg, and 800 mg)

STORAGE

Store in a tightly closed container at room temperature away from heat and direct sunlight.

USES

Ibuprofen is used to treat the inflammation (pain, swelling, stiffness) of certain types of arthritis, gout, bursitis, and tendinitis. It is also used to treat painful menstruation. Ibuprofen has been shown to block production of certain body chemicals, called prostaglandins, that may trigger pain. However, it is not yet fully understood how it does so.

TREATMENT

You should take this medication on an empty stomach 30 to 60 minutes before meals or two hours after meals, so that it gets into your bloodstream quickly. However, to decrease stomach irritation, your doctor may want you to take the medication with food or antacids.

If you are taking ibuprofen to relieve arthritis, you must take it regularly as directed by your doctor. It may take up to two weeks before you feel the full effects of this medication. Ibuprofen does not cure arthritis, but it will help to control the condition as long as you continue to take it.

It is important to take ibuprofen on schedule and not to miss any doses. If you do miss a dose, take it as soon as possible, unless it is almost time for your next dose. In that case, don't take the missed dose at all; just return to your regular dosing schedule. Do not double the next dose.

SIDE EFFECTS

Minor. Bloating, constipation, diarrhea, difficulty in sleeping, dizziness, drowsiness, headache, heartburn, indigestion, light-headedness, loss of appetite, nausea, nervousness, soreness of the mouth, unusual sweating, or vomiting. As your body adjusts to the drug, these side effects should disappear.

To relieve constipation, increase the amount of fiber in your diet (fresh fruits and vegetables, salads, bran, and whole-grain breads), exercise, and drink more water (unless your doctor directs you to do otherwise).

If you become dizzy or light-headed, sit or lie down for a while; get up slowly from a sitting or reclining position, and be careful on stairs.

Major. If any side effects are persistent or particularly bothersome, you should report them to your doctor. IT IS ESPECIALLY IMPORTANT TO TELL YOUR DOCTOR about bloody or black, tarry stools; blurred vision; confusion; depression; difficult or painful urination; palpitations; a problem with hearing; ringing or buzzing in your ears; skin rash, hives, or itching; stomach pain; swelling of the feet; tightness in the chest; unexplained sore throat and fever; unusual bleeding or bruising; unusual fatigue or weakness; unusual weight gain; wheezing or difficulty in breathing; or yellowing of the eyes or skin.

INTERACTIONS

Ibuprofen interacts with several other types of medications:

1. Anticoagulants (blood thinners, such as warfarin) can lead to an increase in bleeding complications.

2. Aspirin, other salicylates, and other anti-inflammatory medications can increase stomach irritation. Aspirin may also decrease the effectiveness of ibuprofen; therefore, it should not be used concurrently with ibuprofen.

3. Ibuprofen can interact with diuretics (water pills).

4. Probenecid may increase blood levels of ibuprofen, which may increase the risk of side effects.

5. The action of beta blockers may be decreased by this drug.

BE SURE TO TELL YOUR DOCTOR about any medications you are currently taking, especially any listed above.

WARNINGS

- Before you start to take this medication, it is important to tell your doctor if you have ever had unusual or allergic reactions to ibuprofen, or to any of the other chemically related drugs (aspirin, other salicylates, diclofenac, diflunisal, fenoprofen, flurbiprofen, indomethacin, ketoprofen, meclofenamate, mefenamic acid, naproxen, oxyphenbutazone, phenylbutazone, piroxicam, sulindac, or tolmetin).
- Tell your doctor if you now have or if you have ever had bleeding problems, colitis, stomach ulcers or other stomach problems, epilepsy, heart disease, high blood pressure, asthma, kidney disease, liver disease, mental illness, or Parkinson's disease.
- If ibuprofen makes you dizzy or drowsy, do not take part in any activity that requires alertness, such as driving a car or operating potentially dangerous machinery.
- Because this drug can prolong bleeding time, tell your doctor or dentist you are taking this drug before having surgery or other medical or dental treatment.
- Stomach problems are more likely to occur if you take aspirin regularly or drink alcohol while being treated with this medication. These should, therefore, be avoided (unless your doctor directs you to do otherwise).
- The elderly may be at increased risk for experiencing side effects of this drug.
- Be sure to tell your doctor if you are pregnant. This type of medication can cause unwanted effects to the heart or blood flow of the fetus. Studies in animals have also shown that this type of medicine, if taken late in pregnancy, may increase the length of pregnancy, prolong labor, or cause other problems during delivery. Also, tell your doctor if you are breast-feeding an infant. Small amounts of ibuprofen can pass into breast milk.

Ifen—see ibuprofen

Iletin I—see insulin

Iletin II—see insulin

Ilosone—see erythromycin

Ilosone Pulvules—see erythromycin

Ilotycin—see erythromycin

Ilozyme—see pancrelipase

---

imipramine

BRAND NAMES (Manufacturers)
imipramine hydrochloride (various manufacturers)
Janimine (Abbott)
Tipramine (Major)
Tofranil (Geigy)
Tofranil-PM (Geigy)
TYPE OF DRUG
Tricyclic antidepressant
INGREDIENT
imipramine
DOSAGE FORMS
Tablets (10 mg, 25 mg, and 50 mg)
Capsules (75 mg, 100 mg, 125 mg, and 150 mg)
STORAGE
Store at room temperature in a tightly closed container.

USES

Imipramine is used to relieve the symptoms of mental depression. This medication belongs to a group of drugs referred to as tricyclic antidepressants. These medicines are thought to relieve depression by increasing the concentration of certain chemicals necessary for nerve transmission in the brain. This medication is also used to treat enuresis (bedwetting) in children six to 12 years of age.

TREATMENT

Imipramine should be taken exactly as your doctor prescribes. It can be taken with water or with food to lessen the chance of stomach irritation, unless your doctor tells you to do otherwise.

If you miss a dose of this medication, take the missed dose as soon as possible, then return to your regular dosing schedule. If, however, the dose you missed was a once-a-day bedtime dose, do not take that dose in the morning; check with your doctor instead. If the dose is taken in the morning, it may cause some unwanted side effects. Never double the dose.

The effects of therapy with this medication may not become apparent for two or three weeks.

SIDE EFFECTS

Minor. Agitation, anxiety, blurred vision, confusion, constipation, cramps, diarrhea, dizziness, drowsiness, dry mouth, fatigue, heartburn, insomnia, loss of appetite, nausea, peculiar tastes in the mouth, restlessness, sweating, vomiting, weakness, or weight gain or loss. As your body adjusts to the medication, these side effects should disappear.

This drug may cause increased sensitivity to sunlight. Therefore, avoid prolonged exposure to sunlight and sunlamps. Wear protective clothing, and use an effective sunscreen.

Dry mouth caused by therapy with this medication can be relieved by chewing sugarless gum or by sucking on ice chips or a piece of hard candy.

To relieve constipation, increase the amount of fiber in your diet (fresh fruits and vegetables, salads, bran, and whole-grain breads), exercise, and drink more water (unless your doctor directs you to do otherwise).

To avoid dizziness or light-headedness when you stand, contract and relax the muscles of your legs for a few moments before rising. Do this by pushing one foot against the floor while raising the other foot slightly, alternating feet so that you are "pumping" your legs in a pedaling motion.

Major. Tell your doctor about any side effects that are persistent or particularly bothersome. IT IS ESPECIALLY IMPORTANT TO TELL YOUR DOCTOR about chest pains, convulsions, difficulty in urinating, enlarged or painful breasts (in both sexes), fainting, fever, fluid retention, hair loss, hallucinations, headaches, impotence, mood changes, mouth sores, nervousness, nightmares, numbness in the fingers or toes, palpitations, ringing in the ears, seizures, skin rash, sleep disorders, sore throat, tremors, uncoordinated movements or balance problems, unusual bleeding or bruising, or yellowing of the eyes or skin.

INTERACTIONS

Imipramine interacts with a number of other types of medications:

1. Extreme drowsiness can occur when this medicine is taken with central nervous system depressants (such as alcohol, antihistamines, barbiturates, benzodiazepine tranquilizers, muscle relaxants, narcotics, pain medications, phenothiazine tranquilizers, and sleeping medications) or with other tricyclic antidepressants.

2. Imipramine may decrease the effectiveness of antiseizure medications and may block the blood-pressure-lowering effects of clonidine and guanethidine.

3. Oral contraceptives (birth control pills) and estrogen-containing drugs can increase the side effects and reduce the effectiveness of the tricyclic antidepressants (including imipramine).

4. Cimetidine can decrease the breakdown of imipramine in the body, thus increasing the possibility of side effects.

5. Tricyclic antidepressants may increase the side effects of thyroid medication and of over-the-counter (nonprescription) cough, cold, allergy, asthma, sinus, and diet medications.

6. The concurrent use of tricyclic antidepressants and monoamine oxidase (MAO) inhibitors should be avoided, because the combination may result in fever, convulsions, or high blood pressure. At least 14 days should separate the use of this drug and the use of an MAO inhibitor.

Before starting to take imipramine, BE SURE TO TELL YOUR DOCTOR about any medications you are currently taking, especially any of those listed above.

WARNINGS

• Tell your doctor if you have had unusual or allergic reactions to any medications, especially to imipramine or any of the other tricyclic antidepressants (such as amitriptyline, doxepin, trimipramine, amoxapine, protriptyline, desipramine, maprotiline, and nortriptyline).

• Tell your doctor if you have a history of alcoholism or if you have ever had asthma, high blood pressure, liver or kidney disease, heart disease, a heart attack, circulatory disease, stomach problems, intestinal problems, difficulty in urinating, enlarged prostate gland, epilepsy, glaucoma, thyroid disease, mental illness, or electroshock therapy.

• If this drug makes you dizzy or drowsy, do not take part in any activity that requires alertness, such as driving a car or operating potentially dangerous machinery.

• Before having surgery or any other medical or dental treatment, tell your doctor or dentist you are taking this drug.

• Do not stop taking this drug suddenly. Stopping it abruptly can cause nausea, headache, stomach upset, fatigue, or a worsening of your condition. Your doctor may want to reduce the dosage gradually.

• The effects of this medication may last as long as seven days after you stop taking it, so continue to observe all precautions during that period.

• Some of these products contain the color additive FD&C Yellow No. 5 (tartrazine), which can cause allergic-type reactions (skin rash, fainting, difficulty in breathing) in certain susceptible individuals.

• The elderly may be at increased risk for experiencing side effects. Report any such effects, especially dizziness, drowsiness, dry mouth, difficulty urinating, or mental confusion to your doctor.

• Be sure to tell your doctor if you are pregnant. Studies in humans have not been conducted, but adverse effects have been observed in the fetuses of animals that were given large doses of this drug during pregnancy. Also, tell your doctor if you are breast-feeding an infant. Small amounts of this drug can pass into breast milk and may cause unwanted effects, such as irritability or sleeping problems, in nursing infants.

imipramine hydrochloride—see imipramine

Imodium—see loperamide

Imuran—see azathioprine

Indameth—see indomethacin

---

indapamide

BRAND NAME (Manufacturer)
Lozol (Rorer)

TYPE OF DRUG
Diuretic and antihypertensive

INGREDIENT
indapamide

DOSAGE FORM
Tablets (2.5 mg)

STORAGE
Store at room temperature in a tightly closed container.

USES
Indapamide is prescribed to treat high blood pressure. It is also used to reduce fluid accumulation in the body caused by conditions such as heart failure, cirrhosis of the liver, kidney disease, and the long-term use of some drugs. This drug reduces fluid accumulation by increasing the elimination of salt and water through the kidneys.

TREATMENT
To decrease stomach irritation, you can take indapamide with a glass of milk or with a meal (unless your doctor directs you to do otherwise). Try to take it at the same time every day. Avoid taking a dose after 6:00 P.M.; otherwise, you may have to get up during the night to urinate.

If you miss a dose of this medication, take the missed dose as soon as possible, unless it is almost time for the next dose. In that case, do not take the missed dose at all; just wait until the next scheduled dose. Do not double the dose.

This medication does not cure high blood pressure, but it will help to control the condition as long as you continue to take it.

SIDE EFFECTS
Minor. Constipation, cramps, diarrhea, dizziness, drowsiness, headache, heartburn, loss of appetite, restlessness, or upset stomach. As your body adjusts to the medication, these side effects should disappear.

This drug can cause increased sensitivity to sunlight. Therefore, avoid prolonged exposure to sunlight and sunlamps. Wear protective clothing, and use an effective sunscreen.

To relieve constipation, increase the amount of fiber in your diet (fresh fruits and vegetables, salads, bran, and whole-grain breads) and exercise more (unless your doctor directs you to do otherwise).

To avoid dizziness or light-headedness when you stand, contract and relax the muscles of your legs for a few moments before rising. Do this by pushing one foot against the floor while raising the other foot slightly, alternating feet so that you are "pumping" your legs in a pedaling motion.

Major. Tell your doctor about any side effects that are persistent or particularly bothersome. IT IS ESPECIALLY IMPORTANT TO TELL YOUR DOCTOR about blurred vision, confusion, difficulty in breathing, dry mouth, excessive thirst, excessive weakness, fever, itching, joint pain, mood changes, muscle pain or spasms, nausea, palpitations, skin rash, sore throat, tingling in the fingers or toes, unusual bleeding or bruising, vomiting, or yellowing of the eyes or skin.

INTERACTIONS
Indapamide interacts with several other types of medications:

1. It may decrease the effectiveness of oral anticoagulants, antigout medications, insulin, oral antidiabetic medicines, and methenamine.

2. Fenfluramine can increase the blood-pressure-lowering effects of indapamide (which can be dangerous).

3. Indomethacin can decrease the blood-pressure-lowering effects of indapamide, thereby counteracting the desired effects.

4. Cholestyramine and colestipol can decrease the absorption of this medication from the gastrointestinal tract. Indapamide should, therefore, be taken one hour before or four hours after a dose of cholestyramine or colestipol (if you have also been prescribed one of these medications).

5. Indapamide may increase the side effects of amphotericin B, calcium, cortisone and cortisone-like steroids (such as dexamethasone, hydrocortisone, prednisone, and prednisolone), digoxin, digitalis, lithium, quinidine, sulfonamide antibiotics, and vitamin D.

BE SURE TO TELL YOUR DOCTOR about any medications you are currently taking, especially any of those listed above.

WARNINGS

- Tell your doctor about unusual or allergic reactions you have had to any medications, especially to indapamide or any other sulfa drugs, including other diuretics, oral antidiabetic medications, and sulfonamide antibiotics.
- Tell your doctor if you now have or if you have ever had kidney disease or problems with urination, diabetes mellitus, gout, liver disease, asthma, pancreatic disease, or systemic lupus erythematosus.
- Indapamide can cause potassium loss. Signs of potassium loss include dry mouth, thirst, weakness, muscle pain or cramps, nausea, and vomiting. If you experience any of these symptoms, call your doctor. To help avoid potassium loss, take this drug with a glass of fresh or frozen orange juice or cranberry juice, or eat a banana every day. The use of a salt substitute also helps to prevent potassium loss. Do not change your diet or use a salt substitute, however, before discussing it with your doctor. Too much potassium can also be dangerous. Your doctor may want to have blood tests performed periodically to monitor your potassium levels.
- In order to avoid dizziness or fainting while taking this medication, try not to stand for long periods of time; avoid drinking excessive amounts of alcohol; and avoid getting overheated (do not perform strenuous exercise in hot weather or take hot baths, showers, or saunas).
- If you have high blood pressure, do not take any over-the-counter (nonprescription) medications for weight control or for allergy, asthma, cough, cold, or sinus problems unless your doctor directs you to do so.
- To prevent dehydration (severe water loss) while taking this medication, check with your doctor if you have any illness that causes severe or continuous nausea, vomiting, or diarrhea.
- This medication can raise blood sugar levels in diabetic patients. Therefore, blood sugar levels should be carefully monitored by blood or urine tests when this medication is being taken.
- Be sure to tell your doctor if you are pregnant. Studies in humans have not been conducted, but adverse effects have been observed in the fetuses of animals that received large doses of this drug during pregnancy. Also, tell your doctor if you are breast-feeding an infant. Although problems in humans have not been reported, small amounts of this drug can pass into breast milk, so caution is warranted.

Inderal—see propranolol

Inderal LA—see propranolol

Inderide—see propranolol and hydrochlorothiazide combination

Inderide LA—see propranolol and hydrochlorothiazide combination

Indocin—see indomethacin

Indocin SR—see indomethacin

Indo-Lemmon—see indomethacin

---

indomethacin

BRAND NAMES (Manufacturers)
Indameth (Major)
Indocin (Merck Sharp & Dohme)
Indocin SR (Merck Sharp & Dohme)
Indo-Lemmon (Lemmon)
indomethacin (various manufacturers)

TYPE OF DRUG
Nonsteroidal anti-inflammatory analgesic

INGREDIENT
indomethacin

DOSAGE FORMS
Capsules (25 mg and 50 mg)
Extended-release capsules (75 mg)
Oral suspension (25 mg per 5-ml spoonful, with 1% alcohol)
Rectal suppositories (50 mg)

STORAGE
Indomethacin capsules, oral suspension, and rectal suppositories should be stored in closed containers at room temperature away from heat and direct sunlight. The rectal suppositories can also be stored in the refrigerator.

USES

Indomethacin is used to treat the inflammation (pain, swelling, and stiffness) of certain types of arthritis, gout, bursitis, and tendinitis. Indomethacin has been shown to block the production of certain body chemicals, called prostaglandins, that may trigger pain. However, it is not yet fully understood how indomethacin works.

TREATMENT

You should take this drug immediately after meals or with food, in order to reduce stomach irritation. Ask your doctor if you can take indomethacin with an antacid.

Do not chew or crush the extended-release capsules; they should be swallowed whole. Breaking the capsule would release the medication all at once—defeating the purpose of the extended-release dosage form.

The suspension form of this medication should be shaken well just before measuring each dose. The contents tend to settle on the bottom of the bottle, so it is necessary to shake the container to distribute the ingredients evenly and equalize the doses. Each dose should be measured carefully with a specially designed 5-ml measuring spoon. An ordinary kitchen teaspoon is not accurate enough.

To use the rectal suppository form of this medication, remove the foil wrapper, and moisten the suppository with water. If the suppository is too soft to insert, refrigerate it for 30 minutes or run cold water over it before removing the foil wrapper. Lie on your left side with your right knee bent. Push the suppository into the rectum, pointed end first. Lie still for a few minutes. Try to avoid having a bowel movement for at least one hour.

It is important to take indomethacin on schedule and not to miss any doses. If you do miss a dose, take the missed dose as soon as possible, unless more than an hour has passed. In that case, do not take the missed dose at all; just return to your regular dosing schedule. Do not double the next dose.

This drug does not cure arthritis, but will help to control the condition as long as you continue to take it. It may take up to four weeks before you feel the full benefits of this medication.

SIDE EFFECTS

Minor. Bloating, constipation, diarrhea, difficulty in sleeping, dizziness, drowsiness, headache, heartburn, indigestion, light-headedness, loss of appetite, nausea, nervousness, soreness of the mouth, unusual sweating, or vomiting. As your body adjusts to the drug, these side effects should disappear.

To relieve constipation, increase the amount of fiber in your diet (fresh fruits and vegetables, salads, bran, and whole-grain breads), exercise, and drink more water (unless your doctor directs you to do otherwise).

If you become dizzy, sit or lie down for a while; get up slowly from a sitting or reclining position, and be careful on stairs.

Major. Tell your doctor about any side effects that are persistent or particularly bothersome. IT IS ESPECIALLY IMPORTANT TO TELL YOUR DOCTOR about bloody or black, tarry stools; blurred vision; confusion; depression; difficult or painful urination; palpitations; a problem with hearing; ringing or buzzing in the ears; skin rash, hives, or itching; stomach pain; swelling of the feet; rectal irritation; tightness in the chest; unexplained sore throat and fever; unusual bleeding or bruising; unusual fatigue or weakness; unusual weight gain; wheezing or difficulty in breathing; or yellowing of the eyes or skin.

INTERACTIONS

Indomethacin interacts with several other types of drugs:

1. Use of anticoagulants (blood thinners, such as warfarin) can lead to an increase in bleeding complications.

2. Anti-inflammatory medications such as aspirin, salicylates, and diflunisal can cause increased stomach irritation when used while taking this drug.

3. Indomethacin can decrease the elimination of lithium from the body, possibly resulting in lithium toxicity.

4. Indomethacin may interfere with the blood-pressure-lowering effects of captopril, enalapril, or beta-blocking medications (acebutolol, atenolol, betaxolol, carteolol, esmolol, labetalol, metoprolol, nadolol, penbutolol, pindolol, propranolol, timolol).

5. Indomethacin can interfere with the diuretic effects of furosemide and thiazide-type diuretics (water pills).

6. Probenecid can increase the amount of indomethacin in the bloodstream when both drugs are being taken.

7. The concurrent use of triamterene and indomethacin can result in kidney problems.

8. Indomethacin can alter the effects of the potassium-sparing diuretics (such as amiloride, spironolactone, or triamterene).

BE SURE TO TELL YOUR DOCTOR about any medications you are currently taking, especially any of those listed above.

WARNINGS

- Tell your doctor if you have ever had unusual or allergic reactions to any medications, especially to indomethacin or any of the other chemically related drugs (including aspirin, other salicylates, diclofenac, diflunisal, fenoprofen, flurbiprofen, ibuprofen, ketoprofen, meclofenamate, mefenamic acid, naproxen, oxyphenbutazone, phenylbutazone, piroxicam, suprofen, or tolmetin).
- Before taking indomethacin, tell your doctor if you now have or if you have ever had bleeding problems, colitis, stomach ulcers or other stomach problems, epilepsy, heart disease, high blood pressure, asthma, kidney disease, liver disease, mental illness, or Parkinson's disease.
- If indomethacin makes you dizzy or drowsy, do not take part in any activity that requires alertness, such as driving a car or operating potentially dangerous machinery.
- If you will be taking this medication for a long period of time, your doctor may want to have your eyes examined periodically by an ophthalmologist. Some visual problems have been known to occur with long-term indomethacin use. Your doctor might want to keep a careful watch for these.
- Stomach problems are more likely to occur if you take aspirin regularly or drink alcohol while being treated with this medication. These should, therefore, be avoided (unless your doctor directs you to do otherwise).
- The elderly may be at increased risk for experiencing side effects of this drug.
- Be sure to tell your doctor if you are pregnant. Studies in animals have shown that indomethacin can cause unwanted effects in offspring, including lower birth weights, slower development of bones, nerve damage, and heart damage. If taken late in pregnancy, the drug can also prolong labor. Studies in humans have not been conducted. Also, tell your doctor if you are breast-feeding. Small amounts of indomethacin can pass into breast milk, so caution is warranted.

Insulatard NPH—see insulin

---

insulin

BRAND NAMES (Manufacturers)

Humulin L (Lilly)
Humulin N (Lilly)
Humulin R (Lilly)
Iletin I (Lilly)
Iletin II (Lilly)
Insulatard NPH (Nordisk-USA)
Mixtard (Nordisk-USA)
Novulin (Squibb-Novo)
Velosulin (Nordisk-USA)

TYPE OF DRUG

Antidiabetic

INGREDIENT

insulin

DOSAGE FORM

Injectable (all types) (40 units/ml, 100 units/ml)
Injectable (regular) (40 units/ml, 100 units/ml, 500 units/ml)

This drug is available only as an injectable (if insulin is taken orally, it is destroyed by stomach acid). Various types of insulin provide different times of onset and different durations of action (see chart on next page).

Insulin Type	Onset of action (in hours)	Duration of action (in hours)
Regular insulin	1/2	6
Insulin zinc suspension, prompt (Semilente)	1/2	14
Isophane insulin (NPH)	1	24
Insulin zinc suspension (Lente)	1	24
Globin zinc insulin	2	24
Protamine zinc insulin (PZI)	6	36
Insulin zinc suspension, extended (Ultralente)	6	36

STORAGE

After opening, keep most forms (except 500 units/ml strength) at room temperature if used in six months. Refrigerate unopened vials. Never freeze insulin.

USES

Insulin is a hormone that is normally produced by the pancreas; it functions in the regulation of blood sugar levels. This medication is used to treat diabetes mellitus (sugar diabetes)—a disorder that results from an inability of the pancreas to produce enough insulin. Injectable insulin is used only to treat those patients whose blood sugar levels cannot be controlled by diet or by oral antidiabetic medications.

TREATMENT

Your doctor, nurse, dietitian, or pharmacist will show you how to inject insulin, using a specially marked hypodermic syringe. This medication is packaged with printed instructions that should be carefully followed.

You may prefer to use presterilized disposable needles and syringes, which are used once and then discarded. If you use a glass syringe and metal needle, you must sterilize them before reuse.

Make sure that the insulin you are using is exactly the kind your doctor ordered and that its expiration date has not passed.

Do not shake the bottle; tip it gently, end to end, to mix. ALWAYS CHECK THE DOSE in the syringe at least twice before injecting it.

Clean the site of the injection thoroughly with an antiseptic, such as rubbing alcohol.

Change the site of the injection daily, and avoid injecting cold insulin.

NEVER use a vial of insulin if there are lumps in it. Make your insulin injection a regular part of your schedule, so that you do not miss any doses. Ask your doctor what to do if you have to take a dose later than the scheduled time.

SIDE EFFECTS

Minor. Insulin can cause redness and rash at the site of injection. Try to rotate injection sites in order to avoid this reaction.

Major. Tell your doctor about any side effects that are persistent or particularly bothersome. IT IS ESPECIALLY IMPORTANT TO TELL YOUR DOCTOR about palpitations, fainting, shortness of breath, skin rash, or sweating.

Too much insulin can cause hypoglycemia (low blood sugar), which can lead to anxiety, chills, cold sweats, drowsiness, fast heart rate, headache, loss of consciousness, nausea, nervousness, tremors, unusual hunger, or unusual weakness. If you experience these symptoms, eat a quick source of sugar (such as table sugar, orange juice, honey, or a nondiet cola). You should also tell your doctor that you have had this reaction.

Too little insulin can cause symptoms of hyperglycemia (high blood sugar), such as confusion, drowsiness, dry skin, fatigue, flushing, frequent urination, fruit-like breath odor, loss of appetite, or rapid breathing. If you experience any of these symptoms, contact your doctor; he or she may want to modify your dosing schedule or change your insulin dosage.

INTERACTIONS

Insulin interacts with several other types of medications:

1. Insulin can increase digoxin's side effects to the heart.

2. Oral contraceptives (birth control pills), adrenocorticosteroids (cortisone-like medicines), danazol, dextrothyroxine, furosemide, ethacrynic acid, thyroid hormone, thiazide diuretics (water pills), phenytoin, or nicotine (from smoking) can increase insulin dosing requirements.

3. Monoamine oxidase (MAO) inhibitors, phenylbutazone, fenfluramine, guanethidine, disopyramide, sulfinpyrazone, tetracycline, alcohol, anabolic steroids, or large doses of aspirin can increase the effects of insulin, leading to hypoglycemia.

4. Beta blockers (acebutolol, atenolol, betaxolol, carteolol, esmolol, labetalol, metoprolol, nadolol, penbutolol, pindolol, propranolol, timolol) may prolong the effects of insulin and mask the signs of hypoglycemia.

BE SURE TO TELL YOUR DOCTOR about any medications you are currently taking, especially any of those listed above.

WARNINGS

- Tell your doctor about unusual or allergic reactions you have had to any medications, especially to insulin.
- Before starting to take this medication, be sure to tell your doctor if you now have or if you have ever had high fevers, infections, kidney disease, liver disease, thyroid disease, or severe nausea and vomiting.
- If your doctor prescribes two types of insulin to achieve better glucose control and recommends mixing the insulin into one syringe, always draw the regular insulin (clear) into the syringe first.
- Some insulin mixtures are stable and won't interact with each other for some time. Others react quickly and require immediate injection. Consult your doctor or pharmacist about this.
- Make sure that your friends and family are aware of the symptoms of an insulin reaction and know what to do should they observe any of the symptoms in you.
- Carry a card or wear a bracelet that identifies you as a diabetic.
- Always have insulin and syringes available.
- When traveling, always carry an ample supply of your diabetic needs and, if possible, a prescription for insulin and

syringes. Carry insulin and syringes on your person; baggage can be lost, delayed, or stolen.

- Do not store insulin in your car's glove compartment.
- To avoid the possibility of hypoglycemia (low blood sugar levels), you should eat on a regular schedule and should avoid skipping meals.
- Before having surgery or other medical or dental treatment, tell your doctor or dentist you are taking insulin.
- Check with your doctor or pharmacist before taking any over-the-counter (nonprescription) cough, cold, diet, allergy, asthma, or sinus medications. Some of these products affect blood sugar levels.
- If you become ill—if you catch a cold or the flu or become nauseated—your insulin requirements may change. Consult your doctor.
- Be sure to tell your doctor if you are pregnant. Insulin dosing requirements often change during pregnancy.

Intal—see cromolyn sodium (inhalation)

Ionamin—see phentermine

Iophen-C—see codeine and iodinated glycerol combination

Iophen DM—see dextromethorphan and iodinated glycerol combination

---

ipecac

BRAND NAME (Manufacturer)
Ipecac (various manufacturers)
Note: This product is available without a prescription.
TYPE OF DRUG
Emetic
INGREDIENT
ipecac
DOSAGE FORM
Oral syrup (with 1.5% or 2% alcohol)
STORAGE
Store at room temperature in a tightly closed container.

USES

Ipecac is for emergency use to treat drug overdose or poisoning. Ipecac works on the stomach and on the vomiting center in the brain to produce vomiting.

TREATMENT

Before administering ipecac, call a poison control center, emergency room, or physician for advice.

It is important to administer ipecac with adequate amounts of water (1/2 glass for infants less than 1 year old; 1 to 2 glasses for children and adults) to ensure that there is adequate fluid in the stomach. If vomiting does not occur within 20 minutes after a second dose has been given, call again IMMEDIATELY for further instructions.

SIDE EFFECTS

Minor. Ipecac can cause diarrhea, drowsiness, or nausea or vomiting that continues for more than 30 minutes. These side effects should disappear within several hours.

Major. Tell your doctor about any side effects that are persistent or particularly bothersome. IT IS ESPECIALLY IMPORTANT TO TELL YOUR DOCTOR about aching or stiffness of the muscles, difficulty in breathing, palpitations, stomach cramps or pain, or weakness.

INTERACTIONS

Ipecac oral syrup should not be administered with milk or with carbonated beverages; these fluids may affect how quickly ipecac works. Activated charcoal absorbs ipecac. If both activated charcoal and ipecac oral syrup are to be used, give the activated charcoal only after successful vomiting has been produced by the ipecac.

WARNINGS

- Vomiting is not the proper treatment in all cases of possible poisoning; ipecac should NOT be used if gasoline, oils, kerosene, acids, alkalies (lye), corrosives, or strychnine has been swallowed, since vomiting of these substances may cause seizures, additional throat burns, or pneumonia.
- Ipecac should probably not be used if the poisoned patient is losing consciousness, has no gag reflex, is in shock, is having seizures, or has heart disease unless directed by a health professional.
- Muscle and heart disorders and at least one death have been reported as a result of the chronic use of ipecac by young women who were using it to induce vomiting in order to lose weight.
- Ipecac is available over-the-counter (nonprescription) and can be purchased from most pharmacies. Mothers should have a one-ounce bottle of ipecac for each child in the house. Always call a poison control center, emergency room, or physician for instructions BEFORE administering ipecac.
- Be sure to tell your doctor if the overdose or poisoning victim is pregnant. Although ipecac appears to be safe, extensive studies in pregnant women have not been conducted.

Ismelin—see guanethidine

Iso-Bid—see isosorbide dinitrate

Isoclor—see pseudoephedrine and chlorpheniramine combination

Isoclor Timesules—see pseudoephedrine and chlorpheniramine combination

Isollyl Improved—see aspirin, caffeine, and butalbital combination

Isonate—see isosorbide dinitrate

---

isoniazid

BRAND NAMES (Manufacturers)
isoniazid (various manufacturers)
Laniazid (Lannett)
Nydrazid (Squibb)
Teebaconin (CMC)

TYPE OF DRUG
Antitubercular
INGREDIENT
isoniazid
DOSAGE FORMS
Tablets (50 mg, 100 mg, and 300 mg)
Oral syrup (50 mg per 5-ml spoonful)
STORAGE
Store at room temperature in a tightly closed, light-resistant container. This medication should never be frozen.

USES

Isoniazid is used to prevent and treat tuberculosis. It acts by severely injuring the cell structure of tuberculosis bacteria, thereby preventing them from growing and multiplying.

TREATMENT

In order to avoid stomach irritation, you can take isoniazid with food or a full glass of water or milk (unless your doctor directs you to do otherwise).

Antacids prevent the absorption of isoniazid from the gastrointestinal tract, so they should not be taken within an hour of a dose of isoniazid.

Each dose of the oral syrup should be measured carefully with a specially designed 5-ml measuring spoon. An ordinary kitchen teaspoon is not accurate enough.

It is important to continue to take this medication for the entire time prescribed by your doctor, even if your symptoms disappear before the end of that period. If you stop taking the drug too soon, your infection could recur.

It is common for therapy to last for at least six months and, at times, for as long as two years.

Try not to miss any doses of this medication. If you do miss a dose, take the missed dose as soon as possible, unless it is almost time for the next dose. In that case, do not take the missed dose at all; just return to your regular dosing schedule. Do not double the next dose.

SIDE EFFECTS

Minor. Abdominal pain, dizziness, heartburn, nausea, or vomiting. These side effects should disappear as your body adjusts to the medication.

If you feel dizzy, sit or lie down for a while; get up slowly from a sitting or reclining position, and be careful on stairs.

Major. Tell your doctor about any side effects that are persistent or particularly bothersome. IT IS ESPECIALLY IMPORTANT TO TELL YOUR DOCTOR about blurred vision, breast enlargement (in both sexes), chills, darkening of the urine, eye pain, fever, malaise, memory impairment, numbness or tingling in the fingers or toes, rash, unusual bleeding or bruising, vision changes, weakness, or yellowing of the eyes or skin.

Your doctor may want to prescribe vitamin B_6 (pyridoxine) to prevent the numbness and tingling. However, do not take vitamin B_6 on your own without consulting your doctor.

INTERACTIONS

Isoniazid interacts with several other types of medications:

1. Concurrent use of isoniazid and alcohol can lead to decreased effectiveness of isoniazid and increased side effects on the liver.
2. The combination of isoniazid and cycloserine can result in dizziness or drowsiness.
3. The combination of isoniazid and disulfiram can lead to dizziness, loss of coordination, irritability, and insomnia.
4. Isoniazid can decrease the breakdown of phenytoin and carbamazepine in the body, which can lead to an increase in side effects from phenytoin and carbamazepine.
5. Isoniazid can increase the breakdown of ketoconazole in the body, which can decrease its effectiveness.
6. In combination, rifampin and isoniazid can increase the risk of liver damage.
7. The effectiveness of isoniazid may be decreased by adrenocorticosteroids (cortisone-like medicines).
8. The side effects of benzodiazepine tranquilizers or meperidine may be increased by isoniazid.

Before starting to take isoniazid, BE SURE TO TELL YOUR DOCTOR about any medications you are currently taking, especially any of those listed above.

WARNINGS

- Tell your doctor about unusual or allergic reactions you have had to any medications, especially to isoniazid, ethionamide, pyrazinamide, or niacin (vitamin B_3).
- Before starting to take this medication, be sure to tell your doctor if you have a history of alcoholism, or if you now have or ever had kidney disease, liver disease, or seizures.
- If this drug makes you dizzy, avoid tasks that require alertness, such as driving a car.
- Your doctor may want you to have periodic eye examinations while taking this medication, especially if you begin to have vison side effects.
- Isoniazid can interact with several foods (skipjack fish, tuna, yeast extracts, sauerkraut juice, sausages, and certain cheeses), leading to severe reactions. You should, therefore, avoid eating these foods while being treated with isoniazid.
- Diabetics using Clinitest urine glucose tests may get erroneously high sugar readings while they are taking isoniazid. Temporarily changing to Clinistix or Tes-Tape urine tests avoids this problem.
- Be sure to tell your doctor if you are pregnant. Although isoniazid appears to be safe during pregnancy, it does cross the placenta. Extensive studies in pregnant women have not been conducted. Also, tell your doctor if you are breast-feeding an infant. Small amounts of isoniazid pass into breast milk.

Isoptin—see verapamil

Isoptin SR—see verapamil

Isopto Carpine—see pilocarpine (ophthalmic)

Isopto Cetamide—see sodium sulfacetamide (ophthalmic)

Isordil Tembids—see isosorbide dinitrate

Isordil Titradose—see isosorbide dinitrate

---

isosorbide dinitrate

BRAND NAMES (Manufacturers)
Dilatrate-SR (Reed & Carnrick)

Iso-Bid (Geriatric)
Isonate (Major)
Isordil Tembids (Wyeth)
Isordil Titradose (Wyeth)
isosorbide dinitrate (various manufacturers)
Isotrate Timecelles (Hauck)
Sorbitrate (ICI Pharma)
Sorbitrate SA (ICI Pharma)

TYPE OF DRUG

Antianginal

INGREDIENT

isosorbide dinitrate

DOSAGE FORMS

Tablets (5 mg, 10 mg, 20 mg, 30 mg, and 40 mg)
Chewable tablets (5 mg and 10 mg)
Sublingual tablets (2.5 mg, 5 mg, and 10 mg)
Sustained-release tablets (40 mg)
Capsules (40 mg)
Sustained-release capsules (40 mg)

STORAGE

Isosorbide dinitrate tablets and capsules should be stored in a cool, dry place. This medication loses potency when exposed to heat or moisture.

USES

Isosorbide dinitrate is a vasodilator that relaxes the muscle of the blood vessels, leading to an increase in the oxygen supply to the heart. It is used to relieve (chewable and sublingual tablets) or to prevent (oral tablets and capsules) angina (chest pain). The chewable and sublingual tablets act quickly; they can be used to relieve chest pain after it has begun. The oral tablets and capsules do not act quickly; they are used only to prevent angina attacks.

TREATMENT

Take the chewable or sublingual forms of this medication at the first sign of an angina attack. DO NOT WAIT for the attack to become severe. Then sit down. These tablets are absorbed more completely through the lining of the mouth than from the stomach. Your mouth should be empty when you take these tablets. Do not eat, drink, or smoke with a tablet in your mouth. If the pain of an attack continues, you can take another tablet after five minutes, and a third tablet after another five minutes. If three tablets provide no relief within 15 minutes, CONTACT YOUR DOCTOR IMMEDIATELY or go to the nearest hospital.

The chewable tablet should be chewed for at least two minutes before swallowing.

Place the sublingual tablet under the tongue or against the cheek and allow it to dissolve—DO NOT CHEW OR SWALLOW IT. Do not swallow until the drug is dissolved, and do not rinse your mouth for several minutes (this gives a greater opportunity for the drug to be absorbed through the lining of the mouth).

The regular tablets and capsules and the sustained-release forms of this medication should be taken with a full glass of water on an empty stomach. The sustained-release forms should be swallowed whole. Breaking, crushing, or chewing these tablets or capsules destroys their sustained-release activity and possibly increases the side effects.

If you are taking this medication on a regular schedule, try not to miss any doses. If you do miss a dose, however, take the missed dose as soon as possible, unless it is within two hours of the next dose (or six hours for the sustained-release forms). In that case, do not take the missed dose at all; just return to your regular dosing schedule. Do not double the next dose.

Some doctors may recommend using this medication to prevent an anginal attack before expected physical or emotional stress. Discuss this with your doctor.

SIDE EFFECTS

Minor. Dizziness, flushing, headache, light-headedness, nausea, or vomiting. These side effects should disappear as your body adjusts to the medication.

If you feel dizzy or light-headed, sit or lie down for a while; get up slowly from a sitting or reclining position, and be careful on stairs. To avoid dizziness or light-headedness when you stand, contract and relax the muscles of your legs for a few moments before rising. Do this by pushing one foot against the floor while raising the other foot slightly, alternating feet so that you are "pumping" your legs in a pedaling motion.

Acetaminophen may help relieve headaches caused by this medication.

Major. Tell your doctor about any side effects that are persistent or particularly bothersome. IT IS ESPECIALLY IMPORTANT TO TELL YOUR DOCTOR about fainting spells, palpitations, rash, restlessness, sweating, or unusual weakness.

INTERACTIONS

Isosorbide dinitrate can interact with other types of drugs:

1. Isosorbide dinitrate, in combination with alcohol, can lead to dizziness and fainting.

2. Over-the-counter (nonprescription) sinus, allergy, cough, cold, asthma, and diet products can block the antiangina effects of isosorbide dinitrate.

BE SURE TO TELL YOUR DOCTOR about any medications you are currently taking, especially any of those listed above.

WARNINGS

- Tell your doctor about unusual or allergic reactions you have had to any medications, especially to isosorbide dinitrate or to any other nitrate-containing drugs (such as nitroglycerin).
- Before starting to take this medication, tell your doctor if you have ever had severe anemia, glaucoma, a heart attack, or thyroid disease.
- Before using this medication to relieve chest pain, be certain that the pain arises from the heart and is not due to a muscle spasm or to indigestion. If your chest pain is not relieved by use of this drug, or if pain arises from a different location or differs in severity, CONSULT YOUR DOCTOR IMMEDIATELY.
- If this drug makes you dizzy or light-headed, do not take part in any activity that requires alertness, such as driving a car or operating potentially dangerous machinery.
- Before having surgery or any other medical or dental treatment, be sure to tell your doctor or dentist that you are taking this medication.
- Tolerance to this medication may develop. If the drug begins to lose its effectiveness, contact your doctor.

• Isosorbide dinitrate should not be discontinued unless you first consult your doctor. Stopping the drug abruptly may lead to further chest pain. Your doctor may, therefore, want to decrease your dosage gradually.
• If you have frequent diarrhea, you may not be absorbing the sustained-release form of this medication. Discuss this with your doctor.
• Be sure to tell your doctor if you are pregnant. Although this drug appears to be safe, extensive studies in pregnant women have not been conducted. Also, tell your doctor if you are breast-feeding an infant. It is not known whether isosorbide dinitrate passes into breast milk.

Isotrate Timecelles—see isosorbide dinitrate

---

isotretinoin

BRAND NAME (Manufacturer)
Accutane (Roche)
TYPE OF DRUG
Acne preparation
INGREDIENT
isotretinoin
DOSAGE FORM
Capsules (10 mg, 20 mg, and 40 mg)
STORAGE
Isotretinoin should be stored at room temperature in a tightly closed, light-resistant container.

USES

This medication is used to treat severe cystic acne. It is not clearly understood how isotretinoin works, but it decreases the production of sebum (a skin oil) and dries up the acne lesions.

TREATMENT

An information leaflet is packaged with this product. Be sure to read it carefully.

Isotretinoin should be taken with meals to obtain maximum benefit.

It may take one to two months before the maximum effects of this medication are observed.

If you miss a dose of this medication, take the missed dose as soon as possible, and then return to your regular dosing schedule. However, if you do not remember until it is time for your next dose, double the next dose, and then return to your regular dosing schedule.

SIDE EFFECTS

Minor. Changes in skin color, drowsiness, dry lips or mouth, fatigue, fluid retention, headache, indigestion, inflammation of the eyelids, inflammation of the lips, irritation of the eyes, or thinning of the hair. These side effects may disappear as your body adjusts to the medication.

You may notice a worsening of your acne for the first few days of treatment.

This medication can cause increased sensitivity to sunlight. Therefore, avoid prolonged exposure to sunlight and sunlamps. You should wear protective clothing and sunglasses, and also use an effective sunscreen.

To relieve mouth dryness, chew sugarless gum or suck on ice chips or a piece of hard candy. If there is no relief within two weeks, consult your doctor.

Major. Tell your doctor about any side effects that are persistent or particularly bothersome. IT IS ESPECIALLY IMPORTANT TO TELL YOUR DOCTOR about black, tarry stools; bruising; burning or tingling sensation of the skin; changes in the menstrual cycle; depression; dizziness; hives; muscle pain; peeling of the palms and soles; rash; visual disturbances; or weight loss.

INTERACTIONS

This medication interacts with the following substances:
1. The concurrent use of alcohol and isotretinoin can lead to an increase in blood lipid (fat) levels, which can be dangerous.
2. Vitamin A and isotretinoin together can result in additive toxic effects.

BE SURE TO TELL YOUR DOCTOR about any medications you are currently taking, especially vitamin A.

WARNINGS

• Tell your doctor about unusual or allergic reactions you have had to any medications, especially to isotretinoin, vitamin A, or the preservative parabens.
• Before starting to take this medication, tell your doctor if you now have or if you have ever had diabetes mellitus (sugar diabetes) or hyperlipidemia (high blood lipid levels).
• If this drug makes you drowsy, do not take part in any activity that requires alertness, such as driving a car or operating potentially dangerous machinery.
• Be sure to tell your doctor if you are pregnant. Isotretinoin has been shown to cause birth defects in humans. An effective form of birth control should be used by women of child-bearing age while they are taking this drug and for at least one month before and after they stop taking it. Within two weeks of starting this drug, women should have a blood pregnancy test. If the test is negative, the drug will be started on the second or third day of the next normal menstrual period. Women should have a pregnancy test each month while they take this medication. All women must also sign an informed-consent sheet. Also, tell your doctor if you are breast-feeding an infant. It is not known whether this drug passes into breast milk.

Janimine—see imipramine

Kaochlor—see potassium chloride

Kaon—see potassium chloride

Kato—see potassium chloride

Kay Ciel—see potassium chloride

K-Dur—see potassium chloride

Keflet—see cephalexin

Keflex—see cephalexin

Kenac—see triamcinolone (topical)

Kenacort—see triamcinolone (systemic)

Kenalog—see triamcinolone (topical)

Kenalog-H—see triamcinolone (topical)

Kerlone—see betaxolol (systemic)

---

ketoprofen

BRAND NAME (Manufacturer)
Orudis (Wyeth)
TYPE OF DRUG
Nonsteroidal anti-inflammatory analgesic
INGREDIENT
ketoprofen
DOSAGE FORM
Capsules (50 mg and 75 mg)
STORAGE
Store at room temperature in a tightly closed container.

USES

Ketoprofen is used to treat rheumatoid arthritis and osteoarthritis. Ketoprofen has been shown to block the production of certain body chemicals, called prostaglandins, that trigger pain and inflammation. However, it is not yet fully understood how ketoprofen works.

TREATMENT

Ketoprofen should be taken immediately after meals or with food in order to reduce stomach irritation. Check with your doctor about taking ketoprofen with an antacid.

It is important to take ketoprofen on schedule and not to miss any doses. If you do miss a dose, take the missed dose as soon as possible, unless it is almost time for the next dose. In that case, do not take the missed dose at all; just return to your regular dosing schedule. Do not double the next dose.

Ketoprofen does not cure arthritis, but it will help to control symptoms as long as you take the drug.

SIDE EFFECTS

Minor. Abdominal pain, changes in taste, constipation, decreased or increased appetite, diarrhea, dizziness, drowsiness, dry mouth, excessive salivation, fatigue, flushing, gas, headache, heartburn, increased heart rate, increased thirst, nausea, nosebleeds, sweating, vomiting, or weight change. These side effects should disappear as your body adjusts to this medication.

Ketoprofen may cause increased sensitivity to sunlight. It is, therefore, important to avoid prolonged exposure to sunlight and sunlamps. Wear protective clothing and sunglasses, and use an effective sunscreen.

To relieve constipation, increase the amount of fiber in your diet (fresh fruits and vegetables, salads, bran, and whole-grain breads), exercise, and drink more water (unless your doctor directs you to do otherwise).

If you become dizzy, sit or lie down; get up slowly from a sitting or reclining position, and be careful on stairs.

Major. Tell your doctor about any side effects that are persistent or particularly bothersome. IT IS ESPECIALLY IMPORTANT TO TELL YOUR DOCTOR about black or tarry stools, chills, confusion, decreased or painful urination, hair loss, itching, memory loss, mouth sores, muscle pains, palpitations, rash, shortness of breath, swelling of the feet, tingling in the fingers or toes, unusual bleeding or bruising, unusual weight gain, visual disturbances, or yellowing of the eyes or skin.

INTERACTIONS

Ketoprofen interacts with several other types of medications:

1. Ketoprofen can increase the risk of bleeding complications with anticoagulants (blood thinners, such as warfarin).
2. Ketoprofen can interfere with the diuretic effects of furosemide and thiazide-type diuretics (water pills).
3. Aspirin can alter the blood levels and elimination of ketoprofen from the body.
4. Ketoprofen can increase the blood levels of probenecid, which can lead to an increased chance of side effects.
5. The action of beta blockers may be affected by this drug.

Before starting ketoprofen, BE SURE TO TELL YOUR DOCTOR about any medications you are currently taking, especially any of those listed above.

WARNINGS

- Tell your doctor about any unusual or allergic reactions you have had to any medications, especially to ketoprofen or to any other chemically related drugs, including aspirin, other salicylates, diclofenac, diflunisal, fenoprofen, flurbiprofen, ibuprofen, indomethacin, meclofenamate, mefenamic acid, naproxen, oxyphenbutazone, phenylbutazone, piroxicam, sulindac, or tolmetin.
- Before taking ketoprofen, tell your doctor if you now have or if you have ever had anemia, bleeding problems, gastrointestinal diseases, heart failure, hypertension, kidney disease, liver disease, or ulcers.
- If ketoprofen makes you dizzy or drowsy, do not take part in any activity that requires alertness, such as driving a car or operating potentially dangerous machinery.
- If vision problems develop while taking this medication, your doctor may refer you to an ophthalmologist.
- Stomach problems are more likely to occur if you take aspirin regularly or drink alcohol while being treated with this medication.
- Before having surgery or any other medical or dental treatment, be sure to tell your doctor or dentist that you are taking this medication. Your doctor or dentist may recommend stopping ketoprofen for several days prior to surgery, to decrease the risk of bleeding complications.
- The elderly may be at increased risk of experiencing some of the side effects of this medication.
- Be sure to tell your doctor if you are pregnant. Although ketoprofen appears to be safe in animals, studies in pregnant women have not been conducted. Ketoprofen should be avoided late in pregnancy because it can alter fetal heart circulation. Also tell your doctor if you are breast-feeding an infant. It is not yet known whether ketoprofen passes into human breast milk.

Kinesed—see atropine, scopolamine, hyoscyamine, and phenobarbital combination

Klonopin—see clonazepam

K-Lor—see potassium chloride

Klor-Con—see potassium chloride

Klorvess—see potassium chloride

Klotrix—see potassium chloride

K-Lyte/Cl—see potassium chloride

Kolyum—see potassium chloride

Kronofed-A Jr.—see pseudoephedrine and chlorpheniramine combination

Kronofed-A Kronocaps—see pseudoephedrine and chlorpheniramine combination

K-Tab—see potassium chloride

Ku-Zyme HP—see pancrelipase

Kwell—see lindane

Kwildane—see lindane

labetalol

BRAND NAMES (Manufacturers)
Normodyne (Schering)
Trandate (Glaxo)
TYPE OF DRUG
Alpha/beta-adrenergic blocking agent
INGREDIENT
labetalol
DOSAGE FORM
Tablets (100 mg, 200 mg, and 300 mg)
STORAGE
Labetalol should be stored at room temperature in a tightly closed container.

USES

Labetalol is used to treat high blood pressure. Labetalol belongs to a group of medicines known as beta-adrenergic blocking agents or, more commonly, beta blockers. These drugs work by controlling impulses along certain nerve pathways.

TREATMENT

Labetalol can be taken either on an empty stomach or with food or milk (as directed by your doctor). In order to become accustomed to taking this medication, try to take it at the same time(s) each day.

If you miss a dose of this medication, take the missed dose as soon as possible, unless it is almost time for your next dose. In that case, do not take the missed dose at all; just wait until the next scheduled dose. Do not double the dose.

Labetalol does not cure high blood pressure but will help control the condition as long as you continue to take it.

SIDE EFFECTS

Minor. Abdominal pain; change in taste; diarrhea; dizziness; drowsiness; dryness of the eyes, mouth, and skin; fainting; fatigue; headache; heartburn; light-headedness; nasal congestion; nausea; numbness or tingling of the fingers or toes; scalp tingling; or vomiting. These side effects should disappear as your body adjusts to this medication.

If you are extra-sensitive to the cold, be sure to dress warmly during cold weather.

Plain, nonmedicated eye drops (artificial tears) may help to relieve eye dryness.

Sucking on ice chips or chewing sugarless gum helps to relieve mouth and throat dryness.

To avoid dizziness or light-headedness when you stand, contract and relax the muscles of your legs for a few moments before rising. Do this by alternately pushing one foot against the floor while raising the other foot slightly, so that you are "pumping" your legs in a pedaling motion.

Major. Tell your doctor about any side effects that are persistent or particularly bothersome. IT IS ESPECIALLY IMPORTANT TO TELL YOUR DOCTOR about cold hands or feet (due to decreased blood circulation to skin, fingers, and toes), confusion, depression, difficult or painful urination, impotence, itching, muscle cramps, rapid weight gain (three to five pounds within a week), rash, sore throat and fever, unusual bleeding or bruising, vision disturbances, wheezing or difficulty in breathing, or yellowing of the eyes or skin.

INTERACTIONS

This medication can interact with a variety of other types of medications:

1. Indomethacin, aspirin, and other salicylates may decrease the blood-pressure-lowering effects of beta blockers.
2. Concurrent use of beta blockers and calcium channel blockers (diltiazem, nifedipine, verapamil) or disopyramide can lead to heart failure or very low blood pressure. However, there may be times when your doctor may decide that multiple medications are necessary.
3. Cimetidine can increase the blood concentrations of labetalol, which can result in greater side effects.
4. Side effects may also be increased when beta blockers are taken with clonidine, digoxin, epinephrine, chlorpromazine furosemide, hydralazine, oral contraceptives (birth control pills), phenylephrine, phenylpropanolamine, phenothiazine tranquilizers, prazosin, reserpine, or monoamine oxidase (MAO) inhibitors. At least 14 days should separate the use of a beta blocker and an MAO inhibitor.
5. Beta blockers may antagonize (work against) the effects of theophylline, aminophylline, albuterol, isoproterenol, metaproterenol, and terbutaline.
6. Beta blockers can also interact with insulin or oral antidiabetic agents, raising or lowering blood sugar levels or masking the symptoms of low blood sugar.
7. Concurrent use of tricyclic antidepressants and labetalol can increase the risk of tremors (trembling or shakiness).
8. Halothane anesthesia and nitroglycerin can increase the blood-pressure-lowering effects of labetalol.
9. Alcohol, barbiturates, and rifampin can decrease blood concentrations of beta blockers, which can result in a decrease of effectiveness.

Before starting labetalol, TELL YOUR DOCTOR about any drugs you are currently taking, especially any listed above.

WARNINGS

- Before you start taking this medication, it is important for you to tell your doctor about any unusual or allergic reaction you have had to any medications, especially to labetalol or to any other beta blocker (acebutolol, atenolol, betaxolol, carteolol, esmolol, metoprolol, nadolol, penbutolol, pindolol, propranolol, timolol).

• Tell your doctor if you now have or if you have ever had asthma, bronchitis, diabetes mellitus, heart block, heart failure, liver disease, pheochromocytoma, poor circulation in fingers and toes, or a slow heartbeat.

• You may want to check your pulse while taking this medication. If your pulse is much slower than your usual rate (or if it is less than 50 beats per minute), check with your doctor. A pulse rate that is too slow may cause circulation problems.

• This drug may affect your body's response to exercise. Ask your doctor how much exercise is appropriate given your state of health.

• Do not stop taking this medicine without first checking with your doctor. Some conditions may become worse when the medicine is stopped suddenly, and the danger of a heart attack is increased in some patients. Your doctor may want you to gradually reduce the amount of medicine you take before stopping completely. Have enough medicine on hand to last through vacations, holidays, and weekends.

• Before undergoing surgery or any other medical or dental treatment, tell your physician or dentist that you are taking this medicine. Often, this medication will be discontinued 48 hours prior to any major surgery.

• Labetalol can cause decreased alertness, dizziness, drowsiness, and light-headedness. Exercise caution while driving a car or using any potentially dangerous machinery.

• While taking this medicine, do not use any over-the-counter (nonprescription) allergy, asthma, cough, cold, sinus, or diet preparation without first checking with your pharmacist or doctor. The combination of these medicines with a beta blocker can result in high blood pressure.

• Be sure to tell your doctor if you are pregnant. Although labetalol appears to be safe in animals, studies in pregnant women have not been conducted. Also, tell your doctor if you are breast-feeding an infant. Small amounts of labetalol may pass into breast milk.

LactiCare-HC—see hydrocortisone (topical)

Lanacort—see hydrocortisone (topical)

Laniazid—see isoniazid

Lanophyllin—see theophylline

Lanophyllin-GG—see theophylline and guaifenesin combination

Lanorinal—see aspirin, caffeine, and butalbital combination

Lanoxicaps—see digoxin

Lanoxin—see digoxin

Lanvisone—see hydrocortisone and iodochlorhydroxyquin combination (topical)

Larodopa—see levodopa

Larotid—see amoxicillin

Lasix—see furosemide

Ledercillin VK—see penicillin VK

Leukeran—see chlorambucil

---

levodopa

BRAND NAMES (Manufacturers)
Dopar (Norwich Eaton)
Larodopa (Roche)
levodopa (various manufacturers)

TYPE OF DRUG
Antiparkinsonism agent

INGREDIENT
levodopa

DOSAGE FORMS
Tablets (100 mg, 250 mg, and 500 mg)
Capsules (100 mg, 250 mg, and 500 mg)

STORAGE
Levodopa tablets and capsules should be stored at room temperature in tightly closed, light-resistant containers.

USES

Levodopa is used to treat the symptoms of Parkinson's disease. It is converted in the body to dopamine, a chemical in the brain that is diminished in patients with Parkinson's disease.

TREATMENT

In order to avoid stomach irritation, you can take levodopa with food or with a full glass of milk or water (unless your doctor directs you to do otherwise).

These tablets and capsules should be swallowed whole for maximum effectiveness—do not crush, break, or chew them.

You may not observe significant benefit from this drug for two to three weeks after starting to take it.

If you miss a dose, take the missed dose as soon as possible, unless it is within two hours of the next scheduled dose. In that case, do not take the missed dose at all; just return to your regular dosing schedule. Do not double the next dose.

SIDE EFFECTS

Minor. Abdominal pain, anxiety, bitter taste in the mouth, constipation, diarrhea, dizziness, dry mouth, fatigue, flushing, gas, headache, hiccups, hoarseness, increased hand tremors, increased sexual interest, increased sweating, insomnia, loss of appetite, nausea, offensive body odor, salivation, vision changes, vomiting, weakness, or weight gain. These side effects may disappear as your body adjusts to the medication.

Levodopa can cause a darkening of your urine or sweat. This is a harmless effect.

To relieve constipation, increase the amount of fiber in your diet (fresh fruits and vegetables, salads, bran, and whole-grain breads), drink more water, and exercise (unless your doctor directs you to do otherwise).

If you feel dizzy, sit or lie down for a while; get up slowly from a sitting or reclining position, and be careful on stairs.

To relieve mouth dryness, chew sugarless gum or suck on ice chips or a piece of hard candy.

Major. Tell your doctor about any side effects that are persistent or particularly bothersome. IT IS ESPECIALLY IMPORTANT TO TELL YOUR DOCTOR about bloody or black, tarry stools; confusion; convulsions; depression; fainting; false sense of well-being; loss of coordination; loss of hair; nightmares; painful erection; palpitations; rapid weight gain (three to five pounds within a week); skin rash; visual disturbances; uncontrolled movements; or unusual weakness.

INTERACTIONS

Levodopa interacts with several other types of medications:

1. The dosage of antihypertensive drugs and oral antidiabetic drugs may require adjustment when levodopa is started.

2. The effectiveness of levodopa may be decreased by benzodiazepine tranquilizers, phenothiazine tranquilizers, haloperidol, thiothixene, phenytoin, papaverine, and reserpine.

3. Methyldopa can increase or decrease the side effects of therapy with levodopa.

4. Use of levodopa and a monoamine oxidase (MAO) inhibitor within 14 days of each other can lead to severe side effects.

5. Levodopa can increase the side effects of tricyclic antidepressants, ephedrine, and amphetamines.

6. Antacids may alter the absorption of levodopa from the gastrointestinal tract.

7. Pyridoxine (vitamin B_6) can decrease the effectiveness of levodopa.

BE SURE TO TELL YOUR DOCTOR about any medications you are currently taking, especially any of those listed above.

WARNINGS

- Tell your doctor about unusual or allergic reactions you have had to any medications, especially to levodopa.
- Before starting to take this medication, be sure to tell your doctor if you now have or if you have ever had asthma, diabetes mellitus, difficulty in urinating, epilepsy, glaucoma, heart disease, hormone disorders, kidney disease, liver disease, lung disease, melanoma (a type of skin cancer), mental disorders, or peptic ulcers.
- Some of these products contain the color additive FD&C Yellow No. 5 (tartrazine), which can cause allergic-type symptoms (difficulty in breathing, faintness, or rash) in certain susceptible individuals.
- If levodopa makes you dizzy or blurs your vision, avoid activities that require alertness, such as driving a car or operating potentially dangerous machinery.
- Notify your doctor if you start to experience any uncontrolled movements of the limbs or face while taking this medication.
- Before having surgery or any other medical or dental treatment, be sure to tell your doctor or dentist that you are taking this medication.
- Levodopa can cause erroneous readings of urine glucose and ketone tests. Diabetic patients should not change their medication dosage unless they first check with their doctor.
- Pyridoxine (vitamin B_6) can decrease the effectiveness of levodopa. Persons taking levodopa should avoid taking this vitamin and should avoid foods rich in pyridoxine (including beans, bacon, avocados, liver, dry skim milk, oatmeal, sweet potatoes, peas, and tuna).
- Be sure to tell your doctor if you are pregnant. Although levodopa appears to be safe in humans, birth defects have been reported in the offspring of animals that received large doses during pregnancy. Also, tell your doctor if you are breast-feeding an infant. Levodopa passes into breast milk and can cause side effects in nursing infants.

Levothroid—see levothyroxine

---

levothyroxine

BRAND NAMES (Manufacturers)

Levothroid (USV)
Levoxine (Daniels)
Synthroid (Flint)
Synthrox (Vortech)
Syroxine (Major)

TYPE OF DRUG

Thyroid hormone

INGREDIENT

levothyroxine

DOSAGE FORM

Tablets (0.025 mg, 0.05 mg, 0.075 mg, 0.1 mg, 0.125 mg, 0.15 mg, 0.175 mg, 0.2 mg, and 0.3 mg)

STORAGE

Levothyroxine tablets should be stored at room temperature in a tightly closed, light-resistant container.

USES

Levothyroxine is prescribed to replace natural thyroid hormones that are absent because of a disorder of the thyroid gland. This product is prepared synthetically (artificially) but is exactly like the natural thyroid hormone that is produced by the human body.

TREATMENT

Levothyroxine tablets should be taken on an empty stomach with a full glass of water. If the drug upsets your stomach, ask your doctor if you can take it with food or milk.

In order to get used to taking this medication, try to take it at the same time each day. Try not to miss any doses. If you do miss a dose of this medication, take it as soon as you remember, unless it is almost time for the next dose. In that case, do not take the missed dose at all; just return to your regular dosing schedule. Do not double the next dose. If you miss more than one or two doses, contact your doctor.

SIDE EFFECTS

Minor. Constipation; dry, puffy skin; fatigue; headache; listlessness; or weight gain. These side effects should disappear as your body adjusts to the medication.

To relieve constipation, increase the amount of fiber in your diet (fresh fruits and vegetables, salads, bran, and whole-grain breads), exercise, and drink more water (unless your doctor directs you to do otherwise).

Major. Tell your doctor about any side effects that are persistent or particularly bothersome. Most of the major side effects associated with this drug are the result of too large a dose. The dosage of this medication may need to be adjusted if you experience any of the following side effects: chest pain, diarrhea, fever, heat intolerance, insomnia, irritability, leg cramps, menstrual irregularities, muscle aches, nervousness, palpitations, shortness of breath, sweating, trembling, or weight loss. CHECK WITH YOUR DOCTOR.

INTERACTIONS

Levothyroxine interacts with several other types of drugs:

1. Dosing requirements for digoxin, insulin, or oral antidiabetic agents may change when levothyroxine is used.

2. The effects of oral anticoagulants (blood thinners, such as warfarin) may be increased by levothyroxine, which could lead to bleeding complications.

3. Cholestyramine and colestipol chemically bind levothyroxine in the gastrointestinal tract, preventing its absorption. Therefore, at least four hours should separate doses of levothyroxine and one of these medications.

4. Oral contraceptives (birth control pills) and estrogen-containing drugs may change dosage requirements for levothyroxine.

5. Phenobarbital may decrease the effects of levothyroxine; but tricyclic antidepressants and over-the-counter (nonprescription) allergy, asthma, cough, cold, sinus, and diet medications may increase its side effects.

BE SURE TO TELL YOUR DOCTOR about any medications you are currently taking, especially any listed above.

WARNINGS

- Tell your doctor about unusual or allergic reactions you have had to any medications, especially to thyroid hormone, levothyroxine, or liothyronine.
- Tell your doctor if you now have or if you have ever had angina pectoris, diabetes mellitus, heart disease, high blood pressure, kidney disease, or an underactive adrenal or pituitary gland.
- If you have an underactive thyroid gland, you may need to take this medication for life. You should not stop taking it unless you first check with your doctor.
- Before having surgery or any other medical or dental treatment, be sure to tell your doctor or dentist that you are taking levothyroxine.
- Over-the-counter (nonprescription) allergy, asthma, cough, cold, sinus, and diet medications can increase the side effects of levothyroxine. Therefore, check with your doctor or pharmacist before taking ANY of these products.
- Although many thyroid products are on the market, they are not all bioequivalent; that is, they may not all be absorbed into the bloodstream at the same rate or have the same overall activity. DON'T CHANGE BRANDS of this drug without first consulting your doctor or pharmacist to make sure you are receiving an equivalent product.
- Some of these products contain the color additive FD&C Yellow No. 5 (tartrazine), which can cause allergic-type reactions (fainting, rash, difficulty in breathing) in certain susceptible individuals.
- Be sure to tell your doctor if you are pregnant. Levothyroxine does not readily cross the placenta, and the drug appears to be safe during pregnancy. However, your dosing requirements of levothyroxine may change during pregnancy. Also, tell your doctor if you are breast-feeding an infant.

Levoxine—see levothyroxine

Librax—see chlordiazepoxide and clidinium combination

Libritabs—see chlordiazepoxide

Librium—see chlordiazepoxide

Lidex—see fluocinonide (topical)

Lidex-E—see fluocinonide (topical)

Lidox—see chlordiazepoxide and clidinium combination

Limbitrol—see chlordiazepoxide and amitriptyline combination

---

lindane

BRAND NAMES (Manufacturers)

G-well (Goldline)
Kwell (Reed & Carnrick)
Kwildane (Major)
lindane (various manufacturers)
Scabene (Stiefel)

TYPE OF DRUG

Pediculicide and scabicide

INGREDIENT

lindane (formerly known as gamma benzene hexachloride)

DOSAGE FORMS

Cream (1%)
Lotion (1%)
Shampoo (1%)

STORAGE

Lindane cream, lotion, and shampoo should be stored at room temperature in tightly closed containers. This medication should never be frozen.

USES

This medication is used to eliminate crab lice, head lice, and scabies. Lindane is a central nervous system (brain and spinal cord) stimulant, which causes convulsions and death of the parasites (at the dosage generally used, it is not harmful to humans).

TREATMENT

Complete directions for the use of these products are supplied by the manufacturers. Be sure to ask your doctor or pharmacist for these directions, and follow the instructions carefully.

If you are applying this medication to another person, you should wear plastic or rubber gloves on your hands in order to avoid absorption of this drug through the skin.

The lotion form of this medication should be shaken well before each dose is measured. The contents of the lotion tend to settle on the bottom of the bottle, so the bottle must be shaken in order to distribute the medication evenly and equalize the doses.

Be sure to rinse off this product according to the directions. If it is not rinsed off COMPLETELY, too much of the medication will be absorbed.

SIDE EFFECTS

Minor. Rash or skin irritation upon application.

Major. Tell your doctor about any side effects that are persistent or particularly bothersome. The serious side effects associated with this medication (clumsiness, convulsions, irritability, muscle cramps, palpitations, restlessness, unsteadiness, unusual nervousness, or vomiting) are due to absorption of this drug through the skin. This should not happen if the product is used according to directions. CONTACT YOUR DOCTOR if you experience any of these symptoms.

INTERACTIONS

Do not use other skin preparations (lotions, ointments, or oils). They increase the absorption of this product through the skin, which can lead to serious side effects.

WARNINGS

- Tell your doctor about unusual or allergic reactions you have had to any medications, especially to lindane.
- This product should NOT be used on the face. If you do get lindane in your eyes, it should be flushed out immediately. In order to decrease the amount of drug absorbed through the skin, avoid using this product on any open wounds, cuts, or sores.
- Lice are easily transmitted from one person to another. All family members (and sexual partners) should be carefully examined. Personal items (clothing, towels) should be machine-washed using the "hot" temperature cycle and then dried. No unusual cleaning measures are required. Combs, brushes, and other washable items may be soaked in boiling water for one hour.
- After using the shampoo for head lice, you must remove the dead nits (eggs). Use a fine-tooth comb to remove them from your hair, or mix a solution of equal parts of water and vinegar and apply it to the affected area. Rub the solution in well. After several minutes, shampoo with your regular shampoo and then brush your hair. This process should remove all nits.
- Be sure to tell your doctor if you are pregnant. Lindane is absorbed through the skin and may cause central nervous system side effects in the mother and in the developing fetus. Also, tell your doctor if you are breast-feeding an infant. Lindane probably passes into breast milk and may cause central nervous system side effects in nursing infants.

Lioresal—see baclofen

---

liothyronine

BRAND NAMES (Manufacturers)

Cyronine (Major)
Cytomel (Smith Kline & French)
liothyronine (various manufacturers)

TYPE OF DRUG

Thyroid hormone

INGREDIENT

liothyronine

DOSAGE FORM

Tablets (5 mcg, 25 mcg, and 50 mcg)

STORAGE

Liothyronine should be stored at room temperature in a tightly closed container.

USES

Liothyronine is a synthetic form of natural thyroid hormone. It has all of the pharmacologic activities of the natural substance. This medication is used to replace thyroid hormone in patients who cannot produce enough of their own.

TREATMENT

Liothyronine can be taken either on an empty stomach or with food or a full glass of water or milk, as directed by your doctor.

In order for you to become accustomed to taking this medication, try to take it at the same time each day.

If you miss a dose of this medication, take the missed dose as soon as possible, unless it is almost time for the next dose. In that case, do not take the missed dose at all; just return to your regular dosing schedule. Do not double the next dose.

SIDE EFFECTS

Minor. Abdominal cramps, diarrhea, headache, insomnia, or nausea. These side effects may disappear as your body adjusts to the medication.

Major. Tell your doctor about any side effects that are persistent or particularly bothersome. Most of the serious side effects of this medication are the result of too high a dose. These include chest pain, fever, intolerance to heat, menstrual irregularities, nervousness, palpitations, skin rash, sweating, tremors, and weight loss. CONTACT YOUR DOCTOR if you experience any of these symptoms.

INTERACTIONS

Liothyronine interacts with several other types of medications:

1. It can increase the effects of oral anticoagulants (blood thinners, such as warfarin), which can lead to bleeding complications.

2. The dosage of digoxin, insulin, or oral antidiabetic medicines may require adjustment when liothyronine is started.

3. Cholestyramine decreases the absorption of liothyronine from the gastrointestinal tract. Therefore, at least four to five hours should separate doses of these medications.

4. Liothyronine may increase the side effects of tricyclic antidepressants.

Before starting to take this medication, BE SURE TO TELL YOUR DOCTOR about any medications you are currently taking, especially any of those listed above.

WARNINGS

- Tell your doctor about unusual or allergic reactions you have had to any medications, especially to liothyronine, thyroid hormone, or levothyroxine.
- Before starting to take this medication, be sure to tell your doctor if you now have or if you have ever had an underac-

tive adrenal gland, diabetes mellitus, heart or blood vessel disease, or an underactive pituitary gland.
• Before having surgery or any other medical or dental treatment, be sure to tell your doctor or dentist that you are taking this medication.
• Because liothyronine is replacing natural thyroid hormone, you may need to take this medication for the rest of your life.
• Do not stop taking this medication unless you first check with your doctor. Stopping this medication may result in worsening of your condition.
• Do not take any over-the-counter (nonprescription) cough, cold, allergy, asthma, sinus, or diet medications without first checking with your doctor or pharmacist. Some of these products can increase the side effects of liothyronine.
• The elderly may be at increased risk of experiencing side effects of this medication.
• Be sure to tell your doctor if you are pregnant. Your dosage of liothyronine may need to be adjusted during pregnancy. Also, tell your doctor if you are breast-feeding an infant. Small amounts of liothyronine pass into breast milk.

Lipo Gantrisin—see sulfonamide antibiotics (oral)

Lipoxide—see chlordiazepoxide

Liquid Pred—see prednisone (systemic)

---

lisinopril

BRAND NAMES (Manufacturers)
Prinivil (Merck Sharp & Dohme)
Zestril (Stuart)
TYPE OF DRUG
Antihypertensive
INGREDIENT
lisinopril
DOSAGE FORM
Tablets (5 mg, 10 mg, 20 mg, and 40 mg)
STORAGE
Store this medication away from heat, direct light, or moisture.

USES

Lisinopril is currently approved for the treatment of hypertension (high blood pressure). It is also being investigated for the treatment of heart failure. Lisinopril is a vasodilator (it widens the blood vessels) that acts by blocking the production of chemicals that may be responsible for constricting blood vessels.

TREATMENT

The duration of action of lisinopril permits once-a-day dosing. Lisinopril can be taken either on an empty stomach or with food if it causes stomach irritation.

If you miss a dose of this medication, take the missed dose as soon as possible, unless it is almost time for the next dose. In that case, do not take the missed dose at all; just wait until the next scheduled dose. Do not double the dose.

In some patients it may require two to four weeks of therapy to achieve maximum therapeutic benefit.

Lisinopril does not cure high blood pressure, but it will help to control the condition as long as you continue to take the medication.

SIDE EFFECTS

Minor. Dizziness; headache; fatigue; diarrhea; nasal congestion; or dry, hacking cough.

To avoid dizziness or light-headedness when you stand, contract and relax the muscles of your legs for a few moments before rising. Do this by pushing one foot against the floor while raising the other foot slightly, alternating feet so that you are "pumping" your legs in a pedaling motion.

Major. Tell your physician about any side effects that are persistent or particularly bothersome. IT IS ESPECIALLY IMPORTANT TO TELL YOUR DOCTOR about chest pain; chills; difficult or painful urination; fever; itching; mouth sores; palpitations; prolonged vomiting or diarrhea; rash; shortness of breath; sore throat; swelling of the face, hands, or feet; tingling in the fingers or toes; unusual bleeding or bruising; or yellowing of the eyes or skin.

INTERACTIONS

1. Lisinopril tends to cause retention of potassium in the body. Many salt substitutes contain potassium chloride and should only be used with the advice of your physician. Caution should also be observed with low-salt foods, some of which may contain significant amounts of potassium. Other medications such as the diuretics (water pills), triamterene, spironolactone, or amiloride may cause potassium retention. Use of these medications together with lisinopril may lead to excessive levels of potassium in the blood.
2. The anti-inflammatory drug indomethacin may reduce the effectiveness of lisinopril.
3. Excessive hypotension (low blood pressure) may occur when starting lisinopril in patients on diuretics.

Before starting to take lisinopril, BE SURE TO TELL YOUR DOCTOR about any medications you are currently taking, especially any of those listed above.

WARNINGS

• Tell your doctor about unusual or allergic reactions you have had to any medications, especially to lisinopril, captopril, or enalapril.
• Tell your doctor if you experience light-headedness, which may be a symptom of excessive hypotension (low blood pressure). This is especially likely to occur during the first few days of therapy. If fainting occurs, stop the drug and consult with your physician.
• Excessive perspiration or dehydration may cause an excessive fall in blood pressure.
• Report any evidence of infections (such as sore throat or fever) to your physician.
• If you have high blood pressure, do not take any over-the-counter (nonprescription) medication for weight control, or for allergy, asthma, sinus, cough, or cold problems unless you first check with your doctor.
• Because lisinopril is eliminated from the body through the kidneys, be sure to report to your physician any symptoms of kidney disease, such as difficulty in urinating.
• Be sure to tell your doctor if you are pregnant or plan to

become pregnant. The safety of lisinopril has not been established in pregnant women. Studies in certain animals, in which administered doses far exceeded those used in humans, have shown a decrease in the number of successful pregnancies. Also tell your doctor if you are breast-feeding an infant. It is not known whether lisinopril passes into breast milk.

Lithane—see lithium

---

lithium

BRAND NAMES (Manufacturers)
Cibalith-S (Ciba)
Eskalith (Smith Kline & French)
Eskalith CR (Smith Kline & French)
Lithane (Miles Pharmaceutical)
lithium carbonate (various manufacturers)
lithium citrate (various manufacturers)
Lithobid (Ciba)
Lithonate (Reid-Rowell)
Lithotabs (Reid-Rowell)

TYPE OF DRUG
Antimanic (mood stabilizer)

INGREDIENT
lithium

DOSAGE FORMS
Tablets (300 mg)
Extended-release tablets (300 mg and 450 mg)
Capsules (150 mg, 300 mg, and 600 mg)
Syrup (300 mg per 5-ml spoonful, with 0.3% alcohol)

STORAGE
Lithium tablets, capsules, and syrup should be stored at room temperature away from heat and direct sunlight. The syrup should not be frozen. Do not store the medication in the bathroom cabinet, because moisture may cause the breakdown of lithium. Do not keep these medications beyond the expiration date.

USES

Lithium is a medication used to control the manic (excited) phase of manic-depressive illness. Manic-depressive patients often experience unstable emotions ranging from excitement to hostility to depression. The mechanism of the mood-stabilizing effect of lithium is unknown, but it appears to work on the central nervous system to control emotions.

TREATMENT

Lithium should be taken exactly as directed by your doctor. The effectiveness of this medication depends upon the amount of lithium in your bloodstream. Therefore, the medication should be taken every day at regularly spaced intervals in order to keep a constant amount of lithium in your bloodstream.

The syrup form must be measured carefully with a specially designed 5-ml measuring spoon. An ordinary kitchen teaspoon is not accurate enough.

If you miss a dose of this medication, take it as soon as possible. However, if it is within two hours (six hours for extended-release tablets) of your next scheduled dose, skip the missed dose and return to your regular schedule. Do not take more than one dose at a time.

An improvement in your condition may not be observed for up to several weeks after you start to take this medication.

SIDE EFFECTS

Minor. Acne, bloating, diarrhea, drowsiness, increased frequency of urination, increased thirst, nausea, trembling of the hands, weight gain, or weakness or tiredness. These side effects should disappear as your body adjusts to this medication.

Major. Blurred vision, clumsiness, confusion, convulsions, difficulty in breathing, dizziness, fainting, palpitations, severe trembling, and slurred speech are possible effects of too much drug in the bloodstream. Dry, rough skin; hair loss; hoarseness; swelling of the feet or lower legs; swelling of the neck; unusual sensitivity to the cold; unusual tiredness; or unusual weight gain may be the result of low thyroid function caused by the medication. CHECK WITH YOUR DOCTOR IMMEDIATELY if any of these side effects appear.

INTERACTIONS

Lithium interacts with a number of other types of medications:

1. Aminophylline, caffeine, verapamil, acetazolamide, sodium bicarbonate, dyphylline, oxtriphylline, and theophylline can increase the elimination of lithium from the body, thus decreasing its effectiveness.

2. Diuretics (water pills), especially hydrochlorothiazide, chlorothiazide, chlorthalidone, triamterene and hydrochlorothiazide combination, and furosemide may cause lithium toxicity by delaying the body's lithium elimination.

3. Chlorpromazine, other phenothiazine tranquilizers, ibuprofen, indomethacin, naproxen, and piroxicam can also slow lithium elimination.

4. Lithium can increase the side effects of haloperidol.

5. Phenytoin, methyldopa, carbamazepine, and tetracycline can increase the side effects of lithium.

6. Drinking large amounts of caffeine-containing coffees, teas, or colas may reduce the effectiveness of lithium by increasing its elimination from the body through the urine.

BE SURE TO TELL YOUR DOCTOR about any medications you are currently taking, especially any of those listed above.

WARNINGS

- Tell your doctor about unusual or allergic reactions you have had to any medications, especially to lithium.
- Tell your doctor if you now have or if you have ever had diabetes mellitus, epilepsy, heart disease, kidney disease, Parkinson's disease, or thyroid disease.
- Elderly patients may be more sensitive to lithium's side effects.
- In order to maintain a constant level of lithium in your bloodstream, it is important to drink two to three quarts of water or other fluids each day and not to change the amount of salt in your diet, unless your doctor directs you to do so.
- The loss of large amounts of body fluid (from prolonged vomiting or diarrhea or from heavy sweating due to hot weather, fever, exercise, saunas, or hot baths) can result in increased lithium levels in the blood, which can lead to an increase in side effects.

• The toxic dose of lithium is very close to the therapeutic dose, so it is extremely important to follow your correct dosing schedule. Diarrhea, drowsiness, lack of coordination, muscular weakness, and vomiting may be signs of toxicity. If these symptoms occur for any length of time or begin shortly after taking a dose, inform your doctor.
• Lithium is not recommended for use during pregnancy, especially during the first three months, because of possible effects on the thyroid and heart of the developing fetus. Also, tell your doctor if you are breast-feeding. Lithium also passes into breast milk and may cause side effects in the nursing infant.

lithium carbonate—see lithium

lithium citrate—see lithium

Lithobid—see lithium

Lithonate—see lithium

Lithotabs—see lithium

Lobac—see chlorzoxazone and acetaminophen combination

Locoid—see hydrocortisone (topical)

Lodrane—see theophylline

Loestrin—see oral contraceptives

Lofene—see diphenoxylate and atropine combination

Logen—see diphenoxylate and atropine combination

Lomanate—see diphenoxylate and atropine combination

Lomotil—see diphenoxylate and atropine combination

---

lomustine

BRAND NAME (Manufacturer)
CeeNU (Bristol)
TYPE OF DRUG
Antineoplastic (anticancer drug)
INGREDIENT
lomustine
DOSAGE FORM
Capsules (10 mg, 40 mg, and 100 mg)
STORAGE
Lomustine should be stored at room temperature in a tightly closed container.

USES

This medication belongs to a group of drugs known as nitrosourea alkylating agents. It is used to treat a variety of cancers. Lomustine is thought to work by binding to the rapidly growing cancer cells, preventing their multiplication and growth.

TREATMENT

To help prevent nausea, you should take lomustine on an empty stomach (unless your doctor directs otherwise).

The patient is usually required to take this medication as a single dose once a week. The total weekly dose consists of a number of capsules of different strengths and colors, which are all taken at the same time. The timing of each weekly dose is very important; be sure you completely understand your doctor's instructions on how and when this medication should be taken.

SIDE EFFECTS

Minor. Nausea and vomiting may occur three to six hours after taking a dose of lomustine; these symptoms usually last less than 24 hours. Lomustine may also cause hair loss, which is reversible when the medication is stopped.
Major. Tell your doctor about any side effects that are persistent or particularly bothersome. IT IS ESPECIALLY IMPORTANT TO TELL YOUR DOCTOR about chills, confusion, decreased coordination, difficult or painful urination, disorientation, fever, itching, loss of appetite, lethargy, mouth sores, sore throat, unusual bleeding or bruising, weakness, or yellowing of the eyes or skin. These side effects may even appear several weeks after the last dose is taken.

INTERACTIONS

Lomustine should not interact with other medications if it is used according to directions.

WARNINGS

• Tell your doctor about unusual or allergic reactions you have had to any medications, especially to lomustine, carmustine, or streptozocin.
• Before starting to take this medication, be sure to tell your doctor if you now have or if you have ever had blood disorders, chronic or recurrent infections, or kidney disease.
• Before having surgery or any other medical or dental treatment, be sure to tell your doctor or dentist that you are taking this medication.
• You should not receive any immunizations or vaccinations while taking this medication. Lomustine blocks the effectiveness of vaccines, which could result in an overwhelming infection if a live-virus vaccine is administered.
• Lomustine can lower your platelet count, which can decrease your body's ability to form blood clots. You should, therefore, be especially careful while brushing your teeth, flossing, or using toothpicks, razors, or fingernail scissors. Try to avoid falls and other injuries. Your doctor may also order periodic laboratory tests to monitor your blood.
• Lomustine can decrease fertility in both men and women.
• Be sure to tell your doctor if you are pregnant. Lomustine has been reported to cause birth defects in both animals and humans whose mothers received the drug during pregnancy. The risks should be discussed with your doctor. Also, tell your doctor if you are breast-feeding an infant. Small amounts of lomustine pass into breast milk.

Loniten—see minoxidil (systemic)

Lonox—see diphenoxylate and atropine combination

Lo/Ovral—see oral contraceptives

loperamide

BRAND NAME (Manufacturer)
Imodium (Janssen)
TYPE OF DRUG
Antidiarrheal
INGREDIENT
loperamide
DOSAGE FORMS
Capsules (2 mg)
Oral liquid (1 mg per 5-ml spoonful)
STORAGE
Loperamide capsules and liquid should be stored at room temperature in tightly closed containers. This medication should never be frozen.

USES

Loperamide is used to treat acute and chronic diarrhea and to reduce the volume of discharge in patients who have ileostomies. It acts by slowing the movement of the gastrointestinal tract and decreasing the passage of water and other substances into the bowel.

TREATMENT

In order to avoid stomach upset, you can take loperamide with food or with a full glass of water or milk.

The oral liquid form of this medication should be measured carefully with a special dropper or with a specially designed 5-ml measuring spoon. An ordinary kitchen teaspoon is not accurate enough.

If you miss a dose of this medication, do not take the missed dose at all; just return to your regular dosing schedule. Do not double the next dose.

SIDE EFFECTS

Minor. Constipation, dizziness, drowsiness, dry mouth, fatigue, loss of appetite, nausea, or vomiting. These effects should disappear as your body adjusts to the drug.

To relieve constipation, exercise and drink more water (unless your doctor directs you to do otherwise).

To reduce mouth dryness, chew sugarless gum or suck on ice chips or a piece of hard candy.

If you feel dizzy or light-headed, sit or lie down for a while; get up from a sitting or lying position slowly, and be careful on stairs.

Major. Tell your doctor about any side effects that are persistent or particularly bothersome. IT IS ESPECIALLY IMPORTANT TO TELL YOUR DOCTOR about abdominal bloating or pain, fever, rash, or sore throat.

INTERACTIONS

Loperamide should not interact with any other drugs.

WARNINGS

- Tell your doctor about unusual or allergic reactions you have had to any medications, especially to loperamide.
- Tell your doctor if you now have or if you have ever had colitis, diarrhea caused by infectious organisms, drug-induced diarrhea, liver disease, dehydration, or conditions in which constipation must be avoided (such as hemorrhoids, diverticulitis, heart or blood vessel disorders, or blood clotting disorders).
- If this drug makes you dizzy or drowsy, do not take part in any activity that requires alertness, such as driving a car or operating potentially dangerous machinery.
- Before having surgery or any other medical or dental treatment, be sure to tell your doctor or dentist that you are taking this medication.
- Check with your doctor if your diarrhea does not subside within two to three days. Unless your doctor prescribes otherwise, do not take this drug for more than ten days at a time.
- While taking this medication, drink lots of fluids to replace those lost because of diarrhea.
- Be sure to tell your doctor if you are pregnant. Although loperamide has been shown to be safe in animals, the effects of this medication during pregnancy have not been thoroughly studied in humans. Also, tell your doctor if you are breast-feeding an infant. It is not known whether loperamide passes into breast milk.

Lopid—see gemfibrozil

Lopressor—see metoprolol

Lopressor HCT—see metoprolol and hydrochlorothiazide combination

Lopurin—see allopurinol

---

lorazepam

BRAND NAMES (Manufacturers)
Alzapam (Major)
Ativan (Wyeth)
lorazepam (various manufacturers)
TYPE OF DRUG
Benzodiazepine sedative/hypnotic
INGREDIENT
lorazepam
DOSAGE FORM
Tablets (0.5 mg, 1 mg, and 2 mg)
STORAGE
This medication should be stored at room temperature in a tightly closed, light-resistant container.

USES

Lorazepam is prescribed to treat symptoms of anxiety and anxiety associated with depression. It is not clear exactly how this medicine works, but it may relieve anxiety by acting as a depressant of the central nervous system (brain and spinal cord). This medication is currently used by many people to relieve nervousness. It is effective for this purpose for short periods, but it is important to try to remove the cause of the anxiety as well.

TREATMENT

Lorazepam should be taken exactly as your doctor directs. It can be taken with food or a full glass of water if stomach upset occurs. Do not take this medication with a dose of antacids, since they may slow its absorption from the gastrointestinal tract.

If you are taking this medication regularly and you miss a dose, take the missed dose immediately if you remember within an hour. If more than an hour has passed, skip the dose you missed and wait for the next scheduled dose. Do not double the dose.

SIDE EFFECTS

Minor. Bitter taste in the mouth, constipation, diarrhea, dizziness, drowsiness (after a night's sleep), dry mouth, fatigue, flushing, headache, heartburn, excessive salivation, loss of appetite, nausea, nervousness, sweating, or vomiting. As your body adjusts to the medication, these side effects should disappear.

To relieve constipation, increase the amount of fiber in your diet (fresh fruits and vegetables, salads, bran, and whole-grain breads), exercise, and drink more water (unless your doctor directs you to do otherwise).

Dry mouth can be relieved by chewing sugarless gum or by sucking on ice chips.

If you feel dizzy, sit or lie down for a while; get up slowly from a sitting or reclining position, and be careful on stairs.

Major. Tell your doctor about any side effects that are persistent or particularly bothersome. IT IS ESPECIALLY IMPORTANT TO TELL YOUR DOCTOR about blurred or double vision, chest pain, depression, difficulty in urinating, fainting, falling, fever, joint pain, hallucinations, memory problems, mouth sores, nightmares, palpitations, rash, shortness of breath, slurred speech, sore throat, uncoordinated movements, unusual excitement, unusual tiredness, or yellowing of the eyes or skin.

INTERACTIONS

Lorazepam interacts with several other types of medications:

1. To prevent oversedation, this drug should not be taken with alcohol, other sedative drugs, or central nervous system depressants (such as antihistamines, barbiturates, muscle relaxants, pain medicines, narcotics, medicines for seizures, and phenothiazine tranquilizers) or with antidepressants.

2. This medication may decrease the effectiveness of carbamazepine, levodopa, and oral anticoagulants (blood thinners) and may increase the effects of phenytoin.

3. Disulfiram, cimetidine, and isoniazid can increase the blood levels of lorazepam, which can lead to toxic effects.

4. Concurrent use of rifampin may decrease the effectiveness of lorazepam.

BE SURE TO TELL YOUR DOCTOR about any medications you are currently taking, especially any listed above.

WARNINGS

- Tell your doctor about unusual or allergic reactions you have had to any medications, especially to lorazepam or other benzodiazepine tranquilizers (such as alprazolam, chlordiazepoxide, clorazepate, diazepam, flurazepam, halazepam, midazolam, oxazepam, prazepam, temazepam, and triazolam).
- Tell your doctor if you now have or if you have ever had liver disease, kidney disease, epilepsy, lung disease, myasthenia gravis, porphyria, mental depression, or mental illness.
- This medicine can cause drowsiness. Avoid tasks that require alertness, such as driving a car or using potentially dangerous machinery.
- This medication has the potential for abuse and must be used with caution. Tolerance may develop quickly; do not increase the dosage without first consulting your doctor. It is also important not to stop this drug suddenly if you have been taking it in large amounts or if you have used it for several weeks. Your doctor may want to reduce the dosage gradually.
- This is a safe drug when used properly. When it is combined with other sedative drugs or alcohol, however, serious side effects can develop.
- Be sure to tell your doctor if you are pregnant. This medicine may increase the chance of birth defects if it is taken during the first three months of pregnancy. In addition, too much use of this medicine during the last six months of pregnancy may cause the fetus to become dependent on it, resulting in withdrawal side effects in the newborn. Also, use of this medicine during the last weeks of pregnancy may cause excessive drowsiness, slowed heartbeat, and breathing difficulties in the newborn. Tell your doctor if you are breastfeeding an infant. This medicine can pass into the breast milk and cause excessive drowsiness, slowed heartbeat, and breathing difficulties in the nursing infant.

Lorelco—see probucol

Lortab 5—see acetaminophen and hydrocodone combination

Lotrimin—see clotrimazole (topical)

Lotrisone—see betamethasone dipropionate and clotrimazole combination

Lo-Trol—see diphenoxylate and atropine combination

---

lovastatin

BRAND NAME (Manufacturer)
Mevacor (Merck Sharp & Dohme)

TYPE OF DRUG
Antihyperlipidemic (lipid-lowering drug)

INGREDIENT
lovastatin

DOSAGE FORM
Tablets (20 mg and 40 mg)

STORAGE
This medication should be stored at room temperature in a tightly closed, light-resistant container. Exposure to heat or moisture may cause this drug to break down.

USES

Lovastatin is used to treat hyperlipidemia (high blood fat levels). It is prescribed in conjunction with nondrug therapies, such as diet modification and regular exercise, in an attempt to regulate lipid and cholesterol levels. Lovastatin chemically interferes with an enzyme in the body that is responsible for synthesizing cholesterol. This enzyme blockade decreases the LDL (low-density lipoprotein) type of cholesterol. This type of cholesterol has been associated with coronary heart disease and atherosclerosis.

TREATMENT

This medication should be taken exactly as prescribed by your doctor. If you are to take the drug once a day, it is best to take the drug in the evening. Lovastatin can be taken with meals or a full glass of water if stomach upset occurs.

While using this medication, try to develop a set schedule for taking it. If you miss a dose and remember within a few hours, take the missed dose and resume your regular schedule. If many hours have passed, skip the dose you missed and then take your next dose as scheduled. Do not double the dose.

SIDE EFFECTS

Minor. Abdominal pain or cramps, constipation, diarrhea, gas, nausea, or stomach pain. These effects may be relieved by taking lovastatin with a meal, adding fiber to your diet, or using mild stool softeners.

Major. Tell your doctor about any side effects that are persistent or particularly bothersome. IT IS ESPECIALLY IMPORTANT TO TELL YOUR DOCTOR about blurred vision (or any other visual changes or difficulties) or muscle pain or tenderness, especially with malaise or fever.

INTERACTIONS

There do not appear to be any significant drug interactions with this medication. However, you should make sure your doctor knows all the medications you are taking.

WARNINGS

- Tell your doctor about unusual or allergic reactions you have had to any medications.
- Tell your doctor if you have ever had liver disease, heart disease, stroke, or disorders of the digestive tract.
- In preliminary studies with lovastatin, some patients were found to develop eye-related problems during treatment. Although these findings are inconclusive, and it has not yet been determined whether lovastatin is involved in such occurrences, it is advisable to have regular checkups with your ophthalmologist and inform him/her of your use of this drug.
- This drug should not be taken if you are pregnant or breast-feeding an infant.

Low-Quel—see diphenoxylate and atropine combination

---

loxapine

BRAND NAMES (Manufacturers)
Loxitane (Lederle)
Loxitane C (Lederle)

TYPE OF DRUG
Antipsychotic

INGREDIENT
loxapine

DOSAGE FORMS
Capsules (5 mg, 10 mg, 25 mg, and 50 mg)
Oral concentrate (25 mg per ml)

STORAGE
Loxapine capsules and oral concentrate should be stored at room temperature (never frozen) in tightly closed containers. If the oral concentrate turns slightly yellowish, the drug is still effective and can be used. However, if the oral concentrate changes color markedly or has particles floating in it, it shouldn't be used; rather, it should instead be discarded down the sink.

USES

Loxapine is prescribed to treat the symptoms of mental illness, such as the emotional symptoms of psychosis. This medication is thought to relieve the symptoms of mental illness by blocking certain chemicals involved with nerve transmission in the brain.

TREATMENT

To avoid stomach irritation, you can take the tablet form of loxapine with a meal or with a glass of water or milk (unless your doctor directs you to do otherwise.)

The oral concentrate form of this medication should be measured carefully with the dropper provided and diluted in eight ounces (a full cup) or more of the orange or grapefruit juice immediately prior to administration.

If you miss a dose of this medication, take the missed dose as soon as possible and return to your regular dosing schedule. If it is almost time for the next dose, however, skip the one you missed and then return to your regular schedule. Do not double the dose unless you are directed to do so by your doctor.

Antacids and antidiarrheal medicines can decrease the absorption of this medication from the gastrointestinal tract. Therefore, at least one hour should separate doses of one of these medicines and loxapine.

The full effects of this medication for the control of emotional or mental symptoms may not become apparent for two weeks after you start to take it.

SIDE EFFECTS

Minor. Blurred vision, constipation, decreased sweating, diarrhea, dizziness, drooling, drowsiness, dry mouth, fatigue, jitteriness, menstrual irregularities, nasal congestion, restlessness, vomiting, or weight gain. As your body adjusts to the medication, these side effects should disappear.

This medication can cause increased sensitivity to sunlight. It is, therefore, important to avoid prolonged exposure to sunlight and sunlamps. Wear protective clothing, and use an effective sunscreen.

If you are constipated, increase the amount of fiber in your diet (fresh fruits and vegetables, salads, bran, and whole-grain breads), exercise, and drink more water (unless your doctor directs you to do otherwise).

To reduce mouth dryness, chew sugarless gum or suck on ice chips or a piece of hard candy.

To avoid dizziness or light-headedness when you stand, contract and relax the muscles of your legs for a few moments before rising. Do this by pushing one foot against the floor while raising the other foot slightly, alternating feet so that you are "pumping" your legs in a pedaling motion.

Major. Tell your doctor about any side effects that are persistent or particularly bothersome. IT IS ESPECIALLY IMPORTANT TO TELL YOUR DOCTOR about breast enlargement (in both sexes); chest pain; convulsions; darkened skin; difficulty in swallowing or breathing; fainting; fever; impotence; involuntary movements of the face, mouth, jaw, or tongue; palpitations; rash; sleep disorders; sore throat; tremors; uncoordinated movements; unusual bleeding or bruising; visual disturbances; or yellowing of the eyes or skin.

INTERACTIONS

Loxapine can interact with a number of other types of medications:

1. It can cause extreme drowsiness when combined with alcohol or other central nervous system depressants (such as barbiturates, benzodiazepine tranquilizers, muscle relaxants, narcotics, and pain medications) or with tricyclic antidepressants.

2. This medication can decrease the effectiveness of amphetamines, guanethidine, anticonvulsants, and levodopa.

3. The side effects of epinephrine, monoamine oxidase (MAO) inhibitors, and tricyclic antidepressants may be increased when combined with this medication. At least 14 days should separate the use of this drug and the use of an MAO inhibitor.

BE SURE TO TELL YOUR DOCTOR about any medications you are currently taking, especially any of those listed above.

WARNINGS

- Tell your doctor about unusual or allergic reactions you have had to any medications, especially to loxapine or to any phenothiazine tranquilizer.
- Tell your doctor if you have a history of alcoholism or if you now have or ever had heart or circulatory disease, epilepsy, glaucoma, liver disease, Parkinson's disease, enlarged prostate gland, or blockage of the urinary tract.
- Avoid drinking alcoholic beverages while taking this medication, in order to prevent oversedation.
- If this medication makes you dizzy or drowsy, do not take part in any activity that requires alertness, such as driving a car or operating potentially dangerous machinery. Be careful on stairs, and avoid getting up suddenly from a lying or sitting position.
- Prior to having surgery or any other medical or dental treatment, be sure to tell your doctor or dentist that you are taking loxapine.
- Some of the side effects caused by this drug can be prevented by taking an antiparkinsonism drug. Discuss this with your doctor.
- This medication can decrease sweating and heat release from the body. Therefore, avoid getting overheated by strenuous exercise in hot weather, and avoid taking hot baths, showers, and saunas.
- This medication has the potential to cause a permanent movement disorder called tardive dyskinesia. Therefore, be sure to report any uncontrolled movements of the body to your doctor.
- Do not stop taking this medication suddenly. If the drug is stopped abruptly, you may experience nausea, vomiting, stomach upset, headache, increased heart rate, insomnia, tremors, or worsening of your condition. Your doctor may want to reduce the dosage gradually.
- If you are planning to have a myelogram, or any other procedure in which dye is injected into the area surrounding the spinal cord, tell your doctor that you are taking this medication.
- Avoid spilling the oral concentrate form of this medication on your skin or clothing; it can cause redness and irritation of the skin.
- While you are taking this prescription medication, do not take any over-the-counter (nonprescription) medication or preparation for weight control or for cough, cold, asthma, allergy, or sinus problems unless you first check with your doctor. The combination of these two types of medications can cause high blood pressure.
- Elderly patients may be at increased risk of experiencing side effects of this medication.
- Be sure to tell your doctor if you are pregnant. Small amounts of this medication will cross the placenta. Although there are reports of safe use of this type of drug during pregnancy, there are also reports of liver disease and tremors in newborn infants whose mothers received this type of medication close to term. Also, tell your doctor if you are breast-feeding an infant. Small amounts of this medication pass into breast milk and may cause unwanted effects in the nursing infant.

Loxitane—see loxapine

Loxitane C—see loxapine

Lozol—see indapamide

Ludiomil—see maprotiline

Luramide—see furosemide

Lysodren—see mitotane

Macrodantin—see nitrofurantoin

Malatal—see atropine, scopolamine, hyoscyamine, and phenobarbital combination

Mandameth—see methenamine

Mandelamine—see methenamine

---

maprotiline

BRAND NAME (Manufacturer)
Ludiomil (Ciba)
TYPE OF DRUG
Tetracyclic antidepressant
INGREDIENT
maprotiline
DOSAGE FORM
Tablets (25 mg, 50 mg, and 75 mg)
STORAGE
Maprotiline tablets should be stored at room temperature in a tightly closed container.

USES

Maprotiline is used to relieve the symptoms of mental depression. This medication is a tetracyclic antidepressant. It is related to a group of drugs referred to as the tricyclic antidepressants. These medicines are thought to relieve depression by increasing the concentration of certain chemicals necessary for nerve transmission in the brain.

TREATMENT

This medication should be taken exactly as your doctor prescribes. It can be taken with water or food to lessen the chance of stomach irritation, unless your doctor tells you to do otherwise.

If you miss a dose of this medication, take the missed dose as soon as possible, then return to your regular dosing schedule. However, if the dose you missed was a once-a-day bedtime dose, do not take that dose in the morning; check with your doctor instead. If the dose is taken in the morning, it may cause some unwanted side effects. Never double the dose.

The effects of therapy with this medication may not become apparent for two or three weeks.

SIDE EFFECTS

Minor. Anxiety, blurred vision, confusion, constipation, diarrhea, dizziness, drowsiness, dry mouth, fatigue, heartburn, insomnia, loss of appetite, nausea, peculiar tastes in the mouth, restlessness, sweating, vomiting, weakness, or weight gain or loss. As your body adjusts to the medication, these side effects should disappear.

This medication can cause increased sensitivity to sunlight. It is, therefore, important to avoid prolonged exposure to sunlight and sunlamps. Wear protective clothing, and use an effective sunscreen.

If you experience dry mouth, it can be relieved by chewing sugarless gum or by sucking on ice chips or a piece of hard candy.

To relieve constipation, increase the amount of fiber in your diet (fresh fruits and vegetables, salads, bran, and whole-grain breads), exercise, and drink more water (unless your doctor directs you to do otherwise).

To avoid dizziness or light-headedness when you stand, contract and relax the muscles of your legs for a few moments before rising. Do this by pushing one foot against the floor while raising the other foot slightly, alternating feet so that you are "pumping" your legs in a pedaling motion.

Major. Tell your doctor about any side effects that are persistent or particularly bothersome. IT IS ESPECIALLY IMPORTANT TO TELL YOUR DOCTOR about agitation, chest pain, convulsions, cramps, difficulty in urinating, enlarged or painful breasts (in both sexes), fainting, fever, fluid retention, hair loss, hallucinations, headaches, impotence, mood changes, mouth sores, nervousness, nightmares, numbness in the fingers or toes, palpitations, ringing in the ears, seizures, skin rash, sleep disorders, sore throat, tremors, uncoordinated movements or balance problems, unusual bleeding or bruising, or yellowing of the eyes or skin.

INTERACTIONS

Maprotiline interacts with other types of medications:

1. Extreme drowsiness can occur when this medicine is taken with central nervous system depressants (such as alcohol, antihistamines, barbiturates, benzodiazepine tranquilizers, muscle relaxants, narcotics, pain medications, phenothiazine tranquilizers, and sleeping medications) or with other antidepressants.

2. Maprotiline may decrease the effectiveness of antiseizure medications and may block the blood-pressure-lowering effects of clonidine and guanethidine.

3. Oral contraceptives (birth control pills) and estrogen-containing drugs can increase the side effects and reduce the effectiveness of tricyclic antidepressants and maprotiline.

4. Tetracyclic antidepressants may increase the side effects of thyroid medication and over-the-counter (nonprescription) allergy, cough, cold, asthma, sinus, and diet medications.

5. The concurrent use of tetracyclic antidepressants and monoamine oxidase (MAO) inhibitors should be avoided, because the combination may result in fever, convulsions, or high blood pressure. At least 14 days should separate the use of this drug and the use of an MAO inhibitor.

Before starting to take maprotiline, BE SURE TO TELL YOUR DOCTOR about any medications you are currently taking, especially any of those listed above.

WARNINGS

- Tell your doctor if you have had unusual or allergic reactions to any medications, especially to maprotiline or any of the tricyclic antidepressants (such as amitriptyline, imipramine, doxepin, trimipramine, amoxapine, protriptyline, desipramine, and nortriptyline).
- Tell your doctor if you have a history of alcoholism or if you have ever had asthma, high blood pressure, liver or kidney disease, heart disease, a heart attack, circulatory disease, stomach problems, intestinal problems, difficulty in urinating, enlarged prostate gland, epilepsy, glaucoma, thyroid disease, mental illness, or electroshock therapy.
- If this drug makes you dizzy or drowsy, do not take part in any activity that requires alertness, such as driving a car or operating potentially dangerous machinery.
- Before having surgery or other medical or dental treatment, tell your doctor or dentist about this drug.
- Do not stop taking this drug suddenly. Abruptly stopping it can cause nausea, headache, stomach upset, fatigue, or a worsening of your condition. Your doctor may want to reduce the dosage gradually.
- The effects of this medication may last as long as seven days after you have stopped taking it, so continue to observe all precautions during that period.
- Elderly patients may be at increased risk of experiencing side effects of this medication.
- Be sure to tell your doctor if you are pregnant. Problems in humans have not been reported; however, studies in animals have shown that this type of medication can cause side effects in the fetus if given to the mother in large doses during pregnancy. Also, tell your doctor if you are breast-feeding an infant. Small amounts of this drug can pass into breast milk and may cause unwanted effects, such as irritability or sleeping problems, in the nursing infant.

Marazide—see benzthiazide

Marbaxin—see methocarbamol

Marnal—see aspirin, caffeine, and butalbital combination

Matulane—see procarbazine

Maxitrol—see dexamethasone, neomycin, and polymyxin B combination

Maxolon—see metoclopramide

Maxzide—see triamterene and hydrochlorothiazide combination

Mazanor—see mazindol

---

mazindol

BRAND NAMES (Manufacturers)
Mazanor (Wyeth)
Sanorex (Sandoz)
TYPE OF DRUG
Anorectic (appetite suppressant)
INGREDIENT
mazindol
DOSAGE FORM
Tablets (1 mg and 2 mg)
STORAGE
Mazindol should be stored at room temperature in a tightly closed container.

USES

Mazindol is used as an appetite suppressant during the first few weeks of dieting, to help establish new eating habits. This medication is thought to relieve hunger by altering nerve impulses to the appetite control center in the brain. Its effectiveness lasts only for short periods (three to 12 weeks), however.

TREATMENT

Mazindol can be taken with a full glass of water one hour before meals (unless your doctor directs you to do otherwise).

If you miss a dose of this medication, take the missed dose as soon as possible, unless it is almost time for your next dose. In that case, do not take the missed dose at all; just return to your regular dosing schedule. Do not double the next dose.

In order to avoid difficulty in falling asleep, the last dose of this medication each day should be taken four to six hours before bedtime (for the 1-mg tablet) or ten to 14 hours before bedtime (for the 2-mg tablet).

SIDE EFFECTS

Minor. Constipation, diarrhea, dizziness, dry mouth, false sense of well-being, fatigue, insomnia, irritability, nausea, nervousness, restlessness, stomach pain, sweating, tremors, unpleasant taste in the mouth, or vomiting. These side effects should disappear as your body adjusts to the drug.

Dry mouth can be relieved by sucking on ice chips or a piece of hard candy or by chewing sugarless gum.

In order to prevent constipation, increase the amount of fiber in your diet (fresh fruits and vegetables, salads, bran, and whole-grain breads), exercise, and drink more water (unless your doctor directs you to do otherwise).

Major. Tell your doctor about any side effects that are persistent or particularly bothersome. IT IS ESPECIALLY IMPORTANT TO TELL YOUR DOCTOR about blurred vision, changes in sexual desire, chest pain, difficulty in urinating, enlarged breasts (in both sexes), fever, hair loss, headaches, impotence, increased blood pressure, menstrual irregularities, mental depression, mood changes, mouth sores, muscle pains, palpitations, rash, sore throat, or unusual bleeding or bruising.

INTERACTIONS

Mazindol interacts with several other types of medications:
1. Use of this medication within 14 days of a monoamine oxidase (MAO) inhibitor (such as isocarboxazid, pargyline, phenelzine, and tranylcypromine) can result in high blood pressure and other side effects.
2. Barbiturate medications and phenothiazine tranquilizers (especially chlorpromazine) can antagonize (act against) the appetite-suppressant activity of this medication.
3. Mazindol can decrease the blood-pressure-lowering effects of antihypertensive medications (especially guanethidine) and may alter insulin and oral antidiabetic medication dosage requirements in diabetic patients.
4. The side effects of other central nervous system stimulants, such as caffeine, over-the-counter (nonprescription) appetite suppressants or sinus, cough, cold, asthma, and allergy preparations, may be increased by the concurrent use of this medication.

Before starting to take mazindol, BE SURE TO TELL YOUR DOCTOR about any medications you are currently taking, especially any of those listed above.

WARNINGS

• Tell your doctor about unusual or allergic reactions you have had to any medications, especially to mazindol or other appetite suppressants (such as benzphetamine, phendimetrazine, diethylpropion, fenfluramine, phenmetrazine, and phentermine) or to epinephrine, norepinephrine, ephedrine, amphetamines, dextroamphetamine, phenylephrine, phenylpropanolamine, pseudoephedrine, albuterol, metaproterenol, or terbutaline.
• Tell your doctor if you have a history of drug abuse or if you have ever had angina, diabetes mellitus, emotional disturbances, glaucoma, heart or cardiovascular disease, high blood pressure, or thyroid disease.
• Mazindol can mask the symptoms of extreme fatigue and can cause dizziness or light-headedness. Your ability to perform tasks that require alertness, such as driving a car or operating potentially dangerous machinery, may be decreased. Appropriate caution should, therefore, be taken.
• Before having surgery or any other medical or dental treatment, be sure to tell your doctor or dentist that you are taking this medication.
• Mazindol is related to amphetamine and may be habit-forming when taken for long periods of time (both physical and psychological dependence can occur). Therefore, you should not increase the dosage of this medication or take it for longer than 12 weeks unless you first consult your doctor. It is also important that you not stop taking this medication abruptly. Fatigue, sleep disorders, mental depression, nausea or vomiting, or stomach cramps or pain can occur while

your body adjusts to discontinuation of this medication. Your doctor may want to decrease the dosage gradually in order to prevent these side effects.

• Mazindol should not be used in children less than 12 years of age.

• There is no specific information about the use of appetite suppressants such as this medication in the elderly.

• Be sure to tell your doctor if you are pregnant. Although studies in humans have not been conducted, it is known that some of the appetite suppressants cause side effects in the offspring of animals that receive large doses of these drugs during pregnancy. Also, tell your doctor if you are breast-feeding an infant. It is not known whether this medication passes into breast milk.

Measurin—see aspirin

---

meclizine

BRAND NAMES (Manufacturers)

Antivert (Roerig)
Antivert/25 (Roerig)
Antivert/50 (Roerig)
Antrizine (Major)
Bonine* (Pfipharmecs)
Dizmiss* (Bowman)
meclizine hydrochloride (various manufacturers)
Motion Cure* (Wisconsin)
Ru-Vert-M (Reid-Provident)
Wehvert* (Hauck)
*Available over-the-counter (without a prescription)

TYPE OF DRUG

Antiemetic

INGREDIENT

meclizine

DOSAGE FORMS

Tablets (12.5 mg, 25 mg, and 50 mg)
Chewable tablets (25 mg)

STORAGE

Store at room temperature in a tightly closed container.

USES

Meclizine is used to provide symptomatic relief of dizziness due to ear infections and to prevent or relieve dizziness, nausea, and vomiting due to motion sickness. It is thought to relieve dizziness and vomiting by altering nerve transmission in the balance and vomiting centers in the brain.

TREATMENT

To avoid stomach upset, you can take meclizine with food or with a full glass of milk or water (unless your doctor directs you to do otherwise).

The chewable tablets should be chewed for at least two minutes in order to obtain the full benefit of this medication.

If you are taking meclizine to prevent motion sickness, you should take it one hour before traveling.

If you miss a dose of this medication, take the missed dose as soon as possible, unless it is almost time for your next dose. In that case, do not take the missed dose at all; just return to your regular dosing schedule. Do not double the next dose.

SIDE EFFECTS

Minor. Confusion; constipation; diarrhea; dizziness; dry mouth, throat, or nose; headache; irritability; loss of appetite; nausea; restlessness; or stomach upset. These side effects should disappear as your body adjusts to the medication.

If you are constipated, increase the amount of fiber in your diet (fresh fruits and vegetables, salads, bran, and whole-grain breads), exercise, and drink more water (unless your doctor tells you not to do so).

Chew sugarless gum or suck on ice chips or a piece of hard candy to reduce mouth dryness.

Major. Tell your doctor about any side effects that are persistent or particularly bothersome. IT IS ESPECIALLY IMPORTANT TO TELL YOUR DOCTOR about blurred vision, change in menstruation, clumsiness, decreased blood pressure, difficult or painful urination, feeling faint, flushing of the face, hallucinations, palpitations, ringing or buzzing in the ears, rash, seizures, shortness of breath, sleeping disorders, sore throat or fever, tightness in the chest, unusual bleeding or bruising, unusual increase in sweating, or unusual tiredness or weakness.

INTERACTIONS

1. Meclizine interacts with several other types of medications: Concurrent use of it with other central nervous system depressants (such as alcohol, barbiturates, benzodiazepine tranquilizers, muscle relaxants, narcotics, pain medications, and phenothiazine tranquilizers) or with tricyclic antidepressants can cause extreme drowsiness.

2. If you take meclizine on a regular basis and also take large amounts of aspirin (for example, for arthritis pain relief), tell your doctor. The effects of too much aspirin (ringing in the ears) may be masked by meclizine.

BE SURE TO TELL YOUR DOCTOR about any medications you are currently taking, especially any of those listed above.

WARNINGS

• Tell your doctor about allergic or unusual reactions you have had to any medications, especially to meclizine, cyclizine, or buclizine.

• Tell your doctor if you now have or if you have ever had asthma, blood vessel disease, glaucoma, high blood pressure, kidney disease, peptic ulcers, enlarged prostate gland, or thyroid disease.

• Meclizine can cause drowsiness or dizziness. Your ability to perform tasks that require alertness, such as driving a car or operating potentially dangerous machinery, may be decreased. Appropriate caution should, therefore, be taken.

• Meclizine should be given to children under age 12 years only under the supervision of a doctor.

• The elderly may be especially sensitive to side effects such as dry mouth.

• Be sure to tell your doctor if you are pregnant. The effects of this medication during pregnancy have not been thoroughly studied in humans. Also, tell your doctor if you are breast-feeding an infant. Small amounts of meclizine pass into breast milk and may cause unusual excitement or irritability in nursing infants.

meclizine hydrochloride—see meclizine

---

meclofenamate

BRAND NAMES (Manufacturers)
meclofenamate sodium (various manufacturers)
Meclomen (Parke-Davis)
TYPE OF DRUG
Nonsteroidal anti-inflammatory analgesic
INGREDIENT
meclofenamate
DOSAGE FORMS
Tablets (50 mg and 100 mg)
Capsules (50 mg and 100 mg)
STORAGE
This medication should be stored in a tightly closed container at room temperature, away from heat and direct sunlight.

USES

Meclofenamate is used as a short-term treatment for the pain and inflammation (pain, swelling, stiffness) of certain types of arthritis, gout, bursitis, and tendinitis. Meclofenamate has been shown to block the production of certain body chemicals, called prostaglandins, that may trigger pain. However, it is not yet fully understood how meclofenamate works.

TREATMENT

If this medication upsets your stomach, you can take it with food, milk, or antacids (unless your doctor recommends otherwise). If stomach irritation continues, check with your doctor.

It is important to take meclofenamate on schedule and not to miss any doses. If you do miss a dose, take it as soon as possible, unless it is almost time for your next dose. In that case, do not take the missed dose at all; just return to your regular dosing schedule. Do not double the next dose.

If you are taking meclofenamate to relieve arthritis, you must take it regularly, as directed by your doctor. It may take up to three weeks before you feel the full benefits of this medication.

This medication does not cure arthritis, but it will help to control the condition as long as you continue to take it.

SIDE EFFECTS

Minor. Bloating, constipation, diarrhea, difficulty in sleeping, dizziness, drowsiness, headache, heartburn, indigestion, light-headedness, loss of appetite, nausea, nervousness, soreness of the mouth, unusual sweating, or vomiting. As your body adjusts to the drug, these side effects should disappear.

To relieve constipation, increase the amount of fiber in your diet (fresh fruits and vegetables, salads, bran, and whole-grain breads), exercise, and drink more water (unless your doctor directs you to do otherwise).

If you become dizzy, sit or lie down for a while; get up slowly from a sitting or reclining position, and be careful on stairs.

Major. If any side effects are persistent or particularly bothersome, you should report them to your doctor. IT IS ESPECIALLY IMPORTANT TO TELL YOUR DOCTOR about bloody or black, tarry stools; blurred vision; confusion; depression; difficult or painful urination; palpitations; a problem with hearing; ringing or buzzing in the ears; severe diarrhea; severe sunburn; shortness of breath; skin rash, hives, or itching; stomach pain; swelling of the feet; tightness in the chest; wheezing or difficulty in breathing; unexplained sore throat and fever; unusual bleeding or bruising; unusual fatigue or weakness; unusual weight gain; or yellowing of the eyes or skin.

INTERACTIONS

Meclofenamate interacts with several other types of medications:

1. Anticoagulants (blood thinners), such as warfarin, taken at the same time as meclofenamate can lead to an increase in bleeding complications.
2. Concurrent use of aspirin, salicylates, or other anti-inflammatory medications can increase stomach irritation.
3. Probenecid may increase blood levels of meclofenamate, which may increase the risk of side effects.
4. The action of beta blockers may be decreased by this drug.
5. This drug can interact with diuretics (water pills).

BE SURE TO TELL YOUR DOCTOR about any medications you are currently taking, especially any of those listed above.

WARNINGS

- Tell your doctor if you have ever had unusual or allergic reactions to meclofenamate or any of the other chemically related drugs (aspirin, other salicylates, diclofenac, diflunisal, fenoprofen, flurbiprofen, ibuprofen, indomethacin, ketoprofen, mefenamic acid, naproxen, oxyphenbutazone, phenylbutazone, piroxicam, sulindac, or tolmetin).
- Before taking meclofenamate, it is important to tell your doctor if you now have or if you have ever had bleeding problems, colitis, stomach ulcers or other stomach problems, epilepsy, heart disease, high blood pressure, asthma, kidney disease, liver disease, mental illness, or Parkinson's disease.
- If this drug makes you dizzy or drowsy, do not take part in any activity that requires alertness, such as driving a car or operating potentially dangerous machinery.
- Because this drug can prolong your bleeding time, it is important to tell your doctor or dentist that you are taking this drug before having surgery or any other medical or dental treatment.
- Stomach problems are more likely to occur if you take aspirin regularly or drink alcohol while being treated with this medication. These should, therefore, be avoided (unless your doctor directs you to do otherwise).
- The elderly may be at increased risk of experiencing side effects from this drug.
- The safety and effectiveness of this drug in children below the age of 14 has not been established.
- Be sure to tell your doctor if you are pregnant. Studies have shown that meclofenamate can cause unwanted effects (including slower development of bones and heart damage) in the offspring of animals that received this drug during pregnancy. If taken late in pregnancy, meclofenamate can

also prolong labor. Also, tell your doctor if you are breast-feeding an infant. Small amounts of meclofenamate pass into breast milk.

meclofenamate sodium—see meclofenamate

Meclomen—see meclofenamate

Medihaler Ergotamine—see ergotamine

Medipren—see ibuprofen

Medrol—see methylprednisolone (systemic)

---

medroxyprogesterone

BRAND NAMES (Manufacturers)
Amen (Carnrick)
Curretab (Reid-Provident)
Cycrin (Ayerst)
medroxyprogesterone acetate (various manufacturers)
Provera (Upjohn)
TYPE OF DRUG
Progesterone
INGREDIENT
medroxyprogesterone
DOSAGE FORM
Tablets (2.5 mg and 10 mg)
STORAGE
These tablets should be stored at room temperature in a tightly closed container.

USES

Medroxyprogesterone is a synthetic progesterone (progesterone is a female hormone that is naturally produced by the body) that is used to treat abnormal menstrual bleeding, difficult menstruation, or lack of menstruation. It can be used for other conditions as determined by your doctor.

TREATMENT

This medication may cause stomach irritation. To avoid or minimize this side effect, you can take medroxyprogesterone with food or immediately after a meal.

If you miss a dose of this medication, take the missed dose as soon as possible, unless it is almost time for the next dose. In that case, do not take the missed dose at all; just return to your regular dosing schedule. Do not double the next dose of the medication.

SIDE EFFECTS

Minor. Acne, dizziness, hair growth, headache, nausea, or vomiting. These side effects should disappear as your body adjusts to the medication.

This medication can increase your sensitivity to sunlight. It is, therefore, important to avoid prolonged exposure to sunlight and sunlamps. Wear protective clothing and sunglasses, and use an effective sunscreen.

This medication may cause tenderness, swelling, or bleeding of the gums. Brushing and flossing your teeth regularly may prevent this. Also, you should see your dentist regularly while you are taking this medicine.

If you feel dizzy or light-headed, sit or lie down for a while; get up slowly from a sitting or reclining position, and be careful on stairs.

Major. Tell your doctor about any side effects that are persistent or particularly bothersome. IT IS ESPECIALLY IMPORTANT TO TELL YOUR DOCTOR about breast tenderness; change in menstrual patterns; chest pain; depression; fainting; hair loss; itching; pain in the calves; rapid weight gain (three to five pounds within a week); rash; slurred speech; sudden, severe headache; swelling of the feet or ankles; unusual vaginal bleeding; or yellowing of the eyes or skin.

INTERACTIONS

Medroxyprogesterone should not interact with other medications if it is used according to directions.

WARNINGS

- Tell your doctor about unusual or allergic reactions you have had to any medications, especially to medroxyprogesterone, progestin, or progesterone.
- Before starting this drug, tell your doctor if you have ever had cancer of the breast or genitals, clotting disorders, diabetes mellitus, depression, epilepsy, gallbladder disease, asthma, heart disease, kidney disease, liver disease, migraines, porphyria, stroke, or vaginal bleeding.
- A package insert should be included with this drug. Read it carefully, and consult your doctor if you have any questions.
- If this drug makes you dizzy or drowsy, do not take part in any activities that require alertness, such as driving a car or operating potentially dangerous machinery.
- Be sure to tell your doctor if you are pregnant. Medroxyprogesterone should not be used during the first four months of pregnancy because it has been shown to cause birth defects. Since hormones have long-term effects on the body, medroxyprogesterone should be stopped at least three months before you attempt to become pregnant. Also, tell your doctor if you are breast-feeding an infant. Small amounts of medroxyprogesterone pass into breast milk.

medroxyprogesterone acetate—see medroxyprogesterone

---

mefenamic acid

BRAND NAME (Manufacturer)
Ponstel (Parke-Davis)
TYPE OF DRUG
Nonsteroidal anti-inflammatory analgesic
INGREDIENT
mefenamic acid
DOSAGE FORM
Capsules (250 mg)
STORAGE
This medication should be stored in a tightly closed container at room temperature away from heat and direct sunlight.

USES

Mefenamic acid is used to treat painful menstruation. Mefenamic acid has been shown to block the production of certain body chemicals, called prostaglandins, that may trigger pain. However, it is not yet fully understood how it works.

TREATMENT

Mefenamic acid should be taken with food or antacids to lessen stomach irritation (unless your doctor recommends otherwise). Take this medication only as directed by your doctor. Do not take more of it or take it more often; and do not take it for longer than seven days at a time, unless your doctor tells you to do so. Taking too much of this medicine or using it for long periods of time may increase your chances of experiencing serious side effects.

It is important to take mefenamic acid on schedule and not to miss any doses. If you do miss a dose, take it as soon as possible, unless it is almost time for your next dose. In that case, do not take the missed dose at all; just return to your regular dosing schedule. Do not double the next dose.

SIDE EFFECTS

Minor. Bloating, constipation, diarrhea, difficulty in sleeping, dizziness, drowsiness, headache, heartburn, indigestion, light-headedness, loss of appetite, nausea, nervousness, soreness of the mouth, unusual sweating, or vomiting. As your body adjusts to the drug, these side effects should disappear.

To relieve constipation, increase the amount of fiber in your diet (fresh fruits and vegetables, salads, bran, and whole-grain breads), exercise, and drink more water (unless your doctor directs you to do otherwise).

If you become dizzy, sit or lie down for a while; get up slowly from a sitting or reclining position, and be careful on stairs.

Major. If any side effects are persistent or particularly bothersome, you should report them to your doctor. IT IS ESPECIALLY IMPORTANT TO TELL YOUR DOCTOR about bloody or black, tarry stools; blurred vision; confusion; depression; difficult or painful urination; palpitations; a problem with hearing; ringing or buzzing in the ears; severe diarrhea; skin rash, hives, or itching; stomach pain; swelling of the feet; tightness in the chest, shortness of breath, or wheezing; unexplained sore throat and fever; unusual bleeding or bruising; unusual fatigue or weakness; unusual weight gain; or yellowing of the eyes or skin.

INTERACTIONS

Mefenamic acid interacts with several other types of medications:

1. Anticoagulants (blood thinners) such as warfarin can lead to an increase in bleeding complications if taken at the same time as mefenamic acid.

2. Concurrent use with aspirin, salicylates, or other anti-inflammatory medications can increase stomach irritation. Aspirin may also decrease the effectiveness of mefenamic acid.

3. Probenecid may increase blood levels of mefenamic acid, which may increase the risk of side effects.

4. The action of beta blockers may be decreased by this medication.

5. The drug can interact with diuretics (water pills).

BE SURE TO TELL YOUR DOCTOR about any medications you are currently taking, especially any listed above.

WARNINGS

- Tell your doctor if you have ever had unusual or allergic reactions to any medications, especially to mefenamic acid or to any of the other chemically related drugs (aspirin, other salicylates, diclofenac, diflunisal, fenoprofen, flurbiprofen, ibuprofen, meclofenamate, indomethacin, ketoprofen, naproxen, oxyphenbutazone, phenylbutazone, piroxicam, sulindac, or tolmetin).
- Before taking mefenamic acid, it is important to tell your doctor if you now have or if you have ever had asthma, bleeding problems, colitis, stomach ulcers or other stomach problems, epilepsy, heart disease, high blood pressure, kidney disease, liver disease, mental illness, or Parkinson's disease.
- If this drug makes you dizzy or drowsy, do not take part in any activity that requires alertness, such as driving a car or operating potentially dangerous machinery.
- Because mefenamic acid can prolong your bleeding time, it is important to tell your doctor or dentist that you are taking this drug before having surgery or any other medical or dental treatment.
- If you experience severe diarrhea while taking this medication, check with your doctor immediately. Do not take this medication again unless you first check with your doctor, because severe diarrhea can occur each time you take it.
- Stomach problems are more likely to occur if you take aspirin regularly or drink alcohol while being treated with this medication. These should, therefore, be avoided (unless your doctor directs you to do otherwise).
- If this drug is to be given to a child under 12 years of age, discuss the risks as well as the benefits with your doctor.
- Be sure to tell your doctor if you are pregnant. This type of medication may cause unwanted effects on the heart or blood flow in the fetus. Also, studies in animals have shown that this type of medicine, if taken late in pregnancy, can increase the length of pregnancy, prolong labor, and cause other problems during delivery. Mefenamic acid has not been shown to cause birth defects in animals; however, studies in humans have not been conducted. Also, tell your doctor if you are breast-feeding. Small amounts of mefenamic acid pass into breast milk.

Mellaril—see thioridazine

---

meperidine

BRAND NAMES (Manufacturers)

Demerol (Winthrop-Breon)
meperidine hydrochloride (various manufacturers)
Pethadol (Halsey)

TYPE OF DRUG

Analgesic

INGREDIENT

meperidine

DOSAGE FORMS

Tablets (50 mg and 100 mg)
Syrup (50 mg per 5-ml spoonful)

STORAGE

Store at room temperature in a tightly closed, light-resistant container. This medication should never be frozen.

USES

Meperidine is a narcotic analgesic (pain reliever) that acts directly on the central nervous system (brain and spinal cord). It is used to relieve moderate to severe pain.

TREATMENT

In order to avoid stomach upset, you can take meperidine with food or milk. It works most effectively if you take it at the onset of pain, rather than waiting until the pain becomes intense.

Measure the syrup form of this medication carefully with a specially designed 5-ml measuring spoon. An ordinary kitchen teaspoon is not accurate enough. Each dose of the syrup should be diluted in four ounces (half a glass) of water in order to avoid the numbness of the mouth and throat that this medication can cause.

If you are taking this medication on a regular schedule and you miss a dose, take the missed dose as soon as possible, unless it is almost time for your next dose. In that case, do not take the missed dose at all; just return to your regular dosing schedule. Do not double the next dose.

SIDE EFFECTS

Minor. Constipation, dizziness, drowsiness, dry mouth, false sense of well-being, flushing, light-headedness, loss of appetite, nausea, rash, or sweating. These side effects should disappear as your body adjusts to the medication.

If you are constipated, increase the amount of fiber in your diet (fresh fruits and vegetables, salads, bran, and whole-grain breads), exercise, and drink more water (unless your doctor directs you to do otherwise).

Chew sugarless gum or suck on ice chips or a piece of hard candy to reduce mouth dryness.

If you feel dizzy or light-headed, sit or lie down for a while; get up from a sitting or lying position slowly, and be careful on stairs.

Major. Tell your doctor about any side effects that are persistent or particularly bothersome. IT IS ESPECIALLY IMPORTANT TO TELL YOUR DOCTOR about anxiety, breathing difficulties, excitation, fatigue, painful or difficult urination, restlessness, sore throat and fever, tremors, or weakness.

INTERACTIONS

Meperidine interacts with several other types of medications:

1. Concurrent use of this medication with other central nervous system depressants (such as alcohol, antihistamines, barbiturates, benzodiazepine tranquilizers, muscle relaxants, and phenothiazine tranquilizers) or with tricyclic antidepressants can cause extreme drowsiness.

2. A monoamine oxidase (MAO) inhibitor taken within 14 days of this medication can lead to unpredictable and severe side effects.

3. The combination of cimetidine and meperidine can cause confusion, disorientation, and shortness of breath.

BE SURE TO TELL YOUR DOCTOR about any medications you are currently taking, especially any listed above.

WARNINGS

- Tell your doctor about unusual or allergic reactions you have had to any drugs, especially to meperidine or to any other narcotic analgesic (such as codeine, hydrocodone, hydromorphone, methadone, morphine, oxycodone, and propoxyphene).
- Tell your doctor if you now have or if you have ever had acute abdominal conditions, asthma, brain disease, colitis, epilepsy, gallstones or gallbladder disease, head injuries, heart disease, kidney disease, liver disease, lung disease, mental illness, emotional disorders, enlarged prostate gland, thyroid disease, or urethral stricture.
- If this drug makes you dizzy or drowsy, do not take part in any activity that requires alertness, such as driving a car or operating potentially dangerous machinery.
- Before having surgery or any other medical or dental treatment, tell your doctor or dentist about this drug.
- Meperidine has the potential for abuse and must be used with caution. Usually, it should not be taken on a regular schedule for longer than ten days (unless your doctor directs you to do so). Tolerance develops quickly; do not increase the dosage or stop taking the drug abruptly unless you first consult your doctor. If you have been taking large amounts of this medication or have been taking it for a long period of time, you may experience withdrawal symptoms (muscle aches, diarrhea, gooseflesh, runny nose, nausea, vomiting, shivering, trembling, stomach cramps, sleep disorders, irritability, weakness, excessive yawning, or sweating) when you stop taking it. Your doctor may, therefore, want to reduce your dosage gradually.
- Tell your doctor if you are pregnant. The effects of this drug during the early stages of pregnancy have not been thoroughly studied in humans. However, the use of meperidine regularly in large doses during the later stages of pregnancy can result in addiction of the fetus, leading to withdrawal symptoms (such as irritability, excessive crying, tremors, fever, vomiting, diarrhea, sneezing, or excessive yawning) at birth. Also, tell your doctor if you are breast-feeding. Small amounts of this drug may pass into breast milk and cause excessive drowsiness in the nursing infant.

meperidine hydrochloride—see meperidine

Mephyton—see vitamin K

Mepro-analgesic—see meprobamate and aspirin combination

---

meprobamate

BRAND NAMES (Manufacturers)
Equanil (Wyeth)
meprobamate (various manufacturers)
Meprospan (Wallace)
Miltown (Wallace)
TYPE OF DRUG
Sedative/hypnotic
INGREDIENT
meprobamate
DOSAGE FORMS
Tablets (200 mg, 400 mg, and 600 mg)
Capsules (400 mg)
Sustained-release capsules (200 mg and 400 mg)

STORAGE
Meprobamate tablets and capsules should be stored at room temperature in tightly closed containers.

USES

Meprobamate is used to relieve anxiety or tension and is also prescribed as a sleeping aid. It is not exactly clear how meprobamate works, but it is thought to act as a central nervous system (brain and spinal cord) depressant.

TREATMENT

In order to avoid stomach irritation, you can take meprobamate with food or with a full glass of water or milk.

The sustained-release capsules should be swallowed whole. Breaking, chewing, or crushing these capsules destroys their sustained-release activity.

If you are taking this medication on a regular schedule and you miss a dose, take the missed dose immediately if you remember within an hour. If more than an hour has passed, skip the dose you missed and wait for the next scheduled dose. Do not double the dose.

SIDE EFFECTS

Minor. Diarrhea, dizziness, drowsiness, dry mouth, headache, nausea, vomiting, or weakness. These side effects should disappear as your body adjusts to the medication.

If you feel dizzy while taking this medication, sit or lie down for a while; get up slowly from a sitting or reclining position, and be careful on stairs.

To relieve mouth dryness, chew sugarless gum or suck on ice chips or a piece of hard candy.

Major. Tell your doctor about any side effects that are persistent or particularly bothersome. IT IS ESPECIALLY IMPORTANT TO TELL YOUR DOCTOR about blurred vision, clumsiness, confusion, convulsions, difficulty in breathing, difficult or painful urination, fainting, false sense of well-being, fever, nightmares, numbness or tingling, palpitations, rapid weight gain (three to five pounds within a week), rash, slurred speech, sore throat, unusual bleeding or bruising, or unusual weakness.

INTERACTIONS

Concurrent use of meprobamate with other central nervous system depressants (such as alcohol, antihistamines, barbiturates, benzodiazepine tranquilizers, muscle relaxants, narcotics, pain medications, phenothiazine tranquilizers, and sleeping medications) or with tricyclic antidepressants can cause extreme drowsiness.

BE SURE TO TELL YOUR DOCTOR about any medications you are currently taking, especially any listed above.

WARNINGS

- Tell your doctor about any unusual or allergic reactions you have had to medications, especially to meprobamate, carbromal, carisoprodol, mebutamate, or tybamate.
- Before starting to take this medication, be sure to tell your doctor if you have a history of drug abuse or if you now have or have ever had epilepsy, kidney disease, liver disease, or porphyria.
- If this drug causes dizziness or drowsiness, avoid tasks that require alertness, such as driving a car or operating potentially dangerous machinery.
- This drug has the potential for abuse and must be used with caution. Tolerance develops quickly; do not increase the dosage unless you first consult your doctor.
- Do not stop taking this drug abruptly if you have been taking it for two or three months. Stopping abruptly can lead to a withdrawal reaction. Your doctor may, therefore, want to reduce your dosage gradually.
- Some of these products contain the color additive FD&C Yellow No. 5 (tartrazine), which can cause allergic-type reactions (rash, fainting, shortness of breath) in certain susceptible individuals.
- Be sure to tell your doctor if you are pregnant. Meprobamate has been reported to cause birth defects when taken during the first three months of pregnancy. Also, tell your doctor if you are breast-feeding an infant. Meprobamate passes into breast milk and can cause excessive drowsiness in the nursing infant.

---

meprobamate and aspirin combination

BRAND NAMES (Manufacturers)
Epromate (Major)
Equagesic (Wyeth)
Equazine M (Rugby)
Mepro-analgesic (United Research)
Meprobamate Compound (Interstate)
Mepro Compound (Schein)
Meproges E (Geneva Generics)
Meprogesic Q (various manufacturers)
Micrainin (Wallace)
TYPE OF DRUG
Sedative and analgesic
INGREDIENTS
meprobamate and aspirin
DOSAGE FORM
Tablets (200 mg meprobamate and 325 mg aspirin)
STORAGE
Meprobamate and aspirin combination tablets should be stored at room temperature in a tightly closed, light-resistant container. Moisture can cause aspirin to decompose.

USES

Meprobamate and aspirin combination is used to relieve tension headaches and pain in muscles or joints associated with tension or anxiety. It is unclear exactly how meprobamate works to relieve anxiety and tension, but it appears to be a central nervous system (brain and spinal cord) depressant.

TREATMENT

In order to avoid stomach irritation, you can take meprobamate and aspirin combination with food or with a full glass of water or milk (unless your doctor directs otherwise).

If you are taking this medication on a regular schedule and you miss a dose, take the missed dose as soon as possible, unless it is almost time for the next dose. In that case, do not take the missed dose at all; just return to your regular dosing schedule. Do not double the next dose.

SIDE EFFECTS

Minor. Abdominal pain, diarrhea, dizziness, drowsiness, dry mouth, fatigue, headache, light-headedness, nausea, vomiting, or weakness. These side effects should disappear as your body adjusts to the medication.

If you feel dizzy or light-headed, sit or lie down for a while; get up slowly from a sitting or reclining position, and be careful on stairs.

Major. Tell your doctor about any side effects that are persistent or particularly bothersome. IT IS ESPECIALLY IMPORTANT TO TELL YOUR DOCTOR about blurred vision, buzzing in the ears, chest tightness, clumsiness, confusion, convulsions, difficult or painful urination, fainting, false sense of well-being, fever, headache, loss of coordination, mental depression, nightmares, numbness or tingling, palpitations, rapid weight gain, shortness of breath, skin rash, slurred speech, sore throat, unusual bleeding or bruising, or unusual weakness.

INTERACTIONS

This medicine interacts with other types of drugs:

1. Concurrent use of meprobamate with other central nervous system depressants (such as alcohol, antihistamines, barbiturates, benzodiazepine tranquilizers, muscle relaxants, narcotics, pain medications, phenothiazine tranquilizers, and sleeping medications) or with tricyclic antidepressants may cause extreme drowsiness.

2. Aspirin can increase the effects of blood thinners, such as warfarin, thereby leading to a possible increase in bleeding complications.

3. The antigout effects of probenecid and sulfinpyrazone may be blocked by aspirin.

4. Aspirin can increase the gastrointestinal side effects of anti-inflammatory medications, including nonsteroidal anti-inflammatory drugs, alcohol, phenylbutazone, and adrenocorticosteroids (cortisone-like medicines).

5. Ammonium chloride, methionine, and furosemide can increase the side effects of aspirin; and acetazolamide, methazolamide, antacids, and phenobarbital can decrease the effectiveness of aspirin.

6. Aspirin can increase the side effects of methotrexate, penicillin, thyroid hormone, phenytoin, sulfinpyrazone, naproxen, valproic acid, insulin, and oral antidiabetic medicines.

7. It can decrease the effects of spironolactone.

Before starting to take this medication, BE SURE TO TELL YOUR DOCTOR about any medications you are currently taking, especially any of those listed above.

WARNINGS

- Tell your doctor about unusual or allergic reactions you have had to any medications, especially to meprobamate, carbromal, carisoprodol, mebutamate, tybamate, aspirin, methyl salicylate (oil of wintergreen), diclofenac, diflunisal, fenoprofen, flurbiprofen, ibuprofen, indomethacin, ketoprofen, meclofenamate, mefenamic acid, naproxen, piroxicam, sulindac, or tolmetin.
- Before starting to take meprobamate and aspirin combination, be sure to tell your doctor if you have a history of drug abuse or if you now have or have ever had asthma, bleeding disorders, congestive heart failure, diabetes, epilepsy, glucose-6-phosphate dehydrogenase (G6PD) deficiency, gout, hemophilia, high blood pressure, kidney disease, liver disease, nasal polyps, peptic ulcers, porphyria, or thyroid disease.
- Before having surgery or any other medical or dental treatment, be sure to tell your doctor or dentist that you are taking aspirin. Treatment with aspirin is usually discontinued five to seven days before surgery, to prevent bleeding complications.
- If this drug makes you dizzy or drowsy, avoid taking part in any activity that requires alertness, such as driving a car or operating potentially dangerous machinery.
- The use of aspirin in children (about 16 years of age or less) with the flu or chicken pox has been associated with a rare, life-threatening condition called Reye's syndrome. Aspirin-containing products should, therefore, not be given to children with signs of infection.
- Diabetic patients should know that large doses of aspirin (greater than eight 325-mg tablets per day) can cause erroneous readings on urine glucose tests. Diabetics should, therefore, check with their doctor before changing their insulin dosage while they are taking this medication.
- Meprobamate is a potentially habit-forming medication. It should, therefore, be used with caution. If this drug is being used for several months, tolerance to it may develop. Do not stop taking the drug unless you first consult your doctor. A withdrawal reaction could result from stopping this medication abruptly. Your doctor may, therefore, want to reduce your dosage of the medication gradually.
- Because this product contains aspirin, additional medications that contain aspirin should not be taken without your doctor's approval. Check the labels on over-the-counter (nonprescription) pain, sinus, allergy, asthma, cough, and cold products to see if they contain aspirin.
- Be sure to tell your doctor if you are pregnant. Meprobamate can cause birth defects if taken during the first three months of pregnancy. In addition, large doses of aspirin taken close to term may prolong labor and may cause bleeding complications in the mother and heart problems in the infant. Also, tell your doctor if you are breast-feeding an infant. Both meprobamate and aspirin pass into breast milk.

Meprobamate Compound—see meprobamate and aspirin combination

Mepro Compound—see meprobamate and aspirin combination

Meproges E—see meprobamate and aspirin combination

Meprogesic Q—see meprobamate and aspirin combination

Meprospan—see meprobamate

---

mesoridazine

BRAND NAME (Manufacturer)

Serentil (Boehringer Ingelheim)

TYPE OF DRUG

Phenothiazine tranquilizer

INGREDIENT
mesoridazine
DOSAGE FORMS
Tablets (10 mg, 25 mg, 50 mg, and 100 mg)
Oral concentrate (25 mg per ml, with 0.61% alcohol)
STORAGE
The tablet form of this medicine should be stored at room temperature in a tightly closed, light-resistant container. The oral concentrate form of this medication should be stored in the refrigerator in a tightly closed, light-resistant container. If the oral concentrate turns slightly yellow, the medicine is still effective and can be used. However, if the oral concentrate changes color markedly or has particles floating in it, it should not be used; rather, it should be discarded down the sink. This medication should never be frozen.

USES
Mesoridazine is prescribed to treat certain types of mental illness, such as psychosis, the manic phase of manic-depressive illness, and severe behavioral problems in children. This medication is thought to relieve the symptoms of mental illness by blocking certain chemicals involved in nerve transmission in the brain. Mesoridazine may also be used to treat anxiety.

TREATMENT
To avoid stomach irritation during treatment with mesoridazine, you can take the tablet form of this medication with a meal or with a glass of water or milk (unless your doctor directs you to do otherwise).

The oral concentrate form of this medication should be measured carefully with the dropper provided and then added to four ounces (½ cup) or more of water, milk, or a carbonated beverage or to applesauce or pudding immediately prior to administration. To prevent possible loss of effectiveness, the medication should not be diluted in tea, coffee, or apple juice.

If you miss a dose of this medication, take the missed dose as soon as possible, unless it is almost time for the next dose. In that case, do not take the missed dose at all; just return to your regular dosing schedule. Do not double the next dose (unless your doctor directs you to do so).

The full effects of this medication for the control of emotional or mental symptoms may not become apparent for two weeks after you start to take it.

SIDE EFFECTS
Minor. Constipation; decreased sweating; diarrhea; discoloration of the urine to red, pink, or red-brown; dizziness; drooling; drowsiness; dry mouth; fatigue; jitteriness; menstrual irregularities; nasal congestion; restlessness; vomiting; or weight gain. As your body adjusts to the medication, these side effects should disappear.

This medication can cause increased sensitivity to sunlight. It is, therefore, important to avoid prolonged exposure to sunlight and sunlamps. Wear protective clothing, and use an effective sunscreen.

If you are constipated, increase the amount of fiber in your diet (fresh fruits and vegetables, salads, bran, and whole-grain breads), exercise, and drink more water (unless your doctor directs you to do otherwise).

Chew sugarless gum or suck on ice chips or a piece of hard candy to reduce mouth dryness.

To avoid dizziness or light-headedness when you stand, contract and relax the muscles of your legs for a few moments before rising. Do this by pushing one foot against the floor while raising the other foot slightly, alternating feet so that you are "pumping" your legs in a pedaling motion.

Major. Tell your doctor about any side effects that are persistent or particularly bothersome. IT IS ESPECIALLY IMPORTANT TO TELL YOUR DOCTOR about blurred vision; breast enlargement (in both sexes); chest pain; convulsions; darkened skin; difficulty in swallowing or breathing; fainting; fever; impotence; involuntary movements of the face, mouth, jaw, or tongue; palpitations; rash; sleep disorders; sore throat; tremors; uncoordinated movements; unusual bleeding or bruising; visual disturbances; or yellowing of the eyes or skin.

INTERACTIONS
Mesoridazine interacts with several other types of medications:

1. It can cause extreme drowsiness when combined with alcohol, other central nervous system depressants (such as barbiturates, benzodiazepine tranquilizers, muscle relaxants, narcotics, and pain medications), or tricyclic antidepressants.

2. Mesoridazine can decrease the effectiveness of amphetamines, guanethidine, and levodopa.

3. The combination of mesoridazine with antiarrhythmic agents such as quinidine may result in impaired heart function.

4. The effects of epinephrine, monoamine oxidase (MAO) inhibitors, propranolol, phenytoin, and tricyclic antidepressants may be increased when combined with this medication.

5. Lithium may increase the side effects and decrease the effectiveness of this medication.

6. Antacids and antidiarrheal medicines may decrease the absorption of mesoridazine from the gastrointestinal tract. Therefore, at least one hour should separate doses of one of these medicines and mesoridazine.

Before starting to take mesoridazine, BE SURE TO TELL YOUR DOCTOR about any medications you are currently taking, especially any of those listed above.

WARNINGS
- Tell your doctor about unusual or allergic reactions you have had to any medications, especially to mesoridazine or any other phenothiazine tranquilizers (such as chlorpromazine, fluphenazine, perphenazine, prochlorperazine, promazine, thioridazine, trifluoperazine, and triflupromazine) or to loxapine.
- Tell your doctor if you have a history of alcoholism or if you now have or have ever had any blood disease, bone marrow disease, brain disease, breast cancer, blockage in the urinary or digestive tract, drug-induced depression, epilepsy, high or low blood pressure, diabetes mellitus, glaucoma, heart or circulatory disease, liver disease, lung disease, Parkinson's disease, peptic ulcers, or an enlarged prostate gland.
- Tell your doctor about any recent exposure to a pesticide or an insecticide. Mesoridazine may increase the side effects from the exposure.
- To prevent oversedation, avoid drinking alcoholic beverages while taking this medication.

• If this medication makes you dizzy or drowsy, do not take part in any activity that requires alertness, such as driving a car or operating potentially dangerous machinery. Be careful on stairs, and avoid getting up suddenly from a lying or sitting position.
• Prior to having surgery or any other medical or dental treatment, be sure to tell your doctor or dentist that you are taking this medication.
• Mesoridazine can decrease sweating and heat release from the body. You should, therefore, avoid becoming overheated by strenuous exercise in hot weather and avoid taking hot baths, showers, and saunas.
• Do not stop taking this medication suddenly. If the drug is stopped abruptly, you may experience nausea, vomiting, stomach upset, headache, increased heart rate, insomnia, tremors, or worsening of your condition. Your doctor may want to reduce the dosage gradually.
• If you are planning to have a myelogram, or any other procedure in which dye is injected into your spinal cord, tell your doctor that you are taking this medication.
• Avoid spilling the oral concentrate form of this medication on your skin or clothing; it may cause redness and irritation of the skin.
• While taking this medication, do not take any over-the-counter (nonprescription) medication for weight control or for cough, cold, allergy, asthma, or sinus problems without first checking with your doctor. The combination of these drugs with mesoridazine may cause high blood pressure.
• Be sure to tell your doctor if you are pregnant. Small amounts of this medication cross the placenta. Although there are reports of safe use of this drug during pregnancy, there are also reports of liver disease and tremors in newborn infants whose mothers received this type of medication close to term. Also, tell your doctor if you are breast-feeding an infant. Small amounts of this medication pass into breast milk and may cause unwanted effects in the nursing infant.

Metahydrin—see trichlormethiazide

Metandren—see methyltestosterone

Metaprel—see metaproterenol

---

metaproterenol

BRAND NAMES (Manufacturers)
Alupent (Boehringer Ingelheim)
Metaprel (Dorsey)
TYPE OF DRUG
Bronchodilator
INGREDIENT
metaproterenol
DOSAGE FORMS
Tablets (10 mg and 20 mg)
Oral syrup (10 mg per 5-ml spoonful)
Inhalation aerosol (each spray delivers 0.65 mg)
Solution for nebulization (0.6% and 5%)
STORAGE
Metaproterenol tablets and oral syrup should be stored at room temperature in tightly closed, light-resistant containers. The solution for nebulization should be stored in the refrigerator. The inhalation aerosol should be stored at room temperature away from excessive heat—the contents are pressurized, and the container can explode if heated. Metaproterenol syrup and solution should not be used if they turn brown or contain particles; such changes indicate that the drug has lost its effectiveness.

USES

Metaproterenol is used to relieve wheezing and shortness of breath caused by lung diseases such as asthma, bronchitis, and emphysema. This drug acts directly on the muscles of the bronchi (breathing tubes) to relieve bronchospasm (muscle contractions of the bronchi), thereby reducing airway resistance and allowing air to move more freely to and from the lungs, which makes breathing easier.

TREATMENT

In order to lessen stomach upset, you can take metaproterenol tablets or oral syrup with food (unless your doctor directs you to do otherwise).

The oral syrup form of this medication should be measured carefully with a specially designed 5-ml measuring spoon. An ordinary kitchen teaspoon is not accurate enough.

The inhalation aerosol form of this medication is usually packaged with an instruction sheet. Read the directions carefully before using this medication. The container should be shaken well just before each use. The contents tend to settle on the bottom, so it is necessary to shake the container to distribute the ingredients evenly and equalize the doses. If more than one inhalation is necessary, wait at least one full minute between doses, so that you receive the full benefit of the first dose.

If you miss a dose of this medication and remember within an hour, take it; then follow your regular schedule for the next dose. If you miss the dose by more than an hour or so, just wait until the next scheduled dose. Do not double the dose.

SIDE EFFECTS

Minor. Anxiety, dizziness, headache, flushing, irritability, insomnia, loss of appetite, muscle cramps, nausea, nervousness, restlessness, sweating, vomiting, weakness, or dryness or irritation of the mouth or throat (from the inhalation aerosol). These side effects should disappear as your body adjusts to the medication.

To help prevent dryness and irritation of the mouth or throat, rinse your mouth with water after each dose of the inhalation aerosol.

In order to avoid difficulty in falling asleep, check with your doctor to see if you can take the last dose of this medication several hours before bedtime each day.

If you feel dizzy, sit or lie down for a while; get up from a sitting or lying position slowly, and be careful on stairs.

Major. Tell your doctor about any side effects that are persistent or particularly bothersome. IT IS ESPECIALLY IMPORTANT TO TELL YOUR DOCTOR about chest pain, difficult breathing, difficult or painful urination, palpitations, rash, or tremors.

INTERACTIONS

Metaproterenol interacts with several other types of medications:

1. Beta blockers (acebutolol, atenolol, betaxolol, carteolol, esmolol, labetalol, metoprolol, nadolol, penbutolol, pindolol, propranolol, timolol) antagonize (act against) this medication, decreasing its effectiveness.

2. Monoamine oxidase (MAO) inhibitors, tricyclic antidepressants, antihistamines, levothyroxine, and over-the-counter (nonprescription) cough, cold, allergy, asthma, diet, and sinus medications may increase the side effects of metaproterenol. At least 14 days should separate the use of this drug and the use of an MAO inhibitor.

3. There may be a change in the dosage requirements of insulin or oral antidiabetic medications when metaproterenol is started.

4. The blood-pressure-lowering effects of guanethidine may be decreased by this medication.

5. The use of metaproterenol with other bronchodilator drugs (either oral or inhaled) can have additive side effects. Discuss this with your doctor.

BE SURE TO TELL YOUR DOCTOR about any medications you are currently taking, especially any of the medications that are listed above.

WARNINGS

- Tell your doctor about unusual or allergic reactions you have had, especially to metaproterenol or any related drug (such as albuterol, amphetamines, ephedrine, epinephrine, isoproterenol, norepinephrine, phenylephrine, phenylpropanolamine, pseudoephedrine, and terbutaline).
- Tell your doctor if you now have or if you have ever had diabetes, glaucoma, high blood pressure, epilepsy, heart disease, enlarged prostate gland, or thyroid disease.
- This medication can cause dizziness. Your ability to perform tasks that require alertness, such as driving a car or operating potentially dangerous machinery, may be decreased. Appropriate caution should, therefore, be taken.
- Before having surgery or any other medical or dental treatment, be sure to tell your doctor or dentist that you are taking this medication.
- Do not exceed the recommended dosage of this medication. Excessive use may lead to an increase in side effects or a loss of effectiveness.
- Try to avoid contact of the aerosol with your eyes.
- Do not puncture, break, or burn the aerosol container. The contents are under pressure and may explode.
- Contact your doctor if you do not respond to the usual dose of this medication. It may be a sign of worsening asthma, which may require additional therapy.
- Be sure to tell your doctor if you are pregnant. The effects of this medication during pregnancy have not been thoroughly studied in humans. Also, tell your doctor if you are breast-feeding an infant. It is not known whether this drug passes into breast milk.

---

methadone

BRAND NAMES (Manufacturers)
Dolophine (Lilly)
methadone hydrochloride (various manufacturers)

TYPE OF DRUG
Analgesic

INGREDIENT
methadone

DOSAGE FORMS
Tablets (5 mg, 10 mg, and 40 mg)
Oral solution (5 mg and 10 mg per 5-ml spoonful, with 8% alcohol)

STORAGE
Methadone analgesic tablets and oral solution should be stored at room temperature in tightly closed, light-resistant containers.

USES

Methadone is a narcotic analgesic (pain reliever) that acts directly on the central nervous system (brain and spinal cord). It is used to relieve moderate to severe pain. It is also used to detoxify narcotic addicts and to provide temporary maintenance treatment for them.

TREATMENT

In order to avoid stomach upset, you can take methadone with food or milk. This medication works most effectively if you take it at the onset of pain, rather than waiting until the pain becomes intense.

Measure the dose of the solution form of this medication carefully with a specially designed 5-ml measuring spoon. An ordinary kitchen teaspoon is not accurate enough.

If you are taking this medication on a regular schedule and you miss a dose, take the missed dose as soon as possible, unless it is almost time for your next dose. In that case, do not take the missed dose at all; just return to your regular dosing schedule. Do not double the next dose.

SIDE EFFECTS

Minor. Constipation, dizziness, drowsiness, dry mouth, false sense of well-being, light-headedness, loss of appetite, nausea, or sweating. These side effects should disappear as your body adjusts to the medication.

If you are constipated, increase the amount of fiber in your diet (fresh fruits and vegetables, salads, bran, and whole-grain breads), exercise, and drink more water (unless your doctor directs you to do otherwise).

Chew sugarless gum or suck on ice chips or a piece of hard candy to reduce mouth dryness.

If you feel dizzy or light-headed, sit or lie down for a while; get up from a sitting or lying position slowly, and be careful on stairs.

Major. Tell your doctor about any side effects that are persistent or particularly bothersome. IT IS ESPECIALLY IMPORTANT TO TELL YOUR DOCTOR about anxiety, breathing difficulties, excitation, fainting, fatigue, flushing, painful or difficult urination, palpitations, pinpoint pupils of eyes, rash, restlessness, sore throat and fever, tremors, or weakness.

INTERACTIONS

Methadone interacts with several other types of medications:

1. Concurrent use of it with other central nervous system depressants (such as alcohol, antihistamines, barbiturates, benzodiazepine tranquilizers, muscle relaxants, and phenothiazine tranquilizers) or with tricyclic antidepressants can cause extreme drowsiness.

2. A monoamine oxidase (MAO) inhibitor taken within 14 days of this medication can lead to unpredictable and severe side effects.

3. Rifampin and phenytoin can decrease the blood levels and effectiveness of methadone.

4. The combination of cimetidine and this medication can cause confusion, disorientation, and shortness of breath.

BE SURE TO TELL YOUR DOCTOR about any medications you are currently taking, especially any listed above.

WARNINGS

- Tell your doctor about unusual or allergic reactions you have had to any medications, especially to methadone or to any other narcotic analgesic (such as codeine, hydrocodone, morphine, oxycodone, and propoxyphene).
- Tell your doctor if you now have or if you have ever had acute abdominal conditions, asthma, brain disease, colitis, epilepsy, gallstones or gallbladder disease, head injuries, heart disease, kidney disease, liver disease, lung disease, mental illness, emotional disorders, enlarged prostate gland, thyroid disease, or urethral stricture.
- If this drug makes you dizzy or drowsy, do not take part in any activity that requires alertness, such as driving a car or operating potentially dangerous machinery.
- Before having surgery or any other medical or dental treatment, be sure to tell your doctor or dentist that you are taking this medication.
- Methadone has the potential for abuse and must be used with caution. Usually, it should not be taken on a regular schedule for longer than ten days (unless your doctor directs you to do so). Tolerance develops quickly; do not increase the dosage or stop taking the drug abruptly unless you first consult your doctor. If you have been taking large amounts of this medication or if you have been taking it for long periods of time, you may experience withdrawal symptoms (muscle aches, diarrhea, gooseflesh, runny nose, nausea, vomiting, shivering, trembling, stomach cramps, sleep disorders, irritability, weakness, excessive yawning, or sweating) when you stop taking it. Your doctor may, therefore, want to reduce the dosage gradually.
- Be sure to tell your doctor if you are pregnant. The effects of this medication during the early stages of pregnancy have not been thoroughly studied in humans. However, regular use of methadone in large doses during the later stages of pregnancy can result in addiction of the fetus, leading to withdrawal symptoms (irritability, excessive crying, tremors, fever, vomiting, diarrhea, sneezing, or excessive yawning) at birth. Also, tell your doctor if you are breast-feeding an infant. Small amounts of this medication may pass into breast milk and cause excessive drowsiness in the nursing infant.

methadone hydrochloride—see methadone

---

methamphetamine

BRAND NAMES (Manufacturers)
Desoxyn (Abbott)
Desoxyn Gradumets (Abbott)

TYPE OF DRUG
Amphetamine

INGREDIENT
methamphetamine

DOSAGE FORMS
Tablets (5 mg)
Sustained-release tablets (5 mg, 10 mg, and 15 mg)

STORAGE
Methamphetamine should be stored at room temperature in a tightly closed container.

USES

This medication is a central nervous system stimulant that increases mental alertness and decreases fatigue. It is used to treat narcolepsy (a disorder involving uncontrollable desires to sleep or actual sleep attacks that occur in a rapid and unpredictable manner) and abnormal behavioral syndrome in children (hyperkinetic syndrome or attention deficit disorder). The way this medication acts to control abnormal behavioral syndrome in children is not clearly understood.

Methamphetamine is also used as an appetite suppressant during the first few weeks of dieting (while you are trying to establish new eating habits). It is thought to relieve hunger by altering nerve impulses to the appetite control center in the brain. Its effectiveness as an appetite suppressant lasts for only short periods (three to 12 weeks), however.

TREATMENT

In order to avoid stomach upset, you can take methamphetamine with food or with a full glass of milk or water (unless your doctor directs you to do otherwise).

If this medication is being used to treat narcolepsy or abnormal behavioral syndrome in children, the first dose each day should be taken soon after awakening. Subsequent doses should be spaced at four- to six-hour intervals.

If this medication has been prescribed as a diet aid, it should be taken one hour before each meal.

The sustained-release form of this medication should be swallowed whole. Breaking, chewing, or crushing these tablets destroys their sustained-release activity and may increase the side effects.

In order to avoid difficulty in falling asleep, the last dose of this medication each day should be taken four to six hours before bedtime (tablets) or ten to 14 hours before bedtime (sustained-release tablets).

If you miss a dose of this drug, take the missed dose as soon as possible, unless it is time for your next dose. In that case, do not take the missed dose at all; just return to your regular dosing schedule. Do not double the next dose.

SIDE EFFECTS

Minor. Abdominal cramps, constipation, diarrhea, dizziness, dry mouth, false sense of well-being, insomnia, irritability, loss of appetite, nausea, restlessness, unpleasant taste in the mouth, or vomiting. These side effects should disappear as your body adjusts to the medication.

In order to prevent constipation, increase the amount of fiber in your diet (fresh fruits and vegetables, salads, bran, and whole-grain breads), exercise, and drink more water (unless your doctor directs you to do otherwise).

Dry mouth can be relieved by sucking on ice chips or a piece of hard candy or by chewing sugarless gum.

If you feel dizzy, sit or lie down for a while; get up from a sitting or lying position slowly, and be careful on stairs.

Major. Tell your doctor about any side effects that are persistent or particularly bothersome. IT IS ESPECIALLY IMPORTANT TO TELL YOUR DOCTOR about blurred vision, confusion, fatigue, headaches, impotence, mental depression, palpitations, rash, sweating, tightness in the chest, tremors, or uncoordinated movements.

INTERACTIONS

Methamphetamine interacts with several other types of medications:

1. Use of it within 14 days of a monoamine oxidase (MAO) inhibitor (isocarboxazid, pargyline, phenelzine, tranylcypromine) can result in high blood pressure and other side effects.

2. Barbiturate medications, phenothiazine tranquilizers (especially chlorpromazine), and tricyclic antidepressants can antagonize (act against) this medication.

3. Amphetamines (such as methamphetamine) can decrease the blood-pressure-lowering effects of antihypertensive medication (especially guanethidine) and may alter insulin and oral antidiabetic medication dosage requirements in diabetic patients.

4. The side effects of other central nervous system stimulants, such as caffeine, over-the-counter (nonprescription) appetite suppressants, and asthma, allergy, cough, sinus, or cold preparations may be increased by methamphetamine.

5. Acetazolamide and sodium bicarbonate can decrease the elimination of methamphetamine from the body, thereby prolonging its action and increasing the risk of side effects.

BE SURE TO TELL YOUR DOCTOR about any medications you are currently taking, especially any of those listed above.

WARNINGS

- Tell your doctor about unusual or allergic reactions you have had to any medications, especially to methamphetamine or other central nervous system stimulants (such as albuterol, amphetamine, dextroamphetamine, ephedrine, isoproterenol, metaproterenol, norepinephrine, phenylephrine, phenylpropanolamine, pseudoephedrine, and terbutaline).
- Tell your doctor if you have a history of drug abuse or if you have ever had problems with agitation, diabetes mellitus, glaucoma, heart or blood vessel disease, high blood pressure, or thyroid disease.
- Methamphetamine can mask the symptoms of extreme fatigue and can cause dizziness. Your ability to perform tasks that require alertness, such as driving a car or operating potentially dangerous machinery, may be decreased. Appropriate caution should, therefore, be taken.
- Before having surgery or any other medical or dental treatment, be sure to tell your doctor or dentist that you are taking this medication.
- Methamphetamine is related to amphetamine and may be habit-forming when taken for long periods of time (both physical and psychological dependence can occur). Therefore, you should not increase the dosage of this medication or take it for longer than 12 weeks, unless you first consult your doctor. It is also important that you not stop taking this medication abruptly; fatigue, sleep disorders, mental depression, nausea, vomiting, stomach cramps, or pain could occur. Your doctor may, therefore, want to reduce your dosage gradually.
- Some of these products contain the color additive FD&C Yellow No. 5 (tartrazine), which can cause allergic-type reactions (rash, fainting, difficulty in breathing) in certain susceptible individuals.
- Long-term methamphetamine use in children may cause unwanted effects on growth. The benefits and risks of the drug should be thoroughly discussed before treatment begins.
- Be sure to tell your doctor if you are pregnant. Although side effects in humans have not been studied, some of the amphetamines can cause heart, brain, and biliary tract abnormalities in the fetuses of animals that receive large doses of these drugs during pregnancy. Also, tell your doctor if you are breast-feeding an infant. Small amounts of this type of drug pass into breast milk and can cause excessive stimulation in nursing infants.

---

methenamine

BRAND NAMES (Manufacturers)

Hiprex (Merrell Dow)
Mandameth (Major)
Mandelamine (Parke-Davis)
methenamine mandelate (various manufacturers)
Urex (Riker)

TYPE OF DRUG

Antibiotic

INGREDIENT

methenamine

DOSAGE FORMS

Tablets (500 mg and 1 g)
Enteric-coated tablets (500 mg and 1 g)
Oral suspension (250 mg and 500 mg per 5-ml spoonful)
Oral granules (1 g packets)

STORAGE

Methenamine tablets, oral suspension, and granules should be stored at room temperature in tightly closed containers. This medication should never be frozen.

USES

Methenamine is used to prevent and treat bacterial infections of the urinary tract. It is chemically converted in the bladder to ammonia and formaldehyde, which kills actively growing bacteria.

TREATMENT

In order to avoid stomach irritation, you should take methenamine with food or with a full glass of water or milk (unless your doctor directs you to do otherwise).

The oral suspension form of this medication should be shaken well just before measuring each dose. The contents tend to settle on the bottom of the bottle, so it is necessary to shake the container to distribute the ingredients evenly and equalize the doses. Each dose should then be measured carefully with a specially designed 5-ml measuring spoon. An ordinary kitchen teaspoon is not accurate enough.

The enteric-coated tablets should be swallowed whole. Breaking, crushing, or chewing these tablets increases their gastrointestinal side effects.

If you are taking the oral granules, the contents of the packet should be dissolved in two to four ounces of water just before you take the dose.

Methenamine works best when the level of medicine in your bloodstream and urine is kept constant. It is best, therefore, to take the doses at evenly spaced intervals day and night. For example, if you are to take four doses a day, the doses should be spaced six hours apart.

Try not to miss any doses of this medication. If you do miss a dose, take it immediately. However, if you do not remember to take the missed dose until it is almost time for your next dose, take the missed dose immediately; space the following dose about halfway through the regular interval between doses; and then continue with your regular dosing schedule.

It is important to continue to take this medication for the entire time prescribed by your doctor (usually seven to 14 days), even if the symptoms disappear before the end of that period. If you stop taking the drug too soon, resistant bacteria are given a chance to continue growing, and the infection could recur.

SIDE EFFECTS

Minor. Abdominal cramps, diarrhea, headache, loss of appetite, nausea, or vomiting. These side effects should disappear as your body adjusts to the medication.

Major. Tell your doctor about any side effects that are persistent or particularly bothersome. IT IS ESPECIALLY IMPORTANT TO TELL YOUR DOCTOR about difficulty in breathing, difficult or painful urination, itching, mouth sores, rapid weight gain (three to five pounds within a week), shortness of breath, or skin rash.

INTERACTIONS

Methenamine interacts with several other types of medications:

1. Sodium bicarbonate, antacids, acetazolamide, and diuretics (water pills) can decrease the effectiveness of methenamine by preventing its conversion to formaldehyde.

2. Methenamine can increase the side effects (to the kidneys) of sulfonamide antibiotics.

Before starting to take methenamine, BE SURE TO TELL YOUR DOCTOR about any medications you are currently taking, especially any of those listed above.

WARNINGS

- Tell your doctor about unusual or allergic reactions you have had to any medications, especially to methenamine.
- Before starting to take methenamine, be sure to tell your doctor if you now have or if you have ever had dehydration, kidney disease, or liver disease.
- Some of these products contain the color additive FD&C Yellow No. 5 (tartrazine), which can cause allergic-type reactions (fainting, rash, shortness of breath) in certain susceptible individuals.
- This medication has been prescribed for your current infection only. Another infection later on, or one that someone else has, may require a different medicine. You should not give your medicine to other people or use it for other infections, unless your doctor specifically directs you to do so.
- If the symptoms of your infection do not improve in several days, CONTACT YOUR DOCTOR. This medication may not be effective for your infection.
- In order for this medication to work properly, it is necessary that your urine remain acidic. You should, therefore, avoid foods that cause the urine to become alkaline (nonacidic), such as citrus fruits and milk products. Your doctor may also want you to take vitamin C (ascorbic acid) to help keep the urine acidic.
- Be sure to tell your doctor if you are pregnant. Although methenamine appears to be safe during pregnancy, it does cross the placenta, and extensive studies have not been conducted. Also, tell your doctor if you are breast-feeding an infant. Small amounts of methenamine pass into breast milk.

methenamine mandelate—see methenamine

---

methocarbamol

BRAND NAMES (Manufacturers)

Delaxin (Ferndale)
Marbaxin (Vortech)
methocarbamol (various manufacturers)
Robaxin (Robins)

TYPE OF DRUG

Muscle relaxant

INGREDIENT

methocarbamol

DOSAGE FORM

Tablets (500 mg and 750 mg)

STORAGE

Methocarbamol should be stored at room temperature in a tightly closed container.

USES

This medication is used to relieve the discomfort of painful muscle aches and spasms. It should be used in conjunction with rest, physical therapy, and other measures that your doctor may prescribe. It is not clear exactly how methocarbamol works, but it is thought to relieve muscle spasms by acting as a central nervous system (brain and spinal cord) depressant.

TREATMENT

Methocarbamol can be taken either on an empty stomach or with food or a full glass of water or milk (as directed by your doctor). These tablets can be crushed and mixed with food or liquid if you have trouble swallowing them.

If you miss a dose of this medication and remember within an hour, take the missed dose immediately. If more than an hour has passed, do not take the missed dose; just return to your regular dosing schedule. Do not double the next dose.

SIDE EFFECTS

Minor. Dizziness, drowsiness, headache, light-headedness, metallic taste in the mouth, nausea, or stomach upset. These side effects should disappear as your body adjusts to the medication.

This medication can cause the urine to darken to brown, black, or green. This is a harmless effect.

If you feel dizzy or light-headed, sit or lie down for a while; get up slowly from a sitting or reclining position, and be careful on stairs.

Major. Tell your doctor about any side effects that are persistent or particularly bothersome. IT IS ESPECIALLY IMPORTANT TO TELL YOUR DOCTOR about fainting, fatigue, fever, flushing, nasal congestion, skin rash, uncoordinated movements, or visual disturbances.

INTERACTIONS

Methocarbamol interacts with several other types of medications:

1. Concurrent use of methocarbamol with other central nervous system depressants (such as alcohol, antihistamines, barbiturates, benzodiazepine tranquilizers, muscle relaxants, narcotics, pain medications, phenothiazine tranquilizers, and sleeping medications) or with tricyclic antidepressants can cause extreme drowsiness.

2. Methocarbamol can decrease the effectiveness of pyridostigmine.

Before starting to take methocarbamol, BE SURE TO TELL YOUR DOCTOR about any medications you are currently taking, especially any of those listed above.

WARNINGS

- Tell your doctor about unusual or allergic reactions you have had to any medications, especially to methocarbamol.
- Before starting to take this medication, be sure to tell your doctor if you now have or if you have ever had brain disease.
- If this drug makes you dizzy or drowsy, avoid taking part in any activity that requires mental alertness, such as driving a car or operating potentially dangerous machinery.
- Be sure to tell your doctor if you are pregnant. Although methocarbamol appears to be safe, extensive studies in humans have not been conducted. Also, tell your doctor if you are breast-feeding an infant. Small amounts of methocarbamol pass into breast milk.

---

methotrexate

BRAND NAME (Manufacturer)
Methotrexate (Lederle)
TYPE OF DRUG
Antineoplastic (anticancer drug), antipsoriatic
INGREDIENT
methotrexate
DOSAGE FORM
Tablets (2.5 mg)
STORAGE
Methotrexate should be stored at room temperature in a tightly closed container.

USES

Methotrexate is used to treat certain types of cancer and severe psoriasis. It works by slowing the growth rate of rapidly proliferating cells.

TREATMENT

In order to avoid stomach irritation, you can take methotrexate with food or with a full glass of water or milk (unless your doctor directs you to do otherwise).

Try not to miss any doses of this medication. If you do miss a dose, take the missed dose as soon as possible, unless it is almost time for the next dose. In that case, do not take the missed dose at all; just return to your regular dosing schedule. Do not double the next dose. If you miss more than two doses in a row, CONTACT YOUR DOCTOR.

SIDE EFFECTS

Minor. Abdominal distress, fatigue, loss of appetite, nasal congestion, nausea, or vomiting. These side effects should disappear as your body adjusts to the medication. Methotrexate also causes hair loss, which is reversible when the medication is stopped.

This medication can increase your sensitivity to sunlight. You should, therefore, try to avoid prolonged exposure to sunlight and sunlamps. Wear protective clothing and sunglasses, and use an effective sunscreen.

Major. Tell your doctor about any side effects that are persistent or particularly bothersome. IT IS ESPECIALLY IMPORTANT TO TELL YOUR DOCTOR about back pain, blurred vision, convulsions, diarrhea, difficult or painful urination, drowsiness, fever, headache, itching, menstrual changes, mouth sores, rash, severe abdominal pain, skin color changes, unusual bleeding or bruising, or yellowing of the eyes or skin.

INTERACTIONS

Methotrexate interacts with several other types of medications:

1. Concurrent use of alcohol and methotrexate can lead to an increased risk of liver damage.

2. Methotrexate can block the effectiveness of antigout medications.

3. Phenylbutazone, probenecid, phenytoin, tetracycline, aspirin, chloramphenicol, salicylates, naproxen, ketoprofen, and sulfonamide antibiotics can increase the blood levels of methotrexate, which can lead to an increase in serious side effects.

4. Methotrexate can increase the effects of the blood thinner warfarin, which can lead to bleeding complications.

5. Folic acid vitamins may decrease the effect of this medication.

Before starting to take methotrexate, BE SURE TO TELL YOUR DOCTOR about any medications you are currently taking, especially any of those listed above.

WARNINGS

- Tell your doctor about unusual or allergic reactions you have had to any medications, especially to methotrexate.
- Before starting to take this medication, be sure to tell your doctor if you now have or if you have ever had blood disorders, gout, infection, kidney disease, liver disease, or inflammation of the gastrointestinal tract.
- If this drug makes you dizzy or drowsy, do not take part in any activity that requires alertness, such as driving a car or operating potentially dangerous machinery.
- While you are taking methotrexate, you should drink plenty of fluids so that you urinate often (unless your doctor

directs you to do otherwise). This helps prevent kidney and bladder problems during therapy.

• You should not be immunized or vaccinated while taking methotrexate. The vaccination or immunization will not be effective and may lead to an infection if a live-virus vaccine is used.

• Methotrexate is a potent medication that can cause serious side effects. Your doctor will, therefore, want to monitor your therapy carefully with blood tests.

• Be sure to tell your doctor if you are pregnant. Methotrexate has been shown to cause birth defects or death of the fetus. Effective contraception should be used during treatment and for at least eight weeks after treatment is stopped. Also, tell your doctor if you are breast-feeding an infant. Methotrexate passes into breast milk and can cause side effects in nursing infants.

---

methyclothiazide

BRAND NAMES (Manufacturers)
Aquatensen (Wallace)
Enduron (Abbott)
Ethon (Major)
methyclothiazide (various manufacturers)

TYPE OF DRUG
Diuretic and antihypertensive

INGREDIENT
methyclothiazide

DOSAGE FORM
Tablets (2.5 mg and 5 mg)

STORAGE
This medication should be stored at room temperature in a tightly closed container.

USES

Methyclothiazide is prescribed to treat high blood pressure. It is also used to reduce fluid accumulation in the body caused by certain conditions, such as heart failure, cirrhosis of the liver, and kidney disease, and by the long-term use of some medications. This medication reduces fluid accumulation by increasing the elimination of salt and water through the kidneys.

TREATMENT

This medication can be taken with a glass of milk or with a meal to decrease stomach irritation (unless your doctor directs you to do otherwise). Try to take it at the same time every day. Avoid taking a dose after 6:00 P.M.; otherwise, you may have to get up during the night to urinate.

If you miss a dose of this medication, take the missed dose as soon as possible, unless it is almost time for the next dose. In that case, do not take the missed dose at all; just wait until the next scheduled dose. Do not double the dose.

This medication does not cure high blood pressure, but it will help to control the condition as long as you continue to take it.

SIDE EFFECTS

Minor. Constipation, cramps, diarrhea, dizziness, drowsiness, headache, heartburn, loss of appetite, restlessness, or upset stomach. As your body adjusts to the medication, these side effects should disappear.

This medication can cause increased sensitivity to sunlight. It is, therefore, important to avoid prolonged exposure to sunlight and sunlamps. Wear protective clothing, and use an effective sunscreen.

To relieve constipation, increase the amount of fiber in your diet (fresh fruits and vegetables, salads, bran, and whole-grain breads) and exercise more (unless your doctor directs you to do otherwise).

To avoid dizziness or light-headedness when you stand, contract and relax the muscles of your legs for a few moments before rising. Do this by pushing one foot against the floor while raising the other foot slightly, alternating feet so that you are "pumping" your legs in a pedaling motion.

Major. Tell your doctor about any side effects that are persistent or particularly bothersome. IT IS ESPECIALLY IMPORTANT TO TELL YOUR DOCTOR about blurred vision, confusion, difficulty in breathing, dry mouth, excessive thirst, excessive weakness, fainting, fever, itching, joint pain, mood changes, muscle pain or spasms, nausea, palpitations, skin rash, sore throat, tingling in the fingers or toes, unusual bleeding or bruising, vomiting, or yellowing of the eyes or skin.

INTERACTIONS

Methyclothiazide interacts with several other types of medications:

1. It may decrease the effectiveness of oral anticoagulants, antigout medications, insulin, oral antidiabetic medicines, and methenamine.

2. Fenfluramine can increase the blood-pressure-lowering effects of methyclothiazide (which can be dangerous).

3. Indomethacin can decrease the blood-pressure-lowering effects of methyclothiazide, thereby counteracting the desired effects.

4. Cholestyramine and colestipol decrease the absorption of this medication from the gastrointestinal tract. Methyclothiazide should, therefore, be taken one hour before or four hours after a dose of cholestyramine or colestipol (if one of those medications has also been prescribed).

5. The side effects of amphotericin B, calcium, cortisone and cortisone-like steroids (such as dexamethasone, hydrocortisone, prednisone, and prednisolone), digitalis, digoxin, lithium, quinidine, sulfonamide antibiotics, and vitamin D may be increased by methyclothiazide.

BE SURE TO TELL YOUR DOCTOR about any medications you are currently taking, especially any listed above.

WARNINGS

• Tell your doctor about unusual or allergic reactions you have had to any medications, especially to methyclothiazide or any other sulfa drug, including other diuretics, oral antidiabetic medications, or sulfonamide antibiotics.

• Before you start taking methyclothiazide, tell your doctor if you now have or if you have ever had kidney disease or problems with urination, diabetes mellitus, gout, liver disease, asthma, pancreatic disease, or systemic lupus erythematosus.

• Methyclothiazide can cause potassium loss. Signs of potassium loss include dry mouth, thirst, weakness, muscle pain or cramps, nausea, and vomiting. If you experience any of these symptoms, call your doctor. To help avoid potassium loss, take this drug with a glass of fresh or frozen orange juice or cranberry juice or eat a banana every day. The use of a salt substitute also helps to prevent potassium loss. Do not change your diet or use a salt substitute, however, before discussing it with your doctor. Too much potassium can also be dangerous. Your doctor may want to have blood tests performed periodically in order to monitor your potassium levels.

• In order to avoid dizziness or fainting while taking this medication, try not to stand for long periods of time; avoid drinking excessive amounts of alcohol; and try not to get overheated (avoid strenuous exercise in hot weather and do not take hot baths, showers, and saunas).

• Do not take any over-the-counter (nonprescription) medications for weight control or for cough, cold, allergy, asthma, or sinus problems, unless your doctor directs you to do so. Some of these products can cause an increase in blood pressure.

• To prevent dehydration (severe water loss) while taking this medication, check with your doctor if you have any illness that causes severe or continuous nausea, vomiting, or diarrhea.

• This medication can raise the blood sugar level in diabetic patients. Therefore, blood sugar levels should be carefully monitored by blood or urine tests when this medication is being taken.

• Be sure to tell your doctor if you are pregnant. Methyclothiazide can cross the placenta and may cause adverse effects in the developing fetus. Also, tell your doctor if you are breast-feeding an infant. Although problems in humans have not been reported, small amounts of this drug can pass into breast milk, so caution is warranted.

---

methyldopa

BRAND NAMES (Manufacturers)
Aldomet (Merck Sharp & Dohme)
methyldopa (various manufacturers)

TYPE OF DRUG
Antihypertensive

INGREDIENT
methyldopa

DOSAGE FORMS
Tablets (125 mg, 250 mg, and 500 mg)
Oral suspension (250 mg per 5-ml spoonful, with 1% alcohol)

STORAGE
Store at room temperature in a tightly closed, light-resistant container. This drug should never be frozen.

USES

Methyldopa is used to treat high blood pressure. It is not clear exactly how methyldopa works, but it is thought to act on the central nervous system (brain and spinal cord) to prevent the release of chemicals responsible for maintaining high blood pressure.

TREATMENT

In order to prevent stomach irritation, you can take methyldopa with food or a full glass of water or milk. In order to become accustomed to taking this medication, try to take it at the same time(s) each day (unless your doctor directs you to do otherwise).

The oral suspension should be shaken well before each dose is measured. The contents tend to settle to the bottom of the bottle, so the bottle should be shaken to distribute the medication evenly and equalize the doses. Each dose should then be measured carefully with a specially designed 5-ml measuring spoon. An ordinary kitchen teaspoon is not accurate enough.

Methyldopa does not cure high blood pressure, but it will help to control the condition as long as you take it.

If you miss a dose of this medication, take the missed dose as soon as possible, unless it is almost time for the next dose. In that case, do not take the missed dose at all; just return to your regular dosing schedule. Do not double the next dose.

SIDE EFFECTS

Minor. Bloating, constipation, diarrhea, dizziness, drowsiness, dry mouth, gas, headache, light-headedness, loss of appetite, nasal congestion, nausea, vomiting, or weakness. These side effects should disappear as your body adjusts to the medication.

To relieve constipation, increase the amount of fiber in your diet (fresh fruits and vegetables, salads, bran, and whole-grain breads), exercise, and drink more water (unless your doctor directs you to do otherwise).

If you feel dizzy or light-headed, sit or lie down for a while; get up slowly from a sitting or reclining position, and be careful on stairs. To avoid dizziness or light-headedness when you stand, contract and relax the muscles of your legs for a few moments before rising. Do this by pushing one foot against the floor while raising the other foot slightly, alternating feet so that you are "pumping" your legs in a pedaling motion.

Major. Tell your doctor about any side effects that are persistent or particularly bothersome. IT IS ESPECIALLY IMPORTANT TO TELL YOUR DOCTOR about abdominal distention, blurred vision, breast enlargement (in both sexes), chest pain, confusion, decreased sexual ability, depression, difficulty in breathing, fainting, fatigue, fever, inflamed salivary glands, insomnia, nightmares, numbness or tingling, rapid weight gain (three to five pounds within a week), severe stomach cramps, sore joints, sore or "black" tongue, tremors, unusual bleeding or bruising, unusual body movements, or yellowing of the eyes or skin.

INTERACTIONS

Methyldopa interacts with several other types of drugs:

1. It can increase or decrease the antiparkinsonism effects of levodopa.

2. The use of a monoamine oxidase (MAO) inhibitor within 14 days of methyldopa can cause headaches, severe hypertension, and hallucinations.

3. The combination of methyldopa and methotrimeprazine can cause a severe drop in blood pressure; methyldopa and haloperidol can cause irritability; methyldopa and phenoxybenzamine can cause urinary retention; and methyldopa and alcohol can cause dizziness and fainting.

4. The effects of methyldopa may be increased by verapamil and fenfluramine.

5. Methyldopa can also increase the side effects of tolbutamide and lithium.

6. Methyldopa may increase the effects of norepinephrine and phenylpropanolamine, which may increase blood pressure.

Before starting to take methyldopa, BE SURE TO TELL YOUR DOCTOR about any medications you are currently taking, especially any of those listed above.

WARNINGS

- Tell your doctor about unusual or allergic reactions you have had to any medications, especially to methyldopa.
- Before starting to take this medication, be sure to tell your doctor if you now have or if you have ever had anemia, angina, kidney disease, liver disease, mental depression, Parkinson's disease, or stroke.
- In order to avoid dizziness or fainting while you are taking this medication, try not to stand for long periods of time; avoid drinking excessive amounts of alcohol; and try not to get overheated (avoid strenuous exercise in hot weather and do not take hot baths, showers, and saunas).
- If this drug makes you dizzy or drowsy, avoid taking part in any activity that requires alertness, such as driving a car or operating potentially dangerous machinery.
- Before surgery or other medical or dental treatment, tell your doctor or dentist you are taking this drug.
- Before taking any over-the-counter (nonprescription) allergy, asthma, sinus, cough, cold, or diet product, check with your doctor or pharmacist. Some of these products can cause an increase in blood pressure.
- Do not stop taking this medication unless you first check with your doctor. If this drug is stopped abruptly, you could experience a sudden rise in blood pressure. Your doctor may, therefore, want to decrease your dosage gradually.
- If you have an unexplained fever, especially during the first two or three weeks after starting to take this medication, CONTACT YOUR DOCTOR. Fever can be a sign of a serious reaction to methyldopa.
- Occasionally, during the second or third month of therapy, drug tolerance may develop. If you notice a decrease in effectiveness of methyldopa, contact your doctor.
- Before donating blood or receiving a blood transfusion, be sure that the doctor knows you are taking this medication. It can cause changes in your blood cells.
- Aldomet suspension contains sodium bisulfite, which may cause allergic-type reactions (hives, itching, wheezing) in certain susceptible persons.
- Be sure to tell your doctor if you are pregnant. Although this drug appears to be safe, extensive studies in women during pregnancy have not been conducted. Also, tell your doctor if you are breast-feeding an infant. Small amounts of methyldopa pass into breast milk.

---

methyldopa and hydrochlorothiazide combination

BRAND NAMES (Manufacturers)
Aldoril (Merck Sharp & Dohme)
methyldopa and hydrochlorothiazide combination (various manufacturers)

TYPE OF DRUG
Antihypertensive and diuretic

INGREDIENTS
methyldopa and hydrochlorothiazide

DOSAGE FORM
Tablets (250 mg methyldopa and 15 mg hydrochlorothiazide; 250 mg methyldopa and 25 mg hydrochlorothiazide; 500 mg methyldopa and 30 mg hydrochlorothiazide; 500 mg methyldopa and 50 mg hydrochlorothiazide)

STORAGE
These tablets should be stored at room temperature in a tightly closed container.

USES

Methyldopa and hydrochlorothiazide combination is used to treat high blood pressure. It is not exactly clear how methyldopa works, but it is thought to act on the central nervous system (brain and spinal cord) to prevent the release of chemicals responsible for maintaining high blood pressure. Hydrochlorothiazide is a diuretic (water pill), which reduces fluid accumulation by increasing the elimination of salt and water through the kidneys.

TREATMENT

To avoid stomach irritation, you can take methyldopa and hydrochlorothiazide combination with food or with a full glass of water or milk (unless your doctor directs you to do otherwise). In order to become accustomed to taking this medication, try to take it at the same time(s) each day. Avoid taking a dose after 6:00 P.M.; otherwise, you may have to get up during the night to urinate.

Methyldopa and hydrochlorothiazide combination does not cure high blood pressure, but it will help to control the condition as long as you continue to take it.

If you miss a dose of this medication, take the missed dose as soon as possible, unless it is almost time for the next dose. In that case, do not take the missed dose at all; just return to your regular dosing schedule. Do not double the next dose.

SIDE EFFECTS

Minor. Bloating, constipation, diarrhea, dizziness, drowsiness, gas, headache, light-headedness, loss of appetite, nasal congestion, or increased urination. These side effects should disappear as your body adjusts to the medication.

This medication can increase your sensitivity to sunlight. You should, therefore, avoid prolonged exposure to sunlight and sunlamps. Wear protective clothing and sunglasses, and use an effective sunscreen.

To relieve constipation, increase the amount of fiber in your diet (fresh fruits and vegetables, salads, bran, and whole-grain breads) and exercise (unless your doctor directs you to do otherwise).

Chew sugarless gum or suck on ice chips or a piece of hard candy to relieve mouth dryness.

If you feel dizzy or light-headed, sit or lie down for a while; get up slowly from a sitting or reclining position, and be careful on stairs. To avoid dizziness or light-headedness when you stand, contract and relax the muscles of your legs for a few moments before rising. Do this by pushing one foot against the floor while raising the other foot slightly, alternating feet so that you are "pumping" your legs in a pedaling motion.

Major. Tell your doctor about any side effects that are persistent or particularly bothersome. IT IS ESPECIALLY IMPORTANT TO TELL YOUR DOCTOR about abdominal distention, blurred vision, breast enlargement (in both sexes), chest pain, confusion, decreased sexual ability, depression, difficulty in breathing, dry mouth, fainting, fatigue, fever, inflamed salivary glands, insomnia, joint pains, muscle pains or spasms, nausea, nightmares, numbness or tingling, rapid weight gain (three to five pounds within a week), severe stomach cramps, sore or "black" tongue, swelling of the feet or ankles, thirst, tremors, unusual bleeding or bruising, unusual body movements, vomiting, weakness, or yellowing of the eyes or skin.

INTERACTIONS

This medicine interacts with other types of drugs:

1. Methyldopa can either increase or decrease the antiparkinsonism effects of levodopa.

2. The use of a monamine oxidase (MAO) inhibitor within 14 days of methyldopa can cause headaches, severe hypertension, and hallucinations.

3. The combination of methyldopa and methotrimeprazine can cause a severe drop in blood pressure; methyldopa and haloperidol can cause irritability; methyldopa and phenoxybenzamine can cause urinary retention; and methyldopa and alcohol can cause dizziness and fainting.

4. The effects of methyldopa may be increased by verapamil and fenfluramine, which may have a negative effect.

5. Methyldopa can increase the side effects of tolbutamide and lithium.

6. Methyldopa may increase the effects of norepinephrine and phenylpropanolamine, which may increase blood pressure.

7. Hydrochlorothiazide can decrease the effectiveness of oral anticoagulants (blood thinners, such as warfarin), antigout medications, insulin, oral antidiabetic medications, and methenamine.

8. Fenfluramine may increase the blood-pressure-lowering effects of hydrochlorothiazide, and indomethacin may decrease its blood-pressure-lowering effects.

9. Cholestyramine and colestipol can decrease the absorption of hydrochlorothiazide from the gastrointestinal tract. Therefore, this medication should be taken one hour before or four hours after a dose of either of these other drugs.

10. The side effects of amphotericin B, calcium, adrenocorticosteroids (cortisone-like medicines), digitalis, digoxin, lithium, quinidine, sulfonamide antibiotics, and vitamin D may be increased by hydrochlorothiazide.

BE SURE TO TELL YOUR DOCTOR about any medications you are currently taking, especially any of those listed above.

WARNINGS

• Tell your doctor about unusual or allergic reactions you have had to medications, especially to methyldopa or hydrochlorothiazide or to any other sulfa medication (diuretics, oral antidiabetic medicines, sulfonamide antibiotics, dapsone, or sulfone).

• Before starting to take this medication, be sure to tell your doctor if you have ever had anemia, angina, diabetes mellitus, gout, kidney disease, liver disease, mental depression, Parkinson's disease, pancreatitis, or stroke.

• A doctor generally does not prescribe this drug or other "fixed-dose" products as the first choice in the treatment of high blood pressure. The patient should initially receive each ingredient singly. If the response is adequate to the dose contained in this product, it can then be substituted. The advantage of a combination product is its increased convenience.

• This medication can cause potassium loss. Signs of potassium loss include dry mouth, thirst, weakness, muscle pain or cramps, nausea, and vomiting. If you experience any of these symptoms, CONTACT YOUR DOCTOR. To help prevent this problem, your doctor may want to have blood tests performed periodically to monitor your potassium levels. To help avoid potassium loss, take this medication with a glass of fresh or frozen orange juice or cranberry juice or eat a banana every day. The use of a salt substitute also helps to prevent potassium loss. Do not change your diet or use a salt substitute, however, until you discuss it with your doctor. Too much potassium can also be dangerous.

• To prevent severe water loss (dehydration) while taking hydrochlorothiazide, check with your doctor if you have any illness that causes severe or continuous nausea, vomiting, or diarrhea.

• Hydrochlorothiazide can raise blood sugar levels in diabetic patients. Blood sugar should, therefore, be monitored carefully when this medication is being taken.

• In order to avoid dizziness or fainting while taking this medication, try not to stand for long periods of time; avoid drinking excessive amounts of alcohol; and try not to get overheated (avoid strenuous exercise in hot weather and do not take hot baths, showers, and saunas).

• If this drug makes you dizzy or drowsy, avoid taking part in any activity that requires alertness, such as driving a car or operating potentially dangerous machinery.

• Before having surgery or any other medical or dental treatment, be sure to tell your doctor or dentist that you are taking this medication.

• Before taking any over-the-counter (nonprescription) allergy, asthma, sinus, cough, cold, or diet product, check with your doctor or pharmacist. Some of these products can cause an increase in blood pressure.

• Do not stop taking this medication unless you first check with your doctor. If this drug is stopped abruptly, you could experience a sudden rise in blood pressure. Your doctor may, therefore, want to decrease your dosage gradually.

• If you have an unexplained fever, especially during the first two to three weeks after starting to take this medication, CONTACT YOUR DOCTOR. Fever can be a sign of a serious reaction to methyldopa.

• Occasionally, tolerance to this medication develops, usually during the second or third month of therapy. If you notice a decrease in effectiveness of this medication, contact your doctor.

• Before donating blood or receiving a blood transfusion, be sure you let the doctor know that you are taking this medication. Methyldopa can cause a change in the blood cells.

• Be sure to tell your doctor if you are pregnant. Methyldopa and hydrochlorothiazide cross the placenta and may cause adverse effects in the developing fetus. Also, tell your doctor if you are breast-feeding an infant. Small amounts of both of these drugs pass into breast milk.

methylphenidate

BRAND NAMES (Manufacturers)
methylphenidate hydrochloride (various manufacturers)
Ritalin (Ciba)
Ritalin-SR (Ciba)

TYPE OF DRUG
Adrenergic

INGREDIENT
methylphenidate

DOSAGE FORMS
Tablets (5 mg, 10 mg, and 20 mg)
Sustained-release tablets (20 mg)

STORAGE
Methylphenidate should be stored at room temperature in tightly closed, light-resistant containers.

USES

Methylphenidate is a central nervous system (brain and spinal cord) stimulant that increases mental alertness and decreases fatigue. It is used in the treatment of narcolepsy (a disorder involving uncontrollable desires to sleep or actual sleep attacks that occur in a rapid and unpredictable manner), mild depression, and abnormal behavioral syndrome in children (hyperkinetic syndrome or attention deficit disorder). The way this medication works in abnormal behavioral syndrome in children is not clearly understood.

TREATMENT

In order to avoid stomach upset, you can take methylphenidate with food or with a full glass of water or milk (unless your doctor directs you to do otherwise).

If methylphenidate is being used to treat narcolepsy or abnormal behavioral syndrome in children, the first dose should be taken soon after awakening.

In order to avoid difficulty in falling asleep, the last dose of the regular tablets should be taken four to six hours before bedtime each day (the sustained-release tablets should be taken at least eight hours before bedtime).

The sustained-release tablets should be swallowed whole. Chewing, crushing, or breaking these tablets destroys their sustained-release activity and may increase the side effects.

If you miss a dose, take the missed dose as soon as possible, unless it is almost time for your next dose. In that case, do not take the missed dose; just return to your regular dosing schedule. Do not double the next dose.

SIDE EFFECTS

Minor. Abdominal pain, dizziness, drowsiness, dry mouth, headache, insomnia, loss of appetite, nausea, nervousness, vomiting, or weakness. These side effects should disappear as your body adjusts to the medication.

Dry mouth can be relieved by sucking on ice chips or a piece of hard candy or by chewing sugarless gum.

If you feel dizzy, sit or lie down for a while; get up from a sitting or lying position slowly, and be careful on stairs.

Major. Tell your doctor about any side effects that are persistent or particularly bothersome. IT IS ESPECIALLY IMPORTANT TO TELL YOUR DOCTOR about chest pain, fever, hair loss, hallucinations, hives, joint pain, mood changes, palpitations, rash, seizures, sore throat, uncoordinated movements, or unusual bleeding or bruising.

INTERACTIONS

Methylphenidate interacts with several other types of medications:

1. Use of it within 14 days of a monoamine oxidase (MAO) inhibitor (such as isocarboxazid, pargyline, phenelzine, tranylcypromine) can result in severe high blood pressure.

2. Methylphenidate can decrease the blood-pressure-lowering effects of antihypertensive medications (especially guanethidine).

3. Acetazolamide and sodium bicarbonate can decrease the elimination of methylphenidate from the body, thereby prolonging its action and increasing the risk of side effects.

4. Methylphenidate can decrease the elimination and increase the side effects of oral anticoagulants (blood thinners, such as warfarin), tricyclic antidepressants (such as amitriptyline, desipramine, imipramine, and nortriptyline), anticonvulsants (such as phenytoin, phenobarbital, and primidone), and phenylbutazone.

Before starting to take this medication, BE SURE TO TELL YOUR DOCTOR about any medications you are currently taking, especially any of those listed above.

WARNINGS

- Tell your doctor about unusual or allergic reactions you have had to any medications, especially to methylphenidate.
- Tell your doctor if you have ever had epilepsy, glaucoma, high blood pressure, motor tics, Tourette's syndrome, anxiety, agitation, depression, or tension.
- Methylphenidate can mask the symptoms of extreme fatigue and can cause dizziness. Your ability to perform tasks that require alertness, such as driving a car or operating potentially dangerous machinery, may be decreased. Appropriate caution should, therefore, be taken. A child taking methylphenidate should be careful while engaging in physical activity.
- Before having surgery or any other medical or dental treatment, be sure to tell your doctor that you are taking this medication.
- Methylphenidate is related to amphetamine and may be habit-forming when taken for long periods of time (both physical and psychological dependence can occur). You should not increase the dosage of this medication or take it for longer than the prescribed time unless you first consult your doctor. It is also important that you not stop taking this medication abruptly; fatigue, sleep disorders, mental depression, nausea, vomiting, or stomach cramps or pain could occur. Your doctor may want to decrease the dosage gradually in order to prevent these side effects.
- Methylphenidate can slow growth in children. Therefore, if this medication is being taken by a child, your doctor may recommend drug-free periods during school holidays and summer vacations. Growth spurts often occur during these drug-free periods.
- Children may be more sensitive to certain side effects such as loss of appetite, stomach pain, trouble sleeping, and weight loss.
- If cocaine is being used now or was used in the past, taking methylphenidate may cause severe nervousness, irritability, trouble sleeping, or possibly irregular heartbeat or seizures.
- Be sure to tell your doctor if you are pregnant. Effects of this drug during pregnancy have not been thoroughly stud-

ied in either humans or animals. Also, tell your doctor if you are breast-feeding an infant. Small amounts of methylphenidate may pass into breast milk.

methylphenidate hydrochloride—see methylphenidate

methylprednisolone (systemic)

BRAND NAMES (Manufacturers)
Medrol (Upjohn)
methylprednisolone (various manufacturers)
TYPE OF DRUG
Adrenocorticosteroid hormone
INGREDIENT
methylprednisolone
DOSAGE FORM
Tablets (2 mg, 4 mg, 8 mg, 16 mg, 24 mg, and 32 mg)
STORAGE
Store at room temperature in a tightly closed container.

USES

Your adrenal glands naturally produce certain cortisone-like chemicals. These chemicals are involved in various regulatory processes in the body (such as those involving fluid balance, temperature, and reactions to inflammation). Methylprednisolone belongs to a group of drugs known as adrenocorticosteroids (or cortisone-like medications). It is used to treat a variety of disorders, including endocrine and rheumatic disorders; asthma; blood diseases; certain cancers; eye disorders; gastrointestinal disturbances, such as ulcerative colitis; respiratory diseases; and inflammations, such as arthritis, dermatitis, and poison ivy. How this drug acts to relieve these disorders is not completely understood.

TREATMENT

In order to prevent stomach irritation, you can take methylprednisolone with food or milk.

If you are taking only one dose of this medication each day, try to take it before 9:00 A.M. This will mimic the body's normal production of this type of chemical.

It is important to try not to miss any doses of methylprednisolone. However, if you do miss a dose of this medication, follow these guidelines:

1. If you are taking it more than once a day, take the missed dose as soon as possible and return to your regular schedule. If it is already time for the next dose, double the dose.

2. If you are taking this medication once a day, take the dose you missed as soon as possible, unless you don't remember until the next day. In that case, do not take the missed dose at all; just follow your regular schedule. Do not double the next dose.

3. If you are taking this drug every other day, take it as soon as you remember. If you missed the scheduled time by a whole day, take it when you remember, and then skip a day before you take the next dose. Do not double the dose.

If you miss more than one dose, CONTACT YOUR DOCTOR.

SIDE EFFECTS

Minor. Dizziness, false sense of well-being, increased appetite, increased susceptibility to infections, increased sweating, indigestion, menstrual irregularities, nausea, reddening of the skin on the face, restlessness, sleep disorders, or weight gain. These side effects should disappear as your body adjusts to the medication.

Major. Tell your doctor about any side effects that are persistent or particularly bothersome. IT IS ESPECIALLY IMPORTANT TO TELL YOUR DOCTOR about abdominal enlargement; abdominal pain; acne or other skin problems; back or rib pain; bloody or black, tarry stools; blurred vision; convulsions; eye pain; fever and sore throat; growth impairment (in children); headaches; impaired healing of wounds; increased thirst and urination; mental depression; mood changes; muscle wasting; muscle weakness; nightmares; rapid weight gain (three to five pounds within a week); rash; shortness of breath; thinning of the skin; unusual bleeding or bruising; and unusual weakness.

INTERACTIONS

Methylprednisolone interacts with several other types of medications:

1. Alcohol, aspirin, and anti-inflammatory medications (diclofenac, diflunisal, fenoprofen, flurbiprofen, ibuprofen, indomethacin, ketoprofen, mefenamic acid, meclofenamate, naproxen, piroxicam, sulindac, or tolmetin) aggravate the stomach problems that are common with use of this medication.

2. The dosage of oral anticoagulants (blood thinners, such as warfarin), oral antidiabetic medications, or insulin may need to be altered when this therapy with systemic methylprednisolone is started or stopped.

3. The loss of potassium caused by methylprednisolone can lead to serious side effects in individuals taking digoxin. Thiazide diuretics (water pills) can increase the potassium loss caused by methylprednisolone.

4. Phenobarbital, phenytoin, rifampin, and ephedrine can increase the elimination of methylprednisolone from the body, thereby decreasing its effectiveness.

5. Oral contraceptives (birth control pills) and estrogen-containing drugs may decrease the elimination of this medication from the body, which can lead to an increase in side effects.

6. Methylprednisolone can increase the elimination of aspirin and isoniazid, thereby decreasing the effectiveness of these two medications.

7. Cholestyramine and colestipol can chemically bind this medication in the stomach and gastrointestinal tract and prevent its absorption.

BE SURE TO TELL YOUR DOCTOR about any medications you are currently taking, especially any of those listed above.

WARNINGS

- Tell your doctor about unusual or allergic reactions you have had to any medications, especially to methylprednisolone or other adrenocorticosteroids (such as betamethasone, cortisone, dexamethasone, hydrocortisone, paramethasone, prednisolone, prednisone, and triamcinolone).
- Tell your doctor if you now have or if you have ever had bone disease, diabetes mellitus, emotional instability, glaucoma, fungal infections, heart disease, high blood pressure, high cholesterol levels, myasthenia gravis, peptic ulcers, osteoporosis, thyroid disease, tuberculosis, ulcerative colitis, kidney disease, or liver disease.

• To help avoid potassium loss while using this drug, take your dose with a glass of fresh or frozen orange juice or eat a banana each day. The use of a salt substitute also helps to prevent potassium loss. Check with your doctor before using a salt substitute.

• If you are using this medication for longer than a week, you may need to have your dosage adjusted if you are subjected to stress, such as serious infections, injury, or surgery. Discuss this with your doctor.

• If you have been taking this drug for more than a week, do not stop taking it suddenly. If it is stopped suddenly, you may experience abdominal or back pain, dizziness, fainting, fever, muscle or joint pain, nausea, vomiting, shortness of breath, or extreme weakness. Your doctor may, therefore, want to reduce the dosage gradually. Never increase the dosage or take the drug for longer than the prescribed time, unless you first consult your doctor.

• While you are taking methylprednisolone, you should not be vaccinated or immunized. This medication decreases the effectiveness of vaccines and can lead to overwhelming infection if a live-virus vaccine is administered.

• Before having surgery or other medical or dental treatment, be sure to tell your doctor or dentist about this drug.

• Because this drug can cause glaucoma and cataracts with long-term use, your doctor may want you to have your eyes examined by an ophthalmologist periodically during treatment.

• If you are taking this medication for prolonged periods, you should wear or carry a notice or identification card stating that you are taking an adrenocorticosteroid.

• This medication can raise blood sugar levels in diabetic patients. Blood sugar levels should, therefore, be monitored carefully with blood or urine tests when this medication is being taken.

• Some of these products contain the color additive FD&C Yellow No. 5 (tartrazine), which can cause allergic-type reactions (rash, wheezing, fainting, shortness of breath) in certain susceptible individuals.

• Be sure to tell your doctor if you are pregnant. This drug crosses the placenta. Although studies in humans have not been conducted, birth defects have been observed in the fetuses of animals that were given large doses of this type of drug during pregnancy. Also, tell your doctor if you are breast-feeding an infant. Small amounts of methylprednisolone pass into breast milk and may cause growth suppression or a decrease in natural adrenocorticosteroid production in the nursing infant.

---

methyltestosterone

BRAND NAMES (Manufacturers)
Android (Brown)
Metandren (Ciba)
methyltestosterone (various manufacturers)
Oreton Methyl (Schering)
Testred (ICN)
Virilon (Star)

TYPE OF DRUG
Androgen

INGREDIENT
methyltestosterone

DOSAGE FORMS
Oral tablets (10 mg and 25 mg)
Buccal tablets (5 mg and 10 mg)
Capsules (10 mg)

STORAGE
Methyltestosterone should be stored at room temperature in a tightly closed container.

USES
This medication is a synthetic androgen (male hormone) that is used to treat conditions such as delayed puberty, eunuchism, or impotence in males whose bodies cannot produce enough testosterone on their own. The medication may be used to treat breast cancer in women whose breast tumor responds to hormone treatment.

TREATMENT
In order to avoid stomach irritation, you can take methyltestosterone oral tablets or capsules with food or with a full glass of water or milk (unless your doctor directs you to do otherwise).

The buccal tablet form of methyltestosterone is meant to be absorbed through the lining of the mouth, rather than swallowed. The tablet should be placed between your gum and cheek and allowed to dissolve slowly. Do not eat, drink, chew, or smoke while the tablet is dissolving.

If you miss a dose of this medication, take the missed dose as soon as possible, unless it is almost time for the next dose. In that case, do not take the missed dose at all; just return to your regular dosing schedule. Do not double the next dose of the medication.

SIDE EFFECTS
Minor. Decrease or increase in sexual desire, diarrhea, headache, loss of appetite, nausea, stomach irritation, sleeping difficulties, or vomiting. These side effects should disappear as your body adjusts to the medication.

Major. Tell your doctor about any side effects that are persistent or particularly bothersome. IT IS ESPECIALLY IMPORTANT TO TELL YOUR DOCTOR about acne; black, bloody, or tarry stools; breast enlargement or tenderness; flushing; frequent or continuous erection; hair loss or growth; hoarseness or deepening of the voice; increased urination; shortness of breath; skin rash; swelling of the hands or feet; sore throat; tiredness; unusual bleeding or bruising; or yellowing of the eyes or skin.

INTERACTIONS
Methyltestosterone interacts with several other types of medications:

1. It can increase the effects of oral anticoagulants (blood thinners, such as warfarin), which can lead to bleeding complications.

2. Diabetic patients should know that methyltestosterone can lower blood sugar levels. The dosage of oral antidiabetic medication or insulin may, therefore, require adjustment when this medication is being taken.

3. Concurrent use of methyltestosterone and adrenocorticosteroids (cortisone-like medications) can lead to fluid retention.

Before starting to take methyltestosterone, BE SURE TO TELL YOUR DOCTOR about any medications you are currently taking, especially any of those listed above.

WARNINGS

• Tell your doctor about unusual or allergic reactions you have had to any medications, especially to methyltestosterone or to any other androgen (such as fluoxymesterone or testosterone).

• Before starting to take this medication, be sure to tell your doctor if you now have or if you have ever had breast cancer, fluid retention, heart disease, hypercalcemia (high blood calcium levels), kidney disease, liver disease, or prostate disorders.

• Although androgens have been used by athletes to increase muscle strength, there is no conclusive evidence that these drugs increase athletic performance. There is also some question as to their safety.

• High-dose methyltestosterone therapy may cause infertility in males.

• Some of these products contain the color additive FD&C Yellow No. 5 (tartrazine), which can cause allergic-type reactions (fainting, rash, shortness of breath) in certain susceptible individuals.

• Be sure to tell your doctor if you are pregnant. If methyltestosterone is taken by a pregnant woman, it can cause masculine characteristics in the developing fetus, such as increased body hair. (Note: This does NOT affect the sex of the fetus, which is determined at conception.) Also, tell your doctor if you are breast-feeding an infant. Methyltestosterone passes into breast milk and can cause masculinization of the nursing infant.

Meticorten—see prednisone (systemic)

---

metoclopramide

BRAND NAMES (Manufacturers)
Maxolon (Beecham)
metoclopramide (various manufacturers)
Reglan (Robins)

TYPE OF DRUG
Dopamine antagonist and antiemetic

INGREDIENT
metoclopramide

DOSAGE FORMS
Tablets (5 mg and 10 mg)
Oral syrup (5 mg per 5-ml spoonful)

STORAGE
Metoclopramide tablets and oral syrup should be stored at room temperature in tightly closed containers. Do not freeze the syrup form of this medication.

USES

This medication is used to relieve the symptoms associated with diabetic gastric stasis or gastric reflux and to prevent nausea and vomiting. Metoclopramide acts directly on the vomiting center in the brain to prevent nausea and vomiting. It also increases the movement of the stomach and intestines.

TREATMENT

To obtain the best results from treatment, you should take metoclopramide tablets or syrup 30 minutes before a meal and at bedtime.

Each dose of the syrup should be measured carefully with a specially designed 5-ml measuring spoon. An ordinary kitchen teaspoon is not accurate enough.

If you miss a dose of this medication, take the missed dose as soon as possible, unless it is almost time for the next dose. In that case, do not take the missed dose at all; just return to your regular dosing schedule. Do not double the next dose.

SIDE EFFECTS

Minor. Diarrhea, dizziness, drowsiness, dry mouth, fatigue, headache, insomnia, nausea, restlessness, or weakness. These side effects should disappear as your body adjusts to the medication.

If you feel dizzy or light-headed, sit or lie down for a while; get up slowly from a sitting or reclining position, and be careful on stairs.

To relieve mouth dryness, chew sugarless gum or suck on ice chips or a piece of hard candy.

Major. Tell your doctor about any side effects that are persistent or particularly bothersome. IT IS ESPECIALLY IMPORTANT TO TELL YOUR DOCTOR about anxiety; confusion; depression; disorientation; involuntary movements of the eyes, face, or limbs; muscle spasms; rash; or trembling of the hands.

INTERACTIONS

Metoclopramide interacts with several types of drugs:

1. Concurrent use of metoclopramide with other central nervous system depressants (such as alcohol, antihistamines, barbiturates, muscle relaxants, narcotics, pain medications, phenothiazine tranquilizers, benzodiazepine tranquilizers, and sleeping medications) or with tricyclic antidepressants can cause extreme drowsiness.

2. Narcotic analgesics may block the effectiveness of metoclopramide.

3. Metoclopramide can block the effectiveness of bromocriptine. It can also decrease the absorption of cimetidine and digoxin from the gastrointestinal tract, decreasing their effectiveness.

4. Metoclopramide can increase the absorption of acetaminophen, tetracycline, levodopa, and alcohol.

5. Diabetic patients should know that dosage requirements of insulin may change when metoclopramide is being taken.

Before starting to take metoclopramide, BE SURE TO TELL YOUR DOCTOR about any medications you are currently taking, especially any of those listed above.

WARNINGS

• Tell your doctor about unusual or allergic reactions you have had to any medications, especially to metoclopramide, procaine, or procainamide.

• Before starting to take metoclopramide, be sure to tell your doctor if you now have or if you have ever had epilepsy, kidney disease, liver disease, intestinal bleeding or blockage, Parkinson's disease, or pheochromocytoma.

• If this drug makes you dizzy or drowsy, do not take part in any activities that require alertness, such as driving a car or operating potentially dangerous machinery.

• Be sure to tell your doctor if you are pregnant. Although this drug appears to be safe, extensive studies in women during pregnancy have not been conducted. Also, tell your doctor if you are breast-feeding an infant. Metoclopramide passes into breast milk.

metolazone

BRAND NAMES (Manufacturers)
Diulo (Searle)
Microx (Pennwalt)
Zaroxolyn (Pennwalt)

TYPE OF DRUG
Diuretic and antihypertensive

INGREDIENT
metolazone

DOSAGE FORM
Tablets (2.5 mg, 5 mg, and 10 mg)

STORAGE
This medication should be stored at room temperature in a tightly closed container.

USES

Metolazone is prescribed to treat high blood pressure. It is also used to reduce fluid accumulation in the body caused by conditions such as heart failure, cirrhosis of the liver, kidney disease, and the long-term use of some medications. Metolazone reduces fluid accumulation by increasing the elimination of salt and water through the kidneys.

TREATMENT

To decrease stomach irritation, you can take this medication with a glass of milk or with a meal (unless your doctor directs you to do otherwise). Try to take it at the same time every day. Avoid taking a dose after 6:00 P.M.; otherwise, you may have to get up during the night to urinate.

If you miss a dose of this medication, take the missed dose as soon as possible, unless it is almost time for the next dose. In that case, do not take the missed dose at all; just wait until the next scheduled dose. Do not double the dose.

This medication does not cure high blood pressure, but it will help to control the condition as long as you take it.

SIDE EFFECTS

Minor. Constipation, cramps, diarrhea, dizziness, drowsiness, headache, heartburn, loss of appetite, restlessness, or upset stomach. As your body adjusts to the medication, these side effects should disappear.

This medication can cause increased sensitivity to sunlight. It is, therefore, important to avoid prolonged exposure to sunlight and sunlamps. Wear protective clothing, and use an effective sunscreen.

To relieve constipation, increase the amount of fiber in your diet (fresh fruits and vegetables, salads, bran, and whole-grain breads) and exercise more (unless your doctor directs you to do otherwise).

To avoid dizziness or light-headedness when you stand, contract and relax the muscles of your legs for a few moments before rising. Do this by pushing one foot against the floor while raising the other foot slightly, alternating feet so that you are "pumping" your legs in a pedaling motion.

Major. Tell your doctor about any side effects that are persistent or particularly bothersome. IT IS ESPECIALLY IMPORTANT TO TELL YOUR DOCTOR about blurred vision, confusion, difficulty in breathing, dry mouth, excessive thirst, excessive weakness, fever, itching, joint pain, mood changes, muscle spasms, nausea, palpitations, skin rash, sore throat, tingling in the fingers or toes, unusual bleeding or bruising, vomiting, or yellowing of the eyes or skin.

INTERACTIONS

Metolazone interacts with several other types of drugs:

1. It may decrease the effectiveness of oral anticoagulants, antigout medications, insulin, oral antidiabetic medicines, and methenamine.

2. Fenfluramine can increase the blood-pressure-lowering effects of metolazone (which can be dangerous).

3. Indomethacin can decrease the blood-pressure-lowering effects of metolazone, thereby counteracting the desired effects.

4. Cholestyramine and colestipol decrease the absorption of this medication from the gastrointestinal tract. Metolazone should, therefore, be taken one hour before or four hours after a dose of cholestyramine or colestipol (if you have also been prescribed one of these medications).

5. The side effects of amphotericin B, calcium, cortisone and cortisone-like steroids (such as dexamethasone, hydrocortisone, prednisone, and prednisolone), digitalis, digoxin, lithium, quinidine, sulfonamide antibiotics, and vitamin D may be increased when these drugs are taken concurrently with metolazone.

Before starting to take metolazone, BE SURE TO TELL YOUR DOCTOR about any medications you are currently taking, especially any of those listed above.

WARNINGS

- Tell your doctor about unusual or allergic reactions you have had to any medications, especially to metolazone or to any other sulfa drugs, including other diuretics, oral antidiabetic medications, or sulfonamide antibiotics.
- Tell your doctor if you now have or if you have ever had kidney disease or problems with urination, diabetes mellitus, gout, liver disease, asthma, pancreatic disease, or systemic lupus erythematosus.
- Metolazone can cause potassium loss. Signs of potassium loss include dry mouth, thirst, weakness, muscle pain or cramps, nausea, and vomiting. If you experience any of these symptoms, call your doctor. To help avoid potassium loss, take this drug with a glass of fresh or frozen orange juice or cranberry juice, or eat a banana every day. The use of a salt substitute also helps to prevent potassium loss. Do not change your diet or use a salt substitute, however, before discussing it with your doctor. Too much potassium can also be dangerous. Your doctor may want to have blood tests performed periodically to monitor your potassium levels.
- Limit your intake of alcoholic beverages while taking this medication, in order to prevent dizziness and light-headedness.
- Do not take any over-the-counter (nonprescription) medications for weight control or for cough, cold, allergy, asthma, or sinus problems unless your doctor directs you to do so. Some of these products can cause an increase in blood pressure.
- To prevent dehydration (severe water loss) while taking this medication, check with your doctor if you have any illness that causes severe or continuous nausea, vomiting, or diarrhea.
- This medication can raise blood sugar levels in diabetic patients. Therefore, blood sugar levels should be carefully monitored by blood or urine tests when this medication is being taken.
- Be sure to tell your doctor if you are pregnant. Metolazone can cross the placenta and may cause adverse effects

in the fetus. Also, tell your doctor if you are breast-feeding an infant. Although problems in humans have not been reported, small amounts of this drug can pass into breast milk, so caution is warranted.

---

metoprolol

BRAND NAME (Manufacturer)
Lopressor (Geigy)
TYPE OF DRUG
Beta-adrenergic blocking agent
INGREDIENT
metoprolol
DOSAGE FORM
Tablets (50 mg and 100 mg)
STORAGE
Metoprolol should be stored at room temperature in a tightly closed, light-resistant container.

USES

Metoprolol is used to treat high blood pressure and angina (chest pain) and to prevent additional heart attacks in heart attack patients. Metoprolol belongs to a group of medicines known as beta-adrenergic blocking agents or, more commonly, beta blockers. These drugs work by controlling nerve impulses along certain nerve pathways.

TREATMENT

Metoprolol can be taken with a glass of water, with meals, immediately following meals, or on an empty stomach, depending on your doctor's instructions. Try to take the medication at the same time(s) each day.

Try not to miss any doses of this medicine. If you do miss a dose of the medication, take the missed dose as soon as possible. However, if the next scheduled dose is within eight hours (if you are taking this medicine only once a day) or within four hours (if you are taking this medicine more than once a day), do not take the missed dose of the medication at all; just return to your regular dosing schedule. Do not double the next dose of the medication.

It is important to remember that metoprolol does not cure high blood pressure, but it will help to control the condition as long as you continue to take it.

SIDE EFFECTS

Minor. Anxiety; cold hands or feet (due to decreased blood circulation to the skin, fingers, and toes); constipation; decreased sexual ability; diarrhea; difficulty in sleeping; drowsiness; dryness of the eyes, mouth, and skin; headache; nausea; nervousness; stomach discomfort; tiredness; or weakness. These side effects should disappear during treatment, as your body adjusts to the medicine.

If you are extra-sensitive to the cold, be sure to dress warmly during cold weather.

To relieve constipation, increase the amount of fiber in your diet (fresh fruits and vegetables, salads, bran, and whole-grain breads) and exercise more (unless your doctor directs you to do otherwise).

Plain, nonmedicated eye drops (artificial tears) may help to relieve eye dryness.

If you experience mouth or throat dryness, you may want to chew sugarless gum or suck on ice chips or a piece of hard candy.

Major. Tell your doctor about any side effects that are persistent or particularly bothersome. IT IS ESPECIALLY IMPORTANT TO TELL YOUR DOCTOR about breathing difficulty or wheezing, confusion, dizziness, fever and sore throat, hair loss, hallucinations, light-headedness, mental depression, nightmares, numbness or tingling of the fingers or toes, rapid weight gain (three to five pounds within a week), reduced alertness, skin rash, swelling, or unusual bleeding or bruising.

INTERACTIONS

Metoprolol interacts with several other types of medications:

1. Indomethacin, aspirin, or other salicylates may decrease the blood-pressure-lowering effects of beta blockers.

2. Concurrent use of beta blockers and calcium channel blockers (diltiazem, nifedipine, verapamil) or disopyramide can lead to heart failure or very low blood pressure.

3. Cimetidine and oral contraceptives (birth control pills) can increase the blood concentrations of metoprolol, which can result in greater side effects.

4. Alcohol, barbiturates, and rifampin can decrease the blood concentrations of metoprolol, which can result in a decrease of effectiveness.

5. Side effects may be increased if beta blockers are taken with clonidine, digoxin, epinephrine, phenylephrine, phenylpropanolamine, phenothiazine tranquilizers, prazosin, or monoamine oxidase (MAO) inhibitors. At least 14 days should separate the use of a beta blocker and the use of an MAO inhibitor.

6. Beta blockers may antagonize (work against) the effects of theophylline, aminophylline, albuterol, isoproterenol, metaproterenol, and terbutaline.

7. Beta blockers can also interact with insulin or oral antidiabetic agents, raising or lowering blood sugar levels and masking the symptoms of low blood sugar.

8. The action of beta blockers may be increased if they are used with chlorpromazine, furosemide, or hydralazine, which may have a negative effect.

BE SURE TO TELL YOUR DOCTOR about any medications you are currently taking, especially any listed above.

WARNINGS

- Tell your doctor if you have ever had unusual or allergic reactions to any medications, especially to metoprolol or any other beta blocker (acebutolol, atenolol, carteolol, esmolol, labetalol, nadolol, penbutolol, pindolol, propranolol, or timolol).
- Tell your doctor if you now have or have ever had allergies, asthma, hay fever, eczema, slow heartbeat, bronchitis, diabetes mellitus, emphysema, heart or blood vessel disease, kidney disease, liver disease, thyroid disease, or poor circulation in the fingers or toes.
- You may want to check your pulse while taking this medication. If your pulse is much slower than your usual rate (or if it is less than 50 beats per minute), check with your doctor. A pulse rate that is too slow may cause circulation problems.
- This medicine may affect your body's response to exercise. Make sure you discuss with your doctor a safe amount of exercise for your medical condition.

• It is important that you do not stop taking this medicine without first checking with your doctor. Some conditions may become worse when the medicine is stopped suddenly, and the danger of a heart attack is increased in some patients. Your doctor may want you to reduce gradually the amount of medicine you take before stopping completely to minimize the potential risks. Make sure that you have enough medicine on hand to last through vacations, holidays, and weekends.

• Before having surgery or any other medical or dental treatment, tell your doctor or dentist that you are taking metoprolol. Often, this medication will be discontinued 48 hours prior to any major surgery.

• Metoprolol can cause dizziness, drowsiness, lightheadedness, or decreased alertness. Exercise caution while driving a car or using any potentially dangerous machinery.

• While taking this medicine, do not use any over-the-counter (nonprescription) allergy, asthma, cough, cold, sinus, or diet preparation without first checking with your pharmacist or doctor. Some of these medicines can result in high blood pressure when taken at the same time as a beta blocker.

• Be sure to tell your doctor if you are pregnant. Animal studies have shown that some beta blockers, when used in very high doses, can cause problems in pregnancy. Adequate studies have not been conducted in humans, but there has been some association between beta blockers used during pregnancy and low birth weight, as well as breathing problems and slow heart rate in newborn infants. However, other reports have shown no effects on newborn infants. Also, tell your doctor if you are breast-feeding an infant. Although this medicine has not been shown to cause problems in breast-fed infants, some of the medicine may pass into breast milk, so caution is warranted.

---

metoprolol and hydrochlorothiazide combination

BRAND NAME (Manufacturer)
Lopressor HCT (Geigy)
TYPE OF DRUG
Beta-adrenergic blocking agent and diuretic
INGREDIENTS
metoprolol and hydrochlorothiazide
DOSAGE FORM
Tablets (50 mg metoprolol and 25 mg hydrochlorothiazide; 100 mg metoprolol and 25 mg hydrochlorothiazide; and 100 mg metoprolol and 50 mg hydrochlorothiazide)
STORAGE
Metoprolol and hydrochlorothiazide combination tablets should be stored at room temperature in a tightly closed, light-resistant container.

USES

Metoprolol and hydrochlorothiazide combination is prescribed to treat high blood pressure. Hydrochlorothiazide is a diuretic (water pill), which reduces fluid accumulation in the body by increasing the elimination of sodium and water through the kidneys. Metoprolol belongs to a group of medications known as beta-adrenergic blocking agents or, more commonly, beta blockers. They work by controlling impulses along certain nerve pathways.

TREATMENT

This medication can be taken with a glass of water, with meals, immediately following meals, or on an empty stomach, depending on your doctor's instructions.

Try to take the medication at the same time(s) each day. Avoid taking a dose after 6:00 P.M.; otherwise, you may have to get up during the night to urinate.

If you miss a dose of this medication, take the missed dose as soon as possible, unless it is almost time for your next dose. In that case, do not take the missed dose at all; just wait until the next scheduled dose. Do not double the dose.

Metoprolol and hydrochlorothiazide combination does not cure high blood pressure, but it will help to control the condition as long as you continue to take it.

SIDE EFFECTS

Minor. Anxiety, cold hands and feet (due to decreased blood circulation to the skin, fingers, and toes), constipation, cramps, decreased sexual ability, diarrhea, difficulty in sleeping, dizziness, drowsiness, dryness of the eyes and skin, gas, headache, heartburn, loss of appetite, nervousness, restlessness, stomach discomfort, sweating, or tiredness. These side effects should disappear as your body adjusts to the medication.

Hydrochlorothiazide can cause increased sensitivity to sunlight. It is, therefore, important to avoid prolonged exposure to sunlight and sunlamps. Wear protective clothing and sunglasses, and use an effective sunscreen.

If you become extra-sensitive to the cold, be sure to dress warmly during cold weather.

Plain, nonmedicated eye drops (artificial tears) may help to relieve eye dryness.

To relieve constipation, increase the amount of fiber in your diet (fresh fruits and vegetables, salads, bran, and whole-grain breads), and exercise (unless your doctor directs you to do otherwise).

To avoid dizziness or light-headedness when you stand, contract and relax the muscles of your legs for a few moments before rising. Do this by alternately pushing one foot against the floor while raising the other foot slightly, so that you are "pumping" your legs in a pedaling motion.

Major. Tell your doctor about any side effects that are persistent or particularly bothersome. IT IS ESPECIALLY IMPORTANT TO TELL YOUR DOCTOR about blurred vision, confusion, depression, difficulty in breathing, dry mouth, excessive thirst, fever, hair loss, hallucinations, itching, joint pain, mood changes, muscle pain or spasms, nausea, nightmares, numbness or tingling in the fingers or toes, palpitations, rapid weight gain (three to five pounds within a week), reduced alertness, ringing in the ears, skin rash, sore throat, swelling, thirst, unusual bleeding or bruising, vomiting, weakness, or yellowing of the eyes or skin.

INTERACTIONS

Metoprolol and hydrochlorothiazide combination can interact with several other types of medications:

1. Indomethacin, aspirin, and other salicylates may decrease the blood-pressure-lowering effects of beta blockers.
2. Concurrent use of metoprolol and calcium channel blockers (diltiazem, nifedipine, verapamil) or disopyramide can lead to heart failure or very low blood pressure.
3. Cimetidine can increase the blood levels of metoprolol, which can result in greater side effects. Side effects may also be increased when metoprolol is taken with clonidine, digoxin, epinephrine, phenylephrine, phenylpropanolamine, phenothiazine tranquilizers, prazosin, reserpine, or monoamine oxidase (MAO) inhibitors. At least 14 days should separate the use of metoprolol and the use of an MAO inhibitor in order to prevent potentially dangerous interactions.
4. Alcohol, barbiturates, and rifampin can decrease the blood concentrations of metoprolol, which can result in a decrease of effectiveness.
5. Metoprolol can antagonize (act against) the effects of theophylline, aminophylline, albuterol, isoproterenol, metaproterenol, and terbutaline.
6. Metoprolol and hydrochlorothiazide combination can interact with insulin and oral antidiabetic agents, raising or lowering blood sugar levels and masking the symptoms of low blood sugar.
7. Hydrochlorothiazide can decrease the effectiveness of oral anticoagulants (blood thinners, such as warfarin), antigout medications, and methenamine.
8. Fenfluramine may increase the blood-pressure-lowering effects of this drug, which can be dangerous.
9. Cholestyramine and colestipol can decrease the absorption of hydrochlorothiazide from the gastrointestinal tract. This drug should, therefore, be taken one hour before or four hours after a dose of cholestyramine or colestipol (if you have also been prescribed one of these drugs).
10. Hydrochlorothiazide may increase the side effects of amphotericin B, calcium, cortisone and cortisone-like steroids (such as dexamethasone, hydrocortisone, prednisone, and prednisolone), digoxin, digitalis, lithium, quinidine, sulfonamide antibiotics, and vitamin D.
11. The action of beta blockers may be increased if they are used with chlorpromazine, furosemide, hydralozine, or oral contraceptives, which may have a negative effect.

Before starting metoprolol and hydrochlorothiazide combination, BE SURE TO TELL YOUR DOCTOR about all of the medications you are currently taking, especially any of the ones listed above.

WARNINGS

• Tell your doctor about unusual or allergic reactions you have had to any medications, especially to metoprolol or any other beta blocker (acebutolol, atenolol, carteolol, esmolol, labetalol, nadolol, penbutolol, pindolol, propranolol, or timolol), to hydrochlorothiazide or other diuretics (such as bendroflumethiazide, benzthiazide, chlorothiazide, chlorthalidone, cyclothiazide, hydroflumethiazide, methyclothiazide, metolazone, polythiazide, quinethazone, trichlormethiazide, and furosemide), or to any sulfa drug (oral antidiabetic medication or sulfonamide antibiotics).

• Tell your doctor if you now have or if you have ever had asthma, diabetes mellitus, heart disease, gout, kidney disease or problems with urination, liver disease, lung disease, pancreatitis, poor circulation in the fingers or toes, systemic lupus erythematosus, or thyroid disease.

• Hydrochlorothiazide can cause potassium loss. Signs of potassium loss include dry mouth, muscle pain or cramps, nausea, thirst, vomiting, and weakness. If you experience any of these symptoms, call your doctor. To help prevent this problem, your doctor may have blood tests performed periodically to monitor your potassium levels. To help avoid potassium loss, take this medication with a glass of fresh or frozen orange juice or cranberry juice, or eat a banana every day. The use of a salt substitute also helps to prevent potassium loss. Do not change your diet, however, until you discuss it with your doctor. Too much potassium may also be dangerous.

• While taking this medication, limit your intake of alcohol in order to prevent dizziness and light-headedness.

• Do not take any over-the-counter (nonprescription) medication for weight control or for allergy, asthma, cough, cold or sinus problems unless you first check with your doctor.

• To prevent severe water loss (dehydration) while taking this medication, check with your doctor if you have any illness that causes severe or continuous nausea, vomiting, or diarrhea.

• This medication can raise blood sugar levels in diabetic patients. Blood sugar levels should be monitored carefully with blood or urine tests when this medication is being taken.

• You may want to check your pulse while taking this medication. If your pulse is much slower than your usual rate (or if it is less than 50 beats per minute), discuss the situation with your doctor. A pulse rate that is too slow may cause circulation problems.

• Metoprolol can affect your body's response to exercise. Make sure you ask your doctor what an appropriate amount of exercise would be for you, taking into account your medical condition.

• Before having surgery or any other medical or dental treatment, tell your doctor or dentist that you are taking this medicine. Often, this medication will be discontinued 48 hours prior to any major surgery.

• This medication can cause dizziness, drowsiness, lightheadedness, or decreased alertness. Therefore, exercise caution while driving a car or operating potentially dangerous machinery.

• A doctor does not usually prescribe a "fixed-dose" drug like this as the first choice in the treatment of high blood pressure. Usually, the patient first receives each ingredient singly. If there is an adequate response to the fixed dose contained in this product, it can then be substituted. The advantage of a combination product is increased convenience and (often) decreased cost.

• It is important that you do not stop taking this medicine unless you first check with your doctor. Some conditions worsen when this medicine is stopped suddenly, and the danger of a heart attack is increased in some patients. Your doctor may, therefore, want you to gradually reduce the amount of medicine you take before stopping completely. Make sure that you have enough medicine on hand to last through vacations, holidays, and weekends.

• Be sure to tell your doctor if you are pregnant. Animal studies have shown that some beta blockers can cause problems in pregnancy when used at very high doses. Adequate studies have not been conducted in humans, but there has been some association between beta blockers used during pregnancy and low birth weight, as well as breathing problems and slow heart rate in newborn infants. However, other reports have shown no effects on newborn infants. Also, tell your doctor if you are breast-feeding an infant. Although problems in humans have not yet been reported, small amounts of metoprolol and hydrochlorothiazide pass into breast milk, so caution is warranted.

Metra—see phendimetrazine

MetroGel—see metronidazole

---

metronidazole

BRAND NAMES (Manufacturers)
Flagyl (Searle)
MetroGel (Curatab)
metronidazole (various manufacturers)
Metryl (Lemmon)
Protostat (Ortho)
Satric (Savage)
TYPE OF DRUG
Antibiotic and antiparasitic
INGREDIENT
metronidazole
DOSAGE FORM
Tablets (250 mg and 500 mg)
Topical gel (0.75%)
STORAGE
Metronidazole should be stored at room temperature in a tightly closed, light-resistant container. The topical gel form of this medication should never be frozen.

USES

Metronidazole is used to treat a wide variety of infections, including infections of the vagina, urinary tract, lower respiratory tract, bones, joints, intestinal tract, and skin. It is also used topically to treat acne rosacea. It acts by killing bacteria or parasites.

TREATMENT

In order to avoid stomach irritation, you should take metronidazole with food or with a full glass of water or milk (unless your doctor directs you to do otherwise).

Metronidazole works best when the level of medicine in your bloodstream is kept constant. It is best, therefore, to take the doses at evenly spaced intervals day and night. For example, if you are to take three doses a day, the doses should be spaced eight hours apart.

Try not to miss any doses of this medication. If you do miss a dose, take the missed dose as soon as possible, unless it is almost time for the next dose. In that case, do not take the missed dose at all; just return to your regular dosing schedule. Do not double the next dose.

It is important to continue to take this medication for the entire time prescribed by your doctor (usually seven to 14 days), even if the symptoms disappear before the end of that period. If you stop taking the drug too soon, resistant bacteria and parasites are given a chance to continue growing, and the infection could recur.

SIDE EFFECTS

Minor. Abdominal cramps, constipation, decreased sexual interest, diarrhea, dizziness, dry mouth, headache, insomnia, irritability, joint pain, loss of appetite, metallic taste in the mouth, nasal congestion, nausea, restlessness, or vomiting. These side effects should disappear as your body adjusts to the medication.

To relieve constipation, increase the amount of fiber in your diet (fresh fruits and vegetables, salads, bran, and whole-grain breads), exercise, and drink more water (unless your doctor directs you to do otherwise).

If you feel dizzy, sit or lie down for a while; get up slowly from a sitting or reclining position, and be careful on stairs.

To relieve mouth dryness, chew sugarless gum or suck on ice chips or a piece of hard candy.

Major. Tell your doctor about any side effects that are persistent or particularly bothersome. IT IS ESPECIALLY IMPORTANT TO TELL YOUR DOCTOR about confusion, convulsions, flushing, hives, itching, joint pain, loss of bladder control, mouth sores, numbness or tingling in the fingers or toes, rash, sense of pressure inside your abdomen, unexplained sore throat and fever, or unusual weakness. Also, if your symptoms of infection seem to be getting worse rather than improving, you should contact your doctor.

INTERACTIONS

Metronidazole interacts with several other types of drugs:

1. Concurrent use of alcohol and metronidazole can lead to a severe reaction (abdominal cramps, nausea, vomiting, headache, and flushing), the severity of which is dependent upon the amount of alcohol ingested.

2. Concurrent use of disulfiram and metronidazole can lead to confusion.

3. The effects of oral anticoagulants (blood thinners, such as warfarin) may be increased by metronidazole, which can lead to bleeding complications.

4 Barbiturates can increase the breakdown of metronidazole, which can decrease its effectiveness.

5. Cimetidine can decrease the breakdown of metronidazole, which can increase the chance of side effects.

BE SURE TO TELL YOUR DOCTOR about any medications you are currently taking, especially any of those listed above.

WARNINGS

- Tell your doctor about unusual or allergic reactions you have had to any medications, especially to metronidazole.
- Before starting to take this medication, be sure to tell your doctor if you now have or if you have ever had blood disorders, a central nervous system (brain or spinal cord) disease, or liver disease.
- When metronidazole is used to treat a vaginal infection, sexual partners should receive concurrent therapy in order to prevent reinfection. In addition, sexual intercourse should be avoided or condoms should be used until treatment is completed.
- This medication has been prescribed for your current infection only. Another infection later on, or one that someone else has, may require different drug therapy. Therefore, you should not give your medicine to other people or use it for other infections, unless your doctor specifically directs you to do so.

• If this drug makes you dizzy, avoid tasks that require alertness, such as driving a car or operating potentially dangerous machinery.
• Before having surgery or any other medical or dental treatment, be sure to tell your doctor or dentist that you are taking this medication.
• Be sure to tell your doctor if you are pregnant. Although metronidazole appears to be safe, it does cross the placenta, and extensive studies in pregnant women have not been conducted. Also, tell your doctor if you are breast-feeding an infant. Metronidazole passes into breast milk.

Metryl—see metronidazole

Mevacor—see lovastatin

---

mexiletine

BRAND NAME (Manufacturer)
Mexitil (Boehringer Ingelheim)
TYPE OF DRUG
Antiarrhythmic
INGREDIENT
mexiletine
DOSAGE FORM
Capsules (150 mg, 200 mg, and 250 mg)
STORAGE
Mexiletine should be stored at room temperature in a tightly closed container. It should not be exposed to high temperatures.

USES

Mexiletine is used to treat arrhythmias (irregular heart rhythms). This medication works through the suppression of irregular heartbeats and the establishment of a more normal rhythm.

TREATMENT

Mexiletine can be taken with meals or an antacid to decrease stomach irritation.

Try to take mexiletine at the same times each day. This medication is most effective when the amount of the drug in your bloodstream is kept at a constant level. Mexiletine should, therefore, be taken at evenly spaced intervals day and night. For example, if you are supposed to take mexiletine three times per day, the doses should be spaced eight hours apart. Your doctor can determine the best dose of mexiletine for you by measuring the amount in your blood. You may need periodic blood tests for this reason.

If you miss a dose of this medication and remember within four hours (if you are taking it three times per day) or within six hours (if you are taking it two times per day), take the missed dose and then return to your regular dosing schedule. If more than that time has passed, do not take the missed dose; just return to your regular dosing schedule. Do not double the next dose.

SIDE EFFECTS

Minor. Abdominal pain, altered taste, changes in appetite, constipation, diarrhea, dizziness, dry skin, fatigue, fluid accumulation, headaches, heartburn, hiccups, hot flashes, light-headedness, nausea, nervousness, sleeping problems, slowed heart rate, sweating, vomiting, or weakness. These side effects should disappear as your body adjusts to the medication.

To relieve constipation, increase the amount of fiber in your diet (fresh fruits and vegetables, salads, bran, and whole-grain breads), exercise, and drink more water (unless your doctor directs you to do otherwise).

If you become dizzy, sit or lie down for a while; get up slowly from a sitting or reclining position, and be careful on stairs.

Major. Tell your doctor about any side effects that are persistent or particularly bothersome. IT IS ESPECIALLY IMPORTANT TO TELL YOUR DOCTOR about black or tarry stools, chest pain, confusion, coordination difficulties, depression, difficult or painful urination, fainting, fever, hair loss, impotence, palpitations, psychological changes, rash, ringing in the ears, seizures, shortness of breath, speech difficulties, tingling or numbness in the hands or feet, trembling of the hands, or visual disturbances.

INTERACTIONS

Mexiletine interacts with several other types of medications:
1. Acetazolamide, sodium bicarbonate, or high doses of antacids can decrease the elimination of mexiletine from the body, which can increase the risks of side effects.
2. Cimetidine can increase the blood levels of mexiletine, which can increase the risks of side effects.
3. Phenytoin, rifampin, and phenobarbital can decrease the blood levels of mexiletine, which can decrease its effectiveness.

Before starting mexiletine, BE SURE TO TELL YOUR DOCTOR about any medications you are currently taking, especially any of those listed above.

WARNINGS

• Tell your doctor about any unusual or allergic reactions you have had to any medications, especially to mexiletine.
• Before taking mexiletine, tell your doctor if you now have or if you have ever had heart block, heart failure, liver disease, low blood pressure, or seizures.
• If this drug makes you dizzy or light-headed, do not take part in any activity that requires alertness, such as driving a car or operating potentially dangerous machinery.
• Before having surgery or any other medical or dental treatment, be sure to tell your doctor or dentist that you are taking mexiletine.
• Do not take any over-the-counter (nonprescription) asthma, allergy, sinus, cough, cold, or diet preparation without first checking with your pharmacist or doctor.
• Do not stop taking this drug without first consulting your doctor. Stopping antiarrhythmics abruptly may cause a serious change in the activity of your heart. Your doctor may, therefore, want to reduce your dosage gradually.
• Be sure to tell your doctor if you are pregnant. Although mexiletine appears to be safe in animals, studies in pregnant women have not been conducted. Also, tell your doctor if you are breast-feeding an infant. Small amounts of mexiletine pass into human breast milk.

Mexitil—see mexiletine

miconazole (vaginal)

BRAND NAMES (Manufacturers)
Monistat 3 (Ortho)
Monistat 7 (Ortho)*
Monistat Dual-Pak (Ortho)
*Available without a prescription.

TYPE OF DRUG
Vaginal antifungal agent

INGREDIENT
miconazole

DOSAGE FORMS
Vaginal cream (2%)
Lotion (2%)
Vaginal suppositories (100 mg and 200 mg)

STORAGE
Store at room temperature in a tightly closed container.

USES

Miconazole is used to treat fungal infections of the vagina. This medication is an antifungal agent that prevents the growth and multiplication of the yeast-like fungus *Candida*.

TREATMENT

Miconazole vaginal cream and suppositories are packaged with detailed directions for use. Follow these instructions carefully. An applicator will probably be provided.

You should wash the vaginal area carefully prior to inserting the cream or suppository.

If you begin to menstruate while being treated with miconazole, continue with your regular dosing schedule.

If you miss a dose, insert the missed dose as soon as possible. However, if you do not remember until the following day, do not insert the missed dose at all; just return to your regular dosing schedule. Do not double the dose.

It is important to continue to insert this medication for the entire time prescribed by your doctor, even if the symptoms disappear before the end of that time. If you stop using the drug too soon, resistant fungi are given a chance to continue growing, and your infection could recur.

Usually, one three-day or one seven-day course of miconazole is sufficient. However, it may be repeated if your doctor determines that *Candida* is still causing your infection.

SIDE EFFECTS

Minor. You may experience vaginal burning, itching, or irritation when this drug is inserted. This sensation should disappear as your body adjusts to the medication.

Do not treat any side effects that occur in the area of the infection unless you first consult your doctor.

Major. Tell your doctor about any side effects that are persistent or particularly bothersome. IT IS ESPECIALLY IMPORTANT TO TELL YOUR DOCTOR about headache, hives, pelvic cramps, or skin rash.

INTERACTIONS

Miconazole (vaginal) does not interact with other medications if it is used according to directions.

WARNINGS

- Tell your doctor about unusual or allergic reactions you have had to any medications, especially to miconazole.
- Tell your doctor if you have had other vaginal infections, especially if they have been resistant to treatment.
- To prevent reinfection, avoid sexual intercourse or ask your partner to use a condom until treatment is complete.
- There may be some vaginal drainage while you are using this medication; therefore, you may want to use a sanitary napkin or panty liner to prevent the staining of clothing.
- Wear cotton panties rather than those made of nylon or other nonporous materials while being treated for a fungal infection of the vagina. Also, in order to prevent reinfection, always wear freshly laundered underclothes.
- If there is no improvement in your condition, or if irritation in the area continues after several days of treatment, CONTACT YOUR DOCTOR. This medication may be causing an allergic reaction, or it may not be effective against the organism causing your infection.
- This drug has been prescribed for you current infection only. Another infection later on, or one that someone else has, may require a different medication. You should not give your medication to other women or use it for other infections, unless your doctor specifically directs you to do so.
- Be sure to tell your doctor if you are pregnant. Small amounts of miconazole are absorbed from the vagina, so caution should be used, especially during the first three months of pregnancy. In addition, your doctor may want to change the instructions on how you are to insert this medication if you are pregnant. Also, tell your doctor if you are breast-feeding an infant. It is not known whether miconazole passes into breast milk.

Micrainin—see meprobamate and aspirin combination

Micro-K—see potassium chloride

Micro-K Extencaps—see potassium chloride

Micronase—see glyburide

Microsulfon—see sulfonamide antibiotics (oral)

Microx—see metolazone

Mictrin—see hydrochlorothiazide

Midamor—see amiloride

Midol 200—see ibuprofen

Millazine—see thioridazine

Miltown—see meprobamate

Minipress—see prazosin

Minocin—see minocycline

minocycline

BRAND NAME (Manufacturer)
Minocin (Lederle)

TYPE OF DRUG
Antibiotic
INGREDIENT
minocycline
DOSAGE FORMS
Capsules (50 mg and 100 mg)
Tablets (50 mg and 100 mg)
Oral suspension (50 mg per 5-ml spoonful, with 5% alcohol)
STORAGE
Minocycline capsules, tablets, and oral suspension should be stored at room temperature in tightly closed, light-resistant containers.

USES

Minocycline is used to treat a wide range of bacterial infections and to prevent meningococcal meningitis. It acts by preventing the growth of bacteria. This drug kills susceptible bacteria, but it is not effective against viruses or fungi.

TREATMENT

To avoid stomach upset, you can take this medication with food (unless your doctor directs you to do otherwise).

The suspension form of this medication should be shaken well just before measuring each dose. The contents tend to settle on the bottom of the bottle, so it is necessary to shake the container to distribute the ingredients evenly and equalize the doses. Each dose should be measured carefully with a specially designed 5-ml measuring spoon. An ordinary kitchen teaspoon is not accurate enough.

Minocycline works best when the level of medicine in your bloodstream is kept constant. It is best, therefore, to take the doses at evenly spaced intervals day and night. For example, if you are to take two doses a day, the doses should be spaced 12 hours apart.

If you miss a dose of this medication, take the missed dose immediately. However, if you do not remember to take the missed dose until it is almost time for your next dose, take it; space the following dose about halfway through the regular interval between doses; then return to your regular dosing schedule. Try not to skip any doses.

It is important to continue to take this medication for the entire time prescribed by your doctor, even if the symptoms disappear before the end of that period. If you stop taking the drug too soon, resistant bacteria are given a chance to continue growing, and the infection could recur.

SIDE EFFECTS

Minor. Diarrhea, dizziness, headache, light-headedness, loss of appetite, nausea, stomach cramps and upset, vomiting, or discoloration of the nails. These side effects should disappear as your body adjusts to the medication.

Minocycline can increase your sensitivity to sunlight. You should, therefore, try to avoid prolonged exposure to sunlight and sunlamps. Wear protective clothing and sunglasses, and use an effective sunscreen.

If you feel dizzy or light-headed, sit or lie down for a while; get up from a sitting or lying position slowly, and be careful on stairs.

Major. Tell your doctor about any side effects that are persistent or particularly bothersome. IT IS ESPECIALLY IMPORTANT TO TELL YOUR DOCTOR about darkened tongue, difficulty in breathing, joint pain, mouth irritation, rash, rectal or vaginal itching, sore throat and fever, unusual bleeding or bruising, or yellowing of the eyes or skin. Also, if your symptoms of infection seem to be getting worse rather than improving, you should contact your doctor.

INTERACTIONS

Minocycline interacts with several other types of drugs:

1. It can increase the absorption of digoxin, which may lead to digoxin toxicity.

2. The gastrointestinal side effects (nausea, vomiting, and stomach upset) of theophylline may be increased by minocycline.

3. The dosage of oral anticoagulants (blood thinners, such as warfarin) may need to be adjusted when this medication is started.

4. Minocycline may decrease the effectiveness of oral contraceptives (birth control pills), and pregnancy could result. You should, therefore, use a different or additional form of birth control while taking minocycline. Discuss this with your doctor.

5. Antacids, calcium channel blockers, and iron may decrease the effects of this drug if they are taken at the same time. Two to three hours should separate doses of these medications and minocycline.

BE SURE TO TELL YOUR DOCTOR about any medications you are currently taking, especially any of those listed above.

WARNINGS

- Tell your doctor about unusual or allergic reactions you have had to any medications, especially to minocycline or to oxytetracycline, doxycycline, or tetracycline.
- Tell your doctor if you now have or if you have ever had kidney or liver disease.
- Minocycline can cause dizziness or light-headedness. Your ability to perform tasks that require alertness, such as driving a car or operating potentially dangerous machinery, may be decreased. Appropriate caution should, therefore, be taken.
- Minocycline can affect tests for syphilis; tell your doctor you are taking this medication if you are also being treated for this disease.
- Make sure that your prescription for this medication is marked with the expiration date. The drug should be discarded after the expiration date. If the drug is used after this date, serious side effects (especially to the kidneys) could result.
- This medication has been prescribed for your current infection only. Another infection later on, or one that someone else has, may require a different medicine. You should not give your medicine to other people or use it for other infections, unless your doctor specifically directs you to do so.
- Be sure to tell your doctor if you are pregnant or if you are breast-feeding an infant. Minocycline crosses the placenta and passes into breast milk. This drug can cause permanent discoloration of the teeth and can inhibit tooth and bone growth if used during their development. In addition, it should not be used for infants or for children less than eight years of age.

Minodyl—see minoxidil (systemic)

minoxidil (systemic)

BRAND NAME (Manufacturer)
Loniten (Upjohn)
Minodyl (Quantum)
TYPE OF DRUG
Antihypertensive
INGREDIENT
minoxidil
DOSAGE FORM
Tablets (2.5 mg and 10 mg)
STORAGE
Minoxidil should be stored at room temperature in a tightly closed container.

USES

In its oral tablet form, minoxidil is used to treat high blood pressure. It lowers blood pressure by dilating (widening) the blood vessels in the body.

TREATMENT

Minoxidil can be taken either on an empty stomach or with food or a full glass of water or milk (as directed by your doctor or pharmacist).

In order to become accustomed to taking this medication, try to take it at the same time(s) each day.

Minoxidil does not cure high blood pressure, but it will help to control the condition as long as you continue to take the medication.

If you miss a dose of this medication, take the missed dose as soon as possible, unless it is almost time for your next dose. In that case, do not take the missed dose at all; just return to your regular dosing schedule. Do not double the next dose.

SIDE EFFECTS

Minor. Fatigue, flushing, headache, nausea, or vomiting. These side effects should disappear as your body adjusts to the medication.
Major. Tell your doctor about any side effects that are persistent or particularly bothersome. IT IS ESPECIALLY IMPORTANT TO TELL YOUR DOCTOR about abnormal hair growth, breast tenderness (in both sexes), chest pain, difficult or painful urination, darkening of the skin, palpitations, rapid weight gain (three to five pounds within a week), skin rash, or unusual bleeding or bruising.

INTERACTIONS

Concurrent use of minoxidil and guanethidine can cause a severe drop in blood pressure.

BE SURE TO TELL YOUR DOCTOR about any medications you are currently taking, especially guanethidine.

WARNINGS

- Tell your doctor about unusual or allergic reactions you have had to any medications, especially to minoxidil.
- Before starting to take this medication, be sure to tell your doctor if you have ever had angina, heart failure, a heart attack, kidney disease, pericardial effusions, pheochromocytoma, or a stroke.
- Do not take any over-the-counter (nonprescription) cough, cold, allergy, asthma, sinus, or diet medication unless you first check with your doctor or pharmacist. Some of these products can increase your blood pressure.
- Do not stop taking minoxidil unless you first check with your doctor. Stopping the drug abruptly may lead to a worsening of your high blood pressure. Your doctor may, therefore, want to reduce your dosage gradually or start you on another medication when you stop taking minoxidil in order to prevent this from occurring.
- Be sure to tell your doctor if you are pregnant. Birth defects have been reported in the offspring of animals that received large doses of minoxidil during pregnancy. Extensive studies in humans have not been conducted. Also, tell your doctor if you are breast-feeding an infant. Minoxidil passes into breast milk, and it is generally recommended that a woman who is taking this medication should not breast-feed an infant.

---

minoxidil (topical)

BRAND NAME (Manufacturer)
Rogaine (Upjohn)
TYPE OF DRUG
Hair growth stimulant
INGREDIENT
minoxidil
DOSAGE FORM
2% solution (20 mg per ml); 60 ml bottle
STORAGE
Minoxidil topical solution should be stored at room temperature in a tightly closed container. It should be kept away from heat or flames because the solution is flammable (it contains alcohol).

USES

Minoxidil topical solution is used to stimulate hair growth in men who are balding. The drug seems to exert its maximum effect at the crown of the head. The exact way that it works is not known, but it may stimulate hair growth by improving the blood supply to the hair follicles.

TREATMENT

Before applying topical minoxidil, the hair and scalp should be dry. To avoid skin irritation from the alcohol contained in this product, wait at least 30 minutes after washing or shaving before applying this medication to the scalp. The evening dose of medication should be applied at least 30 minutes before bedtime for more complete absorption of the medication into the scalp. This will prevent the medication from rubbing onto the pillowcase.

Complete directions for the use of this product are supplied with the medication. Be sure to ask your doctor or pharmacist for these directions, and follow the instructions carefully. The solution is packaged with three applicators that can be used to apply the solution directly to the scalp. Apply 1 ml to the balding areas of the scalp twice daily (in the morning and evening), unless directed to do otherwise by your doctor. Six sprays with either of the spray applicators deliver a 1-ml dose. The rub-on applicator delivers a 1-ml dose when the bottle is squeezed to fill the top chamber to the black line. The full amount in the chamber should then be applied to the scalp. The total daily dosage should not exceed 2 ml. If finger tips are used to apply the solution, wash hands afterwards to avoid spreading the medication to the eyes or other parts of the body.

Two daily applications for up to 4 months may be required before evidence of hair regrowth is observed. The onset and degree of hair regrowth may be variable among different patients treated with this medicine. If hair regrowth occurs, two daily applications are necessary for additional and continued hair growth (unless your doctor directs you to do otherwise).

First hair growth may be soft, downy, colorless hair that is barely visible. After further treatment, the new hair should be the same color and thickness as the other hair on the scalp.

If one or two applications are missed, restart twice daily applications and return to the usual schedule. Do not attempt to make up for missed doses.

It is important to continue to use this medication for the entire time prescribed by your doctor, even if hair growth does not appear within several months.

If there is no hair growth after at least four months or more, consult with your doctor, as this medication may not be effective for you.

SIDE EFFECTS

Minor. Diarrhea, dry skin/scalp, flaking, itching, local redness, nausea, or vomiting. These side effects should disappear as your body adjusts to the medication.

Major. Tell your doctor about any side effects that are persistent or particularly bothersome. IT IS ESPECIALLY IMPORTANT TO TELL YOUR DOCTOR about back pain, chest pain, a cough, a cold, dizziness, faintness, light-headedness, rapid heart beat, fluid retention, headache, weight gain, or worsening of hair loss.

INTERACTIONS

Use of abrasive or medicated cleansers, medicated cleaners, medicated cosmetics, or any topical, alcohol-containing preparations (such as after-shave lotions or cologne) along with topical minoxidil solution can result in excessive skin dryness and irritation.

WARNINGS

- Tell your doctor about unusual or allergic reactions you have had to any medications, especially to minoxidil.
- Before starting to use this medication, be sure to tell your doctor if you now have or if you have ever had heart disease, high blood pressure, or skin problems, such as dermatitis or local abrasions.
- Because this medication contains alcohol, it can cause skin irritation to sensitive areas. You should, therefore, avoid getting this medication in your eyes, nose, or mouth, or in areas surrounding scratches or burns.
- Do not apply minoxidil to other areas of the body because absorption of the drug may be increased and the risk of side effects may become greater; do not use along with other topical medication on your scalp, unless directed to do so by your doctor.
- Avoid inhaling the spray mist.
- If treatment is stopped, new hair growth will probably be shed within a few months.
- More frequent applications or use of larger doses (more than 1 ml twice daily) will not speed up the process of hair growth and may increase the possibility of side effects.

---

misoprostol

BRAND NAME (Manufacturer)
Cytotec
TYPE OF DRUG
Prostaglandin E1 analog (gastrointestinal protective agent)
INGREDIENT
misoprostol
DOSAGE FORM
Tablets (200 mcg)
STORAGE
Store at room temperature in a tightly closed container.

USES

Misoprostol is used to prevent stomach ulcers in people who are taking nonsteroidal anti-inflammatory drugs (NSAIDs). NSAIDs (such as aspirin, carprofen, diclofenac, diflunisal, fenoprofen, flurbiprofen, ibuprofen, indomethacin, ketoprofen, meclofenamate, mefenamic acid, naproxen, phenylbutazone, piroxicam, salsalate, sulindac, or tolmetin) are frequently prescribed to treat pain or arthritis. NSAIDs have been shown to cause ulcers in some patients. Misoprostol belongs to a group of chemicals called prostaglandins, which exert a protective effect on the stomach by decreasing the secretion of acid and increasing the secretion of mucus.

TREATMENT

This medication should be taken with meals and at bedtime, unless otherwise directed by your doctor.

If you miss a dose, take the missed dose as soon as possible, unless it is almost time for your next dose. If that is the case, do not take the missed dose at all; just return to your regular dosing schedule. Never take a double dose.

Misoprostol treatment should continue for as long as you take a NSAID. This medication should be taken exactly as prescribed by your doctor.

SIDE EFFECTS

Minor. Abdominal pain, change in appetite, constipation, diarrhea, flatulence, gas and bloating, heartburn, menstrual cramps and abnormal bleeding, nausea, or vomiting.

Major. Tell your doctor about any side effects that are persistent or particularly bothersome. IT IS ESPECIALLY IMPORTANT TO TELL YOUR DOCTOR ABOUT chest pain, difficulty in breathing, post-menopausal vaginal bleeding, or rash.

INTERACTIONS

- Antacids decrease the absorption of misoprostol into the bloodstream. However, antacids do not appear to decrease the beneficial effects of misoprostol in preventing ulcers. Consult your doctor before using antacids with this product.

Before starting to take misoprostol, BE SURE TO TELL YOUR DOCTOR about any other medications you are currently taking.

WARNINGS

- Misoprostol should not be taken by anyone with a history of allergy to prostaglandins.
- Tell your doctor immediately if you develop a rash while taking this medication.
- Women should notify their doctors immediately if they experience any abnormal vaginal bleeding while taking this medication.
- Women of childbearing age must use extreme caution not to become pregnant while taking misoprostol. This medication may cause miscarriage. Miscarriages caused by misoprostol may be incomplete, which could lead to potentially dangerous bleeding. ANY WOMAN WHO IS PREGNANT OR PLANS TO BECOME PREGNANT SHOULD NOT TAKE MISOPROSTOL. If you are taking misoprostol and discover that you are pregnant, stop taking the drug immediately and call your doctor.

Nursing mothers should not take misoprostol. The body converts it to misoprostol acid, which can pass into breast milk and cause diarrhea in the nursing infant.

---

mitotane

BRAND NAME (Manufacturer)
Lysodren (Bristol)
TYPE OF DRUG
Antineoplastic (anticancer drug)
INGREDIENT
mitotane
DOSAGE FORM
Tablets (500 mg)
STORAGE
Mitotane should be stored at room temperature in a tightly closed, light-resistant container.

USES

This medication is used to treat cancer of the adrenal gland and Cushing's syndrome (overactive adrenal gland) in patients on whom surgery cannot be performed. Mitotane directly suppresses the activity of the adrenal gland.

TREATMENT

Initial therapy with mitotane often occurs in the hospital until the dosage is stabilized. Mitotane is potent medication. The dosage is usually adjusted to an individual's needs and tolerance. Be sure you understand your doctor's instructions on how this medication should be taken.

Mitotane tablets can be taken either on an empty stomach or, to reduce stomach irritation, with food or milk (unless your doctor directs you to do otherwise).

Try not to miss any doses of this medication. If you do miss a dose, take the missed dose as soon as possible, unless it is almost time for the next dose. In that case, do not take the missed dose at all; just return to your regular dosing schedule. Do not double the next dose.

SIDE EFFECTS

Minor. Diarrhea, dizziness, drowsiness, loss of appetite, nausea, or vomiting. These side effects should disappear as your body adjusts to the medication. However, it is important to continue taking this medication despite the nausea and vomiting that may occur.

Mitotane can also cause hair loss (which is reversible when the medication is discontinued).

If you feel dizzy, sit or lie down for a while; get up slowly from a sitting or reclining position, and be careful on stairs.

Major. Tell your doctor about any side effects that are persistent or particularly bothersome. IT IS ESPECIALLY IMPORTANT TO TELL YOUR DOCTOR about blurred vision, depression, difficult or painful urination, fainting, flushing, lethargy, muscle aches, or skin rash.

INTERACTIONS

Mitotane interacts with several other types of medications:

1. Concurrent use of it with central nervous system depressants (such as alcohol, antihistamines, barbiturates, benzodiazepine tranquilizers, muscle relaxants, narcotics, pain medications, phenothiazine tranquilizers, and sleeping medications) or with tricyclic antidepressants can cause extreme drowsiness.

2. Mitotane can decrease the effectiveness of adrenocorticosteroids (cortisone-like medications).

BE SURE TO TELL YOUR DOCTOR about any medications you are currently taking, especially any of those listed above.

WARNINGS

- Tell your doctor about unusual or allergic reactions you have had to any medications, especially to mitotane.
- Before starting to take this medication, be sure to tell your doctor if you now have or if you have ever had chronic infections or liver disease.
- If this medication makes you dizzy, drowsy, or tired or blurs your vision, avoid any activity that requires alertness, such as driving a car or operating potentially dangerous machinery.
- Do not stop taking this medication unless you first check with your doctor. The effects of mitotane on the adrenal glands last several weeks after the drug is stopped.
- Mitotane can impair your body's response to injury, stress, illness, and infection. If you experience injury, stress, illness, or infection while taking this medication, or shortly after you stop taking it (within several weeks), check with your doctor. You may need to take supplemental adrenal hormone during this period.
- Before having surgery or any other medical or dental treatment, be sure to tell your doctor or dentist that you are taking this medication.
- Be sure to tell your doctor if you are pregnant. Extensive studies of mitotane in pregnant women have not been conducted. The risks should be discussed with your doctor. Also, tell your doctor if you are breast-feeding an infant. It is not known whether mitotane passes into breast milk.

Mixtard—see insulin

Modicon—see oral contraceptives

Moduretic—see amiloride and hydrochlorothiazide combination

Monistat 3—see miconazole (vaginal)

Monistat 7—see miconazole (vaginal)

Monistat Dual-Pak—see miconazole (vaginal)

---

morphine

BRAND NAMES (Manufacturers)
morphine sulfate (various manufacturers)
MS Contin (Purdue-Frederick)
MSIR (Purdue-Frederick)
RMS (Upsher-Smith)
Roxanol (Roxane)
Roxanol SR (Roxane)

TYPE OF DRUG
Analgesic

INGREDIENT
morphine

DOSAGE FORMS
Tablets (15 mg and 30 mg)
Sustained-release tablets (30 mg and 60 mg)
Oral solution (10 mg and 20 mg per 5-ml spoonful, with 10% alcohol; 20 mg per ml)
Rectal suppositories (5 mg, 10 mg, and 20 mg)

STORAGE
Morphine tablets and oral solution should be stored at room temperature in tightly closed, light-resistant containers. The rectal suppositories should be stored in the refrigerator.

USES

Morphine is a narcotic analgesic that acts directly on the central nervous system (brain and spinal cord). It is used to relieve moderate to severe pain.

TREATMENT

In order to avoid stomach upset, you can take morphine with food or milk. This medication works most effectively if you take it at the onset of pain, rather than waiting until the pain becomes intense.

The solution form of this medication can be mixed with fruit juices to improve the taste. Measure each dose carefully with a specially designed 5-ml measuring spoon or with the dropper provided. An ordinary kitchen teaspoon is not accurate enough.

The sustained-release tablets should be swallowed whole. Chewing, crushing, or crumbling the tablets destroys their sustained-release activity and possibly increases the side effects.

To use the suppository form of this medication, remove the foil wrapper and moisten the suppository with water (if the suppository is too soft to insert, refrigerate it for half an hour or run cold water over it before removing the wrapper). Lie on your left side with your right knee bent. Push the suppository into the rectum, pointed end first. Lie still for a few minutes. Try to avoid having a bowel movement for at least an hour (to give the medication time to be absorbed).

If you are taking this medication on a regular schedule and you miss a dose, take the missed dose as soon as possible, unless it is almost time for your next dose. In that case, do not take the missed dose at all; just return to your regular dosing schedule. Do not double the next dose.

SIDE EFFECTS

Minor. Constipation, dizziness, drowsiness, dry mouth, false sense of well-being, flushing, light-headedness, loss of appetite, nausea, rash, or sweating. These side effects should disappear as your body adjusts to the medication.

If you are constipated, increase the amount of fiber in your diet (fresh fruits and vegetables, salads, bran, and whole-grain breads), exercise, and drink more water (unless your doctor directs you to do otherwise).

Chew sugarless gum or suck on ice chips or a piece of hard candy to reduce mouth dryness.

If you feel dizzy or light-headed, sit or lie down for a while; get up from a sitting or lying position slowly, and be careful on stairs.

Major. Tell your doctor about any side effects that are persistent or particularly bothersome. IT IS ESPECIALLY IMPORTANT TO TELL YOUR DOCTOR about anxiety, difficulty in breathing, excitation, fainting, fatigue, painful or difficult urination, palpitations, restlessness, sore throat and fever, tremors, or weakness.

INTERACTIONS

Morphine interacts with several other types of drugs:

1. Concurrent use of it with other central nervous system depressants (such as alcohol, antihistamines, barbiturates, benzodiazepine tranquilizers, muscle relaxants, and phenothiazine tranquilizers) or with tricyclic antidepressants can cause extreme drowsiness.

2. A monoamine oxidase (MAO) inhibitor taken within 14 days of this medication can lead to unpredictable and severe side effects.

3. The depressant effects of morphine can be dangerously increased by chloral hydrate, glutethimide, beta blockers, and furazolidone.

4. The combination of cimetidine and morphine can cause confusion, disorientation, and shortness of breath.

BE SURE TO TELL YOUR DOCTOR about any medications you are currently taking, especially any of those listed above.

WARNINGS

- Tell your doctor about unusual or allergic reactions you have had to any medications, especially to morphine or to other narcotic analgesics (such as codeine, hydrocodone, hydromorphone, meperidine, methadone, oxycodone, and propoxyphene).
- Tell your doctor if you now have or if you have ever had acute abdominal conditions, asthma, brain disease, colitis, epilepsy, gallstones or gallbladder disease, head injuries, heart disease, kidney disease, liver disease, lung disease, mental illness, emotional disorders, enlarged prostate gland, thyroid disease, or urethral stricture.
- If this drug makes you dizzy or drowsy, do not take part in any activity that requires alertness, such as driving a car or operating potentially dangerous machinery.
- Before having surgery or any other medical or dental treatment, be sure to tell your doctor or dentist that you are taking this medication.
- Morphine has the potential for abuse and must be used with caution. Usually, it should not be taken on a regular schedule for longer than ten days (unless your doctor directs you to do so). Tolerance develops quickly; do not increase

the dosage or stop taking the drug abruptly, unless you first consult your doctor. If you have been taking large amounts of this medication, or if you have been taking it for long periods of time, you may experience a withdrawal reaction (muscle aches, diarrhea, gooseflesh, runny nose, nausea, vomiting, shivering, trembling, stomach cramps, sleep disorders, irritability, weakness, excessive yawning, or sweating) when you stop taking it. Your doctor may, therefore, want to reduce the dosage gradually.

• Be sure to tell your doctor if you are pregnant. The effects of this medication during the early stages of pregnancy have not been thoroughly studied in humans. However, regular use of morphine in large doses during the later stages of pregnancy can result in addiction of the fetus, leading to withdrawal symptoms (irritability, excessive crying, tremors, fever, vomiting, diarrhea, sneezing, or excessive yawning) at birth. Also, tell your doctor if you are breast-feeding an infant. Small amounts of this medication may pass into breast milk and cause excessive drowsiness in the nursing infant.

morphine sulfate—see morphine

Motion Cure—see meclizine

Motrin—see ibuprofen

Motrin IB—see ibuprofen

MS Contin—see morphine

MSIR—see morphine

multiple sulfonamides—see sulfonamide antibiotics (oral)

Multi-Vita Drops with Fluoride—see vitamins, multiple, with fluoride

Mus-Lax—see chlorzoxazone and acetaminophen combination

Mycadec DM—see pseudoephedrine, carbinoxamine, and dextromethorphan combination

Mycelex—see clotrimazole (topical)

Mycelex-G—see clotrimazole (vaginal)

Mycitracin ophthalmic—see neomycin, polymyxin B, and bacitracin or gramicidin combination (ophthalmic)

My Cort—see hydrocortisone (topical)

Mycostatin—see nystatin

Myco Triacet—see triamcinolone, neomycin, nystatin, and gramicidin combination (topical)

Myfedrine Plus—see pseudoephedrine and chlorpheniramine combination

Myidone—see primidone

Mykinac—see nystatin

Myleran—see busulfan

Myminic—see phenylpropanolamine and chlorpheniramine combination

Myotonachol—see bethanechol

Myproic acid—see valproic acid

Mysoline—see primidone

Mytussin AC—see codeine and guaifenesin combination

---

nadolol

BRAND NAME (Manufacturer)
Corgard (Princeton Pharm.)
TYPE OF DRUG
Beta-adrenergic blocking agent
INGREDIENT
nadolol
DOSAGE FORM
Tablets (20 mg, 40 mg, 80 mg, 120 mg, and 160 mg)
STORAGE
Nadolol should be stored at room temperature in a tightly closed, light-resistant container.

USES

Nadolol is used to treat high blood pressure and angina pectoris (chest pain). It belongs to a group of medicines known as beta-adrenergic blocking agents or, more commonly, beta blockers. These drugs work by controlling nerve impulses along certain nerve pathways.

TREATMENT

Nadolol can be taken with a glass of water, with meals, immediately following meals, or on an empty stomach, depending on your doctor's instructions. Try to take the medication at the same time(s) each day.

Try not to miss any doses of this medicine. If you do miss a dose, take the missed dose as soon as possible. However, if the next scheduled dose is within eight hours (if you are taking this medicine only once a day) or within four hours (if you are taking this medicine more than once a day), do not take the missed dose at all; just return to your regular dosing schedule. Do not double the next dose.

It is important to remember that nadolol does not cure high blood pressure, but will help you to control your condition as long as you continue your drug therapy.

SIDE EFFECTS

Minor. Anxiety; cold hands or feet (due to decreased blood circulation to the skin, fingers, and toes); constipation; decreased sexual ability; diarrhea; difficulty in sleeping; drowsiness; dryness of the eyes, mouth, and skin; headache; nausea; nervousness; stomach discomfort; tiredness; or weakness. These side effects should disappear during treatment, as your body adjusts to the medication.

If you are extra-sensitive to the cold, be sure to dress warmly during cold weather.

To relieve constipation, increase the amount of fiber in your diet (fresh fruits and vegetables, salads, bran, and whole-grain breads), exercise, and drink more water (unless your doctor directs you to do otherwise).

Plain, nonmedicated eye drops (artificial tears) may help to relieve eye dryness.

Sucking on ice chips or chewing sugarless gum helps to relieve mouth or throat dryness.

Major. Tell your doctor about any side effects that are persistent or particularly bothersome. IT IS ESPECIALLY IMPORTANT TO TELL YOUR DOCTOR about breathing difficulty or wheezing, confusion, dizziness, fever and sore throat, hair loss, hallucinations, light-headedness, mental depression, nightmares, numbness or tingling of the fingers or toes, rapid weight gain (three to five pounds within a week), reduced alertness, swelling, skin rash, or unusual bleeding or bruising.

INTERACTIONS

Nadolol interacts with several other types of medications:

1. Indomethacin, aspirin, or other salicylates may decrease the blood-pressure-lowering effects of beta blockers.

2. Concurrent use of beta blockers and calcium channel blockers (diltiazem, nifedipine, verapamil) or disopyramide can potentially lead to heart failure or very low blood pressure.

3. Side effects may be increased when nadolol is taken with cimetidine, clonidine, digoxin, epinephrine, phenylephrine, phenylpropanolamine, phenothiazine tranquilizers, prazosin, or monoamine oxidase (MAO) inhibitors. At least 14 days should separate the use of a beta blocker and an MAO inhibitor.

4. Alcohol, barbiturates, and rifampin may decrease the blood concentrations of beta blockers, which can result in a decrease in effectiveness.

5. Beta blockers may antagonize (work against) the effects of theophylline, aminophylline, albuterol, isoproterenol, metaproterenol, and terbutaline.

6. Beta blockers can also interact with insulin or oral antidiabetic agents, raising or lowering blood sugar levels or masking the symptoms of low blood sugar.

7. The concurrent use of nadolol and reserpine can have additive blood-pressure-lowering effects and can slow the heartbeat.

8. The action of beta blockers may be increased if they are used with chlorpromazine, furosemide, hydralazine, or oral contraceptives (birth control pills), which may have a negative effect.

BE SURE TO TELL YOUR DOCTOR about any medications you are currently taking, especially any of those listed above.

WARNINGS

- Tell your doctor if you have ever had unusual or allergic reactions to any medications, especially to nadolol or any other beta blocker (acebutolol, atenolol, carteolol, esmolol, labetalol, metoprolol, penbutolol, pindolol, propranolol, or timolol).
- Tell your doctor if you now have or if you have ever had allergies, asthma, hay fever, eczema, slow heartbeat, bronchitis, diabetes mellitus, emphysema, heart or blood vessel disease, kidney disease, liver disease, thyroid disease, or poor circulation in the fingers or toes.
- You may want to check your pulse regularly while you are taking this medication. If your pulse is much slower than your usual rate (or if it is less than 50 beats per minute), check with your doctor. A pulse rate that is too slow may cause circulation problems.
- This medicine may affect your body's response to exercise. Make sure you discuss with your doctor a safe amount of exercise for your medical condition.
- It is important that you do not stop taking this medicine without first checking with your doctor. Some conditions may become worse when the medicine is stopped suddenly, and the danger of a heart attack is increased in some patients. Your doctor may want you to gradually reduce the amount of medicine you take before stopping completely. Make sure that you have enough medicine on hand to last through vacations, holidays, and weekends.
- Before having surgery or any other medical or dental treatment, be sure to tell your physician or dentist that you are taking nadolol. Often, this medication will be discontinued 48 hours prior to any major surgery.
- Nadolol can cause dizziness, drowsiness, lightheadedness, or decreased alertness. You should, therefore, use caution while driving a car or operating any potentially dangerous machinery.
- While taking this medicine, do not use any over-the-counter (nonprescription) allergy, asthma, cough, cold, sinus, or diet preparation unless you first check with your pharmacist or doctor. Some of these medicines can result in high blood pressure when combined with a beta blocker.
- Be sure to tell your doctor if you are pregnant. Animal studies have shown that some beta blockers can cause problems in pregnancy when used at very high doses. Adequate studies have not been conducted in humans, but there has been some association between beta blockers used during pregnancy and low birth weight, as well as breathing problems and slow heart rate in newborn infants. However, other reports have shown no effects on newborn infants. Also, tell your doctor if you are breast-feeding an infant. Although this medicine has not been shown to cause problems in breast-fed infants, some of the medicine may pass into breast milk, so caution is warranted.

---

nadolol and bendroflumethiazide combination

BRAND NAME (Manufacturer)
Corzide (Princeton)

TYPE OF DRUG
Beta-adrenergic blocking agent and diuretic

INGREDIENTS
nadolol and bendroflumethiazide

DOSAGE FORM
Tablets (40 mg nadolol and 5 mg bendroflumethiazide; 80 mg nadolol and 5 mg bendroflumethiazide)

STORAGE

Nadolol and bendroflumethiazide combination tablets should be stored at room temperature in a tightly closed container.

USES

Nadolol and bendroflumethiazide combination is prescribed to treat high blood pressure. Bendroflumethiazide is a diuretic (water pill), which reduces fluid accumulation in the body by increasing the elimination of sodium and water through the kidneys. Nadolol belongs to a group of medicines known as beta-adrenergic blocking agents or beta blockers. They work by controlling impulses along certain nerve pathways.

TREATMENT

Nadolol and bendroflumethiazide can be taken with a glass of water, with a meal, immediately after a meal, or on an empty stomach, depending on your doctor's instructions.

Try to take the medication at the same time(s) each day. Avoid taking a dose after 6:00 P.M.; otherwise, you may have to get up during the night to urinate.

If you miss a dose of nadolol and bendroflumethiazide combination, take the missed dose as soon as possible, unless it is almost time for the next dose. In that case, do not take the missed dose of medication at all; just wait until the next scheduled dose. Do not double the dose.

Nadolol and bendroflumethiazide combination does not cure high blood pressure, but it will help to control the condition as long as you continue to take it.

SIDE EFFECTS

Minor. Abdominal discomfort, constipation, diarrhea, dizziness, drowsiness, dry eyes or skin, fatigue, gas, headache, loss of appetite, or stomach discomfort. These minor side effects should disappear as your body adjusts to therapy with this medication.

Bendroflumethiazide can cause increased sensitivity to sunlight. It is, therefore, important to avoid prolonged exposure to sunlight and sunlamps. Wear protective clothing and sunglasses, and use an effective sunscreen.

If you become extra-sensitive to the cold, be sure to dress warmly during cold weather.

Plain, nonmedicated eye drops (artificial tears) may help to relieve eye dryness.

To relieve constipation, increase the amount of fiber in your diet (fresh fruits and vegetables, salads, bran, and whole-grain breads) and exercise more (unless your doctor directs you to do otherwise).

To avoid dizziness or light-headedness when you stand, contract and relax the muscles of your legs for a few moments before rising. Do this by pushing one foot against the floor while raising the other foot slightly, alternating feet so that you are "pumping" your legs in a pedaling motion.

Major. Tell your doctor about any side effects that are persistent or particularly bothersome. IT IS ESPECIALLY IMPORTANT TO TELL YOUR DOCTOR about blurred vision, depression, dry mouth, fever, hair loss, itching, muscle pain or spasm, nausea, numbness or tingling in the fingers or toes, rapid weight gain (three to five pounds within a week), rash, ringing in the ears, shortness of breath, thirst, vomiting, weakness, or yellowing of the eyes or skin.

INTERACTIONS

This medicine interacts with several other types of medications:

1. Indomethacin, aspirin, and other salicylates may decrease the blood-pressure-lowering effects of beta blockers.
2. Concurrent use of nadolol and disopyramide or calcium channel blockers (diltiazem, nifedipine, verapamil) can lead to heart failure or very low blood pressure.
3. Side effects may be increased when nadolol is taken with cimetidine, clonidine, digoxin, epinephrine, hydralazine, oral contraceptives (birth control pills), phenylephrine, phenylpropanolamine, phenothiazine tranquilizers, prazosin, reserpine, or monoamine oxidase (MAO) inhibitors. At least 14 days should separate the use of nadolol and the use of an MAO inhibitor.
4. Nadolol can antagonize (act against) the effects of theophylline, aminophylline, albuterol, isoproterenol, metaproterenol, and terbutaline.
5. Nadolol can also interact with insulin and oral antidiabetic agents, raising or lowering blood sugar levels and masking the symptoms of low blood sugar.
6. Alcohol, barbiturates, and rifampin can decrease the blood concentrations of beta blockers, which can result in a decrease of effectiveness.
7. The action of beta blockers may be increased if they are used with chlorpromazine, furosemide, or hydralazine, which may have a negative effect.
8. Bendroflumethiazide can decrease the effectiveness of oral anticoagulants (blood thinners, such as warfarin), antigout medications, and methenamine.
9. Fenfluramine may increase the blood-pressure-lowering effects of this drug, which can be dangerous.
10. Cholestyramine and colestipol can decrease the absorption of bendroflumethiazide from the gastrointestinal tract; this medication should, therefore, be taken one hour before or four hours after a dose of cholestyramine or colestipol (if you have also been prescribed one of these medications).
11. Bendroflumethiazide may increase the side effects of amphotericin B, calcium, cortisone and cortisone-like steroids (such as dexamethasone, hydrocortisone, prednisolone, and prednisone), digitalis, digoxin, lithium, quinidine, sulfonamide antibiotics, and vitamin D.

Before starting nadolol and bendroflumethiazide combination, BE SURE TO TELL YOUR DOCTOR about any medications you are currently taking, especially any of those listed above.

WARNINGS

- Tell your doctor about unusual or allergic reactions you have had to any medications, especially to nadolol or any other beta blocker (acebutolol, atenolol, carteolol, esmolol, labetalol, metoprolol, penbutolol, pindolol, propranolol, or timolol), to bendroflumethiazide or other diuretics (such as benzthiazide, chlorothiazide, chlorthalidone, cyclothiazide, hydrochlorothiazide, hydroflumethiazide, methyclothiazide, metolozone, polythiazide, quinethazone, trichlormethiazide, and furosemide), or to any other sulfa drug (oral antidiabetic medication, sulfonamide antibiotic).
- Tell your doctor if you now have or if you have ever had asthma, diabetes mellitus, heart disease, gout, kidney disease or problems with urination, liver disease, pancreatitis,

systemic lupus erythematosus, thyroid disease, or poor circulation in the fingers or toes.

• Bendroflumethiazide can cause potassium loss. Signs of potassium loss include dry mouth, thirst, weakness, muscle pain or cramps, nausea, and vomiting. If you experience any of these symptoms, call your doctor. To help prevent this problem, your doctor may have blood tests performed periodically to monitor your potassium levels. To help avoid potassium loss, take this medication with a glass of fresh or frozen orange juice or cranberry juice, or eat a banana every day. The use of a salt substitute also helps to prevent potassium loss. Do not change your diet, however, until you discuss it with your doctor. Too much potassium may also be dangerous.

• While taking this medication, limit your intake of alcohol, in order to prevent dizziness and light-headedness.

• Do not take any over-the-counter (nonprescription) medication for weight control or for allergy, asthma, cough, cold, or sinus problems unless you first check with your doctor.

• To prevent severe water loss (dehydration) while taking this medication, check with your doctor if you have any illness that causes severe or continuous nausea, vomiting, or diarrhea.

• This medication can raise blood sugar levels in diabetic patients. Blood sugar levels should be monitored carefully with blood or urine tests when this medication is being taken.

• You may want to check your pulse while taking this medication. If your pulse is much slower than your usual rate (or if it is less than 50 beats per minute), check with your doctor. A pulse rate that is too slow may cause circulation problems.

• Nadolol can affect your body's response to exercise. Make sure that you ask your doctor what an appropriate amount of exercise would be for you, taking into account your medical condition.

• Before having surgery or any medical or dental treatment, tell your doctor or dentist about this drug. It may be discontinued 48 hours prior to any major surgery.

• This medication can cause dizziness, drowsiness, lightheadedness, or decreased alertness. Exercise caution while driving a car or operating potentially dangerous machinery.

• A doctor does not usually prescribe a "fixed dose" drug like this as the first choice in the treatment of high blood pressure. Usually, the patient first receives each ingredient singly. If there is an adequate response to the fixed dose contained in this product, it can then be substituted. The advantage of a combination product is increased convenience and (often) decreased cost.

• It is important that you do not stop taking this medicine unless you first check with your doctor. Some conditions worsen when this medicine is stopped suddenly, and the danger of a heart attack is increased in some patients. Your doctor may, therefore, want you to gradually reduce the amount of medicine you take before stopping completely. Make sure that you have enough medicine on hand to last through vacations, holidays, and weekends.

• Be sure to tell your doctor if you are pregnant. Animal studies have shown that some beta blockers can cause problems in pregnancy when used at very high doses. Studies have not been conducted in humans, but there has been some association between beta blockers used during pregnancy and low birth weight, as well as breathing problems and slow heart rate in newborn infants. However, other reports have shown no effects on newborn infants. Also, tell your doctor if you are breast-feeding an infant. Although problems in humans have not yet been reported, small amounts of nadolol and bendroflumethiazide pass into breast milk, so caution is warranted.

---

nafcillin

BRAND NAME (Manufacturer)
Unipen (Wyeth)

TYPE OF DRUG
Penicillin antibiotic

INGREDIENT
nafcillin

DOSAGE FORMS
Tablets (500 mg)
Capsules (250 mg)
Oral solution (250 mg per 5-ml spoonful)

STORAGE
Nafcillin tablets and capsules should be stored at room temperature in tightly closed containers. The oral solution should be stored in the refrigerator in a tightly closed container. Any unused portion of the solution should be discarded after 14 days because the drug loses its potency after that time. This medication should never be frozen.

USES

Nafcillin is used to treat a wide variety of bacterial infections, especially those caused by *Staphylococcus* bacteria. It acts by severely injuring the cell membranes of the infecting bacteria, thereby preventing them from growing and multiplying. Nafcillin kills susceptible bacteria, but it is not effective against viruses, parasites, or fungi.

TREATMENT

Nafcillin should be taken on an empty stomach or with a glass of water one hour before or two hours after a meal. This medication should never be taken with fruit juices or carbonated beverages because the acidity of these drinks destroys the drug in the stomach.

The oral solution should be measured carefully with a specially designed 5-ml measuring spoon. An ordinary kitchen teaspoon is not accurate enough.

Nafcillin works best when the level of medicine in your bloodstream is kept constant. It is best, therefore, to take the doses at evenly spaced intervals day and night. For example, if you are taking four doses a day, the doses should be spaced six hours apart.

If you miss a dose of this medication, take the missed dose immediately. However, if you do not remember to take the missed dose until it is almost time for your next dose, take it; space the following dose about halfway through the regular interval between doses; and then return to your regular dosing schedule. Try not to skip any doses.

Take this drug for the entire time prescribed by your doctor (usually seven to 14 days), even if your symptoms disappear before the end of that period. If you stop taking the drug too soon, resistant bacteria are given a chance to continue growing, and the infection could recur.

SIDE EFFECTS

Minor. Diarrhea, heartburn, nausea, or vomiting. These side effects should disappear as your body adjusts to the medication.

Major. Tell your doctor about any side effects that are persistent or particularly bothersome. IT IS ESPECIALLY IMPORTANT TO TELL YOUR DOCTOR about bloating, chills, cough, darkened tongue, difficult or painful urination, difficulty in breathing, fever, irritation of the mouth, muscle aches, rash, rectal or vaginal itching, severe diarrhea, sore throat, or yellowing of the skin or eyes. Also, if your symptoms of infection seem to be getting worse rather than improving, you should contact your doctor.

INTERACTIONS

Nafcillin interacts with several other types of medications:

1. Probenecid can increase the blood concentrations of this medication.

2. Nafcillin may decrease the effectiveness of oral contraceptives (birth control pills), and pregnancy could result. You should, therefore, use another form of birth control while taking this medication. Discuss this with your doctor.

BE SURE TO TELL YOUR DOCTOR about any medications you are currently taking, especially those listed above.

WARNINGS

- Tell your doctor about unusual or allergic reactions you have had to any medications, especially to nafcillin, penicillins, cephalosporin antibiotics, penicillamine, or griseofulvin.
- Tell your doctor if you now have or if you have ever had kidney disease, asthma, or allergies.
- This medication has been prescribed for your current infection only. Another infection later on, or one that someone else has, may require a different medicine. You should not give your medicine to other people or use it for other infections, unless your doctor specifically directs you to do so.
- Diabetics taking nafcillin should know that this drug can cause a false-positive sugar reaction with a Clinitest urine glucose test. To avoid this problem while taking nafcillin, you should switch to Clinistix or Tes-Tape to test your urine for sugar.
- Be sure to tell your doctor if you are pregnant. Although nafcillin appears to be safe during pregnancy, extensive studies in humans have not been conducted. Also, tell your doctor if you are breast-feeding an infant. Small amounts of this medication pass into breast milk and may temporarily alter the bacterial balance in the intestinal tract of the nursing infant, resulting in diarrhea.

Naldecon—see phenylpropanolamine, phenylephrine, chlorpheniramine, and phenyltoloxamine combination

Naldelate—see phenylpropanolamine, phenylephrine, chlorpheniramine, an dphenyltoloxamine combination

Nalfon—see fenoprofen

Nalfon 200—see fenoprofen

Nalgest—see phenylpropanolamine, phenylephrine, chlorpheniramine, and phenyltoloxamine combination

nalidixic acid

BRAND NAME (Manufacturer)
NegGram (Winthrop)

TYPE OF DRUG
Antibiotic

INGREDIENT
nalidixic acid

DOSAGE FORMS
Tablets (250 mg, 500 mg, and 1,000 mg)
Oral suspension (250 mg per 5-ml spoonful)

STORAGE
Nalidixic acid tablets and suspension should be stored at room temperature in tightly closed containers. This medication should never be frozen.

USES

Nalidixic acid is an antibiotic that is used to treat bacterial urinary tract infections. It works by preventing the growth and multiplication of susceptible bacteria. This medication is not effective against viruses, parasites, or fungi.

TREATMENT

In order to avoid stomach irritation, you can take nalidixic acid with food or with a full glass of water or milk (unless your doctor directs you to do otherwise).

The suspension form of this medication should be shaken well just before measuring each dose. The contents tend to settle on the bottom of the bottle, so it is necessary to shake the container to distribute the ingredients evenly and equalize the doses. Each dose should then be measured carefully with a specially designed 5-ml measuring spoon. An ordinary kitchen teaspoon is not accurate enough to ensure that you receive the proper dose.

Nalidixic acid works best when the level of medicine in your bloodstream and urine is kept constant. It is best, therefore, to take the doses at evenly spaced intervals day and night. For example, if you are to take four doses a day, the doses should be spaced six hours apart.

Try not to miss any doses of this medication. If you do miss a dose, take it as soon as you remember. However, if it is almost time for your next dose, take the missed dose immediately; space the following dose about halfway through the regular dosing interval; and then continue with your regular dosing schedule.

It is important to continue to take this medication for the entire time prescribed by your doctor (usually seven to 14 days), even if the symptoms disappear before the end of that period. If you stop taking the drug too soon, resistant bacteria are given a chance to continue growing, and your infection could recur.

SIDE EFFECTS

Minor. Abdominal pain, diarrhea, dizziness, drowsiness, headache, nausea, vomiting, or weakness. These side effects should disappear as your body adjusts to the medication.

This medication can increase your sensitivity to sunlight. You should, therefore, avoid prolonged exposure to sunlight and sunlamps. Wear protective clothing and sunglasses, and use an effective sunscreen.

If you feel dizzy, sit or lie down for a while; get up slowly from a sitting or reclining position, and be careful on stairs.

Major. Tell your doctor about any side effects that are persistent or particularly bothersome. IT IS ESPECIALLY IMPORTANT TO TELL YOUR DOCTOR about convulsions, itching, joint pain, skin rash, tingling sensations, unusual bleeding or bruising, visual disturbances, or yellowing of the eyes or skin.

INTERACTIONS

This drug can interact with several other types of drugs:

1. Nalidixic acid can increase the effects of oral anticoagulants, which can lead to bleeding complications.

2. Nitrofurantoin can reduce the effectiveness of nalidixic acid.

BE SURE TO TELL YOUR DOCTOR about any medications you are currently taking, especially any listed above.

WARNINGS

- Tell your doctor about unusual or allergic reactions you have had to any medications, especially to nalidixic acid or to cinoxacin or norfloxacin.
- Before starting to take this medication, be sure to tell your doctor if you now have or if you have ever had brain disorders, epilepsy, kidney disease, or liver disease.
- If this drug makes you dizzy or drowsy, do not take part in any activity that requires alertness, such as driving a car or operating potentially dangerous machinery.
- This drug has been prescribed for your current infection only. Another infection later on, or one that someone else has, may require a different medicine. You should not give your medication to other people or use it for other infections, unless your doctor specifically directs you to do so.
- Diabetic patients should know that nalidixic acid can cause false-positive readings of Clinitest urine glucose tests. Temporarily changing to Clinistix or Tes-Tape urine glucose tests avoids this problem. CHECK WITH YOUR DOCTOR before adjusting the dosage of your antidiabetic medication.
- If the symptoms of your infection do not improve within several days after starting this medication, CHECK WITH YOUR DOCTOR. Nalidixic acid may not be effective against the organism causing your infection.
- Be sure to tell your doctor if you are pregnant. Although nalidixic acid may cross the placenta, it appears to be safe during pregnancy. However, extensive studies in humans have not been conducted. Also, tell your doctor if you are breast-feeding an infant. Small amounts of nalidixic acid pass into breast milk.

Napamide—see disopyramide

Napril—see pseudoephedrine and chlorpheniramine combination

Naprosyn—see naproxen

---

naproxen

BRAND NAMES (Manufacturers)
Anaprox (Syntex)
Anaprox DS (Syntex)
Naprosyn (Syntex)

TYPE OF DRUG
Nonsteroidal anti-inflammatory analgesic

INGREDIENT
naproxen (Naprosyn)
naproxen as the sodium salt (Anaprox)

DOSAGE FORMS
Tablets (250 mg, 375 mg, and 500 mg [Naprosyn]; 275 mg and 550 mg [Anaprox])
Oral suspension (125 mg per 5-ml spoonful [Naprosyn])

STORAGE
This medication should be stored in a tightly closed container at room temperature, away from heat and direct sunlight.

USES

Naproxen is used to treat the inflammation (pain, swelling, and stiffness) of certain types of arthritis, gout, bursitis, and tendinitis. Naproxen is also used to treat painful menstruation. Naproxen has been shown to block the production of certain body chemicals, called prostaglandins, that may trigger pain. However, it is not yet fully understood how naproxen works.

TREATMENT

You should take this medication on an empty stomach 30 to 60 minutes before meals or two hours after meals, so that it gets into your bloodstream quickly. However, to decrease stomach irritation, your doctor may want you to take the medicine with food or antacids.

It is important to take naproxen on schedule and not to miss any doses. If you do miss a dose, take it as soon as possible, unless it is almost time for your next dose. In that case, do not take the missed dose at all; just return to your regular dosing schedule. Do not double the next dose.

If you are taking naproxen to relieve arthritis, you must take it regularly, as directed by your doctor. It may take up to four weeks before you feel the full benefits of this medication. This medication does not cure arthritis, but it will help to relieve the condition as long as you continue to take it.

SIDE EFFECTS

Minor. Bloating, constipation, diarrhea, difficulty in sleeping, dizziness, drowsiness, headache, heartburn, indigestion, light-headedness, loss of appetite, nausea, nervousness, soreness of the mouth, unusual sweating, and vomiting. As your body adjusts to the medication, these side effects should disappear.

To relieve constipation, increase the amount of fiber in your diet (fresh fruits and vegetables, salads, bran, and whole-grain breads), exercise, and drink more water (unless your doctor directs you to do otherwise).

If you become dizzy, sit or lie down for a while; get up slowly from a sitting or reclining position, and be careful on stairs.

Major. Tell your doctor about any side effects that are persistent or particularly bothersome. IT IS ESPECIALLY IMPORTANT TO TELL YOUR DOCTOR about bloody or black, tarry stools; blurred vision; confusion; depression; palpitations; ringing or buzzing in the ears or a problem with hearing; shortness of breath or wheezing; skin rash, hives, or itching; stomach pain; sudden decrease in amount of urine; swelling of the feet; tightness in the chest; unexplained sore throat and fever; unusual bleeding or bruising; unusual fatigue or weakness; unusual weight gain; or yellowing of the eyes or skin.

INTERACTIONS

Naproxen interacts with several other types of medications:
1. Concurrent use of anticoagulants (blood thinners, such as warfarin) can lead to an increase in bleeding complications.
2. Aspirin, salicylates, or other anti-inflammatory medications can cause increased stomach irritation when used concurrently with naproxen.
3. Naproxen can decrease the elimination of lithium and methotrexate from the body, resulting in possible toxicity from these medications.
4. Naproxen may interfere with the blood-pressure-lowering effects of beta-blocking medications (such as acebutolol, atenolol, betaxolol, carteolol, esmolol, labetalol, metoprolol, nadolol, penbutolol, pindolol, propranolol, and timolol).
5. This medication can also interfere with the diuretic effects of furosemide and thiazide-type diuretics.
6. Probenecid can increase the amount of naproxen in the bloodstream when both drugs are being taken.

Before starting to take this medication, BE SURE TO TELL YOUR DOCTOR about any medications you are currently taking, especially any of those listed above.

WARNINGS

• Before you take this medication, it is important to tell your doctor if you have ever had unusual or allergic reactions to any medications, especially to naproxen or any of the other chemically related drugs (including aspirin, other salicylates, carprofen, diclofenac, diflunisal, fenoprofen, flurbiprofen, indomethacin, ketoprofen, meclofenamate, mefenamic acid, oxyphenbutazone, phenylbutazone, piroxicam, sulindac, or tolmetin).

• Before taking this medication, it is important to tell your doctor if you now have or if you have ever had bleeding problems, colitis, stomach ulcers or other stomach problems, asthma, epilepsy, heart disease, high blood pressure, kidney disease, liver disease, mental illness, or Parkinson's disease.

• If naproxen makes you dizzy or drowsy, do not take part in any activity that requires alertness, such as driving a car or operating potentially dangerous machinery.

• Because this drug can prolong your bleeding time, it is important to tell your doctor or dentist that you are taking this drug before having surgery or any other medical or dental treatment.

• Stomach problems are more likely to occur if you take aspirin regularly or drink alcohol while being treated with this medication. These should, therefore, be avoided (unless your doctor tells you otherwise).

• Be sure to tell your doctor if you are pregnant. Naproxen analgesic may cause unwanted effects on the heart or blood flow of the fetus. Studies in animals have shown that taking naproxen late in pregnancy may increase the length of pregnancy, prolong labor, or cause other problems during delivery. Also, be sure to tell your doctor if you are breast-feeding an infant. Small amounts of this medication can pass into breast milk.

Naptrate—see pentaerythritol tetranitrate

Naqua—see trichlormethiazide

Nardil—see phenelzine

Nasalcrom—see cromolyn sodium (nasal)

Nasalide—see flunisolide (nasal)

Naturetin—see bendroflumethiazide

Navane—see thiothixene

ND Clear T.D.—see pseudoephedrine and chlorpheniramine combination

NegGram—see nalidixic acid

Nembutal—see pentobarbital

---

neomycin, polymyxin B, and bacitracin or gramicidin combination (ophthalmic)

BRAND NAMES (Manufacturers)
AK-Spore (Akorn)
Mycitracin ophthalmic (Upjohn)
neomycin, polymyxin B, and bacitracin or gramicidin combination (various manufacturers)
Neomycin, Polymyxin B, and Gramicidin (Rugby)
Neosporin (Burroughs Wellcome)

TYPE OF DRUG
Ophthalmic antibiotic

INGREDIENTS
neomycin, polymyxin B, and bacitracin (ointment only) or gramicidin (drops only)

DOSAGE FORMS
Ophthalmic drops (1.75 mg neomycin, 10,000 units polymyxin B, and 0.025 mg gramicidin per ml)
Ophthalmic ointment (3.5 mg neomycin, 10,000 units polymyxin B, and 400 units or 500 units bacitracin per gm)

STORAGE
The ophthalmic drops and ointment should be stored at room temperature in tightly closed containers. This medication should never be frozen.

USES

This medication is used to treat bacterial infections of the eye. It is an antibiotic combination that is effective against a wide range of bacteria. The medication acts by preventing the production of nutrients that are required for growth of the infecting bacteria. This medication is not effective against infections caused by viruses or fungi.

TREATMENT

Wash your hands with soap and water before using this medication. In order to prevent contamination of the medication, be careful not to touch the tube portion of the dropper, and do not let the dropper touch your eye.

Note that the bottle of eye drops is not completely full. This is to allow control of the number of drops dispensed. To apply the eye drops, tilt your head back and pull down the lower eyelid with one hand to make a pouch below the eye. Drop the prescribed amount of medicine into this pouch and slowly close your eyes. Try not to blink. Keep your eyes closed, and place one finger at the corner of the eye next to your nose for a minute or two, applying slight pressure (this is done to prevent loss of medication through the duct that drains fluid from the surface of the eye into the nose and throat). Then wipe away any excess with a clean tissue. If you don't think the medicine got into the eye, repeat the process once. If you are using more than one kind of eye drop, wait at least five minutes before applying the other medication(s).

Follow the same general procedure for the ointment. Tilt your head back, pull down your lower eyelid, and squeeze the ointment in a line along the pouch below the eye. Close the eye and place your finger at the corner of the eye near the nose for a minute or two. Do not rub your eyes. Wipe off excess ointment and the tip of the tube with clean tissues.

Since this medication is somewhat difficult to apply, you may prefer to have someone else apply it for you.

If you miss a dose of this medication, insert the drops or apply the ointment as soon as possible, unless it is almost time for the next application. In that case, do not use the missed dose; just return to your regular dosing schedule.

Continue using this medicine for the entire time prescribed by your doctor, even if the symptoms disappear before the end of that period. If you stop too soon, resistant bacteria are given a chance to continue growing, and the infection could recur.

SIDE EFFECTS

Minor. Blurred vision, burning, or stinging. These side effects should disappear as your body adjusts to the drug.

Major. Tell your doctor about any side effects that are persistent or particularly bothersome. IT IS ESPECIALLY IMPORTANT TO TELL YOUR DOCTOR about disturbed or reduced vision and about itching, rash, redness, or swelling in or around your eyes (other than the original symptoms of your infection). Also, if the infection seems to be getting worse rather than improving, contact your doctor.

INTERACTIONS

This medication should not interact with other medications as long as it is used according to directions.

WARNINGS

- Tell your doctor about unusual or allergic reactions you have had to any medications, especially to neomycin, bacitracin, polymyxin B, gramicidin, or any related antibiotics (such as amikacin, colistimethate, colistin, gentamicin, kanamycin, netilmicin, paromomycin, streptomycin, tobramycin, and viomycin).
- Tell your doctor if you now have or if you have ever had kidney disease, an injured cornea, inner ear disease, or myasthenia gravis.
- Do not use this medication for longer than ten consecutive days unless your doctor directs you to do so. Prolonged use of this drug may result in eye damage. If you need to use this medication for six weeks or longer, your doctor may want you to have an eye examination by an ophthalmologist.
- This medication has been prescribed for your current infection only. Another infection later on, or one that someone else has, may require a different medicine. You should not give your medicine to other people or use it for other infections, unless your doctor specifically directs you to do so.
- In order to allow your eye infection to clear, do not apply makeup to the affected eye.
- Be sure to tell your doctor if you are pregnant. The effects of this medication during pregnancy have not been thoroughly studied in humans.

Neomycin, Polymyxin B, and Gramicidin—see neomycin, polymyxin B, and bacitracin or gramicidin combination (ophthalmic)

Neoquess—see atropine, scopolamine, hyoscyamine, and phenobarbital combination

Neosporin—see neomycin, polymyxin B, and bacitracin or gramicidin combination (ophthalmic)

Neotrizine—see sulfonamide antibiotics (oral)

Nervine Nighttime Sleep Aid—see diphenhydramine

New-Decongest—see phenylpropanolamine, phenylephrine, chlorpheniramine, and phenyltoloxamine combination

Niazide—see trichlormethiazide

Nicorette—see nicotine gum

---

nicotine gum

BRAND NAME (Manufacturer)
Nicorette (Merrell Dow)

TYPE OF DRUG
A "stop smoking" aid

INGREDIENT
nicotine

DOSAGE FORM
Chewing gum (2 mg)

STORAGE
This medication should be kept in its original, child-resistant packaging until it is ready to be chewed.

USES

Nicotine gum is used as a temporary aid for smoking cessation programs. It helps control the symptoms of nicotine withdrawal (irritability, headache, fatigue, insomnia) and thus helps you to concentrate on overcoming the psychological and social aspects of your smoking habit.

TREATMENT

Use nicotine gum when you feel the urge to smoke. Keep the gum with you at all times. Place it where you usually keep your cigarettes. Whenever you feel that you want to smoke, put one piece of gum into your mouth. Chew the gum very slowly, until you taste it or feel a slight tingling in your mouth. As soon as you get the taste of the gum, stop chewing. After the taste or tingling is almost gone (after about one minute), chew slowly again until you taste the gum. Then stop chewing again. The gum should be chewed slowly for 30 minutes to release most of the nicotine. You should not expect the gum to give you the same quick satisfaction that smoking does. Do not drink caffeine-containing beverages while chewing a piece of nicotine gum, as this may decrease its effectiveness.

Most people find that ten to 12 pieces of gum per day are enough to control their urge to smoke. Depending on your needs, you can adjust the rate of chewing and the time between pieces. Do not chew more than 30 pieces per day (unless your doctor directs you to do so).

The risk of smoking again is highest in the first few months, so it is important that you follow your smoking cessation program and continue to use nicotine gum as directed during this period. As the urge to smoke decreases, you will find that you use less and less gum.

SIDE EFFECTS

Minor. Because of its nicotine content, the gum does not taste like ordinary chewing gum. It has a peppery taste. During the first several days of chewing the nicotine gum, you may experience mouth sores, jaw muscle aches, and headaches, and you may have an increased amount of saliva in the mouth. These side effects should disappear as you continue to use the gum.

If you chew the gum too fast, you may feel effects similar to those experienced when people inhale a cigarette for the first time or when they smoke too fast. These effects include constipation, coughing, dizziness, dry mouth, gas pains, hiccups, hoarseness, insomnia, light-headedness, nausea, redness of the face, sneezing, stomach pain, stomach upset, throat and mouth irritation, and vomiting. Most of these side effects can be controlled by chewing the gum more slowly.

Major. If any of the side effects are persistent or particularly bothersome, report them to your doctor. IT IS ESPECIALLY IMPORTANT TO TELL YOUR DOCTOR about signs of too much nicotine (cold sweats, confusion, difficulty in breathing, disturbed hearing or vision, faintness, marked weakness, palpitations, or seizures).

If you accidently swallow a piece of gum, you should not experience adverse effects. The nicotine is released by chewing and is absorbed primarily in the mouth.

INTERACTIONS

Smoking cessation, with or without nicotine gum, may affect blood levels of certain medications (including aminophylline, caffeine, glutethimide, imipramine, pentazocine, phenacetin, propoxyphene, and theophylline).

Nicotine can reduce the diuretic effects of furosemide and lessen the blood-pressure-lowering effects of beta blockers.

BE SURE TO TELL YOUR DOCTOR about any medications you are currently taking, especially any listed above.

WARNINGS

- Tell your doctor if you have recently had a heart attack or if you have ever had heart palpitations or arrhythmias, angina, active temporomandibular (jaw) joint disease, cardiovascular disease, endocrine (hormone) disease, thyroid problems, pheochromocytoma, diabetes mellitus, high blood pressure, peptic ulcers, mouth or throat inflammation, or dental problems.
- Be sure to tell your doctor if you are pregnant. Nicotine (from the gum or from cigarette smoke) can cause fetal harm. Also, tell your doctor if you are breast-feeding an infant. Small amounts of nicotine can pass into breast milk.

---

nifedipine

BRAND NAMES (Manufacturers)
Adalat (Miles)
Procardia (Pfizer)
TYPE OF DRUG
Antianginal
INGREDIENT
nifedipine
DOSAGE FORM
Capsules (10 mg and 20 mg)
STORAGE
Nifedipine capsules should be stored at room temperature in a tightly closed, light-resistant container.

USES

This medication is used to treat various types of angina (chest pain). Nifedipine belongs to a group of drugs known as calcium channel blockers. By blocking calcium, nifedipine relaxes and prevents spasms of the blood vessels of the heart and reduces the oxygen needs of the heart muscle.

TREATMENT

Nifedipine should be taken on an empty stomach with a full glass of water one hour before or two hours after a meal (unless your doctor directs you to do otherwise). These capsules should be swallowed whole to obtain maximum benefit.

If you miss a dose of this medication, take the missed dose as soon as possible, unless it is within two hours of your next scheduled dose. In that case, do not take the missed dose at all; just return to your regular dosing schedule. Do not double the next dose.

SIDE EFFECTS

Minor. Bloating, cough, dizziness, flushing, gas, giddiness, headache, heartburn, heat sensation, nasal congestion, nausea, nervousness, sleep disturbances, sweating, or weakness. These side effects should disappear as your body adjusts to the medication.

If you feel dizzy or light-headed, sit or lie down for a while; get up slowly from a sitting or reclining position, and be careful on stairs. To avoid dizziness or light-headedness when you stand, contract and relax the muscles of your legs for a few moments before rising. Do this by pushing one foot against the floor while raising the other foot slightly, alternating feet so that you are "pumping" your legs in a pedaling motion.

Major. Tell your doctor about any side effects that are persistent or particularly bothersome. IT IS ESPECIALLY IMPORTANT TO TELL YOUR DOCTOR about blurred vision, chills, confusion, difficulty in breathing, fainting, fever, fluid retention, impotence, mood changes, muscle cramps, palpitations, rash, sore throat, or tremors.

INTERACTIONS

Nifedipine interacts with several other types of medications:

1. Nifedipine can increase the active blood levels of digoxin, warfarin, phenytoin, and quinine, which can lead to an increase in side effects.

2. The combination of nifedipine and beta blockers (acebutolol, atenolol, betaxolol, carteolol, esmolol, labetalol, metoprolol, nadolol, penbutolol, pindolol, propranolol, or timolol) can lead to a severe drop in blood pressure.

3. Nifedipine can lower quinidine blood levels, which can decrease its effectiveness.

4. Cimetidine can decrease the breakdown of nifedipine in the body, which can increase the risk of side effects.

Before starting to take nifedipine, BE SURE TO TELL YOUR DOCTOR about any medications you are currently taking, especially any of those listed above.

WARNINGS

- Tell your doctor about unusual or allergic reactions you have had to any medications, especially to nifedipine.
- Tell your doctor if you have ever had heart disease, kidney disease, low blood pressure, or liver disease.
- If this drug makes you dizzy or drowsy, do not take part in any activity that requires alertness, such as driving a car or operating potentially dangerous machinery.
- Before having surgery or any other medical or dental treatment, be sure to tell your doctor or dentist that you are taking this medication.
- Do not stop taking this medication unless you first consult your doctor. Stopping this medication abruptly may lead to severe chest pain. Your doctor may, therefore, want to decrease your dosage gradually.
- Be sure to tell your doctor if you are pregnant. Nifedipine has been shown to cause birth defects in the offspring of animals that received large doses of it during pregnancy. This medication has not been studied in pregnant women. Also, tell your doctor if you are breast-feeding an infant. It is not known whether nifedipine passes into breast milk.

Niloric—see ergoloid mesylates

Nilstat—see nystatin

Nitro-Bid—see nitroglycerin (topical)

Nitro-Bid Plateau Caps—see nitroglycerin (systemic)

Nitrocap T.D.—see nitroglycerin (systemic)

Nitrocine—see nitroglycerin (topical)

Nitrocine Timecaps—see nitroglycerin (systemic)

Nitrodisc—see nitroglycerin (topical)

Nitro-Dur—see nitroglycerin (topical)

Nitrofan—see nitrofurantoin

nitrofurantoin

BRAND NAMES (Manufacturers)
Furadantin (Norwich-Eaton)
Furalan (Lannett)
Furan (American Urologicals)
Furanite (Major)
Macrodantin (Norwich-Eaton)
Nitrofan (Major)
nitrofurantoin (various manufacturers)

TYPE OF DRUG
Antibiotic

INGREDIENT
nitrofurantoin

DOSAGE FORMS
Tablets (50 mg and 100 mg)
Capsules (25 mg, 50 mg, and 100 mg)
Oral suspension (25 mg per 5-ml spoonful)

STORAGE
Nitrofurantoin tablets, capsules, and oral suspension should be stored at room temperature in tightly closed, light-resistant containers. Never freeze this medication.

USES

Nitrofurantoin is used to treat bacterial infections of the urinary tract (bladder and kidneys). It kills susceptible bacteria by breaking down their cell membranes and interfering with their production of vital nutrients.

TREATMENT

In order to avoid stomach irritation and to increase the effectiveness of this drug, you can take it with a meal or with a glass of water or milk.

The tablets and capsules should be swallowed whole to obtain maximum benefit.

The oral suspension form of this medication should be shaken well just before measuring each dose. The contents tend to settle on the bottom of the bottle, so it is necessary to shake the container in order to distribute the ingredients evenly and equalize the doses. Each dose of the medication should then be measured carefully with a specially designed 5-ml measuring spoon. An ordinary kitchen teaspoon is not accurate enough to measure your dose of the medication. You can then dilute the dose with water, milk, fruit juice, or infant's formula to mask the unpleasant taste.

Nitrofurantoin works best when the level of medicine in your urine is kept constant. It is best, therefore, to take the doses at evenly spaced invervals day and night. For example, if you are to take three doses a day, the doses should be spaced eight hours apart.

If you miss a dose of this medication, take the missed dose immediately. However, if you do not remember to take the missed dose until it is almost time for your next dose, take it; space the following dose about halfway through the regular interval between doses; then return to your regular dosing schedule. Try not to skip any doses.

It is important to continue to take this medication for the entire time prescribed by your doctor (usually seven to 14 days), even if the symptoms disappear before the end of that period. If you stop taking the drug too soon, resistant bacteria are given a chance to continue growing, and the infection could recur.

SIDE EFFECTS

Minor. Abdominal cramps, diarrhea, dizziness, drowsiness, loss of appetite, nausea, or vomiting. These side effects should disappear as your body adjusts to the medication.

Nitrofurantoin can cause your urine to change color (to rust-yellow or brown). This is a harmless effect, but it may stain your underclothing. The color change will disappear after you stop taking the drug.

If this drug makes you dizzy, sit or lie down; get up slowly, and be careful on stairs.

Major. Tell your doctor about any side effects that are persistent or particularly bothersome. IT IS ESPECIALLY IMPORTANT TO TELL YOUR DOCTOR about chest pain, chills, cough, difficulty in breathing, fainting, fever, hair loss, irritation of the mouth, muscle aches, numbness or tingling, rash, rectal or vaginal itching, unusual bleeding or bruising, weakness, or yellowing of the eyes or skin. Also, if your symptoms or infection seem to be getting worse rather than improving, you should contact your doctor.

INTERACTIONS

Nitrofurantoin interacts with other types of medications:

1. Probenecid and sulfinpyrazone can decrease the effectiveness and increase the side effects of nitrofurantoin.

2. Certain antacids (magnesium trisilicate) can decrease the absorption of nitrofurantoin from the gastrointestinal tract.

Before starting to take nitrofurantoin, BE SURE TO TELL YOUR DOCTOR about any medications you are currently taking, especially any of those listed above.

WARNINGS

- Tell your doctor about unusual or allergic reactions you have had to any medications, especially to nitrofurantoin, nitrofurazone, or furazolidone.
- Be sure to tell your doctor if you now have or if you have ever had anemia, diabetes mellitus, electrolyte abnormalities, glucose-6-phosphate dehydrogenase (G6PD) deficiency, kidney disease, lung disease, nerve damage, or vitamin B deficiencies.
- If this drug makes you dizzy or drowsy, do not take part in any activity that requires alertness, such as driving a car.
- Before surgery or other medical or dental treatment, tell your doctor or dentist you are taking this drug.
- Diabetics should know that nitrofurantoin can cause false-positive results with some urine sugar tests (for example, Clinitest). Be sure to check with your doctor before adjusting your insulin dose.
- This medication has been prescribed for your current infection only. Another infection later on, or one that someone else has, may require a different medicine. You should not give your medicine to other people or use it for other infections, unless your doctor specifically directs you to do so.
- Be sure to tell your doctor if you are pregnant. Nitrofurantoin should not be used close to term. It may cause anemia in the newborn infant. Nitrofurantoin should not be used in an infant less than one month of age. Also, tell your doctor if you are breast-feeding an infant. Nitrofurantoin passes into the breast milk.

Nitrogard—see nitroglycerin (systemic)

Nitroglycerin—see nitroglycerin (systemic)

nitroglycerin (systemic)

BRAND NAMES (Manufacturers)

Nitro-Bid Plateau Caps (Marion)
Nitrocap T.D. (Vortech)
Nitrocine Timecaps (Schwarz Pharma)
Nitrogard (Parke-Davis)
Nitroglycerin (Lilly)
Nitroglyn (Key)
Nitrolin (Henry Schein)
Nitrolingual (Rorer)
Nitrong (Wharton)
Nitrospan (Rorer)
Nitrostat (Parke-Davis)

TYPE OF DRUG

Antianginal

INGREDIENT

nitroglycerin

DOSAGE FORMS

Sustained-release tablets (2.6 mg, 6.5 mg, and 9 mg)
Sustained-release capsules (2.5 mg, 6.5 mg, and 9 mg)
Sublingual tablets (0.15 mg, 0.3 mg, 0.4 mg, and 0.6 mg)
Buccal tablets, controlled release (1 mg, 2 mg, and 3 mg)
Oral spray (6.4 mg per dose)

STORAGE

Nitroglycerin tablets, capsules, and oral spray should be stored in a tightly capped bottle in a cool, dry place.

The sublingual tablets should be kept in their original glass container. A small, temporary supply of tablets can also be stored in a stainless-steel container that is now available. The pendant-type container, which can be worn around your neck, is a convenient storage place for an emergency supply. NEVER store them in the refrigerator or the bathroom medicine cabinet, because the drug may lose its potency.

USES

This medication is used to treat angina (chest pain). Nitroglycerin is a vasodilator, which relaxes the muscles of the blood vessels, causing an increase in the oxygen supply to the heart.

The oral tablets and capsules do not act quickly; they are used to prevent chest pain. The sublingual tablets and oral spray act quickly and can be used to relieve chest pain after it has started.

TREATMENT

You should take the sustained-release tablets or capsules with a full glass of water on an empty stomach one hour before or two hours after a meal. The tablets and capsules should be swallowed whole. Chewing, crushing, or breaking them destroys their sustained-release activity and possibly increases the side effects.

NEVER chew or swallow the sublingual or buccal tablets. The sublingual tablet and oral spray forms of the drug are absorbed directly through the lining of the mouth. The sublingual tablet should be allowed to dissolve under the tongue or against the cheek.

To use the spray, remove the plastic cover on the container. Then, without shaking the container, spray the medication onto or under the tongue. Try not to inhale the spray. Close your mouth after each spray, and try to avoid swallowing right away. Nitroglycerin spray loses its effectiveness if it is swallowed.

Take one tablet or one or two spray doses at the first sign of chest pain. Sit down while you are waiting for the medicine to take effect. Do not eat, drink, or smoke while nitroglycerin is in your mouth. Try not to swallow while nitroglycerin is dissolving, and do not rinse your mouth afterward. Sublingual nitroglycerin or nitroglycerin spray should start working in one to three minutes. If there is no relief, take another tablet in five minutes. IF YOU TAKE THREE TABLETS OR THREE SPRAY DOSES WITHOUT ANY SIGN OF IMPROVEMENT, CALL A DOCTOR IMMEDIATELY OR GO TO A HOSPITAL EMERGENCY ROOM. As a preventive measure, take a nitroglycerin sublingual tablet or a spray dose five or ten minutes before heavy exercise, exposure to high altitudes or extreme cold, or any other potentially stressful situation. Be sure to carry some nitroglycerin sublingual tablets or oral spray with you at ALL times.

The buccal tablet should be placed between the upper lip and the gum on either side of the front teeth or between the cheek and the gum. The tablet is held in place by a sticky gel seal that develops once the tablet is in contact with saliva. If you wear dentures, the tablet can be placed anywhere between the cheek and the gum. Avoid drinking hot liquids or touching the tablet with your tongue. This can cause the tablet to dissolve faster and could increase the risk of side effects. If the tablet is swallowed by mistake, replace it with another tablet. Nitroglycerin buccal tablets lose their effectiveness when swallowed. Try not to take the buccal tablet at bedtime in order to avoid inadvertently swallowing and choking on the tablet while you are sleeping.

If you miss a dose of the sustained-release tablets or capsules, take the missed dose as soon as possible, unless it is more than halfway through the interval between doses. In that case, do not take the missed dose at all; just return to your regular dosing schedule. Do not double the next dose.

SIDE EFFECTS

Minor. Dizziness, flushing of the face, headache, lightheadedness, nausea, vomiting, or weakness. These side effects should disappear as your body adjusts to the medication.

If you feel dizzy or light-headed, sit or lie down for a while; get up slowly from a sitting or reclining position, and be careful on stairs. To avoid dizziness or light-headedness when you stand, contract and relax the muscles of your legs for a few moments before rising. Do this by pushing one foot against the floor while raising the other foot slightly, alternating feet so that you are "pumping" your legs in a pedaling motion.

Acetaminophen may help to relieve headaches.

Major. Tell your doctor about any side effects that are persistent or particularly bothersome. IT IS ESPECIALLY IMPORTANT TO TELL YOUR DOCTOR about diarrhea, fainting, palpitations, rash, or sweating.

INTERACTIONS

Nitroglycerin can interact with other types of medications:

1. The combination of alcohol and nitroglycerin can lead to dizziness and fainting.

2. Nitroglycerin can increase the side effects of the tricyclic antidepressants.

Before starting to take nitroglycerin, BE SURE TO TELL YOUR DOCTOR about any medications you are currently taking, especially tricyclic antidepressants.

WARNINGS

- Tell your doctor about unusual or allergic reactions you have had to any medications, especially to nitroglycerin or isosorbide dinitrate.
- Before starting to take this medication, be sure to tell your doctor if you now have or if you have ever had anemia, glaucoma, a head injury, low blood pressure, or thyroid disease or if you have recently had a heart attack.
- If this drug makes you dizzy or light-headed, do not take part in any activity that requires alertness, such as driving a car or operating potentially dangerous machinery.
- Before surgery or other medical or dental treatment, tell your doctor or dentist you are taking this drug.
- Tolerance may develop to this medication within one to three months. If it seems to lose its effectiveness, contact your doctor.
- You should not discontinue use of nitroglycerin (if you have been taking it on a regular basis) unless you first consult your doctor. Stopping the drug abruptly may lead to further chest pain. Your doctor may, therefore, want to decrease your dosage gradually.
- If you have frequent diarrhea, you may not be absorbing the sustained-release form of this medication. Discuss this with your doctor.
- While taking this medication, do not take any over-the-counter (nonprescription) asthma, allergy, sinus, cough, cold, or diet preparations unless you first check with your doctor or pharmacist. Some of these drugs decrease the effectiveness of nitroglycerin.
- The cotton plug should be removed when the bottle is first opened; it should NOT be replaced (the cotton absorbs some of the medication, decreasing its potency).
- Nitroglycerin is highly flammable. Do not use it in places where it might be ignited.
- Be sure to tell your doctor if you are pregnant. Although this drug appears to be safe, extensive studies in pregnant women have not been conducted. Also, tell your doctor if you are breast-feeding an infant. It is not known whether nitroglycerin passes into breast milk.

---

nitroglycerin (topical)

BRAND NAMES (Manufacturers)

Deponit (Wyeth)
Nitro-Bid (Marion)
Nitrocine (Schwarz Pharma)
Nitrodisc (Searle)
Nitro-Dur (Key)
nitroglycerin (various manufacturers)
Nitroglycerin Transdermal System (Bolar)
Nitrol (Adria)
Nitrong (Wharton)
Nitrostat (Parke-Davis)
Transderm-Nitro (Ciba)

TYPE OF DRUG

Antianginal

INGREDIENT
nitroglycerin
DOSAGE FORMS
Ointment (2%)
Transdermal system (the patch delivers 2.5 mg, 5 mg, 7.5 mg, 10 mg, or 15 mg per 24 hours)
STORAGE
Nitroglycerin ointment and patches should be stored at room temperature in their original containers. The ointment container should always be tightly capped.

USES

Nitroglycerin is used to prevent angina (chest pain). It is a vasodilator, which relaxes the muscles of the blood vessels, causing an increase in the oxygen supply to the heart. The ointment and patches do not act quickly—they should not be used to treat chest pain that has already started.

TREATMENT

The ointment comes with an applicator with which the prescribed dosage can be easily measured and applied. Before a new dose is applied, the previous dose should be thoroughly removed. Each dose should be applied to a new site on the skin. Do not rub or massage the ointment into the skin. Just spread the ointment in a thin, even layer, covering an area of about the same size each time. Avoid contact of the ointment with other parts of the body, since it is absorbed wherever it touches the skin. Either use plastic or rubber gloves to apply the ointment, or wash your hands immediately after application. Cover the ointment only if directed to do so by your doctor.

The transdermal system (patches) allows controlled, continuous release of nitroglycerin. Patches are convenient and easy to use. For best results, apply the patch to a hairless or clean-shaven area of skin, avoiding scars and wounds. Choose a site (such as the chest or upper arm) that is not subject to excessive movement. It is all right to bathe or shower with a patch in place. In the event that a patch becomes dislodged, discard and replace it. Replace a patch by applying a new unit before removing the old one. This allows for uninterrupted drug therapy, and skin irritation is minimized since the site is changed each time. If redness or irritation develops at the application site, consult your physician. Some people are sensitive to the materials used to make the patches. Do not trim or cut the patches. This alters the dose of the medication.

If you miss an application of this medication, apply the missed dose as soon as possible, unless it is more than halfway through the interval between doses. In that case, do not apply the missed dose at all; just return to your regular dosing schedule. Do not double the next dose.

SIDE EFFECTS

Minor. Dizziness, flushing of the face, headache, lightheadedness, nausea, vomiting, or weakness. These side effects should disappear as your body adjusts to the drug.

If you feel dizzy or light-headed, sit or lie down for a while; get up slowly, and be careful on stairs. To avoid dizziness or light-headedness when you stand, contract and relax the muscles of your legs for a few moments before rising. Do this by pushing one foot against the floor while raising the other foot slightly, alternating feet so that you are "pumping" your legs in a pedaling motion.

Acetaminophen may help to relieve headaches.

Major. Tell your doctor about any side effects that are persistent or particularly bothersome. IT IS ESPECIALLY IMPORTANT TO TELL YOUR DOCTOR about fainting, palpitations, rash, or sweating.

INTERACTIONS

Nitroglycerin can interact with other types of medications:
1. The combination of alcohol and nitroglycerin can lead to dizziness and fainting.
2. Nitroglycerin can increase the side effects of the tricyclic antidepressants.

Before starting to take nitroglycerin, BE SURE TO TELL YOUR DOCTOR about any medications you are currently taking, especially tricyclic antidepressants.

WARNINGS

- Tell your doctor about unusual or allergic reactions you have had to any medications, especially to nitroglycerin or isosorbide dinitrate.
- Before starting to take this medication, be sure to tell your doctor if you now have or if you have ever had anemia, glaucoma, a head injury, low blood pressure, or thyroid disease or if you have recently had a heart attack.
- If this drug makes you dizzy or light-headed, do not take part in any activity that requires alertness, such as driving a car or operating potentially dangerous machinery.
- Before having surgery or any other medical or dental treatment, be sure to tell your doctor or dentist that you are taking this medication.
- Tolerance to this medication may develop within one to three months. If it seems to lose its effectiveness, contact your doctor.
- You should not discontinue use of nitroglycerin unless you first consult your doctor. Stopping the drug abruptly may lead to further chest pain. Your doctor may, therefore, want to decrease your dosage gradually.
- While taking this medication, do not take any over-the-counter (nonprescription) asthma, allergy, sinus, cough, cold, or diet preparations unless you first check with your doctor or pharmacist. Some of these drugs decrease the effectiveness of nitroglycerin.
- Nitroglycerin is highly flammable. Do not use it in places where it might be ignited.
- Be sure to tell your doctor if you are pregnant. Although this drug appears to be safe, extensive studies in pregnant women have not been conducted. Also, tell your doctor if you are breast-feeding an infant. It is not known whether nitroglycerin passes into breast milk.

Nitroglycerin Transdermal System—see nitroglycerin (topical)

Nitroglyn—see nitroglycerin (systemic)

Nitrol—see nitroglycerin (topical)

Nitrolin—see nitroglycerin (systemic)

Nitrolingual—see nitroglycerin (systemic)

Nitrong—see nitroglycerin (systemic) and nitroglycerin (topical)

Nitrospan—see nitroglycerin (systemic)

Nitrostat—see nitroglycerin (systemic) and nitroglycerin (topical)

Noctec—see chloral hydrate

Nolex LA—see phenylpropanolamine and guaifenesin combination

Nolvadex—see tamoxifen

Noraminic—see phenylpropanolamine and chlorpheniramine combination

Norcet—see acetaminophen and hydrocodone combination

Nordette—see oral contraceptives

Nordryl—see diphenhydramine

---

norfloxacin

BRAND NAME (Manufacturer)
Noroxin (Merck Sharp & Dohme)
TYPE OF DRUG
Antibiotic
INGREDIENT
norfloxacin
DOSAGE FORM
Tablets (400 mg)
STORAGE
Norfloxacin should be stored at room temperature in a tightly closed container.

USES

Norfloxacin is an antibiotic that is used to treat bacterial urinary tract infections. It works by interfering with the reproduction of the bacteria. Norfloxacin kills susceptible bacteria but is not effective against viruses, parasites, or fungi.

TREATMENT

In order to obtain the maximum benefit from norfloxacin, it is best to take this drug on an empty stomach (one hour before or two hours after a meal) with a full glass of water. Antacids can decrease the absorption of this medication. Therefore, antacids should not be taken within two hours (before or after) of a dose of norfloxacin, unless otherwise directed by your doctor.

Norfloxacin works best when the level of medicine in your urine is kept constant. It is best, therefore, to take the doses at evenly spaced intervals day and night. For example, if you are to take two doses a day, the doses should be spaced 12 hours apart.

Try not to miss any doses of this medication. If you do miss a dose, take it as soon as you remember. However, if you do not remember to take the missed dose until it is almost time for your next dose, take it; space the following dose about halfway through the regular interval between doses; then continue with your regular dosing schedule.

It is important to continue to take this medication for the entire time prescribed by your doctor (usually five to 14 days), even if the symptoms disappear before the end of that period. If you stop taking the drug too soon, resistant bacteria are given a chance to continue growing, and your infection could recur.

SIDE EFFECTS

Minor. Abdominal pain, constipation, diarrhea, dizziness, dry mouth, fatigue, gas, headache, heartburn, nausea, sleeping problems, or vomiting. These side effects should disappear as your body adjusts to this medication.

If you are constipated, increase the amount of fiber in your diet (fresh fruits and vegetables, salads, bran, and whole-grain breads), exercise, and drink more water (unless your doctor directs you to do otherwise).

To reduce mouth dryness, chew sugarless gum or suck on ice chips or hard candy.

If you feel dizzy or light-headed, sit or lie down for a while; get up slowly from a sitting or reclining position, and be careful on stairs.

Major. Tell your doctor about any side effects that are persistent or particularly bothersome. IT IS ESPECIALLY IMPORTANT TO TELL YOUR DOCTOR about depression, difficult or painful urination, rash, visual disturbances, or yellowing of the skin or eyes. Also, if the symptoms of your infection seem to be getting worse rather than improving, contact your doctor.

INTERACTIONS

Norfloxacin can interact with several other types of drugs:

1. Probenecid can block the excretion of norfloxacin into the urinary tract, decreasing its effectiveness in treating infections located there.

2. Antacids can decrease the absorption of norfloxacin from the gastrointestinal tract.

3. Nitrofurantoin may antagonize (act against) the effectiveness of norfloxacin.

Before starting norfloxacin, BE SURE TO TELL YOUR DOCTOR about any medications you are currently taking, especially any of those listed above.

WARNINGS

• Tell your doctor about unusual or allergic reactions you have had to any medications, especially to norfloxacin or to the related antibiotics cinoxacin and nalidixic acid.

• Before starting norfloxacin, tell your doctor if you now have or if you have ever had liver disease or seizures.

• If this drug makes you dizzy, do not take part in any activity that requires alertness, such as driving a car or operating potentially dangerous machinery.

• In order to prevent the formation of crystals in the kidneys, try to drink plenty of fluids (at least eight glasses of water or fruit juice each day) while you are taking this medication (unless your doctor directs you to do otherwise).

• This medication has been prescribed for your current infection only. A subsequent infection, or one that someone else has, may require a different medicine. Do not give your medicine to other people or use it to treat other infections, unless your doctor directs you to do so.

• Be sure to tell your doctor if you are pregnant. Studies in pregnant women have not been conducted. However, lameness has occurred in the immature offspring of animals that received large doses of norfloxacin during pregnancy. Also, tell your doctor if you are breast-feeding an infant. It is not yet known if norfloxacin passes into breast milk.

Norgesic—see orphenadrine, aspirin, and caffeine combination

Norgesic Forte—see orphenadrine, aspirin, and caffeine combination

Norinyl—see oral contraceptives

Norlestrin—see oral contraceptives

Normatane Elixir—see phenylpropanolamine, phenylephrine, and brompheniramine combination

Normatane Expectorant—see phenylephrine, phenylpropanolamine, brompheniramine, and guaifenesin combination

Nor-Mil—see diphenoxylate and atropine combination

Normodyne—see labetalol

Noroxin—see norfloxacin

Norpace—see disopyramide

Norpace CR—see disopyramide

Norpanth—see propantheline

Norpramin—see desipramine

Nor-Tet—see tetracycline

nortriptyline

BRAND NAMES (Manufacturers)
Aventyl (Lilly)
Pamelor (Sandoz)

TYPE OF DRUG
Tricyclic antidepressant

INGREDIENT
nortriptyline

DOSAGE FORMS
Capsules (10 mg, 25 mg, and 75 mg)
Oral solution (10 mg per 5-ml spoonful, with 4% alcohol)

STORAGE
Store at room temperature in a tightly closed container.

USES

Nortriptyline is used to relieve the symptoms of mental depression. This medication belongs to a group of drugs referred to as the tricyclic antidepressants. These medicines are thought to relieve depression by increasing the concentration of certain chemicals necessary for nerve transmission in the brain.

TREATMENT

This medication should be taken exactly as your doctor prescribes. It can be taken with water or with food to lessen the chance of stomach irritation, unless your doctor tells you to do otherwise.

If you miss a dose of this medication, take the missed dose as soon as possible, and then return to your regular dosing schedule. However, if the dose you missed was a once-a-day bedtime dose, do not take that dose in the morning; check with your doctor instead. If the dose is taken in the morning, it may cause unwanted side effects. Never double the dose.

The effects of therapy with this medication may not become apparent for two or three weeks.

SIDE EFFECTS

Minor. Anxiety, blurred vision, confusion, constipation, cramps, diarrhea, dizziness, drowsiness, dry mouth, fatigue, heartburn, insomnia, loss of appetite, nausea, peculiar tastes in the mouth, restlessness, sweating, vomiting, weakness, or weight gain or loss. As your body adjusts to the medication, these side effects should disappear.

This medication may increase your sensitivity to sunlight. You should, therefore, avoid prolonged exposure to sunlight or sunlamps. Wear protective clothing and use sunscreen.

Dry mouth caused by therapy with this medication can be relieved by chewing sugarless gum or by sucking on ice chips or a piece of hard candy.

To relieve constipation, increase the amount of fiber in your diet (fresh fruits and vegetables, salads, bran, and whole-grain breads), and drink more water (unless your doctor directs you to do otherwise).

To avoid dizziness or light-headedness when you stand, contract and relax the muscles of your legs for a few moments before rising. Do this by pushing one foot against the floor while raising the other foot slightly, alternating feet so that you are "pumping" your legs in a pedaling motion.

Major. Tell your doctor about any side effects that are persistent or particularly bothersome. IT IS ESPECIALLY IMPORTANT TO TELL YOUR DOCTOR about agitation, chest pain, convulsions, difficulty in urinating, enlarged or painful breasts (in both sexes), fainting, fever, fluid retention, hair loss, hallucinations, headaches, impotence, mood changes, mouth sores, nervousness, nightmares, numbness in the fingers or toes, palpitations, ringing in the ears, seizures, skin rash, sleep disorders, sore throat, swelling, tremors, uncoordinated movements or balance problems, unusual bleeding or bruising, or yellowing of the eyes or skin.

INTERACTIONS

Nortriptyline interacts with several other types of medications:

1. Extreme drowsiness can occur when this drug is taken with central nervous system depressants (such as alcohol, antihistamines, barbiturates, benzodiazepine tranquilizers, muscle relaxants, narcotics, pain medications, phenothiazine tranquilizers, and sleeping medications) or other tricyclic antidepressants.

2. Nortriptyline may decrease the effectiveness of antiseizure medications and may block the blood-pressure-lowering effects of clonidine and guanethidine.
3. Birth control pills and estrogen-containing drugs can increase the side effects and reduce the effectiveness of the tricyclic antidepressants (including nortriptyline).
4. Tricyclic antidepressants may increase the side effects of thyroid medication and over-the-counter (nonprescription) cough, cold, asthma, allergy, sinus, and diet medications.
5. The concurrent use of tricyclic antidepressants and monoamine oxidase (MAO) inhibitors should be avoided because the combination may result in fever, convulsions, or high blood pressure. At least 14 days should separate the use of this drug and the use of an MAO inhibitor.
6. Cimetidine can decrease the elimination of nortriptyline from the body, increasing the possibility of side effects.

Before starting to take nortriptyline, BE SURE TO TELL YOUR DOCTOR about any medications you are currently taking, especially any of those listed above.

WARNINGS

• Tell your doctor if you have had unusual or allergic reactions to any medications, especially to nortriptyline or any of the other tricyclic antidepressants (amitriptyline, imipramine, doxepin, trimipramine, amoxapine, protriptyline, desipramine, or maprotiline).
• Tell your doctor if you have a history of alcoholism or if you have ever had asthma, high blood pressure, liver or kidney disease, heart disease, a heart attack, circulatory disease, stomach problems, intestinal problems, difficulty in urinating, enlarged prostate gland, epilepsy, glaucoma, thyroid disease, mental illness, or electroshock therapy.
• If this drug makes you dizzy or drowsy, do not take part in any activity that requires alertness, such as driving a car or operating potentially dangerous machinery.
• Before having surgery or other medical or dental treatment, be sure to tell your doctor or dentist about this drug.
• Do not stop taking this drug suddenly. Abruptly stopping it can cause nausea, headache, stomach upset, fatigue, or a worsening of your condition. Your doctor may want to reduce the dosage gradually.
• The effects of nortriptyline may last as long as seven days after you have stopped taking it, so continue to observe all precautions during that period.
• Be sure to tell your doctor if you are pregnant. Problems in humans have not been reported; however, studies in animals have shown that this type of medication can cause side effects in the fetus when given to the mother in large doses during pregnancy. Also, tell your doctor if you are breast-feeding an infant. Small amounts of this drug can pass into breast milk and may cause unwanted effects, such as irritability or sleeping problems, in nursing infants.

Nortussin with Codeine—see codeine and guaifenesin combination

Novafed A—see pseudoephedrine and chlorpheniramine combination

Novulin—see insulin

Nuprin—see ibuprofen

Nutracort—see hydrocortisone (topical)

Nydrazid—see isoniazid

---

nystatin

BRAND NAMES (Manufacturers)
Mycostatin (Squibb)
Mykinac (NMC)
Nilstat (Lederle)
nystatin (various manufacturers)
Nystex (Savage)
O-V Statin (Squibb)
TYPE OF DRUG
Antifungal
INGREDIENT
nystatin
DOSAGE FORMS
Oral tablets (500,000 units)
Oral suspension (100,000 units per ml with not more than 1.0% alcohol)
Oral lozenges (200,000 units)
Vaginal tablets (100,000 units)
Topical cream, ointment, and powder (100,000 units per gram)
STORAGE
Nystatin should be stored at room temperature (never frozen) in a tightly closed, light-resistant container.

USES

Nystatin is used to treat fungal infections of the throat, gastrointestinal tract, skin, and vagina. By chemically binding to the cell membranes of fungal organisms, this medication causes the cell contents to leak out, which kills the fungi.

TREATMENT

You can take the oral tablet form of nystatin either on an empty stomach or with food or milk (as directed by your doctor).

The oral suspension should be shaken well just before using each dose. The contents tend to settle on the bottom of the bottle, so it is necessary to shake the container to distribute the ingredients evenly and equalize the doses.

Each dose of the oral suspension should then be measured carefully with a specially designed 5-ml measuring spoon. An ordinary kitchen teaspoon is not accurate enough. Place half of the dose in each side of your mouth. Try to hold the suspension in the mouth or swish it through the mouth for as long as possible before swallowing it.

The oral lozenge form should be allowed to dissolve slowly in the mouth.

The vaginal tablets are packaged with instructions and an applicator for inserting the tablets into the vagina. Read the instructions carefully before using this product.

Occasionally, the vaginal tablets are prescribed to be taken orally (to treat mouth or throat infections). The tablets are sucked on to increase contact time with the mouth and throat.

The region where you are to apply the topical cream, ointment, or powder should be washed carefully and patted dry.

A sufficient amount of medication should then be applied to the affected area. An occlusive dressing (like kitchen plastic wrap) should NOT be applied over the medication (unless your doctor directs you to do so).

If you are using the powder form to treat a foot infection, sprinkle liberally into your shoes and socks.

Try not to miss any doses of this medication. If you do miss a dose, take (or apply) the missed dose as soon as possible, unless it is almost time for the next dose. In that case, do not take (or apply) the missed dose at all; just return to your regular dosing schedule. Do not double the next dose of this medication.

It is important to continue to take this medication for the entire time prescribed by your doctor (usually seven to 14 days), even if the symptoms disappear before the end of that period. If you stop taking the drug too soon, resistant fungi are given a chance to continue growing, and your infection could recur.

SIDE EFFECTS

Minor. Oral forms: diarrhea, nausea, or vomiting. Topical and vaginal forms: itching. These side effects should disappear as your body adjusts to the drug.

Major. Tell your doctor about any side effects that are persistent or particularly bothersome. IT IS ESPECIALLY IMPORTANT TO TELL YOUR DOCTOR about a rash. Also, if symptoms of your infection seem to be getting worse rather than improving, tell your doctor.

INTERACTIONS

Nystatin should not interact with other medications if it is used according to directions.

WARNINGS

- Tell your doctor about unusual or allergic reactions you have had to any medications, especially to nystatin.
- If you are using this drug to treat a vaginal infection, avoid sexual intercourse or ask your partner to wear a condom until treatment has been completed. These measures help prevent reinfection. Use the vaginal tablets continuously, even during a menstrual period. Unless instructed otherwise by your doctor, do not douche during treatment or until three weeks after you stop using the vaginal tablets. Wear cotton panties, rather than nylon or other nonporous materials, when you are being treated for fungal infections of the vagina. There may be some vaginal drainage while using the vaginal tablets, so you may wish to use a sanitary napkin or panty liner to prevent the soiling of your underwear.
- This medication has been prescribed for your current infection only. Another infection later on, or one that someone else has, may require a different medicine. You should not give your medicine to other people or use it for other infections, unless your doctor specifically directs you to do so.
- If the symptoms of infection do not begin to improve two or three days after starting nystatin, CONTACT YOUR DOCTOR. This medication may not be effective against the organism causing your infection.
- Be sure to tell your doctor if you are pregnant. Although nystatin appears to be safe during pregnancy, extensive studies in humans have not been conducted. Also, tell your doctor if you are breast-feeding an infant. It is not known whether this medication passes into breast milk.

Nystex—see nystatin

Nytol—see diphenhydramine

Obalan—see phendimetrazine

Obe-Nix—see phentermine

Obephen—see phentermine

Obermine—see phentermine

Obestin-30—see phentermine

Ocusert Pilo-20—see pilocarpine (ophthalmic)

Ocusert Pilo-40—see pilocarpine (ophthalmic)

---

omeprazole

BRAND NAME (Manufacturer)
Prilosec (MSD)
TYPE OF DRUG
Gastric acid secretion inhibitor
INGREDIENT
omeprazole
DOSAGE FORM
Delayed-release capsules (20 mg)
STORAGE
Omeprazole should be stored at room temperature in a tightly closed container.

USES

Omeprazole is prescribed to treat peptic ulcer disease, gastroesophageal reflux, and hypersecretory syndromes. This drug suppresses the secretion of acid in the stomach.

TREATMENT

Omeprazole capsules should not be opened, chewed, or crushed. They should be taken with a glass of water on an empty stomach. It is best to take the dose one hour before meals or two hours after meals.

Try to take the medication at the same time(s) each day. If you miss a dose of the medication, take the missed dose as soon as possible, then return to your regular dosing schedule. If it is almost time for the next dose, however, skip the one you missed and return to your regular schedule. Do not double the next dose (unless your doctor directs you to do so) of the medication.

It is important that you take this medication for as long as prescribed by your doctor since it may take a long time for your ulcers to heal.

SIDE EFFECTS

Minor. Abdominal pain, burning sensation in mouth, constipation, diarrhea, dizziness, dry mouth, fatigue, headache, or palpitations.

To relieve constipation while you are being treated with this medication, exercise and drink more water, unless your doctor directs you to do otherwise.

To avoid dizziness when you stand, contract and relax the muscles of your legs for a few moments before rising. Do this by pushing one foot against the floor while raising the other foot slightly, alternating feet so that you are "pumping" your legs in a pedaling motion.

To relieve dry mouth, chew sugarless gum or suck on ice chips or a piece of hard candy.

Major. Tell your doctor about any side effects that are persistent or particularly bothersome. IT IS ESPECIALLY IMPORTANT TO TELL YOUR DOCTOR about itching, numbness or tingling of fingers or toes, rash, or yellowing of the eyes and skin.

INTERACTIONS

Omeprazole may increase the effects of diazepam, warfarin, phenytoin, and antipyrine.

Be sure to tell your doctor about any medications you are currently taking, especially any of the ones listed above.

WARNINGS

- Tell your doctor about unusual or allergic reactions you have had to any medications, especially to omeprazole.
- Tell your doctor if you now have or if you have ever had thyroid disease, liver disease, Addison's disease, or Cushing's disease.
- This medication may cause dizziness and lightheadedness, so use caution while driving a car or operating potentially dangerous equipment.
- Long-term and high-dose treatment with omeprazole has been associated with higher incidences of gastric tumors. Consult your doctor if you need to take high doses of omeprazole for a long time.
- Be sure to tell your doctor if you are pregnant or breastfeeding. Adequate human studies have not been conducted with omeprazole.

Omnipen—see ampicillin

Ophthacet—see sodium sulfacetamide (ophthalmic)

Optimine—see azatadine

Oragest T.D.—see phenylpropanolamine and chlorpheniramine combination

---

oral contraceptives

BRAND NAMES (Manufacturers)

Brevicon (Syntex)
Demulen (Searle)
Enovid-E (Searle)
Loestrin (Parke-Davis)
Lo/Ovral (Wyeth)
Modicon (Ortho)
Nordette (Wyeth)
Norinyl (Syntex)
Norlestrin (Parke-Davis)
Ortho-Novum (Ortho)
Ovcon (Mead Johnson)
Ovral (Wyeth)
Ovulen (Searle)
Tri-Levlen (Berlex)
Tri-Norinyl (Syntex)
Triphasil-21 (Wyeth)

TYPE OF DRUG

Oral contraceptive

INGREDIENTS

Estrogens and progestins

DOSAGE FORM

Tablets (in packages of 21 or 28 tablets; when 28 tablets are present, seven of the tablets either are placecebos or contain iron)

STORAGE

Oral contraceptives should be stored at room temperature. They should be kept in their original container, which is designed to help you keep track of your dosing schedule.

USES

Oral contraceptives change the hormone balance of the body to prevent pregnancy.

TREATMENT

To avoid stomach irritation, you can take oral contraceptives with food or with a full glass of water or milk.

In order to become accustomed to taking this medication, try to take it at the same time every day.

Use a supplemental method of birth control for the first week after you start taking oral contraceptives (the medication takes time to become fully effective).

Even if you do not start to menstruate on schedule at the end of the pill cycle, begin the next cycle of pills at the prescribed time. Many women taking oral contraceptives have irregular menstruation.

If you miss a dose of this medication and you are on a 21-day schedule, take the missed dose as soon as you remember. If you don't remember until the next day, take the dose of that day plus the one you missed; then return to your regular dosing schedule. If you miss two days' doses, you should take two tablets a day for the next two days; then return to your regular dosing schedule. You should also use another form of birth control during those four days. If you miss your dose three days in a row, you should stop taking this drug and use a different method of birth control until you check with your doctor. Your doctor may want you to start a new package seven days after the last tablet was missed and use an additional method of birth control until the start of your next period. If you are on the 28-day schedule and you miss taking any one of the first 21 tablets, you should follow the instructions for the 21-day schedule. If you missed taking any of the last seven tablets, there is no danger of pregnancy, but you should take the first pill of the next month's cycle on the regularly scheduled day.

SIDE EFFECTS

Minor. Abdominal cramps, acne, backache, bloating, change in appetite, changes in sexual desire, diarrhea, dizziness, fatigue, headache, nasal congestion, nausea, nervousness, vaginal irritation, or vomiting. These side effects should disappear as your body adjusts to the medication.

This medication can increase your sensitivity to sunlight. Avoid prolonged exposure to sunlight and sunlamps. wear protective clothing and sunglasses, and use an effective sunscreen.

If you feel dizzy, sit or lie down for a while; get up slowly from a sitting or reclining position, and be careful on stairs.
Major. Tell your doctor about any side effects that are persistent or particularly bothersome. IT IS ESPECIALLY IMPORTANT TO TELL YOUR DOCTOR about abdominal pain; breakthrough vaginal bleeding (spotting); changes in menstrual flow; chest pain; depression; difficult or painful urination; enlarged or tender breasts; hearing changes; increase or decrease in hair growth; migraine headaches; numbness or tingling; pain in your calves; rash; skin color changes; swelling of the feet, ankles, or lower legs; unusual bleeding or bruising; vaginal itching; weight changes; or yellowing of the eyes or skin.

INTERACTIONS

These drugs interact with several other types of drugs:
1. Pain relievers, antimigraine preparations, rifampin, barbiturates, phenylbutazone, phenytoin, primidone, carbamazepine, isoniazid, neomycin, griseofulvin, penicillins, tetracycline, chloramphenicol, sulfonamide antibiotics, nitrofurantoin, and ampicillin can decrease the effectiveness of oral contraceptives.
2. Oral contraceptives can reduce the effectiveness of oral anticoagulants (blood thinners, such as warfarin), anticonvulsants, tricyclic antidepressants, antihypertensive agents, oral antidiabetic agents, and vitamins.
3. Oral contraceptives can increase the blood levels of caffeine, diazepam, chlordiazepoxide, metoprolol, propranolol, adrenocorticosteroids (cortisone-like medications), imipramine, clomipramine, phenytoin, and phenylbutazone, which can lead to an increase in side effects.
4. Oral contraceptives can decrease the blood levels and, therefore, the effectiveness of lorazepam and oxazepam.

Before starting to take oral contraceptives, BE SURE TO TELL YOUR DOCTOR about any medications you are currently taking, especially any of those listed above.

WARNINGS

- Tell your doctor about unusual or allergic reactions you have had to any medications, especially to estrogens, progestins, or progesterones.
- Before starting to take this medication, be sure to tell your doctor if you now have or if you have ever had asthma, bleeding problems, breast cancer, clotting disorders, diabetes mellitus, endometriosis, epilepsy, gallbladder disease, heart disease, high blood pressure, kidney disease, liver disease, mental depression, migraine headaches, porphyria, strokes, thyroid disease, uterine tumors, vaginal bleeding, or vitamin deficiencies.
- Some women who have used an oral contraceptive have had difficulty becoming pregnant after discontinuing use. Most of these women had had scanty or irregular periods before starting oral contraceptives. Possible subsequent difficulty in becoming pregnant is a matter you should discuss with your doctor before using an oral contraceptive.
- Every prescription comes with a booklet that explains birth control pills. Read this booklet carefully. It contains exact directions on how to use this medicine correctly and describes the risks involved.
- Women over 30 years of age and women who smoke while taking this medication have an increased risk of developing serious heart or blood vessel side effects.
- If this drug makes you dizzy, avoid taking part in any activity that requires alertness, such as driving a car or operating potentially dangerous machinery.
- Oral contraceptives can change the clotting properties of blood. Before surgery or other medical or dental treatment, tell your doctor or dentist you are taking this drug.
- This type of drug has been suspected of causing cancer. If you have a family history of cancer, you should consult your doctor before taking oral contraceptives.
- Be sure to tell your doctor if you are pregnant. Oral contraceptives have been associated with birth defects in animals and in humans. Because hormones have long-term effects on the body, oral contraceptives should be stopped at least three months prior to becoming pregnant. Another method of birth control should be used for those three months. Also, tell your doctor if you are breast-feeding an infant. This medication passes into breast milk.

Oramide—see tolbutamide

Oraminic—see phenylpropanolamine and chlorpheniramine combination

Orasone—see prednisone (systemic)

Oretic—see hydrochlorothiazide

Oreton Methyl—see methyltestosterone

Oridol C—see codeine and iodinated glycerol combination

Oridol DM—see dextromethorphan and iodinated glycerol combination

Orinase—see tolbutamide

Ormazine—see chlorpromazine

Ornade—see phenylpropanolamine and chlorpheniramine combination

---

orphenadrine, aspirin, and caffeine combination

BRAND NAMES (Manufacturers)
Norgesic (Riker)
Norgesic Forte (Riker)
Orphengesic (various manufacturers)

TYPE OF DRUG
Muscle relaxant and analgesic

INGREDIENTS
orphenadrine, aspirin, and caffeine

DOSAGE FORM
Tablets (25 mg orphenadrine, 385 mg aspirin, and 30 mg caffeine [Norgesic]; 50 mg orphenadrine, 770 mg aspirin, and 60 mg caffeine [Norgesic Forte])

STORAGE
This medication should be stored at room temperature in a tightly closed, light-resistant container.

USES

Orphenadrine, aspirin, and caffeine combination drug is used to relax muscles and to relieve the pain of sprains, strains, and other muscle injuries. Orphenadrine acts as a central nervous system (brain and spinal cord) depressant, which blocks reflexes involved in producing and maintaining muscle spasms. It does not act directly on tense muscles. Caffeine is a central nervous system stimulant that acts by constricting the blood vessels in the head. This may help relieve headaches. Aspirin is a pain reliever.

TREATMENT

These tablets should be taken with a full glass of water. To avoid stomach irritation, you can also take this medication with food or milk (unless your doctor directs otherwise).

If you miss a dose of this medication and remember within an hour, take the missed dose and then return to your regular dosing schedule. If it has been longer than an hour, do not take the missed dose at all; just return to your regular dosing schedule. Do not double the next dose.

SIDE EFFECTS

Minor. Blurred vision, confusion, constipation, diarrhea, dizziness, drowsiness, dry mouth, headache, indigestion, insomnia, nausea, nervousness, vomiting, or weakness. These side effects should disappear as your body adjusts to the medication.

If you are constipated, increase the amount of fiber in your diet (fresh fruits and vegetables, salads, bran, and whole-grain breads), exercise, and drink more water (unless your doctor directs you to do otherwise).

If you feel dizzy or light-headed, sit or lie down for a while; get up slowly from a sitting or reclining position, and be careful on stairs.

To relieve mouth dryness, suck on ice chips or a piece of hard candy or chew sugarless gum.

Major. Tell your doctor about any side effects that are persistent or particularly bothersome. IT IS ESPECIALLY IMPORTANT TO TELL YOUR DOCTOR about bloody or black, tarry stools; chest tightness; difficulty in breathing; difficulty in urinating; hearing loss; palpitations; rash; ringing in the ears; or severe abdominal pain.

INTERACTIONS

This medication interacts with several other types of drugs:

1. Orphenadrine can cause extreme drowsiness when combined with other central nervous system depressants (such as alcohol, antihistamines, barbiturates, benzodiazepine tranquilizers, phenothiazine tranquilizers, narcotics, and sleeping medications) or with tricyclic antidepressants.
2. Orphenadrine can cause confusion, anxiety, and tremors when combined with propoxyphene.
3. Aspirin can increase the active blood levels of methotrexate, oral antidiabetic agents, and oral anticoagulants (blood thinners, such as warfarin), which can lead to an increase in side effects.
4. The antigout activity of probenecid and sulfinpyrazone are decreased by aspirin.
5. The gastrointestinal side effects of anti-inflammatory medications may be increased by aspirin.

Before starting to take this medication, BE SURE TO TELL YOUR DOCTOR about any medications you are currently taking, especially any of those listed above.

WARNINGS

- Tell your doctor about unusual or allergic reactions you have had to any drugs, especially to orphenadrine, caffeine, aspirin, other salicylates, methyl salicylate, or nonsteroidal anti-inflammatory agents (such as diclofenac, diflunisal, fenoprofen, flurbiprofen, ibuprofen, indomethacin, ketoprofen, meclofenamate, naproxen, oxyphenbutazone, phenylbutazone, piroxicam, sulindac, and tolmetin).
- Tell your doctor if you now have or if you have ever had anemia, bladder obstruction, glaucoma, gout, kidney disease, liver disease, myasthenia gravis, peptic ulcers, an enlarged prostate gland, an intestinal obstruction, or bleeding problems.
- This medication should not be taken as a substitute for rest, physical therapy, or other measures recommended by your doctor to treat your condition.
- If this medication makes you dizzy or drowsy or blurs your vision, do not take part in any activity that requires alertness, such as driving a car or operating potentially dangerous machinery, while you are taking it.
- Before having surgery or other medical or dental treatment, tell your doctor or dentist about this drug. Treatment with aspirin-containing drugs is usually discontinued several days before any major surgery, to prevent bleeding complications.
- Because this product contains aspirin, additional medications that contain aspirin should not be taken without your doctor's approval. Check the labels on over-the-counter (nonprescription) pain, sinus, allergy, asthma, cough, and cold products to see if they contain aspirin.
- The use of aspirin in children (about 16 years of age or less) with the flu or chicken pox has been associated with a rare, life-threatening condition called Reye's syndrome. Aspirin-containing products should, therefore, not be given to children who are exhibiting signs of infection.
- Diabetic patients should be aware that large doses of aspirin (more than six 385-mg tablets or three 770-mg tablets per day) may interfere with urine sugar testing. Diabetics should, therefore, check with their doctor before changing their insulin dose.
- Be sure to tell your doctor if you are pregnant. Aspirin can prolong labor if it is taken by the mother close to term and can cause heart problems in newborn infants. Also, tell your doctor if you are breast-feeding an infant. It is not known whether orphenadrine passes into breast milk, but small quantities of aspirin and caffeine are able to pass into breast milk.

Orphengesic—see orphenadrine, aspirin, and caffeine combination

Ortega-Otic M—see hydrocortisone, polymyxin B, and neomycin combination (otic)

Ortho-Novum—see oral contraceptives

Orudis—see ketoprofen

Oto—see antipyrine, benzocaine, oxyquinoline, and glycerin combination

Otocort—see hydrocortisone, polymyxin B, and neomycin combination (otic)

Otomycin-Hpn Otic—see hydrocortisone, polymyxin B, and neomycin combination (otic)

Otoreid-HC—see hydrocortisone, polymyxin B, and neomycin combination (otic)

Ovcon—see oral contraceptives

Ovral—see oral contraceptives

O-V Statin—see nystatin

Ovulen—see oral contraceptives

---

oxacillin

BRAND NAMES (Manufacturers)
Bactocill (Beecham)
Prostaphlin (Bristol)
TYPE OF DRUG
Penicillin antibiotic
INGREDIENT
oxacillin
DOSAGE FORMS
Capsules (250 mg and 500 mg)
Oral solution (250 mg per 5-ml spoonful)
STORAGE
Oxacillin capsules should be stored at room temperature in a tightly closed container. The oral solution should be stored in the refrigerator in a tightly closed container. Any unused portion of the solution should be discarded after 14 days. This medication should never be frozen.

USES

Oxacillin is used to treat a wide variety of bacterial infections, especially those involving *Staphylococcus* bacteria. It acts by severely injuring the cell membranes of the infecting bacteria, thereby preventing them from growing and multiplying. Oxacillin kills susceptible bacteria, but it is not effective against viruses, parasites, or fungi.

TREATMENT

Oxacillin should be taken on an empty stomach or with a glass of water one hour before or two hours after a meal. This medication should never be taken with fruit juices or carbonated beverages, because the acidity of these drinks destroys the drug in the stomach.

The oral solution should be measured carefully with a specially designed 5-ml measuring spoon. An ordinary kitchen teaspoon is not accurate enough.

Oxacillin works best when the level of medicine in your bloodstream is kept constant. It is best, therefore, to take the doses at evenly spaced intervals day and night. For example, if you are taking four doses a day, the doses should be spaced six hours apart.

If you miss a dose of this medication, take the missed dose immediately. If you do not remember to take the missed dose until it is almost time for your next dose, take it immediately, space the following dose about halfway through the regular interval between doses, and then return to your regular dosing schedule. Try not to skip any doses.

It is important to continue to take this medication for the entire time prescribed by your doctor (usually seven to 14 days), even if the symptoms of infection disappear before the end of that period. If you stop taking the drug too soon, resistant bacteria are given a chance to continue growing, and the infection could recur.

SIDE EFFECTS

Minor. Diarrhea, heartburn, nausea, or vomiting. These side effects should disappear as your body adjusts to the drug.
Major. Tell your doctor about any side effects that are persistent or particularly bothersome. IT IS ESPECIALLY IMPORTANT TO TELL YOUR DOCTOR about bloating, chills, cough, darkened tongue, difficulty in breathing, difficult or painful urination, fever, irritation of the mouth, muscle aches, rash, rectal or vaginal itching, severe diarrhea, sore throat, or yellowing of the eyes or skin. Also, if your symptoms of infection seem to be getting worse rather than improving, you should contact your doctor.

INTERACTIONS

Oxacillin interacts with other types of medications:
1. Probenecid can increase the blood concentrations of this medication.
2. Oxacillin may decrease the effectiveness of birth control pills, and pregnancy could result. You should, therefore, use another form of birth control while taking this drug. Discuss alternatives with your doctor.

BE SURE TO TELL YOUR DOCTOR about any medications you are currently taking, especially any listed above.

WARNINGS

- Tell your doctor about unusual or allergic reactions you have had to any medications, especially to oxacillin, other penicillins, cephalosporin antibiotics, penicillamine, or griseofulvin.
- Tell your doctor if you now have or if you have ever had kidney disease, asthma, or allergies.
- This medication has been prescribed for your current infection only. Another infection later on, or one that someone else has, may require a different medicine. Therefore, you should not give your medicine to other people or use it for other infections, unless your doctor specifically directs you to do so.
- Diabetics taking oxacillin should know that this drug can cause a false-positive sugar reaction with a Clinitest urine glucose test. To avoid this problem while taking oxacillin, you should switch to Clinistix or Tes-Tape to test your urine for sugar.
- Be sure to tell your doctor if you are pregnant. Although oxacillin appears to be safe during pregnancy, extensive studies in humans have not been conducted. Also, tell your doctor if you are breast-feeding an infant. Small amounts of this medication pass into breast milk and may temporarily alter the bacterial balance in the intestinal tract of the nursing infant, resulting in diarrhea.

---

oxazepam

BRAND NAME (Manufacturer)
Serax (Wyeth)

TYPE OF DRUG
Benzodiazepine sedative/hypnotic
INGREDIENT
oxazepam
DOSAGE FORMS
Capsules (10 mg, 15 mg, and 30 mg)
Tablets (15 mg)
STORAGE
This medication should be stored at room temperature in a tightly closed, light-resistant container.

USES

Oxazepam is prescribed to treat symptoms of anxiety and sometimes to treat anxiety associated with depression or alcohol withdrawal. It is not clear exactly how this medicine works, but it may relieve anxiety by acting as a depressant of the central nervous system (brain and spinal cord). Oxazepam is currently used by many people to relieve nervousness. It is effective for this purpose for short periods, but it is important to try to remove the cause of the anxiety as well.

TREATMENT

This medication should be taken exactly as directed by your doctor. It can be taken with food or a full glass of water if stomach upset occurs. Do not take oxazepam with a dose of antacids, since they may slow its absorption.

If you are taking this drug regularly and you miss a dose, take the missed dose immediately if remembered within an hour. If more than an hour has passed, skip the dose you missed and wait for the next scheduled dose. Do not double the dose.

SIDE EFFECTS

Minor. Bitter taste in the mouth, constipation, depression, diarrhea, dizziness, drowsiness (after a night's sleep), dry mouth, excessive salivation, fatigue, flushing, headache, heartburn, loss of appetite, nausea, nervousness, sweating, or vomiting. These side effects should disappear as your body adjusts to the medication.

To relieve constipation, increase the amount of fiber in your diet (fresh fruits and vegetables, salads, bran, and whole-grain breads), exercise, and drink more water (unless your doctor directs you to do otherwise).

Dry mouth can be relieved by chewing sugarless gum or by sucking on ice chips.

If you feel dizzy, sit or lie down for a while; get up slowly from a sitting or reclining position, and be careful on stairs.
Major. Tell your doctor about any side effects that are persistent or particularly bothersome. IT IS ESPECIALLY IMPORTANT TO TELL YOUR DOCTOR about blurred or double vision, chest pain, difficulty in urinating, fainting, falling, fever, hallucinations, joint pain, mouth sores, nightmares, palpitations, rash, severe depression, shortness of breath, slurred speech, sore throat, uncoordinated movements, unusual excitement, unusual tiredness, or yellowing of the eyes or skin.

INTERACTIONS

Oxazepam interacts with several other types of medications:
1. To prevent oversedation, this drug should not be taken with alcohol, other sedative drugs, or central nervous system depressants (such as antihistamines, barbiturates, muscle relaxants, pain medicines, narcotics, medicines for seizures, and phenothiazine tranquilizers) or with antidepressants.
2. This medication may decrease the effectiveness of carbamazepine, levodopa, and oral anticoagulants (blood thinners) and may increase the effects of phenytoin.
3. Disulfiram and isoniazid can increase the blood levels of oxazepam, which can lead to toxic effects.
4. Concurrent use of rifampin may decrease the effectiveness of oxazepam.

BE SURE TO TELL YOUR DOCTOR about any medications you are currently taking, especially any listed above.

WARNINGS

- Tell your doctor about unusual or allergic reactions you have had to any medications, especially to oxazepam or other benzodiazepine tranquilizers (such as alprazolam, chlordiazepoxide, clorazepate, diazepam, flurazepam, halazepam, lorazepam, midazolam, prazepam, temazepam, or triazolam).
- Tell your doctor if you have ever had kidney, liver, or lung disease; epilepsy; myasthenia gravis; porphyria; or mental illness or depression.
- This medicine can cause drowsiness. Avoid tasks that require mental alertness, such as driving a car or using potentially dangerous machinery.
- Oxazepam has the potential for abuse and must be used with caution. Tolerance may develop quickly; do not increase the dosage without first consulting your doctor. It is also important not to stop taking this drug suddenly if you have been taking it in large amounts, or if you have used it for several weeks. Your doctor may want to reduce the dosage gradually.
- This is a safe drug when used properly. When it is combined with other sedative drugs or alcohol, however, serious side effects can develop.
- Be sure to tell your doctor if you are pregnant. This medicine may increase the chance of birth defects if it is taken during the first three months of pregnancy. In addition, too much use of this medicine during the last six months of pregnancy may cause the baby to become dependent on it. This may result in withdrawal side effects in the newborn. Also, use of this medicine during the last weeks of pregnancy may cause excessive drowsiness, slowed heartbeat, and breathing difficulties in the newborn. Tell your doctor if you are breast-feeding. Oxazepam may pass into breast milk and cause excessive drowsiness, slowed heartbeat, and breathing difficulties in the nursing infant.

---

oxtriphylline

BRAND NAMES (Manufacturers)
Choledyl (Parke-Davis)
Choledyl SA (Parke-Davis)
oxtriphylline (various manufacturers)
TYPE OF DRUG
Bronchodilator
INGREDIENT
oxtriphylline
DOSAGE FORMS
Tablets (100 mg and 200 mg)

Sustained-release tablets (400 mg and 600 mg)
Oral pediatric liquid (50 mg per 5-ml spoonful)
Oral elixir (100 mg per 5-ml spoonful, with 20% alcohol)

STORAGE

Oxtriphylline tablets, liquid, and elixir should be stored at room temperature in tightly closed containers. This medication should never be frozen.

USES

This medication is used to treat breathing problems (wheezing and shortness of breath) caused by asthma, bronchitis, or emphysema. It relaxes the smooth muscle of the bronchial airways (breathing tubes), which opens the air passages to the lungs and allows air to move in and out more easily.

TREATMENT

Oxtriphylline should be taken on an empty stomach 30 to 60 minutes before or two hours after a meal. If this medication causes stomach irritation, however, you can take it with food or with a full glass of water or milk (unless your doctor directs you to do otherwise).

Antidiarrheal medications prevent the absorption of oxtriphylline. Therefore, at least one hour should separate doses of these two types of medications.

The sustained-release tablets should be swallowed whole (if the tablet is scored for breaking, you can break it along these lines). Chewing, crushing, or crumbling the tablets destroys their sustained-release activity and possibly increases the side effects.

Each dose of the oral liquid should be measured carefully with a specially designed 5-ml measuring spoon. An ordinary kitchen teaspoon is not accurate enough.

Oxtriphylline works best when the level of the medicine in your bloodstream is kept constant. It is best, therefore, to take the doses at evenly spaced intervals day and night. For example, if you are to take four doses a day, the doses should be spaced six hours apart.

Try not to miss any doses of this medication. If you do miss a dose, take the missed dose as soon as possible, unless it is almost time for the next dose. In that case, do not take the missed dose at all; just return to your regular dosing schedule. Do not double the next dose.

SIDE EFFECTS

Minor. Diarrhea, dizziness, flushing, headache, heartburn, increased urination, insomnia, irritability, loss of appetite, nausea, nervousness, stomach pain, or vomiting. These side effects should disappear as your body adjusts to the medication.

If you feel dizzy or light-headed, sit or lie down for a while; get up slowly from a sitting or reclining position, and be careful on stairs.

Major. Tell your doctor about any side effects that are persistent or particularly bothersome. IT IS ESPECIALLY IMPORTANT TO TELL YOUR DOCTOR about bloody or black, tarry stools; confusion; convulsions; difficulty in breathing; fainting; muscle twitches; palpitations; rash; severe abdominal pain; or unusual weakness.

INTERACTIONS

Oxtriphylline interacts with several other types of drugs:

1. It can increase the diuretic effects of furosemide.
2. Reserpine, in combination with oxtriphylline, can cause a rapid heart rate.
3. Beta blockers (acebutolol, atenolol, betaxolol, carteolol, esmolol, labetalol, metoprolol, nadolol, penbutolol, pindolol, propranolol, timolol) can block the effectiveness of oxtriphylline.
4. Phenobarbital and rifampin can increase the elimination of oxtriphylline from the body, decreasing its effectiveness.
5. Cimetidine, erythromycin, oral contraceptives (birth control pills), troleanodomycin, allopurinol, and thiabendazole can decrease the elimination of oxtriphylline from the body, increasing its side effects.

Before you start to take this medication, BE SURE TO TELL YOUR DOCTOR about any medications you are currently taking, especially any of those listed above.

WARNINGS

- Tell your doctor about unusual or allergic reactions you have had to any medications, especially to oxtriphylline, aminophylline, caffeine, dyphylline, theophylline, or theobromine.
- Tell your doctor if you now have or if you have ever had fibrocystic breast disease, heart disease, kidney disease, low or high blood pressure, liver disease, stomach ulcers, thyroid disease, or an enlarged prostate gland.
- Cigarette or marijuana smoking may affect this drug's action. BE SURE TO TELL YOUR DOCTOR if you smoke. Also, do not suddenly stop smoking without informing your doctor.
- High fever, diarrhea, the flu, and influenza vaccinations can also affect the actions of this drug. Therefore, tell your doctor about episodes of high fever or prolonged diarrhea. Before having any vaccinations, especially those to prevent the flu, be sure to tell the person administering the vaccine that you are taking this medication.
- Avoid drinking large amounts of caffeine-containing beverages (coffee, cocoa, tea, and cola drinks), and avoid eating large amounts of chocolate. These products may increase the side effects of oxtriphylline.
- Do not change your diet without first consulting your doctor. The action of this drug may be affected by charbroiled foods or a high-protein, low-carbohydrate diet.
- Before having surgery or other medical or dental treatment, be sure to tell your doctor or dentist about this drug.
- Before taking any over-the-counter (nonprescription) asthma, allergy, cough, cold, sinus, or diet medication, ask your doctor or pharmacist whether it will interact with oxtriphylline. These products may add to the side effects of oxtriphylline.
- Be sure to tell your doctor if you are pregnant. Although oxtriphylline appears to be safe during pregnancy, extensive studies in humans have not been conducted. Also, tell your doctor if you are breast-feeding an infant. Small amounts of oxtriphylline pass into breast milk and may cause irritability, fretfulness, or insomnia in nursing infants.

---

oxybutynin

BRAND NAME (Manufacturer)

Ditropan (Marion)

TYPE OF DRUG
Antispasmodic
INGREDIENT
oxybutynin
DOSAGE FORMS
Tablets (5 mg)
Oral syrup (5 mg per 5-ml spoonful)
STORAGE
Oxybutynin tablets and syrup should be stored at room temperature in tightly closed containers.

USES

Oxybutynin is used to relieve the symptoms associated with urinary incontinence (inability to control the bladder) or urinary frequency. It works directly on the muscle of the bladder, increasing bladder capacity and thereby delaying the desire to urinate.

TREATMENT

Oxybutynin can be taken either on an empty stomach with water only or, to reduce stomach irritation, with food or milk (as directed by your doctor).

Each dose of the oral syrup should be measured carefully with a specially designed 5-ml measuring spoon. An ordinary kitchen teaspoon is not accurate enough.

If you miss a dose of this medication, take the missed dose as soon as possible, unless it is almost time for the next dose. In that case, do not take the missed dose at all; just return to your regular dosing schedule. Do not double the next dose.

SIDE EFFECTS

Minor. Bloating, blurred vision, constipation, decreased sweating, dizziness, drowsiness, dry mouth, insomnia, nausea, vomiting, or weakness. These side effects should disappear as your body adjusts to the medication.

This medication can also cause increased sensitivity of your eyes to sunlight. Sunglasses may help relieve the discomfort caused by bright lights.

To relieve constipation, increase the amount of fiber in your diet (fresh fruits and vegetables, salads, bran, and whole-grain breads) and exercise (unless your doctor directs you to do otherwise).

If you feel dizzy, sit or lie down for a while; get up slowly from a sitting or reclining position, and be careful on stairs.

To help relieve mouth dryness, chew sugarless gum or suck on ice chips or a piece of hard candy.

Major. Tell your doctor about any side effects that are persistent or particularly bothersome. IT IS ESPECIALLY IMPORTANT TO TELL YOUR DOCTOR about decreased sexual ability, difficult or painful urination, eye pain, itching, palpitations, or skin rash.

INTERACTIONS

Oxybutynin should not interact with other medications if it is used according to directions.

WARNINGS

- Tell your doctor about unusual or allergic reactions you have had to any medications, especially to oxybutynin.
- Before starting to take this medication, be sure to tell your doctor if you now have or if you have ever had bleeding disorders, glaucoma, heart disease, hiatal hernia, high blood pressure, intestinal blockage, kidney disease, liver disease, myasthenia gravis, enlarged prostate gland, thyroid disease, toxemia of pregnancy, ulcerative colitis, or urinary retention.
- If this drug makes you dizzy or blurs your vision, avoid taking part in any activity that requires alertness, such as driving a car or operating potentially dangerous machinery.
- This medication can decrease sweating and heat release from the body. You should, therefore, try not to become overheated (avoid strenuous exercise in hot weather, and do not take hot baths, showers, and saunas).
- Be sure to tell your doctor if you are pregnant. Although oxybutynin appears to be safe during pregnancy, extensive studies in humans have not been conducted. Also, tell your doctor if you are breast-feeding. This drug may decrease milk production. It is not known whether oxybutynin passes into breast milk.

oxycodone hydrochloride, oxycodone terephthalate, and aspirin—see aspirin and oxycodone combination

oxycodone hydrochloride with acetaminophen—see acetaminophen and oxycodone combination

Oxydess II—see dextroamphetamine

---

oxymetholone

BRAND NAME (Manufacturer)
Anadrol-50 (Syntex)
TYPE OF DRUG
Anabolic hormone
INGREDIENT
oxymetholone
DOSAGE FORM
Tablets (50 mg)
STORAGE
Store at room temperature in a tightly closed container.

USES

This medication is used to treat anemia and osteoporosis (bone loss). Oxymetholone belongs to a group of drugs known as anabolic hormones (steroids). It works by promoting the buildup of body tissues, including red blood cells and bone.

TREATMENT

You can take oxymetholone either on an empty stomach or, to reduce stomach irritation, with food or milk (as directed by your doctor).

If you miss a dose of this medication, take the missed dose as soon as possible, unless it is almost time for your next dose. In that case, do not take the missed dose at all; just return to your regular dosing schedule. Do not double the next dose.

SIDE EFFECTS

Minor. Chills, decreased sexual ability, diarrhea, increased or decreased sexual desire, stomach upset, or trouble sleeping. These side effects should disappear as your body adjusts to the medication.

Major. Tell your doctor about any side effects that are persistent or particularly bothersome. IT IS ESPECIALLY IMPORTANT TO TELL YOUR DOCTOR about acne or oily skin; bloody or black, tarry stools; breath odor; deepening of the voice (in women); depression; enlarged or painful breasts (in both sexes); increased or decreased hair growth; headaches; loss of appetite; menstrual irregularities; muscle cramps; sore throat or fever; swelling of the feet or legs; unusual bleeding or bruising; weakness; weight gain or loss; or yellowing of the eyes or skin.

INTERACTIONS

Oxymetholone interacts with several other types of drugs:

1. It can increase the effects of oral anticoagulants (blood thinners, such as warfarin), which can lead to bleeding complications.

2. Diabetic patients should know that oxymetholone can decrease blood glucose levels. The dosage of oral antidiabetic medications or insulin may, therefore, need to be adjusted when this medication is being taken.

BE SURE TO TELL YOUR DOCTOR about any medications you are currently taking, especially any of those listed above.

WARNINGS

- Tell your doctor about unusual or allergic reactions you have had to any medications, especially to oxymetholone or to other anabolic hormones (such as dromostanolone, nandrolone, oxandrolone, or stanozolol).
- Before starting to take this medication, be sure to tell your doctor if you now have or if you have ever had breast cancer, heart disease, hypercalcemia (high blood calcium levels), kidney disease, liver disease, prostate cancer, or an enlarged prostate gland.
- To obtain maximum benefit from this medication, eat a well-balanced diet that provides adequate protein and calories.
- Athletes sometimes use anabolic steroids to increase performance. However, there is conflicting and inconclusive evidence as to whether these drugs increase muscle strength. There is also some question as to their safety.
- Be sure to tell your doctor if you are pregnant. Oxymetholone crosses the placenta and can cause masculine characteristics, such as increased body hair, in the developing fetus. (Note: This drug does NOT affect the sex of the fetus, which is determined at conception.) Also, tell your doctor if you are breast-feeding an infant. It is not known whether oxymetholone passes into breast milk.

---

oxytetracycline

BRAND NAMES (Manufacturers)

E.P. Mycin (Edwards)
oxytetracycline hydrochloride (various manufacturers)
Terramycin (Pfizer)
Uri-Tet (American Urologicals)

TYPE OF DRUG

Tetracycline antibiotic

INGREDIENT

oxytetracycline

DOSAGE FORMS

Tablets (250 mg)
Capsules (250 mg)

STORAGE

Oxytetracycline should be stored at room temperature in a tightly closed, light-resistant container.

USES

Oxytetracycline is used to treat acne and a wide variety of bacterial infections. It acts by inhibiting the growth of bacteria. Bacteria may be partly responsible for the development of acne lesions. Oxytetracycline kills susceptible bacteria, but it is not effective against viruses or fungi.

TREATMENT

Ideally, this medication should be taken on an empty stomach one hour before or two hours after a meal. It should be taken with a full glass of water in order to avoid irritation of the throat or esophagus (tube leading to the stomach). If this drug causes stomach upset, however, you can take it with food or water (unless your doctor directs otherwise).

Avoid consuming any dairy products, including milk and cheese, within two hours of any dose of this drug. Avoid taking antacids or laxatives containing aluminum, calcium, or magnesium within an hour or two of a dose. Avoid taking any medication containing iron within three hours of a dose. These products chemically bind oxytetracycline and prevent the drug from being absorbed into the body.

Oxytetracycline works best when the level of medicine in your bloodstream is kept constant. It is best, therefore, to take the doses at evenly spaced intervals day and night. For example, if you are to take four doses a day, the doses should be spaced six hours apart.

If you miss a dose of this medication, take the missed dose immediately. However, if you do not remember to take the missed dose until it is almost time for your next dose, take it; space the following dose about halfway through the regular interval between doses; then return to your regular dosing schedule. Try not to skip any doses.

It is important to continue to take this medication for the entire time prescribed by your doctor, even if the symptoms disappear before the end of that period. If you stop taking the drug too soon, resistant bacteria are given a chance to continue growing, and the infection could recur.

SIDE EFFECTS

Minor. Diarrhea, dizziness, loss of appetite, nausea, stomach cramps and upset, vomiting, or discoloration of the nails. These side effects should disappear as your body adjusts to the medication.

Oxytetracycline can increase your sensitivity to sunlight. You should, therefore, avoid prolonged exposure to sunlight and sunlamps. Wear protective clothing and sunglasses, and use an effective sunscreen.

Major. Tell your doctor about any side effects that are persistent or particularly bothersome. IT IS ESPECIALLY IMPORTANT TO TELL YOUR DOCTOR about darkened tongue, difficulty in breathing, joint pain, mouth irritation, rash, rectal or vaginal itching, sore throat and fever, unusual bleeding or bruising, or yellowing of the eyes or skin. Also, if your symptoms of infection seem to be getting worse rather than improving, contact your doctor.

INTERACTIONS

Oxytetracycline interacts with several other types of drugs:

1. It can increase the absorption of digoxin, which may lead to digoxin toxicity.

2. The gastrointestinal side effects (nausea, vomiting, stomach upset) of theophylline may be increased by oxytetracycline.

3. The dosage of oral anticoagulants (blood thinners, such as warfarin) may need to be adjusted when this medication is started.

4. Oxytetracycline may decrease the effectiveness of oral contraceptives (birth control pills), and pregnancy could result. You should, therefore, use another form of birth control while taking oxytetracycline. Consult your doctor.

BE SURE TO TELL YOUR DOCTOR about any medications you are currently taking, especially any listed above.

WARNINGS

- Tell your doctor about unusual or allergic reactions you have had to any medications, especially to oxytetracycline or to tetracycline, doxycycline, or minocycline.
- Tell your doctor if you now have or if you have ever had kidney or liver disease.
- Oxytetracycline can affect tests for syphilis; tell your doctor you are taking this medication if you are also being treated for this disease.
- Make sure that your prescription for oxytetracycline is marked with the expiration date. The drug should be discarded after the expiration date. If the medication is used after it has expired, serious side effects (especially to the kidneys) could result.
- This medication has been prescribed for your current infection only. Another infection later on, or one that someone else has, may require a different medicine. Therefore, you should not give your medicine to other people or use it for other infections, unless your doctor specifically directs you to do so.
- Be sure to tell your doctor if you are pregnant or if you are breast-feeding an infant. Oxytetracycline crosses the placenta and passes into breast milk. This medication can cause permanent discoloration of the teeth and can inhibit tooth and bone growth if used during their development. In addition, oxytetracycline should not be used for infants or for children less than eight years of age because of the potential risks involved.

oxytetracycline hydrochloride—see oxytetracycline

Pamelor—see nortriptyline

Pamprin-IB—see ibuprofen

Panasol-S—see prednisone (systemic)

Pancrease—see pancrelipase

---

pancreatin

BRAND NAMES (Manufacturers)

Pancreatin Enseals* (Lilly)

Pancreatin Tablets* (Lilly)

*Available over-the-counter (without a prescription)

TYPE OF DRUG

Digestive enzymes

INGREDIENTS

pancreatin, lipase, protease, and amylase

DOSAGE FORMS

Pancreatin Tablets (pancreatin 325 mg; lipase 650 units; protease 8,125 units; amylase 8,125 units)

Pancreatin Enseals (pancreatin 1000 mg; lipase 2000 units; protease 25,000 units; amylase 25,000 units)

STORAGE

Store at room temperature in a tightly closed container.

USES

This medication is a combination of specific digestive (pancreatic) enzymes obtained from pigs or cows. These enzymes aid in the digestion and absorption of fats and starch. Pancreatin is used in the treatment of various pancreatic enzyme deficiencies resulting from conditions such as pancreatitis, cystic fibrosis, or gastrointestinal bypass surgery.

TREATMENT

In order to obtain the maximum benefit from this medication, you should take pancreatin just before or with meals or snacks. The tablets can be crushed and mixed with food.

If you miss a dose of this medication, do not take the missed dose at all; just return to your regular dosing schedule. Do not double the next dose.

SIDE EFFECTS

Minor. Diarrhea, nausea, or stomach cramps. These side effects should disappear as your body adjusts to the medication.

Major. Tell your doctor about any side effects that are persistent or particularly bothersome. IT IS ESPECIALLY IMPORTANT TO TELL YOUR DOCTOR about bloody urine, hives, joint pain, skin rash, or swelling of the feet or legs.

INTERACTIONS

Pancreatin can decrease the absorption of iron from the gastrointestinal tract, which may lead to nutritional deficiency. Your doctor may want to prescribe iron supplements if this becomes a problem. Cimetidine or antacids are often prescribed concurrently with pancreatin in order to maximize its effectiveness. However, calcium- or magnesium-containing antacids should be avoided—they decrease this medication's effectiveness. You should discuss these effects with your doctor.

WARNINGS

- Tell your doctor about unusual or allergic reactions you have had to any medications, especially to pancreatin, pancrelipase, or any other digestive enzymes.
- Patients who have allergies to pork or beef products may also be allergic to pancreatin, since it is obtained from pigs and cows.
- Be sure to tell your doctor if you are pregnant. Although pancreatin appears to be safe during pregnancy, extensive studies have not been conducted. Also, tell your doctor if you are breast-feeding an infant. It is not known whether pancreatin passes into breast milk.

Pancreatin Enseals—see pancreatin

Pancreatin Tablets—see pancreatin

---

pancrelipase

BRAND NAMES (Manufacturers)
Cotazym-S (Organon)
Festal II* (Hoechst-Roussel)
Ilozyme (Adria)
Ku-Zyme HP (Kremers-Urban)
Pancrease (McNeil)
Viokase (Robins)
*Available over-the-counter (without a prescription)

TYPE OF DRUG
Digestive enzymes

INGREDIENTS
lipase, protease, and amylase

DOSAGE FORMS
Tablets (in various strengths)
Capsules (in various strengths)
Powder packets (in various strengths)

STORAGE
Pancrelipase tablets, capsules, and powder should be stored at room temperature in tightly closed containers.

USES

This medication is a combination of digestive (pancreatic) enzymes obtained from pigs. These enzymes aid in the digestion and absorption of starch and fats. Pancrelipase is used to treat pancreatic enzyme deficiencies resulting from conditions such as pancreatitis, cystic fibrosis, or gastrointestinal bypass surgery.

TREATMENT

In order to obtain the maximum benefit, you should take pancrelipase just before or with meals or snacks. The powder can be added to food; the tablets can also be crushed and mixed with food.

If you are taking the capsules containing the enteric-coated microspheres, swallow the capsule whole. Chewing, crushing, or breaking the capsules decreases their effectiveness and increases the side effects. However, if you have difficulty swallowing the capsules, you can open them and sprinkle the contents on a small amount of liquid or soft food, which you should then swallow without chewing. DO NOT mix this medication with alkaline foods (such as dairy products)—they can reduce its effectiveness.

If you miss a dose of this medication, do not take the missed dose at all; just return to your regular dosing schedule. Do not double the next dose.

SIDE EFFECTS

Minor. Diarrhea, nausea, or stomach cramps. These side effects should disappear as your body adjusts to the medication.

Major. Tell your doctor about any side effects that are persistent or particularly bothersome. IT IS ESPECIALLY IMPORTANT TO TELL YOUR DOCTOR about bloody urine, hives, joint pain, skin rash, or swelling of the feet or legs.

INTERACTIONS

Pancrelipase can decrease the absorption of iron from the gastrointestinal tract, which may lead to nutritional deficiency. Your doctor may want to prescribe iron supplements if this becomes a problem. Cimetidine or antacids are often prescribed concurrently with pancrelipase, in order to maximize its effectiveness. However, calcium- or magnesium-containing antacids should be avoided—they decrease this medication's effectiveness. You should discuss these effects with your doctor.

WARNINGS

- Tell your doctor about unusual or allergic reactions you have had to any medications, especially to pancrelipase, pancreatin, or any other digestive enzymes.
- Patients who have allergies to pork products may also be allergic to pancrelipase, since it is obtained from pigs.
- The powder form and the powder from opened capsules of this medication can be very irritating to the nose and throat. Avoid inhaling the particles.
- Be sure to tell your doctor if you are pregnant. Although pancrelipase appears to be safe during pregnancy, extensive studies have not been conducted. Also, tell your doctor if you are breast-feeding an infant. It is not known whether pancrelipase passes into breast milk.

Panmycin—see tetracycline

Panwarfin—see warfarin

---

papaverine

BRAND NAMES (Manufacturers)
Cerespan (Rorer)
papaverine hydrochloride (various manufacturers)
Pavabid HP Capsulet (Marion)
Pavabid Plateau (Marion)
Pavacen Cenules (Central)
Pavagen (Rugby)
Pavarine Spancaps (Vortech)
Pavased (Hauck)
Pavatym (Everett)
Paverolan Lanacaps (Lannett)

TYPE OF DRUG
Vasodilator

INGREDIENT
papaverine

DOSAGE FORMS
Tablets (30 mg, 60 mg, 100 mg, 150 mg, 200 mg, and 300 mg)
Sustained-release capsules (150 mg)
Sustained-release tablets (200 mg)

STORAGE
Papaverine should be stored at room temperature in a tightly closed container.

USES

Papaverine is used to treat circulation disorders. It is a vasodilator that acts directly on the muscle tissues of blood vessels to increase blood supply to various parts of the body.

TREATMENT

In order to avoid stomach irritation, you can take papaverine with food or with a full glass of water or milk. Ask your doctor if you can take it with an antacid.

The sustained-release capsules should be swallowed whole. Breaking, crushing, or chewing these capsules destroys their sustained-release activity and possibly increases the side effects.

If you miss a dose of this medication, take the missed dose as soon as possible, unless it is almost time for the next dose. In that case, do not take the missed dose at all; just return to your regular dosing schedule. Do not double the next dose.

SIDE EFFECTS

Minor. Abdominal distress, blurred vision, constipation, diarrhea, dizziness, drowsiness, fatigue, flushing, headache, loss of appetite, nausea, or sweating. These side effects should disappear as your body adjusts to the medication.

If you feel dizzy, sit or lie down for a while; get up slowly from a sitting or reclining position, and be careful on stairs.

To relieve constipation, increase the amount of fiber in your diet (fresh fruits and vegetables, salads, bran, and whole-grain breads), exercise, and drink more water (unless your doctor directs you to do otherwise).

Major. Tell your doctor about any side effects that are persistent or particularly bothersome. IT IS ESPECIALLY IMPORTANT TO TELL YOUR DOCTOR about depression, difficulty in breathing, palpitations, rash, unusual bleeding or bruising, or yellowing of the eyes or skin.

INTERACTIONS

Concurrent use of papaverine and levodopa can lead to decreased effectiveness of levodopa.

Before starting to take papaverine, BE SURE TO TELL YOUR DOCTOR about any medications you are currently taking, especially levodopa.

WARNINGS

- Tell your doctor about unusual or allergic reactions you have had to any medications, especially to papaverine.
- Be sure to tell your doctor if you have ever had angina, glaucoma, heart block, liver disease, low or high blood pressure, a heart attack, or Parkinson's disease.
- A government panel has recently reviewed the effectiveness of this medication in the treatment of hardening of the arteries and leg cramps and in the prevention of stroke. This drug may not be as effective as once thought. Discuss this with your physician.
- Before taking any over-the-counter (nonprescription) cough, cold, allergy, asthma, sinus, or diet medication, check with your doctor or pharmacist. Some of these products can decrease the effectiveness of papaverine.
- If this drug makes you dizzy or drowsy, do not take part in any activity that requires alertness, such as driving a car or operating potentially dangerous machinery.
- The beneficial effects of this medication may be decreased by the nicotine in cigarettes. Try to stop smoking.
- To prevent dizziness and fainting while taking this medication, avoid drinking large quantities of alcohol, and try not to get overheated (avoid strenuous exercise in hot weather and do not take hot baths, showers, and saunas).
- Be sure to tell your doctor if you are pregnant. Although papaverine appears to be safe, extensive studies in pregnant women have not been conducted. Also, tell your doctor if you are breast-feeding. It is not known whether papaverine passes into breast milk.

papaverine hydrochloride—see papaverine

Paracet Forte—see chlorzoxazone and acetaminophen combination

---

pargyline

BRAND NAME (Manufacturer)
Eutonyl Filmtabs (Abbott)
TYPE OF DRUG
Monoamine oxidase (MAO) inhibitor and antihypertensive
INGREDIENT
pargyline
DOSAGE FORM
Tablets (10 mg and 25 mg)
STORAGE
Store at room temperature in a tightly closed container.

USES

Pargyline belongs to a group of drugs known as monoamine oxidase (MAO) inhibitors. It is used to treat high blood pressure. It is not exactly clear how this medication works, but it is thought to decrease the activity of the chemicals responsible for increasing blood pressure.

TREATMENT

Pargyline can be taken either on an empty stomach or, to avoid stomach irritation, with food or milk (unless your doctor directs you to do otherwise).

In order to become accustomed to taking this medication, try to take the dose(s) at the same time(s) each day. If you are taking a single daily dose, it is best to take the dose in the morning (to avoid sleeping difficulties).

If you miss a dose of this medication and remember within two hours, take the missed dose immediately. If more than two hours has passed, do not take the missed dose at all; just return to your regular dosing schedule. Do not double the next dose.

Pargyline does not cure high blood pressure, but it will help to control the condition as long as you continue to take the medication.

SIDE EFFECTS

Minor. Constipation, dizziness, drowsiness, dry mouth, headache, increased appetite and weight gain, insomnia, nausea, restlessness, or sweating. These side effects should disappear as your body adjusts to the medication.

Pargyline can increase your sensitivity to sunlight. You should, therefore, avoid prolonged exposure to sunlight and sunlamps. Wear protective clothing and sunglasses, and use an effective sunscreen.

To relieve constipation, increase the amount of fiber in your diet (fresh fruits and vegetables, salads, bran, and whole-grain breads), and drink more water (unless your doctor directs you to do otherwise).

If you feel dizzy, sit or lie down for a while; get up slowly from a sitting or reclining position, and be careful on stairs.

To help relieve mouth dryness, chew sugarless gum or suck on ice chips or a piece of hard candy.

Major. Tell your doctor about any side effects that are persistent or particularly bothersome. IT IS ESPECIALLY IMPORTANT TO TELL YOUR DOCTOR about blurred vision, difficulty in urinating, fainting, fever, hallucinations, muscle aches or twitching, swelling of the feet or legs, or yellowing of the eyes or skin.

If you experience a severe headache, stiff neck, chest pain, palpitations, or vomiting while taking this medication, CONTACT YOUR DOCTOR OR AN EMERGENCY ROOM IMMEDIATELY. These symptoms may be the result of a food or drug interaction.

INTERACTIONS

Pargyline interacts with a number of drugs and foods:

1. Concurrent use of pargyline and central nervous system depressants (such as alcohol, barbiturates, benzodiazepine tranquilizers, muscle relaxants, narcotics, pain medications, phenothiazine tranquilizers, and sleeping medications) or tricyclic antidepressants can lead to extreme drowsiness.

2. The dosage of anticonvulsant medications may need to be adjusted when pargyline is being taken.

3. Use of pargyline within 14 days of either another monoamine oxidase inhibitor or carbamazepine, cyclobenzaprine, methyldopa, guanethidine, reserpine, levodopa, meperidine or another narcotic, an amphetamine, ephedrine, methylphenidate, phenylpropanolamine, pseudoephedrine, or a tricyclic antidepressant can lead to serious (sometimes fatal) side effects.

4. Tyramine-containing foods and beverages (aged cheeses, sour cream, yogurt, pickled herring, chicken livers, canned figs, raisins, bananas, avocados, soy sauce, broad bean pods, yeast extracts, beer, and certain wines), excessive amounts of caffeine-containing beverages (coffee, tea, cocoa, and cola), and chocolate can also cause serious reactions in patients on pargyline therapy.

5. Pargyline can increase the blood-sugar-lowering effects of insulin and oral antidiabetic medications.

Before starting to take pargyline, BE SURE TO TELL YOUR DOCTOR about any medications you are currently taking, especially any of those listed above. Be sure you are aware of the foods (listed in item number four above) that interact with this medication.

WARNINGS

- Tell your doctor about unusual or allergic reactions you have had to any medications, especially to pargyline.
- Before starting to take this medication, be sure to tell your doctor if you now have or if you have ever had asthma, bronchitis, diabetes mellitus, epilepsy, glaucoma, severe headaches, heart or blood vessel disease, kidney disease, liver disease, mental disorders, Parkinson's disease, pheochromocytoma, or thyroid disease.
- If this drug makes you dizzy or drowsy, do not take part in any activity that requires alertness, such as driving a car or operating potentially dangerous machinery.
- Before having surgery or any other medical or dental treatment, be sure to tell your doctor or dentist that you are taking this medication.
- Check with your doctor or pharmacist before taking any nonprescription asthma, allergy, cough, cold, diet, or sinus preparation. Concurrent use of some of these products with pargyline can lead to serious side effects.
- The 25-mg tablets contain FD&C Yellow No. 5 (tartrazine), which can cause allergic-type reactions (fainting, shortness of breath, rash) in certain individuals.
- If you have angina, do not increase your amount of physical activity unless you check with your doctor. Pargyline can decrease the symptoms of angina without decreasing the risks of strenuous exercise.
- Be sure to tell your doctor if you are pregnant. Although pargyline appears to be safe during pregnancy, extensive studies have not been conducted. Also, tell your doctor if you are breast-feeding an infant. It is not known whether pargyline passes into breast milk.

Parlodel—see bromocriptine

Parlodel SnapTabs—see bromocriptine

Parmine—see phentermine

Pathocil—see dicloxacillin

Pavabid—see papaverine

Pavabid Plateau—see papaverine

Pavacen Cenules—see papaverine

Pavagen—see papaverine

Pavarine Spancaps—see papaverine

Pavased—see papaverine

Pavatym—see papaverine

Paverolan Lanacaps—see papaverine

Paxipam—see halazepam

PCE Dispertab—see erythromycin

Pedia Care 2—see pseudoephedrine and chlorpheniramine combination

Pediamycin—see erythromycin

Pediazole—see erythromycin and sulfisoxazole combination

Pedi-Cort V—see hydrocortisone and iodochlorhydroxyquin combination (topical)

---

pemoline

BRAND NAME (Manufacturer)
Cylert (Abbott)

TYPE OF DRUG
Stimulant
INGREDIENT
pemoline
DOSAGE FORMS
Tablets (18.75 mg, 37.5 mg, and 75 mg)
Chewable tablets (37.5 mg)
STORAGE
Pemoline should be stored at room temperature in a tightly closed container.

USES

Pemoline is a central nervous system (brain and spinal cord) stimulant that is used to treat attention deficit disorders (hyperkinetic syndrome). It is not yet clear how pemoline works to improve behavioral disorders in children, but it seems to decrease hyperactivity and increase attention span.

TREATMENT

Pemoline can be taken either on an empty stomach or with food or milk (as directed by your doctor). The chewable tablet form of this medication can be either chewed or swallowed whole.

If you miss a dose of this medication, take the missed dose as soon as possible, unless it is almost time for the next dose. In that case, do not take the missed dose at all; just return to your regular dosing schedule. Do not double the next dose of this medication.

You may not observe the full therapeutic benefits of this medication for three to four weeks.

SIDE EFFECTS

Minor. Dizziness, drowsiness, headache, insomnia, irritability, loss of appetite, nausea, stomachache, or weight loss. These side effects should disappear as your body adjusts to the drug.

If you feel dizzy, sit or lie down for a while; get up slowly from a sitting or reclining position, and be careful on stairs.

Major. Tell your doctor about any side effects that are persistent or particularly bothersome. IT IS ESPECIALLY IMPORTANT TO TELL YOUR DOCTOR about convulsions; depression; hallucinations; palpitations; skin rash; unusual movements of the tongue, lips, face, hands, or feet; or yellowing of the eyes or skin.

INTERACTIONS

Pemoline should not interact with other medications if it is used according to the directions given to you by your doctor or pharmacist.

WARNINGS

- Tell your doctor about unusual or allergic reactions you have had to any medications, especially to pemoline.
- Before starting to take this medication, be sure to tell your doctor if you now have or if you have ever had kidney disease, liver disease, or mental disorders.
- If this drug makes you dizzy or drowsy, do not take part in any activity that requires alertness, such as driving a car or operating potentially dangerous machinery. Children who are taking this drug should be cautious while playing.
- This medication has the potential for abuse and must be used with caution. It should, therefore, not be taken in larger doses or for longer periods than prescribed by your doctor. In addition, you should not stop taking pemoline unless you first check with your doctor. Stopping the drug abruptly can lead to a withdrawal reaction. Your doctor may, therefore, want to reduce the dosage gradually.
- Your doctor may want to interrupt pemoline therapy occasionally for short periods ("drug holidays") to see if the symptoms of the attention deficit disorder have disappeared.
- Be sure to tell your doctor if you are pregnant. Although pemoline appears to be safe, extensive studies in humans during pregnancy have not been conducted. Also, tell your doctor if you are breast-feeding an infant. It is not known whether pemoline passes into breast milk.

Penapar-VK—see penicillin VK

Penecort—see hydrocortisone (topical)

---

penicillamine

BRAND NAMES (Manufacturers)
Cuprimine (Merck Sharp & Dohme)
Depen Titratable Tablets (Wallace)
TYPE OF DRUG
Chelator and antirheumatic
INGREDIENT
penicillamine
DOSAGE FORMS
Tablets (250 mg)
Capsules (125 mg and 250 mg)
STORAGE
Store at room temperature in a tightly closed container.

USES

This drug is used to treat Wilson's disease (high blood copper levels), severe rheumatoid arthritis, and cystinuria (high urine levels of cystine). Penicillamine binds to copper and cystine, which prevents their harmful effects on the body. It is not clearly understood how penicillamine relieves rheumatoid arthritis.

TREATMENT

In order to obtain the maximum benefit from penicillamine, you should take it on an empty stomach one hour before or two hours after a meal. To ensure maximal absorption of this drug, each dose should be separated from doses of other medications and from food and milk by at least an hour.

If you miss a dose of this medication, take the missed dose as soon as possible, unless it is almost time for the next dose. In that case, do not take the missed dose at all; just return to your regular dosing schedule. Do not double the next dose.

The full benefits of this medication may not become apparent for as long as three months after beginning therapy.

SIDE EFFECTS

Minor. Altered taste sensations, diarrhea, loss of appetite, nausea, stomach upset, or vomiting. These side effects should disappear as your body adjusts to the medication.

Major. Tell your doctor about any side effects that are persistent or particularly bothersome. IT IS ESPECIALLY IM-

PORTANT TO TELL YOUR DOCTOR about breast enlargement (in both sexes), difficult or painful urination, difficulty in breathing, joint pain, loss of hair, mouth sores, ringing in the ears, skin rash, sore throat, tingling sensations in the fingers or toes, unusual bleeding or bruising, or wheezing.

INTERACTIONS

Penicillamine interacts with several other types of medications:

1. The absorption of penicillamine from the gastrointestinal tract can be decreased by iron or antacids.

2. Penicillamine can decrease the blood levels and beneficial effects of digoxin.

3. Concurrent use of penicillamine and gold salts, hydroxychloroquine, phenylbutazone, oxyphenbutazone, or anticancer drugs can lead to increased side effects to the blood and kidneys.

BE SURE TO TELL YOUR DOCTOR about any medications you are currently taking, especially any of those listed above.

WARNINGS

- Tell your doctor about unusual or allergic reactions you have had to any medications, especially to penicillamine or penicillin or cephalosporin antibiotics.
- Before starting to take this medication, be sure to tell your doctor if you now have or if you have ever had blood disorders or kidney disease.
- Do not stop taking this drug unless you first check with your doctor. Stopping the drug and restarting it at a later time can lead to increased side effects.
- Penicillamine can decrease the body's ability to repair wounds, so try to avoid injuring yourself while you are taking this medication. This warning is especially important for diabetic patients.
- Before having surgery or any other medical or dental treatment, be sure to tell your doctor or dentist that you are taking this drug.
- Your doctor may want you to take pyridoxine (vitamin B_6) to prevent some of the side effects (for example, tingling sensations) of penicillamine.
- Be sure to tell your doctor if you are pregnant. Penicillamine has been reported to cause birth defects in both animals and humans. Also, tell your doctor if you are breast-feeding an infant. It is not known whether penicillamine passes into breast milk.

---

penicillin G

BRAND NAMES (Manufacturers)

penicillin G potassium (various manufacturers)
Pentids (Squibb)

TYPE OF DRUG

Penicillin antibiotic

INGREDIENT

penicillin G potassium

DOSAGE FORMS

Tablets (200,000 units; 250,000 units; 400,000 units; 500,000 units; and 800,000 units)
Oral solution (200,000 units and 400,000 units per 5-ml spoonful)

STORAGE

Penicillin G tablets should be stored at room temperature in a tightly closed container. The oral solution should be stored in the refrigerator in a tightly closed container. Any unused portion of the solution should be discarded after 14 days because the drug loses its potency after that time. This medication should never be frozen.

USES

Penicillin G is used to treat a wide variety of bacterial infections, including infections of the middle ear, the respiratory tract, and the urinary tract. It acts by severely injuring the cell membranes of infecting bacteria, thereby preventing them from growing and multiplying. Penicillin G kills susceptible bacteria, but it is not effective against viruses, parasites, or fungi.

TREATMENT

Penicillin G should be taken on an empty stomach or with a glass of water one hour before or two hours after a meal. This medication should never be taken with fruit juices or carbonated beverages because the acidity of these drinks destroys the drug in the stomach.

The oral solution should be measured carefully with a specially designed 5-ml measuring spoon. An ordinary kitchen teaspoon is not accurate enough.

Penicillin G works best when the level of medicine in your bloodstream is kept constant. It is best, therefore, to take the doses at evenly spaced intervals day and night. For example, if you are taking four doses a day, the doses should be spaced six hours apart.

If you miss a dose of this medication, take the missed dose immediately. However, if you do not remember to take the missed dose until it is almost time for the next dose, take it; space the following dose about halfway through the regular interval between doses; then return to your regular dosing schedule. Try not to skip any doses.

It is important to continue to take this medication for the entire time prescribed by your doctor (usually seven to 14 days), even if the symptoms of infection disappear before the end of that period. If you stop taking the drug too soon, resistant bacteria are given a chance to continue growing, and the infection could recur.

SIDE EFFECTS

Minor. Diarrhea, heartburn, nausea, or vomiting. These side effects should disappear as your body adjusts to the medication.

Major. Tell your doctor about any side effects that are persistent or particularly bothersome. IT IS ESPECIALLY IMPORTANT TO TELL YOUR DOCTOR about bloating, chills, cough, darkened tongue, difficulty in breathing, fever, irritation of the mouth, muscle aches, rash, rectal or vaginal itching, severe diarrhea, or sore throat. Also, if your infection seems to be getting worse rather than improving, you should contact your physician.

INTERACTIONS

Penicillin G antibiotic interacts with several other types of medications:

1. Probenecid can increase the blood concentrations of this medication.
2. Oral neomycin may decrease the absorption of penicillin from the gastrointestinal tract.
3. Penicillin G may decrease the effectiveness of oral contraceptives (birth control pills), and pregnancy could result. You should, therefore, use a different or additional form of birth control while taking this medication. Discuss this with your doctor.

BE SURE TO TELL YOUR DOCTOR about any medications you are currently taking, especially any of those listed above.

WARNINGS

- Tell your doctor about unusual or allergic reactions you have had to any medications, especially to penicillins or other penicillin antibiotics (such as ampicillin and amoxicillin), cephalosporin antibiotics, penicillamine, or griseofulvin.
- Tell your doctor if you now have or if you have ever had kidney disease, asthma, or allergies.
- This medication has been prescribed for your current infection only. Another infection later on, or one that a family member or friend has, may require a different medicine. You should not give your medicine to other people or use it for other infections, unless your doctor specifically directs you to do so.
- Diabetics taking penicillin should know that this drug can cause a false-positive sugar reaction with a Clinitest urine glucose test. To avoid this problem while taking penicillin, you should switch to Clinistix or Tes-Tape to test your urine for sugar.
- Some of these products contain the color additive FD&C Yellow No. 5 (tartrazine), which can cause allergic-type reactions (shortness of breath, wheezing, rash, fainting) in certain susceptible individuals.
- Be sure to tell your doctor if you are pregnant. Although penicillin appears to be safe during pregnancy, extensive studies in humans have not been conducted. Also, tell your doctor if you are breast-feeding an infant. Small amounts of this drug pass into breast milk and may temporarily alter the bacterial balance in the intestinal tract of a nursing infant, resulting in diarrhea.

penicillin G potassium—see penicillin G

---

penicillin VK

BRAND NAMES (Manufacturers)

Beepen-VK (Beecham)
Betapen-VK (Bristol)
Ledercillin VK (Lederle)
Penapar-VK (Parke-Davis)
penicillin VK (various manufacturers)
Pen-Vee K (Wyeth)
Robicillin VK (Robins)
Suspen (Circle)
Uticillin VK (Upjohn)
V-Cillin K (Lilly)
Veetids (Squibb)

TYPE OF DRUG

Penicillin antibiotic

INGREDIENT

penicillin potassium phenoxymethyl

DOSAGE FORMS

Tablets (125 mg, 250 mg, and 500 mg)
Oral solution (125 mg and 250 mg per 5-ml spoonful)

STORAGE

Penicillin VK tablets should be stored at room temperature in a tightly closed container. The oral solution should be stored in the refrigerator in a tightly closed container. Any unused portion of the solution should be discarded after 14 days because the drug loses its potency after that time. This medication should never be frozen.

USES

Penicillin VK is used to treat a wide variety of bacterial infections, including infections of the middle ear, the respiratory tract, and the urinary tract. It acts by severely injuring the cell membranes of infecting bacteria, thereby preventing them from growing and multiplying. Penicillin VK kills susceptible bacteria, but it is not effective against viruses, parasites, or fungi.

TREATMENT

Penicillin VK should be taken on an empty stomach or with a glass of water one hour before or two hours after a meal. This medication should never be taken with fruit juices or carbonated beverages because the acidity of these drinks destroys the drug in the stomach.

The oral solution should be measured carefully with a specially designed 5-ml measuring spoon. An ordinary kitchen teaspoon is not accurate enough.

Penicillin VK works best when the level of medicine in your bloodstream is kept constant. It is best, therefore, to take the doses at evenly spaced intervals day and night. For example, if you are taking four doses a day, the doses should be spaced six hours apart.

If you miss a dose of this medication, take the missed dose immediately. However, if you do not remember to take the missed dose until it is almost time for the next dose, take it; space the following dose about halfway through the regular interval between doses; then return to your regular dosing schedule. Try not to skip any doses.

It is important to continue to take this medication for the entire time prescribed by your doctor (usually seven to 14 days), even if the symptoms of infection disappear before the end of that period. If you stop taking the drug too soon, resistant bacteria are given a chance to continue growing, and the infection could recur.

SIDE EFFECTS

Minor. Diarrhea, heartburn, nausea, or vomiting. These side effects should disappear as your body adjusts to the drug.

Major. Tell your doctor about any side effects that are persistent or particularly bothersome. IT IS ESPECIALLY IMPORTANT TO TELL YOUR DOCTOR about bloating, chills, cough, darkened tongue, difficulty in breathing, fever, irritation of the mouth, muscle aches, rash, rectal or vaginal itching, severe diarrhea, or sore throat. Also, if the infection seems to be getting worse rather than improving, you should contact your physician.

INTERACTIONS

Penicillin VK interacts with several other types of drugs:

1. Probenecid can increase the blood concentrations of this medication.

2. Oral neomycin may decrease the absorption of penicillin from the gastrointestinal tract.

3. Penicillin VK may decrease the effectiveness of oral contraceptives (birth control pills), and pregnancy could result. You should, therefore, use a different or additional form of birth control while taking this medication. Discuss this with your doctor.

BE SURE TO TELL YOUR DOCTOR about any medications you are currently taking, especially any of those listed above.

WARNINGS

• Tell your doctor about unusual or allergic reactions you have had to any medications, especially to penicillin or other penicillin antibiotics (such as ampicillin and amoxicillin), cephalosporin antibiotics, penicillamine, or griseofulvin.

• Tell your doctor if you now have or if you have ever had kidney disease, asthma, or allergies.

• This medication has been prescribed for your current infection only. Another infection later on, or one that someone else has, may require a different medicine. You should not give your medicine to other people or use it for other infections, unless your doctor specifically directs you to do so.

• Diabetics taking penicillin should know that this drug can cause a false-positive sugar reaction with a Clinitest urine glucose test. To avoid this problem while taking penicillin, you should switch to Clinistix or Tes-Tape to test your urine for sugar.

• Be sure to tell your doctor if you are pregnant. Although penicillin appears to be safe during pregnancy, extensive studies in humans have not been conducted. Also, tell your doctor if you are breast-feeding an infant. Small amounts of this medication pass into breast milk and may temporarily alter the bacterial balance in the intestinal tract of a nursing infant, resulting in diarrhea.

---

pentaerythritol tetranitrate

BRAND NAMES (Manufacturers)

Duotrate Plateau Caps (Jones Medical)
Naptrate (Vortech)
Pentylan (Lannett)
Peritrate (Parke-Davis)
Peritrate SA (Parke-Davis)
P.E.T.N. (various manufacturers)

TYPE OF DRUG

Antianginal

INGREDIENT

pentaerythritol tetranitrate

DOSAGE FORMS

Tablets (10 mg, 20 mg, 40 mg, and 80 mg)
Sustained-release tablets (80 mg)
Sustained-release capsules (30 mg, 45 mg, and 80 mg)

STORAGE

Pentaerythritol tetranitrate should be stored at room temperature in tightly closed containers. This medication loses potency if exposed to heat or moisture.

USES

Pentaerythritol tetranitrate is used to prevent angina (chest pain). It dilates (widens) blood vessels, which increases the oxygen supply to the heart, thereby preventing chest pain. It is not effective in relieving pain once an angina attack has begun.

TREATMENT

To ensure that the maximum amount of medication is absorbed into the bloodstream, you should take pentaerythritol tetranitrate on an empty stomach at least 30 minutes before or one hour after a meal with a glass of water (unless your doctor directs you to do otherwise).

The sustained-release tablets or capsules should be swallowed whole. Chewing, crushing, or breaking these tablets or capsules destroys their sustained-release activity and possibly increases the side effects.

If you miss a dose of this medication and remember within two hours (six hours for the sustained-release tablets or capsules), take the missed dose immediately and then return to your regular dosing schedule. If more than two hours have passed (six hours for the sustained-release tablets or capsules), do not take the missed dose at all; just return to your regular dosing schedule. Never double the dose (unless your doctor specifically directs you to do so).

SIDE EFFECTS

Minor. Dizziness, flushing or redness of the face and neck, headache, light-headedness, nausea, or vomiting. These effects should disappear as your body adjusts to the drug.

If you feel dizzy or light-headed, sit or lie down for a while; get up slowly from a sitting or reclining position, and be careful on stairs.

Acetaminophen may help relieve mild headaches.

Major. Tell your doctor about any side effects that are persistent or particularly bothersome. IT IS ESPECIALLY IMPORTANT TO TELL YOUR DOCTOR about fainting, palpitations, or skin rash.

INTERACTIONS

Alcohol can increase the blood-pressure-lowering effects of pentaerythritol tetranitrate, which can lead to serious side effects. You should, therefore, avoid drinking alcoholic beverages while taking this medication.

WARNINGS

• Tell your doctor about unusual or allergic reactions you have had to any medications, especially to pentaerythritol tetranitrate or to any other nitrate product (such as erythrityl tetranitrate, isosorbide dinitrate, or nitroglycerin).

• Before you take this drug, be sure to tell your doctor if you have ever had anemia, a heart attack, or thyroid disease.

• If this medication makes you dizzy or light-headed, avoid taking part in any activity that requires alertness, such as driving a car or operating potentially dangerous machinery.

• Tolerance to this drug can develop after prolonged use. If you begin to notice a decrease in effectiveness, contact your doctor. Do not increase the dosage of this drug unless you first check with your doctor. Also, stopping the drug abruptly can lead to a worsening in your condition. Your doctor may, therefore, want to reduce your dosage gradually.

• Before taking any over-the-counter (nonprescription) cough, cold, allergy, asthma, sinus, or diet preparation, check with your doctor. Some of these products can reduce the effectiveness of pentaerythritol tetranitrate.

• If you find whole or partially dissolved sustained-release tablets or capsules in your stool, contact your doctor. This indicates that you are not digesting and absorbing the tablets or capsules completely.

• Be sure to tell your doctor if you are pregnant. Although pentaerythritol tetranitrate appears to be safe during pregnancy, extensive studies in humans have not been conducted. Also, tell your doctor if you are breast-feeding an infant. It is not known whether pentaerythritol tetranitrate passes into breast milk.

---

pentazocine

BRAND NAME (Manufacturer)
Talwin NX (Winthrop)
TYPE OF DRUG
Analgesic
INGREDIENTS
pentazocine and naloxone
DOSAGE FORM
Tablets (50 mg pentazocine and 0.5 mg naloxone)
STORAGE
Pentazocine tablets should be stored at room temperature in a tightly closed, light-resistant container.

USES

Pentazocine is a narcotic analgesic that acts directly on the central nervous system (brain and spinal cord) to relieve moderate to severe pain. Naloxone is added to this compound to prevent abuse. It is not absorbed from the gastrointestinal tract, but it does block the action of pentazocine if the drug is injected into the body.

TREATMENT

In order to avoid stomach upset, you can take pentazocine with food or with a full glass of milk or water.

This medication works most effectively if you take it at the onset of pain, rather than waiting until the pain becomes intense.

If you are taking this medication on a regular schedule and you miss a dose, take the missed dose as soon as possible, unless it is almost time for your next dose. In that case, do not take the missed dose at all; just return to your regular dosing schedule. Do not double the next dose.

SIDE EFFECTS

Minor. Constipation, dizziness, drowsiness, dry mouth, false sense of well-being, flushing, light-headedness, loss of appetite, nausea, rash, or sweating. These side effects should disappear as your body adjusts to the medication.

If you are constipated, increase the amount of fiber in your diet (fresh fruits and vegetables, salads, bran, and whole-grain breads), exercise, and drink more water (unless your doctor directs you to do otherwise).

Chew sugarless gum or suck on ice chips or a piece of hard candy to reduce mouth dryness.

If you feel dizzy or light-headed, sit or lie down for a while; get up slowly from a sitting or lying position, and be careful on stairs.

Major. Tell your doctor about any side effects that are persistent or particularly bothersome. IT IS ESPECIALLY IMPORTANT TO TELL YOUR DOCTOR about anxiety, difficulty in breathing, excitation, fatigue, painful or difficult urination, palpitations, rash, restlessness, sore throat and fever, tremors, or weakness.

INTERACTIONS

Pentazocine interacts with several other types of drugs:

1. Concurrent use of it with other central nervous system depressants (such as alcohol, antihistamines, barbiturates, benzodiazepine tranquilizers, muscle relaxants, and phenothiazine tranquilizers) or with tricyclic antidepressants can cause extreme drowsiness.

2. A monoamine oxidase (MAO) inhibitor taken within 14 days of this drug can lead to unpredictable and severe side effects.

3. The combination of cimetidine and this medication may cause confusion, disorientation, and shortness of breath.

BE SURE TO TELL YOUR DOCTOR about any medications you are currently taking, especially any of those listed above.

WARNINGS

• Tell your doctor about unusual or allergic reactions you have had to any medications, especially to pentazocine or to other narcotic analgesics (such as codeine, hydrocodone, hydromorphone, meperidine, methadone, morphine, oxycodone, and propoxyphene).

• Tell your doctor if you now have or if you have ever had acute abdominal conditions, asthma, brain disease, colitis, epilepsy, gallstones or gallbladder disease, head injuries, heart disease, kidney disease, liver disease, lung disease, mental illness, emotional disorders, enlarged prostate gland, thyroid disease, or urethral stricture.

• If this drug makes you dizzy or drowsy, do not take part in any activity that requires alertness, such as driving a car or operating potentially dangerous machinery.

• Before having surgery or any other medical or dental treatment, be sure to tell your doctor or dentist that you are taking this medication.

• Because this product contains pentazocine, it has the potential for abuse and must be used with caution. Usually, it should not be taken on a regular schedule for longer than ten days, unless your doctor directs you to do so. Tolerance develops quickly; do not increase the dosage or stop taking the drug abruptly, unless you first consult your doctor. If you have been taking large amounts of this medication, or have been taking it for long periods, you may experience a withdrawal reaction (muscle aches, diarrhea, gooseflesh, runny nose, nausea, vomiting, shivering, trembling, stomach cramps, sleep disorders, irritability, weakness, excessive yawning, or sweating) when you stop taking it. Your doctor may, therefore, want to reduce the dosage gradually.

• Be sure to tell your doctor if you are pregnant. The effects of this medication during the early stages of pregnancy have not been thoroughly studied in humans. However, pentazocine, used regularly in large doses during the later stages of pregnancy, may result in addiction of the fetus—leading to withdrawal symptoms (irritability, excessive crying, tremors, fever, vomiting, diarrhea, sneezing, or excessive yawning) at birth. Also, tell your doctor if you are breast-feeding an infant. Small amounts of this medication may pass into breast milk and cause excessive drowsiness in the nursing infant.

Pentids—see penicillin G

---

pentobarbital

BRAND NAMES (Manufacturers)
Nembutal (Abbott)
pentobarbital sodium (various manufacturers)
TYPE OF DRUG
Sedative/hypnotic
INGREDIENT
pentobarbital
DOSAGE FORMS
Capsules (50 mg and 100 mg)
Oral elixir (20 mg per 5-ml spoonful, with 18% alcohol)
Suppositories (30 mg, 60 mg, 120 mg, and 200 mg)
STORAGE
Pentobarbital capsules and oral elixir should be stored at room temperature in tightly closed containers. The suppositories should be stored in the refrigerator. Pentobarbital should never be frozen.

USES

This medication belongs to a group of drugs known as barbiturates, which are central nervous system (brain and spinal cord) depressants. It is used as a sleeping aid in the treatment of insomnia.

TREATMENT

You can take pentobarbital at bedtime. The capsules can be taken with water, food, or milk.

Each dose of the oral elixir form of this medication should be measured carefully with a specially designed 5-ml measuring spoon. An ordinary kitchen teaspoon is not accurate enough. The elixir can be taken by itself or mixed with water, milk, or fruit juice.

To insert the suppository form of this medication, first unwrap it and moisten it slightly with water (if the suppository is too soft to insert, run cold water over it or refrigerate it for 30 minutes before you unwrap it). Lie down on your left side, with your right knee bent. Push the suppository well into the rectum with your finger. Try to avoid having a bowel movement for at least an hour so that the medication can be absorbed.

You should not use this drug as a sleeping aid for more than two weeks. With prolonged use, pentobarbital loses its ability to induce and sustain sleep.

SIDE EFFECTS

Minor. Constipation, diarrhea, dizziness, drowsiness, a "hangover" feeling, headache, nausea, stomach upset, or vomiting. These side effects should disappear as your body adjusts to the medication.

If you feel dizzy or light-headed, sit or lie down for a while; get up slowly from a sitting or reclining position, and be careful on stairs.

To relieve constipation, increase the amount of fiber in your diet (fresh fruits and vegetables, salads, bran, and whole-grain breads), exercise, and drink more water (unless your doctor directs you to do otherwise).

Major. Tell your doctor about any side effects that are persistent or particularly bothersome. IT IS ESPECIALLY IMPORTANT TO TELL YOUR DOCTOR about chest tightness, confusion, depression, difficulty in breathing, excitation, fatigue, feeling faint, hives or itching, loss of coordination, muscle or joint pain, skin rash, slurred speech, sore throat, unusual bleeding or bruising, unusual weakness, or yellowing of the eyes or skin.

INTERACTIONS

Pentobarbital interacts with several other types of drugs:

1. Concurrent use of it with other central nervous system depressants (such as alcohol, antihistamines, benzodiazepine tranquilizers, muscle relaxants, narcotics, pain medications, and phenothiazine tranquilizers) or with tricyclic antidepressants can cause extreme drowsiness.

2. Valproic acid, chloramphenicol, and monoamine oxidase (MAO) inhibitors can prolong the effects of pentobarbital.

3. Pentobarbital can decrease the blood levels and, therefore, the effectiveness of oral anticoagulants (blood thinners, such as warfarin), digitoxin, tricyclic antidepressants, doxycycline, cortisone-like medicines, metronidazole, quinidine, estrogens, birth control pills, phenytoin, acetaminophen, and carbamazepine.

4. The combination of pentobarbital and furosemide can cause low blood pressure and fainting.

5. Pentobarbital can increase the side effects of cyclophosphamide or large doses of acetaminophen.

Before starting to take pentobarbital, BE SURE TO TELL YOUR DOCTOR about any medications you are currently taking, especially any of those listed above.

WARNINGS

- Tell your doctor about unusual or allergic reactions you have had to any medications, especially to pentobarbital or to other barbiturates (such as amobarbital, butabarbital, mephobarbital, metharbital, phenobarbital, primidone, and secobarbital).
- Before starting to take this medication, be sure to tell your doctor if you now have or if you have ever had acute or chronic (long-term) pain, Addison's disease (an underactive adrenal gland), diabetes mellitus, kidney disease, liver disease, lung disease, mental depression, porphyria, or thyroid disease.
- Since this medication makes you drowsy, do not take part in any activity that requires alertness, such as driving a car or operating potentially dangerous machinery.
- This drug has the potential for abuse and must be used with caution. Tolerance develops quickly; do not increase the dosage or stop taking this drug without consulting your doctor.
- If you have been taking pentobarbital for a long time or have been taking large doses, you may experience anxiety, muscle twitching, tremors, weakness, dizziness, nausea,

vomiting, insomnia, or blurred vision when you stop taking it. To avoid this reaction, your doctor may want to reduce your dosage gradually.

• Be sure to tell your doctor if you are pregnant. Barbiturates cross the placenta, and there has been an association between birth defects and the use of this class of drugs during pregnancy. Such drugs may also lead to an increase in bleeding complications in the newborn. The risks should be discussed with your doctor. In addition, if pentobarbital is used for prolonged periods during the last three months of pregnancy, there is a chance that the infant will be born addicted to the medication and will experience a withdrawal reaction (convulsions or irritability) at birth. Also, tell your doctor if you are breast-feeding an infant. Small amounts of pentobarbital pass into breast milk and may cause excessive drowsiness or breathing problems in nursing infants.

pentobarbital sodium—see pentobarbital

---

pentoxifylline

BRAND NAME (Manufacturer)
Trental (Hoechst-Roussel)
TYPE OF DRUG
hemorrheologic
INGREDIENT
pentoxifylline
DOSAGE FORM
Controlled-release tablets (400 mg)
STORAGE
Store at room temperature in a tightly closed container.

USES

Pentoxifylline is used to treat intermittent claudication (leg pain caused by poor blood circulation) or peripheral vascular disease. It increases the flow of blood to areas of reduced circulation by decreasing the viscosity (stickiness) of blood.

TREATMENT

To avoid stomach irritation, pentoxifylline should be taken with meals.

The tablets should be swallowed whole; chewing, crushing, or breaking them will destroy the controlled-release activity and increase the risk of side effects.

If you miss a dose of pentoxifylline, take the missed dose as soon as possible, unless it is almost time for the next dose. In that case, do not take the missed dose at all; just wait until the next scheduled dose. Do not double the dose.

The benefits from pentoxifylline may be seen within two to four weeks after starting the medication.

SIDE EFFECTS

Minor. Abdominal pain, altered taste, belching, bloating, constipation, diarrhea, dizziness, drowsiness, dry mouth, excessive salivation, flushing, gas, headache, heartburn, insomnia, nasal congestion, nausea, nosebleeds, trembling of the hands, vomiting, or weight change. As your body adjusts to pentoxifylline, these side effects should disappear.

If you are constipated, increase the amount of fiber in your diet (fresh fruits and vegetables, salads, bran, and whole-grain breads), exercise, and drink more water (unless your doctor directs you to do otherwise).

To reduce mouth dryness, chew sugarless gum or suck on ice chips or hard candy.

If you feel dizzy or light-headed, lie or sit down for a while; get up slowly from a sitting or reclining position, and be careful on stairs.

Major. Tell your doctor about any side effects that are persistent or particularly bothersome. IT IS ESPECIALLY IMPORTANT TO TELL YOUR DOCTOR about chest pain, confusion, earache, flu-like symptoms, itching, palpitations, rash, shortness of breath, sore throat, unusual bleeding or bruising, unusual weight gain, visual disturbances, or yellowing of the eyes or skin.

INTERACTIONS

Pentoxifylline interacts with other types of medications:

1. Anticoagulants (blood thinners, such as warfarin) in combination with pentoxifylline can increase the risk of bleeding complications.

2. Pentoxifylline can add to the blood-pressure-lowering effects of antihypertensive medications.

BE SURE TO TELL YOUR DOCTOR about any medications you are currently taking, especially anticoagulants or antihypertensives.

WARNINGS

• Before you take this medication, it is important to tell your doctor if you have ever had unusual or allergic reactions to any medications, especially to pentoxifylline or chemically related compounds, such as caffeine, dyphylline, oxtriphylline, theophylline, and aminophylline.

• Tell your doctor if you now have or if you have ever had liver disease, kidney disease, or peptic ulcer disease.

• Before having surgery or any other medical or dental treatment, be sure to tell your doctor or dentist that you are taking this drug. Pentoxifylline can increase bleeding complications.

• If pentoxifylline makes you dizzy or drowsy, do not take part in any activity that requires alertness, such as driving a car or operating potentially dangerous machinery.

• Be sure to tell your doctor if you are pregnant. Although pentoxifylline appears to be safe in animals, studies in pregnant women have not been conducted. Also, tell your doctor if you are breast-feeding an infant. Small amounts of pentoxifylline pass into human breast milk.

Pentylan—see pentaerythritol tetranitrate

Pen-Vee K—see penicillin VK

Pepcid—see famotidine

Percocet—see acetaminophen and oxycodone combination

Percodan—see aspirin and oxycodone combination

Percodan-Demi—see aspirin and oxycodone combination

Periactin—see cyproheptadine

Peridex—see chlorhexidene gluconate

Peritrate—see pentaerythritol tetranitrate

Peritrate SA—see pentaerythritol tetranitrate

Permitil—see fluphenazine

perphenazine

BRAND NAMES (Manufacturers)
Trilafon (Schering)
Trilafon Repetabs (Schering)
TYPE OF DRUG
Phenothiazine tranquilizer
INGREDIENT
perphenazine
DOSAGE FORMS
Tablets (2 mg, 4 mg, 8 mg, and 16 mg)
Oral concentrate (16 mg per 5-ml spoonful, with less than 0.1% alcohol)
STORAGE
The tablet forms of this medication should be stored at room temperature in tightly closed, light-resistant containers. The oral concentrate form of this medication may be stored in the refrigerator in a tightly closed, light-resistant container. If the oral concentrate turns slightly yellow, the medicine is still effective and can be used. However, if it changes color markedly or has particles floating in it, it should not be used; rather, it should be discarded down the sink. This medication should never be frozen.

USES

Perphenazine is prescribed to treat the symptoms of certain types of mental illness, such as psychosis, the manic phase of manic-depressive illness, and severe behavioral problems in children. This medication is thought to relieve the symptoms of mental illness by blocking certain chemicals involved with the transmission of nerve impulses in the brain.

TREATMENT

To avoid stomach irritation, you can take the tablet form of this medication with a meal or with a glass of water or milk (unless your doctor directs you to do otherwise).

The oral concentrate form of this medication should be measured carefully with the dropper provided, then added to four ounces (1/2 cup) or more of water, milk, or a carbonated beverage or to applesauce or pudding immediately prior to administration. To prevent possible loss of effectiveness, the medication should not be diluted in tea, coffee, or apple juice.

Antacids and antidiarrheal medicines may decrease the absorption of this medication from the gastrointestinal tract. Therefore, at least an hour should separate doses of one of these medicines and perphenazine.

If you miss a dose, take the missed dose as soon as possible, then return to your regular dosing schedule. If it is almost time for the next dose, however, skip the one you missed and return to your regular schedule. Do not double the next dose (unless your doctor directs you to do so).

The full effects of this medication for the control of emotional or mental symptoms may not become apparent for two weeks after you start to take it.

SIDE EFFECTS

Minor. Blurred vision, constipation, decreased sweating, diarrhea, dizziness, drooling, drowsiness, dry mouth, fatigue, jitteriness, menstrual irregularities, nasal congestion, restlessness, vomiting, or weight gain. As your body adjusts to the medication, these side effects should disappear.

Perphenazine can also cause discoloration of the urine—a harmless side effect. The urine may become red, pink, or red-brown.

This medication can cause increased sensitivity to sunlight. It is, therefore, important to avoid prolonged exposure to sunlight and sunlamps. Wear protective clothing and sunglasses, and use an effective sunscreen.

If you are constipated, increase the amount of fiber in your diet (fresh fruits and vegetables, salads, bran, and whole-grain breads), exercise, and drink more water (unless your doctor directs you to do otherwise).

Chew sugarless gum or suck on ice chips or a piece of hard candy to reduce mouth dryness.

To avoid dizziness or light-headedness when you stand, contract and relax the muscles of your legs for a few moments before rising. Do this by pushing one foot against the floor while raising the other foot slightly, alternating feet so that you are "pumping" your legs in a pedaling motion.

Major. Tell your doctor about any side effects that are persistent or particularly bothersome. IT IS ESPECIALLY IMPORTANT TO TELL YOUR DOCTOR about breast enlargement (in both sexes); chest pain; convulsions; darkened skin; difficulty in swallowing or breathing; fainting; fever; impotence; involuntary movements of the face, mouth, jaw, or tongue; palpitations; rash; sleep disorders; sore throat; tremors; uncoordinated movements; unusual bleeding or bruising; visual disturbances; weakness; or yellowing of the eyes or skin.

INTERACTIONS

Perphenazine interacts with several other types of drugs:

1. It can cause extreme drowsiness when combined with alcohol or other central nervous system (brain and spinal cord) depressants, such as barbiturates, benzodiazepine tranquilizers, muscle relaxants, narcotics, and pain medications or with tricyclic antidepressants.

2. Perphenazine can decrease the effectiveness of amphetamines, guanethidine, anticonvulsants, and levodopa.

3. The side effects of epinephrine, monoamine oxidase (MAO) inhibitors, propranolol, phenytoin, and tricyclic antidepressants may be increased by this medication. At least 14 days should separate the use of this drug and the use of an MAO inhibitor.

4. Lithium may increase the side effects and decrease the effectiveness of this medication.

Before starting to take perphenazine, BE SURE TO TELL YOUR DOCTOR about any medications you are currently taking, especially any of those listed above.

WARNINGS

- Tell your doctor about unusual or allergic reactions you have had to any medications, especially to perphenazine or other phenothiazine tranquilizers (such as chlorpromazine, fluphenazine, mesoridazine, prochlorperazine, promazine, thioridazine, trifluoperazine, and triflupromazine) or to loxapine.

- Tell your doctor if you have a history of alcoholism or if you now have or have ever had blood disease, bone marrow disease, brain disease, breast cancer, blockage in the urinary or digestive tracts, drug-induced depression, epilepsy, high or low blood pressure, diabetes mellitus, glaucoma, heart or circulatory disease, liver disease, lung disease, Parkinson's disease, peptic ulcers, or an enlarged prostate gland.
- Tell your doctor about any recent exposure to a pesticide or an insecticide. Perphenazine may increase the side effects from the exposure.
- To prevent oversedation, avoid drinking alcoholic beverages while taking this medication.
- If this drug makes you dizzy or drowsy, do not take part in any activity that requires alertness, such as driving a car or operating dangerous machinery. Be careful on stairs and avoid getting up suddenly from a lying or sitting position.
- Before having surgery or any other medical or dental treatment, be sure to tell your doctor or dentist that you are taking this medication.
- Some of the side effects caused by this drug can be prevented by taking an antiparkinsonism drug. Discuss this with your doctor.
- This medication can decrease sweating and heat release from the body. You should, therefore, try not to get overheated (avoid exercising strenuously in hot weather and taking hot baths, showers, and saunas).
- Do not stop taking this medication suddenly. If the drug is stopped abruptly, you may experience nausea, vomiting, stomach upset, headache, increased heart rate, insomnia, tremors, or a worsening of your condition. Your doctor may want to reduce the dosage gradually.
- If you are planning to have a myelogram or any other procedure in which dye will be injected into your spinal cord, tell your doctor that you are taking this medication.
- Avoid spilling the oral concentrate form on your skin or clothing; it may cause redness and irritation of the skin.
- While taking this medication, do not take any over-the-counter (nonprescription) medication for weight control or for cough, cold, allergy, asthma, or sinus problems without first checking with your doctor.
- Be sure to tell your doctor if you are pregnant. Small amounts of this medication cross the placenta. Although there are reports of safe use of this drug during pregnancy, there are also reports of liver disease and tremors in newborn infants whose mothers received this type of medication close to term. Also, tell your doctor if you are breast-feeding an infant. Small amounts of this medication pass into breast milk and may cause unwanted effects in the nursing infant.

---

perphenazine and amitriptyline combination

BRAND NAMES (Manufacturers)

Etrafon (Schering)
Triavil (Merck Sharp & Dohme)

TYPE OF DRUG

Phenothiazine tranquilizer and tricyclic antidepressant

INGREDIENTS

perphenazine and amitriptyline

DOSAGE FORM

Tablets (2 mg perphenazine and 10 mg amitriptyline; 2 mg perphenazine and 25 mg amitriptyline; 4 mg perphenazine and 10 mg amitriptyline; 4 mg perphenazine and 25 mg amitriptyline; and 4 mg perphenazine and 50 mg amitriptyline)

STORAGE

Store at room temperature in a tightly closed, light-resistant container.

USES

Perphenazine and amitriptyline combination is used to relieve anxiety or depression. Amitriptyline belongs to a group of drugs referred to as tricyclic antidepressants. These medicines are thought to relieve depression by increasing the concentration of certain chemicals in the brain. Perphenazine is a phenothiazine tranquilizer. It is thought to relieve the symptoms of mental illness by blocking certain chemicals involved with nerve transmission in the brain.

TREATMENT

This medication should be taken exactly as your doctor prescribes. In order to avoid stomach irritation, you can take the tablets with food or with a full glass of water or milk (unless your doctor directs you to do otherwise).

Antacids and antidiarrheal medicines may decrease the absorption of this medication from the gastrointestinal tract. Therefore, at least one hour should separate doses of perphenazine and amitriptyline combination and one of these medicines.

If you miss a dose of this medication, take the missed dose as soon as possible, unless it is within two hours of your next scheduled dose. In that case, do not take the missed dose at all; just return to your regular dosing schedule. Do not double the next dose.

The full benefits of this medication for the control of emotional or mental symptoms may not become apparent for two weeks after you start to take it.

SIDE EFFECTS

Minor. Bloating, blurred vision, constipation, cramps, decreased or increased sweating, diarrhea, dizziness, drowsiness, dry mouth, fatigue, headache, heartburn, insomnia, loss of appetite, nasal congestion, nausea, peculiar tastes in the mouth, restlessness, stomach upset, vomiting, weakness, or weight gain or loss. These side effects should disappear as your body adjusts to the medication.

This medication can increase your sensitivity to sunlight. You should, therefore, avoid prolonged exposure to sunlight and sunlamps. Wear protective clothing and sunglasses, and use an effective sunscreen.

This drug combination may cause a discoloration of the urine. This is a harmless effect.

If you experience dry mouth, you might want to try chewing sugarless gum or sucking on ice chips or a piece of hard candy.

To relieve constipation, increase the amount of fiber in your diet (fresh fruits and vegetables, salads, bran, and

whole-grain breads), exercise, and drink more water (unless your doctor directs you to do otherwise).

To avoid dizziness and light-headedness when you stand, contract and relax the muscles of your legs for a few moments before rising. Do this by pushing one foot against the floor while raising the other foot slightly, alternating feet so that you are "pumping" your legs in a pedaling motion.

Major. Tell your doctor about any side effects that are persistent or particularly bothersome. IT IS ESPECIALLY IMPORTANT TO TELL YOUR DOCTOR about agitation, confusion, convulsions, difficult or painful urination, enlarged or painful breasts (in both sexes), fainting, fever, hair loss, hallucinations, chest tightness, impotence, menstrual irregularities, mood changes, mouth sores, nervousness, nightmares, numbness in fingers or toes, palpitations, rash, ringing in the ears, sore throat, tremors, uncoordinated movements or balance problems, unusual bleeding or bruising, or yellowing of the eyes or skin.

INTERACTIONS

This drug interacts with several other types of drugs:

1. Extreme drowsiness can occur if this medication is taken with central nervous system depressants (such as alcohol, antihistamines, barbiturates, benzodiazepine tranquilizers, muscle relaxants, narcotics, pain medications, and sleeping medications) or with other antidepressants.

2. Amitriptyline may decrease the effectiveness of antiseizure medications and block the blood-pressure-lowering effects of clonidine and guanethidine.

3. Estrogens and oral contraceptives (birth control pills) can increase the side effects and reduce the effectiveness of amitriptyline.

4. Amitriptyline may increase the side effects of thyroid medication and of over-the-counter (nonprescription) cough, cold, allergy, asthma, sinus, and diet medications.

5. The concurrent use of this medication with monoamine oxidase (MAO) inhibitors should be avoided, because the combination may result in fever, convulsions, or high blood pressure. At least 14 days should separate the use of this drug and the use of an MAO inhibitor.

6. Perphenazine can decrease the effectiveness of amphetamines, guanethidine, anticonvulsants, and levodopa.

7. The side effects of epinephrine and propranolol may be increased by perphenazine.

Before starting to take this medication, BE SURE TO TELL YOUR DOCTOR about any medications you are currently taking, especially any of those listed above.

WARNINGS

• Tell your doctor about unusual or allergic reactions you have had to any medications, especially to perphenazine or other phenothiazine tranquilizers (such as chlorpromazine, mesoridazine fluphenazine, promazine, thioridazine, and prochlorperazine), or to amitriptyline or other tricyclic antidepressants (such as desipramine, doxepin, imipramine, and nortriptyline).

• Tell your doctor if you have ever had asthma, breast cancer, brain disease, diabetes mellitus, electroshock therapy, epilepsy, glaucoma, heart disease, a heart attack, liver disease, lung disease, kidney disease, thyroid disease, intestinal or urinary tract blockage, low or high blood pressure, Parkinson's disease, peptic ulcers, or an enlarged prostate.

• The effects of this medication may last as long as seven days after you have stopped taking it, so continue to observe all precautions during that period.

• To prevent oversedation, avoid drinking alcoholic beverages while taking this medication.

• If this medication makes you dizzy or drowsy, do not take part in any activity that requires alertness, such as driving a car or operating potentially dangerous machinery. Be careful on stairs, and avoid getting up suddenly from a lying or sitting position.

• Prior to having surgery or any other medical or dental treatment, be sure to tell your doctor or dentist that you are taking this medication.

• This medication can decrease sweating and heat release from the body. You should, therefore, try not to get overheated (avoid exercising strenuously in hot weather and taking hot baths, showers, and saunas).

• Do not stop taking this medication suddenly. If the drug is stopped abruptly, you may experience nausea, vomiting, stomach upset, headache, increased heart rate, insomnia, tremors, or a worsening of your condition. Your doctor may, therefore, want to reduce the dosage gradually.

• If you are planning to have a myelogram, or any other procedure in which dye will be injected into your spinal cord, tell your doctor that you are taking this medication.

• While taking this medication, do not take any over-the-counter (nonprescription) medication for weight control or for cough, cold, asthma, allergy, or sinus problems without first checking with your doctor. The combination of these medications with perphenazine and amitriptyline may cause high blood pressure.

• Be sure to tell your doctor if you are pregnant. Small amounts of this medication cross the placenta. Although there are reports of safe use of this drug during pregnancy, there are also reports of liver disease and tremors in newborn infants whose mothers received this type of medication close to term. Also, tell your doctor if you are breast-feeding an infant. Small amounts of this medication pass into breast milk and may cause unwanted effects in the nursing infant.

Persantine—see dipyridamole

Pertofrane—see desipramine

Pethadol—see meperidine

P.E.T.N.—see pentaerythritol tetranitrate

Pharma-Cort—see hydrocortisone (topical)

Phenameth—see promethazine

Phenaphen-650 with Codeine—see acetaminophen and codeine combination

Phenaphen with Codeine—see acetaminophen and codeine combination

Phenazine VC with Codeine—see phenylephrine, promethazine, and codeine combination

Phenazodine—see phenazopyridine

phenazopyridine

BRAND NAMES (Manufacturers)
Azo-Standard* (Webcon)
Baridium* (Pfeiffer)
Di-Azo* (Kay)
Eridium* (Hauck)
Geridium (Goldline)
Phenazodine (Lannett)
phenazopyridine hydrochloride (various manufacturers)
Pyridiate (various manufacturers)
Pyridium (Parke-Davis)
Urodine (various manufacturers)
Urogesic (Edwards)
*Available (100-mg tablets) without a prescription.
TYPE OF DRUG
Urinary tract analgesic
INGREDIENT
phenazopyridine
DOSAGE FORM
Tablets (100 mg and 200 mg)
STORAGE
Phenazopyridine tablets should be stored at room temperature in a tightly closed, light-resistant container.

USES

Phenazopyridine is used for the symptomatic relief of the burning, pain, and discomfort caused by urinary tract infections or irritations. It is excreted in the urine, where it exerts a topical analgesic effect on the urinary tract. This medication is not useful for other types of pain.

TREATMENT

Phenazopyridine tablets should be taken with a full glass of water, either with meals or immediately after a meal.

If you miss a dose of this medication, take the missed dose as soon as possible, unless it is almost time for the next dose. In that case, do not take the missed dose at all; just return to your regular dosing schedule. Do not double the next dose.

SIDE EFFECTS

Minor. Dizziness, headache, indigestion, nausea, stomach cramps, or vomiting. These side effects should disappear as your body adjusts to the medication.

This drug causes urine to become orange-red. This is not harmful, but it may stain your clothing. The urine will return to normal soon after the drug is discontinued.

If you feel dizzy, sit or lie down for a while; get up slowly from a sitting or reclining position, and be careful on stairs.

Major. Tell your doctor about any side effects that are persistent or particularly bothersome. IT IS ESPECIALLY IMPORTANT TO TELL YOUR DOCTOR about a bluish color of the skin or fingernails, rash, unusual fatigue, or yellowing of the eyes or skin.

INTERACTIONS

Phenazopyridine should not interact with other medications as long as it is used according to directions.

WARNINGS

• Tell your doctor about unusual or allergic reactions you have had to any medications, especially to phenazopyridine.

• Tell your doctor if you have ever had kidney disease or hepatitis.

• If this drug makes you dizzy, do not take part in any activity that requires alertness, such as driving a car.

• Diabetic patients using this medication may get delayed reactions or false-positive readings for sugar or ketones with urine tests. Clinitest is not affected by this medication, but the other urine sugar tests are.

• Be sure to tell your doctor if you are pregnant. Although phenazopyridine appears to be safe in animals, extensive studies in humans have not been conducted. Also, tell your doctor if you are breast-feeding an infant. It is not known whether phenazopyridine passes into breast milk.

phenazopyridine hydrochloride—see phenazopyridine

---

phendimetrazine

BRAND NAMES (Manufacturers)
Adipost (Ascher)
Adphen (Ferndale)
Anorex (Dunhall)
Bontril PDM (Carnrick)
Bontril Slow-Release (Carnrick)
Dyrexan-OD (Trimen)
Metra (Forest)
Obalan (Lannett)
phendimetrazine tartrate (various manufacturers)
Plegine (Ayerst)
Prelu-2 (Boehringer Ingelheim)
Slyn-LL (Edwards)
Statobex (Lemmon)
Trimcaps (Maynard)
Trimstat (Laser)
Trimtabs (Maynard)
Weh-less (Hauck)
Weightrol (Vortech)
TYPE OF DRUG
Anorectic
INGREDIENT
phendimetrazine
DOSAGE FORMS
Tablets (35 mg)
Capsules (35 mg)
Sustained-release capsules (105 mg)
STORAGE
Phendimetrazine should be stored at room temperature in a tightly closed, light-resistant container.

USES

Phendimetrazine is used as an appetite suppressant during the first few weeks of dieting to help establish new eating habits. This medication is thought to relieve hunger by altering nerve impulses to the appetite control center in the brain. Its effectiveness lasts only for short periods (three to 12 weeks), however.

TREATMENT

You can take phendimetrazine with a full glass of water one hour before meals (unless your doctor directs otherwise).

The sustained-release form of this medication should be swallowed whole. Breaking, chewing, or crushing these capsules destroys their sustained-release activity and may increase the side effects.

In order to avoid difficulty in falling asleep, the last dose of this medication each day should be taken four to six hours (regular tablets) or ten to 14 hours (sustained-release capsules) before bedtime.

If you miss a dose of this medication, take the missed dose as soon as possible, unless it is almost time for your next dose. In that case, do not take the missed dose at all; just return to your regular dosing schedule. Do not double the next dose.

SIDE EFFECTS

Minor. Blurred vision, constipation, diarrhea, dizziness, dry mouth, false sense of well-being, fatigue, insomnia, irritability, nausea, nervousness, restlessness, stomach pain, sweating, unpleasant taste in the mouth, or vomiting. These side effects should disappear as your body adjusts to the medication.

Dry mouth can be relieved by sucking on ice chips or a piece of hard candy or by chewing sugarless gum.

In order to prevent constipation, increase the amount of fiber in your diet (fresh fruits and vegetables, salads, bran, and whole-grain breads), exercise, and drink more water (unless your doctor tells you not to do so).

Major. Tell your doctor about any side effects that are persistent or particularly bothersome. IT IS ESPECIALLY IMPORTANT TO TELL YOUR DOCTOR about changes in sexual desire, chest pain, difficulty in urinating, enlarged breasts (in either sex), fever, hair loss, headaches, impotence, menstrual irregularities, mental depression, mood changes, mouth sores, muscle pains, palpitations, rash, sore throat, tremors, or unusual bleeding or bruising.

INTERACTIONS

Phendimetrazine interacts with several other types of drugs:

1. Use of it within 14 days of a monoamine oxidase (MAO) inhibitor (isocarboxazid, pargyline, phenelzine, tranylcypromine) can result in high blood pressure and other side effects.

2. Phenothiazine tranquilizers (especially chlorpromazine) can antagonize (act against) the appetite-suppressant activity of this medication.

3. Phendimetrazine can decrease the blood-pressure-lowering effects of antihypertensive medications (especially guanethidine) and may alter insulin and oral antidiabetic medication dosage requirements in diabetic patients.

4. The side effects of other central nervous system stimulants, such as caffeine and over-the-counter (nonprescription) cough, allergy, asthma, sinus, diet, or cold preparations, may be increased by this medication.

Before starting to take phendimetrazine, BE SURE TO TELL YOUR DOCTOR about any medications you are currently taking, especially any of those listed above.

WARNINGS

- Tell your doctor about unusual or allergic reactions you have had to any medications, especially to phendimetrazine or other appetite suppressants (such as benzphetamine, phenmetrazine, diethylpropion, fenfluramine, mazindol, and phentermine) or to epinephrine, norepinephrine, ephedrine, amphetamines, dextroamphetamine, phenylephrine, phenylpropanolamine, pseudoephedrine, albuterol, metaproterenol, or terbutaline.
- Tell your doctor if you have a history of drug abuse or if you now have or have ever had angina, diabetes mellitus, emotional disturbances, glaucoma, heart or cardiovascular disease, high blood pressure, or thyroid disease.
- Phendimetrazine can mask the symptoms of extreme fatigue and can cause dizziness or light-headedness. Your ability to perform tasks that require alertness, such as driving a car or operating potentially dangerous machinery, may be decreased. Appropriate caution should, therefore, be taken.
- Before having surgery or other medical or dental treatment, tell your doctor or dentist you are taking this drug.
- Phendimetrazine is related to amphetamine and may be habit-forming when taken for long periods of time (both physical and psychological dependence can occur). You should not increase the dosage of this medication or take it for longer than 12 weeks without first consulting your doctor. It is also important that you not stop taking this medication abruptly—fatigue, sleep disorders, mental depression, nausea, vomiting, or stomach cramps or pain could occur. Your doctor may, therefore, want to decrease your dosage gradually.
- Be sure to tell your doctor if you are pregnant. Although studies of phendimetrazine in humans have not been conducted, some of the appetite suppressants have been shown to cause side effects in the fetuses of animals that received large doses during pregnancy. Also, tell your doctor if you are breast-feeding an infant. It is not known whether this medication passes into breast milk.

phendimetrazine tartrate—see phendimetrazine

---

phenelzine

BRAND NAME (Manufacturer)
Nardil (Parke-Davis)

TYPE OF DRUG
Monoamine oxidase (MAO) inhibitor

INGREDIENT
phenelzine

DOSAGE FORM
Tablets (15 mg)

STORAGE
Phenelzine should be stored at room temperature in a tightly closed, light-resistant container.

USES

This medication is used to treat depression. Phenelzine belongs to a group of drugs known as monoamine oxidase (MAO) inhibitors. It is not clearly understood how it works, but it is thought to increase the amounts of certain chemicals in the brain that act to relieve depression.

TREATMENT

You can take phenelzine either on an empty stomach or, to avoid stomach irritation, with food or milk (as directed by your doctor).

If you are taking a single daily dose, it is best to take the dose in the morning in order to avoid sleeping difficulties.

If you miss a dose of this medication and remember within two hours, take the missed dose immediately and then return to your regular dosing schedule. If more than two hours has passed, do not take the missed dose at all; just return to your regular dosing schedule. Do not double the next dose.

The full therapeutic benefits of this medication may not be observed for up to four weeks after you start to take it.

SIDE EFFECTS

Minor. Constipation, diarrhea, dizziness, drowsiness, dry mouth, fatigue, headache, insomnia, nausea, restlessness, stomach upset, sweating, or weakness. These side effects should disappear as your body adjusts to the medication.

Phenelzine can increase your sensitivity to sunlight. Avoid prolonged exposure to sunlight and sunlamps. Wear protective clothing and sunglasses, and use an effective sunscreen.

If you feel dizzy, sit or lie down for a while; get up slowly from a sitting or reclining position, and be careful on stairs.

To relieve constipation, increase the amount of fiber in your diet (fresh fruits and vegetables, salads, bran, and whole-grain breads) and drink more water (unless your doctor directs you to do otherwise).

To relieve mouth dryness, chew sugarless gum or suck on ice chips or a piece of hard candy.

Major. Tell your doctor about any side effects that are persistent or particularly bothersome. IT IS ESPECIALLY IMPORTANT TO TELL YOUR DOCTOR about anxiety, blurred vision, changes in sexual ability, chills, confusion, convulsions, darkened tongue, difficult or painful urination, fainting, false sense of well-being, hallucinations, jitteriness, mental disorders, rapid weight gain (three to five pounds within a week), uncoordinated movements, or yellowing of the eyes or skin.

If you experience a severe headache, stiff neck, chest pains, palpitations, or vomiting while taking this medication, CONTACT YOUR DOCTOR OR AN EMERGENCY ROOM IMMEDIATELY. These symptoms may be the result of a food or drug interaction.

INTERACTIONS

Phenelzine interacts with a number of drugs and foods:

1. Concurrent use of phenelzine with central nervous system depressants (such as alcohol, barbiturates, benzodiazepine tranquilizers, muscle relaxants, narcotics, pain medications, phenothiazine tranquilizers, and sleeping medications) or with tricyclic antidepressants can lead to extreme drowsiness.

2. The dosage of anticonvulsant medications may need to be adjusted when phenelzine is started.

3. The use of phenelzine within 14 days of either another monoamine oxidase inhibitor or carbamazepine, cyclobenzaprine, methyldopa, guanethidine, reserpine, levodopa, meperidine or another narcotic, amphetamines, ephedrine, methylphenidate, phenylpropanolamine, pseudoephedrine, or a tricyclic antidepressant can lead to serious (sometimes fatal) side effects.

4. Tyramine-containing foods and beverages (aged cheeses, sour cream, yogurt, pickled herring, chicken livers, canned figs, raisins, bananas, avocados, soy sauce, broad bean pods, yeast extracts, beer, and certain wines), excessive amounts of caffeine-containing beverages (coffee, tea, cocoa, and cola), or chocolate can also cause serious reactions in patients on phenelzine therapy.

5. Phenelzine can increase the blood-sugar-lowering effects of insulin and oral antidiabetic medications.

Before starting to take this medication, BE SURE TO TELL YOUR DOCTOR about any medications you are currently taking, especially any of those listed above. Be sure you are aware of the foods that interact with phenelzine.

WARNINGS

- Tell your doctor about unusual or allergic reactions you have had to any medications, especially to phenelzine.
- Before starting to take this medication, be sure to tell your doctor if you now have or if you have ever had asthma, bronchitis, diabetes mellitus, epilepsy, glaucoma, severe headaches, heart or blood vessel disease, kidney disease, liver disease, mental disorders, Parkinson's disease, pheochromocytoma, or thyroid disease.
- If this drug makes you dizzy or drowsy, do not take part in any activity that requires alertness, such as driving a car or operating potentially dangerous machinery.
- Before having surgery or any other medical or dental treatment, be sure to tell your doctor or dentist that you are taking this medication.
- Check with your doctor or pharmacist before taking any over-the-counter (nonprescription) asthma, allergy, cough, cold, diet, or sinus preparations. Concurrent use of some of these products with phenelzine can lead to serious side effects.
- If you also have angina, do not increase your amount of physical activity unless you first check with your doctor. Phenelzine can decrease the symptoms of angina without decreasing the risks of strenuous exercise.
- Be sure to tell your doctor if you are pregnant. Studies in animals have shown that phenelzine can cause birth defects if it is taken in high doses during pregnancy. Studies in humans have not been conducted. Also, tell your doctor if you are breast-feeding an infant. Small amounts of phenelzine may pass into breast milk.

Phenergan—see promethazine

Phenergan VC with Codeine—see phenylephrine, promethazine, and codeine combination

Phenergan with Codeine—see promethazine and codeine combination

Phenetron—see chlorpheniramine

---

phenmetrazine

BRAND NAME (Manufacturer)
Preludin Endurets (Boehringer Ingelheim)
TYPE OF DRUG
Anorectic
INGREDIENT
phenmetrazine

DOSAGE FORM
Sustained-release tablets (75 mg)

STORAGE
Phenmetrazine should be stored at room temperature in tightly closed, light-resistant containers.

USES

Phenmetrazine is used as an appetite suppressant during the first few weeks of dieting to help establish new eating habits. This medication is thought to relieve hunger by altering nerve impulses to the appetite control center in the brain. Its effectiveness lasts only for short periods (three to 12 weeks), however.

TREATMENT

You can take phenmetrazine with a full glass of water one hour before meals (unless your doctor directs you to do otherwise).

This medication should be swallowed whole. Breaking, chewing, or crushing these tablets destroys their sustained-release activity and may increase the side effects.

In order to avoid difficulty in falling asleep, the last dose of this medication each day should be taken ten to 14 hours before bedtime.

If you miss a dose of this medication, take the missed dose as soon as possible, unless it is almost time for your next dose. In that case, do not take the missed dose at all; just return to your regular dosing schedule. Do not double the next dose.

SIDE EFFECTS

Minor. Blurred vision, constipation, diarrhea, dizziness, dry mouth, false sense of well-being, fatigue, insomnia, irritability, nausea, nervousness, restlessness, stomach pain, sweating, unpleasant taste in the mouth, or vomiting. These side effects should disappear as your body adjusts to the drug.

If you experience mouth dryness, try sucking on ice chips or a piece of hard candy or chewing sugarless gum.

In order to prevent constipation, increase the amount of fiber in your diet (fresh fruits and vegetables, salads, bran, and whole-grain breads), exercise, and drink more water (unless your doctor tells you not to do so).

Major. Tell your doctor about any side effects that are persistent or particularly bothersome. IT IS ESPECIALLY IMPORTANT TO TELL YOUR DOCTOR about changes in sexual desire, chest pain, difficulty in urinating, enlarged breasts (in both sexes), fever, hair loss, headaches, impotence, menstrual irregularities, mental depression, mood changes, mouth sores, muscle pains, palpitations, rash, sore throat, tremors, or unusual bleeding or bruising.

INTERACTIONS

Phenmetrazine interacts with several other types of drugs:

1. Use of it within 14 days of a monoamine oxidase (MAO) inhibitor (isocarboxazid, pargyline, phenelzine, tranylcypromine) can result in high blood pressure and other side effects.

2. Tricyclic antidepressants and phenothiazine tranquilizers (especially chlorpromazine) can antagonize (act against) the appetite-suppressant activity of this medication.

3. Phenmetrazine can decrease the blood-pressure-lowering effects of antihypertensive medications (especially guanethidine) and may alter insulin and oral antidiabetic medication dosage requirements in diabetic patients.

4. The side effects of other central nervous system stimulants, such as caffeine or over-the-counter (nonprescription) diet, cough, cold, sinus, asthma, or allergy preparations, may be increased by this medication.

BE SURE TO TELL YOUR DOCTOR about any medications you are currently taking, especially any of those listed above.

WARNINGS

- Tell your doctor about unusual or allergic reactions you have had to any medications, especially to phenmetrazine or other appetite suppressants (such as benzphetamine, phendimetrazine, diethylpropion, fenfluramine, mazindol, and phentermine), or to epinephrine, norepinephrine, ephedrine, amphetamines, dextroamphetamine, phenylephrine, phenylpropanolamine, pseudoephedrine, albuterol, metaproterenol, or terbutaline.
- Tell your doctor if you have a history of drug abuse or if you now have or have ever had angina, diabetes mellitus, emotional disturbances, glaucoma, heart or cardiovascular disease, high blood pressure, or thyroid disease.
- Phenmetrazine can mask the symptoms of extreme fatigue and can cause dizziness or light-headedness. Your ability to perform tasks that require alertness, such as driving a car or operating potentially dangerous machinery, may be decreased. Appropriate caution should, therefore, be taken.
- Before having surgery or any other medical or dental treatment, be sure to tell your doctor or dentist that you are taking this medication.
- Phenmetrazine is related to amphetamine and may be habit-forming when taken for long periods of time (both physical and psychological dependence can occur). Therefore, you should not increase your dosage of this medication or take it for longer than 12 weeks, unless you first consult your doctor. It is also important that you not stop taking this medication abruptly—fatigue, sleep disorders, mental depression, nausea or vomiting, or stomach cramps or pain could occur. Your doctor may, therefore, want to decrease the dosage gradually in order to prevent or minimize these side effects.
- Phenmetrazine 75-mg sustained-release tablets contain the color additive FD&C Yellow No. 5 (tartrazine), which can cause allergic-type reactions (fainting, shortness of breath, or rash) in certain susceptible individuals.
- Be sure to tell your doctor if you are pregnant. Although studies of phenmetrazine in humans have not been conducted, some of the appetite suppressants have been shown to cause side effects in the fetuses of animals that received large doses during pregnancy. Also, tell your doctor if you are breast-feeding an infant. It is not known whether this medication passes into breast milk.

---

phenobarbital

BRAND NAMES (Manufacturers)
Barbita (Vortech)
phenobarbital (various manufacturers)
Solfoton (Poythress)

TYPE OF DRUG
Barbiturate sedative and anticonvulsant
INGREDIENT
phenobarbital
DOSAGE FORMS
Tablets (8 mg, 16 mg, 32 mg, 65 mg, and 100 mg)
Capsules (16 mg)
Oral liquid (15 mg and 20 mg per 5-ml spoonful, with 13.5% alcohol)
STORAGE
Phenobarbital tablets and capsules should be stored at room temperature in tightly closed containers. The oral liquid should be stored at room temperature in a tightly closed, light-resistant container. Phenobarbital liquid should not be used if the solution becomes cloudy—it is no longer effective. This medication should never be frozen.

USES

Phenobarbital is used to control convulsions, to relieve anxiety or tension, and to promote sleep. Phenobarbital belongs to a group of drugs known as barbiturates. The barbiturates are central nervous system (brain and spinal cord) depressants.

TREATMENT

In order to avoid stomach irritation, you should take phenobarbital with food or with a full glass of water or milk.

The oral liquid should be measured carefully with a specially designed 5-ml measuring spoon. An ordinary kitchen teaspoon is not accurate enough. The liquid dose can be taken by itself or diluted with water, milk, or fruit juice.

If phenobarbital is being taken as a sleeping aid, take it 30 to 60 minutes before you want to go to sleep.

If you are taking this medication for the treatment of seizures, phenobarbital works best when the level of medicine in your bloodstream is kept constant. It is best, therefore, to take the doses at evenly spaced intervals day and night. For example, if you are to take three doses a day, the doses should be spaced eight hours apart.

If you are taking this medication on a regular basis and you miss a dose, take the missed dose as soon as you remember. However, if it is almost time for your next dose, do not take the missed dose at all; just return to your regular dosing schedule. Do not double the next dose. If you are taking this medication to control seizures and you miss more than two doses, contact your doctor.

SIDE EFFECTS

Minor. Constipation, diarrhea, dizziness, drowsiness, a "hangover" feeling, headache, nausea, stomach upset, or vomiting. These side effects should disappear as your body adjusts to the medication.

If you feel dizzy or light-headed, sit or lie down for a while; get up slowly from a sitting or reclining position, and be careful on stairs.

To relieve constipation, increase the amount of fiber in your diet (fresh fruits and vegetables, salads, bran, and whole-grain breads), exercise, and drink more water (unless your doctor directs you to do otherwise).

Major. Tell your doctor about any side effects that are persistent or particularly bothersome. IT IS ESPECIALLY IMPORTANT TO TELL YOUR DOCTOR about chest tightness, confusion, depression, difficulty in breathing, excitation, fatigue, feeling faint, hives or itching, loss of coordination, muscle or joint pain, skin rash, slurred speech, sore throat, unusual bleeding or bruising, unusual weakness, or yellowing of the eyes or skin.

INTERACTIONS

Phenobarbital interacts with other types of medications:

1. Concurrent use of it with other central nervous system depressants (such as alcohol, antihistamines, benzodiazepine tranquilizers, muscle relaxants, narcotics, pain medications, phenothiazine tranquilizers, and sleeping medications) or with tricyclic antidepressants can cause extreme drowsiness.

2. Valproic acid, chloramphenicol, and monoamine oxidase (MAO) inhibitors can prolong the effects of the barbiturates.

3. Phenobarbital can increase the elimination from the body (thereby decreasing the effectiveness) of oral anticoagulants (blood thinners, such as warfarin), digitoxin, tricyclic antidepressants, cortisone-like medications, doxycycline, metronidazole, quinidine, oral contraceptives (birth control pills), estrogen-containing drugs, phenytoin, acetaminophen, and carbamazepine.

4. Phenobarbital can decrease the absorption of griseofulvin from the gastrointestinal tract.

5. The combination of phenobarbital and furosemide can cause low blood pressure and fainting.

6. Phenobarbital can increase the side effects of cyclophosphamide or large doses of acetaminophen.

BE SURE TO TELL YOUR DOCTOR about any medications you are currently taking, especially any listed above.

WARNINGS

• Tell your doctor about unusual or allergic reactions you have had to any medications, especially to phenobarbital or other barbiturates (such as amobarbital, butabarbital, mephobarbital, pentobarbital, primidone, and secobarbital).

• Tell your doctor if you now have or if you have ever had acute or chronic (long-term) pain, Addison's disease (caused by an underactive adrenal gland), diabetes mellitus, kidney disease, liver disease, lung disease, mental depression, porphyria, or thyroid disease.

• Before having surgery or any other medical or dental treatment, be sure to tell your doctor or dentist that you are taking this medication.

• If this medication makes you dizzy or drowsy, do not take part in any activity that requires alertness, such as driving a car or operating potentially dangerous machinery.

• This drug has the potential for abuse and must be used with caution. Tolerance to the medication develops quickly; do not increase the dosage or stop taking this drug unless you first consult your doctor. If you have been taking this drug for a long time or have been taking large doses of it, you may experience anxiety, muscle twitching, tremors, weakness, dizziness, nausea, vomiting, insomnia, or blurred vision when you stop taking it. Your doctor may, therefore, want to reduce your dosage of this medication gradually.

• Some of these products contain the color additive FD&C Yellow No. 5 (tartrazine), which can cause allergic-type reactions (rash, fainting, difficulty in breathing) in certain susceptible individuals.

• Be sure to tell your doctor if you are pregnant. Phenobarbital crosses the placenta, and birth defects have been associated with the use of this medication during pregnancy. If phenobarbital is used during the last three months of pregnancy, there is a chance that the infant will be born addicted to the medication and will experience a withdrawal reaction (seizures or irritability) at birth. The infant could also be born with bleeding problems. The risks and benefits of treatment should be discussed with your doctor. Also, tell your doctor if you are breast-feeding an infant. Small amounts of phenobarbital pass into breast milk and may cause excessive drowsiness in the nursing infant.

---

phentermine

BRAND NAMES (Manufacturers)
Adipex-P (Lemmon)
Dapex (Ferndale)
Fastin (Beecham)
Ionamin (Pennwalt)
Obe-Nix (Holloway)
Obephen (Hauck)
Obermine (Forest)
Obestin-30 (Ferndale)
Parmine (Parmed)
phentermine hydrochloride (various manufacturers)
Phentrol (Vortech)
Wilpowr (Foy)

TYPE OF DRUG
Anorectic

INGREDIENT
phentermine

DOSAGE FORMS
Tablets (8 mg, 30 mg, and 37.5 mg)
Capsules (15 mg, 18.75 mg, 30 mg, and 37.5 mg)
Timed-release capsules (15 mg and 30 mg)

STORAGE
Phentermine should be stored at room temperature in tightly closed, light-resistant containers.

USES

Phentermine is used as an appetite suppressant during the first few weeks of dieting, to help establish new eating habits. This medication is thought to relieve hunger by altering nerve impulses to the appetite control center in the brain. Its effectiveness lasts only for short periods (three to 12 weeks), however.

TREATMENT

You can take phentermine tablets, capsules, or timed-release capsules with a full glass of water one hour before meals (unless your doctor directs you to do otherwise).

The timed-release form of this medication should be swallowed whole. Breaking, chewing, or crushing these capsules destroys their timed-release activity and may increase side effects.

In order to avoid difficulty in falling asleep, the last daily dose of this medication should be taken four to six hours (regular tablets and capsules) or ten to 14 hours (timed-release capsules) before bedtime.

If you miss a dose of this medication, be sure to take the missed dose as soon as possible, unless it is almost time for your next dose. In that case, do not take the missed dose at all; just return to your regular dosing schedule. Do not double the next dose of the medication.

SIDE EFFECTS

Minor. Blurred vision, constipation, diarrhea, dizziness, dry mouth, false sense of well-being, fatigue, insomnia, irritability, nausea, nervousness, restlessness, stomach pain, sweating, unpleasant taste in the mouth, or vomiting. These side effects should disappear as your body adjusts to the drug.

Dry mouth can be relieved by sucking on ice chips or a piece of hard candy or by chewing sugarless gum.

In order to prevent constipation, increase the amount of fiber in your diet (fresh fruits and vegetables, salads, bran, and whole-grain breads), exercise, and drink more water (unless your doctor tells you not to do so).

Major. Tell your doctor about any side effects that are persistent or particularly bothersome. IT IS ESPECIALLY IMPORTANT TO TELL YOUR DOCTOR about changes in sexual desire, chest pain, difficulty in urinating, enlarged breasts (in both sexes), fever, hair loss, headaches, impotence, menstrual irregularities, mental depression, mood changes, mouth sores, muscle pains, palpitations, rash, sore throat, or tremors.

INTERACTIONS

Phentermine interacts with several other types of medications:

1. Use of it within 14 days of a monoamine oxidase (MAO) inhibitor (isocarboxazid, pargyline, phenelzine, tranylcypromine) can result in high blood pressure and other side effects.

2. Barbiturate medications and phenothiazine tranquilizers (especially chlorpromazine) can antagonize (act against) the appetite-suppressant activity of this medication.

3. Phentermine can decrease the blood-pressure-lowering effects of antihypertensive medications (especially guanethidine) and may alter insulin and oral antidiabetic medication dosage requirements in diabetic patients.

4. The side effects of other central nervous system stimulants, such as caffeine or over-the-counter (nonprescription) cough, cold, sinus, asthma, diet, or allergy preparations, may be increased by this medication.

BE SURE TO TELL YOUR DOCTOR about any medications you are currently taking, especially any of those listed above.

WARNINGS

• Tell your doctor about unusual or allergic reactions you have had to any medications, especially to phentermine or other appetite suppressants (such as benzphetamine, phendimetrazine, diethylpropion, fenfluramine, mazindol, and phenmetrazine), or to epinephrine, norepinephrine, ephedrine, amphetamines, dextroamphetamine, phenylephrine, phenylpropanolamine, pseudoephedrine, albuterol, metaproterenol, or terbutaline.

• Tell your doctor if you have a history of drug abuse or if you now have or have ever had angina, diabetes mellitus, emotional disturbances, glaucoma, heart or cardiovascular disease, high blood pressure, or thyroid disease.

• Phentermine can mask the symptoms of extreme fatigue and can cause dizziness or light-headedness. Your ability to perform tasks that require alertness, such as driving a car or operating potentially dangerous machinery, may be decreased. Appropriate caution should, therefore, be taken.
• Before having surgery or other medical or dental treatment, tell your doctor or dentist you are taking this drug.
• Phentermine is related to amphetamine and may be habit-forming when taken for long periods of time (both physical and psychological dependence can occur). You should, therefore, not increase the dosage of this medication or take it for longer than 12 weeks without first consulting your doctor. It is also important that you not stop taking this medication abruptly—fatigue, sleep disorders, mental depression, nausea, vomiting, or stomach cramps or pain could occur. Your doctor may, therefore, want to decrease your dosage gradually.
• Be sure to tell your doctor if you are pregnant. Although studies of phentermine in humans have not been conducted, some of the appetite suppressants have been shown to cause side effects in the fetuses of animals that received large doses during pregnancy. Also, tell your doctor if you are breast-feeding an infant. It is not known whether this medication passes into breast milk.

phentermine hydrochloride—see phentermine

Phentrol—see phentermine

---

phenylbutazone

BRAND NAMES (Manufacturers)
Azolid (U.S.V.)
Butazolidin (Geigy)
phenylbutazone (various manufacturers)
TYPE OF DRUG
Nonsteroidal anti-inflammatory analgesic
INGREDIENT
phenylbutazone
DOSAGE FORMS
Tablets (100 mg)
Capsules (100 mg)
STORAGE
Phenylbutazone tablets and capsules should be stored at room temperature in tightly closed containers.

USES

Phenylbutazone is used to reduce inflammation (pain, redness, and swelling) due to arthritis or thrombophlebitis. It is not clearly understood how phenylbutazone works, but it is thought to act by interfering with the body's inflammatory mechanism or by decreasing the sensitivity of the body's pain mechanism.

TREATMENT

In order to avoid stomach upset, you can take phenylbutazone with food or with a full glass of water or milk. Ask your doctor if you can take phenylbutazone with an antacid.

Phenylbutazone tablets should be swallowed whole. Do not break or crush them.

If you miss a dose of this medication and you are taking it once or twice a day, take the missed dose as soon as possible, unless it is almost time for the next dose. In that case, do not take the missed dose at all; just return to your regular dosing schedule. Do not double the next dose.

If you are taking phenylbutazone three or more times per day and you miss a dose, take the missed dose right away (if you remember within an hour of the correct time); then take the next dose as scheduled. If more than an hour has passed, however, do not take the missed dose at all; just return to your regular schedule. Do not double the next dose of this medication.

SIDE EFFECTS

Minor. Abdominal pain, bloating, constipation, diarrhea, drowsiness, gas, headache, heartburn, indigestion, irritability, nausea, numbness, vomiting, or weakness. These side effects should disappear as your body adjusts to the medication.

To relieve constipation, increase the amount of fiber in your diet (fresh fruits and vegetables, salads, bran, and whole-grain breads), exercise, and drink more water (unless your doctor directs you to do otherwise).

Major. Tell your doctor about any side effects that are persistent or particularly bothersome. IT IS ESPECIALLY IMPORTANT TO TELL YOUR DOCTOR about bloody or black, tarry stools; blurred vision; confusion; depression; difficulty in breathing; difficulty in hearing; difficult or painful urination; fatigue; fever; itching; mouth sores; rash; ringing in the ears; severe abdominal pain; sore throat; swelling of the ankles; tremors; unusual bleeding or bruising; weight gain of more than three pounds within a week; or yellowing of the eyes or skin.

INTERACTIONS

Phenylbutazone interacts with several other types of medications:

1. It can increase the kidney side effects of penicillamine; increase skin reactions to chloroquine, gold compounds, and hydroxychloroquine; and increase the effects on the blood of antineoplastic agents (anticancer medicines), chloramphenicol, colchicine, gold compounds, pyrimethamine, and trimethoprim.
2. The gastrointestinal side effects of phenylbutazone analgesic can be increased by the use of alcohol or anti-inflammatory medications.
3. Phenylbutazone can decrease the blood levels and effectiveness of digitoxin, hexobarbital, and cortisone.
4. Cholestyramine can decrease the absorption of phenylbutazone from the gastrointestinal tract, which can decrease its effectiveness.
5. The active blood levels and side effects of oral anticoagulants (blood thinners, such as warfarin), insulin, oral antidiabetic medicines, sulfonamide antibiotics, sodium valproate, methotrexate, sulfonylurea drugs, and phenytoin can be increased by phenylbutazone.
6. Phenylbutazone can decrease the elimination of lithium through the kidneys, which can lead to an increased risk of side effects.

Before starting to take this medication, BE SURE TO TELL YOUR DOCTOR about any medications you are currently taking, especially any of those listed above.

WARNINGS

- Tell your doctor about unusual or allergic reactions you have had to any medications, especially to phenylbutazone or other nonsteroidal anti-inflammatory medications (such as aspirin, diclofenac, diflunisal, fenoprofen, flurbiprofen, ibuprofen, indomethacin, ketoprofen, meclofenamate, mefenamic acid, naproxen, oxyphenbutazone, sulfinpyrazone, sulindac, or tolmetin).
- Tell your doctor if you now have or if you have ever had anemia, blood disorders, heart disease, hypertension, inflamed salivary glands, kidney disease, liver disease, mouth sores, pancreatitis, peptic ulcers, polymyalgia rheumatica, stomach problems, temporal arteritis, or thyroid disease.
- Use of this drug has been associated with leukemia, although there is no definite proof that it causes the disease.
- If phenylbutazone makes you dizzy or drowsy, do not take part in any activity that requires alertness, such as driving a car or operating potentially dangerous machinery.
- Because phenylbutazone can prolong your bleeding time, tell your doctor or dentist that you are taking this drug before having surgery or any other medical or dental treatment.
- This medication can cause serious blood disorders. Therefore, it should never be used for trivial aches or pains.
- This drug should be used for a short time only. Follow your doctor's directions exactly, and never exceed the recommended dosage.
- Some of these products contain the color additive FD&C Yellow No. 5 (tartrazine), which can cause allergic-type reactions (shortness of breath, rash, or fainting) in certain susceptible individuals.
- Be sure to tell your doctor if you are pregnant. Although studies in humans have not been conducted, unwanted effects have been observed in the offspring of animals that received large doses of this drug during pregnancy. If taken late in pregnancy, phenylbutazone can also prolong labor. Also, tell your doctor if you are breast-feeding an infant. Small doses of phenylbutazone pass into breast milk.

---

phenylephrine, phenylpropanolamine, brompheniramine, and guaifenesin combination

BRAND NAME (Manufacturer)
Normatane Expectorant (Vortech)

TYPE OF DRUG
Adrenergic (decongestant), antihistamine, and expectorant

INGREDIENTS
phenylephrine, phenylpropanolamine, brompheniramine, guaifenesin, and alcohol

DOSAGE FORM
Oral expectorant (5 mg phenylephrine, 5 mg phenylpropanolamine, 2 mg brompheniramine, and 100 mg guaifenesin per 5-ml spoonful, with 3.5% alcohol)

STORAGE
Phenylephrine, phenylpropanolamine, brompheniramine, and guaifenesin combination should be stored at room temperature (never frozen) in a tightly closed container.

USES

This drug combination is used to relieve the coughing and congestion of allergy and the common cold.

Phenylephrine and phenylpropanolamine belong to a group of drugs known as adrenergic agents (decongestants). They act by constricting (narrowing) blood vessels in the nasal passages, thereby reducing swelling and congestion.

Brompheniramine belongs to a group of drugs known as antihistamines, which are used to relieve or prevent symptoms of allergy. Antihistamines block the actions of histamine, which is a chemical released by the body during an allergic reaction.

Guaifenesin is an expectorant, a drug that loosens bronchial secretions.

TREATMENT

In order to avoid stomach upset, you can take phenylephrine, phenylpropanolamine, brompheniramine, and guaifenesin combination with food or with a full glass of milk or water (unless your doctor directs you to do otherwise).

The expectorant should be measured carefully with a specially designed 5-ml measuring spoon. An ordinary kitchen teaspoon is not accurate enough.

If you miss a dose of this medication, take the missed dose as soon as possible, unless it is almost time for your next dose. In that case, do not take the missed dose at all; just return to your regular dosing schedule. Do not double the next dose.

SIDE EFFECTS

Minor. Anxiety; blurred vision; constipation; diarrhea; dizziness; drowsiness; dry mouth, nose, and throat; heartburn; insomnia; irritability; loss of appetite; nasal congestion; nausea; restlessness; reduced sweating; vomiting; or weakness. These side effects should disappear as your body adjusts to the medication.

This medication can increase your sensitivity to sunlight. Avoid prolonged exposure to sunlight and sunlamps, wear protective clothing, and use an effective sunscreen.

If you are constipated, increase the amount of fiber in your diet (fresh fruits and vegetables, salads, bran, and whole-grain breads), exercise, and drink more water (unless your doctor directs you to do otherwise).

Chew sugarless gum or suck on ice chips or a piece of hard candy to reduce mouth dryness.

If you feel dizzy or light-headed, sit or lie down for a while; get up slowly from a sitting or reclining position, and be careful on stairs.

In order to avoid difficulty in falling asleep, take the last dose of this medication several hours before bedtime.

Major. Tell your doctor about any side effects that are persistent or particularly bothersome. IT IS ESPECIALLY IMPORTANT TO TELL YOUR DOCTOR about chest pain, confusion, convulsions, difficult or painful urination, difficulty in breathing, fainting, hallucinations, headaches, loss of coordination, mood changes, nosebleeds, palpitations, rash, severe abdominal pain, sore throat, or unusual bleeding or bruising.

INTERACTIONS

This combination medication interacts with several other types of medications:

1. Concurrent use of it with central nervous system depressants (such as alcohol, barbiturates, benzodiazepine tranquilizers, muscle relaxants, narcotics, pain medications, and phenothiazine tranquilizers) or with tricyclic antidepressants can cause extreme drowsiness.

2. Monoamine oxidase (MAO) inhibitors (isocarboxazid, pargyline, phenelzine, tranylcypromine) and tricyclic antidepressants can increase the side effects of this medication. At least 14 days should separate the use of this drug and the use of an MAO inhibitor.

3. The side effects of the antihistamine part of this medication may be increased by quinidine, procainamide, haloperidol, and phenothiazine tranquilizers, and the side effects of the decongestant component can be increased by digoxin or over-the-counter (nonprescription) diet, allergy, asthma, cough, cold, or sinus preparations.

4. The blood-pressure-lowering effects of guanethidine may be decreased by phenylephrine, phenylpropanolamine, brompheniramine, and guaifenesin combination.

BE SURE TO TELL YOUR DOCTOR about any medications you are currently taking, especially any of those listed above.

WARNINGS

- Tell your doctor about unusual or allergic reactions you have had to any medications, especially to brompheniramine or other antihistamines (such as azatadine, chlorpheniramine, carbinoxamine, clemastine, cyproheptadine, dexchlorpheniramine, dimenhydrinate, diphenhydramine, diphenylpyraline, doxylamine, hydroxyzine, promethazine, pyrilamine, trimeprazine, tripelennamine, and triprolidine); to phenylpropanolamine, phenylephrine, or other adrenergic agents (such as albuterol, amphetamines, ephedrine, epinephrine, isoproterenol, metaproterenol, norepinephrine, pseudoephedrine, and terbutaline); or to guaifenesin.
- Tell your doctor if you now have or if you have ever had diabetes mellitus, epilepsy, glaucoma, heart or blood vessel disease, hiatal hernia, high blood pressure, myasthenia gravis, obstructed bladder or intestinal tract, peptic ulcers, enlarged prostate gland, or thyroid disease.
- Because phenylephrine, phenylpropanolamine, brompheniramine, and guaifenesin combination can reduce sweating and heat release from the body, you should avoid excessive work and exercise in hot weather, and do not take hot baths, showers, and saunas.
- While you are taking phenylephrine, phenylpropanolamine, brompheniramine, and guaifenesin combination, drink at least eight glasses of water a day to help loosen bronchial secretions.
- This medication can cause drowsiness. Exercise caution when performing tasks that require alertness, such as driving a car or operating potentially dangerous machinery.
- Be sure to tell your doctor if you are pregnant. The effects of this medication during pregnancy have not been thoroughly studied in humans. Also, tell your doctor if you are breast-feeding an infant. Small amounts of this medication pass into breast milk and may cause unusual excitement or irritability in nursing infants.

phenylephrine, promethazine, and codeine combination

BRAND NAMES (Manufacturers)

Phenazine VC with Codeine (Halsey)
Phenergan VC with Codeine (Wyeth)
Prometh VC with Codeine (Barre)

TYPE OF DRUG

Adrenergic (decongestant), antihistamine, and cough suppressant combination

INGREDIENTS

phenylephrine, promethazine, and codeine

DOSAGE FORM

Oral syrup (5 mg phenylephrine, 6.25 mg promethazine, and 10 mg codeine per 5-ml spoonful, with 7% alcohol)

STORAGE

Phenylephrine, promethazine, and codeine combination should be stored at room temperature (never frozen) in a tightly closed, light-resistant container.

USES

This combination medication is used to provide symptomatic relief of coughs due to colds, minor upper respiratory tract infections, and allergy.

Phenylephrine belongs to a group of drugs known as adrenergic agents (decongestants), which constrict blood vessels in the nasal passages to reduce swelling and congestion.

Promethazine belongs to a group of drugs known as antihistamines, which block the actions of histamine, a chemical released by the body during an allergic reaction. It is used to relieve or prevent symptoms of allergy.

Codeine is a narcotic cough suppressant that acts on the cough reflex center in the brain.

TREATMENT

To avoid stomach upset, you can take this medication with food or with a full glass of milk or water (unless your doctor directs you to do otherwise).

The oral syrup should be shaken well just before measuring each dose. The contents tend to settle on the bottom of the bottle, so it is necessary to shake the container to distribute the ingredients evenly and equalize the doses. Each dose should then be measured carefully with a specially designed 5-ml measuring spoon. An ordinary kitchen teaspoon is not accurate enough for measuring your dosage.

If you miss a dose of this medication, take the missed dose as soon as possible, unless it is almost time for your next dose. In that case, do not take the missed dose at all; just return to your regular dosing schedule. Do not double the next dose.

SIDE EFFECTS

Minor. Blurred vision, constipation, diarrhea, dizziness, dry mouth, heartburn, insomnia, loss of appetite, confusion, nasal congestion, nausea, nervousness, rash, restlessness, sweating, vomiting, or weakness. These side effects should disappear as your body adjusts to the medication.

This medication can cause increased sensitivity to sunlight. It is, therefore, important to avoid prolonged exposure to sunlight and sunlamps. Wear protective clothing, and use an effective sunscreen.

If you are constipated, increase the amount of fiber in your diet (fresh fruits and vegetables, salads, bran, and whole-grain breads), exercise, and drink more water (unless your doctor directs you to do otherwise).

Chew sugarless gum or suck on ice chips or a piece of hard candy to reduce mouth dryness.

If you feel dizzy or light-headed, sit or lie down for a while; get up slowly from a sitting or reclining position, and be careful on stairs.

In order to avoid difficulty in falling asleep, check with your doctor to see if you can take the last dose of this medication several hours before bedtime each day.

Major. Tell your doctor about any side effects that are persistent or particularly bothersome. IT IS ESPECIALLY IMPORTANT TO TELL YOUR DOCTOR about convulsions, difficult or painful urination, difficulty in breathing, disturbed coordination, excitation, fainting, headaches, muscle spasms, nightmares, nosebleeds, severe abdominal pain, or sore throat or fever.

INTERACTIONS

This medication interacts with other types of drugs:

1. Concurrent use of this medication with central nervous system depressants (such as alcohol, barbiturates, benzodiazepine tranquilizers, muscle relaxants, narcotics, pain medications, and phenothiazine tranquilizers) or with tricyclic antidepressants can cause extreme drowsiness.

2. This medication can decrease the effectiveness of amphetamines, guanethidine, anticonvulsants, and levodopa.

3. The side effects of monoamine oxidase (MAO) inhibitors (isocarboxazid, pargyline, phenelzine, tranylcypromine) and tricyclic antidepressants may also be increased. At least 14 days should separate the use of this drug and the use of an MAO inhibitor.

BE SURE TO TELL YOUR DOCTOR about any medications you are currently taking, especially any of those listed above.

WARNINGS

- Tell your doctor about unusual or allergic reactions you have had to any medications, especially to promethazine or other antihistamines (such as azatadine, brompheniramine, carbinoxamine, clemastine, cyproheptadine, chlorpheniramine, dexbrompheniramine, dimenhydrinate, diphenhydramine, diphenylpyraline, doxylamine, hydroxyzine, pyrilamine, trimeprazine, tripelennamine, and triprolidine); to phenothiazine tranquilizers, phenylephrine, or other adrenergic agents (such as albuterol, amphetamines, ephedrine, epinephrine, isoproterenol, metapro terenol, norepinephrine, pseudoephedrine, phenylpropanolamine, and terbutaline); or to codeine or any other narcotic cough suppressant or pain medication.
- Tell your doctor if you now have or if you have ever had asthma, brain disease, blockage of the urinary or digestive tract, diabetes mellitus, colitis, gallbladder disease, glaucoma, heart or blood vessel disease, high blood pressure, kidney disease, liver disease, lung disease, peptic ulcers, enlarged prostate gland, or thyroid disease.
- This medication can cause drowsiness. Your ability to perform tasks that require alertness, such as driving a car or operating potentially dangerous machinery, may be decreased. Appropriate caution should, therefore, be taken.
- Because this product contains codeine, there is a potential for abuse, so it must be used with caution. This medication usually should not be taken for longer than ten days at a time since a tolerance may develop quickly. Do not increase the dosage unless you first consult your doctor.
- Before having surgery or any other medical or dental treatment, be sure to tell your doctor or dentist that you are taking this medication.
- Be sure to tell your doctor if you are pregnant. The effects of this medication during the early stages of pregnancy have not been thoroughly studied in humans. However, regular use of codeine during the later stages of pregnancy may lead to addiction of the fetus, resulting in withdrawal symptoms (irritability, excessive crying, tremors, fever, vomiting, diarrhea, sneezing, or excessive yawning) in the newborn infant. Also, tell your doctor if you are breast-feeding an infant. Small amounts of this medication pass into breast milk and may cause unusual excitement or irritability in nursing infants.

---

phenylpropanolamine and caramiphen combination

BRAND NAMES (Manufacturers)

Detuss (various manufacturers)
Tussadon (Rugby)
Tuss-Allergine Modified T.D. (Rugby)
Tuss-Genade Modified Capsules (Goldline)
Tussogest (Major)
Tuss-Ornade (Smith Kline & French)

TYPE OF DRUG

Adrenergic (decongestant) and cough suppressant

INGREDIENTS

phenylpropanolamine and caramiphen

DOSAGE FORMS

Sustained-release capsules (75 mg phenylpropanolamine and 40 mg caramiphen)
Oral liquid (12.5 mg phenylpropanolamine and 6.7 mg caramiphen per 5-ml spoonful, with 5% alcohol)

STORAGE

Phenylpropanolamine and caramiphen combination capsules or oral liquid should be stored at room temperature in a tightly closed container. This medication should never be frozen.

USES

This drug combination is used to relieve the coughing and congestion associated with the common cold.

Phenylpropanolamine belongs to a group of drugs known as adrenergic agents (decongestants). They act by constricting (narrowing) blood vessels in the nasal passages, thereby reducing swelling and congestion.

Caramiphen is a nonnarcotic cough suppressant that acts at the cough center in the brain.

TREATMENT

In order to avoid stomach upset during treatment, you can take phenylpropanolamine and caramiphen combination with food or with a full glass of milk or water (unless your doctor directs you to do otherwise).

The sustained-release capsules should be swallowed whole. Breaking, chewing, or crushing these capsules destroys their sustained-release activity and may increase the side effects.

The oral liquid form should be measured carefully with a specially designed 5-ml measuring spoon. An ordinary kitchen teaspoon is not accurate enough.

If you miss a dose of this medication, take the missed dose as soon as possible, unless it is almost time for your next dose. In that case, do not take the missed dose at all; just return to your regular dosing schedule. Do not double the next dose.

SIDE EFFECTS

Minor. Blurred vision, constipation, diarrhea, dizziness, heartburn, insomnia, irritability, loss of appetite, nasal congestion, nausea, nervousness, restlessness, upset stomach, or vomiting. These side effects should disappear as your body adjusts to the medication.

If you are constipated, increase the amount of fiber in your diet (fresh fruits and vegetables, salads, bran, and whole-grain breads), exercise, and drink more water (unless your doctor directs you to do otherwise).

Chew sugarless gum or suck on ice chips or a piece of hard candy to reduce mouth dryness.

If you feel dizzy or light-headed, sit or lie down for a while; get up slowly from a sitting or reclining position, and be careful on stairs.

In order to avoid difficulty in falling asleep, take the last dose of this medication several hours before bedtime.

Major. Tell your doctor about any side effects that are persistent or particularly bothersome. IT IS ESPECIALLY IMPORTANT TO TELL YOUR DOCTOR about chest pain, difficult or painful urination, fainting, headaches, nosebleeds, palpitations, or uncoordinated body movements.

INTERACTIONS

Phenylpropanolamine and caramiphen combination interacts with several other types of medications:

1. Monoamine oxidase (MAO) inhibitors (isocarboxazid, pargyline, phenelzine, tranylcypromine) can increase the side effects of this medication. At least 14 days should separate the use of this drug and the use of an MAO inhibitor.

2. The blood-pressure-lowering effects of guanethidine may be decreased by this medication.

3. The side effects of phenylpropanolamine may be increased by digoxin or over-the-counter (nonprescription) diet, allergy, asthma, cough, cold, or sinus preparations.

BE SURE TO TELL YOUR DOCTOR about any medications you are currently taking, especially any of those listed above.

WARNINGS

- Tell your doctor about unusual or allergic reactions you have had to any medications, especially to caramiphen or phenylpropanolamine or to other adrenergic agents (such as albuterol, amphetamines, ephedrine, epinephrine, isoproterenol, metaproterenol, norepinephrine, pseudoephedrine, and terbutaline).
- Tell your doctor if you now have or if you have ever had asthma, diabetes mellitus, glaucoma, heart or blood vessel disease, high blood pressure, an enlarged prostate gland, or thyroid disease.
- Be sure to tell your doctor if you are pregnant. The effects of this medication during pregnancy have not been thoroughly studied in humans. Also, tell your doctor if you are breast-feeding an infant. Small amounts of this medication may pass into breast milk.

---

phenylpropanolamine and chlorpheniramine combination

BRAND NAMES (Manufacturers)

Allerest 12-Hour* (Pharmacraft)
Condrin-LA (Hauck)
Conex D.A.* (Forest)
Contac 12-Hour* (Smith Kline Consumer)
Dehist* (Forest)
Demazin* (Schering)
Drize (Ascher)
Dura-Vent/A (Dura)
Genamin* (Goldline)
Gencold* (Goldline)
Histabid Duracaps (Glaxo)
Myminic* (My-K Labs)
Noraminic* (Vortech)
Oragest T.D. (Major)
Oraminic (Vortech)
Ornade (Smith Kline & French)
phenylpropanolamine HCl and chlorpheniramine maleate (Cord)
Resaid S.R. (Geneva Generics)
Rhinolar-Ex 12 (McGregor)
Ru-Tuss II (Boots)
Triaminic* (Dorsey)
Triaminic-12* (Sandoz)
Trind* (Mead Johnson Nutrition)
Triphenyl (Rugby)
*Available over-the-counter (without a prescription)

TYPE OF DRUG

Adrenergic (decongestant) and antihistamine

INGREDIENTS

phenylpropanolamine and chlorpheniramine

DOSAGE FORMS

Oral tablets (25 mg or 37.5 mg phenylpropanolamine and 4 mg chlorpheniramine)
Sustained-release tablets (25 mg phenylpropanolamine and 4 mg chlorpheniramine)
Sustained-release capsules (75 mg phenylpropanolamine and 4 mg, 8 mg, 10 mg, or 12 mg chlorpheniramine)
Oral syrup (12.5 mg phenylpropanolamine and 2 mg chlorpheniramine per 5-ml spoonful, with 5% or 7.5% alcohol)

STORAGE

Phenylpropanolamine and chlorpheniramine combination tablets, capsules, and oral syrup should be stored at room temperature (never frozen) in tightly closed containers.

USES

This drug combination is used to relieve the symptoms of upper respiratory tract infections, hay fever and other allergies, and sinusitis (inflammation of the sinuses).

Phenylpropanolamine belongs to a group of drugs known as adrenergic agents (decongestants). They act by constricting (narrowing) blood vessels in the nasal passages, thereby reducing swelling and congestion.

Chlorpheniramine belongs to a group of drugs known as antihistamines, which block the action of histamine, a chemical released by the body during an allergic reaction. It is used to relieve or prevent symptoms of allergy.

TREATMENT

In order to avoid stomach upset, you can take phenylpropanolamine and chlorpheniramine combination with food or with a full glass of milk or water (unless your doctor directs you to do otherwise).

The oral syrup form of this medication should be measured carefully with a specially designed 5-ml measuring spoon. An ordinary kitchen teaspoon is not accurate enough.

The sustained-release tablets and capsules should be swallowed whole. Breaking, chewing, or crushing these tablets or capsules destroys their sustained-release activity and may increase the side effects.

If you miss a dose of this medication, take the missed dose as soon as possible, unless it is almost time for your next dose. In that case, do not take the missed dose at all; just return to your regular dosing schedule. Do not double the next dose.

SIDE EFFECTS

Minor. Anxiety; blurred vision; constipation; diarrhea; dizziness; drowsiness; dry mouth, nose, and throat; heartburn; insomnia; irritability; loss of appetite; nasal congestion; nausea; restlessness; decreased sweating; vomiting; or weakness. These side effects should disappear as your body adjusts to the medication.

This medication can increase your sensitivity to sunlight. Avoid prolonged exposure to sunlight and sunlamps, wear protective clothing, and use an effective sunscreen.

If you are constipated, increase the amount of fiber in your diet (fresh fruits and vegetables, salads, bran, and whole-grain breads), exercise, and drink more water (unless your doctor directs you to do otherwise).

Chew sugarless gum or suck on ice chips or a piece of hard candy to reduce mouth dryness.

If you feel dizzy or light-headed, sit or lie down for a while; get up slowly from a sitting or reclining position, and be careful on stairs.

In order to avoid difficulty in falling asleep, take the last dose of this medication several hours before bedtime.

Major. Tell your doctor about any side effects that are persistent or particularly bothersome. IT IS ESPECIALLY IMPORTANT TO TELL YOUR DOCTOR about chest pain, convulsions, difficult or painful urination, difficulty in breathing, fainting, hallucinations, headaches, loss of coordination, confusion, mood changes, nosebleeds, palpitations, rash, severe abdominal pain, sore throat, or unusual bleeding or bruising.

INTERACTIONS

This drug interacts with several other types of drugs:

1. Concurrent use of it with central nervous system depressants (such as alcohol, barbiturates, benzodiazepine tranquilizers, muscle relaxants, narcotics, pain medications, and phenothiazine tranquilizers) or with tricyclic antidepressants can cause extreme drowsiness.

2. Monoamine oxidase (MAO) inhibitors (isocarboxazid, pargyline, phenelzine, tranylcypromine) and tricyclic antidepressants can increase the side effects of this medication. At least 14 days should separate the use of this drug and the use of an MAO inhibitor.

3. The side effects of the antihistamine part of this medication may be increased by quinidine, procainamide, haloperidol, and phenothiazine tranquilizers; and the side effects of the decongestant component may be increased by digoxin or over-the-counter (nonprescription) diet, allergy, asthma, cough, cold, or sinus preparations.

4. The blood-pressure-lowering effects of guanethidine may be decreased by this medication.

BE SURE TO TELL YOUR DOCTOR about any medications you are currently taking, especially any listed above.

WARNINGS

- Tell your doctor about unusual or allergic reactions you have had to any medications, especially to chlorpheniramine or other antihistamines (such as azatadine, brompheniramine, carbinoxamine, clemastine, cyproheptadine, dexchlorpheniramine, dimenhydrinate, diphenhydramine, diphenylpyraline, doxylamine, hydroxyzine, promethazine, pyrilamine, trimeprazine, tripelennamine, and triprolidine) or to phenylpropanolamine or other adrenergic agents (such as albuterol, amphetamines, ephedrine, epinephrine, isoproterenol, metaproterenol, norepinephrine, pseudoephedrine, and terbutaline).
- Tell your doctor if you now have or if you have ever had diabetes mellitus, epilepsy, glaucoma, heart or blood vessel disease, hiatal hernia, high blood pressure, myasthenia gravis, obstructed bladder or intestinal tract, peptic ulcers, enlarged prostate gland, or thyroid disease.
- Because this drug can reduce sweating and heat release from the body, avoid excessive work or exercise in hot weather, and do not take hot baths, showers, or saunas.
- This medication can cause drowsiness. Exercise caution when performing tasks that require alertness, such as driving a car or operating potentially dangerous machinery.
- Be sure to tell your doctor if you are pregnant. The effects of this medication during pregnancy have not been thoroughly studied in humans. Also, tell your doctor if you are breast-feeding an infant. Small amounts of this medication pass into breast milk and may cause unusual excitement or irritability in nursing infants.

---

phenylpropanolamine and guaifenesin combination

BRAND NAMES (Manufacturers)

Banex-LA (Lu Chem)

Dura-Vent (Dura)
Entex L.A. (Norwich-Eaton)
Guipax (Vitarine)
Nolex LA (Carnrick)
Rymed-TR (Edwards)
Tega D&E (Ortega)

TYPE OF DRUG
Adrenergic (decongestant) and expectorant

INGREDIENTS
phenylpropanolamine and guaifenesin

DOSAGE FORM
Sustained-release tablets (75 mg phenylpropanolamine and 400 mg or 600 mg guaifenesin)

STORAGE
Phenylpropanolamine and guaifenesin combination tablets and capsules should be stored at room temperature in tightly closed containers.

USES

This drug combination is used to relieve the coughing and congestion associated with colds, sinusitis (inflammation of the sinuses), sore throat, bronchitis, and asthma.

Phenylpropanolamine belongs to a group of drugs known as adrenergic agents (decongestants). They act by constricting (narrowing) blood vessels in the nasal passages, thereby reducing swelling and congestion.

Guaifenesin is an expectorant, a drug that loosens bronchial secretions.

TREATMENT

In order to avoid stomach upset, you can take phenylpropanolamine and guaifenesin combination with food or with a full glass of milk or water (unless your doctor directs you to do otherwise).

These sustained-release tablets should be swallowed whole. Breaking, chewing, or crushing them destroys their sustained-release activity and may increase side effects.

If you miss a dose of this medication, take the missed dose as soon as possible, unless it is almost time for your next dose. In that case, do not take the missed dose at all; just return to your regular dosing schedule. Do not double the next dose.

SIDE EFFECTS

Minor. Insomnia, nervousness, or restlessness. These side effects should disappear as your body adjusts to the medication.

In order to help you avoid difficulty in falling asleep, take the last dose of this medication several hours before bedtime.

Major. Tell your doctor about any side effects that are persistent or particularly bothersome. IT IS ESPECIALLY IMPORTANT TO TELL YOUR DOCTOR about fainting, headaches, nosebleeds, or palpitations.

INTERACTIONS

Phenylpropanolamine and guaifenesin combination interacts with several other types of medications:

1. Monoamine oxidase (MAO) inhibitors (isocarboxazid, pargyline, phenelzine, tranylcypromine) can increase the side effects of this medication. At least 14 days should separate the use of this drug and the use of an MAO inhibitor.

2. The blood-pressure-lowering effects of guanethidine may be decreased by this medication.

3. The side effects of the decongestant component of this medication can be increased by digoxin or by over-the-counter (nonprescription) allergy, asthma, cough, cold, diet, or sinus preparations.

BE SURE TO TELL YOUR DOCTOR about any medications you are currently taking, especially any listed above.

WARNINGS

- Tell your doctor about unusual or allergic reactions you have had to any medications, especially to guaifenesin or phenylpropanolamine or to other adrenergic agents (such as albuterol, amphetamines, ephedrine, epinephrine, isoproterenol, metaproterenol, norepinephrine, pseudoephedrine, and terbutaline).
- Tell your doctor if you now have or if you have ever had diabetes mellitus, glaucoma, heart or blood vessel disease, high blood pressure, enlarged prostate, or thyroid disease.
- While you are taking phenylpropanolamine and guaifenesin combination, drink at least eight glasses of water a day to help loosen bronchial secretions.
- Be sure to tell your doctor if you are pregnant. The effects of this medication during pregnancy have not been thoroughly studied in humans. Also, tell your doctor if you are breast-feeding an infant. Small amounts of this medication may pass into breast milk.

phenylpropanolamine HCl and chlorpheniramine maleate—see phenylpropanolamine and chlorpheniramine combination

---

phenylpropanolamine, phenylephrine, and brompheniramine combination

BRAND NAMES (Manufacturers)
Bromatapp (various manufacturers)
Bromophen T.D. (Rugby)
brompheniramine, phenylephrine, and phenylpropanolamine (Lederle)
Dimetapp Extentabs* (Robins)
Normatane Elixir (Vortech)
Tamine SR (Geneva Generics)
Veltap Elixir (Lannett)
*Recently reformulated Dimetapp does not contain phenylephrine and is available without a prescription.

TYPE OF DRUG
Adrenergic (decongestant) and antihistamine

INGREDIENTS
phenylpropanolamine, phenylephrine, and brompheniramine

DOSAGE FORMS
Sustained-release tablets (15 mg phenylpropanolamine, 15 mg phenylephrine, and 12 mg brompheniramine; recently reformulated Dimetapp Extentabs contain 75 mg phenylpropanolamine and 12 mg brompheniramine, but no phenylephrine)

Oral elixir (5 mg phenylpropanolamine, 5 mg phenylephrine, 4 mg brompheniramine per 5-ml spoonful, with 2.3% or 3% alcohol)

STORAGE

The tablets and oral elixir should be stored at room temperature in tightly closed, light-resistant containers. This medication should never be frozen.

USES

This drug combination is used to relieve the symptoms of upper respiratory tract infections, hay fever and other allergies, and sinusitis (inflammation of the sinuses).

Phenylpropanolamine and phenylephrine belong to a group of drugs known as adrenergic agents (decongestants). They act by constricting (narrowing) blood vessels in the nasal passages, thereby reducing swelling and congestion.

Brompheniramine belongs to a group of drugs known as antihistamines, which block the actions of histamine, a chemical released by the body during an allergic reaction. It is used to relieve or prevent symptoms of allergy.

TREATMENT

This medication may cause stomach upset. In order to avoid this side effect, you can take phenylpropanolamine, phenylephrine, and brompheniramine combination with food or with a full glass of milk or water (unless your doctor directs you to do otherwise).

The oral elixir form of this medication should be measured carefully with a specially designed 5-ml measuring spoon. An ordinary kitchen teaspoon is not accurate enough.

The sustained-release tablets should be swallowed whole. Breaking, chewing, or crushing these tablets destroys their sustained-release activity and may increase the side effects.

If you miss a dose of this medication, take the missed dose as soon as possible, unless it is almost time for your next dose. In that case, do not take the missed dose at all; just return to your regular dosing schedule. Do not double the next dose.

SIDE EFFECTS

Minor. Anxiety; blurred vision; constipation; diarrhea; dizziness; drowsiness; dry mouth, nose, and throat; heartburn; insomnia; irritability; loss of appetite; nasal congestion; nausea; restlessness; decreased sweating; vomiting; or weakness. These side effects should disappear as your body adjusts to the medication.

If you are constipated, increase the amount of fiber in your diet (fresh fruits and vegetables, salads, bran, and whole-grain breads), and drink more water (unless your doctor directs you to do otherwise).

Chew sugarless gum or suck on ice chips or a piece of hard candy to reduce mouth dryness.

This medication can increase your sensitivity to sunlight. Avoid prolonged exposure to sunlight and sunlamps, wear protective clothing, and use an effective sunscreen.

If you feel dizzy or light-headed, sit or lie down for a while; get up slowly from a sitting or reclining position, and be careful on stairs.

In order to avoid difficulty in falling asleep, take the last dose of this medication several hours before bedtime.

Major. Tell your doctor about any side effects that are persistent or particularly bothersome. IT IS ESPECIALLY IMPORTANT TO TELL YOUR DOCTOR about chest pain, confusion, convulsions, difficult or painful urination, difficulty in breathing, fainting, hallucinations, headaches, loss of coordination, mood changes, nosebleeds, palpitations, rash, severe abdominal pain, sore throat, or unusual bleeding or bruising.

INTERACTIONS

Phenylpropanolamine, phenylephrine, and brompheniramine combination interacts with several other types of medications:

1. Concurrent use of it with central nervous system depressants (such as alcohol, barbiturates, benzodiazepine tranquilizers, muscle relaxants, narcotics, pain medications, and phenothiazine tranquilizers) or with tricyclic antidepressants can cause extreme drowsiness.

2. Monoamine oxidase (MAO) inhibitors (isocarboxazid, pargyline, phenelzine, tranylcypromine) and tricyclic antidepressants can increase the side effects of this medication. At least 14 days should separate the use of this drug and the use of an MAO inhibitor.

3. The side effects of the antihistamine part of this medication may be increased by quinidine, procainamide, haloperidol, and phenothiazine tranquilizers; and the side effects of the decongestant component may be increased by digoxin or by over-the-counter (nonprescription) allergy, asthma, cough, cold, diet, or sinus preparations.

4. The blood-pressure-lowering effects of guanethidine may be decreased by this medication.

BE SURE TO TELL YOUR DOCTOR about any medications you are currently taking, especially any of those listed above.

WARNINGS

- Tell your doctor about unusual or allergic reactions you have had to any medications, especially to brompheniramine, to other antihistamines (such as azatadine, chlorpheniramine, carbinoxamine, clemastine, cyproheptadine, dexchlorpheniramine, dimenhydrinate, diphenhydramine, diphenylpyraline, doxylamine, hydroxyzine, promethazine, pyrilamine, trimeprazine, tripelennamine, and triprolidine), or to phenylpropanolamine, phenylephrine, or other adrenergic agents (such as albuterol, amphetamines, ephedrine, epinephrine, isoproterenol, metaproterenol, norepinephrine, pseudoephedrine, and terbutaline).
- Tell your doctor if you now have or if you have ever had diabetes mellitus, epilepsy, glaucoma, heart or blood vessel disease, hiatal hernia, high blood pressure, myasthenia gravis, obstructed bladder or intestinal tract, peptic ulcers, enlarged prostate gland, or thyroid disease.
- Because this drug can reduce sweating and heat release from the body, avoid excessive work and exercise in hot weather, and do not take hot baths, showers, and saunas.
- This medication can cause drowsiness. Your ability to perform tasks that require alertness, such as driving a car or operating potentially dangerous machinery, may be decreased. Appropriate caution should, therefore, be taken.
- Be sure to tell your doctor if you are pregnant. The effects of this medication during pregnancy have not been thoroughly studied in humans. Also, tell your doctor if you are

breast-feeding an infant. Small amounts of this medication pass into breast milk and may cause unusual excitement or irritability in nursing infants.

---

phenylpropanolamine, phenylephrine, chlorpheniramine, and phenyltoloxamine combination

BRAND NAMES (Manufacturers)
Amaril D Spantab (Vortech)
Decongestabs (various manufacturers)
Histamic (Lexis)
Naldecon (Bristol)
Naldelate (various manufacturers)
Nalgest (Major)
New-Decongest (Goldline)
Tri-Phen-Chlor (Rugby)

TYPE OF DRUG
Adrenergic (decongestant) and antihistamine

INGREDIENTS
phenylpropanolamine, phenylephrine, chlorpheniramine, and phenyltoloxamine

DOSAGE FORMS
Sustained-release tablets (40 mg phenylpropanolamine, 10 mg phenylephrine, 5 mg chlorpheniramine, and 15 mg phenyltoloxamine)
Sustained-release capsules (50 mg phenylpropanolamine, 25 mg phenylephrine, 12 mg chlorpheniramine, and 30 mg phenyltoloxamine)
Oral syrup (20 mg phenylpropanolamine, 5 mg phenylephrine, 2.5 mg chlorpheniramine, and 7.5 mg phenyltoloxamine per 5-ml spoonful)
Oral pediatric drops (5 mg phenylpropanolamine, 1.25 mg phenylephrine, 0.5 mg chlorpheniramine, and 2 mg phenyltoloxamine per ml)

STORAGE
Store at room temperature in a tightly closed container. This medication should never be frozen.

USES

This drug combination is used to relieve symptoms of upper respiratory tract infections, hay fever and other allergies, and sinusitis (inflammation of the sinuses).

Phenylpropanolamine and phenylephrine belong to a group of drugs known as adrenergic agents (decongestants). They act by constricting (narrowing) blood vessels in the nasal passages, thereby reducing swelling and congestion.

Chlorpheniramine and phenyltoloxamine belong to a group of drugs known as antihistamines, which block the actions of histamine, a chemical released by the body during an allergic reaction. They are, therefore, used to relieve or prevent the symptoms of allergy.

TREATMENT

In order to avoid stomach upset, you can take phenylpropanolamine, phenylephrine, chlorpheniramine, and phenyltoloxamine combination with food or with a full glass of milk or water (unless your doctor directs you to do otherwise).

The oral pediatric drops should be measured carefully with the dropper provided.

The oral syrup form of this medication should be measured carefully with a specially designed 5-ml measuring spoon. An ordinary kitchen teaspoon is not accurate enough for measuring your dosage of this medication.

The sustained-release tablets and capsules should be swallowed whole. Breaking, chewing, or crushing them destroys their sustained-release activity and may increase the side effects.

If you miss a dose, take it as soon as possible, unless it is almost time for your next dose. In that case, do not take the missed dose at all; just return to your regular dosing schedule. Do not double the next dose.

SIDE EFFECTS

Minor. Anxiety; blurred vision; constipation; diarrhea; dizziness; drowsiness; dry mouth, nose, and throat; heartburn; insomnia; irritability; loss of appetite; nasal congestion; reduced sweating; restlessness; vomiting; or weakness. These side effects should disappear as your body adjusts to the medication.

This medication can increase your sensitivity to sunlight. Avoid prolonged exposure to sunlight and sunlamps, wear protective clothing, and use an effective sunscreen.

If you are constipated, increase the amount of fiber in your diet (fresh fruits and vegetables, salads, bran, and whole-grain breads), exercise, and drink more water (unless your doctor directs you to do otherwise).

If you experience dry mouth or throat, you should try chewing sugarless gum or sucking on ice chips or a piece of hard candy to reduce mouth dryness.

If you feel dizzy or light-headed, sit or lie down for a while; get up slowly from a sitting or reclining position, and be careful on stairs.

In order to avoid difficulty in falling asleep, take the last dose of this medication several hours before bedtime.

Major. Tell your doctor about any side effects that are persistent or particularly bothersome. IT IS ESPECIALLY IMPORTANT TO TELL YOUR DOCTOR about chest pain, confusion, convulsions, difficult or painful urination, difficulty in breathing, fainting, hallucinations, headaches, loss of coordination, mood changes, nosebleeds, palpitations, rash, severe abdominal pain, sore throat, or unusual bleeding or bruising.

INTERACTIONS

This medication interacts with several other types of drugs:

1. Concurrent use of this medication with central nervous system depressants (such as alcohol, barbiturates, benzodiazepine tranquilizers, muscle relaxants, narcotics, pain medications, and phenothiazine tranquilizers) or with tricyclic antidepressants can cause extreme drowsiness.

2. Monoamine oxidase (MAO) inhibitors (isocarboxazid, pargyline, phenelzine, tranylcypromine) and tricyclic antidepressants can increase the side effects of this medication. At least 14 days should separate the use of this drug and the use of an MAO inhibitor.

3. The side effects of the antihistamine part of this medication may be increased by quinidine, procainamide, haloperidol, and phenothiazine tranquilizers; and the side effects of the decongestant component may be increased by digoxin or by over-the-counter (nonprescription) allergy, asthma, cough, cold, diet, or sinus preparations.

4. The blood-pressure-lowering effects of guanethidine may be decreased by this medication.

BE SURE TO TELL YOUR DOCTOR about any medications you are currently taking, especially any of the medications that are listed above.

WARNINGS

• Tell your doctor about unusual or allergic reactions you have had to any medications, especially to chlorpheniramine, phenyltoloxamine, or any other antihistamine (such as azatadine, brompheniramine, carbinoxamine, clemastine, cyproheptadine, dexchlorpheniramine, dimenhydrinate, diphenhydramine, diphenylpyraline, doxylamine, hydroxyzine, promethazine, pyrilamine, trimeprazine, tripelennamine, and triprolidine), or to phenylpropanolamine, phenylephrine, or any other adrenergic agent (such as albuterol, amphetamines, ephedrine, epinephrine, isoproterenol, metaproterenol, norepinephrine, pseudoephedrine, and terbutaline).

• Tell your doctor if you now have or if you have ever had diabetes mellitus, epilepsy, glaucoma, heart or blood vessel disease, hiatal hernia, high blood pressure, myasthenia gravis, obstructed bladder or intestinal tract, peptic ulcers, enlarged prostate gland, or thyroid disease.

• Because this drug can reduce sweating and heat release from the body, you should avoid excessive work or exercise in hot weather and you should not take hot baths, showers, and saunas while taking this medication.

• This medication can cause drowsiness. Your ability to perform tasks that require alertness, such as driving a car or operating potentially dangerous machinery, may be decreased. Appropriate caution should, therefore, be taken.

• Be sure to tell your doctor if you are pregnant. The effects of this medication during pregnancy have not been thoroughly studied in humans. Also, tell your doctor if you are breast-feeding an infant. Small amounts of this medication pass into breast milk and may cause unusual excitement or irritability in nursing infants.

---

phenytoin

BRAND NAMES (Manufacturers)

Dilantin (Parke-Davis)
Dilantin Infatab (Parke-Davis)
Dilantin Kapseal (Parke-Davis)
Diphenylan (Lannett)
phenytoin (various manufacturers)

TYPE OF DRUG

Anticonvulsant

INGREDIENT

phenytoin

DOSAGE FORMS

Capsules (30 mg and 100 mg)
Chewable tablets (50 mg)
Oral suspension (30 mg and 125 mg per 5-ml spoonful, with 0.6% alcohol)

STORAGE

Phenytoin capsules, tablets, and oral suspension should be stored at room temperature in tightly closed, light-resistant containers. This medication should never be frozen.

USES

Phenytoin is used to control certain types of convulsions, or seizures. It is not clear exactly how phenytoin works to control convulsions, but it appears to prevent the spread of seizure activity in the brain. Phenytoin may also be used to treat other conditions as determined by your physician.

TREATMENT

In order to avoid stomach irritation, and to increase this drug's absorption, you can take phenytoin with food or with a full glass of water or milk (unless your doctor directs you to do otherwise).

The tablet form of this medication should be chewed before swallowing.

The suspension form of this medication should be shaken well just before measuring each dose. The contents tend to settle on the bottom of the bottle, so it is necessary to shake the container to distribute the ingredients evenly and equalize the doses. Each dose should then be measured carefully with a specially designed 5-ml measuring spoon. An ordinary kitchen teaspoon is not accurate enough.

Phenytoin works best when the level of medicine in your bloodstream is kept constant. It is best, therefore, to take the doses at evenly spaced intervals day and night. For example, if you are taking three doses a day, the doses should be spaced eight hours apart.

If you miss a dose of this medication, take the missed dose as soon as possible, unless it is almost time for the next dose. In that case, do not take the missed dose at all; just return to your regular dosing schedule. Do not double the next dose. If you miss two or more doses in a row, contact your doctor.

SIDE EFFECTS

Minor. Constipation, drowsiness (mild), headache, insomnia, nausea, or vomiting. These side effects should disappear as your body adjusts to the medication.

To relieve constipation, increase the amount of fiber in your diet (fresh fruits and vegetables, salads, bran, and whole-grain breads), exercise, and drink more water (unless your doctor directs you to do otherwise).

Major. Tell your doctor about any side effects that are persistent or particularly bothersome. IT IS ESPECIALLY IMPORTANT TO TELL YOUR DOCTOR about blurred vision, chest pain, confusion, dizziness, change in facial features, gum enlargement, increased hair growth, joint pain, muscle twitching, nervousness, numbness, rash, slurred speech, sore throat, swollen glands, uncoordinated movements, unusual bleeding or bruising, change in the color of your urine, or yellowing of the eyes or skin.

INTERACTIONS

Phenytoin interacts with a number of other types of drugs:

1. The effectiveness of phenytoin can be decreased by alcohol, barbiturates, folic acid, tricyclic antidepressants, reserpine, molindone, benzodiazepine tranquilizers, chloral hydrate, rifampin, phenothiazine tranquilizers, and haloperidol.

2. Phenytoin can decrease the effectiveness of calcifediol, warfarin, quinidine, disopyramide, dexamethasone, doxycycline, levodopa, and oral contraceptives (birth control pills).
3. The active blood levels and side effects of phenytoin can be increased by chloramphenicol, cimetidine, warfarin, disulfiram, isoniazid, oxyphenbutazone, phenylbutazone, ibuprofen, amiodarone, trimethoprim, sulfonamide antibiotics, tolbutamide, chlordiazepoxide, chlorpromazine, diazepam, estrogens, ethosuximide, methylphenidate, and prochlorperazine.
4. Valproic acid can either increase or decrease the effects of phenytoin.
5. The dosage of oral antidiabetic medications may need to be adjusted when phenytoin is started.
6. Phenytoin may decrease the absorption of furosemide from the gastrointestinal tract, decreasing its effectiveness.
7. Antacids, calcium, oxacillin, sucralfate, medicines for diarrhea, and antineoplastics (anticancer drugs) may decrease the gastrointestinal absorption and effectiveness of phenytoin. Do not take phenytoin within two to three hours of taking an antacid or antidiarrheal.

Before starting to take phenytoin, BE SURE TO TELL YOUR DOCTOR about any medications you are currently taking, especially any of those listed above.

WARNINGS

• Tell your doctor about unusual or allergic reactions you have had to any medications, especially to phenytoin, ethotoin, or mephenytoin.

• Before starting to take this medication, be sure to tell your doctor if you now have or if you have ever had blood disorders, diabetes mellitus, or liver disease.

• If this drug makes you dizzy or drowsy, do not take part in any activity that requires alertness, such as driving a car or operating potentially dangerous machinery. Children should be careful while playing.

• Before surgery or other medical or dental treatment, tell your doctor or dentist you are taking phenytoin.

• Do not stop taking this medication unless you first consult your doctor. If this drug is stopped abruptly, you may experience uncontrollable seizures. Your doctor may, therefore, want to reduce your dosage gradually. Be sure you have enough on hand for holidays and vacations.

• Although several generic versions of this drug are available, you should not switch from one brand to another without your doctor's careful assessment and complete approval. If you have your medication refilled and it looks different, be sure to consult with your pharmacist.

• Therapy with phenytoin may cause your gums to enlarge enough to cover your teeth. This can be minimized, at least partially, by frequent brushing and massaging of the gums with the rubber tip of a good toothbrush.

• Be sure to tell your doctor if you are pregnant. Birth defects have been reported more often in infants whose mothers have seizure disorders. It is unclear if the increased risk of birth defects is associated with the seizure disorders or with the anticonvulsant medications, such as phenytoin, that are used to treat them. The risks and benefits of treatment should, therefore, be discussed throughly with your doctor. Also, tell your doctor if you are breast-feeding an infant. Phenytoin anticonvulsant passes into breast milk and can cause extreme drowsiness in the nursing infant.

Phyllocontin—see aminophylline

Pilocar—see pilocarpine (ophthalmic)

---

pilocarpine (ophthalmic)

BRAND NAMES (Manufacturers)
Adsorbocarpine (Alcon)
Akarpine (Akorn)
Isopto Carpine (Alcon)
Ocusert Pilo-20 (Alza)
Ocusert Pilo-40 (Alza)
Pilocar (Iolab Pharm.)
pilocarpine hydrochloride (various manufacturers)

TYPE OF DRUG
Antiglaucoma ophthalmic solution

INGREDIENT
pilocarpine

DOSAGE FORMS
Ophthalmic drops (0.25%, 0.5%, 1%, 2%, 3%, 4%, 5%, 6%, 8%, and 10%)
Ocular therapeutic system (oval ring of plastic that contains pilocarpine. The ring is placed in the eye, and the drug is released gradually over a period of seven days.)

STORAGE
Pilocarpine eye drops should be stored at room temperature in a tightly closed container. This medication should never be frozen. If it discolors or turns brown, it should be discarded. A color change signifies a loss of potency.

The ocular therapeutic system form of this medication should be stored in the refrigerator in its original container.

USES

Pilocarpine (ophthalmic) is used to reduce the increased pressure in the eye caused by glaucoma or other eye conditions. When pilocarpine is applied to the eye, it constricts the pupil and increases the flow of fluid (aqueous humor) out of the eye, thereby reducing the pressure.

TREATMENT

Wash your hands with soap and water before applying this medication. In order to avoid contamination of the eye drops, be careful not to touch the tube portion of the dropper or let it touch your eye; DO NOT wipe off or rinse the dropper after you use it.

To apply the eye drops, tilt your head back and pull down your lower eyelid with one hand to make a pouch below the eye. Drop the prescribed amount of medicine into this pouch and slowly close your eyes. Try not to blink. Keep your eyes closed, and place one finger at the corner of the eye next to your nose for a minute or two, applying a slight pressure (to prevent loss of medication through the duct that drains fluid from the surface of the eye into the nose and throat). Wipe away any excess with a clean tissue. If you think the medicine did not get into the eye, repeat the process once. Since the drops are somewhat difficult to apply, you may want someone to apply them for you.

If more than one type of eye drop has been prescribed, wait at least five minutes after instilling pilocarpine before using any other eye medicine (this is done in order to give the pilocarpine a chance to work).

The ocular therapeutic system comes packaged with detailed instructions for insertion and removal. Follow these directions carefully. Damaged or deformed ocular therapeutic systems should not be placed or retained in the eye. Use a new system instead.

If you miss a dose of this medication, apply the missed dose as soon as possible, unless it is almost time for the next dose. In that case, do not apply the missed dose at all; just return to your regular dosing schedule. Do not double the next dose.

SIDE EFFECTS

Minor. Blurred vision, browache, headache, or twitching of the eyelids. These side effects should disappear as your body adjusts to the medication.

Major. Tell your doctor about any side effects that are persistent or particularly bothersome. IT IS ESPECIALLY IMPORTANT TO TELL YOUR DOCTOR about diarrhea, difficult or painful urination, flushing, muscle tremors, nausea, nearsightedness, palpitations, shortness of breath, stomach cramps, or sweating.

INTERACTIONS

This medication should not interact with other drugs as long as it is applied according to directions.

WARNINGS

- Tell your doctor about unusual or allergic reactions you have had to any medications, especially to pilocarpine.
- Tell your doctor if you now have or if you have ever had asthma, epilepsy, heart disease, peptic ulcers, thyroid disease, Parkinson's disease, or blockage of the urinary tract.
- This drug can cause difficulty in adjusting to low light levels. Caution should be exercised during night driving and while performing hazardous tasks in poor light.
- Be sure to tell your doctor if you are pregnant. The effects of this drug during pregnancy have not been thoroughly studied in humans, but small amounts of pilocarpine may be absorbed into the bloodstream. Also, tell your doctor if you are breast-feeding an infant. Small amounts of pilocarpine may pass into breast milk.

pilocarpine hydrochloride—see pilocarpine (ophthalmic)

---

pindolol

BRAND NAME (Manufacturer)
Visken (Sandoz)

TYPE OF DRUG
Beta-adrenergic blocking agent

INGREDIENT
pindolol

DOSAGE FORM
Tablets (5 mg and 10 mg)

STORAGE
Pindolol should be stored at room temperature in a tightly closed, light-resistant container.

USES

Pindolol is used to treat high blood pressure. It belongs to a group of medicines known as beta-adrenergic blocking agents or, more commonly, beta blockers. These drugs work by controlling nerve impulses along certain nerve pathways.

TREATMENT

This medicine can be taken with a glass of water, with meals, immediately following meals, or on an empty stomach (depending on your doctor's instructions). Try to take the medication at the same time(s) each day.

Try not to miss any doses of this medicine. If you do miss a dose, take the missed dose as soon as possible, unless it is within eight hours (if you are taking this medicine once a day) or within four hours (if you are taking this medicine more than once a day) of your next scheduled dose. In that case, do not take the missed dose at all; just return to your regular dosing schedule. Do not double the next dose.

It is important to remember that pindolol does not cure high blood pressure, but it will help to control the condition as long as you continue to take it.

SIDE EFFECTS

Minor. Anxiety; constipation; decreased sexual ability; diarrhea; difficulty in sleeping; drowsiness; dryness of the eyes, mouth, and skin; headache; nausea; tiredness; or weakness. These side effects should disappear as your body adjusts to the medicine.

To relieve constipation, increase the amount of fiber in your diet (fresh fruits and vegetables, salads, bran, and whole-grain breads) unless your doctor directs you to do otherwise.

If you are extra-sensitive to the cold, be sure to dress warmly during cold weather.

Plain, nonmedicated eye drops (artificial tears) may help to relieve eye dryness.

Sucking on ice chips or chewing sugarless gum helps to relieve mouth or throat dryness.

Major. Tell your doctor about any side effects that are persistent or particularly bothersome. IT IS ESPECIALLY IMPORTANT TO TELL YOUR DOCTOR about cold hands or feet (due to decreased blood circulation to skin, fingers, and toes), confusion, dizziness, fever and sore throat, hair loss, hallucinations, light-headedness, mental depression, nightmares, numbness or tingling of the fingers or toes, rapid weight gain (three to five pounds within a week), reduced alertness, skin rash, swelling, unusual bleeding or bruising, or wheezing or difficulty in breathing.

INTERACTIONS

Pindolol interacts with a number of other types of drugs:

1. Indomethacin, aspirin, or other salicylates may decrease the blood-pressure-lowering effects of the beta blockers.

2. Concurrent use of beta blockers and calcium channel blockers (diltiazem, nifedipine, verapamil) or disopyramide can lead to heart failure or very low blood pressure.

3. Cimetidine and oral contraceptives (birth control pills) can increase the blood concentrations of pindolol, which can result in greater side effects.

4. Side effects may also be increased when beta blockers are taken with clonidine, digoxin, epinephrine, phenylephrine, phenylpropanolamine, phenothiazine tranquilizers, prazosin, or monoamine oxidase (MAO) inhibitors. At least 14 days should separate use of a beta blocker and the use of an MAO inhibitor.

5. Beta blockers may antagonize (work against) the effects of theophylline, aminophylline, albuterol, isoproterenol, metaproterenol, and terbutaline.

6. Beta blockers can also interact with insulin or oral antidiabetic agents, raising or lowering blood sugar levels or masking the symptoms of low blood sugar.

7. The concurrent use of pindolol and reserpine can have additive blood-pressure-lowering effects.

8. The action of beta blockers may be increased if they are used with chlorpromazine, furosemide, or hydralazine.

9. Alcohol, barbiturates, and rifampin can decrease the blood concentrations of pindolol, which can result in a decrease in effectiveness.

BE SURE TO TELL YOUR DOCTOR about any medications you are currently taking, especially any listed above.

WARNINGS

• Before starting to take this drug, it is important to tell your doctor if you have ever had unusual or allergic reactions to any beta-blocking medication (acebutolol, atenolol, betaxolol, carteolol, esmolol, labetalol, metoprolol, nadolol, penbutolol, propranolol, timolol).

• Tell your doctor if you now have or if you have ever had allergies, asthma, hay fever, eczema, slow heartbeat, bronchitis, diabetes mellitus, emphysema, heart or blood vessel disease, kidney disease, liver disease, thyroid disease, or poor circulation in the fingers or toes.

• You may want to check your pulse while taking this medication. If your pulse is much slower than your usual rate (or if it is less than 50 beats per minute), check with your doctor. A pulse rate that is too slow may cause circulation problems.

• This medicine may affect your body's response to exercise. Make sure you discuss with your doctor a safe amount of exercise for your medical condition.

• It is important that you do not stop taking this medicine unless you first check with your doctor. Some conditions may become worse when the medicine is stopped suddenly, and the danger of a heart attack is increased in some patients. Your doctor may want you to reduce gradually the amount of medicine you take before stopping completely. Make sure that you have enough medicine on hand to last through vacations, holidays, and weekends.

• Before having surgery or any other medical or dental treatment, tell your physician or dentist that you are taking pindolol. Often, this medication will be discontinued 48 hours prior to any major surgery.

• Pindolol can cause dizziness, drowsiness, lightheadedness, or decreased alertness. You should, therefore, exercise caution while driving a car or using potentially dangerous machinery.

• While taking this medicine, do not use any over-the-counter (nonprescription) allergy, asthma, cough, cold, sinus, or diet preparations unless you first check with your pharmacist or doctor. Some of these medicines can result in high blood pressure if taken in conjunction with a beta blocker.

• Be sure to tell your doctor if you are pregnant. Animal studies have shown that some beta blockers can cause problems in pregnancy when used at very high doses. Adequate studies have not been conducted in humans, but there has been some association between beta blockers used during pregnancy and low birth weight, as well as breathing problems and slow heart rate in newborn infants. However, other reports have shown no effects on newborn infants. Also, tell your doctor if you are breast-feeding. Although pindolol has not been shown to cause problems in breast-fed infants, some of the medicine may pass into breast milk.

---

piroxicam

BRAND NAME (Manufacturer)
Feldene (Pfizer)
TYPE OF DRUG
Nonsteroidal anti-inflammatory analgesic
INGREDIENT
piroxicam
DOSAGE FORM
Capsules (10 mg and 20 mg)
STORAGE
Store in a tightly closed container at room temperature away from heat and direct sunlight.

USES

Piroxicam is used to treat the inflammation (pain, swelling, and stiffness) of certain types of arthritis, gout, bursitis, and tendinitis. Piroxicam has been shown to block the production of certain body chemicals, called prostaglandins, that may trigger pain. However, it is not fully understood how piroxicam works.

TREATMENT

You should take this medication on an empty stomach 30 to 60 minutes before meals or two hours after meals, so that it gets into your bloodstream quickly. To decrease stomach irritation, your doctor may want you to take the medicine with food or antacids.

It is important to take piroxicam on schedule and not to miss any doses. If you do miss a dose, take the missed dose as soon as possible. However, if you are taking this drug once a day and are six hours late OR if you take this drug twice a day and are two hours late, do not take the missed dose at all; just return to your regular dosing schedule. Do not double the next dose.

If you are taking piroxicam to relieve arthritis, you must take it regularly, as directed by your doctor. It may take up to three months before you feel the full benefits of this medication. Piroxicam does not cure arthritis, but it will help to control the condition as long as you continue to take it.

SIDE EFFECTS

Minor. Abdominal bloating, constipation, difficulty in sleeping, dizziness, drowsiness, headache, heartburn, indigestion, light-headedness, loss of appetite, nausea, nervousness, soreness of the mouth, unusual sweating, or vomiting. As your body adjusts to the drug, these should disappear.

To relieve constipation, increase the amount of fiber in your diet (fresh fruits and vegetables, salads, bran, and whole-grain breads), exercise, and drink more water (unless your doctor directs you to do otherwise).

If you become dizzy, sit or lie down; get up slowly from a sitting or reclining position, and be careful on stairs.

Major. Tell your doctor about any side effects that are persistent or particularly bothersome. IT IS ESPECIALLY IMPORTANT TO TELL YOUR DOCTOR about bloody or black, tarry stools; blurred vision; confusion; depression; difficult or painful urination; a problem with hearing; palpitations; ringing or buzzing in the ears; skin rash, hives, or itching; stomach pain; swelling of the feet; tightness in the chest; unexplained sore throat and fever; unusual bleeding or bruising; unusual fatigue or weakness; unusual weight gain; wheezing or difficulty in breathing; or yellowing of the eyes or skin.

INTERACTIONS

Piroxicam interacts with several types of medications:

1. Anticoagulants (blood thinners, such as warfarin) can lead to an increase in bleeding complications.

2. Aspirin, salicylates, or other anti-inflammatory medications can increase stomach irritation.

3. Probenecid may increase blood levels of piroxicam, which may increase the risks of side effects.

4. The action of beta blockers may be decreased by this drug.

5. This drug may interact with diuretics (water pills).

BE SURE TO TELL YOUR DOCTOR about any medications you are currently taking, especially any listed above.

WARNINGS

• Before you take this drug, tell your doctor if you have ever had unusual or allergic reactions to piroxicam or any of the other chemically related drugs (including aspirin or other salicylates, diclofenac, diflunisal, fenoprofen, flurbiprofen, ibuprofen, indomethacin, ketoprofen, meclofenamate, mefenamic acid, naproxen, oxyphenbutazone, phenylbutazone, sulindac, or tolmetin).

• Tell your doctor if you have ever had asthma, bleeding problems, colitis, epilepsy, heart disease, high blood pressure, kidney disease, liver disease, mental illness, Parkinson's disease, or stomach ulcers or other stomach problems.

• If this drug makes you dizzy or drowsy, do not take part in any activity that requires alertness, such as driving a car or operating potentially dangerous machinery.

• This drug can prolong bleeding time. Therefore, before having surgery or any other medical or dental treatment, it is important for you to tell your doctor or dentist that you are taking this medication.

• Stomach problems are more likely to occur if you take aspirin regularly or drink alcohol while being treated with this medication. These should, therefore, be avoided (unless your doctor directs you to do otherwise).

• Be sure to tell your doctor if you are pregnant. Although studies in humans have not been conducted, unwanted cardiac (heart) side effects have been observed in the offspring of animals that received this type of drug during pregnancy. If taken late in pregnancy, it can also prolong labor. Also, tell your doctor if you are breast-feeding an infant. Small amounts of piroxicam can pass into breast milk.

Plegine—see phendimetrazine

Poladex T.D.—see dexchlorpheniramine

Polaramine—see dexchlorpheniramine

Polaramine Repetabs—see dexchlorpheniramine

Polargen—see dexchlorpheniramine

Polycillin—see ampicillin

Polyflex—see chlorzoxazone and acetaminophen combination

Polymox—see amoxicillin

Poly-Vi-Flor—see vitamins, multiple, with fluoride

Polyvitamins with Fluoride Drops—see vitamins, multiple with fluoride

Polyvite with Fluoride Drops—see vitamins, multiple, with fluoride

Pondimin—see fenfluramine

Ponstel—see mefenamic acid

Potachlor—see potassium chloride

Potasalan—see potassium chloride

Potassine—see potassium chloride

---

potassium chloride

BRAND NAMES (Manufacturers)
Cena-K (Century)
Kaochlor (Adria)
Kaon (Adria)
Kato (ICN)
Kay Ciel (Forest)
K-Dur (Key)
K-Lor (Abbott)
Klor-Con (Upsher-Smith)
Klorvess (Sandoz)
Klotrix (Mead Johnson)
K-Lyte/Cl (Mead Johnson)
Kolyum (Pennwalt)
K-Tab (Abbott)
Micro-K (Robins)
Micro-K Extencaps (Robins)
Potachlor (Bay Labs)
Potasalan (Lannett)
Potassine (Recsei)
potassium chloride (various manufacturers)
Rum-K (Fleming)
Slow-K (Ciba)

TYPE OF DRUG
Potassium replacement

INGREDIENT
potassium chloride

DOSAGE FORMS
Effervescent tablets (20 mEq, 25 mEq, and 50 mEq)
Sustained-release tablets (6.7 mEq, 8 mEq, 10 mEq, and 20 mEq)
Enteric-coated tablets (4 mEq and 13 mEq)
Sustained-release capsules (8 mEq and 10 mEq)
Oral liquid (10 mEq, 15 mEq, 20 mEq, 30 mEq, and 40 mEq per 15-ml spoonful, with alcohol varying from 0% to 5%)
Oral powder (15 mEq, 20 mEq, and 25 mEq per packet)

STORAGE
Store at room temperature in a tightly closed container.

USES

This medication is used to prevent or treat potassium deficiency, especially potassium deficiency that is caused by the use of diuretics (water pills).

TREATMENT

In order to avoid stomach irritation, you should take potassium chloride with food or immediately after a meal. In order to become accustomed to taking this medication, try to take it at the same time(s) each day.

Each dose of the liquid form of this medication should be measured carefully with a specially designed measuring spoon. An ordinary teaspoon is not accurate enough.

If you are taking the liquid, powder, or effervescent tablet form,dilute each dose in at least four ounces (1/2 cup) of cold water or juice. Be sure the medication has dissolved completely and has stopped fizzing before you drink it. Then sip it slowly. DO NOT use tomato juice to dissolve this medication (unless your doctor directs you to do so). Tomato juice contains a great deal of sodium.

The sustained-release tablets and capsules should be swallowed whole. Chewing, crushing, or breaking these tablets or capsules destroys their sustained-release activity and possibly increases the side effects.

If you miss a dose of this medication, take the missed dose as soon as possible, unless it is within two hours of the next scheduled dose. In that case, do not take the missed dose at all; just return to your regular dosing schedule. Do not double the next dose.

SIDE EFFECTS

Minor. Diarrhea, nausea, stomach pains, or vomiting. These should disappear as your body adjusts to the drug.

Major. Tell your doctor about any side effects that are persistent or particularly bothersome. IT IS ESPECIALLY IMPORTANT TO TELL YOUR DOCTOR about anxiety; bloody or black, tarry stools; confusion; difficulty in breathing; numbness or tingling in the arms, legs, or feet; palpitations; severe abdominal pain; or unusual weakness.

INTERACTIONS

This drug interacts with several other types of drugs:

1. The combination of potassium chloride with amiloride, spironolactone, or triamterene can lead to hyperkalemia (high levels of potassium in the bloodstream).

2. The combination of digoxin and high doses of potassium chloride can lead to heart problems.

Before starting to take potassium chloride, BE SURE TO TELL YOUR DOCTOR about any medications you are currently taking, especially any of those listed above.

WARNINGS

- Tell your doctor about unusual or allergic reactions you have had to any medications, especially to potassium.
- Before starting to take this medication, be sure to tell your doctor if you now have or if you have ever had Addison's disease, dehydration, heart disease, heat cramps, hyperkalemia, intestinal blockage, kidney disease, myotonia congenita, or peptic ulcers.
- Ask your doctor about using a salt substitute instead of potassium chloride; salt substitutes are similar, but less expensive and more convenient. However, salt substitutes should only be used with your doctor's approval. Too much potassium can be dangerous.
- If you are taking the sustained-release tablets and you find something that looks like a tablet in your stool, there is no reason for concern; the potassium chloride has been absorbed from the tablet. The drug is "held" in a wax core designed to release the medication slowly. This wax core is eliminated in the stool after the drug has been absorbed.
- Some of these products contain the color additive FD&C Yellow No. 5 (tartrazine), which can cause allergic-type reactions (rash, shortness of breath, or fainting) in certain susceptible individuals.
- Be sure to tell your doctor if you are pregnant. Although this drug appears to be safe, extensive studies in pregnant women have not been conducted. Also, tell your doctor if you are breast-feeding an infant. Small amounts of potassium pass into breast milk.

---

prazepam

BRAND NAME (Manufacturer)
Centrax (Parke-Davis)

TYPE OF DRUG
Benzodiazepine sedative/hypnotic

INGREDIENT
prazepam

DOSAGE FORMS
Capsules (5 mg, 10 mg, and 20 mg)
Tablets (10 mg)

STORAGE
This medication should be stored at room temperature in a tightly closed, light-resistant container.

USES

Prazepam is prescribed to treat symptoms of anxiety. It is not clear exactly how this medicine works, but it may relieve anxiety by acting as a depressant of the central nervous system. This drug is currently used by many people to relieve nervousness. It is effective for this purpose for short periods, but it is important to try to remove the cause of the anxiety as well.

TREATMENT

Prazepam should be taken exactly as directed by your doctor. It can be taken with food or a full glass of water if stomach upset occurs. Do not take this medication with a dose of antacids, since they may retard its absorption.

If you are taking this medication regularly and you miss a dose, take the missed dose immediately if you remember within an hour. If more than an hour has passed, skip the dose you missed and wait for the next scheduled dose. Do not double the next dose.

SIDE EFFECTS

Minor. Bitter taste in mouth, constipation, diarrhea, dizziness, drowsiness (after a night's sleep), dry mouth, excessive salivation, fatigue, flushing, headache, heartburn, loss of appetite, nausea, nervousness, sweating, or vomiting. As your body adjusts to the medicine, these side effects should disappear.

To relieve constipation during therapy with this medication, increase the amount of fiber in your diet (fresh fruits and vegetables, salads, bran, and whole-grain breads), exercise, and drink more water (unless your doctor directs you to do otherwise).

Dry mouth can be relieved by chewing sugarless gum or by sucking on ice chips.

If you feel dizzy, sit or lie down for a while; get up slowly from a sitting or reclining position, and be careful on stairs.

Major. Tell your doctor about any side effects that are persistent or particularly bothersome. IT IS ESPECIALLY IMPORTANT TO TELL YOUR DOCTOR about blurred or double vision, chest pain, depression, difficulty in urinating, fainting, falling, fever, joint pain, hallucinations, mouth sores, nightmares, palpitations, rash, shortness of breath, slurred speech, sore throat, uncoordinated movements, unusual excitement, unusual tiredness, or yellowing of the eyes or skin.

INTERACTIONS

Prazepam interacts with a number of other types of medications:

1. To prevent oversedation, this drug should not be taken with alcohol, other sedative drugs, central nervous system depressants (such as antihistamines, barbiturates, muscle relaxants, pain medicines, narcotics, medicines for seizures, and phenothiazine tranquilizers), or antidepressants.

2. This medication may decrease the effectiveness of levodopa.

3. This drug may increase the effects of phenytoin.

4. Disulfiram, isoniazid, and cimetidine can increase the blood levels of prazepam, which can lead to toxic effects.

5. Concurrent use of rifampin or carbamazepine may decrease the effectiveness of prazepam.

BE SURE TO TELL YOUR DOCTOR about any medications you are currently taking, especially any of those listed above.

WARNINGS

- Tell your doctor about any unusual or allergic reactions that you have had to any medications, especially to prazepam or to other benzodiazepine tranquilizers (such as alprazolam, chlordiazepoxide, clorazepate, diazepam, flurazepam, halazepam, lorazepam, oxazepam, temazepam, and triazolam).
- Tell your doctor if you now have or if you have ever had liver disease, kidney disease, epilepsy, lung disease, myasthenia gravis, porphyria, mental depression, or mental illness.
- This medicine can cause drowsiness. Your ability to perform tasks that require alertness, such as driving a car or using potentially dangerous machinery, may be decreased. Appropriate caution should, therefore, be taken.
- Prazepam has the potential for abuse and must be used with caution. Tolerance may develop quickly; do not increase the dosage without first consulting your doctor. It is also important not to stop this drug suddenly if you have been taking it in large amounts or if you have used it for several weeks. Your doctor may reduce the dosage gradually.
- This is a safe drug when used properly. When it is combined with other sedative drugs or alcohol, however, serious side effects can develop.
- Be sure to tell your doctor if you are pregnant. This type of medicine may increase the chance of birth defects if it is taken during the first three months of pregnancy. In addition, too much use of this medicine during the last six months of pregnancy may result in addiction of the fetus, leading to withdrawal side effects in the newborn. Also, use of this medicine during the last weeks of pregnancy may cause excessive drowsiness, slowed heartbeat, and breathing difficulties in the infant. Tell your doctor if you are breast-feeding an infant. This medicine can pass into the breast milk and cause excessive drowsiness, slowed heartbeat, and breathing difficulties in nursing infants.

---

prazosin

BRAND NAME (Manufacturer)
Minipress (Pfizer)
TYPE OF DRUG
Antihypertensive
INGREDIENT
prazosin
DOSAGE FORM
Capsules (1 mg, 2 mg, and 5 mg)
STORAGE
Prazosin capsules should be stored at room temperature in a tightly closed, light-resistant container.

USES

Prazosin is used to treat high blood pressure. It is a vasodilator that relaxes the muscle tissue of the blood vessels, which in turn lowers blood pressure.

TREATMENT

To avoid stomach irritation, you can take prazosin with food or with a full glass of water or milk. In order to become accustomed to taking this medication, try to take it at the same time(s) each day.

The first dose of this medication can cause fainting. Therefore, it is often recommended that this dose be taken at bedtime.

If you miss a dose of this medication, take the missed dose as soon as possible, unless it is almost time for the next dose. In that case, do not take the missed dose at all; just return to your regular dosing schedule. Do not double the next dose.

Prazosin does not cure high blood pressure, but it will help to control the condition as long as you continue to take the medication.

The effects of this medication may not become apparent for two weeks.

SIDE EFFECTS

Minor. Abdominal pain, constipation, diarrhea, dizziness, drowsiness, dry mouth, frequent urination, headache, impotence, nasal congestion, nausea, nervousness, sweating, tiredness, vomiting, or weakness. These side effects should disappear as your body adjusts to the medication.

To relieve constipation, increase the amount of fiber in your diet (fresh fruits and vegetables, salads, bran, and whole-grain breads), exercise, and drink more water (unless your doctor directs you to do otherwise).

To relieve mouth dryness, chew sugarless gum or suck on ice chips or a piece of hard candy.

If you feel dizzy or light-headed, sit or lie down for a while; get up slowly from a sitting or reclining position, and be careful on stairs. To avoid dizziness or light-headedness when you stand, contract and relax the muscles of your legs for a few moments before rising. Do this by pushing one foot against the floor while raising the other foot slightly, alternating feet so that you are "pumping" your legs in a pedaling motion.

Major. Tell your doctor about any side effects that are persistent or particularly bothersome. IT IS ESPECIALLY IMPORTANT TO TELL YOUR DOCTOR about blurred vision; chest pain; constant erection; depression; difficulty in breathing; difficulty in urinating; fainting; hallucinations; itching; loss of hair; nosebleeds; palpitations; rapid weight gain (three to five pounds within a week); rash; ringing in the ears; swelling of the feet, legs, or ankles; or tingling of the fingers or toes.

INTERACTIONS

Prazosin can interact with other types of medications:

1. The combination of prazosin and alcohol or verapamil can lead to a severe drop in blood pressure and fainting.

2. The severity and duration of the blood-pressure-lowering effects of the first dose of prazosin may be enhanced by a beta blocker.

BE SURE TO TELL YOUR DOCTOR about any medications you are currently taking, especially any of those listed above.

WARNINGS

- Tell your doctor about unusual or allergic reactions you have had to any medications, especially to prazosin or terazosin.
- Before starting to take this medication, be sure to tell your doctor if you now have or if you have ever had angina (chest pain) or kidney disease.
- Because initial therapy with this drug may cause dizziness or fainting, your doctor will probably start you on a low dosage and increase the dosage gradually.
- If this drug makes you dizzy or drowsy or blurs your vision, do not take part in any activity that requires alertness, such as driving a car or operating potentially dangerous machinery.
- In order to avoid dizziness or fainting while taking this drug, try not to stand for long periods of time, avoid drinking excessive amounts of alcohol, and try not to get overheated (avoid exercising strenuously in hot weather and taking hot baths, showers, and saunas).
- Before taking any over-the-counter (nonprescription) sinus, allergy, asthma, cough, cold, or diet preparation, check with your doctor or pharmacist. Some of these products can cause an increase in blood pressure.
- Do not stop taking this medication unless you first check with your doctor. If you stop taking this drug abruptly, you may experience a sudden rise in blood pressure. Your doctor may, therefore, want to decrease your dosage gradually.
- Be sure to tell your doctor if you are pregnant. Although this drug appears to be safe, there have been only limited studies in pregnant women. Also, tell your doctor if you are breast-feeding an infant. Small amounts of prazosin pass into breast milk.

Prednicen-M—see prednisone (systemic)

---

prednisolone (systemic)

BRAND NAMES (Manufacturers)
Delta-Cortef (Upjohn)
prednisolone (various manufacturers)
Prelone (Muro)

TYPE OF DRUG
Adrenocorticosteroid hormone

INGREDIENT
prednisolone

DOSAGE FORMS
Tablets (5 mg)
Oral syrup (15 mg per 5-ml spoonful, with 5% alcohol)

STORAGE
Prednisolone tablets and oral syrup should be stored at room temperature (never frozen) in a tightly closed container.

USES

Your adrenal glands naturally produce certain cortisone-like chemicals. These chemicals are involved in various regulatory processes in the body (such as those involving fluid balance, temperature, and reaction to inflammation). Prednisolone belongs to a group of drugs known as adrenocorticosteroids (or cortisone-like medications). It is used to treat a variety of disorders, including endocrine and rheumatic disorders; asthma; blood diseases; certain cancers; eye disorders; gastrointestinal disturbances, such as ulcerative colitis; respiratory diseases; and inflammations, such as arthritis, dermatitis, and poison ivy. How this drug acts to relieve these disorders is not completely understood.

TREATMENT

In order to prevent stomach irritation, you can take prednisolone with food or milk.

Each dose of the oral syrup form should be measured carefully with a specially designed 5-ml measuring spoon. An ordinary kitchen teaspoon is not accurate enough.

If you are taking only one dose of this medication each day, try to take it before 9:00 A.M. This will mimic the body's normal production of this type of chemical.

It is important to try not to miss any doses of prednisolone. However, if you do miss a dose, follow these guidelines:

1. If you are taking it more than once a day, take the missed dose as soon as possible and return to your regular dosing schedule. If it is already time for the next dose, double it.

2. If you are taking this medication once a day, take the dose you missed as soon as possible, unless you don't remember until the next day. In that case, do not take the missed dose at all; just follow your regular dosing schedule. Do not double the next dose.
3. If you are taking this drug every other day, take it as soon as you remember. If you missed the scheduled time by a whole day, take it when you remember, then skip a day before you take the next dose. Do not double the next dose.

If you miss more than one dose of prednisolone, CONTACT YOUR DOCTOR.

SIDE EFFECTS

Minor. Dizziness, false sense of well-being, increased appetite, increased sweating, indigestion, menstrual irregularities, nausea, reddening of the skin on the face, restlessness, sleep disorders, or weight gain. These side effects should disappear as your body adjusts to the medication.

Major. Tell your doctor about any side effects that are persistent or particularly bothersome. IT IS ESPECIALLY IMPORTANT TO TELL YOUR DOCTOR about abdominal enlargement; abdominal pain; acne or other skin problems; back or rib pain; bloody or black, tarry stools; blurred vision; convulsions; eye pain; fever and sore throat; growth impairment (in children); headaches; impaired healing of wounds; increased thirst and urination; mental depression; mood changes; muscle wasting or weakness; rapid weight gain (three to five pounds within a week); rash; shortness of breath; thinning of the skin; unusual bruising or bleeding; or unusual weakness.

INTERACTIONS

Prednisolone interacts with several other types of medications:

1. Alcohol, aspirin, and anti-inflammatory medications (such as diclofenac, diflunisal, fenoprofen, flurbiprofen, ibuprofen, indomethacin, ketoprofen, meclofenamate, mefenamic acid, naproxen, piroxicam, sulindac, and tolmetin) aggravate the stomach problems that are common with use of this medication.
2. The dosage of oral anticoagulants (blood thinners, such as wafarin), oral antidiabetic drugs, or insulin may need to be adjusted when this medication is being taken.
3. The loss of potassium caused by prednisolone can lead to serious side effects in individuals taking digoxin.
4. Thiazide diuretics (water pills) can increase the potassium loss caused by this medication.
5. Phenobarbital, phenytoin, rifampin, or ephedrine can increase the elimination of prednisolone from the body, thereby decreasing its effectiveness.
6. Oral contraceptives (birth control pills) and estrogen-containing drugs may decrease the elimination of this drug from the body, which can lead to an increase in side effects.
7. Prednisolone can increase the elimination of aspirin and isoniazid, thereby decreasing the effectiveness of these two medications.
8. Cholestyramine and colestipol can chemically bind this medication in the stomach and gastrointestinal tract, preventing its absorption.

BE SURE TO TELL YOUR DOCTOR about any medications you are currently taking, especially any of the medications listed above.

WARNINGS

- Tell your doctor about unusual or allergic reactions you have had to any medications, especially to prednisolone or other adrenocorticosteroids (such as betamethasone, cortisone, dexamethasone, hydrocortisone, methylprednisolone, prednisone, and triamcinolone).
- Tell your doctor if you now have or if you have ever had bone disease, diabetes mellitus, emotional instability, glaucoma, fungal infections, heart disease, high blood pressure, high cholesterol levels, myasthenia gravis, peptic ulcers, osteoporosis, thyroid disease, tuberculosis, ulcerative colitis, kidney disease, or liver disease.
- To help avoid potassium loss while you are using this medication, you can take your dose of the drug with a glass of fresh or frozen orange juice, or eat a banana each day. The use of a salt substitute also helps prevent potassium loss. Check with your doctor, however, before making any dietary changes or using a salt substitute.
- If you are using this medication for longer than a week, you may need to have your dosage adjusted if you are subjected to stress, which you might experience as a result of serious infections, injury, or surgery. Discuss this with your doctor.
- If you have been taking this drug for more than a week, do not stop taking it suddenly. If it is stopped abruptly, you may experience abdominal or back pain, dizziness, fainting, fever, muscle or joint pain, nausea, vomiting, shortness of breath, or extreme weakness. Your doctor may, therefore, want to reduce the dosage gradually. Never increase the dosage or take the drug for longer than the prescribed time unless you first consult your doctor.
- While you are taking this drug, you should not be vaccinated or immunized. Prednisolone decreases the effectiveness of vaccines and can lead to overwhelming infection if a live-virus vaccine is administered.
- Before having surgery or any other medical or dental treatment, be sure to tell your doctor or dentist that you are taking this medication.
- Because this drug can cause glaucoma and cataracts with long-term use, your doctor may want you to have your eyes examined by an ophthalmologist periodically during treatment.
- If you are taking prednisolone for prolonged periods, you should wear or carry an identification card or notice stating that you are taking an adrenocorticosteroid.
- This medication can raise blood sugar levels in diabetic patients. Blood sugar levels should, therefore, be monitored carefully with blood or urine tests when this medication is being taken.
- Some of these products contain the color additive FD&C Yellow No. 5 (tartrazine), which can cause allergic-type reactions (shortness of breath, wheezing, rash, fainting) in certain susceptible individuals.
- Be sure to tell your doctor if you are pregnant. This drug crosses the placenta, and its safety in humans is not established. Birth defects have been observed in the fetuses of animals who were given large doses of this type of drug during pregnancy. Also, tell your doctor if you are breast-feeding an infant. Small amounts of this drug pass into breast milk and may cause growth suppression or a decrease in natural adrenocorticosteroid hormone production in the nursing infant.

prednisone (systemic)

BRAND NAMES (Manufacturers)
Deltasone (Upjohn)
Liquid Pred (Muro)
Meticorten (Schering)
Orasone (Reid-Rowell)
Panasol-S (Seatrace)
Prednicen-M (Central)
prednisone (various manufacturers)

TYPE OF DRUG
Adrenocorticosteroid hormone

INGREDIENT
prednisone

DOSAGE FORMS
Tablets (1 mg, 2.5 mg, 5 mg, 10 mg, 20 mg, 25 mg, and 50 mg)
Oral syrup (5 mg per 5-ml spoonful, with 5% alcohol)
Oral solution (5 mg per 5-ml spoonful, with 5% alcohol)
Oral intensol solution (5 mg per ml, with 30% alcohol)

STORAGE
Prednisone tablets, oral syrup, and oral solution should be stored at room temperature (never frozen) in tightly closed containers.

USES

Your adrenal glands naturally produce certain cortisone-like chemicals. These chemicals are involved in various regulatory processes in the body (such as those involving fluid balance, temperature, and reaction to inflammation). Prednisone belongs to a group of drugs known as adrenocorticosteroids (or cortisone-like medications). It is used to treat a variety of disorders, including endocrine and rheumatic disorders; asthma; blood diseases; certain cancers; eye disorders; gastrointestinal disturbances, such as ulcerative colitis; respiratory diseases; and inflammations, such as arthritis, dermatitis, and poison ivy. How this drug acts to relieve these disorders is not completely understood.

TREATMENT

In order to prevent stomach irritation, you can take prednisone with food or milk.

If you are taking only one dose of this medication each day, try to take it before 9:00 A.M. This will mimic the body's normal production of this type of chemical.

The oral syrup or solution form of this medication should be measured carefully with a specially designed dropper (intensol solution) or 5-ml measuring spoon. An ordinary kitchen teaspoon is not accurate enough.

It is important to try not to miss any doses of prednisone. However, if you do miss a dose of this medication, follow these guidelines:

1. If you are taking it more than once a day, take the missed dose as soon as possible and return to your regular dosing schedule. If it is already time for the next dose, double it.
2. If you are taking this medication once a day, take the dose you missed as soon as possible, unless you don't remember until the next day. In that case, do not take the missed dose at all; just follow your regular dosing schedule. Do not double the next dose.
3. If you are taking this drug every other day, take it when you remember. If you missed the scheduled dose by a whole day, take it; then skip a day before you take the next dose. Do not double the dose.

If you miss more than one dose of prednisone, CONTACT YOUR DOCTOR.

SIDE EFFECTS

Minor. Dizziness, false sense of well-being, increased appetite, increased sweating, indigestion, menstrual irregularities, nausea, reddening of the skin on the face, restlessness, sleep disorders, or weight gain. These side effects should disappear as your body adjusts to the medication.

Major. Tell your doctor about any side effects that are persistent or particularly bothersome. IT IS ESPECIALLY IMPORTANT TO TELL YOUR DOCTOR about abdominal enlargement; abdominal pain; acne or other skin problems; back or rib pain; bloody or black, tarry stools; blurred vision; convulsions; eye pain; fever and sore throat; growth impairment (in children); headaches; impaired healing of wounds; increased thirst and urination; mental depression; mood changes; muscle wasting or weakness; rapid weight gain (three to five pounds within a week); rash; shortness of breath; thinning of the skin; unusual bruising or bleeding; or unusual weakness.

INTERACTIONS

Prednisone interacts with several other types of medications:

1. Alcohol, aspirin, and anti-inflammatory medications (such as diclofenac diflunisal, fenoprofen, flurbiprofen, ibuprofen, indomethacin, ketoprofen, meclofenamate, mefenamic acid, naproxen, piroxicam, sulindac, or tolmetin) aggravate the stomach problems that are common with use of this medication.
2. The dosage of oral anticoagulants (blood thinners, such as warfarin), oral antidiabetic drugs, or insulin may need to be adjusted when this medication is being taken.
3. The loss of potassium caused by prednisone can lead to serious side effects in individuals taking digoxin.
4. Thiazide diuretics (water pills) can increase the potassium loss caused by this medication.
5. Phenobarbital, phenytoin, rifampin, and ephedrine can increase the elimination of prednisone from the body, thereby decreasing its effectiveness.
6. Oral contraceptives (birth control pills) and estrogen-containing drugs may decrease the elimination of this drug from the body, which can lead to an increase in side effects.
7. Prednisone can increase the elimination of aspirin and isoniazid, decreasing the effectiveness of these two drugs.
8. Cholestyramine and colestipol can chemically bind this medication in the stomach and gastrointestinal tract, preventing its absorption.

BE SURE TO TELL YOUR DOCTOR about any medications you are currently taking, especially any listed above.

WARNINGS

- Tell your doctor about unusual or allergic reactions you have had to any medications, especially to prednisone or other adrenocorticosteroids (such as betamethasone, cortisone, dexamethasone, hydrocortisone, methylprednisolone, prednisolone, and triamcinolone).
- Tell your doctor if you now have or if you have ever had bone disease, diabetes mellitus, emotional instability, glaucoma, fungal infections, heart disease, high blood pressure,

high cholesterol levels, kidney disease, liver disease, myasthenia gravis, peptic ulcers, osteoporosis, thyroid disease, tuberculosis, or ulcerative colitis.

• To help avoid potassium loss while using this drug, take your dose with a glass of fresh or frozen orange juice or eat a banana each day. The use of a salt substitute also helps prevent potassium loss. Check with your doctor before making any dietary changes.

• If you are using this medication for longer than a week, you may need to have your dosage adjusted if you are subjected to stress, such as serious infections, injury, or surgery. Discuss this with your doctor.

• If you have been taking this drug for more than a week, do not stop taking it suddenly. If it is stopped abruptly, you may experience abdominal or back pain, dizziness, fainting, fever, muscle or joint pain, nausea, vomiting, shortness of breath, or extreme weakness. Your doctor may, therefore, want to reduce the dosage gradually. Never increase the dosage or take the drug for longer than the prescribed time unless you first consult your doctor.

• While you are taking this drug, you should not be vaccinated or immunized. This medication decreases the effectiveness of vaccines and can lead to overwhelming infection if a live-virus vaccine is administered.

• Before surgery or other medical or dental treatment, tell your doctor or dentist you are taking this drug.

• Because this drug can cause glaucoma and cataracts with long-term use, your doctor may want you to have your eyes examined by an ophthalmologist periodically during treatment.

• If you are taking this medication for prolonged periods, you should wear or carry an identification card or notice stating that you are taking an adrenocorticosteroid.

• This drug can raise blood sugar levels in diabetic patients. Blood sugar should, therefore, be monitored carefully with blood or urine tests when this drug is started.

• Be sure to tell your doctor if you are pregnant. Prednisone crosses the placenta, and its safety in human pregnancy has not been established. Birth defects have been observed in the fetuses of animals that were given large doses of this drug during pregnancy. Also, tell your doctor if you are breast-feeding an infant. Small amounts of this drug pass into breast milk and may cause growth suppression or a decrease in natural adrenocorticosteroid production in the nursing infant.

Prelone—see prednisolone (systemic)

Prelu-2—see phendimetrazine

Preludin Endurets—see phenmetrazine

Premarin—see estrogens, conjugated

Prilosec—see omeprazole

---

primidone

BRAND NAMES (Manufacturers)
Myidone (Major)
Mysoline (Wyeth-Ayerst)
primidone (various manufacturers)

TYPE OF DRUG
Anticonvulsant

INGREDIENT
primidone

DOSAGE FORMS
Tablets (50 mg and 250 mg)
Oral suspension (250 mg per 5-ml spoonful)

STORAGE
Primidone tablets and oral suspension should be stored at room temperature in tightly closed containers. This medication should never be frozen.

USES

Primidone is used to treat various seizure disorders. This drug is converted in the body to phenobarbital. It is not clear exactly how primidone or phenobarbital acts to decrease the number of seizures, but both drugs are central nervous system (brain and spinal cord) depressants.

TREATMENT

In order to avoid stomach irritation, you can take primidone with food or with a full glass of water or milk (unless your doctor directs you to do otherwise).

The oral suspension form of this medication should be shaken well just before measuring each dose. The contents tend to settle on the bottom of the bottle, so it is necessary to shake the container to distribute the ingredients evenly and equalize the doses. Each dose should then be measured carefully with a specially designed 5-ml measuring spoon. An ordinary kitchen teaspoon is not accurate enough.

Primidone works best when the level of medicine in your bloodstream is kept constant. It is best, therefore, to take the doses at evenly spaced intervals day and night. For example, if you are to take three doses a day, the doses should be spaced eight hours apart.

It is important to try not to miss any doses of this medication. If you do miss a dose and remember within two hours, take the missed dose immediately. If more than two hours has passed, do not take the missed dose at all; just return to your regular dosing schedule. Do not double the next dose. If you miss two or more consecutive doses, contact your doctor as soon as possible.

SIDE EFFECTS

Minor. Dizziness, drowsiness, fatigue, loss of appetite, nausea, or vomiting. These side effects should disappear as your body adjusts to the medication.

If you feel dizzy, sit or lie down for a while; get up slowly from a sitting or reclining position, and be careful on stairs.

Major. Tell your doctor about any side effects that are persistent or particularly bothersome. IT IS ESPECIALLY IMPORTANT TO TELL YOUR DOCTOR about blurred vision, emotional disturbances, irritability, loss of coordination, or skin rash.

INTERACTIONS

Primidone interacts with several other types of medications:

1. Concurrent use of primidone with other central nervous system depressants (such as alcohol, antihistamines, barbiturates, benzodiazepine tranquilizers, muscle relaxants, narcotics, pain medications, phenothiazine tranquilizers, and sleeping medications) or with tricyclic antidepressants can lead to extreme drowsiness.

2. The blood levels and therapeutic effects of oral anticoagulants (blood thinners, such as warfarin), adrenocorticosteroids (cortisone-like medications), digitoxin, phenytoin, doxycycline, and tricyclic antidepressants can be decreased by primidone.

3. Primidone can decrease the absorption of griseofulvin from the gastrointestinal tract, thereby decreasing its effectiveness.

Before starting to take primidone, BE SURE TO TELL YOUR DOCTOR about any medications you are currently taking, especially any of those listed above.

WARNINGS

- Tell your doctor about unusual or allergic reactions you have had to any medications, especially to primidone, phenobarbital, or other barbiturates (such as amobarbital, butabarbital, mephobarbital, pentobarbital, and secobarbital).
- Before starting to take primidone, be sure to tell your doctor if you now have or if you have ever had asthma, kidney disease, liver disease, or porphyria.
- If this drug makes you dizzy or drowsy, do not take part in any activity that requires alertness, such as driving a car or operating potentially dangerous machinery.
- Before having surgery or any other medical or dental treatment, be sure to tell your doctor or dentist that you are taking primidone.
- Do not stop taking this medication unless you first check with your doctor. Stopping the drug abruptly can lead to a worsening of your condition. Your doctor may, therefore, want to reduce your dosage gradually or start you on another drug when primidone is stopped.
- Be sure to tell your doctor if you are pregnant. An increased risk of birth defects in infants of mothers with seizure disorders has been reported. It is unclear whether this increased risk is associated with the disorders or with the anticonvulsant medications, such as primidone, that are used to treat them. Such drugs may also lead to bleeding complications in the newborn. The risks and benefits of treatment should be discussed with your doctor. Also, tell your doctor if you are breast-feeding an infant. Primidone passes into breast milk and can cause extreme drowsiness in nursing infants.

Principen—see ampicillin

Prinivil—see lisinopril

Probalan—see probenecid

Pro-Banthine—see propantheline

---

probenecid

BRAND NAMES (Manufacturers)
Benemid (Merck Sharp & Dohme)
Probalan (Lannett)
probenecid (various manufacturers)

TYPE OF DRUG
Uricosuric (antigout preparation)

INGREDIENT
probenecid

DOSAGE FORM
Tablets (500 mg)

STORAGE
Probenecid should be stored at room temperature in a tightly closed container.

USES

Probenecid is used to prevent gout attacks. It increases the elimination of uric acid (the chemical responsible for the symptoms of gout) through the kidneys. Probenecid is also occasionally used in combination with penicillin or ampicillin to increase the length of time that the antibiotics remain in the bloodstream.

TREATMENT

In order to avoid stomach irritation, you may take probenecid with a full glass of water or milk. You should also drink at least ten to 12 full eight-ounce glasses of liquids (not alcoholic beverages) each day to prevent formation of uric acid kidney stones.

If you miss a dose of this medication, take the missed dose as soon as possible, unless it is almost time for the next dose. In that case, do not take the missed dose at all; just return to your regular dosing schedule. Do not double the next dose.

SIDE EFFECTS

Minor. Dizziness, frequent urination, headache, loss of appetite, nausea, rash, sore gums, or vomiting. These side effects should disappear as your body adjusts to the medication.

If you feel dizzy, sit or lie down for a while; get up slowly from a sitting or reclining position, and be careful on stairs.

Major. Tell your doctor about any side effects that are persistent or particularly bothersome. IT IS ESPECIALLY IMPORTANT TO TELL YOUR DOCTOR about fatigue, fever, flushing, lower back pain, painful or difficult urination, sore throat, unusual bleeding or bruising, or yellowing of the eyes or skin.

INTERACTIONS

Probenecid interacts with several other types of drugs:

1. Aspirin and pyrazinamide antagonize (act against) the antigout effects of probenecid.

2. The blood levels of methotrexate, sulfonamide antibiotics, nitrofurantoin, oral antidiabetic medicines, ketoprofen, naproxen, indomethacin, rifampin, sulindac, dapsone, and clofibrate can be increased by probenecid, which can lead to an increase in side effects.

3. Alcohol, chlorthalidone, ethacrynic acid, furosemide, or thiazide diuretics (water pills) can increase blood uric acid levels, which can decrease the effectiveness of probenecid.

Before starting to take probenecid, BE SURE TO TELL YOUR DOCTOR about any medications you are taking, especially any of those listed above.

WARNINGS

- Tell your doctor about unusual or allergic reactions you have had to any medications, especially to probenecid.

• Before starting to take probenecid, be sure to tell your doctor if you now have or if you have ever had blood diseases, diabetes mellitus, glucose-6-phosphate dehydrogenase (G6PD) deficiency, kidney stones, peptic ulcers, or porphyria.
• Diabetics using Clinitest urine glucose tests may get erroneously high readings of blood sugar levels while they are taking this drug. Temporarily changing to Clinistix or Tes-Tape urine tests will avoid this problem.
• If probenecid makes you dizzy, do not take part in any activity that requires alertness, such as driving a car or operating potentially dangerous machinery.
• Avoid taking large amounts of vitamin C while on probenecid. Vitamin C can increase the risk of kidney stone formation.
• Probenecid is not effective during an attack of gout. It is used to prevent attacks.
• Be sure to tell your doctor if you are pregnant. Although probenecid appears to be safe, it does cross the placenta. Extensive studies in pregnant women have not been conducted. Also, tell your doctor if you are breast-feeding an infant. It is not known whether probenecid passes into breast milk.

---

probucol

BRAND NAME (Manufacturer)
Lorelco (Merrell Dow)
TYPE OF DRUG
Antihyperlipidemic (lipid-lowering drug)
INGREDIENT
probucol
DOSAGE FORM
Tablets (250 mg and 500 mg)
STORAGE
Probucol should be stored at room temperature in a tightly closed, light-resistant container.

USES

This medication is used to treat hypercholesterolemia (high blood cholesterol levels) in patients who have not responded to diet, weight reduction, exercise, and control of blood sugar. It is not clear how probucol lowers blood cholesterol levels, but it is thought to decrease the body's own production of cholesterol.

TREATMENT

Probucol should be taken with meals, in order to maximize its effectiveness.

If you miss a dose of this medication, take the missed dose as soon as possible, unless it is almost time for the next dose. In that case, do not take the missed dose at all; just return to your regular dosing schedule. Do not double the next dose.

The therapeutic benefits of this medication may not become apparent for up to three months after it is started.

SIDE EFFECTS

Minor. Diarrhea, dizziness, gas, headache, insomnia, nausea, stomach upset, or vomiting. These side effects should disappear as your body adjusts to the medication.

If you feel dizzy, sit or lie down for a while; get up slowly from a sitting or reclining position, and be careful on stairs.

Major. Tell your doctor about any side effects that are persistent or particularly bothersome. IT IS ESPECIALLY IMPORTANT TO TELL YOUR DOCTOR about blurred vision; bloody or black, tarry stools; chest pain; impotence; palpitations; rash; ringing in the ears; sweating; tingling sensations; or unusual bleeding or bruising.

INTERACTIONS

The effectiveness of chenodiol, used to treat gallstone disease, may be decreased by concurrent probucol therapy. Before starting to take probucol, BE SURE TO TELL YOUR DOCTOR about any medications you are currently taking, especially chenodiol.

WARNINGS

• Tell your doctor about unusual or allergic reactions you have had to any medications, especially to probucol.
• Before starting this drug, tell your doctor if you now have or have ever had biliary tract disorders, gallstones or gallbladder disease, heart disease, or liver disease.
• Do not stop taking this medication unless you first check with your doctor. Stopping the drug abruptly may lead to a rapid increase in blood lipid (fats) and cholesterol levels. Your doctor may, therefore, want to start you on a special diet or another medication when probucol treatment is stopped.
• Be sure to tell your doctor if you are pregnant. Although probucol appears to be safe during pregnancy, extensive studies in humans have not been conducted. If you and your doctor decide that you should stop the drug for a planned pregnancy, some form of birth control should be used for at least six months after probucol therapy is stopped to ensure that the drug has been completely eliminated from the body. Also, tell your doctor if you are breast-feeding an infant. It is not known whether probucol passes into breast milk.

---

procainamide

BRAND NAMES (Manufacturers)
procainamide hydrochloride (various manufacturers)
Procamide SR (Reid-Rowell)
Procan-SR (Parke-Davis)
Promine (Major)
Pronestyl (Princeton Pharm)
Rhythmin (Sidmak)
TYPE OF DRUG
Antiarrhythmic
INGREDIENT
procainamide
DOSAGE FORMS
Tablets (250 mg, 375 mg, 500 mg)
Sustained-release tablets (250 mg, 500 mg, 750 mg, 1,000 mg)
Capsules (250 mg, 375 mg, 500 mg)
STORAGE
Procainamide tablets and capsules should be stored in tightly closed containers in a cool, dry place. Exposure to moisture causes deterioration of this medication.

USES

Procainamide is used to treat heart arrhythmias. It corrects irregular heartbeats and helps to achieve a more normal rhythm.

TREATMENT

To increase absorption, take procainamide with a full glass of water on an empty stomach one hour before or two hours after a meal. However, if it upsets your stomach, ask your doctor if you can take it with food or milk.

Try to take it at the same time(s) each day. Procainamide works best when the amount of drug in your bloodstream is kept at a constant level. This medication should, therefore, be taken at evenly spaced intervals day and night. For example, if you are to take this medication four times per day, the doses should be spaced six hours apart.

The sustained-release tablets should be swallowed whole. Breaking, chewing, or crushing these tablets destroys their sustained-release activity and possibly increases the side effects.

If you miss a dose of this medication and remember within two hours, take the missed dose immediately. If more than two hours have passed (four hours for the sustained-release tablets), do not take the missed dose; just return to your regular dosing schedule. Do not double the next dose of this medication.

SIDE EFFECTS

Minor. Bitter taste in the mouth, diarrhea, dizziness, dry mouth, loss of appetite, nausea, stomach upset, or vomiting. These side effects should disappear as your body adjusts to the medication.

If you feel dizzy, sit or lie down for a while; get up slowly from a sitting or reclining position, and be careful on stairs.

To relieve mouth dryness, chew sugarless gum or suck on ice chips or a piece of hard candy.

Major. Tell your doctor about any side effects that are persistent or particularly bothersome. IT IS ESPECIALLY IMPORTANT TO TELL YOUR DOCTOR about chest pain, chills, confusion, depression, fainting, fatigue, fever, giddiness, hallucinations, itching, joint pain, palpitations, rash, sore throat, unusual bleeding or bruising, or weakness.

INTERACTIONS

Procainamide interacts with several other types of medications:

1. The combination of digoxin and procainamide can lead to an increase in side effects to the heart.

2. Procainamide can block the effectiveness of neostigmine, pyridostigmine, and prostigmine.

3. Cimetidine, ranitidine, and amiodarone can increase the blood levels of procainamide, which can lead to an increase in side effects.

Before starting to take procainamide, BE SURE TO TELL YOUR DOCTOR about any medications you are currently taking, especially any of those listed above.

WARNINGS

- Tell your doctor about unusual or allergic reactions you have had to any medications, especially to procainamide, procaine, lidocaine, benzocaine, or tetracaine.
- Before starting this medication, be sure to tell your doctor if you now have or if you have ever had asthma, heart block, kidney disease, liver disease, myasthenia gravis, or systemic lupus erythematosus.
- If this drug makes you dizzy, do not take part in any activity that requires alertness, such as driving a car or operating potentially dangerous machinery.
- Before having surgery or any other medical or dental treatment, be sure to tell your doctor or dentist that you are taking this medication.
- Do not stop taking this drug without first consulting your doctor. Stopping procainamide abruptly may cause a serious change in the activity of your heart. Your doctor may, therefore, want to reduce your dosage gradually.
- If you are taking Procan-SR and you occasionally notice something in your stool that looks like a tablet, it does not mean that the drug is not being absorbed. The drug is "held" in a wax core designed to release the medication slowly. The wax core is eliminated in the stool after the drug has been absorbed.
- Some of these products contain the color additive FD&C Yellow No. 5 (tartrazine), which can cause allergic-type symptoms (rash, shortness of breath, fainting) in certain susceptible individuals.
- Be sure to tell your doctor if you are pregnant. Although this drug appears to be safe, extensive studies in pregnant women have not been conducted. Also, tell your doctor if you are breast-feeding an infant. It is not known whether procainamide passes into breast milk.

procainamide hydrochloride—see procainamide

Procamide SR—see procainamide

Procan-SR—procainamide

---

procarbazine

BRAND NAME (Manufacturer)
Matulane (Roche)
TYPE OF DRUG
Antineoplastic (anticancer drug)
INGREDIENT
procarbazine
DOSAGE FORM
Capsules (50 mg)
STORAGE
Procarbazine capsules should be stored at room temperature in a tightly closed, light-resistant container.

USES

This medication belongs to a group of drugs known as alkylating agents. It is used to treat a variety of cancers. Procarbazine is thought to work by binding to the rapidly growing cancer cells, thereby preventing their multiplication and growth.

TREATMENT

In order to prevent stomach irritation, you can take procarbazine with food or milk (unless your doctor directs you to do otherwise).

The timing of the dose of this medication is important. Be sure you completely understand your doctor's instructions on how and when this medication should be taken.

If you miss a dose of this medication and remember within a short period of time, take the missed dose immediately. If more than several hours has passed, check with your doctor to find out when the dose should be taken.

SIDE EFFECTS

Minor. Constipation, diarrhea, dizziness, drowsiness, dry mouth, headache, insomnia, loss of appetite, nausea, or vomiting. These side effects may disappear as your body adjusts to the medication. However, it is important to continue taking this medication despite any nausea and vomiting that occur.

Procarbazine can also cause hair loss (which is reversible when the medication is stopped).

This medication can increase your sensitivity to sunlight. You should, therefore, avoid prolonged exposure to sunlight and sunlamps. Wear protective clothing and sunglasses, and use an effective sunscreen.

To relieve constipation, increase the amount of fiber in your diet (fresh fruits and vegetables, salads, bran, and whole-grain breads), exercise, and drink more water (unless your doctor directs you to do otherwise).

If you feel dizzy, sit or lie down for a while; get up slowly from a sitting or reclining position, and be careful on stairs.

To help relieve mouth dryness, chew sugarless gum or suck on ice chips or a piece of hard candy.

Major. Tell your doctor about any side effects that are persistent or particularly bothersome. IT IS ESPECIALLY IMPORTANT TO TELL YOUR DOCTOR about unusual bleeding or bruising; bloody or black, tarry stools; blurred vision; changes in hearing ability; chest pain; chills; confusion; convulsions; darkening of the skin; depression; difficulty in swallowing; fainting; flushing; fever; hallucinations; itching; joint pain; lethargy; loss of coordination; menstrual irregularities; mouth sores; muscle pains; nervousness; nightmares; skin rash; slurred speech; sore throat; sweating; tingling sensations; tremors; weakness; or yellowing of the eyes or skin.

INTERACTIONS

Procarbazine interacts with several other types of medications:

1. Concurrent use of it with central nervous system depressants (such as alcohol, antihistamines, barbiturates, benzodiazepine tranquilizers, muscle relaxants, narcotics, pain medications, and phenothiazine tranquilizers) or with tricyclic antidepressants can lead to extreme drowsiness.

2. Diabetic patients should know that procarbazine can increase the blood-sugar-lowering effects of insulin and oral antidiabetic medications. Dosages of these medications may need to be adjusted when procarbazine is being taken.

3. The combination of procarbazine with guanethidine, levodopa, methyldopa, or reserpine can result in excitation and high blood pressure.

4. Concurrent use of procarbazine with tricyclic antidepressants, monoamine oxidase (MAO) inhibitors, amphetamines, decongestants, or phenothiazine tranquilizers can lead to severe reactions. Tricyclic antidepressants should be stopped seven days before starting procarbazine therapy, and MAO inhibitors should be stopped 14 days prior to starting therapy with procarbazine.

5. Ingestion of alcohol while taking procarbazine can result in fainting, flushing, headache, nausea, vomiting, and weakness.

Before starting to take procarbazine, BE SURE TO TELL YOUR DOCTOR about any medications you are currently taking, especially any of those listed above.

WARNINGS

- Tell your doctor about unusual or allergic reactions you have had to any medications, especially to procarbazine.
- Before starting to take this medication, be sure to tell your doctor if you now have or if you have ever had blood disorders, chronic or recurrent infections, diabetes mellitus, kidney disease, or liver disease.
- If this drug makes you dizzy or drowsy or blurs your vision, avoid taking part in any activity that requires alertness, such as driving a car or operating potentially dangerous machinery.
- Before having surgery or any other medical or dental treatment, be sure to tell your doctor or dentist that you are taking this medication.
- You should not receive any immunizations or vaccinations while taking this medication. Procarbazine blocks the effectiveness of vaccines and may result in an overwhelming infection if a live-virus vaccine is administered.
- Procarbazine can lower your platelet count, thereby decreasing your body's ability to form blood clots. You should, therefore, be especially careful while brushing your teeth, flossing, or using toothpicks, razors, or fingernail scissors. Try to avoid falls and other injuries.
- While you are taking procarbazine, avoid eating foods containing tyramine (certain cheeses, soy sauce, fava beans, chicken liver, avocados, bananas, canned figs, raisins, beer, and certain wines). The combination can lead to severe hypertensive (high blood pressure) reactions.
- Procarbazine can decrease fertility in both men and women.
- Be sure to tell your doctor if you are pregnant. Birth defects have been reported in the offspring of both humans and animals that received procarbazine during pregnancy. The risks should be discussed with your doctor. Also, tell your doctor if you are breast-feeding an infant. It is not known whether procarbazine passes into breast milk.

Procardia—see nifedipine

---

prochlorperazine

BRAND NAMES (Manufacturers)

Compazine (Smith Kline & French)
Compazine Spansules (Smith Kline & French)
prochlorperazine maleate (various manufacturers)

TYPE OF DRUG

Phenothiazine tranquilizer and antiemetic

INGREDIENT

prochlorperazine

DOSAGE FORMS

Tablets (5 mg, 10 mg, and 25 mg)

Sustained-release capsules (10 mg, 15 mg, and 30 mg)
Suppositories (2.5 mg, 5 mg, and 25 mg)
Oral syrup (5 mg per 5-ml spoonful)

STORAGE

The tablet and capsule forms of this medication should be stored at room temperature in tightly closed, light-resistant containers. The oral syrup and suppository forms may be stored in the refrigerator in tightly closed, light-resistant containers. If the oral syrup turns slightly yellow, the medicine is still effective and can be used. However, if it changes color markedly, or has particles floating in it, it should not be used; rather, it should be discarded down the sink. Prochlorperazine should never be frozen.

USES

Prochlorperazine is prescribed to treat the symptoms of certain types of mental illness, such as the emotional symptoms of psychosis, the manic phase of manic-depressive illness, and severe behavioral problems in children. This medication is thought to relieve the symptoms of mental illness by blocking certain chemicals involved with nerve transmission in the brain. Prochlorperazine is also frequently used to treat nausea and vomiting (this medication works at the vomiting center in the brain to relieve nausea and vomiting).

TREATMENT

To avoid stomach irritation, you can take the tablet or capsule form of this medication with a meal or with a glass of water or milk (unless your doctor directs you to do otherwise).

Antacids and antidiarrheal medicines may decrease the absorption of this medication from the gastrointestinal tract. Therefore, at least one hour should separate doses of one of these medicines and prochlorperazine.

The sustained-release capsules should be swallowed whole; do not crush, break, or open them. Breaking the capsules releases the medication all at once, destroying their sustained-release activity.

Measure the oral syrup carefully with a specially designed 5-ml measuring spoon. An ordinary kitchen teaspoon is not accurate enough.

To use the suppository form of this medication, remove the foil wrapper (if the suppository is too soft to insert, refrigerate it for half an hour or run cold water over it before removing the wrapper), and moisten the suppository with water. Lie on your left side with your right knee bent. Push the suppository into the rectum, pointed end first. Lie still for a few minutes. Try to avoid having a bowel movement for at least an hour (to give the medication time to be absorbed).

If you miss a dose of this medication, take the missed dose as soon as possible, unless it is almost time for your next dose. In that case, do not take the missed dose at all; just return to your regular schedule. Do not double the dose (unless your doctor directs you to do so).

The full effects of this medication for the control of emotional or mental symptoms may not become apparent for two weeks after you start to take it.

SIDE EFFECTS

Minor. Blurred vision, constipation, decreased sweating, diarrhea, dizziness, drooling, drowsiness, dry mouth, fatigue, jitteriness, menstrual irregularities, nasal congestion, restlessness, vomiting, or weight gain. As your body adjusts to the medication, these side effects should disappear.

Prochlorperazine can also cause discoloration of the urine to red, pink, or red-brown. This is a harmless effect.

This medication can cause increased sensitivity to sunlight. It is, therefore, important to avoid prolonged exposure to sunlight and sunlamps. Wear protective clothing and sunglasses, and use an effective sunscreen.

If you are constipated, increase the amount of fiber in your diet (fresh fruits and vegetables, salads, bran, and whole-grain breads), exercise, and drink more water (unless your doctor directs you to do otherwise).

Chew sugarless gum or suck on ice chips or a piece of hard candy to reduce mouth dryness.

To avoid dizziness or light-headedness when you stand, contract and relax the muscles of your legs for a few moments before rising. Do this by pushing one foot against the floor while raising the other foot slightly, alternating feet so that you are "pumping" your legs in a pedaling motion.

Major. Tell your doctor about any side effects that are persistent or particularly bothersome. IT IS ESPECIALLY IMPORTANT TO TELL YOUR DOCTOR about unusual bleeding or bruising; breast enlargement (in both sexes); chest pain; convulsions; darkened skin; difficulty in swallowing or breathing; fainting; fever; impotence; involuntary movements of the face, mouth, jaw, or tongue; palpitations; rash; sleep disorders; sore throat; tremors; uncoordinated movements; visual disturbances; or yellowing of the eyes or skin.

INTERACTIONS

Prochlorperazine interacts with several other types of medications:

1. It can cause extreme drowsiness when combined with alcohol or other central nervous system depressants (drugs that slow the activity of the brain and spinal cord), such as barbiturates, benzodiazepine tranquilizers, muscle relaxants, narcotics, and pain medications, or with tricyclic antidepressants.

2. Prochlorperazine can decrease the effectiveness of amphetamines, guanethidine, anticonvulsants, and levodopa.

3. The side effects of epinephrine, monoamine oxidase (MAO) inhibitors, propranolol, phenytoin, and tricyclic antidepressants may be increased by this medication. At least 14 days should separate the use of this drug and the use of an MAO inhibitor.

4. Lithium may increase the side effects, and decrease the effectiveness, of this medication.

5. Thiazide diuretics can enhance the blood-pressure-lowering side effects of prochlorperazine.

Before starting to take prochlorperazine, BE SURE TO TELL YOUR DOCTOR about any medications you are currently taking, especially any of those listed above.

WARNINGS

- Tell your doctor about unusual or allergic reactions you have had to any medications, especially to prochlorperazine or other phenothiazine tranquilizers (such as chlorpromazine, fluphenazine, mesoridazine, perphenazine, promazine, thioridazine, trifluoperazine, and triflupromazine) or to loxapine.

• Tell your doctor if you have a history of alcoholism or if you now have or have ever had any blood disease, bone marrow disease, brain disease, breast cancer, blockage in the urinary or digestive tracts, drug-induced depression, epilepsy, high or low blood pressure, diabetes mellitus, glaucoma, heart or circulatory disease, liver disease, lung disease, Parkinson's disease, peptic ulcers, or an enlarged prostate gland.
• Tell your doctor about any recent exposure to a pesticide or an insecticide. Prochlorperazine may increase the side effects from the exposure.
• To prevent oversedation, avoid drinking alcoholic beverages while taking this medication.
• If this medication makes you dizzy or drowsy, do not take part in any activity that requires alertness, such as driving a car or operating potentially dangerous machinery. Be careful on stairs, and avoid getting up suddenly from a lying or sitting position.
• Prior to having surgery or any other medical or dental treatment, be sure to tell your doctor or dentist that you are taking this medication.
• Some of the side effects caused by this drug can be prevented by taking an antiparkinsonism drug. Discuss this with your doctor.
• This medication can decrease sweating and heat release from the body. You should, therefore, try not to get overheated (avoid exercising strenuously in hot weather, and avoid taking hot baths, showers, and saunas).
• Do not stop taking prochlorperazine suddenly if you have been taking it for a prolonged period. If the drug is stopped abruptly, you may experience nausea, vomiting, stomach upset, headache, increased heart rate, insomnia, tremors, or a worsening of your condition. Your doctor may want to reduce the dosage gradually.
• If you are planning to have a myelogram, or any other procedure in which dye will be injected into your spinal cord, tell your doctor that you are taking this medication.
• Avoid spilling the oral syrup form of this medication on your skin or clothing; it may cause redness and irritation of the skin.
• While taking this medication, do not take any over-the-counter (nonprescription) medication for weight control or for cough, cold, allergy, asthma, or sinus problems unless you first check with your doctor. The combination of these medications with prochlorperazine may cause high blood pressure.
• Be sure to tell your doctor if you are pregnant. Small amounts of this medication cross the placenta. Although there are reports of safe use of this drug during pregnancy, there are also reports of liver disease and tremors in newborn infants whose mothers received this type of medication close to term. Also, tell your doctor if you are breast-feeding an infant. Small amounts of this medication pass into breast milk and may cause unwanted effects in the nursing infant.

prochlorperazine maleate—see prochlorperazine

Proklar—see sulfonamide antibiotics (oral)

Prolixin—see fluphenazine

Proloprim—see trimethoprim

promazine

BRAND NAME (Manufacturer)
Sparine (Wyeth-Ayerst)
TYPE OF DRUG
Phenothiazine tranquilizer
INGREDIENT
promazine
DOSAGE FORM
Tablets (25 mg, 50 mg, and 100 mg)
STORAGE
This medication should be stored at room temperature in a tightly closed, light-resistant container.

USES

Promazine is prescribed to treat the symptoms of certain types of mental illness, such as emotional symptoms of psychosis, the manic phase of manic-depressive illness, and severe behavioral problems in children. It is thought to relieve symptoms of mental illness by blocking certain chemicals involved with nerve transmission in the brain.

TREATMENT

To avoid stomach irritation, you can take this medication with a meal or with a glass of water or milk (unless your doctor directs you to do otherwise).

If you miss a dose of this medication, take the missed dose as soon as possible, unless it is almost time for your next dose. In that case, do not take the missed dose at all; just return to your regular dosing schedule. Do not double the dose (unless your doctor directs you to do so).

Antacids and antidiarrheal medicines may decrease the absorption of this medication from the gastrointestinal tract. Therefore, at least one hour should separate doses of one of these medicines and promazine.

The full effects of this medication for the control of emotional or mental symptoms may not become apparent until two weeks after you start to take it.

SIDE EFFECTS

Minor. Blurred vision, constipation, decreased sweating, diarrhea, dizziness, drooling, drowsiness, dry mouth, fatigue, jitteriness, menstrual irregularities, nasal congestion, restlessness, vomiting, or weight gain. As your body adjusts to the medication, these side effects should disappear.

Promazine can also cause discoloration of the urine to red, pink, or red-brown. This is a harmless effect.

This medication can cause increased sensitivity to sunlight. It is, therefore, important to avoid prolonged exposure to sunlight and sunlamps. Wear protective clothing and sunglasses, and use an effective sunscreen.

If you are constipated, increase the amount of fiber in your diet (raw fruits and vegetables, salads, bran, and whole-grain breads), exercise, and drink more water (unless your doctor directs you to do otherwise).

Chew sugarless gum or suck on ice chips or a piece of hard candy to reduce mouth dryness.

To avoid dizziness or light-headedness when you stand, contract and relax the muscles of your legs for a few moments before rising. Do this by pushing one foot against the floor while raising the other foot slightly, alternating feet so that you are "pumping" your legs in a pedaling motion.

Major. Tell your doctor about any side effects that are persistent or particularly bothersome. IT IS ESPECIALLY IMPORTANT TO TELL YOUR DOCTOR about unusual bleeding or bruising; breast enlargement (in both sexes); chest pain; convulsions; darkened skin; difficulty in swallowing or breathing; fainting; fever; impotence; involuntary movements of the face, mouth, jaw, or tongue; palpitations; rash; sleep disorders; sore throat; tremors; uncoordinated movements; visual disturbances; or yellowing of the eyes or skin.

INTERACTIONS

This medication interacts with a number of other types of medications:

1. It can cause extreme drowsiness when combined with alcohol or other central nervous system depressants (drugs that slow the activity of the brain and spinal cord), such as barbiturates, benzodiazepine tranquilizers, muscle relaxants, narcotics, and pain medications, or with tricyclic antidepressants.

2. Promazine can decrease the effectiveness of amphetamines, guanethidine, anticonvulsants, and levodopa.

3. The side effects of epinephrine, monoamine oxidase (MAO) inhibitors, propranolol, phenytoin, and tricyclic antidepressants may be increased by this medication.

4. Lithium may increase the side effects and decrease the effectiveness of this medication.

Before starting to take promazine, BE SURE TO TELL YOUR DOCTOR about any medications you are currently taking, especially any of those listed above.

WARNINGS

- Tell your doctor about unusual or allergic reactions you have had to any medications, especially to promazine or other phenothiazine tranquilizers (such as chlorpromazine, fluphenazine, mesoridazine, perphenazine, prochlorperazine, thioridazine, trifluoperazine, and triflupromazine) or to loxapine.
- Tell your doctor if you have a history of alcoholism or if you now have or have ever had any blood disease, bone marrow disease, brain disease, breast cancer, blockage in the urinary or digestive tracts, drug-induced depression, epilepsy, high or low blood pressure, diabetes mellitus, glaucoma, heart or circulatory disease, liver disease, lung disease, Parkinson's disease, peptic ulcers, or an enlarged prostate gland.
- Tell your doctor about any recent exposure to a pesticide or an insecticide. Promazine may increase the side effects from the exposure.
- To prevent oversedation, avoid drinking alcoholic beverages while taking this medication.
- If this medication makes you dizzy or drowsy, do not take part in any activity that requires alertness, such as driving a car or operating potentially dangerous machinery. Be careful on stairs, and avoid getting up suddenly from a lying or sitting position.
- Prior to having surgery or any other medical or dental treatment, be sure to tell your doctor or dentist that you are taking this medication.
- Some of the side effects caused by this drug can be prevented by taking an antiparkinsonism drug. Discuss this with your doctor.
- This medication can decrease sweating and heat release from the body. You should, therefore, try not to get overheated (avoid strenuous exercise in hot weather and do not take hot baths, showers, and saunas).
- Do not stop taking this medication suddenly. If the drug is stopped abruptly, you may experience nausea, vomiting, stomach upset, headache, increased heart rate, insomnia, tremors, or a worsening of your condition. Your doctor may, therefore, want to reduce the dosage gradually.
- If you are planning to have a myelogram, or any other procedure in which dye will be injected into the space surrounding your spinal cord, tell your doctor that you are taking this medication.
- While taking this medication, do not take any over-the-counter (nonprescription) medication for weight control or for cough, cold, allergy, asthma, or sinus problems unless you first check with your doctor. The combination of these medications may cause high blood pressure.
- Be sure to tell your doctor if you are pregnant. Small amounts of this medication cross the placenta. Although there are reports of safe use of this drug during pregnancy, there are also reports of liver disease and tremors in newborn infants whose mothers received this medication close to term. Also, tell your doctor if you are breast-feeding an infant. Small amounts of this medication pass into breast milk and may cause unwanted effects in nursing infants.

---

promethazine

BRAND NAMES (Manufacturers)
Phenameth (Major)
Phenergan (Wyeth-Ayerst)
promethazine (various manufacturers)
Prothazine (Vortech)

TYPE OF DRUG
antihistamine and antiemetic

INGREDIENT
promethazine

DOSAGE FORMS
Tablets (12.5 mg, 25 mg, and 50 mg)
Oral syrup (6.25 mg per 5-ml spoonful, with 7% alcohol; 25 mg per 5-ml spoonful, with 1.5% alcohol)
Rectal suppositories (12.5 mg, 25 mg, and 50 mg)

STORAGE
Promethazine tablets and oral syrup should be stored at room temperature (never frozen) in tightly closed, light-resistant containers. The suppositories should be kept in the refrigerator in a tightly closed container.

USES

Promethazine is prescribed for a wide range of conditions. Promethazine belongs to a group of drugs known as antihistamines, which block the action of histamine, a chemical that is released by the body during an allergic reaction. It is, therefore, used to treat or prevent symptoms of allergy or hay fever. Promethazine also (1) works at the vomiting center in the brain and can be used for the prevention or treatment of nausea and vomiting; (2) is a central nervous system (brain and spinal cord) depressant, which produces light sleep or mild sedation; and (3) prevents motion sickness.

TREATMENT

To avoid stomach irritation, you can take the tablet or oral syrup form of this medication with a meal or with a glass of water or milk (unless your doctor directs otherwise).

Measure the oral syrup carefully with a specially designed 5-ml measuring spoon. An ordinary kitchen teaspoon is not accurate enough.

To use the suppository, remove the foil wrapper (if the suppository is too soft to insert, refrigerate it for half an hour or run cold water over it before removing the wrapper), and moisten the suppository with water. Lie on your left side with your right knee bent. Push the suppository into the rectum, pointed end first. Lie still for a few minutes. Try to avoid having a bowel movement for at least an hour (to give the medication time to be absorbed).

If you are taking this medication regularly and you miss a dose, take the missed dose as soon as possible, unless it is almost time for the next dose. In that case, do not take the missed dose at all; just return to your regular schedule. Do not double the next dose (unless your doctor directs you to do so).

SIDE EFFECTS

Minor. Blurred vision, diarrhea, dizziness, drowsiness, dry mouth, light-headedness, nausea, or vomiting. These side effects should disappear as your body adjusts to this drug.

This medication can cause increased sensitivity to sunlight. It is, therefore, important to avoid prolonged exposure to sunlight and sunlamps. Wear protective clothing and sunglasses, and use an effective sunscreen.

To reduce mouth dryness, chew sugarless gum or suck on ice chips or hard candy.

To avoid dizziness or light-headedness when you stand, contract and relax the muscles of your legs for a few moments before rising. Do this by alternately pushing one foot against the floor while raising the other foot slightly, so that you are "pumping" your legs in a pedaling motion.

Major. Tell your doctor about any side effects that are persistent or particularly bothersome. IT IS ESPECIALLY IMPORTANT TO TELL YOUR DOCTOR about confusion; disorientation; involuntary movements of the face, mouth, jaw, or tongue; rash; uncoordinated movements; unusual bleeding or bruising; or yellowing of the eyes or skin.

INTERACTIONS

Promethazine interacts with other types of medications:

1. Promethazine can cause extreme drowsiness when combined with alcohol or other central nervous system depressants (drugs that slow the activity of the brain and spinal cord), such as barbiturates, benzodiazepine tranquilizers, muscle relaxants, narcotics, and pain medications or with tricyclic antidepressants.

2. Promethazine can decrease the effectiveness of amphetamines, guanethidine, anticonvulsants, and levodopa.

3. The side effects of epinephrine, monoamine oxidase (MAO) inhibitors, propranolol, and tricyclic antidepressants may be increased by this medication. At least 14 days should separate the use of this medication and the use of an MAO inhibitor.

Before starting promethazine, BE SURE TO TELL YOUR DOCTOR about any of the medications you are currently taking, especially any of those listed above.

WARNINGS

- Tell your doctor about any unusual or allergic reactions you have had to any medications, especially to promethazine or any chemically related phenothiazine drug (chlorpromazine, fluphenazine, mesoridazine, perphenazine, prochlorperazine, promazine, thioridazine, trifluoperazine, triflupromazine).
- Before starting promethazine, tell your doctor if you now have or if you have ever had asthma, blockage of the urinary or digestive tract, diabetes mellitus, enlarged prostate gland, epilepsy, glaucoma, heart disease, liver disease, peptic ulcers, or sleep apnea.
- To prevent oversedation, avoid drinking alcoholic beverages while taking this medication.
- If this medication makes you dizzy or drowsy, do not take part in any activity that requires alertness, such as driving a car or operating potentially dangerous machinery. Be careful on stairs, and avoid getting up suddenly from a reclining or sitting position.
- Prior to having surgery or any other medical or dental treatment, be sure to tell your doctor or dentist that you are taking this medication.
- Be sure to tell your doctor if you are pregnant. Small amounts of this medication cross the placenta. Although there are reports of safe use of this drug during pregnancy, there are also reports of liver disease and tremors in newborns whose mothers received this medication close to term. Also, tell your doctor if you are breast-feeding. Small amounts of this medication pass into breast milk and may cause unwanted effects in nursing infants, such as sudden infant death syndrome (SIDS) or sleep apnea.

---

promethazine and codeine combination

BRAND NAMES (Manufacturers)

Phenergan with Codeine (Wyeth-Ayerst)
Prometh with Codeine (Goldline)
Prothazine DC (Vortech)

TYPE OF DRUG

Antihistamine and cough suppressant

INGREDIENTS

promethazine and codeine

DOSAGE FORM

Oral syrup (6.25 mg promethazine and 10 mg codeine per 5-ml spoonful, with 7% alcohol)

STORAGE

This medication should be stored at room temperature in a tightly closed, light-resistant container. This medication should never be frozen.

USES

This drug combination is used to provide symptomatic relief of coughs due to colds, minor upper respiratory tract infections, or allergy.

Promethazine belongs to a group of drugs known as antihistamines, which block the actions of histamine, a chemical released by the body during an allergic reaction. It is used to relieve or prevent symptoms of allergy.

Codeine is a narcotic cough suppressant that acts at the cough reflex center in the brain.

TREATMENT

To avoid stomach upset, you can take this medication with food or with a full glass of milk or water (unless your doctor directs you to do otherwise).

The oral syrup should be shaken well just before measuring each dose. The contents tend to settle on the bottom of the bottle, so it is necessary to shake the container to distribute the ingredients evenly and equalize the doses. Each dose should then be measured carefully with a specially designed 5-ml measuring spoon. An ordinary kitchen teaspoon is not accurate enough.

If you miss a dose of this medication, take the missed dose as soon as possible, unless it is almost time for your next dose. In that case, do not take the missed dose at all; just return to your regular dosing schedule. Do not double the next dose.

SIDE EFFECTS

Minor. Blurred vision; constipation; diarrhea; dizziness; dry mouth, throat, or nose; irritability; loss of appetite; confusion; nausea; restlessness; stomach upset; or unusual increase in sweating. These side effects should disappear as your body adjusts to the medication.

This medication can cause increased sensitivity to sunlight. Avoid prolonged exposure to sunlight, wear protective clothing and sunglasses, and use an effective sunscreen.

If you are constipated, increase the amount of fiber in your diet (fresh fruits and vegetables, salads, bran, and whole-grain breads), exercise, and drink more water (unless your doctor tells you not to do so).

Chew sugarless gum or suck on ice chips or a piece of hard candy to reduce mouth dryness.

If you feel dizzy or light-headed, sit or lie down for a while; get up slowly from a sitting or reclining position, and be careful on stairs.

Major. Tell your doctor about any side effects that are persistent or particularly bothersome. IT IS ESPECIALLY IMPORTANT TO TELL YOUR DOCTOR about convulsions, difficulty in breathing, difficult or painful urination, disturbed coordination, excitation, fainting, headaches, muscle spasms, nightmares, nosebleeds, palpitations, rash, ringing or buzzing in the ears, severe abdominal pain, sore throat or fever, or yellowing of the eyes or skin.

INTERACTIONS

This medicine interacts with other types of drugs:

1. Concurrent use of it with central nervous system depressants (drugs that slow the activity of the brain and spinal cord), such as alcohol, barbiturates, benzodiazepine tranquilizers, muscle relaxants, narcotics, pain medications, and phenothiazine tranquilizers, or with tricyclic antidepressants can cause extreme drowsiness.

2. This medication can decrease the effectiveness of amphetamines, guanethidine, anticonvulsants, and levodopa.

3. This combination medication can increase the side effects of monoamine oxidase (MAO) inhibitors (isocarboxazid, pargyline, phenelzine, tranylcypromine) and tricyclic antidepressants. At least 14 days should separate the use of this drug and the use of an MAO inhibitor.

BE SURE TO TELL YOUR DOCTOR about any medications you are currently taking, especially any listed above.

WARNINGS

- Tell your doctor about unusual or allergic reactions you have had to any medications, especially to promethazine or other antihistamines; to phenothiazine tranquilizers; to codeine; or to any other narcotic cough suppressant or pain medication.
- Tell your doctor if you now have or if you have ever had asthma, brain disease, blockage of the urinary or digestive tract, diabetes mellitus, colitis, gallstones or gallbladder disease, glaucoma, heart or blood vessel disease, high blood pressure, kidney disease, liver disease, lung disease, peptic ulcers, enlarged prostate gland, or thyroid disease.
- This medication can cause drowsiness. Your ability to perform tasks that require alertness, such as driving a car or operating potentially dangerous machinery, may be decreased. Appropriate caution should, therefore, be taken.
- Before having surgery or any other medical or dental treatment, be sure to tell your doctor or dentist that you are taking this medication.
- Because this product contains codeine, it has the potential for abuse and must be used with caution. Usually, it should not be taken on a regular schedule for longer than ten days at a time. Tolerance develops quickly; do not increase the dosage or stop taking the drug abruptly, unless you first consult your doctor. If you have been taking large amounts of this medication or have been taking it for a long period of time, you may experience a withdrawal reaction (muscle aches, diarrhea, gooseflesh, runny nose, nausea, vomiting, shivering, trembling, stomach cramps, sleep disorders, irritability, weakness, excessive yawning, or sweating) when you stop taking it. Your doctor may, therefore, want to reduce the dosage gradually.
- Be sure to tell your doctor if you are pregnant. The effects of this medication during the early stages of pregnancy have not been thoroughly studied in humans. However, regular use of codeine during the later stages of pregnancy may lead to addiction of the fetus, resulting in withdrawal symptoms (irritability, excessive crying, tremors, fever, vomiting, diarrhea, sneezing, yawning) in the newborn infant. There are also reports of liver disease and tremors in newborns whose mothers received this medication close to term. Also, tell your doctor if you are breast-feeding an infant. Small amounts of this medication pass into breast milk and may cause unusual excitement or irritability in nursing infants as well as other unwanted effects such as sudden infant death syndrome (SIDS) or sleep apnea.

Prometh VC with Codeine—see phenylephrine, promethazine, and codeine combination

Prometh with Codeine—see promethazine and codeine combination

Promine—see procainamide

Pronestyl—see procainamide

Propacet 100—see acetaminophen and propoxyphene combination

propantheline

BRAND NAMES (Manufacturers)
Norpanth (Vortech)
Pro-Banthine (Searle)
propantheline bromide (various manufacturers)
TYPE OF DRUG
Anticholinergic (antiulcer drug)
INGREDIENT
propantheline
DOSAGE FORM
Tablets (7.5 mg and 15 mg)
STORAGE
Store at room temperature in a tightly closed container.

USES

Propantheline is used to treat peptic ulcers. It is thought to reduce the amount of acid formed in the stomach. It also relieves cramping and spasms of the gastrointestinal tract and bladder.

TREATMENT

In order to obtain the maximum benefit, you should take propantheline 30 minutes before meals and at bedtime (unless your doctor directs you to do otherwise).

If you miss a dose of this medication, do not take the missed dose at all; just return to your regular dosing schedule. Do not double the next dose.

SIDE EFFECTS

Minor. Bloating, blurred vision, constipation, decreased sweating, dizziness, drowsiness, dry mouth, headache, increased sensitivity of the eyes to sunlight, nausea, nervousness, taste disorders, or vomiting. These side effects should disappear as your body adjusts to the medication.

To relieve constipation, exercise and drink more water (unless your doctor directs you to do otherwise).

If you feel dizzy, sit or lie down for a while; change positions slowly, and be careful on stairs.

To help relieve mouth dryness, chew sugarless gum or suck on ice chips or a piece of hard candy.

Sunglasses may help to relieve the sensitivity of your eyes to sunlight.

Major. Tell your doctor about any side effects that are persistent or particularly bothersome. IT IS ESPECIALLY IMPORTANT TO TELL YOUR DOCTOR about decreased sexual ability, difficulty in urinating, eye pain, itching, palpitations, or skin rash.

INTERACTIONS

Propantheline interacts with several other types of drugs:

1. Amantadine, antihistamines, disopyramide, haloperidol, monoamine oxidase (MAO) inhibitors, phenothiazine tranquilizers, procainamide, quinidine, and tricyclic antidepressants can increase the side effects of propantheline. At least 14 days should separate the use of this drug and the use of an MAO inhibitor.

2. Antacids and antidiarrheal medications can reduce the absorption of propantheline from the gastrointestinal tract, which can decrease its effectiveness. Therefore, at least two hours should separate doses of one of these types of medications and propantheline.

BE SURE TO TELL YOUR DOCTOR about any medications you are currently taking, especially any of those listed above.

WARNINGS

- Tell your doctor about unusual or allergic reactions you have had to any medications, especially to propantheline.
- Before starting this medication, be sure to tell your doctor if you now have or if you have ever had glaucoma, heart disease, hiatal hernia, high blood pressure, intestinal blockage, kidney disease, liver disease, lung disease, myasthenia gravis, enlarged prostate gland, thyroid disease, ulcerative colitis, or urinary retention.
- This medication can decrease sweating and heat release from the body. You should, therefore, try not to get overheated (avoid strenuous exercise in hot weather, and do not take hot baths, showers, and saunas).
- If this medication makes you dizzy or drowsy or blurs your vision, avoid taking part in any activity that requires alertness, such as driving a car or operating potentially dangerous equipment.
- Be sure to tell your doctor if you are pregnant. Although propantheline appears to be safe during pregnancy, extensive studies in humans have not been conducted. Also, tell your doctor if you are breast-feeding an infant. It is not known whether propantheline passes into breast milk.

propantheline bromide—see propantheline

---

propoxyphene

BRAND NAMES (Manufacturers)
Darvon (Lilly)
Darvon-N (Lilly)
Dolene (Lederle)
propoxyphene hydrochloride (various manufacturers)
TYPE OF DRUG
Analgesic
INGREDIENT
propoxyphene
DOSAGE FORMS
Capsules (32 mg and 65 mg)
Tablets (100 mg)
Suspension (10 mg per ml)
STORAGE
This medication should be stored at room temperature (never frozen) in tightly closed containers.

USES

Propoxyphene is a narcotic analgesic that acts on the central nervous system (brain and spinal cord) to relieve mild to moderate pain.

TREATMENT

In order to avoid stomach upset, you can take propoxyphene with food or milk.

The suspension form of this medication should be shaken well just before measuring each dose. The contents tend to settle on the bottom of the bottle, so it is necessary to shake the container to distribute the ingredients evenly and equalize the doses. Each dose should be measured carefully with a specially designed 5-ml measuring spoon. An ordinary kitchen teaspoon is not accurate enough.

This medication works best if taken at the first sign of pain. Do not wait for the pain to become severe.

If your doctor has prescribed this medication to be taken on a regular schedule and you miss a dose, take the missed dose as soon as possible, unless it is almost time for your next dose. In that case, do not take the missed dose at all; just return to your regular dosing schedule. Do not double the next dose.

SIDE EFFECTS

Minor. Blurred vision, constipation, dizziness, drowsiness, indigestion, light-headedness, nausea, nervousness, restlessness, vomiting, or weakness. As your body adjusts to the medication, these side effects should disappear.

If you are constipated, increase the amount of fiber in your diet (fresh fruits and vegetables, salads, bran, and whole-grain breads), exercise, and drink more water (unless your doctor directs you to do otherwise).

If you feel dizzy or light-headed, sit or lie down for a while; get up slowly from a sitting or reclining position, and be careful on stairs.

Major. Tell your doctor about any side effects that are persistent or particularly bothersome. IT IS ESPECIALLY IMPORTANT TO TELL YOUR DOCTOR about confusion, convulsions, darkening of the urine, depression, difficulty in breathing, hallucinations, palpitations, ringing in the ears, skin rash, yellow stools, or yellowing of the eyes or skin.

INTERACTIONS

Propoxyphene can interact with several types of drugs:

1. Concurrent use of it with other central nervous system depressants (such as antihistamines, barbiturates, tranquilizers, sleeping medications, muscle relaxants, and other pain medications) or with tricyclic antidepressants can cause extreme drowsiness.

2. Propoxyphene can increase carbamazepine blood levels, which in turn can result in greater side effects.

3. A monoamine oxidase (MAO) inhibitor taken within 14 days of this medication can lead to unpredictable and severe side effects.

4. Propoxyphene also interacts with alcohol, increasing its intoxicating effects. You should, therefore, avoid drinking alcoholic beverages while taking this medicine.

BE SURE TO TELL YOUR DOCTOR about any medications you are currently taking, especially any of those listed above.

WARNINGS

- Tell your doctor about unusual or allergic reactions you have had to any medications, especially to propoxyphene or to other narcotic analgesics (such as codeine, hydrocodone, hydromorphone, meperidine, methadone, morphine, and oxycodone).
- Tell your doctor if you now have or if you have ever had acute abdominal conditions, asthma, brain disease, colitis, epilepsy, gallstones or gallbladder disease, head injuries, heart disease, kidney disease, liver disease, lung disease, mental illness, emotional disorders, enlarged prostate gland, thyroid disease, or urethral stricture.
- If this drug makes you dizzy or drowsy, do not take part in any activity that requires alertness, such as driving a car.
- Before having surgery or any other medical or dental treatment, be sure to tell your doctor or dentist that you are taking this medication.
- Propoxyphene has the potential for abuse and must be used with caution. Usually, you should not take it on a regular schedule for longer than ten days (unless your doctor directs you to do so). Tolerance develops quickly; do not increase the dosage or stop taking the drug abruptly, unless you first consult your doctor. If you have been taking large amounts of this medication or have been taking it for long periods of time, you may experience a withdrawal reaction (muscle aches, diarrhea, gooseflesh, runny nose, nausea, vomiting, shivering, trembling, stomach cramps, sleep disorders, irritability, weakness, excessive yawning, or sweating) when you stop taking it. Your doctor may, therefore, want to reduce the dosage gradually.
- Be sure to tell your doctor if you are pregnant. The effects of this medication during the early stages of pregnancy have not been thoroughly studied in humans. However, regular use of propoxyphene in large doses during the later stages of pregnancy can result in addiction of the fetus, leading to withdrawal symptoms (irritability, excessive crying, tremors, fever, vomiting, diarrhea, sneezing, or excessive yawning) at birth. Also, tell your doctor if you are breast-feeding an infant. Small amounts of this medication may pass into breast milk and cause excessive drowsiness in the nursing infant.

propoxyphene hydrochloride—see propoxyphene

propoxyphene hydrochloride compound—see aspirin, caffeine, and propoxyphene combination

propoxyphene hydrochloride with acetaminophen—see acetaminophen and propoxyphene combination

---

propranolol

BRAND NAMES (Manufacturers)

Inderal (Wyeth-Ayerst)
Inderal LA (Wyeth-Ayerst)
propranolol (various manufacturers)

TYPE OF DRUG

Beta-adrenergic blocking agent

INGREDIENT

propranolol

DOSAGE FORMS

Tablets (10 mg, 20 mg, 40 mg, 60 mg, 80 mg, and 90 mg)
Extended-release capsules (80 mg, 120 mg, and 160 mg)
Oral solution (4 mg and 8 mg per ml)
Oral concentrated solution (80 mg per ml)

STORAGE

Store at room temperature in a tightly closed, light-resistant container. The solutions should never be frozen.

USES

Propranolol is used to treat high blood pressure, angina pectoris (chest pain), and irregular heartbeats. It is also useful in preventing migraine headaches and preventing additional heart attacks in heart attack patients. Propranolol belongs to a group of medicines known as beta-adrenergic blocking agents or, more commonly, beta blockers. These drugs work by controlling nerve impulses along certain nerve pathways.

TREATMENT

Propranolol can be taken with a glass of water, with meals, immediately following meals, or on an empty stomach (depending on your doctor's instructions). Try to take the medication at the same time(s) each day.

The extended-release capsules should be swallowed whole. Do not chew or crush them. Breaking the capsule releases the medication all at once—defeating the purpose of extended-release capsules.

The oral solution should be measured with a specially designed 5-ml measuring spoon. An ordinary kitchen teaspoon is not accurate enough.

The oral concentrated solution must be mixed in four ounces (1/2 cup) of water, juice, or soda before drinking. The cup should be refilled with more of the liquid, which must be drunk to ensure that the entire dose is taken. This form may also be mixed with applesauce or pudding.

It is important to remember that propranolol does not cure high blood pressure, but it will help to control the condition as long as you continue to take it.

Try not to miss any doses of this medicine. If you do miss a dose, take the missed dose as soon as possible, unless it is within eight hours (if you are taking this medicine only once a day) or within four hours (if you are taking this medicine more than once a day) of your next scheduled dose. In that case, do not take the missed dose at all; just return to your regular dosing schedule. Do not double the next dose of the medication.

SIDE EFFECTS

Minor. Anxiety; constipation; decreased sexual ability; diarrhea; difficulty in sleeping; drowsiness; dryness of the eyes, mouth, and skin; headache; nausea; nervousness; stomach discomfort; tiredness; or weakness. These side effects should disappear during treatment, as your body adjusts to the medicine.

To relieve constipation, increase the amount of fiber in your diet (fresh fruits and vegetables, salads, bran, and whole-grain breads) and drink more water (unless your doctor directs you to do otherwise).

If you are extra-sensitive to the cold, be sure to dress warmly during cold weather.

Plain, nonmedicated eye drops (artificial tears) may help to relieve eye dryness.

Sucking on ice chips or chewing sugarless gum helps to relieve mouth and throat dryness.

Major. Tell your doctor about any side effects that are persistent or particularly bothersome. IT IS ESPECIALLY IMPORTANT TO TELL YOUR DOCTOR about breathing difficulty or wheezing, cold hands or feet (due to decreased blood circulation to skin, fingers, and toes), confusion, depression, dizziness, hair loss, hallucinations, lightheadedness, nightmares, numbness or tingling of the fingers or toes, rapid weight gain (three to five pounds within a week), reduced alertness, swelling, sore throat and fever, skin rash, or unusual bleeding or bruising.

INTERACTIONS

Propranolol interacts with a number of other types of medications:

1. Indomethacin, aspirin, or other salicylates may decrease the blood-pressure-lowering effects of beta blockers.

2. Concurrent use of beta blockers and calcium channel blockers (diltiazem, nifedipine, verapamil) or disopyramide can lead to heart failure or very low blood pressure.

3. Cimetidine and oral contraceptives (birth control pills) can increase the blood concentrations of propranolol, which can result in greater side effects.

4. Side effects may also be increased when beta blockers are taken with clonidine, digoxin, epinephrine, phenylephrine, phenylpropanolamine, phenothiazine tranquilizers, prazosin, reserpine, or monoamine oxidase (MAO) inhibitors. At least 14 days should separate the use of a beta blocker and an MAO inhibitor.

5. Barbiturates, alcohol, and rifampin can increase the breakdown of propranolol in the body, which can lead to a decrease in its effectiveness.

6. Beta blockers may antagonize (work against) the effects of theophylline, aminophylline, albuterol, isoproterenol, metaproterenol, and terbutaline.

7. Beta blockers can also interact with insulin or oral antidiabetic agents, raising or lowering blood sugar levels or masking the symptoms of low blood sugar.

8. The action of beta blockers may be excessively increased if they are used with chlorpromazine, furosemide, or hydralazine.

BE SURE TO TELL YOUR DOCTOR about any medications you are currently taking, especially any of those listed above.

WARNINGS

- Before starting to take this medication, it is important to tell your doctor if you have ever had unusual or allergic reactions to any beta blocker (acebutolol, atenolol, betaxolol, carteolol, esmolol, labetalol, metoprolol, nadolol, penbutolol, pindolol, propranolol, timolol).
- Tell your doctor if you now have or if you have ever had allergies, asthma, hay fever, eczema, slow heartbeat, bronchitis, diabetes mellitus, emphysema, heart or blood vessel disease, kidney disease, liver disease, thyroid disease, or poor circulation in the fingers or toes.
- You may want to check your pulse while taking this medication. If your pulse is much slower than your usual rate (or if it is less than 50 beats per minute), check with your doctor. A pulse rate that is too slow may cause circulation problems.
- This medicine may affect your body's response to exercise. Make sure you ask your doctor what an appropriate amount of exercise would be for you, taking into account your medical condition.
- It is important that you do not stop taking this medicine without first checking with your doctor. Some conditions may become worse when the medicine is stopped suddenly, and the danger of a heart attack is increased in some patients. Your doctor may want you to gradually reduce the amount of medicine you take before stopping completely. Make sure that you have enough medicine on hand to last through vacations, holidays, and weekends.
- Before having surgery or any other medical or dental treatment, tell your physician or dentist that you are taking

this medicine. Often, this medication will be discontinued 48 hours prior to any major surgery.

• Propranolol can cause dizziness, drowsiness, light-headedness, and decreased alertness. Use caution while driving a car or operating dangerous machinery.

• While taking this medicine, do not use any over-the-counter (nonprescription) allergy, asthma, cough, cold, sinus, or diet preparations without first checking with your pharmacist or doctor. The combination of these medicines with a beta blocker can result in high blood pressure.

• Be sure to tell your doctor if you are pregnant. Animal studies have shown that some beta blockers can cause problems in pregnancy when used at very high doses. Adequate studies have not been done in humans, but there has been some association between use of beta blockers during pregnancy and low birth weight, as well as breathing problems and slow heart rate in newborn infants. However, other reports have shown no effects in newborn infants. Also, tell your doctor if you are breast-feeding an infant. Although this medicine has not been shown to cause problems in breast-fed infants, some of the medicine may pass into breast milk, so caution is warranted.

---

propranolol and hydrochlorothiazide combination

BRAND NAMES (Manufacturers)
Inderide (Wyeth-Ayerst)
Inderide LA (Wyeth-Ayerst)

TYPE OF DRUG
Beta-adrenergic blocking agent and diuretic

INGREDIENTS
propranolol and hydrochlorothiazide

DOSAGE FORMS
Tablets (40 mg propranolol and 25 mg hydrochlorothiazide; 80 mg propranolol and 25 mg hydrochlorothiazide)
Long-acting capsules (80 mg propranolol and 50 mg hydrochlorothiazide; 120 mg propranolol and 50 mg hydrochlorothiazide; and 160 mg propranolol and 50 mg hydrochlorothiazide)

STORAGE
Store at room temperature in a tightly closed, light-resistant container.

USES

This drug is prescribed to treat high blood pressure. Hydrochlorothiazide is a diuretic (water pill), which reduces fluid accumulation in the body by increasing the elimination of salt and water through the kidneys. Propranolol belongs to a group of drugs known as beta-adrenergic blocking agents or, more commonly, beta blockers. They work by controlling nerve impulses along certain nerve pathways.

TREATMENT

This medication can be taken with a glass of water, with meals, immediately following meals, or on an empty stomach (depending on your doctor's instructions).

Try to take the medication at the same time(s) each day. Avoid taking a dose after 6:00 P.M.; otherwise, you may have to get up during the night to urinate.

If you miss a dose of this medication, take the missed dose as soon as possible, unless it is almost time for your next dose. In that case, do not take the missed dose at all; just wait until the next scheduled dose. Do not double the dose.

Propranolol and hydrochlorothiazide combination does not cure high blood pressure, but it will help to control the condition as long as you continue to take it.

SIDE EFFECTS

Minor. Anxiety, constipation, cramps, decreased sexual ability, diarrhea, difficulty in sleeping, drowsiness, dizziness, dryness of the eyes and skin, headache, heartburn, loss of appetite, nervousness, stomach discomfort, restlessness, or tiredness. These side effects should disappear as your body adjusts to the medication.

Hydrochlorothiazide can cause increased sensitivity to sunlight. It is, therefore, important to avoid prolonged exposure to sunlight and sunlamps. Wear protective clothing and sunglasses, and use an effective sunscreen.

If you become extra-sensitive to the cold, be sure to dress warmly during cold weather.

To relieve constipation, increase the amount of fiber in your diet (fresh fruits and vegetables, salads, bran, and whole-grain breads) unless your doctor directs you to do otherwise.

Plain, nonmedicated eye drops (artificial tears) may help to relieve eye dryness.

To avoid dizziness or light-headedness when you stand, contract and relax the muscles of your legs for a few moments before rising from a sitting or reclining position. Do this by pushing one foot against the floor while raising the other foot slightly, alternating feet so that you are "pumping" your legs in a pedaling motion.

Major. Tell your doctor about any side effects that are persistent or particularly bothersome. IT IS ESPECIALLY IMPORTANT TO TELL YOUR DOCTOR about blurred vision, cold hands and feet (due to decreased blood circulation to skin, fingers, and toes), confusion, depression, difficulty in breathing, dry mouth, excessive thirst, excessive weakness, fever, hair loss, hallucinations, itching, joint pain, mood changes, muscle spasms, nausea, nightmares, numbness or tingling in the fingers or toes, palpitations, rapid weight gain (three to five pounds within a week), reduced alertness, skin rash, sore throat, swelling, unusual bleeding or bruising, vomiting, or yellowing of the eyes or skin.

INTERACTIONS

This medicine interacts with other types of drugs:

1. Indomethacin, aspirin, and other salicylates may decrease the blood-pressure-lowering effects of beta blockers.

2. Concurrent use of propranolol and calcium channel blockers (diltiazem, nifedipine, verapamil) or disopyramide can lead to heart failure or very low blood pressure.

3. Cimetidine and oral contraceptives (birth control pills) can increase the blood levels of propranolol, which can result in greater side effects. Side effects may also be increased when propranolol is taken with clonidine, digoxin, epinephrine, phenylephrine, phenylpropanolamine, phenothiazine tranquilizers, prazosin, reserpine, or monoamine

oxidase (MAO) inhibitors. At least 14 days should separate the use of propranolol and an MAO inhibitor.
4. Barbiturates, alcohol, and rifampin can increase the breakdown of propranolol, which can lead to a decrease in its effectiveness.
5. The action of beta blockers may be increased if they are used with chlorpromazine, furosemide, or hydralazine, which may have a negative effect.
6. Propranolol can antagonize (act against) the effects of theophylline, aminophylline, albuterol, isoproterenol, metaproterenol, and terbutaline.
7. Propranolol can also interact with insulin and oral antidiabetic agents, raising or lowering blood sugar levels and masking the symptoms of low blood sugar.
8. Hydrochlorothiazide can decrease the effectiveness of oral anticoagulants (blood thinners, such as warfarin), antigout medications, and methenamine.
9. Antihypertensive medications may increase the blood-pressure-lowering effects of propranolol and hydrochlorothiazide combination, which can be dangerous.
10. Cholestyramine and colestipol can decrease the absorption of hydrochlorothiazide from the gastrointestinal tract; therefore, hydrochlorothiazide should be taken one hour before or four hours after a dose of cholestyramine or colestipol if one of these medications has also been prescribed for you.
11. Hydrochlorothiazide may increase the side effects of amphotericin B, calcium, cortisone and cortisone-like steroids (such as dexamethasone, hydrocortisone, prednisone, and prednisolone), digoxin, digitoxin, lithium, quinidine, sulfonamide antibiotics, and vitamin D.

BE SURE TO TELL YOUR DOCTOR about any medications you are currently taking, especially any of those listed above.

WARNINGS

- Tell your doctor about unusual or allergic reactions you have had to medications, especially to propranolol or any other beta blocker (such as acebutolol, atenolol, betaxolol, carteolol, esmolol, labetalol, metoprolol, nadolol, penbutolol, pindolol, or timolol), to hydrochlorothiazide or other diuretics (such as bendroflumethiazide, benzthiazide, chlorothiazide, chlorthalidone, cyclothiazide, hydroflumethiazide methyclothiazide, metolazone, polythiazide, quinethazone, trichlormethiazide, and furosemide), or to any sulfa drug (oral antidiabetic medication and sulfonamide antibiotic).
- Tell your doctor if you have ever had asthma, diabetes mellitus, heart disease, gout, kidney disease or problems with urination, liver disease, pancreatitis, systemic lupus erythematosus, thyroid disease, or poor circulation in the fingers or toes.
- Hydrochlorothiazide can cause potassium loss. Signs of potassium loss include dry mouth, thirst, weakness, muscle pain or cramps, nausea, and vomiting. If you experience any of these symptoms, call your doctor. To help prevent this problem, your doctor may have blood tests performed periodically to monitor your potassium levels. To help avoid potassium loss, take this medication with a glass of fresh or frozen orange juice or cranberry juice, or eat a banana every day. The use of a salt substitute also helps to prevent potassium loss. Do not change your diet, however, until you discuss it with your doctor. Too much potassium may also be dangerous.
- While you are taking this medication, limit your intake of alcohol, in order to prevent dizziness and light-headedness.
- Do not take any over-the-counter (nonprescription) medication for weight control or for allergy, asthma, cough, cold, or sinus problems unless you first check with your doctor.
- To prevent severe water loss (dehydration) while taking this medication, check with your doctor if you have any illness that causes severe or continuous nausea, vomiting, or diarrhea.
- This medication can raise blood sugar levels in diabetic patients. Blood sugar levels should be monitored carefully with blood or urine tests when this medication is being taken.
- You may want to check your pulse while taking this medication. If your pulse is much slower than your usual rate (or if it is less than 50 beats per minute), check with your doctor. A pulse rate that is too slow may cause circulation problems.
- Propranolol can affect your body's response to exercise. Make sure you ask your doctor what an appropriate amount of exercise would be for you, taking into account your medical condition.
- Before having surgery or any other medical or dental treatment, tell your doctor or dentist that you are taking this medicine. Often, this medication will be discontinued 48 hours prior to any major surgery.
- This medication can cause dizziness, drowsiness, lightheadedness, or decreased alertness. Therefore, you must exercise caution while driving a car or operating potentially dangerous machinery.
- It is important that you do not stop taking this medicine unless you first check with your doctor. Some conditions worsen when this medicine is stopped suddenly, and the danger of a heart attack is increased in some patients. Your doctor may, therefore, want you to gradually reduce the amount of medicine you take before stopping completely. Make sure that you have enough medicine on hand to last through vacations, holidays, and weekends.
- A doctor does not usually prescribe a "fixed-dose" drug like this as the first choice in the treatment of high blood pressure. Usually, the patient first receives each ingredient singly. If there is an adequate response to the fixed dose contained in this product, it can then be substituted. The advantage of a combination product is increased convenience and (often) decreased cost.
- Be sure to tell your doctor if you are pregnant. Animal studies have shown that some beta blockers can cause problems in pregnancy when used at very high doses. Adequate studies have not been conducted in humans, but there has been some association between beta blockers used during pregnancy and low birth weight, as well as breathing problems and slow heart rate in newborn infants. However, other reports have shown no such effects in newborn infants. Hydrochlorothiazide has been associated with jaundice, blood problems, and low potassium in the newborn. Also, tell your doctor if you are breast-feeding an infant. Although problems in humans have not been reported, small amounts of propranolol and hydrochlorothiazide pass into breast milk, so caution is warranted.

Prostaphlin—see oxacillin

Prothazine—see promethazine

Prothazine DC—see promethazine and codeine combination

Protostat—see metronidazole

protriptyline

BRAND NAME (Manufacturer)
Vivactil (Merck Sharp & Dohme)
TYPE OF DRUG
Tricyclic antidepressant
INGREDIENT
protriptyline
DOSAGE FORM
Tablets (5 mg and 10 mg)
STORAGE
Store at room temperature in a tightly closed container.

USES

Protriptyline is used to relieve the symptoms of mental depression. This medication belongs to a group of drugs referred to as the tricyclic antidepressants. These medicines are thought to relieve depression by increasing the concentration of certain chemicals necessary for the transmission of nerve impulses in the brain. This drug may also be used in the treatment of certain sleep disorders.

TREATMENT

This medication should be taken exactly as your doctor prescribes. You can take it with water or with food to lessen the chance of stomach irritation, unless your doctor tells you to do otherwise.

If you miss a dose of this medication, take the missed dose as soon as possible, then return to your regular dosing schedule. However, if the dose you missed was a once-a-day bedtime dose, do not take that dose in the morning; check with your doctor instead. If the dose is taken in the morning, it may cause some unwanted side effects. Never double the dose.

The effects of therapy with this medication may not become apparent for two or three weeks.

SIDE EFFECTS

Minor. Anxiety, blurred vision, constipation, cramps, diarrhea, dizziness, drowsiness, dry mouth, fatigue, headache, heartburn, insomnia, loss of appetite, nausea, peculiar tastes in the mouth, restlessness, sweating, vomiting, weakness, or weight gain or loss. As your body adjusts to the medication, these side effects should disappear.

This medication may increase your sensitivity to sunlight. You should, therefore, avoid prolonged exposure to sunlight and sunlamps. Wear protective clothing, and use an effective sunscreen.

If you experience dry mouth, you should try chewing sugarless gum or sucking on ice chips or a piece of hard candy.

To relieve constipation, increase the amount of fiber in your diet (fresh fruits and vegetables, salads, bran, and whole-grain breads), exercise, and drink more water (unless your doctor directs you to do otherwise).

To avoid dizziness or light-headedness when you stand, contract and relax the muscles of your legs for a few moments before rising. You can accomplish this by pushing one foot against the floor while raising the other foot slightly, alternating feet so that you are "pumping" your legs in a pedaling motion.

Major. Tell your doctor about any side effects that are persistent or particularly bothersome. IT IS ESPECIALLY IMPORTANT TO TELL YOUR DOCTOR about agitation, bleeding, chest pain, confusion, convulsions, difficulty in urinating, enlarged or painful breasts (in both sexes), fainting, fever, fluid retention, hair loss, hallucinations, headaches, impotence, mood changes, mouth sores, nervousness, nightmares, nosebleeds, numbness in the fingers or toes, palpitations, ringing in the ears, seizures, skin rash, sleep disorders, sore throat, tremors, uncoordinated movements or balance problems, or yellowing of the eyes or skin.

INTERACTIONS

Protriptyline interacts with a number of other types of medications:

1. Extreme drowsiness can occur when this medicine is taken with central nervous system depressants (medicines that slow the activity of the brain and spinal cord), including alcohol, antihistamines, barbiturates, benzodiazepine tranquilizers, muscle relaxants, narcotics, pain medications, phenothiazine tranquilizers, and sleeping medications, or with other tricyclic antidepressants.

2. Protriptyline may decrease the effectiveness of antiseizure medications and may block the blood-pressure-lowering effects of clonidine and guanethidine.

3. Oral contraceptives (birth control pills) or estrogen-containing drugs can increase the side effects and reduce the effectiveness of tricyclic antidepressants (including protriptyline).

4. Tricyclic antidepressants may increase the side effects of thyroid medication and over-the-counter (nonprescription) cough, cold, allergy, asthma, sinus, and diet medications.

5. The concurrent use of tricyclic antidepressants and monoamine oxidase (MAO) inhibitors should be undertaken very carefully, because the combination may result in fever, convulsions, or high blood pressure.

Before starting to take protriptyline, BE SURE TO TELL YOUR DOCTOR about any medications you are currently taking, especially any of those listed above.

WARNINGS

- Tell your doctor if you have had unusual or allergic reactions to any medications, especially to protriptyline or other tricyclic antidepressants (such as amitriptyline, imipramine, doxepin, trimipramine, amoxapine, desipramine, maprotiline, and nortriptyline).
- Tell your doctor if you have a history of alcoholism or if you have ever had asthma, high blood pressure, liver or kidney disease, heart disease, a heart attack, circulatory disease, stomach problems, intestinal problems, difficulty in urinating, enlarged prostate gland, epilepsy, glaucoma, thyroid disease, mental illness, or electroshock therapy.
- If this drug makes you dizzy or drowsy, do not take part in

any activity that requires alertness, such as driving a car or operating potentially dangerous machinery.

• Before having surgery or any other medical or dental treatment, be sure to tell your doctor or dentist that you are taking this medication.

• Do not stop taking this drug suddenly. Stopping abruptly can cause nausea, headache, stomach upset, fatigue, or a worsening of your condition. Your doctor may want to reduce the dosage gradually.

• The effects of this medication may last as long as seven days after you have stopped taking it, so continue to observe all precautions during that period.

• Be sure to tell your doctor if you are pregnant. The safe use of this medication in human pregnancy has not been established. Side effects have been observed in the fetuses of animals that received this type of medication in large doses during pregnancy. Also, tell your doctor if you are breast-feeding an infant. Small amounts of this drug can pass into breast milk and may cause unwanted effects, such as irritability or sleeping problems, in nursing infants.

Proventil—see albuterol

Provera—see medroxyprogesterone

Prozac—see fluoxetine

Pseudo-Car DM—see pseudoephedrine, carbinoxamine, and dextromethorphan combination

---

pseudoephedrine and azatadine combination

BRAND NAME (Manufacturer)
Trinalin Repetabs (Schering)

TYPE OF DRUG
Adrenergic (decongestant) and antihistamine

INGREDIENTS
pseudoephedrine and azatadine

DOSAGE FORM
Sustained-release tablets (120 mg pseudoephedrine and 1 mg azatadine)

STORAGE
Pseudoephedrine and azatadine combination tablets should be stored at room temperature in a tightly closed container.

USES

Pseudoephedrine and azatadine combination medication is used to relieve the symptoms of upper respiratory tract infections, hay fever and other allergies, and sinusitis (inflammation of the sinuses).

Pseudoephedrine belongs to a group of drugs known as adrenergic agents (decongestants). They act by constricting (narrowing) blood vessels in the nasal passages to reduce swelling and congestion.

Azatadine belongs to a group of drugs known as antihistamines, which block the action of histamine, a chemical released by the body during an allergic reaction. It is, therefore, used to relieve or prevent symptoms of allergy.

TREATMENT

In order to avoid stomach upset, you can take pseudoephedrine and azatadine combination with food or with a full glass of milk or water (unless your doctor directs you to do otherwise).

The sustained-release tablets should be swallowed whole. Breaking, chewing, or crushing these tablets destroys their sustained-release activity and may increase the side effects.

If you miss a dose of this medication, take the missed dose as soon as possible, unless it is almost time for your next dose. In that case, do not take the missed dose at all; just return to your regular dosing schedule. Do not double the next dose.

SIDE EFFECTS

Minor. Anxiety; blurred vision; constipation; diarrhea; dizziness; drowsiness; dry mouth, nose, and throat; heartburn; insomnia; irritability; loss of appetite; nasal congestion; nausea; restlessness; decreased sweating; vomiting; or weakness. These side effects should disappear as your body adjusts to the medication.

This medication can increase your sensitivity to sunlight. Avoid prolonged exposure to sunlight and sunlamps. Wear protective clothing, and use an effective sunscreen.

If you are constipated, increase the amount of fiber in your diet (fresh fruits and vegetables, salads, bran, and whole-grain breads), exercise, and drink more water (unless your doctor directs you to do otherwise).

Chew sugarless gum or suck on ice chips or a piece of hard candy to reduce mouth dryness.

If you feel dizzy or light-headed, sit or lie down for a while; get up slowly from a sitting or reclining position, and be careful on stairs.

In order to avoid difficulty in falling asleep, take the last dose of this medication several hours before bedtime.

Major. Tell your doctor about any side effects that are persistent or particularly bothersome. IT IS ESPECIALLY IMPORTANT TO TELL YOUR DOCTOR about chest pain, confusion, convulsions, difficult or painful urination, difficulty in breathing, fainting, hallucinations, headaches, loss of coordination, mood changes, nosebleeds, palpitations, rash, severe abdominal pain, sore throat, or unusual bleeding or bruising.

INTERACTIONS

Pseudoephedrine and azatadine combination can interact with several other types of medications:

1. Concurrent use of this medication with central nervous system depressants (drugs that slow the activity of the brain and spinal cord), such as alcohol, barbiturates, benzodiazepine tranquilizers, muscle relaxants, narcotics, pain medications, and phenothiazine tranquilizers, or with tricyclic antidepressants can cause extreme drowsiness.

2. Monoamine oxidase (MAO) inhibitors (isocarboxazid, pargyline, phenelzine, tranylcypromine) and tricyclic antidepressants can increase the side effects of this drug. At least 14 days should separate the use of this drug and the use of an MAO inhibitor.

3. The action of oral anticoagulants (blood thinners) may be decreased by the antihistamine component of this drug.

4. Procarbazine may interact with the antihistamine component of this drug.

5. The side effects of the antihistamine component of this medication may be increased by quinidine, procainamide, haloperidol, and phenothiazine tranquilizers.
6. The side effects of the decongestant component of this drug may be increased by digoxin or over-the-counter (nonprescription) asthma, allergy, cough, cold, diet, or sinus preparations.
7. The blood-pressure-lowering effects of guanethidine may be decreased by this medication.

BE SURE TO TELL YOUR DOCTOR about any medications you are currently taking, especially any of the medications that are listed above.

WARNINGS

• Tell your doctor about unusual or allergic reactions you have had to any medications, especially to azatadine or other antihistamines (such as brompheniramine, carbinoxamine, chlorpheniramine, clemastine, cyproheptadine, dexchlorpheniramine, dimenhydrinate, dimethindene, diphenhydramine, diphenylpyraline, doxylamine, hydroxyzine, promethazine, pyrilamine, trimeprazine, tripelennamine, and triprolidine) or to pseudoephedrine or other adrenergic agents (such as albuterol, amphetamines, ephedrine, epinephrine, isoproterenol, metaproterenol, norepinephrine, phenylpropanolamine, and terbutaline).

• Tell your doctor if you now have or if you have ever had diabetes mellitus, epilepsy, glaucoma, heart or blood vessel disease, hiatal hernia, high blood pressure, myasthenia gravis, obstructed bladder or intestinal tract, peptic ulcers, enlarged prostate gland, or thyroid disease.

• This drug can reduce sweating and heat release from the body. Avoid excessive work and exercise in hot weather, and do not take hot baths, showers, and saunas.

• This medication can cause drowsiness. Your ability to perform tasks that require alertness, such as driving a car or operating potentially dangerous machinery, may be decreased. Appropriate caution should, therefore, be taken.

• Be sure to tell your doctor if you are pregnant. The effects of this medication during pregnancy have not been thoroughly studied in humans. Also, tell your doctor if you are breast-feeding an infant. Small amounts of this medication pass into breast milk and may cause unusual excitement or irritability in nursing infants.

---

pseudoephedrine and carbinoxamine combination

BRAND NAMES (Manufacturers)
Carbodec (Rugby)
Cardec-S (various manufacturers)
Rondec (Ross)

TYPE OF DRUG
Adrenergic (decongestant) and antihistamine

INGREDIENTS
pseudoephedrine and carbinoxamine

DOSAGE FORMS
Tablets (60 mg pseudoephedrine and 4 mg carbinoxamine)
Oral syrup (60 mg pseudoephedrine and 4 mg carbinoxamine per 5-ml spoonful)
Oral drops (25 mg pseudoephedrine and 2 mg carbinoxamine per ml)

STORAGE
Pseudoephedrine and carbinoxamine combination tablets, oral syrup, and oral drops should be stored at room temperature in tightly closed containers. No form of this medication should ever be frozen.

USES

This drug combination is used to relieve symptoms of upper respiratory tract infections, hay fever and other allergies, and sinusitis (inflammation of the sinuses).

Pseudoephedrine belongs to a group of drugs known as adrenergic agents (decongestants). They act by constricting (narrowing) blood vessels in the nasal passages to reduce swelling and congestion.

Carbinoxamine belongs to a group of drugs known as antihistamines, which block the actions of histamine, a chemical released by the body during an allergic reaction. It is, therefore, used to relieve or prevent symptoms of allergy.

TREATMENT

In order to avoid stomach upset, you can take pseudoephedrine and carbinoxamine combination with food or with a full glass of water (unless your doctor directs you to do otherwise).

The oral drops should be measured carefully with the dropper provided.

The oral syrup form of this medication should be measured carefully with a specially designed 5-ml measuring spoon. An ordinary kitchen teaspoon is not accurate enough.

If you miss a dose of this medication, take the missed dose as soon as possible, unless it is almost time for your next dose. In that case, do not take the missed dose at all; just return to your regular dosing schedule. Do not double the next dose.

SIDE EFFECTS

Minor. Anxiety; blurred vision; constipation; diarrhea; dizziness; drowsiness; dry mouth, nose, and throat; heartburn; insomnia; irritability; loss of appetite; nasal congestion; nausea; restlessness; decreased sweating; vomiting; or weakness. These side effects should disappear as your body adjusts to the medication.

This medication can increase your sensitivity to sunlight. You should, therefore, avoid prolonged exposure to sunlight and sunlamps. Wear protective clothing, and use an effective sunscreen.

If you are constipated, increase the amount of fiber in your diet (fresh fruits and vegetables, salads, bran, and whole-grain breads), exercise, and drink more water (unless your doctor directs you to do otherwise).

Chew sugarless gum or suck on ice chips or a piece of hard candy to reduce mouth dryness.

If you feel dizzy or light-headed, sit or lie down for a while; get up slowly from a sitting or reclining position, and be careful on stairs.

In order to avoid difficulty in falling asleep, take the last dose of this medication several hours before bedtime.

Major. Tell your doctor about any side effects that are persistent or particularly bothersome. IT IS ESPECIALLY IM-

PORTANT TO TELL YOUR DOCTOR about chest pain, confusion, convulsions, difficult or painful urination, difficulty in breathing, fainting, hallucinations, headaches, loss of coordination, mood changes, nosebleeds, palpitations, rash, severe abdominal pain, sore throat, or unusual bleeding or bruising.

INTERACTIONS

Pseudoephedrine and carbinoxamine combination interacts with several other types of medications:

1. Concurrent use of it with central nervous system depressants (drugs that slow the activity of the brain and spinal cord), such as alcohol, barbiturates, benzodiazepine tranquilizers, muscle relaxants, narcotics, pain medications, and phenothiazine tranquilizers, or with tricyclic antidepressants can cause extreme drowsiness.

2. Monoamine oxidase (MAO) inhibitors (isocarboxazid, pargyline, phenelzine, tranylcypromine) and tricyclic antidepressants can increase the side effects of this drug. At least 14 days should separate the use of this drug and the use of an MAO inhibitor.

3. The action of oral anticoagulants may be decreased by the antihistamine component of this drug.

4. Procarbazine may interact with the antihistamine component of this drug.

5. The side effects of the antihistamine component of this medication may be increased by quinidine, procainamide, haloperidol, and phenothiazine tranquilizers.

6. The side effects of the decongestant component of this drug may be increased by digoxin or over-the-counter (nonprescription) asthma, allergy, cough, cold, diet, or sinus preparations.

7. The blood-pressure-lowering effects of guanethidine may be decreased by this medication.

BE SURE TO TELL YOUR DOCTOR about any medications you are currently taking, especially any listed above.

WARNINGS

• Tell your doctor about unusual or allergic reactions you have had to any medications, especially to carbinoxamine or other antihistamines (such as azatadine, chlorpheniramine, clemastine, cyproheptadine, dexchlorpheniramine, dimenhydrinate, dimethindene, diphenhydramine, diphenylpyraline, doxylamine, hydroxyzine, promethazine, pyrilamine, trimeprazine, tripelennamine, and triprolidine) or to pseudoephedrine or other adrenergic agents (such as albuterol, amphetamines, ephedrine, epinephrine, isoproterenol, metaproterenol, norepinephrine, phenylpropanolamine, and terbutaline).

• Tell your doctor if you now have or if you have ever had diabetes mellitus, epilepsy, glaucoma, heart or blood vessel disease, hiatal hernia, high blood pressure, myasthenia gravis, obstructed bladder or intestinal tract, peptic ulcers, enlarged prostate gland, or thyroid disease.

• Because this drug can reduce sweating and heat release from the body, you should avoid excessive work and exercise in hot weather, and do not take hot baths, showers, and saunas.

• This medication can cause drowsiness. Your ability to perform tasks that require alertness, such as driving a car or operating potentially dangerous machinery, may be decreased. Appropriate caution should, therefore, be taken.

• Be sure to tell your doctor if you are pregnant. The effects of this medication during pregnancy have not been thoroughly studied in humans. Also, tell your doctor if you are breast-feeding an infant. Small amounts of this medication pass into breast milk and may cause unusual excitement or irritability in nursing infants.

---

pseudoephedrine and chlorpheniramine combination

BRAND NAMES (Manufacturers)

Anamine T.D. (Mayrand)
Brexin L.A. (Savage)
Chlorafed (Half-Strength) (Hauck)
Chlorafed Timecelles (Hauck)
Chlor-Trimeton Decongestant* (Schering)
Chlor-Trimeton Decongestant Repetabs* (Schering)
Codimal-L.A. (Central)
Co-Pyronil 2* (Dista)
Dallergy-D* (Laser)
Deconamine (Berlex)
Deconamine SR (Berlex)
Dorcol Children's Liquid Cold Formula* (Sandoz)
Duralex (American Urologicals)
Fedahist* (Kremers Urban)
Histalet (Reid-Rowell)
Isoclor (Fisons)
Isoclor Timesules* (Fisons)
Kronofed-A Jr. (Ferndale)
Kronofed-A Kronocaps (Ferndale)
Myfedrine Plus* (P.B.I.)
Napril* (Randob)
ND Clear T.D. (Seatrace)
Novafed A (Lakeside)
PediaCare 2 Liquid (McNeil Consumer)
Pseudo-Hist* (Abana)
Ryna* (Wallace)
Sudafed Plus* (Burroughs Wellcome)
T-Dry Jr (T.E. Williams)
*Available over-the-counter (without a prescription)

TYPE OF DRUG

Adrenergic (decongestant) and antihistamine

INGREDIENTS

Pseudoephedrine and chlorpheniramine

DOSAGE FORMS

Tablets (30 mg pseudoephedrine and 4 mg chlorpheniramine; 60 mg pseudoephedrine and 4 mg chlorpheniramine)
Capsules (30 mg pseudoephedrine and 4 mg chlorpheniramine; 30 mg pseudoephedrine and 2 mg chlorpheniramine)
Sustained-release capsules (60 mg pseudoephedrine and 4 mg chlorpheniramine; 65 mg pseudoephedrine and 10 mg chlorpheniramine; 120 mg pseudoephedrine and 8 mg chlorpheniramine; and 120 mg pseudoephedrine and 12 mg chlorpheniramine)
Oral elixir (30 mg pseudoephedrine and 2 mg chlorpheniramine per 5-ml spoonful, with 5% alcohol)
Oral syrup (15 mg pseudoephedrine and 1 mg chlorphen-

iramine; 15 mg pseudoephedrine and 2 mg chlorpheniramine; 30 mg pseudoephedrine and 2 mg chlorpheniramine; and 45 mg pseudoephedrine and 3 mg chlorpheniramine per 5-ml spoonful)

STORAGE

Pseudoephedrine and chlorpheniramine combination tablets, capsules, elixir, and syrup should be stored at room temperature in tightly closed containers. This medication should never be frozen.

USES

This drug combination is used to relieve the symptoms of upper respiratory tract infections, hay fever and other allergies, and sinusitis (inflammation of the sinuses).

Pseudoephedrine belongs to a group of drugs known as adrenergic agents (decongestants). They act by constricting (narrowing) blood vessels in the nasal passages to reduce swelling and congestion.

Chlorpheniramine belongs to a group of drugs known as antihistamines, which block the actions of histamine, a chemical released by the body during an allergic reaction. It is, therefore, used to relieve or prevent symptoms of allergy.

TREATMENT

In order to avoid stomach upset, you can take pseudoephedrine and chlorpheniramine combination with food or with a full glass of milk or water (unless your doctor directs you to do otherwise).

The oral syrup and elixir forms of this medication should be measured carefully with a specially designed 5-ml measuring spoon. An ordinary kitchen teaspoon is not accurate enough.

The sustained-release capsules should be swallowed whole. Breaking, chewing, or crushing these capsules destroys their sustained-release activity and may increase the side effects.

If you miss a dose of this medication, take the missed dose as soon as possible, unless it is almost time for your next dose. In that case, do not take the missed dose at all; just return to your regular dosing schedule. Do not double the next dose.

SIDE EFFECTS

Minor. Anxiety; blurred vision; constipation; diarrhea; dizziness; drowsiness; dry mouth, nose, and throat; heartburn; insomnia; irritability; loss of appetite; nasal congestion; nausea; restlessness; decreased sweating; vomiting; or weakness. These side effects should gradually disappear as your body adjusts to this medication.

This medication can increase your sensitivity to sunlight. You should, therefore, avoid prolonged exposure to sunlight and sunlamps. Wear protective clothing, and use an effective sunscreen.

If you are constipated, increase the amount of fiber in your diet (fresh fruits and vegetables, salads, bran, and whole-grain breads), exercise, and drink more water (unless your doctor directs you to do otherwise).

Chew sugarless gum or suck on ice chips or a piece of hard candy to reduce mouth dryness.

If you feel dizzy or light-headed, sit or lie down for a while; get up slowly from a sitting or reclining position, and be careful on stairs.

In order to avoid difficulty in falling asleep, take the last dose of this medication several hours before bedtime.

Major. Tell your doctor about any side effects that are persistent or particularly bothersome. IT IS ESPECIALLY IMPORTANT TO TELL YOUR DOCTOR about chest pain, confusion, convulsions, difficult or painful urination, difficulty in breathing, fainting, hallucinations, headaches, loss of coordination, mood changes, palpitations, rash, severe abdominal pain, sore throat, or unusual bleeding or bruising.

INTERACTIONS

Pseudoephedrine and chlorpheniramine combination interacts with several other types of medications:

1. Concurrent use of this medication with central nervous system depressants (drugs that slow the activity of the brain and spinal cord), such as alcohol, barbiturates, benzodiazepine tranquilizers, muscle relaxants, narcotics, pain medications, and phenothiazine tranquilizers, or with tricyclic antidepressants can cause extreme drowsiness.

2. Monoamine oxidase (MAO) inhibitors (isocarboxazid, pargyline, phenelzine, tranylcypromine) and tricyclic antidepressants can increase the side effects of this medication. At least 14 days should separate the use of this drug and the use of an MAO inhibitor.

3. The action of oral anticoagulants may be decreased by the antihistamine component of this drug.

4. Procarbazine may interact with the antihistamine component of this drug.

5. The side effects of the antihistamine component of this medication may be increased by quinidine, procainamide, haloperidol, or phenothiazine tranquilizers.

6. The side effects of the decongestant component may be increased by digoxin or over-the-counter (nonprescription) asthma, allergy, cough, cold, diet, or sinus preparations.

7. The blood-pressure-lowering effects of guanethidine may be decreased by this medication.

BE SURE TO TELL YOUR DOCTOR about any medications you are currently taking, especially any listed above.

WARNINGS

- Tell your doctor about unusual or allergic reactions you have had to any medications, especially to chlorpheniramine or to other antihistamines (such as azatadine, brompheniramine, carbinoxamine, clemastine, cyproheptadine, dexchlorpheniramine, dimenhydrinate, dimethindene, diphenhydramine, diphenylpyraline, doxylamine, hydroxyzine, promethazine, pyrilamine, trimeprazine, tripelennamine, and triprolidine) or to pseudoephedrine or other adrenergic agents (such as albuterol, amphetamines, ephedrine, epinephrine, isoproterenol, metaproterenol, norepinephrine, phenylpropanolamine, and terbutaline).
- Tell your doctor if you now have or if you have ever had diabetes mellitus, epilepsy, glaucoma, heart or blood vessel disease, hiatal hernia, high blood pressure, myasthenia gravis, obstructed bladder or intestinal tract, peptic ulcers, enlarged prostate gland, or thyroid disease.
- Because this drug can reduce sweating and heat release from the body, you should avoid excessive work or exercise in hot weather, and do not take hot baths, showers, and saunas.
- This medication can cause drowsiness. Your ability to

perform tasks that require alertness, such as driving a car or operating potentially dangerous machinery, may be decreased. Appropriate caution should, therefore, be taken.

• Be sure to tell your doctor if you are pregnant. The effects of this medication during pregnancy have not been thoroughly studied in humans. Also, tell your doctor if you are breast-feeding an infant. Small amounts of this medication pass into breast milk and may cause unusual excitement or irritability in nursing infants.

---

pseudoephedrine and dexbrompheniramine combination

BRAND NAMES (Manufacturers)
dexbrompheniramine and pseudoephedrine (Baxter)
Disophrol* (Schering)
Disophrol Chronotabs* (Schering)
Drixoral* (Schering)
*Available over-the-counter (without a prescription)

TYPE OF DRUG
Adrenergic (decongestant) and antihistamine

INGREDIENTS
pseudoephedrine and dexbrompheniramine

DOSAGE FORMS
Tablets (60 mg pseudoephedrine and 2 mg dexbrompheniramine)
Sustained-release tablets (120 mg pseudoephedrine and 6 mg dexbrompheniramine)

STORAGE
Pseudoephedrine and dexbrompheniramine combination tablets should be stored at room temperature in a tightly closed container.

USES

This drug combination is used to relieve the symptoms of upper respiratory tract infections, hay fever and other allergies, and sinusitis (inflammation of the sinuses).

Pseudoephedrine belongs to a group of drugs known as adrenergic agents (decongestants). They act by constricting (narrowing) blood vessels in the nasal passages to reduce swelling and congestion.

Dexbrompheniramine belongs to a group of drugs known as antihistamines, which block the actions of histamine, a chemical released by the body during an allergic reaction. It is, therefore, used to relieve or prevent symptoms of allergy.

TREATMENT

To avoid stomach upset, you can take pseudoephedrine and dexbrompheniramine combination with food or with a full glass of milk or water (unless your doctor directs you to do otherwise).

The sustained-release form of this medication should be swallowed whole. Breaking, chewing, or crushing these tablets destroys their sustained-release activity and may increase the side effects of the medication.

If you miss a dose of this medication, take the missed dose as soon as possible, unless it is almost time for your next dose. In that case, do not take the missed dose at all; just return to your regular dosing schedule. Do not double the next dose.

SIDE EFFECTS

Minor. Anxiety; blurred vision; constipation; decreased sweating; diarrhea; dizziness; drowsiness; dry mouth, nose, and throat; heartburn; insomnia; irritability; loss of appetite; nasal congestion; nausea; restlessness; vomiting; or weakness. These side effects should disappear as your body adjusts to the medication.

This medication can increase your sensitivity to sunlight. You should, therefore, avoid prolonged exposure to sunlight and sunlamps. Wear protective clothing, and use an effective sunscreen.

If you are constipated, increase the amount of fiber in your diet (fresh fruits and vegetables, salads, bran, and whole-grain breads), exercise, and drink more water (unless your doctor directs you to do otherwise).

Chew sugarless gum or suck on ice chips or a piece of hard candy to reduce mouth dryness.

If you feel dizzy or light-headed, sit or lie down for a while; get up slowly from a sitting or reclining position, and be careful on stairs. In order to avoid difficulty in falling asleep, take the last dose of this medication several hours before bedtime.

Major. Tell your doctor about any side effects that are persistent or particularly bothersome. IT IS ESPECIALLY IMPORTANT TO TELL YOUR DOCTOR about chest pain, confusion, convulsions, difficult or painful urination, difficulty in breathing, fainting, hallucinations, headaches, loss of coordination, mood changes, nosebleeds, palpitations, rash, severe abdominal pain, sore throat, or unusual bleeding or bruising.

INTERACTIONS

This medicine interacts with several other types of drugs:

1. Concurrent use of it with central nervous system depressants (such as alcohol, barbiturates, benzodiazepine tranquilizers, muscle relaxants, narcotics, pain medications, and phenothiazine tranquilizers) or with tricyclic antidepressants can cause extreme drowsiness.

2. Monoamine oxidase (MAO) inhibitors (isocarboxazid, pargyline, phenelzine, tranylcypromine) and tricyclic antidepressants can increase the side effects of this medication. At least 14 days should separate the use of this drug and the use of an MAO inhibitor.

3. The action of oral anticoagulants may be decreased by the antihistamine component of this drug.

4. Procarbazine may interact with the antihistamine component of this drug.

5. The side effects of the antihistamine part of this medication may be increased by quinidine, procainamide, haloperidol, or phenothiazine tranquilizers.

6. The side effects of the decongestant component may be increased by digoxin or over-the-counter (nonprescription) asthma, allergy, cough, cold, diet, or sinus preparations.

7. The blood-pressure-lowering effects of guanethidine may be decreased by this medication.

BE SURE TO TELL YOUR DOCTOR about any medications you are currently taking, especially any of those listed above.

WARNINGS

• Tell your doctor about unusual or allergic reactions you have had to any medications, especially to dexbrompheniramine or other antihistamines (such as azatadine, brompheniramine, carbinoxamine, chlorpheniramine, clemastine, cyproheptadine, dexchlorpheniramine, dimenhydrinate, dimethindene, diphenhydramine, diphenylpyraline, doxylamine, hydroxyzine, promethazine, pyrilamine, trimeprazine, tripelennamine, and triprolidine) or to pseudoephedrine or other adrenergic agents (such as albuterol, amphetamines, ephedrine, epinephrine, isoproterenol, metaproterenol, norepinephrine, phenylpropanolamine, and terbutaline).
• Tell your doctor if you now have or if you have ever had diabetes mellitus, epilepsy, glaucoma, heart or blood vessel disease, hiatal hernia, high blood pressure, myasthenia gravis, obstructed bladder or intestinal tract, peptic ulcers, enlarged prostate gland, or thyroid disease.
• Because this drug can reduce sweating and heat release from the body, avoid excessive work and exercise in hot weather, and do not take hot baths, showers, and saunas.
• This medication can cause drowsiness. Your ability to perform tasks that require alertness, such as driving a car or operating potentially dangerous machinery, may be decreased. Appropriate caution should, therefore, be taken.
• Be sure to tell your doctor if you are pregnant. The effects of this medication during pregnancy have not been thoroughly studied in humans. Also, tell your doctor if you are breast-feeding an infant. Small amounts of this medication pass into breast milk and may cause unusual excitement or irritability in nursing infants.

---

pseudoephedrine, carbinoxamine, and dextromethorphan combination

BRAND NAMES (Manufacturers)
Carbodec DM (Rugby)
Cardec DM (various manufacturers)
Mycadec DM (My-K Labs)
Pseudo-Car DM (Geneva Generics)
Rondec DM (Ross)
Tussafed (Everett)

TYPE OF DRUG
Adrenergic (decongestant), antihistamine, and cough suppressant

INGREDIENTS
pseudoephedrine, carbinoxamine, and dextromethorphan

DOSAGE FORMS
Oral syrup (60 mg pseudoephedrine, 4 mg carbinoxamine, and 15 mg dextromethorphan per 5-ml spoonful)
Oral drops (25 mg pseudoephedrine, 2 mg carbinoxamine, and 4 mg dextromethorphan per 1-ml dropperful)

STORAGE
Pseudoephedrine, carbinoxamine, and dextromethorphan combination oral syrup and oral drops should be stored at room temperature in a tightly closed, light-resistant glass container. Avoid exposing these medications to excessive heat.

USES

This drug combination is used to relieve coughs and the symptoms of upper respiratory tract infections, hay fever and other allergies, and sinusitis (inflammation of the sinuses).

Pseudoephedrine belongs to a group of drugs known as adrenergic agents (decongestants). They act by constricting (narrowing) blood vessels in the nasal passages to reduce swelling and congestion.

Carbinoxamine belongs to a group of drugs known as antihistamines, which block the actions of histamine, a chemical released by the body during an allergic reaction. It is, therefore, used to relieve or prevent symptoms of allergy.

Dextromethorphan is a cough suppressant, which acts at the cough reflex center in the brain.

TREATMENT

In order to avoid stomach upset, you can take this medicine with food or with a full glass of water (unless your doctor directs you to do otherwise).

The oral drops should be measured carefully with the dropper provided. The oral syrup should be measured carefully with a specially designed 5-ml measuring spoon. An ordinary kitchen teaspoon is not accurate enough.

If you miss a dose of this medication, take the missed dose as soon as possible, unless it is almost time for your next dose. In that case, do not take the missed dose at all; just return to your regular dosing schedule. Do not double the next dose.

SIDE EFFECTS

Minor. Abdominal pain, blurred vision, decreased sweating, diarrhea, dizziness, drowsiness, dry mouth, headache, heartburn, loss of appetite, nausea, nervousness, sleeping problems, vomiting, or weakness. These side effects should disappear as your body adjusts to the medication.

Chew sugarless gum or suck on ice chips or hard candy to reduce mouth dryness.

If you feel dizzy or light-headed, sit or lie down for a while; get up slowly from a sitting or reclining position, and be careful on stairs.

This medication can increase your sensitivity to sunlight. You should, therefore, avoid prolonged exposure to sunlight and sunlamps. Wear protective clothing, and use an effective sunscreen.

In order to avoid difficulty in falling asleep, you should take the last dose of this medication several hours before bedtime.

Major. Tell your doctor about any side effects that are persistent or particularly bothersome. IT IS ESPECIALLY IMPORTANT TO TELL YOUR DOCTOR about chest pain, difficult or painful urination, difficulty in breathing, hallucinations, pallor, palpitations, seizures, or tremors.

INTERACTIONS

This medication can interact with several types of drugs:

1. Concurrent use of it with central nervous system depressants (drugs that slow the activity of the brain and spinal cord), such as alcohol, barbiturates, benzodiazepine tranquilizers, muscle relaxants, narcotics, pain medications, and phenothiazine tranquilizers, or with tricyclic antidepressants can cause extreme drowsiness.

2. Monoamine oxidase (MAO) inhibitors (isocarboxazid, pargyline, phenelzine, tranylcypromine), beta blockers (acebutolol, atenolol, betaxolol, carteolol, esmolol, labetalol, metoprolol, nadolol, penbutolol, pindolol, propranolol, timolol), and tricyclic antidepressants can increase the side effects of this drug. At least 14 days should separate the use of this drug and the use of an MAO inhibitor.

3. The side effects of the antihistamine part of this medication may be increased by quinidine, procainamide, haloperidol, and phenothiazine tranquilizers.

4. The side effects of the decongestant component may be increased by digoxin or over-the-counter (nonprescription) asthma, allergy, cough, cold, diet, or sinus preparations.

5. The blood-pressure-lowering effects of guanethidine, methyldopa, and reserpine may be decreased by this drug.

Before starting pseudoephedrine, carbinoxamine, and dextromethorphan combination, BE SURE TO TELL YOUR DOCTOR about any medications you are curently taking, especially any of those listed above.

WARNINGS

• Tell your doctor about unusual or allergic reactions you have had to any medications, especially to carbinoxamine or other antihistamines (such as azatadine, chlorpheniramine, clemastine, cyproheptadine, dexchlorpheniramine, dimenhydrinate, dimethindene, diphenhydramine, diphenylpyraline, doxylamine, hydroxyzine, promethazine, pyrilamine, trimeprazine, tripelennamine, and triprolidine), to pseudoephedrine or other adrenergic agents (such as albuterol, amphetamines, ephedrine, epinephrine, isoproterenol, metaproterenol, norepinephrine, phenylpropanolamine, and terbutaline), or to dextromethorphan.

• Tell your doctor if you have ever had diabetes mellitus, glaucoma, heart or blood vessel disease, high blood pressure, myasthenia gravis, obstructed bladder or intestinal tract, peptic ulcers, enlarged prostate, or thyroid disease.

• Because this drug can reduce sweating and heat release from the body, you should avoid excessive work and exercise in hot weather, and do not take hot baths, showers, and saunas.

• This medication can cause drowsiness. Your ability to perform tasks that require alertness, such as driving a car or operating potentially dangerous machinery, may be decreased. Appropriate caution should, therefore, be taken.

• Be sure to tell your doctor if you are pregnant. The safe use of this medication in human pregnancy has not been established. Also, tell your doctor if you are breast-feeding an infant. Small amounts of this medication pass into human breast milk and may cause unusual excitement or irritability in nursing infants.

---

pseudoephedrine, triprolidine, and codeine combination

BRAND NAMES (Manufacturers)

Actagen-C Cough Syrup (Goldline)
Actifed with Codeine (Burroughs Wellcome)
Allerfrin with Codeine (Rugby)
Triacin-C (various manufacturers)
Trifed-C (Geneva Generics)

TYPE OF DRUG

Adrenergic (decongestant), antihistamine, and cough suppressant

INGREDIENTS

pseudoephedrine, triprolidine, and codeine

DOSAGE FORM

Oral syrup (30 mg pseudoephedrine, 1.25 mg triprolidine, and 10 mg codeine per 5-ml spoonful, with 4.3% alcohol)

STORAGE

This medication should be stored at room temperature (never frozen) in a tightly closed container.

USES

It is used to provide symptomatic relief of coughs due to colds, minor upper respiratory infections, and allergy.

Pseudoephedrine belongs to a group of drugs known as adrenergic agents (decongestants). They act by constricting (narrowing) blood vessels in the nasal passages, thereby reducing swelling and congestion.

Triprolidine belongs to a group of drugs known as antihistamines, which block the action of histamine, a chemical released by the body during an allergic reaction. It is used to relieve or prevent symptoms of allergy.

Codeine is a narcotic cough suppressant, which acts at the cough reflex center in the brain.

TREATMENT

To avoid stomach upset, you can take this medication with food or with a full glass of milk or water (unless your doctor directs you to do otherwise).

The oral syrup should be measured carefully with a specially designed 5-ml measuring spoon. An ordinary kitchen teaspoon is not accurate enough.

If you miss a dose of this medication, take the missed dose as soon as possible, unless it is almost time for your next dose. In that case, do not take the missed dose at all; just return to your regular dosing schedule. Do not double the next dose.

SIDE EFFECTS

Minor. Blurred vision; constipation; diarrhea; dizziness; dry mouth, throat, or nose; irritability; loss of appetite; nausea; restlessness; stomach upset; unusual increase in sweating; or vomiting. These side effects should disappear as your body adjusts to the medication.

This medication can cause increased sensitivity to sunlight. It is, therefore, important to avoid prolonged exposure to sunlight and sunlamps. Wear protective clothing, and use an effective sunscreen.

If you are constipated, increase the amount of fiber in your diet (fresh fruits and vegetables, salads, bran, and whole-grain breads), exercise, and drink more water (unless your doctor directs you to do otherwise).

Chew sugarless gum or suck on ice chips or a piece of hard candy to reduce mouth dryness.

If you feel dizzy or light-headed, sit or lie down for a while; get up slowly from a sitting or reclining position, and be careful on stairs.

Major. Tell your doctor about any side effects that are persistent or particularly bothersome. IT IS ESPECIALLY IMPORTANT TO TELL YOUR DOCTOR about chest pain, confusion, difficult or painful urination, feeling faint, headaches, palpitations, rash, ringing or buzzing in the ears, severe abdominal pain, sore throat, or unusual bleeding or bruising.

INTERACTIONS

This medicine interacts with several other types of drugs:

1. Concurrent use of it with other central nervous system depressants (drugs that slow the activity of the brain and spinal cord), such as alcohol, barbiturates, benzodiazepine tranquilizers, muscle relaxants, narcotics, pain medications, and phenothiazine tranquilizers, or with tricyclic antidepressants can cause extreme drowsiness.

2. Monoamine oxidase (MAO) inhibitors (isocarboxazid, pargyline, phenelzine, tranylcypromine) and tricyclic antidepressants can increase the side effects of this medication. At least 14 days should separate the use of this drug and the use of an MAO inhibitor.

3. The action of oral anticoagulants may be decreased by the antihistamine component of this drug.

4. Procarbazine may interact with the antihistamine component of this drug.

5. The side effects of the antihistamine component of this medication may be increased by quinidine, procainamide, haloperidol, or phenothiazine tranquilizers.

6. The blood-pressure-lowering effects of guanethidine, methyldopa, and reserpine may be decreased by this medication.

7. The side effects of the decongestant component of this medication may be increased by digoxin or over-the-counter (nonprescription) allergy, asthma, cough, cold, diet, or sinus preparations.

BE SURE TO TELL YOUR DOCTOR about any medications you are currently taking, especially any of those listed above.

WARNINGS

- Tell your doctor about unusual or allergic reactions you have had to any medications, especially to triprolidine or other antihistamines (such as azatadine, brompheniramine, carbinoxamine, clemastine, cyproheptadine, chlorpheniramine, dexbrompheniramine, dimenhydrinate, dimethindene, diphenhydramine, diphenylpyraline, doxylamine, hydroxyzine, promethazine, pyrilamine, trimeprazine, and tripelennamine), to pseudoephedrine or other adrenergic agents (such as albuterol, amphetamines, ephedrine, epinephrine, isoproterenol, metaproterenol, norepinephrine, phenylephrine, phenylpropanolamine, and terbutaline), or to codeine or any other narcotic cough suppressant or pain medication.
- Tell your doctor if you now have or if you have ever had asthma, brain disease, blockage of the urinary or digestive tract, diabetes mellitus, colitis, gallbladder disease, glaucoma, heart or blood vessel disease, high blood pressure, kidney disease, liver disease, lung disease, peptic ulcers, enlarged prostate gland, or thyroid disease.
- This medicine can cause drowsiness. Exercise caution while performing tasks that require alertness, such as driving a car or operating potentially dangerous machinery.
- While you are taking this medication, drink at least eight glasses of water a day to help loosen bronchial secretions.
- Because this product contains codeine, it has the potential for abuse and must be used with caution. Usually, it should not be taken on a regular schedule for longer than ten days at a time. Tolerance develops quickly; do not increase the dosage or stop taking the drug abruptly, unless you first consult your doctor. If you have been taking large amounts of this medication, or if you have been taking it for long periods of time, you may experience a withdrawal reaction (muscle aches, diarrhea, gooseflesh, runny nose, nausea, vomiting, shivering, trembling, stomach cramps, sleep disorders, irritability, weakness, excessive yawning, or sweating) when you stop taking it. Your doctor may, therefore, want to reduce the dosage gradually.
- Before surgery or other medical or dental treatment, tell your doctor or dentist you are taking this drug.
- Be sure to tell your doctor if you are pregnant. The effects of this drug during the early stages of pregnancy have not been thoroughly studied in humans. However, the regular use of codeine during the later stages of pregnancy may lead to addiction of the fetus, resulting in withdrawal symptoms (irritability, excessive crying, tremors, fever, vomiting, diarrhea, sneezing, or excessive yawning) in the newborn. Also, tell your doctor if you are breast-feeding. Small amounts of this drug pass into breast milk and may cause unusual excitement or irritability in nursing infants.

Pseudo-Hist—see pseudoephedrine and chlorpheniramine combination

Pyridamole—see dipyridamole

Pyridiate—see phenazopyridine

Pyridium—see phenazopyridine

Questran—see cholestyramine

Quiagen—see theophylline and guaifenesin combination

Quibron—see theophylline and guaifenesin combination

Quibron-300—see theophylline and guaifenesin combination

Quibron-T—see theophylline

Quinaglute Dura-Tabs—see quinidine

Quinatime—see quinidine

Quinidex Extentabs—see quinidine

---

quinidine

BRAND NAMES (Manufacturers)

Cardioquin (Purdue Frederick)
Cin-Quin (Reid-Rowell)
Duraquin (Parke-Davis)

Quinaglute Dura-Tabs (Berlex)
Quinatime (CMC)
Quinidex Extentabs (Robins)
quinidine gluconate (various manufacturers)
quinidine sulfate (various manufacturers)
Quinora (Key)
Quin-Release (Major)

TYPE OF DRUG
Antiarrhythmic

INGREDIENT
quinidine

DOSAGE FORMS
Tablets (100 mg, 200 mg, 275 mg, and 300 mg)
Sustained-release tablets (300 mg, 324 mg, and 330 mg)
Capsules (200 mg and 300 mg)

STORAGE
Quinidine tablets and capsules should be stored at room temperature in tightly closed, light-resistant containers.

USES

Quinidine is used to treat heart arrhythmias. It corrects irregular heartbeats and helps to achieve a more normal rhythm.

TREATMENT

To increase absorption of the drug, take quinidine on an empty stomach with a full glass of water one hour before or two hours after a meal. To lessen stomach upset, ask your doctor if you can take it with food or milk.

Try to take it at the same time(s) each day. Quinidine works best when the amount of the drug in your bloodstream is kept constant. This medication should, therefore, be taken at evenly spaced intervals day and night. For example, if you are to take quinidine four times per day, the doses should be spaced six hours apart.

The sustained-release tablets should be swallowed whole. Breaking, chewing, or crushing them destroys their sustained-release activity and may increase side effects.

If you miss a dose of this medication and remember within two hours, take the missed dose immediately and then return to your regular dosing schedule. If more than two hours have passed (four hours for the sustained-release tablets), do not take the missed dose at all; just return to your regular dosing schedule. Do not double the next dose.

SIDE EFFECTS

Minor. Abdominal pain, bitter taste in mouth, confusion, cramping, diarrhea, flushing, headache, loss of appetite, nausea, restlessness, or vomiting. These side effects should disappear as your body adjusts to the medication.

Major. Tell your doctor about any side effects that are persistent or particularly bothersome. IT IS ESPECIALLY IMPORTANT TO TELL YOUR DOCTOR about blurred vision, difficulty in breathing, dizziness, fainting, fever, headache, light-headedness, palpitations, ringing in the ears, sore throat, or unusual bleeding or bruising.

INTERACTIONS

Quinidine interacts with several foods and medications:

1. It can increase the effects of warfarin, which can lead to bleeding complications.

2. Acetazolamide, cimetidine, thiazide diuretics (water pills), sodium bicarbonate, antacids, and citrus fruit juices can increase the blood levels and thus the possibility of side effects of quinidine.

3. Nifedipine, phenobarbital, phenytoin, and rifampin can decrease blood levels of quinidine.

4. The combination of quinidine and phenothiazine tranquilizers, reserpine, nifedipine, amiodarone, or other antiarrhythmic agents can lead to cardiac side effects.

5. Quinidine can increase blood levels of digoxin, leading to serious side effects.

BE SURE TO TELL YOUR DOCTOR about any medications you are currently taking, especially any listed above.

WARNINGS

- Tell your doctor about unusual or allergic reactions you have had to any drugs, especially to quinidine or quinine.
- Before starting to take this medication, be sure to tell your doctor if you have ever had heart block, hypokalemia (low blood levels of potassium), kidney disease, liver disease, lung disease, myasthenia gravis, psoriasis, or thyroid disease.
- Although many quinidine products are on the market, they are not all bioequivalent; that is, they may not all be absorbed into the bloodstream at the same rate or have the same overall pharmacologic activity. Do not change brands of this drug without consulting your doctor or pharmacist.
- Do not take any over-the-counter (nonprescription) products for asthma, allergy, sinus, cough, cold, or weight reduction unless you first check with your doctor or pharmacist.
- If this drug makes you dizzy or light-headed, do not take part in any activity that requires alertness, such as driving a car or operating potentially dangerous machinery.
- Before having surgery or other medical or dental treatment, tell your doctor or dentist you are taking this drug.
- Do not stop taking this drug without first consulting your doctor. Stopping quinidine abruptly may cause a serious change in the activity of your heart. Your doctor may, therefore, want to reduce your dosage gradually.
- Be sure to tell your doctor if you are pregnant. Although this drug appears to be safe, extensive studies in pregnant women have not been conducted. Also, tell your doctor if you are breast-feeding an infant. Small amounts of quinidine pass into breast milk.

quinidine gluconate—see quinidine

quinidine sulfate—see quinidine

Quinora—see quinidine

Quin-Release—see quinidine

Racet—see hydrocortisone and iodochlorhydroxyquin combination

Racet SE—see hydrocortisone (topical)

---

ranitidine

BRAND NAMES (Manufacturers)
Zantac (Glaxo)
Zantac (Roche)

TYPE OF DRUG
Gastric acid secretion inhibitor (decreases stomach acid)
INGREDIENT
ranitidine
DOSAGE FORMS
Tablets (150 mg and 300 mg)
Oral syrup (15 mg per ml)
STORAGE
Ranitidine should be stored at room temperature in a tightly closed, light-resistant container.

USES

Ranitidine is used to treat duodenal and gastric ulcers. It is also used in the long-term treatment of excessive stomach acid secretion, in the prevention of recurrent ulcers, and in the treatment of reflex esophagitis (inflammation of the esophagus). Ranitidine works by blocking the effects of histamine on the stomach, thereby reducing stomach acid secretion.

TREATMENT

You can take ranitidine either on an empty stomach or with food or milk.

Antacids can block the absorption of ranitidine. If you are taking antacids as well as ranitidine, at least one hour should separate doses of the two medications.

If you miss a dose of this medication, take the missed dose as soon as possible, unless it is almost time for the next dose. In that case, do not take the missed dose at all; just return to your regular dosing schedule. Do not double the next dose.

SIDE EFFECTS

Minor. Constipation, diarrhea, dizziness, headache, nausea, or stomach upset. These side effects should disappear as your body adjusts to the medication.

To relieve constipation, exercise and drink more water (unless your doctor directs you to do otherwise).

If you feel dizzy while taking this medication, sit or lie down for a while; get up slowly from a sitting or reclining position, and be careful on stairs.

Major. Tell your doctor about any side effects that are persistent or particularly bothersome. IT IS ESPECIALLY IMPORTANT TO TELL YOUR DOCTOR about confusion, decreased sexual ability, unusual bleeding or bruising, or weakness.

INTERACTIONS

Ranitidine can interact with other types of medications:

1. Ranitidine may increase the blood-sugar-lowering effects of glipizide.

2. Ranitidine can decrease the elimination of warfarin from the body, which can increase the risk of bleeding complications.

3. Ranitidine can increase blood levels of procainamide.

4. Ranitidine may cause a false positive result with the Multistix urine protein test. Testing with sulfasalicylic acid is recommended.

BE SURE TO TELL YOUR DOCTOR about any medications you are currently taking, especially any listed above.

WARNINGS

• Tell your doctor about unusual or allergic reactions you have had to any medications, especially to ranitidine.

• Tell your doctor if you now have or if you have ever had kidney or liver disease.

• Ranitidine should be taken continuously for as long as your doctor prescribes. Stopping therapy early may be a cause of ineffective therapy.

• Cigarette smoking may block the beneficial effects of ranitidine.

• If this drug makes you dizzy, do not take part in any activity that requires alertness, such as driving a car or operating potentially dangerous machinery.

• Be sure to tell your doctor if you are pregnant. Ranitidine appears to be safe during pregnancy; however, extensive testing has not been conducted. Also, tell your doctor if you are breast-feeding an infant. Small amounts of ranitidine pass into breast milk.

Rectacort—see hydrocortisone, benzyl benzoate, bismuth resorcin compound, bismuth subgallate, zinc oxide, and Peruvian balsam combination (topical)

Reglan—see metoclopramide

Rela—see carisoprodol

Relaxadon—see atropine, scopolamine, hyoscyamine, and phenobarbital combination

Renoquid—see sulfonamide antibiotics (oral)

Reposans-10—see chlordiazepoxide

Resaid S.R.—see phenylpropanolamine and chlorpheniramine combination

---

reserpine

BRAND NAMES (Manufacturers)
reserpine (various manufacturers)
Serpalan (Lannett)
Serpasil (Ciba)
TYPE OF DRUG
Antihypertensive
INGREDIENT
reserpine
DOSAGE FORMS
Tablets (0.1 mg, 0.25 mg, and 1 mg)
Sustained-release capsules (0.5 mg)
STORAGE
Reserpine tablets and capsules should be stored at room temperature in tightly closed, light-resistant containers.

USES

Reserpine is used to treat high blood pressure. It works by depleting certain chemicals from the nervous system that are responsible for maintaining high blood pressure.

TREATMENT

To avoid stomach irritation, you can take reserpine with food or with a full glass of water or milk (unless your doctor directs otherwise). Try to take reserpine at the same time(s) each day, to become accustomed to taking it.

The sustained-release form of this medication should be swallowed whole. Chewing, crushing, or breaking these capsules destroys their sustained-release activity and possibly increases the side effects.

Reserpine does not cure hypertension, but it will help to control the condition as long as you continue to take it.

If you miss a dose of this medication, take the missed dose as soon as possible, unless it is almost time for the next dose. In that case, do not take the missed dose at all; just return to your regular dosing schedule. Do not double the next dose.

SIDE EFFECTS

Minor. Abdominal pain, constipation, decrease in sexual desire, diarrhea, dizziness, dry mouth, headache, impotence, loss of appetite, nasal congestion, nausea, nosebleeds, vomiting, or weight gain. These side effects should disappear as your body adjusts to the medication.

To relieve constipation, increase the amount of fiber in your diet (fresh fruits and vegetables, salads, bran, and whole-grain breads), exercise, and drink more water (unless your doctor directs you to do otherwise).

If you feel dizzy, sit or lie down for a while; get up slowly from a sitting or reclining position, and be careful on stairs.

To relieve mouth dryness, chew sugarless gum or suck on ice chips or a piece of hard candy.

Major. Tell your doctor about any side effects that are persistent or particularly bothersome. IT IS ESPECIALLY IMPORTANT TO TELL YOUR DOCTOR about anxiety; black, tarry stools; chest pain; depression; difficulty in urinating; drowsiness; enlarged breasts (in both sexes); fainting; fatigue; flushing of the skin; hearing loss; itching; muscle aches; nervousness; nightmares; palpitations; pinpoint pupils of eyes; rapid weight gain (three to five pounds within a week); rash; severe dizziness; shortness of breath; tremors; unusual bleeding or bruising; or weakness.

INTERACTIONS

Reserpine interacts with several other types of medications:

1. Concurrent use of reserpine with central nervous system depressants, such as alcohol, antihistamines, barbiturates, benzodiazepine tranquilizers, muscle relaxants, narcotics, pain medications, phenothiazine tranquilizers, and sleeping medications, or with tricyclic antidepressants can cause extreme drowsiness.

2. Reserpine can increase the side effects of digoxin, beta blockers, and quinidine and can decrease the effectiveness of levodopa.

3. Methotrimeprazine can increase the blood-pressure-lowering effects of reserpine, which can be dangerous.

4. Tricyclic antidepressants can decrease the blood-pressure-lowering effects of reserpine.

5. Concurrent use of reserpine and monoamine oxidase (MAO) inhibitors can lead to severe side effects. At least 14 days should separate the use of this drug and the use of an MAO inhibitor.

Before starting reserpine, BE SURE TO TELL YOUR DOCTOR about any drugs you are taking, especially those listed above.

WARNINGS

- Tell your doctor about unusual or allergic reactions you have had to any medications, especially to reserpine or to any rauwolfia alkaloids.
- Before starting to take this medication, be sure to tell your doctor if you now have or if you have ever had arrhythmias, epilepsy, gallstones or gallbladder disease, heart disease, kidney disease, lung disease, mental depression, Parkinson's disease, peptic ulcers, pheochromocytoma, or ulcerative colitis.
- Reserpine should not be used within two weeks of electroshock therapy.
- If this drug makes you dizzy or drowsy, do not take part in any activity that requires alertness, such as driving a car or operating potentially dangerous machinery.
- Before having surgery or any other medical or dental procedure, tell your doctor or dentist you are taking this drug.
- Before taking any over-the-counter (nonprescription) cough, cold, sinus, asthma, allergy, or diet medication, consult your doctor or pharmacist. Some of these products may increase your blood pressure.
- Be sure to tell your doctor if you are pregnant. Reserpine has been reported to cause birth defects in infants whose mothers received the drug during pregnancy. Also, tell your doctor if you are breast-feeding. Reserpine can pass into breast milk and cause side effects in the nursing infant.

Respbid—see theophylline

Restoril—see temazepam

Retin-A—see tretinoin

Rhinolar-Ex 12—see phenylpropanolamine and chlorpheniramine combination

Rhulicort—see hydrocortisone (topical)

Rhythmin—see procainamide

Ridaura—see auranofin

Rifadin—see rifampin

---

rifampin

BRAND NAMES (Manufacturers)
Rifadin (Merrell Dow)
Rimactane (Ciba)

TYPE OF DRUG
Antibiotic

INGREDIENT
rifampin

DOSAGE FORM
Capsules (150 mg and 300 mg)

STORAGE
Rifampin should be stored at room temperature in a tightly closed, light-resistant container.

USES

Rifampin is an antibiotic that is used to treat tuberculosis and to prevent meningococcal meningitis. Rifampin works by preventing the growth and multiplication of susceptible bacteria. Rifampin, however, is not effective against viruses, parasites, or fungi.

TREATMENT

Rifampin should be taken with a full glass of water on an empty stomach one hour before or two hours after a meal. If this medication causes stomach irritation, however, check with your doctor to see if you can take it with food.

Try not to miss any doses of this medication. If you do miss a dose, take the missed dose as soon as possible, unless it is almost time for your next dose. In that case, do not take the missed dose at all; just return to your regular dosing schedule. Do not double the next dose.

Continue to take this medication for the entire time prescribed by your doctor (which may be months to years), even if the symptoms disappear before the end of that period. If you stop taking the drug too soon, resistant bacteria are given a chance to continue growing, and your infection could recur.

SIDE EFFECTS

Minor. Diarrhea, dizziness, drowsiness, gas, headache, heartburn, loss of appetite, nausea, stomach irritation, or vomiting. These side effects should disappear as your body adjusts to the medication.

If you feel dizzy, sit or lie down for a while; get up slowly from a sitting or reclining position, and be careful on stairs.

Major. Tell your doctor about any side effects that are persistent or particularly bothersome. IT IS ESPECIALLY IMPORTANT TO TELL YOUR DOCTOR about confusion, difficult or painful urination, fatigue, fever, flushing, itching, muscle weakness, numbness, skin rash, uncoordinated movements, visual disturbances, or yellowing of the eyes or skin. Also, if your symptoms of infection seem to be worsening rather than improving, tell your doctor.

INTERACTIONS

Rifampin interacts with several other types of medications:

1. Concurrent use with p-aminosalicylic acid may decrease the blood levels and effectiveness of rifampin.

2. Rifampin can decrease the blood levels and effectiveness of metoprolol, propranolol, verapamil, aminophylline, theophylline, oxtriphylline, quinidine, adrenocorticosteroids (cortisone-like medicines), progestins, clofibrate, methadone, oral anticoagulants (blood thinners, such as warfarin), oral antidiabetic medicines, barbiturates, benzodiazepine tranquilizers, dapsone, digitoxin, and trimethoprim.

3. Concurrent use of rifampin with alcohol or isoniazid can lead to an increased risk of liver damage.

4. Rifampin may decrease the effectiveness of oral contraceptives (birth control pills), and pregnancy could result. You should, therefore, use a different or additional form of birth control while taking rifampin. Discuss this with your doctor.

Before starting to take rifampin, BE SURE TO TELL YOUR DOCTOR about any medications you are currently taking, especially any of those listed above.

WARNINGS

- Tell your doctor about unusual or allergic reactions you have had to any medications, especially to rifampin.
- Before starting to take this medication, be sure to tell your doctor if you have a history of alcoholism or liver disease.
- Rifampin has been prescribed for your current infection only. Another infection later on, or one that someone else has, may require a different medicine. You should not give your medicine to other people or use it for other infections, unless your doctor specifically directs you to do so.
- If this drug makes you dizzy or drowsy, do not take part in any activity that requires alertness, such as driving a car or operating potentially dangerous machinery.
- Rifampin can cause reddish-orange to reddish-brown discoloration of your urine, feces, saliva, sputum, sweat, and tears. This is a harmless effect. The drug may also permanently discolor soft contact lenses. You might want to stop wearing them while you are taking this medication. Discuss this with your ophthalmologist.
- Do not stop taking this medication unless you first check with your doctor. Stopping the drug and restarting it at a later time can lead to an increase in side effects.
- Be sure to tell your doctor if you are pregnant. Although rifampin appears to be safe in humans, birth defects have been reported in the offspring of animals that received large doses of the drug during pregnancy. Also, tell your doctor if you are breast-feeding an infant. Small amounts of rifampin pass into breast milk.

Rimactane—see rifampin

Ritalin—see methylphenidate

Ritalin-SR—see methylphenidate

---

ritodrine

BRAND NAME (Manufacturer)
Yutopar (Astra)

TYPE OF DRUG
Beta-adrenergic receptor agonist (labor inhibitor)

INGREDIENT
ritodrine

DOSAGE FORM
Tablets (10 mg)

STORAGE
Ritodrine should be stored at room temperature in a tightly closed container.

USES

Ritodrine is used to prevent premature labor. It belongs to a group of drugs called beta-adrenergic nerve receptor stimulants. It prevents premature labor by relaxing uterine muscle, thus decreasing the strength and frequency of uterine contractions.

TREATMENT

Ritodrine treatment is usually begun intravenously. Once the contractions stop, the medication is generally continued orally (in tablet form).

Ritodrine tablets can be taken either on an empty stomach or with food or milk (as directed by your doctor).

BE SURE YOU UNDERSTAND YOUR DOCTOR'S INSTRUCTIONS on how this medication should be taken.

It is important to try not to miss any doses of this medication. If you do miss a dose and remember within an hour, take the missed dose immediately. If more than an hour has passed, do not take the missed dose at all; just return to your regular dosing schedule. Do not double the next dose of the medication.

SIDE EFFECTS

Minor. Nausea or jitteriness. These side effects should disappear as your body adjusts to the medication.
Major. Tell your doctor about any side effects that are persistent or particularly bothersome. IT IS ESPECIALLY IMPORTANT TO TELL YOUR DOCTOR about palpitations, shortness of breath, skin rash, tremors, or vomiting.

INTERACTIONS

This medication interacts with a number of types of medications:
1. Beta blockers (acebutolol, atenolol, betaxolol, carteolol, esmolol, labetalol, metoprolol, nadolol, penbutolol, pindolol, propranolol, timolol) decrease the effectiveness of ritodrine.
2. Concurrent use of ritodrine and adrenocorticosteroids (cortisone-like medicines) can lead to additional side effects in the mother or newborn.

BE SURE TO TELL YOUR DOCTOR about any medications you are currently taking, especially any of those listed above.

WARNINGS

• Be sure to tell your doctor about any unusual or allergic reactions that you have had to any medications, especially to ritodrine.
• Before starting to take ritodrine, be sure to tell your doctor if you now have or if you have ever had diabetes mellitus, eclampsia or pre-eclampsia, heart disease, high blood pressure, pulmonary hypertension, or thyroid disease.
• Do not take any over-the-counter (nonprescription) cough, cold, allergy, asthma, sinus, or diet medication, unless you first check with your doctor or pharmacist. Some of these products decrease the effectiveness of ritodrine.
• You should CHECK WITH YOUR DOCTOR IMMEDIATELY for further instructions if your contractions begin again or if your water bag breaks while you are taking this medication.

RMS—see morphine

Robaxin—see methocarbamol

Robicillin VK—see penicillin VK

Robimycin—see erythromycin

Robitet Robicaps—see tetracycline

Robitussin A-C—see codeine and guaifenesin combination

Rocaltrol—see calcitriol

Rogaine—see minoxidil (topical)

Rondec—see pseudoephedrine and carbinoxamine combination

Rondec-DM—see pseudoephedrine, carbinoxamine, and dextromethorphan combination

Roxanol—see morphine

Roxanol SR—see morphine

Rufen—see ibuprofen

Rum-K—see potassium chloride

Ru-Tuss II—see phenylpropanolamine and chlorpheniramine combination

Ru-Vert-M—see meclizine

Rymed-TR—see phenylpropanolamine and guaifenesin combination

Ryna—see pseudoephedrine and chlorpheniramine combination

Sandimmune—see cyclosporine

Sanorex—see mazindol

S.A.S.-500—see sulfasalazine

Satric—see metronidazole

Scabene—see lindane

---

scopolamine (transdermal)

BRAND NAME (Manufacturer)
Transderm-Scop (Ciba)
TYPE OF DRUG
Antiemetic and antivertigo
INGREDIENT
scopolamine
DOSAGE FORM
Transdermal system (the patch delivers 0.5 mg of scopolamine over three days)
STORAGE
The patches should be stored at room temperature in their original containers away from direct heat and light.

USES

Scopolamine is used to prevent nausea and vomiting associated with motion sickness. Scopolamine is one of a group of substances known as belladonna alkaloids. Transdermal scopolamine is a small patch that is applied to the skin. Transdermal application (i.e. application of medicine through the skin) delivers reduced doses of scopolamine, which are large enough to be effective but small enough to decrease the risk of adverse side effects.

TREATMENT

The transdermal system (patches) allows controlled continuous release of scopolamine. Patches are easy to use and convenient. For best results, wash and dry hands thoroughly before handling. Apply the disc to the hairless area of the skin behind the ear at least four hours before the antiemetic effect is required. Do not place over any cuts or irritations. Wash hands thoroughly after handling the disc to prevent direct contact of the medication with the eyes. The medication should last up to three days. If treatment is needed for more than three days, discard the used disc, and replace with a new disc behind the other ear. It is all right to bathe or shower with a patch in place. If the disc becomes displaced at any time during treatment, it should be discarded, and a fresh one placed on the hairless area behind the other ear. If redness or irritation develops at the application site, consult your physician. Do not trim or cut the patches. This alters the dose of the medication.

SIDE EFFECTS

Minor. Blurred vision and dilation of pupils; drowsiness; or dryness of mouth, nose, and throat.

To relieve mouth dryness, chew sugarless gum or suck on ice chips or hard candy.

If you feel dizzy or light-headed, sit or lie down for a while; get up slowly from a sitting or reclining position, and be careful on stairs.

Major. Tell your doctor about any side effects that are persistent or particularly bothersome. IT IS ESPECIALLY IMPORTANT TO TELL YOUR DOCTOR ABOUT blurred vision (severe); confusion (severe); convulsions; difficulty in breathing; dizziness; drowsiness (severe); dry mouth, nose, or throat (severe); eye pain (severe); fast heart beat; fever; rash; slurred speech; unusual excitement or restlessness; unusual warmth; dryness; or flushing of the skin.

INTERACTIONS

Scopolamine can interact with other types of medications:

1. It can cause additive drowsiness when combined with alcohol or other central nervous system depressants (such as antihistamines, barbiturates, benzodiazepine tranquilizers, muscle relaxants, narcotics, and pain medications) or with tricyclic antidepressants.

2. It can cause additive anticholinergic effects (such as dryness of mouth, nose, and throat, or difficulty in urinating) when combined with drugs such as belladonna alkaloids, antidepressants, and antihistamines.

Before starting to take scopolamine, BE SURE TO TELL YOUR DOCTOR about any medications you are currently taking, especially any of those listed above.

WARNINGS

- Tell your doctor about unusual or allergic reactions you have had to any medications, especially to scopolamine.
- Tell your doctor if you now have or if you have ever had blockage of the urinary tract, stomach, or intestinal tract.
- Tell your doctor if you now have or if you have ever had metabolic, liver, or kidney disease.
- Tell your doctor if you have glaucoma (increased pressure in the eyeball).
- This medication may cause drowsiness or blurred vision. Make sure you know how you react to this medication before you attempt activities such as driving a car or operating potentially dangerous equipment.
- Patients who use the patch for more than three days are more likely to experience dizziness, headache, nausea, or vomiting for a short time following discontinuation.
- Do not use the transdermal system on children.
- Elderly patients may be especially susceptible to the central nervous system effects (confusion, sedation, memory impairment, unusual excitement) of scopolamine.
- Be sure to tell your doctor if you are pregnant. Extensive studies in pregnant women have not been conducted. Also, tell your doctor if you are breast-feeding. It is not known whether scopolamine passes into breast milk.

---

secobarbital

BRAND NAMES (Manufacturers)

secobarbital sodium (various manufacturers)
Seconal (Lilly)

TYPE OF DRUG

Barbiturate sedative/hypnotic

INGREDIENT

secobarbital

DOSAGE FORMS

Tablets (100 mg)
Capsules (50 mg and 100 mg)

STORAGE

Secobarbital tablets and capsules should be stored at room temperature in tightly closed containers.

USES

Secobarbital belongs to a group of drugs known as barbiturates, which are central nervous system depressants (drugs that slow the activity of the brain and spinal cord). This medication is used as a sleeping aid in the treatment of insomnia.

TREATMENT

You can take secobarbital at bedtime. The tablets and capsules can be taken with water, food, or milk.

You should not use this drug as a sleeping aid for more than two weeks. With prolonged use, secobarbital loses its ability to induce and sustain sleep.

SIDE EFFECTS

Minor. Constipation, diarrhea, dizziness, drowsiness, a "hangover" feeling, headache, nausea, nightmares, stomach upset, or vomiting. These side effects should disappear as your body adjusts to the medication.

If you feel dizzy or light-headed, sit or lie down for a while; get up slowly from a sitting or reclining position, and be careful on stairs.

To relieve constipation, increase the amount of fiber in your diet (fresh fruits and vegetables, salads, bran, and whole-grain breads), exercise, and drink more water (unless your doctor directs you to do otherwise).

Major. Tell your doctor about any side effects that are persistent or particularly bothersome. IT IS ESPECIALLY IMPORTANT TO TELL YOUR DOCTOR about chest tightness, confusion, depression, difficulty in breathing, excitation, fatigue, feeling faint, fever, hives or itching, loss of coordination, muscle or joint pain, skin rash, slurred speech, sore throat, unusual bleeding or bruising, unusual weakness, or yellowing of the eyes or skin.

INTERACTIONS

Secobarbital interacts with several other types of medications:

1. Concurrent use of this barbiturate medication with other central nervous system depressants (such as alcohol, antihistamines, benzodiazepine tranquilizers, muscle relaxants, narcotics, pain medications, and phenothiazine tranquilizers) or with tricyclic antidepressants can cause extreme drowsiness.
2. Valproic acid, chloramphenicol, and monoamine oxidase (MAO) inhibitors can prolong the effects of secobarbital.
3. Secobarbital can decrease the blood levels and effectiveness of oral anticoagulants (blood thinners, such as warfarin), digoxin, tricyclic antidepressants, cortisone-like medicines, doxycycline, quinidine, estrogens, oral contraceptives (birth control pills), phenytoin, acetaminophen, and carbamazepine.
4. The combination of secobarbital and furosemide can cause low blood pressure and fainting.
5. Secobarbital can increase the side effects of cyclophosphamide or large doses of acetaminophen.

Before starting secobarbital, BE SURE TO TELL YOUR DOCTOR about any medications you are currently taking, especially any of those listed above.

WARNINGS

- Tell your doctor about unusual or allergic reactions you have had to any medications, especially to secobarbital or to other barbiturates (such as amobarbital, butabarbital, mephobarbital, metharbital, pentobarbital, phenobarbital, and primidone).
- Tell your doctor if you now have or if you have ever had acute or chronic (long-term) pain, Addison's disease (caused by an underactive adrenal gland), diabetes mellitus, kidney disease, liver disease, lung disease, mental depression, porphyria, or thyroid disease.
- If this medication makes you dizzy or drowsy during the day, do not take part in any activity that requires alertness, such as driving a car or operating potentially dangerous machinery.
- Children, the elderly, and very ill patients are more likely to experience unusual excitement, confusion, or mental depression.
- Secobarbital has the potential for abuse and must be used with caution. Tolerance to the medication develops quickly; do not increase the dosage or stop taking this drug unless you first consult your doctor. If you have been taking secobarbital for a long time or have been taking large doses, you may experience anxiety, muscle twitching, tremors, weakness, dizziness, nausea, vomiting, insomnia, or blurred vision when you stop taking it. To avoid or minimize this reaction, your doctor may want to reduce your dosage gradually.
- Be sure to tell your doctor if you are pregnant. Barbiturates cross the placenta, and there has been an association between birth defects and the use of this class of drugs during pregnancy. Such drugs may also lead to bleeding complications in the newborn. The risks involved with secobarbital therapy should be discussed with your doctor. In addition, if secobarbital is used for long periods during the last three months of pregnancy, there is a chance that the infant will be born addicted to the medication and will experience a withdrawal reaction (convulsions, irritability) at birth. Also, tell your doctor if you are breast-feeding an infant. Small amounts of secobarbital pass into breast milk and may cause excessive drowsiness and breathing problems in nursing infants.

secobarbital sodium—see secobarbital

Seconal—see secobarbital

Sectral—see acebutolol

Seldane—see terfenadine

---

selegiline

BRAND NAME (Manufacturer)
Eldepryl (Somerset)

TYPE OF DRUG
Antiparkinson agent

INGREDIENT
selegiline

DOSAGE FORM
Tablets (5 mg)

STORAGE
Selegiline should be stored at room temperature in a tightly closed container.

USES

This medication is used either alone or in combination with levodopa or levodopa/carbidopa to treat the symptoms of Parkinson's disease. This drug helps to increase and extend the beneficial effects of levodopa. Recent studies suggest that selegiline may help to slow the progression of Parkinson's disease when taken early in the course of the disease. This drug has also been used to treat depression.

TREATMENT

This medication should be taken exactly as your doctor prescribes. You can take it with food to lessen the chance of stomach irritation, unless your doctor tells you otherwise.

If you miss a dose of this medication, take the missed dose as soon as possible, then return to your regular dosing schedule. However, if you do not remember the missed dose until late afternoon or evening, skip the missed dose. If the drug is taken late in the afternoon, it may cause some unwanted side effects. Never double the dose.

The full effects of this medication may not be apparent for two to three days. At that time, your doctor may change your dose of levodopa or levodopa/carbidopa.

SIDE EFFECTS

Minor. Dizziness, drowsiness, dryness of mouth, headache, heartburn, light-headedness, nausea, nervousness, restlessness, stomach pain, trouble sleeping, or vomiting. These side effects should lessen or disappear as your body adjusts to the medication.

Dry mouth can be relieved by chewing sugarless gum or by sucking on ice chips or a piece of hard candy.

To avoid dizziness or light-headedness when you stand, contract and relax the muscles of your legs for a few moments before rising. Do this by pushing one foot against the floor while raising the other foot slightly, alternating feet so that you are "pumping" your legs in a pedaling motion.

Major. Tell your doctor about any side effects that are persistent or particularly bothersome. IT IS ESPECIALLY IMPORTANT TO TELL YOUR DOCTOR about blood in your urine; chest pain; convulsions; dark or tarry stools; difficulty in breathing; difficulty in speaking; difficulty in urination; fast heartbeat; feelings of euphoria; hallucinations; mood changes; persistent restlessness; severe stomach pain; stiff neck; or uncontrolled movements of your arms, legs, or face.

INTERACTIONS

When taken in the recommended dose at the times directed by your doctor, selegiline should not interact with many types of medications or foods.

Be sure to tell your doctor if you have received the drug meperidine anytime within the two to three weeks before starting selegiline therapy.

Be sure to tell your doctor about any medications, including over-the-counter products, you are currently taking.

WARNINGS

- Tell your doctor if you have had unusual or allergic reactions to any medications, especially to selegiline or to any monoamine oxidase (MAO) inhibitors (such as tranylcypromine, phenelzine, or isocarboxazid).
- Tell your doctor if you have a history of stomach problems, intestinal problems, asthma, high blood pressure, or seizure disorders.
- If this drug makes you dizzy or drowsy, do not take part in any activity that requires alertness, such as driving a car or operating potentially dangerous equipment.
- Before having surgery or any other medical or dental treatment, tell your doctor or dentist that you are taking this medication.
- Your doctor may give you a list of foods that you should either avoid or limit in your diet. These foods or beverages may include those containing caffeine (coffee, tea, cola, or chocolate) or those containing a substance called tyramine (found in certain cheeses and meats).
- Be sure to tell your doctor if you are pregnant. This drug has not caused adverse effects to the fetus in animal studies, and problems in humans have not been reported. Also, tell your doctor if you are breast-feeding an infant. It is not known whether selegiline passes into breast milk.

Sensacort—see hydrocortisone (topical)

Septra—see sulfamethoxazole and trimethoprim combination

Septra DS—see sulfamethoxazole and trimethoprim combination

Ser-A-Gen—see hydralazine, hydrochlorothiazide, and reserpine combination

Seralazide—see hydralazine, hydrochlorothiazide, and reserpine combination

Ser-Ap-Es—see hydralazine, hydrochlorothiazide, and reserpine combination

Serax—see oxazepam

Serentil—see mesoridazine

Serophene—see clomiphene

Serpalan—see reserpine

Serpasil—see reserpine

Serpazide—see hydralazine, hydrochlorothiazide, and reserpine combination

Sinequan—see doxepin

Sleep-Eze 3—see diphenhydramine

Slo-bid Gyrocaps—see theophylline

Slo-Phyllin—see theophylline

Slo-Phyllin-GG—see theophylline and guaifenesin combination

Slow-K—see potassium chloride

Slyn-LL—see phendimetrazine

Sodium Sulamyd—see sodium sulfacetamide (ophthalmic)

---

sodium sulfacetamide (ophthalmic)

BRAND NAMES (Manufacturers)

AK-Sulf (Akorn)
AK-Sulf Forte (Akorn)
Bleph-10 (Allergan)
Cetamide (Alcon)
Isopto Cetamide (Alcon)
Ophthacet (Vortech)
Sodium Sulamyd (Schering)
sodium sulfacetamide (various manufacturers)
Sulf-10 (Iolab Pharm.)
Sulfair 15 (Pharmafair)
Sulten-10 (Bausch & Lomb)

TYPE OF DRUG

Ophthalmic antibiotic

INGREDIENT

sodium sulfacetamide

DOSAGE FORMS

Ophthalmic drops (10%, 15%, and 30%)
Ophthalmic ointment (10%)

STORAGE

Sodium sulfacetamide drops and ointment should be stored

at room temperature in tightly closed containers. This medication should never be frozen. If the eye drops discolor or turn brown, they should be discarded. A change in color signifies a loss of potency.

USES

Sodium sulfacetamide is used to treat bacterial eye infections and corneal ulcers. Sodium sulfacetamide is an antibiotic that is effective against a wide range of bacteria. It acts by preventing production of the nutrients that are required for growth of the infecting bacteria. This medication, however, is not effective against infections that are caused by viruses or fungi.

TREATMENT

Wash your hands with soap and water before applying this medication. To avoid contamination of the eye drops or ointment, be careful not to touch the tube of the dropper or the tip of the ointment tube or let them touch your eyes; DO NOT wipe off or rinse the dropper after use.

To apply the drops, tilt your head back and pull down the lower eyelid with one hand to make a pouch below the eye. Drop the prescribed amount of medicine into this pouch and slowly close your eyes. Try not to blink. Keep your eyes closed, and place one finger at the corner of the eye next to your nose for a minute or two, applying a slight pressure (this is done to prevent loss of medication through the duct that drains fluid from the surface of the eye into the nose and throat). Then wipe away any excess with a clean tissue.

To apply the ointment, tilt the head back, pull down the lower lid to form a pouch below the eye, and squeeze a small amount of ointment (approximately 1/8 to 1/4 inch) in a line along the pouch. Close the eyes, and place your finger at the corner of the eye next to your nose for a minute or two. Do not rub your eyes. Wipe off excess ointment with a clean tissue.

Since this medication is somewhat difficult to apply, you may want to have someone else apply it for you.

It is important to continue to take this medication for the entire time prescribed by your doctor, even if the symptoms disappear before the end of that period. If you stop applying the drug too soon, resistant bacteria are given a chance to continue growing, and the infection could recur.

If you miss a dose of this medication, apply the missed dose as soon as possible, unless it is almost time for your next dose. In that case, do not apply the missed dose at all; just return to your regular dosing schedule. Do not use twice as much medication at the next dose.

SIDE EFFECTS

Minor. Sodium sulfacetamide may cause blurred vision or burning or stinging in the eyes immediately after it is applied (especially the 30% solution). This effect should last only a few minutes.

Major. Tell your doctor about any side effects that are persistent or particularly bothersome. IT IS ESPECIALLY IMPORTANT TO TELL YOUR DOCTOR about signs of irritation in the eyes (such as redness, swelling, or itching) that last more than several minutes, chills, fever, itching, or difficulty in breathing. Also, if your symptoms of infection seem to be getting worse rather than improving, you should contact your doctor.

INTERACTIONS

This drug is incompatible with silver preparations.

WARNINGS

- Tell your doctor about unusual or allergic reactions you have had to any medications, especially to sodium sulfacetamide or to any other sulfa medication (diuretics, oral antidiabetic medications, sulfonamide antibiotics).
- This medication may cause allergic-type symptoms, such as hives, itching, wheezing, or anaphylaxis, in sulfite-sensitive patients.
- Sodium sulfacetamide may cause eye sensitivity to bright light; wearing sunglasses may lessen this problem.
- This medication has been prescribed for your current infection only. Another infection later on, or one that someone else has, may require a different medicine. You should not give your medicine to other people or use it for other infections, unless your doctor specifically directs you to do so.
- In order to allow your eye infection to clear, do not apply makeup to the affected eye.
- If there is no change in your condition two or three days after starting to take this medication, contact your doctor. The medication may not be effective for your particular infection.
- Be sure to tell your doctor if you are pregnant. The safe use of this medication in human pregnancy has not been established. Although an ophthalmic, if large amounts of this drug are applied for prolonged periods, some of it may be absorbed into the bloodstream. Also, tell your doctor if you are breast-feeding an infant. If this drug is absorbed, small amounts may pass into the breast milk and may temporarily alter the bacterial balance in the intestinal tract of the nursing infant, resulting in diarrhea.

Sofarin—see warfarin

Solfoton—see phenobarbital

Soma—see carisoprodol

Sominex 2—see diphenhydramine

Somophyllin—see aminophylline

Somophyllin-DF—see aminophylline

Somophyllin-T—see theophylline

Sonazine—see chlorpromazine

Soprodol—see carisoprodol

Sorbitrate—see isosorbide dinitrate

Sorbitrate SA—see isosorbide dinitrate

Spancap No. 1—see dextroamphetamine

Sparine—see promazine

Spasmolin—see atropine, scopolamine, hyoscyamine, and phenobarbital combination

Spasmophen—see atropine, scopolamine, hyoscyamine, and phenobarbital combination

Spasquid—see atropine, scopolamine, hyoscyamine, and phenobarbital combination

Spironazide—see spironolactone and hydrochlorothiazide combination

---

spironolactone

BRAND NAMES (Manufacturers)
Alatone (Major)
Aldactone (Searle)
spironolactone (various manufacturers)
TYPE OF DRUG
Diuretic and antihypertensive
INGREDIENT
spironolactone
DOSAGE FORM
Tablets (25 mg, 50 mg, and 100 mg)
STORAGE
Spironolactone should be stored at room temperature in a tightly closed, light-resistant container.

USES

Spironolactone is prescribed to treat high blood pressure. It is also used to reduce fluid accumulation in the body caused by conditions such as heart failure, cirrhosis of the liver, kidney disease, and the long-term use of some medications. Spironolactone reduces fluid accumulation by increasing the elimination of salt and water through the kidneys. It may be used in combination with other diuretics to prevent potassium loss. Since spironolactone blocks the effects of a chemical (aldosterone) released from the adrenal gland, it can also be used to diagnose and treat an overactive adrenal gland.

TREATMENT

To decrease stomach irritation, you can take spironolactone with a glass of milk or with a meal (unless your doctor directs you to do otherwise). Try to take it at the same time every day. Avoid taking a dose after 6:00 P.M.; otherwise, you may have to get up during the night to urinate.

If you miss a dose of this medication, take the missed dose as soon as possible, unless it is almost time for the next dose. In that case, do not take the missed dose at all; just wait until the next scheduled dose. Do not double the dose.

This medication does not cure high blood pressure, but it will help to control the condition as long as you take it.

SIDE EFFECTS

Minor. Cramping, diarrhea, dizziness, drowsiness, dry mouth, headache, increased urination, nausea, rash, restlessness, vomiting, or weakness. As your body adjusts to the medication, these side effects should disappear.

Dry mouth can be relieved by chewing sugarless gum or by sucking on ice chips or a piece of hard candy.

To avoid dizziness or light-headedness when you stand, contract and relax the muscles of your legs for a few moments before rising. Do this by pushing one foot against the floor while raising the other foot slightly, alternating feet so that you are "pumping" your legs in a pedaling motion.

Major. Tell your doctor about any side effects that are persistent or particularly bothersome. IT IS ESPECIALLY IMPORTANT TO TELL YOUR DOCTOR about anxiety; clumsiness; confusion; deepening of the voice (in women); enlarged breasts (in both sexes); fever; impotence; increased hair growth; menstrual disturbances; muscle cramps; numbness or tingling in the hands, feet, or lips; palpitations; postmenopausal bleeding; rapid weight gain (three to five pounds within a week); stomach cramps; uncoordinated movements; or unusual tiredness or weakness.

INTERACTIONS

Spironolactone interacts with several foods and medications:

1. Concurrent use of spironolactone with amiloride, triamterene, potassium salts, low-salt milk, salt substitutes, captopril, or laxatives can cause serious side effects from hyperkalemia (high levels of potassium in the blood).
2. Spironolactone may increase the side effects of lithium, digoxin, digitoxin, and ammonium chloride.
3. The effectiveness of oral anticoagulants (blood thinners, such as warfarin) may be decreased by this medication.
4. Aspirin may decrease the diuretic effects of spironolactone.

Before starting to take spironolactone, BE SURE TO TELL YOUR DOCTOR about any medications you are currently taking, especially any of those listed above.

WARNINGS

• Tell your doctor about unusual or allergic reactions you have had to any medications, especially to spironolactone or to any other diuretic.
• Tell your doctor if you now have or if you have ever had kidney or urination problems, heart disease, hyperkalemia (high blood levels of potassium), liver disease, menstrual abnormalities, breast enlargement, or diabetes mellitus.
• Spironolactone can cause hyperkalemia. Signs of hyperkalemia include palpitations; confusion; numbness or tingling in the hands, feet, or lips; anxiety; or unusual tiredness or weakness. However, do not alter your diet in an effort to avoid this problem, unless your doctor tells you to do so. Elderly patients may be more susceptible to hyperkalemia.
• There are several "generic brands" of this drug. Consult your pharmacist about these items; some of them are not equivalent to the brand-name medications.
• Limit your intake of alcoholic beverages in order to prevent dizziness and light-headedness while taking this medication.
• Do not take any over-the-counter (nonprescription) medication for weight control or for allergy, asthma, cough, cold, or sinus problems unless you first check with your doctor. Some of these products can increase blood pressure.
• To prevent severe water loss (dehydration) while taking this medication, check with your doctor if you have any illness that causes severe or continuous nausea, vomiting, or diarrhea.
• Be sure to tell your doctor if you are pregnant. This drug crosses the placenta, and its safety in human pregnancy has not been established. Adverse effects have been observed in

the fetuses of animals that were given large doses of this drug during pregnancy. Also, tell your doctor if you are breast-feeding an infant. Small amounts of this drug pass into breast milk.

---

spironolactone and hydrochlorothiazide combination

BRAND NAMES (Manufacturers)
Alazide (Major)
Aldactazide (Searle)
Spironazide (Henry Schein)
spironolactone and hydrochlorothiazide (various manufacturers)
Spirozide (Rugby)

TYPE OF DRUG
Diuretic and antihypertensive

INGREDIENTS
spironolactone and hydrochlorothiazide

DOSAGE FORM
Tablets (25 mg spironolactone and 25 mg hydrochlorothiazide; 50 mg spironolactone and 50 mg hydrochlorothiazide)

STORAGE
Store at room temperature in a tightly closed, light-resistant container.

USES

Spironolactone and hydrochlorothiazide combination is prescribed to treat high blood pressure. It is also used to reduce fluid acccumulation in the body caused by conditions such as heart failure, cirrhosis of the liver, kidney disease, and the long-term use of some medications. This medication reduces fluid accumulation by increasing the elimination of salt and water through the kidneys. Spironolactone is combined with hydrochlorothiazide to prevent potassium loss from the body.

TREATMENT

To decrease stomach irritation, you can take this medication with a glass of milk or with a meal (unless your doctor directs you to do otherwise). Try to take it at the same time every day. Avoid taking a dose after 6:00 P.M.; otherwise, you may have to get up during the night to urinate.

If you miss a dose of this medication, take the missed dose as soon as possible, unless it is almost time for the next dose. In that case, do not take the missed dose at all; just wait until the next scheduled dose. Do not double the dose.

This medication does not cure high blood pressure, but it will help to control the condition as long as you take it.

SIDE EFFECTS

Minor. Constipation, cramping, diarrhea, dizziness, headache, increased urination, loss of appetite, lack of energy, light-headedness, restlessness, or unusual sweating. These side effects should disappear as your body adjusts to this medication.

This medication can increase your sensitivity to sunlight. You should, therefore, avoid prolonged exposure to sunlight and sunlamps. Wear protective clothing, and use an effective sunscreen.

To relieve constipation, increase the amount of fiber in your diet (fresh fruits and vegetables, salads, bran, and whole-grain breads) and exercise more (unless your doctor directs you to do otherwise).

To avoid dizziness or light-headedness when you stand, contract and relax the muscles of your legs for a few moments before rising. Do this by pushing one foot against the floor while raising the other foot slightly, alternating feet so that you are "pumping" your legs in a pedaling motion.

Major. Tell your doctor about any side effects that are persistent or particularly bothersome. IT IS ESPECIALLY IMPORTANT TO TELL YOUR DOCTOR about anxiety; blurred vision; breast tenderness or enlargement (in both sexes); clumsiness; confusion; deepening of the voice (in women); drowsiness; dry mouth; impotence; increased hair growth; irregular menstrual periods or vaginal bleeding; joint pain; mood changes; muscle cramps; nausea; numbness or tingling in the hands, feet, or lips; palpitations; rapid weight gain (three to five pounds within a week); rash; sore throat and fever; swelling; thirst; unusual bleeding or bruising; unusual tiredness or weakness; vomiting; or yellowing of the eyes or skin.

INTERACTIONS

Spironolactone and hydrochlorothiazide combination interacts with several foods and medications:

1. Concurrent use of it with triamterene, amiloride, potassium salts, low-salt milk, salt substitutes, captopril, or laxatives can cause serious side effects from hyperkalemia (high levels of potassium in the blood).

2. This drug may decrease the effectiveness of oral anticoagulants, antigout medications, insulin, oral antidiabetic medicines, and methenamine.

3. Fenfluramine may increase the blood-pressure-lowering effects of this drug.

4. Indomethacin and aspirin may decrease the blood-pressure-lowering effects of this medication.

5. Cholestyramine and colestipol can decrease the absorption of this medication from the gastrointestinal tract. Therefore, spironolactone and hydrochlorothiazide combination should be taken one hour before or four hours after a dose of cholestyramine or colestipol if either of these medications has also been prescribed for you.

6. Spironolactone and hydrochlorothiazide may increase the side effects of amphotericin B, ammonium chloride, calcium, cortisone and cortisone-like steroids (such as dexamethasone, hydrocortisone, prednisone, and prednisolone), digoxin, digitoxin, digitalis, lithium, quinidine, sulfonamide antibiotics, and vitamin D.

BE SURE TO TELL YOUR DOCTOR about any medications you are currently taking, especially any listed above.

WARNINGS

- Tell your doctor about unusual or allergic reactions you have had to any medications, especially to spironolactone or hydrochlorothiazide or to any other sulfa drug, including other diuretics (water pills), oral antidiabetic medications, or sulfonamide antibiotics.

• Before you start taking this medication, tell your doctor if you now have or if you have ever had kidney disease or problems with urination, diabetes mellitus, gout, liver disease, asthma, pancreas disease, systemic lupus erythematosus, hyperkalemia, menstrual abnormalities, breast enlargement, acidosis, or hypercalcemia.
• This drug can occasionally cause potassium loss from the body. Signs of potassium loss include dry mouth, muscle pain or cramps, nausea, thirst, vomiting, and weakness. If you experience any of these symptoms, call your doctor.
• Spironolactone can cause hyperkalemia. Signs of hyperkalemia include anxiety; confusion; numbness or tingling in the hands, feet, or lips; palpitations; or unusual tiredness or weakness. Do not alter your diet in an attempt to avoid this problem unless you first consult your doctor. Elderly patients may be more susceptible to hyperkalemia.
• There are several "generic brands" of this drug. Consult your pharmacist about these items. Some of them are not equivalent to the brand-name medications.
• Limit your intake of alcoholic beverages to prevent dizziness and light-headedness while taking this drug.
• Do not take any over-the-counter (nonprescription) medication for weight control or for allergy, asthma, cough, cold, or sinus problems unless you first check with your doctor.
• To prevent severe water loss (dehydration), check with your doctor if you develop any illness that causes severe or continuous nausea, vomiting, or diarrhea.
• This medication can raise blood sugar levels in diabetic patients. Blood sugar should be monitored carefully with blood or urine tests when this drug is being taken.
• A doctor does not usually prescribe a "fixed-dose" drug like this as the first choice in the treatment of high blood pressure. Usually, the patient first receives each ingredient singly. If there is an adequate response to the fixed dose contained in this product, it can then be substituted. The advantages of a combination product are increased convenience and (often) decreased cost.
• Be sure to tell your doctor if you are pregnant. This drug crosses the placenta, and its safety in human pregnancy has not been established. Adverse effects have been observed in the fetuses of animals that were given large doses of this drug during pregnancy. Also, tell your doctor if you are breast-feeding an infant. Small amounts of this medication pass into breast milk.

Spirozide—see spironolactone and hydrochlorothiazide combination

S-P-T—see thyroid hormone

Statobex—see phendimetrazine

Stelazine—see trifluoperazine

StuartNatal 1 + 1—see vitamins, prenatal

---

sucralfate

BRAND NAME (Manufacturer)
Carafate (Marion)

TYPE OF DRUG
Antiulcer

INGREDIENT
sucralfate

DOSAGE FORM
Tablets (1 g)

STORAGE
Sucralfate should be stored at room temperature in a tightly closed container.

USES

Sucralfate is used for the short-term treatment of ulcers. This medication binds to the surface of the ulcer, thereby protecting it from stomach acid and promoting healing.

TREATMENT

In order to obtain maximum benefit from this drug, you should swallow it whole with a full glass of water. Take it on an empty stomach one hour before or two hours after a meal and at bedtime. Do not take antacids within 30 minutes before or one hour after taking sucralfate.

Continue to take sucralfate for the full length of time prescribed by your doctor, even if your symptoms disappear. Your ulcer may not yet be healed. However, do not take it for more than eight weeks without your doctor's authorization.

If you miss a dose of this medication, take the missed dose as soon as possible, unless it is almost time for the next dose. In that case, do not take the missed dose at all; just return to your regular dosing schedule. Do not double the next dose.

SIDE EFFECTS

Minor. Back pain, constipation, diarrhea, dizziness, drowsiness, dry mouth, indigestion, nausea, or stomach pain. These side effects should disappear as your body adjusts to the medication.

To relieve constipation, exercise and drink more water (unless your doctor directs you to do otherwise).

If you feel dizzy, sit or lie down for a while; get up slowly from a sitting or reclining position, and be careful on stairs.

To relieve mouth dryness, chew sugarless gum or suck on ice chips or a piece of hard candy.

Major. Tell your doctor about any side effects that are persistent or particularly bothersome. IT IS ESPECIALLY IMPORTANT TO TELL YOUR DOCTOR about itching or rash. Also, if your condition does not improve or seems to be getting worse, you should contact your doctor.

INTERACTIONS

Sucralfate may prevent the absorption of tetracycline, digoxin, phenytoin, ranitidine, and fat-soluble vitamins (vitamins A, D, E, and K) from the gastrointestinal tract. At least one hour should separate doses of any of these medications and sucralfate.

BE SURE TO TELL YOUR DOCTOR about any medications you are currently taking, especially any listed above.

WARNINGS

• Tell your doctor about unusual or allergic reactions you have had to any medications, especially to sucralfate.
• Tell your doctor if you now have or if you have ever had kidney disease.
• If sucralfate makes you dizzy or drowsy, do not take part

in any activity that requires alertness, such as driving a car or operating potentially dangerous machinery.

• Be sure to tell your doctor if you are pregnant. Although sucralfate appears to be safe, extensive studies in pregnant women have not been conducted. Also, tell your doctor if you are breast-feeding an infant. It is not known whether sucralfate passes into breast milk.

Sudafed Plus—see pseudoephedrine and chlorpheniramine combination

Sulf-10—see sodium sulfacetamide (ophthalmic)

sulfacytine—see sulfonamide antibiotics (oral)

sulfadiazine—see sulfonamide antibiotics (oral)

Sulfa-Gyn—see sulfathiazole, sulfacetamide, and sulfabenzamide combination

Sulfair 15—see sodium sulfacetamide (ophthalmic)

sulfamethiazole—see sulfonamide antibiotics (oral)

sulfamethoxazole—see sulfonamide antibiotics (oral)

---

sulfamethoxazole and phenazopyridine combination

BRAND NAME (Manufacturer)
Azo Gantanol (Roche)
TYPE OF DRUG
Antibiotic and urinary tract analgesic
INGREDIENTS
sulfamethoxazole and phenazopyridine
DOSAGE FORM
Tablets (500 mg sulfamethoxazole and 100 mg phenazopyridine)
STORAGE
Sulfamethoxazole and phenazopyridine combination tablets should be stored at room temperature in a tightly closed, light-resistant container.

USES

This medication is used to treat painful infections of the urinary tract.

Sulfamethoxazole is a sulfonamide antibiotic. It acts by preventing production of the nutrients that are required for growth of the infecting bacteria. Phenazopyridine is excreted in the urine, where it exerts a topical analgesic (pain-relieving) effect on the urinary tract. This medication is not useful for any pain other than that of a urinary tract infection.

TREATMENT

It is best to take this medication with a full glass of water on an empty stomach, either one hour before or two hours after a meal. However, if it causes stomach upset, check with your doctor to see if you can take it with food or milk.

This medication works best when the level of medicine in your blood and urine is kept constant. It is best, therefore, to take the doses at evenly spaced intervals day and night. For example, if you are to take two doses a day, the doses should be spaced 12 hours apart.

If you miss a dose of this medication, take the missed dose immediately. However, if you do not remember to take the missed dose until it is almost time for your next dose, take the missed dose immediately; space the following dose about halfway through the regular interval between doses; and then return to your regular dosing schedule. Try not to skip any doses.

It is important to continue to take this medication for the entire time prescribed by your doctor (usually seven to 14 days), even if the symptoms disappear before the end of that period. If you stop taking the drug too soon, resistant bacteria are given a chance to continue growing, and the infection could recur.

SIDE EFFECTS

Minor. Abdominal pain, diarrhea, dizziness, dry mouth, headache, indigestion, insomnia, loss of appetite, nausea, or vomiting. These side effects should disappear as your body adjusts to the medication.

Sulfamethoxazole can cause increased sensitivity to sunlight. It is, therefore, important to avoid prolonged exposure to sunlight and sunlamps. Wear protective clothing and sunglasses, and use an effective sunscreen. However, a sunscreen containing para-aminobenzoic acid (PABA) interferes with the antibacterial activity of this medication and should NOT be used.

Phenazopyridine causes your urine to become orange-red in color. This is not harmful. However, it may stain your clothing. The urine will return to its normal color soon after the drug is discontinued.

If you feel dizzy during treatment with this drug, sit or lie down for a while; get up slowly from a sitting or reclining position, and be careful on stairs.

Sucking on ice chips or a piece of hard candy or chewing sugarless gum helps to relieve mouth dryness.

Major. Tell your doctor about any side effects that are persistent or particularly bothersome. IT IS ESPECIALLY IMPORTANT TO TELL YOUR DOCTOR about aching joints and muscles, back pain, bloating, blood in the urine, chest pain, chills, confusion, convulsions, depression, difficult or painful urination, difficulty in breathing, difficulty in swallowing, fever, hallucinations, hives, itching, loss of coordination, pale skin, rash or peeling skin, ringing in the ears, sore throat, swelling of the front part of the neck, swollen ankles, unusual bleeding or bruising, unusual tiredness, or yellowing of the eyes or skin. Also, if your symptoms of infection seem to be getting worse rather than improving, you should contact your doctor.

INTERACTIONS

This medicine interacts with other types of drugs:

1. Sulfamethoxazole can increase the blood levels of oral anticoagulants (blood thinners, such as warfarin), oral antidiabetic agents, aspirin, methotrexate, thiopental, and phenytoin, which can lead to serious side effects.

2. Methenamine can increase the side effects to the kidneys caused by sulfamethoxazole.

3. Probenecid, phenylbutazone, oxyphenbutazone, and sulfinpyrazone can increase the blood levels of sulfamethoxazole, which can lead to an increase in side effects.

Before starting to take this medication, BE SURE TO TELL YOUR DOCTOR about any medications you are currently taking, especially any of those listed above.

WARNINGS

• Tell your doctor about unusual or allergic reactions you have had to any medications, especially to phenazopyridine, sulfamethoxazole, or any other sulfa drug (other sulfonamide antibiotics, diuretics, dapsone, sulfoxone, oral antidiabetic medications, oral antiglaucoma medication, acetazolamide).

• Tell your doctor if you now have or if you have ever had glucose-6-phosphate dehydrogenase (G6PD) deficiency, kidney disease, liver disease, or porphyria.

• This medication has been prescribed for your current infection only. Another infection later on, or one that someone else has, may require a different medicine. You should not give your medicine to other people or use it for other infections, unless your doctor specifically directs you to do so.

• This medication should be taken with plenty of water, orange juice, or cranberry juice in order to avoid kidney stone formation.

• If this drug makes you dizzy, do not take part in any activity that requires alertness, such as driving a car or operating potentially dangerous machinery.

• Diabetic patients using this medication (phenazopyridine) may get delayed reactions or false-positive readings for sugar or ketones with urine tests. Clinitest is not affected by this medication, but the other urine sugar tests may be.

• If there is no improvement in your condition several days after starting this medication, check with your doctor. This medication may not be effective against the particular type of bacteria causing your infection.

• Before having surgery or any other medical or dental treatment, be sure to tell your doctor or dentist that you are taking this medication.

• Be sure to tell your doctor if you are pregnant. Small amounts of sulfamethoxazole cross the placenta. Although this medication appears to be safe during pregnancy, extensive studies in humans have not been conducted. Also, tell your doctor if you are breast-feeding an infant. Small amounts of this medication pass into breast milk and may temporarily alter the bacterial balance in the intestinal tract of the nursing infant, resulting in diarrhea. This medication should not be used in an infant less than two months of age (in order to avoid side effects involving the liver).

---

sulfamethoxazole and trimethoprim combination

BRAND NAMES (Manufacturers)

Bactrim (Roche)
Bactrim DS (Roche)
Bethaprim DS (Major)
Cotrim (Lemmon)
Cotrim DS (Lemmon)
Cotrim Pediatric (Lemmon)
Septra (Burroughs Wellcome)
Septra DS (Burroughs Wellcome)
sulfamethoxazole and trimethoprim (various manufacturers)
Sulfatrim (various manufacturers)
Sulfatrim DS (various manufacturers)

TYPE OF DRUG

Antibiotic

INGREDIENTS

sulfamethoxazole and trimethoprim

DOSAGE FORMS

Tablets (400 mg sulfamethoxazole and 80 mg trimethoprim)
Double-strength (DS) tablets (800 mg sulfamethoxazole and 160 mg trimethoprim)
Oral suspension (200 mg sulfamethoxazole and 40 mg trimethoprim per 5-ml spoonful)

STORAGE

Sulfamethoxazole and trimethoprim combination tablets and oral suspension should be stored at room temperature in tightly closed, light-resistant containers. The oral suspension does not need to be refrigerated. This medication should never be frozen.

USES

Sulfamethoxazole and trimethoprim combination is used to treat a broad range of infections, including urinary tract infections, certain respiratory and gastrointestinal infections, and otitis media (middle ear infection). Sulfamethoxazole and trimethoprim acts by preventing production of the nutrients that are required for growth of the infecting bacteria.

TREATMENT

It is best to take this medication with a full glass of water on an empty stomach, either one hour before or two hours after a meal. However, if it causes stomach upset, check with your doctor to see if you can take it with food or milk.

The oral suspension form of this medication should be shaken well just before measuring each dose. The contents tend to settle on the bottom of the bottle, so it is necessary to shake the container to distribute the ingredients evenly and equalize the doses. Each dose should then be measured carefully with a specially designed 5-ml measuring spoon. An ordinary kitchen teaspoon is not accurate enough.

This medication works best when the level of medicine in your bloodstream (and urine) is kept constant. It is best, therefore, to take the doses at evenly spaced intervals day and night. For example, if you are to take two doses a day, the doses should be spaced 12 hours apart. Try not to skip any doses.

If you miss a dose of this medication, take the missed dose immediately. However, if you do not remember to take the missed dose until it is almost time for your next dose, take the missed dose immediately; space the following dose about halfway through the regular interval between doses (wait about six hours if you are taking two doses a day); and then return to your regular dosing schedule.

It is important to continue to take this medication for the entire time prescribed by your doctor (usually seven to 14 days), even if the symptoms disappear before the end of that period. If you stop taking the drug too soon, resistant bacteria are given a chance to continue growing, and the infection could recur.

SIDE EFFECTS

Minor. Abdominal pain, diarrhea, dizziness, headache, loss of appetite, nausea, sore mouth, or vomiting. These side effects should disappear as your body adjusts to the drug.

Sulfamethoxazole can cause increased sensitivity to sunlight. It is, therefore, important to avoid prolonged exposure to sunlight and sunlamps. Wear protective clothing and sunglasses, and use an effective sunscreen. However, a sunscreen containing para-aminobenzoic acid (PABA) interferes with the antibacterial activity of this medication and should NOT be used.

If you feel dizzy, sit or lie down for a while; get up slowly from a sitting or reclining position, and be careful on stairs.

Major. Tell your doctor about any side effects that are persistent or particularly bothersome. IT IS ESPECIALLY IMPORTANT TO TELL YOUR DOCTOR about bloody urine, convulsions, difficult or painful urination, difficulty in breathing, difficulty in swallowing, fever, hallucinations, itching, joint pain, lower back pain, pale skin, rash, ringing in the ears, sore throat, swelling of the front part of the neck, swollen or inflamed tongue, tingling in the hands or feet, unusual bleeding or bruising, unusual fatigue, or yellowing of the eyes or skin. Also, if your infection seems to be getting worse rather than improving, contact your doctor.

INTERACTIONS

This medicine interacts with other types of drugs:

1. Sulfamethoxazole can increase the blood levels of oral anticoagulants (blood thinners, such as warfarin), oral antidiabetic agents, methotrexate, aspirin, thiopental, and phenytoin, which can lead to serious side effects.

2. Methenamine can increase the side effects to the kidneys caused by sulfamethoxazole.

3. Probenecid, phenylbutazone, oxyphenbutazone, and sulfinpyrazone can increase the blood levels of sulfamethoxazole, which can lead to an increase in side effects.

4. Rifampin can increase the elimination of trimethoprim from the body, decreasing its antibacterial effects.

5. Concurrent use of trimethoprim with antineoplastic agents (anticancer drugs) can increase the risk of developing blood disorders.

6. Trimethoprim can decrease the elimination of phenytoin from the body and increase the chance of side effects.

BE SURE TO TELL YOUR DOCTOR about any medications you are currently taking, especially any listed above.

WARNINGS

- Tell your doctor about unusual or allergic reactions you have had to any medications, especially to trimethoprim, sulfamethoxazole, or other sulfa drugs (other sulfonamide antibiotics, diuretics, dapsone, sulfoxone, oral antidiabetic medications, oral antiglaucoma medication, or acetazolamide).
- Tell your doctor if you now have or if you have ever had glucose-6-phosphate dehydrogenase (G6PD) deficiency, kidney disease, liver disease, porphyria, or megaloblastic anemia (folate-deficiency anemia).
- This medication has been prescribed for your current infection only. Another infection later on, or one that someone else has, may require a different medicine. You should not give your medicine to other people or use it for other infections, unless your doctor specifically directs you to do so.
- This medication should be taken with plenty of water, orange juice, or cranberry juice in order to avoid kidney stone formation.
- If this drug makes you dizzy, do not take part in any activity that requires alertness, such as driving a car or operating potentially dangerous machinery.
- If there is no improvement in your condition several days after starting to take this medication, check with your doctor. This medication may not be effective against the bacteria causing your infection.
- Before having surgery or any other medical or dental treatment, be sure to tell your doctor or dentist that you are taking this medication.
- Be sure to tell your doctor if you are pregnant. Small amounts of sulfamethoxazole and trimethoprim cross the placenta. Although these drugs appear to be safe during pregnancy, extensive studies in humans have not been conducted. Trimethoprim has been shown to cause birth defects in the offspring of animals that received very large doses during pregnancy. Tell your doctor if you are breast-feeding an infant. Small amounts of sulfamethoxazole pass into breast milk and may temporarily alter the bacterial balance in the intestinal tract of the nursing infant, resulting in diarrhea. Also, small amounts of trimethoprim pass into breast milk, and there is a chance that it may cause anemia in the nursing infant. This combination medication should not be used in an infant less than two months of age (to avoid side effects involving the liver).

---

sulfasalazine

BRAND NAMES (Manufacturers)

Azaline (Major)
Azulfidine (Pharmacia)
Azulfidine EN-tabs (Pharmacia)
S.A.S.-500 (Rowell)
sulfasalazine (various manufacturers)

TYPE OF DRUG

Sulfonamide and anti-inflammatory

INGREDIENT

sulfasalazine

DOSAGE FORMS

Tablets (500 mg)
Enteric-coated tablets (500 mg)
Oral suspension (250 mg per 5-ml spoonful)

STORAGE

Store at room temperature in a tightly closed, light-resistant container. This medication should never be frozen.

USES

This medication is used to treat inflammatory bowel disease (regional enteritis or ulcerative colitis). In the intestine, sulfasalazine is converted to 5-aminosalicylic acid, an aspirin-like drug, which acts to relieve inflammation.

TREATMENT

In order to avoid stomach irritation while you are being treated with this medication, you should take your doses with a full glass of water, with food, or after meals (unless your doctor directs you to do otherwise).

The enteric-coated tablets should be swallowed whole. The enteric coating is added to lessen stomach irritation. Chewing, breaking, or crushing these tablets destroys the coating.

The suspension form of this medication should be shaken well just before measuring each dose. The contents tend to settle on the bottom of the bottle, so it is necessary to shake the container to distribute the ingredients evenly and equalize the doses. Each dose should then be measured carefully with a specially designed 5-ml measuring spoon. An ordinary kitchen teaspoon is not accurate enough.

If you miss a dose of this medication, take the missed dose as soon as possible, unless it is almost time for the next dose. In that case, do not take the missed dose at all; just return to your regular dosing schedule. Do not double the next dose.

SIDE EFFECTS

Minor. Diarrhea, dizziness, drowsiness, headache, insomnia, loss of appetite, nausea, stomach upset, or vomiting. These should disappear as your body adjusts to the drug.

This medication can increase your sensitivity to sunlight. You should, therefore, avoid prolonged exposure to sunlight and sunlamps. Wear protective clothing and sunglasses, and use an effective sunscreen. However, a sunscreen containing para-aminobenzoic acid (PABA) interferes with the action of this drug and should not be used.

Sulfasalazine can discolor contact lenses. You may want to stop wearing them while taking this medication. Discuss this with your ophthalmologist.

Sulfasalazine can cause your urine to change to an orange-yellow color. This is a harmless effect.

If you feel dizzy, sit or lie down for a while; get up slowly from a sitting or reclining position, and be careful on stairs.

Major. Tell your doctor about any side effects that are persistent or particularly bothersome. IT IS ESPECIALLY IMPORTANT TO TELL YOUR DOCTOR about blood in the urine, convulsions, depression, difficulty in swallowing, difficult or painful urination, fatigue, fever, hallucinations, hearing loss, itching, joint pain, lower back pain, mouth sores, pale skin, rash or peeling skin, ringing in the ears, sore throat, swelling of the front part of the neck, tingling sensations, unusual bleeding or bruising, or yellowing of the eyes or skin.

INTERACTIONS

Sulfasalazine interacts with several other types of drugs:

1. It can increase the side effects of oral anticoagulants (blood thinners, such as warfarin), oral antidiabetic agents, methotrexate, aspirin, phenytoin, and thiopental.

2. The blood levels and effectiveness of digoxin and folic acid are decreased by concurrent use of sulfasalazine.

3. Probenecid, oxyphenbutazone, phenylbutazone, methenamine, and sulfinpyrazone can increase the blood levels and side effects of sulfasalazine.

Before starting to take sulfasalazine, BE SURE TO TELL YOUR DOCTOR about any medications you are currently taking, especially any of those listed above.

WARNINGS

• Tell your doctor about unusual or allergic reactions you have had to any medications, especially to sulfasalazine, aspirin or other salicylates, or any sulfa drug (diuretics, oral antidiabetic medications, sulfonamide antibiotics, oral antiglaucoma medication, acetazolamide, sulfoxone, dapsone).

• Before starting to take this medication, be sure to tell your doctor if you now have or if you have ever had blood disorders, blockage of the urinary tract or intestine, glucose-6-phosphate dehydrogenase (G6PD) deficiency, kidney disease, liver disease, or porphyria.

• To help prevent the formation of kidney stones, try to drink at least eight to 12 glasses of water or fruit juice each day while you are taking this medication (unless your doctor directs you to do otherwise).

• Before having surgery or other medical or dental treatment, tell your doctor or dentist you are taking this drug.

• If your condition does not improve within a month or two after starting to take sulfasalazine, check with your doctor. It may be necessary to change your medication.

• Be sure to tell your doctor if you are pregnant. Although sulfasalazine appears to be safe during most of pregnancy, extensive studies in humans have not been conducted. There is also concern that if this drug is taken during the ninth month of pregnancy, it may cause liver or brain disorders in the newborn infant. Also, tell your doctor if you are breast-feeding an infant. Small amounts of sulfasalazine pass into breast milk.

---

sulfathiazole, sulfacetamide, and sulfabenzamide combination

BRAND NAMES (Manufacturers)

Sulfa-Gyn (Mayrand)
Sultrin Triple Sulfa (Ortho)
Triple Sulfa (various manufacturers)
Trysul (Savage)

TYPE OF DRUG

Antibiotic

INGREDIENTS

sulfathiazole, sulfacetamide, and sulfabenzamide

DOSAGE FORMS

Vaginal tablets (172.5 mg sulfathiazole, 143.75 mg sulfacetamide, and 184 mg sulfabenzamide)
Vaginal cream (3.42% sulfathiazole, 2.86% sulfacetamide, and 3.7% sulfabenzamide)

STORAGE

This medication should be stored at room temperature (never frozen) in tightly-closed, light-resistant containers.

USES

Sulfathiazole, sulfacetamide, and sulfabenzamide are sulfonamide antibiotics used to treat vaginal infections. They work by blocking production of nutrients needed by the infecting bacteria, thus killing the bacteria.

TREATMENT

This product is packaged with instructions and an applicator. Read the instructions carefully before inserting the vaginal cream or tablets. Wash the applicator with warm water and soap, and dry it thoroughly after each use.

It is important to continue to take this medication for the entire time prescribed by your doctor, even if your symptoms disappear before the end of that period. If you stop taking the drug too soon, resistant bacteria are given a chance to continue growing, and your infection could recur.

If you miss a dose of this medication, insert the missed dose as soon as possible, unless it is almost time for the next dose. In that case, do not insert the missed dose at all; just return to your regular dosing schedule. Do not double the next dose.

SIDE EFFECTS

Minor. This medication can cause a mild, temporary burning or stinging sensation after the first few applications. As your body adjusts to the drug, this should disappear.

Major. Tell your doctor about any side effects that are persistent or particularly bothersome. IT IS ESPECIALLY IMPORTANT TO TELL YOUR DOCTOR about itching, rash, redness, swelling, or any other signs of irritation that were not present before you started taking this medication.

INTERACTIONS

This medication should not interact with other medications if it is used according to directions.

WARNINGS

• Tell your doctor about unusual or allergic reactions you have had to any medications, especially to sulfathiazole, sulfacetamide, sulfabenzamide, or any other sulfa drug, including sulfonamide antibiotics, diuretics (water pills), oral antidiabetic medicines, oral antiglaucoma medication, dapsone, sulfone, and sulfoxone.

• Before starting to take this medication, tell your doctor if you now have or if you have ever had kidney disease.

• You should not use tampons while using this medication.

• During intercourse, your partner should wear a condom to prevent reinfection. Ask your doctor if your partner needs to be treated at the same time as you.

• This medication has been prescribed for your current infection only. Another infection later on, or one that someone else has, may require a different medicine. You should not give your medicine to other people or use it for other infections, unless your doctor specifically directs you to do so.

• If symptoms do not begin to improve within several days after starting this drug, CONTACT YOUR DOCTOR. This drug may not be effective for your infection.

• If you are pregnant or breast-feeding, ASK YOUR DOCTOR if you should continue to use this drug.

Sulfatrim—see sulfamethoxazole and trimethoprim combination

Sulfatrim DS—see sulfamethoxazole and trimethoprim combination

---

sulfinpyrazone

BRAND NAMES (Manufacturers)
Anturane (Ciba)
sulfinpyrazone (various manufacturers)

TYPE OF DRUG
Antigout and antiplatelet

INGREDIENT
sulfinpyrazone

DOSAGE FORMS
Tablets (100 mg)
Capsules (200 mg)

STORAGE
Sulfinpyrazone tablets and capsules should be stored at room temperature in tightly closed containers.

USES

Sulfinpyrazone is used to treat gout. It acts by increasing the elimination of uric acid (the chemical responsible for gout) through the kidneys. It is also used to prevent further heart attacks in patients who have had a recent attack. It prevents the formation of certain types of blood clots.

TREATMENT

In order to prevent stomach irritation, you should take sulfinpyrazone with food, milk, or antacids (unless your doctor directs you to do otherwise).

Sulfinpyrazone does not cure gout, but it will help to control blood uric acid levels as long as you continue to take the medication.

If you miss a dose of this medication, take the missed dose as soon as possible, unless it is almost time for your next dose. In that case, do not take the missed dose at all; just return to your regular dosing schedule. Do not double the next dose.

SIDE EFFECTS

Minor. Diarrhea, nausea, stomach upset, or vomiting. These side effects should disappear as your body adjusts to the medication.

Major. Tell your doctor about any side effects that are persistent or particularly bothersome. IT IS ESPECIALLY IMPORTANT TO TELL YOUR DOCTOR about back pain; bloody or black, tarry stools; convulsions; difficult or painful urination; fever; sore throat; skin rash; or unusual bleeding or bruising.

INTERACTIONS

Sulfinpyrazone interacts with other types of medications:

1. Aspirin can increase uric acid levels, thereby decreasing the therapeutic effects of sulfinpyrazone.

2. Sulfinpyrazone can increase the side effects of sulfonamide antibiotics, oral antidiabetic medications, oral anticoagulants (blood thinners, such as warfarin), and nitrofurantoin.

3. Alcohol, pyrazinamide, and diuretics (water pills) can increase the blood levels of uric acid, thereby decreasing the effectiveness of sulfinpyrazone.

Before starting to take this medication, BE SURE TO TELL YOUR DOCTOR about any medications you are currently taking, especially any of those listed above.

WARNINGS

• Tell your doctor about unusual or allergic reactions you have had to any medications, especially to sulfinpyrazone, dipyrone, oxyphenbutazone, or phenylbutazone.

• Before starting to take this medication, be sure to tell your doctor if you have ever had blood disorders, kidney disease, peptic ulcers, or stomach or intestinal inflammation.

• Before taking any over-the-counter (nonprescription) medication, check the label to see if it contains aspirin. Aspirin can decrease the effectiveness of sulfinpyrazone.

• Sulfinpyrazone is not an analgesic (pain reliever) and does not relieve an acute gout attack. It is used to prevent future gout attacks.

• In order to prevent the formation of kidney stones, try to drink at least eight to 12 glasses of water or fruit juice each day while taking this medication (unless your doctor directs you to do otherwise).

• Before having surgery or other medical or dental treatment, tell your doctor or dentist you are taking this drug. Treatment with sulfinpyrazone is usually discontinued several days prior to surgery, to prevent bleeding complications.

• Be sure to tell your doctor if you are pregnant. Although this medication appears to be safe during pregnancy, extensive studies in humans have not been conducted. Also, tell your doctor if you are breast-feeding an infant. It is not known whether sulfinpyrazone passes into breast milk.

---

sulfisoxazole and phenazopyridine combination

BRAND NAMES (Manufacturers)
Azo Gantrisin (Roche)
Azo-Sulfisoxazole (various manufacturers)

TYPE OF DRUG
Antibiotic and urinary tract analgesic

INGREDIENTS
sulfisoxazole and phenazopyridine

DOSAGE FORM
Tablets (500 mg sulfisoxazole and 50 mg phenazopyridine)

STORAGE
Sulfisoxazole and phenazopyridine combination tablets should be stored at room temperature in a tightly closed, light-resistant container.

USES

Sulfisoxazole and phenazopyridine combination is used to treat painful infections of the urinary tract. Sulfisoxazole is a sulfonamide antibiotic, which acts by preventing production of nutrients that are required for growth of infecting bacteria. Phenazopyridine is excreted in the urine, where it exerts a topical analgesic (pain-relieving) effect on the urinary tract. This medication is not useful for any pain other than that of a urinary tract infection.

TREATMENT

It is best to take this medication with a full glass of water on an empty stomach, either one hour before or two hours after a meal. However, if it causes stomach upset, check with your doctor to see if you can take it with food or milk.

This medication works best when the level of medication in your blood and urine is kept constant. It is best, therefore, to take the doses at evenly spaced intervals day and night. For example, if you are to take two doses a day, the doses should be spaced 12 hours apart.

If you miss a dose of this medication, take the missed dose immediately. However, if you do not remember to take the missed dose until it is almost time for your next dose, take the missed dose immediately; space the following dose about halfway through the regular interval between doses; and then return to your regular dosing schedule. Try not to skip any doses.

It is important to continue to take this medication for the entire time prescribed by your doctor (usually seven to 14 days), even if your symptoms disappear before the end of that period. If you stop taking the drug too soon, resistant bacteria are given a chance to continue growing, and the infection could recur.

SIDE EFFECTS

Minor. Abdominal pain, diarrhea, dizziness, dry mouth, headache, indigestion, insomnia, loss of appetite, nausea, or vomiting. These side effects should disappear as your body adjusts to the medication.

Sulfisoxazole can cause increased sensitivity to sunlight. It is, therefore, important to avoid prolonged exposure to sunlight and sunlamps. Wear protective clothing and sunglasses, and use an effective sunscreen. However, a sunscreen containing para-aminobenzoic acid (PABA) interferes with the antibacterial activity of this medication and should NOT be used.

Phenazopyridine causes your urine to become orange-red in color. This is not harmful; however, it may stain your clothing. The urine will return to its normal color soon after the drug is discontinued.

If you feel dizzy, sit or lie down for a while; get up slowly from a sitting or reclining position, and be careful on stairs.

Sucking on ice chips or a piece of hard candy or chewing sugarless gum helps to relieve mouth dryness.

Major. Tell your doctor about any side effects that are persistent or particularly bothersome. IT IS ESPECIALLY IMPORTANT TO TELL YOUR DOCTOR about aching joints and muscles, back pain, bloating, blood in the urine, chest pain, chills, confusion, convulsions, depression, difficulty in breathing, difficulty in swallowing, difficult or painful urination, fever, hallucinations, hives, itching, loss of coordination, pale skin, rash or peeling skin, ringing in the ears, sore throat, swelling of the front part of the neck, swollen ankles, unusual bleeding or bruising, unusual tiredness, or yellowing of the eyes or skin. Also, if your symptoms of infection seem to be getting worse rather than improving, you should contact your doctor.

INTERACTIONS

This drug interacts with several types of drugs:

1. Sulfisoxazole can increase the blood levels of oral anticoagulants (blood thinners, such as warfarin), oral antidiabetic agents, methotrexate, aspirin, thiopental, and phenytoin, which can lead to serious side effects.
2. Methenamine can increase the side effects to the kidneys caused by sulfisoxazole.
3. Probenecid, oxyphenbutazone, phenylbutazone, and sulfinpyrazone can increase the blood levels of sulfisoxazole, which can lead to an increase in side effects.

Before starting to take this medication, BE SURE TO TELL YOUR DOCTOR about any medications you are currently taking, especially any of those listed above.

WARNINGS

• Tell your doctor about any reactions you have had to drugs, especially to phenazopyridine, sulfisoxazole, or any other sulfa drug (other sulfonamide antibiotics, diuretics, dapsone, sulfoxone, oral antidiabetic medications, oral antiglaucoma medications, acetazolamide).

• Tell your doctor if you now have or if you have ever had glucose-6-phosphate dehydrogenase (G6PD) deficiency, kidney disease, liver disease, or porphyria.

• This medication has been prescribed for your current infection only. Another infection later on, or one that someone else has, may require a different medicine. You should not give your medicine to other people or use it for other infections, unless your doctor specifically directs you to do so.

• This medication should be taken with plenty of water, orange juice, or cranberry juice in order to prevent kidney stone formation.

• If this drug makes you dizzy, do not take part in any activity that requires alertness, such as driving a car or operating potentially dangerous machinery.

• Diabetic patients using this medication, which contains phenazopyridine may get delayed reactions or false-positive readings for sugar or ketones with urine tests. Clinitest is not affected by this medication, but the other urine sugar tests may be. Discuss this with your doctor.

• If there is no improvement in your condition several days after starting to take this medication, check with your doctor. This medication may not be effective against the bacteria causing your infection.

• Before having surgery or any other medical or dental treatment, be sure to tell your doctor or dentist that you are taking this medication.

• Be sure to tell your doctor if you are pregnant. Small amounts of sulfisoxazole cross the placenta. Although this medication appears to be safe during pregnancy, extensive studies in humans have not been conducted. Also, tell your doctor if you are breast-feeding an infant. Small amounts of this medication pass into breast milk and may temporarily alter the bacterial balance in the intestinal tract of a nursing infant, resulting in diarrhea. This medication should not be used in an infant less than two months of age (in order to avoid side effects involving the liver).

---

sulfonamide antibiotics (oral)

BRAND NAMES (Manufacturers)

Gamazole (Major)
Gantanol (Roche)
Gantanol DS (Roche)
Gantrisin (Roche)
Gulfasin (Major)
Lipo Gantrisin (Roche)
Microsulfon (CMC)
multiple sulfonamides (various manufacturers)
Neotrizine (Lilly)
Proklar (O'Neal)
Renoquid (Glenwood)
sulfacytine (various manufacturers)
sulfadiazine (various manufacturers)
sulfamethizole (various manufacturers)
sulfamethoxazole (various manufacturers)
sulfisoxazole (various manufacturers)
Terfonyl (Squibb)
Thiosulfil (Ayerst)
Thiosulfil Forte (Ayerst)
Triple Sulfa (systemic) (various manufacturers)
Urobak (Shionogi USA)

TYPE OF DRUG

Anti-infective

INGREDIENTS AND DOSAGE FORMS

sulfacytine (Renoquid)
Tablets (250 mg)
sulfadiazine (Microsulfon)
Tablets (500 mg)
sulfamethiazole (Proklar, Thiosulfil, Thiosulfil Forte)
Tablets (250 mg and 500 mg)
sulfamethoxazole (Gamazole, Gantanol, Gantanol DS, Urobak)
Tablets (500 mg and 1 g)
Suspension (500 mg per 5-ml spoonful)
sulfisoxazole (Gantrisin, Gulfasin, Lipo-Gantrisin)
Tablets (500 mg)
Syrup (500 mg per 5-ml spoonful)
Pediatric suspension (500 mg per 5-ml spoonful)
Emulsion, long-acting (1 g per 5-ml spoonful)
multiple sulfonamides (Neotrizine, Sul-Trio MM #2, Terfonyl, Triple Sulfa)
Tablets (167 mg sulfadiazine, 167 mg sulfamerazine, and 167 mg sulfamethazine)
Suspension (167 mg sulfadiazine, 167 mg sulfamerazine, and 167 mg sulfamethazine per 5-ml spoonful, with 2% alcohol)

STORAGE

Store at room temperature in the original container.

USES

Sulfonamide antibiotics are a family of related drugs that have activity against many types of bacteria. This group of medications is often used to treat urinary tract infections, as well as other infections. These medications kill the bacteria responsible for the infection.

TREATMENT

Sulfonamide antibiotics should be taken with a full glass of water on an empty stomach (either one hour before or two hours after a meal). Several additional glasses of water should also be taken every day (unless your doctor directs you to do otherwise). Drinking extra water helps to prevent kidney damage.

Sulfonamide antibiotics work best when the level of the medicine in your bloodstream is kept constant. It is best, therefore, to take the doses at evenly spaced intervals day and night. For example, if you are to take four doses a day, the doses should be spaced about six hours apart.

If the liquid suspension or emulsion form of the sulfonamides has been prescribed for you, be sure to shake the bottle well. The contents tend to settle on the bottom of the bottle, so it is necessary to shake the container to distribute the ingredients evenly and equalize the doses. Be sure to use specially marked droppers or spoons to accurately measure the correct amount of liquid. Household teaspoons vary in size and may not give you the correct dosage.

If you miss a dose, take the missed dose as soon as possible, unless it is almost time for your next dose. In that case, if you are taking two doses a day, space the missed dose and the following dose five to six hours apart; if you are taking three or more doses a day, space the missed dose and the following dose two to four hours apart, or double the next dose. Then return to your regular dosing schedule.

It is very important to continue to take these medications for the entire time prescribed by your doctor (usually ten days), even if the symptoms disappear before the end of that period. If you stop taking the drug too soon, resistant bacteria are given a chance to continue growing, and your infection could recur.

SIDE EFFECTS

Minor. Diarrhea, dizziness, headache, loss of appetite, nausea, or vomiting. As your body adjusts to the medication, these side effects should disappear.

These medications can also cause a brown discoloration of the urine, which is harmless.

These drugs can increase your sensitivity to sunlight. You should, therefore, avoid prolonged exposure to sunlight and sunlamps. Wear protective clothing and sunglasses; and use an effective sunscreen, but not one that contains para-aminobenzoic acid (PABA). PABA interferes with the antibacterial activity of this medication.

Major. Tell your doctor about any side effects that are persistent or particularly bothersome. IT IS ESPECIALLY IMPORTANT TO TELL YOUR DOCTOR about aching of joints and muscles; blood in the urine; difficulty in swallowing; itching; lower back pain; pain while urinating; pale skin; redness, blistering, or peeling of the skin; skin rash; sore throat and fever; swelling of the front part of the neck; unusual bleeding or bruising; unusual tiredness; or yellowing of the eyes or skin. Also, if your symptoms of infection seem to be getting worse rather than improving, you should contact your doctor.

INTERACTIONS

Sulfonamides interact with several types of drugs:

1. Aminobenzoic acid can decrease the effectiveness of the sulfonamides.

2. The activity and side effects of anticoagulants (blood thinners, such as warfarin), oral antidiabetic medications, methotrexate, aspirin, phenytoin, and thiopental may be increased when sulfonamides are also taken.

3. Oxyphenbutazone, phenylbutazone, methenamine, probenecid, and sulfinpyrazone can increase the toxicity of the sulfonamides.

BE SURE TO TELL YOUR DOCTOR about any medications you are currently taking, especially any listed above.

WARNINGS

• Before starting to take this medication, tell your doctor about any unusual or allergic reactions you have had to any medications, especially to sulfonamide antibiotics or other sulfa drugs, including diuretics (water pills), dapsone, sulfoxone, oral antidiabetics, and oral antiglaucoma medication.

• Tell your doctor if you now have or if you have ever had glucose-6-phosphate dehydrogenase (G6PD) deficiency, liver disease, porphyria, or kidney disease.

• Before having surgery or any other medical or dental treatment, be sure to tell your doctor or dentist that you are taking a sulfonamide antibiotic.

• This medication has been prescribed for your current infection only. Another infection later on, or one that someone else has, may require a different medicine. You should not give your medicine to other people or use it for other infections, unless your doctor specifically directs you to do so.

• Be sure to tell your doctor if you are pregnant. These medications, if given to a woman late in pregnancy, can be toxic to the infant. Also, tell your doctor if you are breastfeeding an infant. Sulfonamides can pass into breast milk and may cause side effects in a small number of nursing infants—those who have glucose-6-phosphate dehydrogenase (G6PD) deficiency. In addition, you should not give sulfonamides to an infant less than one month of age, unless your doctor specifically directs you to do so.

---

sulindac

BRAND NAME (Manufacturer)
Clinoril (Merck Sharp & Dohme)

TYPE OF DRUG
Nonsteroidal anti-inflammatory analgesic

INGREDIENT
sulindac

DOSAGE FORM
Tablets (150 mg and 200 mg)

STORAGE
This medication should be stored in a closed container at room temperature away from heat and direct sunlight.

USES

Sulindac is used to treat the inflammation (pain, swelling, and stiffness) of certain types of arthritis, gout, bursitis, and tendinitis. Sulindac has been shown to block the production of certain body chemicals, called prostaglandins, that may trigger pain. However, it is not fully understood how sulindac works.

TREATMENT

You should take this medication on an empty stomach 30 to 60 minutes before meals or two hours after meals, so that it gets into your bloodstream quickly. However, to decrease stomach irritation, your doctor may want you to take the medicine with food or antacids.

It is important to take sulindac on schedule and not to miss any doses. If you do miss a dose, take it as soon as possible, unless it is almost time for your next dose. In that case, do not take the missed dose at all; just return to your regular dosing schedule. Do not double the next dose.

If you are taking sulindac to relieve arthritis, you must take it regularly, as directed by your doctor. It may take up to three weeks for you to feel the full benefits of this medication. Sulindac does not cure arthritis, but it will help to control the condition as long as you continue to take it.

SIDE EFFECTS

Minor. Bloating, constipation, diarrhea, difficulty in sleeping, dizziness, drowsiness, headache, heartburn, indigestion, light-headedness, loss of appetite, nausea, nervousness, soreness of the mouth, unusual sweating, or vomiting. As your body adjusts to the medication, these side effects should disappear.

To relieve constipation, increase the amount of fiber in your diet (fresh fruits and vegetables, salads, bran, and whole-grain breads), exercise, and drink more water (unless your doctor directs you to do otherwise).

If you become dizzy or light-headed while taking this drug, sit or lie down for a while; get up slowly from a sitting or reclining position, and be careful on stairs.

Major. Tell your doctor about any side effects that are persistent or particularly bothersome. IT IS ESPECIALLY IMPORTANT TO TELL YOUR DOCTOR about bloody or black, tarry stools; blurred vision; chills; confusion; depression; difficulty in breathing; difficulty in hearing; difficult or painful urination; palpitations; ringing or buzzing in the ears; skin rash, hives, or itching; stomach pain; swelling; tightness in the chest; unexplained sore throat and fever; unusual bleeding or bruising; unusual fatigue or weakness; unusual weight gain; vaginal bleeding; wheezing; or yellowing of the eyes or skin.

INTERACTIONS

Sulindac interacts with several types of medications:

1. The combination of anticoagulants (blood thinners, such as warfarin) and sulindac can lead to an increase in bleeding complications.

2. Aspirin, salicylates, or other anti-inflammatory medications can cause an increase in stomach irritation.

3. Probenecid can increase the amount of sulindac in the bloodstream when the drugs are taken concurrently.

4. The action of beta blockers may be decreased by this drug.

5. This drug may interact with diuretics (water pills).

BE SURE TO TELL YOUR DOCTOR about any medications you are currently taking, especially any of those listed above.

WARNINGS

- Tell your doctor if you have ever had unusual or allergic reactions to sulindac or any of the other chemically related drugs (including aspirin and other salicylates, diclofenac, diflunisal, fenoprofen, flurbiprofen, ibuprofen, indomethacin, ketoprofen, meclofenamate, mefenamic acid, naproxen, oxyphenbutazone, phenylbutazone, piroxicam, or tolmetin).
- Tell your doctor if you have ever had asthma, bleeding problems, colitis, stomach ulcers or other stomach problems, epilepsy, heart disease, high blood pressure, kidney disease, liver disease, mental illness, or Parkinson's disease.
- If sulindac makes you dizzy or drowsy, do not take part in any activity that requires alertness, such as driving a car or operating potentially dangerous machinery.
- Because this drug can prolong your bleeding time, tell your doctor or dentist you are taking this drug before having surgery or any other medical or dental treatment.
- Stomach problems are more likely to occur if you take aspirin or other salicylates regularly or drink alcoholic beverages while being treated with this medication. These should be avoided (unless your doctor directs you to do otherwise).
- Be sure to tell your doctor if you are pregnant. The safe use of this medication in human pregnancy has not been established. Side effects have been observed in the development of bones and organs in the offspring of animals that received sulindac during pregnancy. If taken late in pregnancy, this type of drug can also prolong labor. Also, tell your doctor if you are breast-feeding an infant. Small amounts of sulindac can pass into breast milk.

Sulten-10—see sodium sulfacetamide (ophthalmic)

Sultrin Triple Sulfa—see sulfathiazole, sulfacetamide, and sulfabenzamide combination

Sumycin—see tetracycline

Surmontil—see trimipramine

Susano—see atropine, scopolamine, hyoscyamine, and phenobarbital combination

Suspen—see penicillin VK

Sustaire—see theophylline

Symmetrel—see amantadine

Synacort—see hydrocortisone (topical)

Synalar—see fluocinolone (topical)

Synalar-HP—see fluocinolone (topical)

Synalgos-DC—see aspirin, caffeine, dihydrocodeine, and promethazine combination

Synemol—see fluocinolone (topical)

Synkayvite—see vitamin K

Synophylate-GG—see theophylline and guaifenesin combination

Synthroid—see levothyroxine

Synthrox—see levothyroxine

Syroxine—see levothyroxine

Tagamet—see cimetidine

Talwin NX—see pentazocine

Tamine SR—see phenylpropanolamine, phenylephrine, and brompheniramine combination

---

tamoxifen

BRAND NAME (Manufacturer)

Nolvadex (Stuart)

TYPE OF DRUG

Antiestrogen and antineoplastic (anticancer drug)

INGREDIENT
tamoxifen
DOSAGE FORM
Tablets (10 mg)
STORAGE
Tamoxifen should be stored at room temperature in a tightly closed, light-resistant container.

USES

This medication is used to treat advanced breast cancer in postmenopausal women. Tamoxifen is a nonsteroidal antiestrogen drug. It is unclear how tamoxifen works, but it may block estrogen binding to breast tissue, thereby slowing tumor growth.

TREATMENT

Tamoxifen can be taken either on an empty stomach or with food or a glass of milk, unless your doctor directs you to do otherwise.

If you miss a dose of this medication, take the missed dose as soon as possible, unless it is almost time for the next dose. In that case, do not take the missed dose at all; just return to your regular dosing schedule. Do not double the next dose of this medication.

SIDE EFFECTS

Minor. Distaste for food, dizziness, headache, hot flashes, light-headedness, nausea, vaginal itching, or vomiting. These side effects should disappear as your body adjusts to the medication.

It is important to continue taking this medication despite any nausea or vomiting that may occur. If you vomit immediately after taking a dose, call your doctor; you may have to repeat the dose.

You may experience an increase in bone and tumor pain when tamoxifen is first started. The pain generally subsides rapidly but may require the temporary use of analgesics (pain relievers).

If you feel dizzy or light-headed, sit or lie down for a while; get up slowly from a sitting or reclining position, and be careful on stairs.

Major. Tell your doctor about any side effects that are persistent or particularly bothersome. IT IS ESPECIALLY IMPORTANT TO TELL YOUR DOCTOR about blurred vision, chills, depression, fever, rapid weight gain (three to five pounds within a week), rash, sore throat, unusual weakness, or vaginal bleeding or discharge.

INTERACTIONS

Tamoxifen should not interact with other medications as long as it is used according to directions.

WARNINGS

• Tell your doctor about unusual or allergic reactions you have had to any medications, especially to tamoxifen.

• Before starting to take this medication, be sure to tell your doctor if you now have or if you have ever had blood disorders or visual disturbances.

Taractan—see chlorprothixene

Tavist—see clemastine

Tavist-1—see clemastine

T-Dry Jr.—see pseudoephedrine and chlorpheniramine combination

Tebamide—see trimethobenzamide

Teebaconin—see isoniazid

Tega D&E—see phenylpropanolamine and guaifenesin combination

Tegopen—see cloxacillin

Tegretol—see carbamazepine

Tegretol Chewable—see carbamazepine

Telachlor S.R.—see chlorpheniramine

Teldrin—see chlorpheniramine

---

temazepam

BRAND NAMES (Manufacturers)
Restoril (Sandoz)
temazepam (various manufacturers)
TYPE OF DRUG
Benzodiazepine sedative/hypnotic
INGREDIENT
temazepam
DOSAGE FORM
Capsules (15 mg and 30 mg)
STORAGE
This medication should be stored at room temperature in a tightly closed, light-resistant container.

USES

Temazepam is prescribed to treat insomnia, including problems with falling asleep, waking during the night, and early morning wakefulness. It is not clear exactly how this medicine works, but it may relieve insomnia by acting as a depressant of the central nervous system (brain and spinal cord).

TREATMENT

This medicine should be taken 30 to 60 minutes before bedtime. It can be taken with food or a full glass of water if stomach upset occurs. Do not take this medication with antacids, since they may retard its absorption from the gastrointestinal tract.

If you are taking this medication regularly and you miss a dose, take the missed dose immediately if you remember within an hour. If more than an hour has passed, do not take the missed dose at all; just wait for the next scheduled dose. Do not double the dose.

SIDE EFFECTS

Minor. Bitter taste in the mouth, constipation, diarrhea, dizziness, drowsiness (after a night's sleep), dry mouth, excessive salivation, fatigue, flushing, headache, heartburn, loss of appetite, nausea, nervousness, sweating, or vomiting. As your body adjusts to the medication, these side effects should disappear.

To relieve constipation, increase the amount of fiber in your diet (fresh fruits and vegetables, salads, bran, and whole-grain breads), exercise, and drink more water (unless your doctor directs you to do otherwise).

Dry mouth can be relieved by chewing sugarless gum or by sucking on ice chips.

If you feel dizzy, sit or lie down for a while; get up slowly from a sitting or reclining position, and be careful on stairs.

Major. Tell your doctor about any side effects that are persistent or particularly bothersome. IT IS ESPECIALLY IMPORTANT TO TELL YOUR DOCTOR about blurred or double vision, chest pain, depression, difficulty in urinating, fainting, falling, fever, joint pain, hallucinations, mouth sores, nightmares, palpitations, rash, severe depression, shortness of breath, slurred speech, sore throat, uncoordinated movements, unusual excitement, unusual tiredness, or yellowing of the eyes or skin.

INTERACTIONS

Temazepam interacts with several other types of drugs:

1. To prevent oversedation, this drug should not be taken with alcohol, other sedative drugs, or central nervous system depressants (such as antihistamines, barbiturates, muscle relaxants, pain medications, narcotics, antiseizure medications, and phenothiazine tranquilizers) or with antidepressants.

2. Temazepam may decrease the effectiveness of carbamazepine, levodopa, and oral anticoagulants (blood thinners) and may increase the effects of phenytoin.

3. Disulfiram, cimetidine, oral contraceptives (birth control pills), and isoniazid can increase the blood levels of temazepam, which can lead to toxic effects.

4. Concurrent use of rifampin may decrease the effectiveness of temazepam.

BE SURE TO TELL YOUR DOCTOR about any medications you are currently taking, especially any of those listed above.

WARNINGS

• Tell your doctor about unusual or allergic reactions you have had to any medications, especially to temazepam or other benzodiazepine tranquilizers (such as alprazolam, chlordiazepoxide, clorazepate, diazepam, flurazepam, halazepam, lorazepam, oxazepam, prazepam, and triazolam).

• Tell your doctor if you now have or if you have ever had liver disease, kidney disease, epilepsy, lung disease, myasthenia gravis, porphyria, mental depression, or mental illness.

• This medicine can cause drowsiness. Avoid tasks that require alertness, such as driving a car or operating potentially dangerous machinery.

• Temazepam has the potential for abuse and must be used with caution. Tolerance may develop quickly; do not increase the dosage without first consulting your doctor. It is also important not to stop taking this drug suddenly if you have been taking it in large amounts or if you have used it for several weeks. Your doctor may want to reduce the dosage gradually.

• This is a safe drug when used properly. When it is combined with other sedative drugs or alcohol, however, serious side effects may develop.

• Be sure to tell your doctor if you are pregnant. This type of medicine may increase the chance of birth defects if it is taken during the first three months of pregnancy. In addition, use of this medicine during the last six months of pregnancy may result in addiction of the fetus, leading to withdrawal side effects in the newborn. Also, use of this medicine during the last weeks of pregnancy may cause excessive drowsiness, slowed heartbeat, and breathing difficulties in the infant. Tell your doctor if you are breast-feeding an infant. This medicine can pass into breast milk and cause excessive drowsiness, slowed heartbeat, and breathing difficulties in nursing infants.

Tenoretic—see atenolol and chlorthalidone combination

Tenormin—see atenolol

Tenuate—see diethylpropion

Tenuate Dospan—see diethylpropion

Tepanil—see diethylpropion

Tepanil Ten-Tab—see diethylpropion

Teramycin—see oxytetracycline

---

terbutaline

BRAND NAMES (Manufacturers)
Brethaire (Geigy)
Brethine (Geigy)
Bricanyl (Lakeside)

TYPE OF DRUG
Bronchodilator

INGREDIENT
terbutaline

DOSAGE FORMS
Tablets (2.5 mg and 5 mg)
Inhalation aerosol (each spray delivers 0.2 mg)

STORAGE
Terbutaline tablets should be stored at room temperature in a tightly closed, light-resistant container. The inhalation aerosol should be stored at room temperature away from excessive heat.

USES

Terbutaline is used to relieve wheezing and shortness of breath caused by lung diseases such as asthma, bronchitis, and emphysema. This drug acts directly on the muscles of the bronchi (breathing tubes) to relieve bronchospasm (muscle contractions of the bronchi), which in turn reduces airway resistance—making breathing easier.

TREATMENT

In order to lessen stomach upset, you can take terbutaline with food (unless your doctor directs you to do otherwise).

The inhalation aerosol form of this medication is usually packaged with an instruction sheet. Read the directions carefully before using the medication. The contents should be shaken well just before each use. The contents tend to settle on the bottom, so it is necessary to shake the bottle to distribute the ingredients evenly and equalize the doses. If more than one inhalation is necessary, wait at least one full minute between doses in order to receive the full benefit of the first dose.

If you miss a dose of this medication and remember within an hour, take the missed dose immediately and then return to your regular schedule. If more than an hour has passed, do not take the missed dose at all; just return to your regular dosing schedule. Do not double the next dose of this medication.

SIDE EFFECTS

Minor. Anxiety, bad taste in mouth, dizziness, headache, flushing, irritability, insomnia, loss of appetite, nausea, nervousness, restlessness, sweating, vomiting, or weakness. These side effects should disappear as your body adjusts to the medication.

To prevent dryness or irritation of the mouth or throat, rinse your mouth with water after each dose.

In order to avoid difficulty in falling asleep, check with your doctor to see if you can take the last dose of this medication several hours before bedtime each day.

If you feel dizzy, sit or lie down for a while; get up from a sitting or lying position slowly, and be careful on stairs.

Major. Tell your doctor about any side effects that are persistent or particularly bothersome. IT IS ESPECIALLY IMPORTANT TO TELL YOUR DOCTOR about chest pain, difficult or painful urination, increased wheezing or difficulty in breathing, muscle cramps, palpitations, or tremors.

INTERACTIONS

Terbutaline interacts with other types of medications:

1. The beta blockers (acebutolol, atenolol, betaxolol, carteolol, esmolol, labetalol, metoprolol, nadolol, penbutolol, pindolol, propranolol, timolol) antagonize (act against) this medication, decreasing its effectiveness.

2. Monoamine oxidase (MAO) inhibitors; tricyclic antidepressants; antihistamines; levothyroxine; and over-the-counter (nonprescription) cough, cold, allergy, asthma, diet, and sinus medications may increase the side effects of terbutaline. At least 14 days should separate the use of this drug and the use of an MAO inhibitor.

3. There may be a change in the dosage requirements of insulin or oral antidiabetic medications when terbutaline is started.

4. The blood-pressure-lowering effects of guanethidine may be decreased by this medication.

5. The use of terbutaline with other bronchodilator drugs (either oral or inhalant drugs) can have additive side effects. Discuss this with your doctor.

BE SURE TO TELL YOUR DOCTOR about any medications you are currently taking, especially any of those listed above.

WARNINGS

- Tell your doctor about unusual or allergic reactions you have had to any medications, especially to terbutaline or any related drug (albuterol, amphetamines, ephedrine, epinephrine, isoproterenol, norepinephrine, phenylephrine, phenylpropanolamine, pseudoephedrine, metaproterenol).
- Tell your doctor if you now have or if you have ever had diabetes, glaucoma, high blood pressure, epilepsy, heart disease, enlarged prostate gland, or thyroid disease.
- This medication can cause dizziness. Your ability to perform tasks that require alertness, such as driving a car may be decreased. Appropriate caution should be taken.
- Before having surgery or any other medical or dental treatment, be sure to tell your doctor or dentist that you are taking this medication.
- Avoid allowing the aerosol inhalation to come in contact with eyes.
- Do not puncture, break, or burn the aerosol inhalation container. The contents are under pressure and may explode.
- Do not exceed the recommended dosage of this medication; excessive use may lead to an increase in side effects or a loss of effectiveness. Contact your doctor if you do not respond to the usual dose of this medication. It may be a sign of worsening asthma, which may require additional therapy.
- Be sure to tell your doctor if you are pregnant. Although terbutaline appears to be safe during pregnancy, extensive studies in humans have not been conducted. Thus, terbutaline should only be administered during pregnancy if the benefits to the mother clearly outweigh potential risks to the fetus. Also, tell your doctor if you are breast-feeding an infant. Small amounts of terbutaline pass into breast milk.

---

terfenadine

BRAND NAME (Manufacturer)
Seldane (Merrell Dow)
TYPE OF DRUG
Antihistamine
INGREDIENT
terfenadine
DOSAGE FORM
Tablets (60 mg)
STORAGE
Terfenadine should be stored at room temperature in a tightly closed container. The tablets should not be exposed to high temperatures (above 104°F), direct sunlight, or moisture during storage.

USES

Terfenadine is used to treat the symptoms of allergy, including sneezing, runny nose, itching, and tearing. It belongs to a group of drugs known as antihistamines, which act by blocking the action of histamine, a chemical that is released by the body during an allergic reaction.

TREATMENT

Terfenadine can be taken either on an empty stomach or with food or milk (unless your doctor directs otherwise).

Terfenadine should be taken only as needed to control the symptoms of allergy.

If you miss a dose of this medication and you are taking it on a regular schedule, take the missed dose as soon as possible, unless it is almost time for your next dose. In that case, do not take the missed dose at all; just return to your regular dosing schedule. Do not double the next dose.

SIDE EFFECTS

Minor. Abdominal pain; cough; dizziness; drowsiness; dry mouth, nose, or throat; fatigue; headache; increased appetite; insomnia; nausea; nervousness; nosebleeds; sore throat; sweating; vomiting; or weakness. These side effects should disappear as your body adjusts to this medication.

To reduce mouth dryness, chew sugarless gum or suck on ice chips or hard candy.

If you feel dizzy or light-headed, sit or lie down for a while; get up slowly from a sitting or reclining position, and be careful on stairs.

Major. Tell your doctor about any side effects that are persistent or particularly bothersome. IT IS ESPECIALLY IMPORTANT TO TELL YOUR DOCTOR about depression, hair loss, itching, menstrual disorders, muscle or bone pain, nightmares, palpitations, shortness of breath, tingling of your fingers or toes, tremors, urinary frequency, visual disturbances, or yellowing of the skin or eyes.

INTERACTIONS

Although it appears that terfenadine is not likely to interact with other drugs, it is still very important to tell your doctor about all of the medications you are taking before starting terfenadine.

WARNINGS

- Tell your doctor about unusual or allergic reactions you have had to any medications, especially to terfenadine.
- Before starting terfenadine, tell your doctor if you now have or if you have ever had asthma.
- Terfenadine causes less drowsiness than other antihistamines. However, until you see how terfenadine affects you, be cautious about performing tasks that require alertness, such as driving a car or operating potentially dangerous machinery.
- Be sure to tell your doctor if you are pregnant. Although terfenadine appears to be safe in animals, safety in human pregnancy has not been established. Also, tell your doctor if you are breast-feeding an infant. The effects of terfenadine on nursing infants are not yet known.

Terfonyl—see sulfonamide antibiotics (oral)

---

terpin hydrate and codeine combination

BRAND NAME (Manufacturer)
terpin hydrate with codeine (various manufacturers)
TYPE OF DRUG
Expectorant and cough suppressant
INGREDIENTS
terpin hydrate and codeine
DOSAGE FORM
Oral elixir (85 mg terpin hydrate and 10 mg codeine per 5-ml spoonful, with 40% alcohol)
STORAGE
Terpin hydrate and codeine elixir should be stored at room temperature in a tightly closed, light-resistant container. This medication should never be frozen. If crystals form in the bottle, they can be dissolved by warming the closed container in warm water and then gently shaking it.

USES

This medication is used to relieve coughs due to colds. Terpin hydrate is an expectorant, which is used to promote discharge of mucus from the respiratory tract. Codeine is a narcotic cough suppressant, which acts on the cough reflex center in the brain.

TREATMENT

You can take terpin hydrate and codeine elixir either on an empty stomach or, to avoid stomach irritation, with food or milk (as directed by your doctor).

Each dose should be measured carefully with a specially designed 5-ml measuring spoon. An ordinary kitchen teaspoon is not accurate enough.

To help loosen the mucus in the bronchi, you should drink a glass of water after each dose.

If you miss a dose of this medication, take the missed one as soon as possible, unless it is almost time for the next dose. In that case, do not take the missed dose at all; just return to your regular dosing schedule. Do not double the next dose.

SIDE EFFECTS

Minor. Constipation, dizziness, drowsiness, nausea, restlessness, stomach upset, vomiting, or weakness. These should disappear as your body adjusts to the drug.

If you feel dizzy, sit or lie down for a while; get up slowly from a sitting or reclining position, and be careful on stairs.

To relieve constipation, increase the amount of fiber in your diet (fresh fruits and vegetables, salads, bran, and whole-grain breads), exercise, and drink more water (unless your doctor directs you to do otherwise).

Major. Tell your doctor about any side effects that are persistent or particularly bothersome. IT IS ESPECIALLY IMPORTANT TO TELL YOUR DOCTOR about blurred vision; cold, clammy skin; confusion; convulsions; difficulty in breathing; or fainting.

INTERACTIONS

This drug interacts with several other drugs:

1. Concurrent use of it with other central nervous system depressants (drugs that slow the activity of the brain and spinal cord), such as alcohol, barbiturates, benzodiazepine tranquilizers, muscle relaxants, other narcotics, pain medications, phenothiazine tranquilizers, and sleeping medications, or with tricyclic antidepressants can lead to extreme drowsiness.

2. Use of a monoamine oxidase (MAO) inhibitor within 14 days of use of terpin hydrate and codeine combination can lead to serious side effects.

BE SURE TO TELL YOUR DOCTOR about any medications you are currently taking, especially any listed above.

WARNINGS

- Tell your doctor about unusual or allergic reactions you have had to any medications, especially to terpin hydrate or codeine or to other narcotics (such as hydrocodone, hydromorphone, meperidine, methadone, opium, oxycodone, propoxyphene, and pentazocine).

• Before starting to take this medication, be sure to tell your doctor if you now have or if you have ever had asthma, brain disease, epilepsy, gallstones or gallbladder disease, gastrointestinal disease, heart disease, kidney disease, liver disease, lung disease, mental disorders, enlarged prostate gland, or thyroid disease.

• If this drug makes you dizzy or drowsy, do not take part in any activity that requires alertness, such as driving a car or operating potentially dangerous machinery.

• While you are taking terpin hydrate and codeine combination, drink at least eight glasses of water a day (to help loosen bronchial secretions).

• If your cough lasts longer than seven days or if you develop other symptoms such as a fever or sore throat, call your doctor.

• Because this product contains codeine, it has the potential for abuse and must be used with caution. Tolerance may develop quickly; you should not use it in higher doses or for longer periods than recommended by your doctor. If you have been taking it for longer than several weeks, do not stop taking it unless you first check with your doctor. Stopping the drug abruptly can lead to a withdrawal reaction (body aches, diarrhea, gooseflesh, vomiting, restlessness, runny nose, sneezing, execessive yawning, sweating, or trembling). Your doctor may, therefore, want to reduce your dosage gradually.

• Be sure to tell your doctor if you are pregnant. Large amounts of codeine taken during pregnancy can lead to addiction of the developing fetus, resulting in withdrawal reactions in the newborn infant. In addition, it is wise to avoid alcohol during pregnancy. Also, tell your doctor if you are breast-feeding an infant. Codeine and alcohol pass into breast milk and can cause extreme drowsiness in the nursing infant.

terpin hydrate with codeine—see terpin hydrate and codeine combination

Testred—see methyltestosterone

Tetracap—see tetracycline

---

tetracycline

BRAND NAMES (Manufacturers)
Achromycin V (Lederle)
Nor-Tet (Vortech)
Panmycin (Upjohn)
Robitet Robicaps (Robins)
Sumycin (Squibb)
Tetracap (Circle)
tetracycline hydrochloride (various manufacturers)
Tetracyn (Pfizer)
Tetralan (Lannett)
Tetram (Dunhall)

TYPE OF DRUG
Tetracycline antibiotic

INGREDIENT
tetracycline

DOSAGE FORMS
Tablets (250 mg and 500 mg)
Capsules (100 mg, 250 mg, and 500 mg)
Oral suspension (125 mg per 5-ml spoonful)

STORAGE
Tetracycline tablets, capsules, and oral suspension should be stored at room temperature in tightly closed, light-resistant containers. Any unused portion of the suspension should be discarded after 14 days because the drug loses its potency after that period. Discard any medication that is outdated or no longer needed. This medication should never be frozen.

USES

Tetracycline is used to treat acne (bacteria may be partly responsible for the development of acne lesions) and a wide variety of bacterial infections. It acts by inhibiting the growth of bacteria. Tetracycline kills susceptible bacteria, but it is not effective against viruses or fungi.

TREATMENT

Ideally, this medication should be taken on an empty stomach one hour before or two hours after a meal. It should be taken with a full glass of water in order to avoid irritating the throat or esophagus (swallowing tube). If this drug causes stomach upset, however, you can take it with food (unless your doctor directs you to do otherwise).

Avoid consuming dairy products (milk, cheese, etc.) within two hours of any dose of this drug. Avoid taking antacids and laxatives that contain aluminum, calcium, or magnesium within an hour or two of a dose. Avoid taking any medication containing iron within three hours of a dose. These products, including vitamins, chemically bind tetracycline in the stomach and gastrointestinal tract, preventing the drug from being absorbed into the body.

The oral suspension form of this medication should be shaken well just before measuring each dose. The contents tend to settle on the bottom of the bottle, so it is necessary to shake the container to distribute the ingredients evenly and equalize the doses. Each dose should then be measured carefully with a specially designed 5-ml measuring spoon. An ordinary kitchen teaspoon is not accurate enough. The oral suspension form of this medication should not be mixed with any other substance, unless your doctor directs you to do so.

Tetracycline works best when the level of medicine in your bloodstream is kept constant. It is best, therefore, to take the doses at evenly spaced intervals day and night. For example, if you are to take four doses a day, the doses should be spaced six hours apart.

If you miss a dose of this medication, take the missed dose immediately. However, if you do not remember to take the missed dose until it is almost time for your next dose, take it; space the following dose about halfway through the regular interval between doses; and then return to your regular dosing schedule. Try not to skip any doses.

It is important to continue to take this medication for the entire time prescribed by your doctor, even if the symptoms disappear before the end of that period. If you stop taking the drug too soon, resistant bacteria are given a chance to continue growing, and the infection could recur.

SIDE EFFECTS

Minor. Diarrhea, discoloration of the nails, dizziness, loss of appetite, nausea, stomach cramps and upset, or vomiting. These side effects should disappear as your body adjusts to the medication.

Tetracycline can increase your sensitivity to sunlight. You should, therefore, avoid prolonged exposure to sunlight or sunlamps. Wear protective clothing and sunglasses, and use an effective sunscreen.

Major. Tell your doctor about any side effects that are persistent or particularly bothersome. IT IS ESPECIALLY IMPORTANT TO TELL YOUR DOCTOR about darkened tongue, difficulty in breathing, joint pain, mouth irritation, rash, rectal or vaginal itching, sore throat and fever, unusual bleeding or bruising, or yellowing of the eyes or skin. Also, if your symptoms of infection seem to be getting worse rather than improving, you should contact your doctor.

INTERACTIONS

Tetracycline interacts with other types of medications:

1. It can increase the absorption of digoxin, which may lead to digoxin toxicity.

2. The gastrointestinal side effects (nausea, vomiting, or stomach upset) of theophylline may be increased by tetracycline.

3. The dosage of oral anticoagulants (blood thinners, such as warfarin) may need to be adjusted when this medication is started.

4. Tetracycline may decrease the effectiveness of oral contraceptives (birth control pills), and pregnancy could result. You should, therefore, use a different or additional form of birth control while taking tetracycline. Discuss this with your doctor.

BE SURE TO TELL YOUR DOCTOR about any medications that you are currently taking, especially any of the medications that are listed above.

WARNINGS

- Tell your doctor about unusual or allergic reactions you have had to any medications, especially to tetracycline or to oxytetracycline, doxycycline, or minocycline.
- Tell your doctor if you now have or if you have ever had kidney or liver disease.
- Tetracycline can affect tests for syphilis; tell your doctor you are taking this drug if you are being treated for syphilis.
- Make sure that your prescription for this drug is marked with the expiration date. The drug should be discarded after the expiration date. If tetracycline is used after it has expired, serious side effects (especially to the kidneys) could result.
- This medication has been prescribed for your current infection only. Another infection later on, or one that someone else has, may require a different medicine. You should not give your medicine to other people or use it for other infections, unless your doctor specifically directs you to do so.
- Be sure to tell your doctor if you are pregnant or if you are breast-feeding an infant. Tetracycline crosses the placenta and passes into breast milk. If used during tooth development, this drug can cause permanent tooth discoloration. It can also inhibit tooth and bone growth in the fetus. It should not be used in pregnant or nursing women, infants, or children less than eight years of age.

tetracycline hydrochloride—see tetracycline

Tetracyn—see tetracycline

Tetralan—see tetracycline

Tetram—see tetracycline

Texacort—see hydrocortisone (topical)

T-Gen—see trimethobenzamide

T-Gesic—see acetaminophen and hydrocodone combination

Thalitone—see chlorthalidone

Theo-24—see theophylline

Theobid—see theophylline

Theochron—see theophylline

Theoclear—see theophylline

Theocolate—see theophylline and guaifenesin combination

Theo-Dur—see theophylline

Theolair—see theophylline

Theolate—see theophylline and guaifenesin combination

Theon—see theophylline

theophylline

BRAND NAMES (Manufacturers)

Accurbron (Merrell Dow)
Aerolate (Fleming)
Aquaphyllin (Ferndale)
Asmalix (Century)
Bronkodyl (Breon)
Constant-T (Geigy)
Elixicon (Berlex)
Elixomin (Cenci)
Elixophyllin (Berlex)
Lanophyllin (Lannett)
Lodrane (Poythress)
Quibron-T (Mead Johnson)
Respbid (Boehringer Ingelheim)
Slo-bid Gyrocaps (Rorer)
Slo-Phyllin (Rorer)
Somophyllin-T (Fisons)
Sustaire (Pfipharmics)
Theo-24 (Searle)

Theobid (Glaxo)
Theochron (Forest)
Theoclear (Central)
Theo-Dur (Key)
Theolair (Riker)
Theon (Bock)
theophylline (various manufacturers)
Theospan (Laser)
Theostat (Laser)
Theo-Time (Major)
Theovent (Schering)
Uniphyl (Purdue Frederick)

TYPE OF DRUG
Bronchodilator

INGREDIENT
theophylline

DOSAGE FORMS
Tablets (100 mg, 125 mg, 200 mg, 225 mg, 250 mg, and 300 mg)
Capsules (100 mg, 200 mg, and 250 mg)
Sustained-release tablets and capsules (50 mg, 60 mg, 65 mg, 75 mg, 100 mg, 125 mg, 130 mg, 200 mg, 250 mg, 260 mg, 300 mg, 400 mg, and 500 mg)
Oral liquid (80 mg, 150 mg, and 160 mg per 15-ml spoonful, some with alcohol of varying amounts, including 1%, 7.5%, and 20%)
Oral suspension (300 mg per 15-ml spoonful)

STORAGE
Theophylline tablets, capsules, liquid, and suspension should be stored at room temperature. It should also be kept in tightly closed, light-resistant containers. This medication should never be frozen. Discard any outdated medication.

USES

Theophylline is prescribed to treat breathing problems (wheezing and shortness of breath) caused by asthma, bronchitis, or emphysema. It relaxes the smooth muscle of the bronchial airways (breathing tubes), which opens the air passages to the lungs and allows air to move in and out more easily.

TREATMENT

Theophylline should be taken on an empty stomach 30 to 60 minutes before a meal or two hours after a meal. If this medication causes stomach irritation, however, you can take it with food or with a full glass of water or milk (unless your doctor directs you to do otherwise).

Antidiarrheal medications and some antacids prevent the absorption of theophylline from the gastrointestinal tract. Therefore, at least one hour should separate doses of one of these medications and theophylline.

The sustained-release tablets and capsules should be swallowed whole. Chewing, crushing, or crumbling the tablets or capsules destroys their sustained-release activity and possibly increases the side effects. If the tablet is scored for breaking, you can break it along these lines. If the regular capsules are too large to swallow, they can be opened and the contents mixed with jam, jelly, or applesauce. The mixture should then be swallowed without chewing.

The theophylline sprinkle capsules can also be taken whole, or the capsule can be opened and the beads sprinkled on a spoonful of soft food, such as applesauce or pudding. The sprinkles should be swallowed immediately without chewing the beads. The contents of the capsule should not be subdivided in order to ensure equal doses.

If you are using the suspension form of this medication, the bottle should be shaken well just before measuring each dose. The contents tend to settle on the bottom of the bottle, so it is necessary to shake the container to distribute the medication evenly and equalize the doses. Each dose of the oral liquid or suspension should be measured carefully with a 5-ml measuring spoon or a dose cup designed for that purpose. Ordinary kitchen spoons are not accurate enough to ensure that you receive the proper dose.

Theophylline works best when the level of the medicine in your bloodstream is kept constant. It is best, therefore, to take it at evenly spaced intervals day and night. For example, if you are to take four doses a day, the doses should be spaced six hours apart. Try to take your medication at the same time(s) each day.

Try not to miss any doses of this medication. If you do miss a dose, take the missed dose as soon as possible, unless it is almost time for the next dose. In that case, do not take the missed dose at all; just return to your regular dosing schedule. Do not double the next dose.

SIDE EFFECTS

Minor. Diarrhea, dizziness, flushing, headache, heartburn, increased urination, insomnia, irritability, loss of appetite, nausea, nervousness, stomach pain, or vomiting. These side effects should disappear as your body adjusts to the medication.

If you feel dizzy or light headed, sit or lie down for a while; get up slowly from a sitting or reclining position, and be careful on stairs.

Major. Tell your doctor about any side effects that are persistent or particularly bothersome. IT IS ESPECIALLY IMPORTANT TO TELL YOUR DOCTOR about black, tarry stools; confusion; convulsions; difficulty in breathing; fainting; muscle twitches; palpitations; rash; severe abdominal pain; or unusual weakness.

INTERACTIONS

Theophylline interacts with several other types of drugs:

1. It can increase the diuretic effect of furosemide.

2. Concurrent use of reserpine and theophylline can cause a rapid heart rate.

3. Beta blockers (acebutolol, atenolol, betaxolol, carteolol, esmolol, labetalol, metoprolol, nadolol, penbutolol, pindolol, propranolol, timolol) can decrease the effectiveness of theophylline.

4. Theophylline can increase the side effects of over-the-counter (nonprescription) sinus, cough, cold, asthma, allergy, and diet products; digoxin; and oral anticoagulants (blood thinners, such as warfarin).

5. Theophylline can decrease the effectiveness of phenytoin and lithium.

6. Phenobarbital, carbamazepine, and rifampin can increase the elimination of theophylline from the body, decreasing its effectiveness.

7. Cimetidine, erythromycin, troleandomycin, oral contraceptives (birth control pills), allopurinol, and thiabendazole can decrease the elimination of theophylline from the body and increase its side effects.

8. Verapamil can cause an increase in the effects of theophylline.

Before you start to take this medication, BE SURE TO TELL YOUR DOCTOR about any medications you are currently taking, especially any of those listed above.

WARNINGS

- Tell your doctor about unusual or allergic reactions you have had to any medications, especially to theophylline, aminophylline, caffeine, dyphylline, oxtriphylline, or theobromine.
- Tell your doctor if you now have or if you have ever had an enlarged prostate gland, fibrocystic breast disease, heart disease, kidney disease, low or high blood pressure, liver disease, stomach ulcers, or thyroid disease.
- Cigarette or marijuana smoking may affect this drug's action. BE SURE TO TELL YOUR DOCTOR if you smoke. Also, do not quit smoking without informing your doctor.
- High fever, diarrhea, the flu, and influenza vaccinations can affect the action of this drug. Therefore, be sure to tell your doctor if you experience any episodes of high fever or prolonged diarrhea while taking this drug. Before having any vaccinations, especially those to prevent the flu, BE SURE TO TELL YOUR DOCTOR that you are taking this medication.
- Avoid drinking large amounts of caffeine-containing beverages (coffee, cocoa, tea, or cola drinks), and avoid eating large amounts of chocolate. These products may increase the side effects of theophylline.
- Do not change your diet without first consulting your doctor. A high-protein, low-carbohydrate diet or charbroiled foods may affect the action of this drug.
- Before having surgery or any other medical or dental treatment, be sure to tell your doctor or dentist that you are taking this medication.
- Before taking any over-the-counter (nonprescription) asthma, allergy, cough, cold, sinus, or diet product, ask your doctor or pharmacist. These products may add to the side effects of theophylline.
- Do not change brands or dosage forms of this medication without your doctor's permission. If your medication refill looks different, check with your doctor or pharmacist.
- The elderly and young children may be more sensitive to the effects of theophylline.
- Your doctor may require you to have periodic blood tests to be sure your medication is working properly.
- Be sure to tell your doctor if you are pregnant. Although theophylline appears to be safe during pregnancy, extensive studies in humans have not been conducted. Also, tell your doctor if you are breast-feeding an infant. Small amounts of theophylline pass into breast milk and may cause irritability, fretfulness, or insomnia in nursing infants.

---

theophylline and guaifenesin combination

BRAND NAMES (Manufacturers)

Asbron G (Sandoz)
Bronchial (various manufacturers)
Glyceryl-T (Rugby)
Lanophyllin-GG (Lannett)
Quiagen (Goldline)
Quibron (Bristol Labs)
Quibron 300 (Bristol Labs)
Slo-Phyllin GG (Rorer)
Synophylate-GG (Central)
Theocolate (My-K Labs)
Theolate (various manufacturers)

TYPE OF DRUG

Bronchodilator and expectorant

INGREDIENTS

theophylline and guaifenesin

DOSAGE FORMS

Tablets (137 mg or 138 mg theophylline and 100 mg guaifenesin)
Capsules (150 mg theophylline and 90 mg guaifenesin; 300 mg theophylline and 180 mg guaifenesin)
Oral liquid (100 mg theophylline and 100 mg guaifenesin; 137 mg theophylline and 100 mg guaifenesin; and 150 mg theophylline and 90 mg guaifenesin per 15-ml spoonful, some with alcohol [10% or 15%])

STORAGE

Theophylline and guaifenesin combination tablets, capsules, and oral liquid should be stored at room temperature in tightly closed containers. This medication should never be frozen. Discard any outdated medication or medication that is no longer needed.

USES

Theophylline and guaifenesin combination medication is prescribed to treat breathing problems (wheezing and shortness of breath) caused by asthma, bronchitis, or emphysema. Theophylline relaxes the smooth muscle of the bronchial airways (breathing tubes), which opens up the air passages, allowing air to move more easily to and from the lungs. Guaifenesin is an expectorant that is used to loosen phlegm, thin bronchial secretions, and promote discharge of mucus from the respiratory tract.

TREATMENT

Theophylline and guaifenesin should be taken on an empty stomach 30 to 60 minutes before a meal or two hours after a meal. If this medication causes stomach irritation, however, you can take it with food or with a full glass of water or milk (unless your doctor directs you to do otherwise).

Antidiarrheal medications and some antacids prevent the absorption of theophylline. Therefore, at least one hour should separate doses of these two types of medication.

The dose of the oral liquid should be measured carefully with a 5-ml measuring spoon or a dose cup designed for that purpose. An ordinary kitchen teaspoon is not accurate enough.

Theophylline works best when the concentration of medicine in your bloodstream is kept constant. It is best, therefore, to take the doses at evenly spaced intervals day and night. For example, if you are to take four doses a day, the doses should be spaced six hours apart.

Try not to miss any doses of this medication. If you do miss a dose, take the missed dose as soon as possible, unless it is almost time for the next dose. Do not take more than the recommended dose.

SIDE EFFECTS

Minor. Diarrhea, dizziness, flushing, headache, heartburn, increased urination, insomnia, irritability, loss of appetite, nausea, nervousness, paleness, stomach pain, or vomiting. These side effects should disappear as your body adjusts to the medication.

If you feel dizzy or light-headed, sit or lie down for a while; get up slowly from a sitting or reclining position, and be careful on stairs.

This medication may cause you to cough more frequently. Coughing is your body's way of discharging the mucus from the respiratory tract. This medication loosens and thins the mucus in your respiratory tract, making your cough more productive.

Major. Tell your doctor about any side effects that are persistent or particularly bothersome. IT IS ESPECIALLY IMPORTANT TO TELL YOUR DOCTOR about black, tarry stools; confusion; convulsions; difficulty in breathing; fainting; muscle twitches; palpitations; rash; severe abdominal pain; or unusual weakness.

INTERACTIONS

Theophylline interacts with several other types of drugs:

1. It can increase the effects (diuresis, or increased urination) of furosemide.

2. Concurrent use of reserpine and theophylline can cause a rapid heart rate.

3. Beta blockers (acebutolol, atenolol, betaxolol, carteolol, esmolol, labetalol, metoprolol, nadolol, penbutolol, pindolol, propranolol, timolol) can decrease the effectiveness of theophylline.

4. Theophylline can increase the side effects of over-the-counter (nonprescription) sinus, cough, cold, asthma, allergy, and diet products; digoxin; and oral anticoagulants (blood thinners, such as warfarin).

5. Theophylline can decrease the effectiveness of phenytoin and lithium.

6. Phenobarbital, carbamazepine, and rifampin can increase the elimination of theophylline from the body, decreasing its effectiveness.

7. Cimetidine, erythromycin, troleandomycin, oral contraceptives (birth control pills), allopurinol, and thiabendazole can decrease the elimination of theophylline from the body and increase its side effects.

Before starting to take this medication, BE SURE TO TELL YOUR DOCTOR about any medications you are currently taking, especially any of those listed above.

WARNINGS

- Tell your doctor about unusual or allergic reactions you have had to any medications, especially to theophylline, aminophylline, caffeine, dyphylline, oxtriphylline, theobromine, or guaifenesin.
- Tell your doctor if you now have or if you have ever had an enlarged prostate gland, fibrocystic breast disease, heart disease, kidney disease, low or high blood pressure, liver disease, stomach ulcers, or thyroid disease.
- Cigarette or marijuana smoking may affect this drug's action. BE SURE TO TELL YOUR DOCTOR if you smoke. Also, do not suddenly stop smoking without informing your doctor.
- High fever, diarrhea, the flu, or an influenza vaccination can also affect the action of this drug. You should tell your doctor about episodes of high fever or prolonged diarrhea. Before having any vaccinations, especially those to prevent the flu, BE SURE TO TELL YOUR DOCTOR that you are taking this medication.
- Avoid drinking large amounts of caffeine-containing beverages (coffee, cocoa, tea, or cola drinks), and avoid eating large amounts of chocolate. These products may increase the side effects of theophylline.
- While you are taking this medication, drink at least eight glasses of water a day to help loosen bronchial secretions (unless your doctor directs you to do otherwise).
- Do not change brands of this medication without your doctor's permission. If you receive a refill, and the medication looks different, consult your doctor or pharmacist.
- Do not change your diet without first consulting your doctor. A high-protein, low-carbohydrate diet or charbroiled foods can affect the action of this drug.
- Before having surgery or any other medical or dental treatment, be sure to tell your doctor or dentist that you are taking this medication.
- Your doctor may want you to have regular blood tests done to make sure this medication is working properly.
- Elderly patients and young children are more sensitive to the effects of this medication.
- Be sure to tell your doctor if you are pregnant. Although theophylline appears to be safe during pregnancy, extensive studies in humans have not been conducted. Also, tell your doctor if you are breast-feeding. Small amounts of theophylline pass into breast milk and may cause irritability, fretfulness, and insomnia in nursing infants.

Theospan—see theophylline

Theostat—see theophylline

Theo-Time—see theophylline

Theovent—see theophylline

---

thioridazine

BRAND NAMES (Manufacturers)

Mellaril (Sandoz)
Millazine (Major)
thioridazine hydrochloride (various manufacturers)

TYPE OF DRUG

Phenothiazine tranquilizer

INGREDIENT

thioridazine

DOSAGE FORMS

Tablets (10 mg, 15 mg, 25 mg, 50 mg, 100 mg, 150 mg, and 200 mg)
Oral concentrate (30 mg and 100 mg per ml, with 3% and 4.2% alcohol, respectively)
Oral suspension (25 mg and 100 mg per 5-ml spoonful)

STORAGE

The tablet form of this medication should be stored at room temperature in a tightly closed, light-resistant container. The oral concentrate and oral suspension forms of this medication should be stored in the refrigerator in tightly closed, light-resistant containers. If the oral concentrate or suspension turns slightly yellowish, the medication is still effective and can be used. However, if it changes color markedly or has particles floating in it, it should not be used; rather, it should be discarded down the sink. This medication should never be frozen.

USES

Thioridazine is prescribed to treat the symptoms of certain types of mental illness, such as emotional symptoms of psychosis, the manic phase of manic-depressive illness, and severe behavioral problems in children. It may also be used for moderate to marked depression or sleep disturbances in adults. This medication is thought to relieve the symptoms of mental illness by blocking certain chemicals involved with nerve transmission in the brain. Thioridazine may also be used to treat anxiety.

TREATMENT

In order to avoid stomach irritation, you can take this medication with a meal or with a glass of water or milk (unless your doctor directs you to do otherwise).

Antacids and antidiarrheal medicines may decrease the absorption of this medication from the gastrointestinal tract. Therefore, at least one hour should separate doses of one of these medicines and thioridazine.

The oral suspension form of this medication should be shaken well just before measuring each dose. The contents tend to settle on the bottom of the bottle, so it is necessary to shake the container to distribute the ingredients evenly and equalize the doses. Each dose should then be measured carefully with a specially designed 5-ml measuring spoon. An ordinary kitchen teaspoon is not accurate enough.

The oral concentrate form of this medication should be measured carefully with the dropper provided, then added to four ounces (1/2 cup) or more of water, milk, or a carbonated beverage or to applesauce or pudding immediately prior to administration. To prevent possible loss of effectiveness, the medication should not be diluted in tea, coffee, or apple juice.

If you miss a dose of this medication, take the missed dose as soon as possible, unless it is almost time for your next dose. In that case, do not take the missed dose at all; just return to your regular dosing schedule. Do not double the next dose (unless your doctor directs you to do so).

The full effects of this medication for the control of emotional or mental symptoms may not become apparent for at least two weeks after you start to take it.

SIDE EFFECTS

Minor. Blurred vision, constipation, decreased sweating, diarrhea, dizziness, drooling, drowsiness, dry mouth, fatigue, jitteriness, menstrual irregularities, nasal congestion, restlessness, vomiting, and weight gain. As your body adjusts to the medication, these side effects should disappear.

This medication can cause increased sensitivity to sunlight. It is, therefore, important to avoid prolonged exposure to sunlight and sunlamps. Wear protective clothing and sunglasses, and use an effective sunscreen.

Thioridazine can also cause discoloration of the urine to red, pink, or red-brown. This is a harmless effect.

If you are constipated, increase the amount of fiber in your diet (fresh fruits and vegetables, salads, bran, and whole-grain breads), exercise, and drink more water (unless your doctor directs you to do otherwise).

Chew sugarless gum or suck on ice chips or a piece of hard candy to reduce mouth dryness.

To avoid dizziness or light-headedness when you stand, contract and relax the muscles of your legs for a few moments before rising. Do this by pushing one foot against the floor while raising the other foot slightly, alternating feet so that you are "pumping" your legs in a pedaling motion.

Major. Tell your doctor about any side effects that are persistent or particularly bothersome. IT IS ESPECIALLY IMPORTANT TO TELL YOUR DOCTOR about breast enlargement (in both sexes); chest pain; convulsions; darkened skin; difficulty in swallowing or breathing; fainting; fever; impotence; involuntary movements of the face, mouth, jaw, or tongue; palpitations; rash; sleep disorders; sore throat; tremors; uncoordinated movements; unusual bleeding or bruising; visual disturbances; or yellowing of the eyes or skin.

INTERACTIONS

Thioridazine interacts with several other types of medications:

1. It can cause extreme drowsiness when combined with alcohol or other central nervous system depressants (drugs that slow the activity of the brain and spinal cord), such as barbiturates, benzodiazepine tranquilizers, muscle relaxants, narcotics, and pain medications, or with tricyclic antidepressants.

2. Thioridazine can decrease the effectiveness of amphetamines, guanethidine, anticonvulsants, and levodopa.

3. The side effects of epinephrine, monoamine oxidase (MAO) inhibitors, metoprolol, propranolol, phenytoin, and tricyclic antidepressants may be increased by this medication. At least 14 days should separate the use of this drug and the use of an MAO inhibitor.

4. Lithium may increase the side effects and decrease the effectiveness of this medication.

5. False positive pregnancy tests may occur. If you think you may be pregnant, call your doctor.

Before starting to take thioridazine, BE SURE TO TELL YOUR DOCTOR about any medications you are currently taking, especially any of those listed above.

WARNINGS

- Tell your doctor about unusual or allergic reactions you have had to any medications, especially to thioridazine or any other phenothiazine tranquilizers (such as chlorpromazine, fluphenazine, mesoridazine, perphenazine, prochlorperazine, promazine, trifluoperazine, and triflupromazine) or to loxapine.
- Tell your doctor if you have a history of alcoholism or if you now have or have ever had any blood disease, bone marrow disease, brain disease, breast cancer, blockage in the urinary or digestive tracts, drug-induced depression, epilepsy, high or low blood pressure, diabetes mellitus, glaucoma, heart or circulatory disease, liver disease, lung disease, Parkinson's disease, peptic ulcers, or an enlarged prostate gland.
- Tell your doctor about any recent exposure to a pesticide

or an insecticide. Thioridazine may increase the side effects from the exposure.

- To prevent oversedation, avoid drinking alcoholic beverages while taking this medication.
- If this medication makes you dizzy or drowsy, do not take part in any activity that requires alertness, such as driving a car or operating potentially dangerous machinery. Be careful on stairs, and avoid getting up suddenly from a lying or sitting position.
- Prior to having surgery or any other medical or dental treatment, be sure to tell your doctor or dentist that you are taking thioridazine.
- Some of the side effects caused by this drug can be prevented by taking an antiparkinsonism drug. Discuss this with your doctor.
- This medication can decrease sweating and heat release from the body. You should, therefore, try not to become overheated (avoid exercising strenuously in hot weather, and do not take hot baths, showers, and saunas).
- Do not stop taking this medication suddenly. If the drug is stopped abruptly, you may experience nausea, vomiting, stomach upset, headache, increased heart rate, insomnia, tremors, or a worsening of your condition. Your doctor may want to reduce the dosage gradually.
- If you are planning to have a myelogram, or any other procedure in which dye will be injected into your spinal cord, tell your doctor that you are taking this medication.
- Avoid spilling the oral concentrate or suspension form of this medication on your skin or clothing; either may cause redness and irritation of the skin.
- While taking this medication, do not take any over-the-counter (nonprescription) drugs for weight control or for cough, cold, allergy, asthma, or sinus problems unless you first check with your doctor. Concurrent use of any of these drugs and thioridazine may cause high blood pressure.
- Your doctor may schedule regular office visits for your first few months of therapy with this medication in order to monitor your progress and possibly adjust your dosage.
- Your doctor may want to schedule you for an eye examination if you take thioridazine for longer than a year. Prolonged use of this drug can cause visual disturbances.
- Be sure to tell your doctor if you are pregnant. Small amounts of this medication cross the placenta. Although there are reports of safe use of this drug during pregnancy, there are also reports of liver disease and tremors in newborn infants whose mothers received this type of medication close to term. Also, tell your doctor if you are breast-feeding. Small amounts of this medication pass into breast milk and may cause unwanted effects in nursing infants.

thioridazine hydrochloride—see thioridazine

Thiosulfil—see sulfonamide antibiotics (oral)

Thiosulfil Forte—see sulfonamide antibiotics (oral)

---

thiothixene

BRAND NAME (Manufacturer)
Navane (Roerig)

TYPE OF DRUG
Antipsychotic

INGREDIENT
thiothixene

DOSAGE FORMS
Capsules (1 mg, 2 mg, 5 mg, 10 mg, and 20 mg)
Oral concentrate (5 mg per ml, with 7% alcohol)

STORAGE
Thiothixene capsules should be stored at room temperature in a tightly closed, light-resistant container. The oral concentrate should be stored in the refrigerator in a tightly closed, light-resistant container. This medication should never be frozen. Discard any medication that is outdated or no longer needed.

USES

Thiothixene is prescribed to treat the symptoms of certain types of mental illness, such as emotional symptoms of psychosis. It is thought to relieve the symptoms of mental illness by blocking certain chemicals involved with nerve transmission in the brain.

TREATMENT

To avoid stomach irritation, you can take the capsule form of thiothixene with a meal or with a glass of water or milk (unless your doctor directs you to do otherwise).

The oral concentrate form of this medication should be measured carefully with the dropper provided and then added to four ounces (1/2 cup) or more of water, milk, or a carbonated beverage or to applesauce or pudding immediately prior to administration. To prevent possible loss of effectiveness, this medication should not be diluted in tea, coffee, or apple juice.

Antacids and antidiarrheal medicines decrease the absorption of this medication from the gastrointestinal tract. Therefore, at least one hour should separate doses of one of these medicines and thiothixene.

If you miss a dose of this medication, take the missed dose as soon as possible and then return to your regular dosing schedule. If it is almost time for the next dose, however, skip the one you missed and return to your regular schedule. Do not double the dose (unless so directed by your doctor).

The full effects of this medication for the control of emotional or mental symptoms may not become apparent for at least two weeks after you start to take it.

SIDE EFFECTS

Minor. Blurred vision, constipation, decreased sweating, diarrhea, dizziness, drooling, drowsiness, dry mouth, fatigue, jitteriness, menstrual irregularities, nasal congestion, restlessness, vomiting, or weight gain. As your body adjusts to the medication, these side effects should disappear.

This medication can cause increased sensitivity to sunlight. It is, therefore, important to avoid prolonged exposure to sunlight and sunlamps. Wear protective clothing, and use an effective sunscreen.

Thiothixene can cause discoloration of the urine to red, pink, or red-brown. This is a harmless effect.

If you are constipated, increase the amount of fiber in your diet (fresh fruits and vegetables, salads, bran, and whole-grain breads), exercise, and drink more water (unless your doctor directs you to do otherwise).

To reduce mouth dryness, chew sugarless gum or suck on ice chips or a piece of hard candy.

To avoid dizziness or light-headedness when you stand, contract and relax the muscles of your legs for a few moments before rising. Do this by pushing one foot against the floor while raising the other foot slightly, alternating feet so that you are "pumping" your legs in a pedaling motion.

Major. Tell your doctor about any side effects that are persistent or particularly bothersome. IT IS ESPECIALLY IMPORTANT TO TELL YOUR DOCTOR about breast enlargement (in both sexes); chest pain; convulsions; darkened skin; difficulty in swallowing or breathing; fainting; fever; impotence; involuntary movements of the face, mouth, jaw, or tongue; palpitations; rash; sleep disorders; sore throat; tremors; uncoordinated movements; unusual bleeding or bruising; visual disturbances; or yellowing of the eyes or skin.

INTERACTIONS

Thiothixene interacts with other types of medications:

1. It can cause extreme drowsiness when combined with alcohol or other central nervous system depressants (drugs that slow the activity of the brain and spinal cord), such as barbiturates, benzodiazepine tranquilizers, muscle relaxants, narcotics, and pain medications, or with tricyclic antidepressants.

2. Thiothixene can decrease the effectiveness of amphetamines, guanethidine, anticonvulsants, and levodopa.

3. The side effects of epinephrine, monoamine oxidase (MAO) inhibitors, and tricyclic antidepressants may be increased by this medication. At least 14 days should separate the use of this drug and the use of an MAO inhibitor.

4. Lithium may increase the side effects and decrease the effectiveness of thiothixene.

5. False positive pregnancy tests may occur. If you think you may be pregnant, call your doctor.

BE SURE TO TELL YOUR DOCTOR about any medications you are currently taking, especially any of those listed above.

WARNINGS

• Tell your doctor about unusual or allergic reactions you have had to any medications, especially to thiothixene, chlorprothixene, or any phenothiazine tranquilizer.

• Tell your doctor if you have a history of alcoholism or if you now have or have ever had blood disease, bone marrow disease, brain disease, breast cancer, blockage in the urinary or digestive tract, drug-induced depression, epilepsy, high or low blood pressure, diabetes mellitus, glaucoma, heart or circulatory disease, liver disease, lung disease, Parkinson's disease, peptic ulcers, or an enlarged prostate gland.

• Avoid drinking alcoholic beverages while taking this medication, in order to prevent oversedation.

• If this drug makes you dizzy or drowsy, do not take part in any activity that requires alertness, such as driving a car or operating potentially dangerous machinery. Be careful on stairs, and avoid getting up suddenly from a lying or sitting position.

• Prior to having surgery or any other medical or dental treatment, be sure to tell your doctor or dentist that you are taking this medication.

• Some of the side effects caused by this drug can be prevented by taking an antiparkinsonism drug. Discuss this with your doctor.

• This medication can decrease sweating and heat release from the body. You should, therefore, try not to become overheated (avoid exercising strenuously in hot weather, and do not take hot baths, showers, and saunas).

• Do not stop taking this medication suddenly. If the drug is stopped abruptly you may experience nausea, vomiting, stomach upset, headache, increased heart rate, insomnia, tremors, or worsening of your condition. Your doctor may want to reduce the dosage gradually.

• If you are planning to have a myelogram, or any other procedure in which dye is injected into the space surrounding the spinal cord, tell your doctor that you are taking this medication.

• Avoid spilling the oral concentrate form of this medication on your skin or clothing; it can cause redness and irritation of the skin.

• While taking this medication, do not take any over-the-counter (nonprescription) medication for weight control or for cough, cold, allergy, asthma, or sinus problems unless you first check with your doctor. The combination of these medications may cause high blood pressure.

• Your doctor may schedule regular office visits during your first few months of therapy with this medication in order to monitor your progress and possibly adjust the dosage.

• Be sure to tell your doctor if you are pregnant. Small amounts of this medication cross the placenta. Although there are reports of safe use of this drug during pregnancy, there are also reports of liver disease and tremors in newborn infants whose mothers received this type of medication close to term. Also, tell your doctor if you are breast-feeding. Small amounts of this medication pass into breast milk and may cause unwanted effects in nursing infants.

Thiuretic—see hydrochlorothiazide

Thorazine—see chlorpromazine

Thorazine Spansules—see chlorpromazine

Thor-Prom—see chlorpromazine

Thyrar—see thyroid hormone

---

thyroid hormone

BRAND NAMES (Manufacturers)

Armour Thyroid (USV)
S-P-T (Fleming)
Thyrar (USV)
Thyroid Strong (Marion)

TYPE OF DRUG

Thyroid hormone

INGREDIENT

thyroid hormone

DOSAGE FORMS

Tablets (16 mg, 32 mg, 65 mg, 98 mg, 130 mg, 195 mg, 260 mg, and 325 mg)
Enteric-coated tablets (65 mg and 130 mg)

Sugar-coated tablets (32 mg, 65 mg, 130 mg, and 195 mg)
Capsules (65 mg, 130 mg, 195 mg, and 325 mg)

Note that 16 mg = 1/4 grain (gr); 32 mg = 1/2 gr; 65 mg = 1 gr; 98 mg = 1 1/2 gr; 130 mg = 2 gr; 195 mg = 3 gr; 260 mg = 4 gr; and 325 mg = 5 gr.

STORAGE

Store at room temperature in a tightly closed, light-resistant container. Discard outdated medication.

USES

This medication is prescribed to replace natural thyroid hormones that are absent because of a thyroid gland disorder. This product is obtained from animal thyroid glands.

TREATMENT

Thyroid hormone tablets should be taken on an empty stomach with a full glass of water. If this medication upsets your stomach, however, you can check with your doctor to see if you can take the medication with food or milk.

In order to get used to taking this medication, try to take it at the same time each day. Try not to miss any doses. If you do miss a dose of this medication, take it as soon as you remember, unless it is almost time for the next dose. In that case, do not take the missed dose at all; just return to your regular dosing schedule. Do not double the next dose. If you miss more than one or two doses of this medication, check with your doctor.

SIDE EFFECTS

Minor. Constipation, dry puffy skin, fatigue, headache, listlessness, muscle aches, or weight gain. These side effects should disappear as your body adjusts to the medication.

To relieve constipation, increase the amount of fiber in your diet (fresh fruits and vegetables, salads, bran, and whole-grain breads), exercise, and drink more water (unless your doctor directs you to do otherwise).

Major. Tell your doctor about any side effects that are persistent or particularly bothersome. Most of the major side effects associated with this drug are the result of too large a dose. The dosage of this medication may need to be adjusted if you experience any of the following side effects: chest pain, diarrhea, fever, heat intolerance, insomnia, irritability, leg cramps, menstrual irregularities, nervousness, palpitations, shortness of breath, sweating, trembling, or weight loss. CHECK WITH YOUR DOCTOR.

INTERACTIONS

Thyroid hormone interacts with other types of medications:

1. Dosing requirements for digoxin, insulin, or oral antidiabetic agents may change when this medication is used.

2. The effects of oral anticoagulants (blood thinners, such as warfarin) may be increased by thyroid hormone, which could lead to bleeding complications.

3. Cholestyramine and colestipol chemically bind thyroid hormone in the gastrointestinal tract, preventing its absorption. Therefore, at least four hours should separate doses of thyroid hormone and one of these medications.

4. Oral contraceptives (birth control pills) and estrogen-containing drugs may change your dosing requirements for thyroid hormone.

5. Phenobarbital may decrease the effectiveness of thyroid hormone.

6. Phenytoin, tricyclic antidepressants, and over-the-counter (nonprescription) allergy, asthma, cough, cold, sinus, or diet medications may increase the side effects of thyroid hormone.

BE SURE TO TELL YOUR DOCTOR about any medications you are currently taking, especially any listed above.

WARNINGS

- Tell your doctor about unusual or allergic reactions you have had to any medications, especially to thyroid hormone or to beef or pork products.
- Tell your doctor if you now have or if you have ever had angina pectoris, diabetes mellitus, heart disease, high blood pressure, kidney disease, or an underactive adrenal or pituitary gland.
- If you have an underactive thyroid gland, you may need to take this medication for life. You should not stop taking it unless you first check with your doctor.
- Patients with certain heart diseases may experience chest pain or shortness of breath while on this medication. Check with your doctor if you experience such effects. Do not overdo physical work or exercise.
- Before having surgery or any other medical or dental treatment, be sure to tell your doctor or dentist that you are taking thyroid hormone.
- Over-the-counter (nonprescription) allergy, asthma, cough, cold, sinus, and diet medications can increase the side effects of thyroid hormone. Therefore, be sure to check with your doctor or pharmacist before taking ANY of these preparations.
- Although many thyroid products are on the market, they are not all bioequivalent—that is, they may not all be absorbed into the bloodstream at the same rate or have the same overall activity. DO NOT CHANGE BRANDS of this drug without first consulting your doctor or pharmacist to make sure you are receiving an equivalent product.
- Be sure to tell your doctor if you are pregnant. Thyroid hormone does not readily cross the placenta, and the drug appears to be safe during pregnancy. However, your dosing requirements of thyroid hormone may change during pregnancy. Also, tell your doctor if you are breast-feeding an infant. Small amounts of thyroid hormone pass into breast milk.

Thyroid Strong—see thyroid hormone

Tigan—see trimethobenzamide

Timolide—timolol and hydrochlorothiazide combination

---

timolol (ophthalmic)

BRAND NAME (Manufacturer)

Timoptic (Merck Sharp & Dohme)

TYPE OF DRUG

Antiglaucoma ophthalmic solution

INGREDIENT

timolol

DOSAGE FORM

Ophthalmic drops (0.25% and 0.5%)

STORAGE

Timolol ophthalmic drops should be stored at room temperature in a tightly closed container. This medication should never be frozen. If this medication discolors or turns brown, it should be discarded—a color change indicates a loss of potency.

USES

Timolol (ophthalmic) is used to reduce pressure in the eye caused by glaucoma or other eye conditions. This medication belongs to a group of drugs known as beta blockers. When applied to the eye, timolol reduces pressure within the eye by decreasing eye fluid (aqueous humor) production and perhaps by increasing the outflow of fluid from the eye.

TREATMENT

Wash your hands with soap and water before applying this medication. In order to avoid contamination of the eye drops, be careful not to touch the tube portion of the dropper or let it touch your eye, and do not wipe off or rinse the dropper after you use it.

To apply the ophthalmic drops, tilt your head back and pull down your lower eyelid with one hand to make a pouch below the eye. Drop the prescribed amount of medicine into this pouch and slowly close your eyes. Try not to blink. Keep your eyes closed, and place one finger at the corner of the eye next to your nose for a minute or two, applying a slight pressure (this is done to prevent loss of medication through the duct that drains fluid from the surface of the eye into the nose and throat). Then wipe away any excess medication with a clean tissue. Since applying the medication is somewhat difficult to do, you may want to have someone else apply the ophthalmic drops for you.

If you miss a dose of this medication, apply the missed dose as soon as possible, unless it is almost time for your next dose. In that case, do not apply the missed dose at all; just return to your regular dosing schedule. If the medication is used only once a day, and you do not remember missing a dose until the next day, skip the missed dose. Do not double the next dose.

SIDE EFFECTS

Minor. When you first apply this medication, it may sting your eyes. This should stop in a few minutes.

Major. Tell your doctor about any side effects that are persistent or particularly bothersome. IT IS ESPECIALLY IMPORTANT TO TELL YOUR DOCTOR about itching, skin rash, hives, or irritation of the eye that lasts more than a few minutes after application. Major side effects are rare when this product is used correctly. However, rare occurrences of anxiety, bronchospasm, confusion, depression, dizziness, drowsiness, generalized rash, indigestion, loss of appetite, nausea, weakness, and a slight reduction of the resting heart rate have been observed in some users of this drug. If you have any of these symptoms, contact your doctor.

INTERACTIONS

Timolol (ophthalmic) may increase the side effects of reserpine and oral beta blockers.

Before starting to take timolol (ophthalmic), BE SURE TO TELL YOUR DOCTOR about any medications you are currently taking, especially reserpine or oral beta blockers.

WARNINGS

- Tell your doctor about unusual or allergic reactions you have had to any medications, especially to timolol or to any other beta blockers (acebutolol, atenolol, betaxolol, carteolol, esmolol, labetalol, metoprolol, nadolol, penbutolol, pindolol, propranolol).
- Tell your doctor if you now have or if you have ever had asthma, diabetes mellitus, heart disease, or myasthenia gravis.
- Your doctor should check your eye pressure regularly to be sure the glaucoma is under control.
- Be sure to tell your doctor if you are pregnant. Small amounts of timolol may be absorbed into the bloodstream, and its safety in human pregnancy has not been established. Birth defects have been observed in the fetuses of animals that were given large oral doses of this type of drug during pregnancy. Also, tell your doctor if you are breast-feeding an infant. If this drug reaches the bloodstream and passes into the breast milk, it can cause a slowed heart rate in the nursing infant.

---

timolol (systemic)

BRAND NAME (Manufacturer)
Blocadren (Merck Sharp & Dohme)

TYPE OF DRUG
Beta-adrenergic blocking agent

INGREDIENT
timolol

DOSAGE FORM
Tablets (5 mg, 10 mg, and 20 mg)

STORAGE
Timolol should be stored at room temperature in a tightly closed, light-resistant container.

USES

Timolol is used to treat high blood pressure and to prevent additional heart attacks in heart attack patients. This drug belongs to a group of medicines known as beta-adrenergic blocking agents or, more commonly, beta blockers. These drugs work by controlling nerve impulses along certain nerve pathways.

TREATMENT

Timolol tablets can be taken with a glass of water, with meals, immediately following meals, or on an empty stomach, depending on your doctor's instructions for taking your medication. You should try to take your dose(s) of the medication at the same time(s) each day.

Try not to miss any doses of this medication. If you do miss a dose, take the missed dose as soon as possible. However, if the next scheduled dose is within eight hours (if you are taking this medicine only once a day) or within four hours (if you are taking this medicine more than once a day), do not take the missed dose at all; just return to your regular dosing schedule. Do not double the next dose that you take of this medication.

It is important to remember that timolol does not cure high blood pressure, but it will help to control the condition as long as you continue to take it.

SIDE EFFECTS

Minor. Anxiety; constipation; decreased sexual ability; diarrhea; difficulty in sleeping; drowsiness; dryness of the eyes, mouth, and skin; headache; nausea; nervousness; stomach discomfort; tiredness; or weakness. These side effects should disappear during treatment, as your body adjusts to the medicine.

If you are extra-sensitive to the cold, be sure to dress warmly during cold weather.

To relieve constipation, increase the fiber in your diet (fresh fruits and vegetables, salads, bran, and whole-grain breads) unless your doctor directs otherwise.

Plain, nonmedicated eye drops (artificial tears) may help to relieve eye dryness.

Sucking on ice chips or chewing sugarless gum helps to relieve mouth and throat dryness.

Major. Tell your doctor about any side effects that are persistent or particularly bothersome. IT IS ESPECIALLY IMPORTANT TO TELL YOUR DOCTOR about cold hands or feet (due to decreased blood circulation to skin, fingers, and toes), confusion, depression, dizziness, fever and sore throat, hair loss, hallucinations, light-headedness, nightmares, numbness or tingling of the fingers or toes, rapid weight gain (three to five pounds within a week), reduced alertness, skin rash, swelling, unusual bleeding or bruising, or wheezing or difficulty in breathing.

INTERACTIONS

Timolol interacts with several other types of drugs:

1. Indomethacin has been shown to decrease the blood-pressure-lowering effects of the beta blockers. This may also happen with aspirin or other salicylates.

2. Concurrent use of beta blockers and calcium channel blockers (diltiazem, nifedipine, verapamil) or disopyramide can lead to heart failure or very low blood pressure.

3. Cimetidine and oral contraceptives (birth control pills) can increase the blood concentrations of timolol, which can result in greater side effects.

4. Side effects may also be increased when beta blockers are taken with clonidine, digoxin, epinephrine, phenylephrine, phenylpropanolamine, phenothiazine tranquilizers, prazosin, reserpine, or monoamine oxidase (MAO) inhibitors. At least 14 days should separate the use of a beta blocker and the use of an MAO inhibitor.

5. Alcohol, barbiturates, and rifampin can decrease the blood concentrations of beta blockers, which can result in a decrease in effectiveness.

6. Beta blockers may antagonize (work against) the effects of theophylline, aminophylline, albuterol, isoproterenol, metaproterenol, and terbutaline.

7. Beta blockers can also interact with insulin or oral antidiabetic agents, raising or lowering blood sugar levels or masking the symptoms of low blood sugar.

8. The action of beta blockers may be increased if they are used with chlorpromazine, furosemide, or hydralazine.

BE SURE TO TELL YOUR DOCTOR about any medications you are currently taking, especially any listed above.

WARNINGS

- Before starting to take this medication, it is important to tell your doctor if you have ever had unusual or allergic reactions to timolol or to any beta blocker (acebutolol, atenolol, betaxolol, carteolol, esmolol, labetalol, metoprolol, nadolol, penbutolol, pindolol, propranolol).
- Tell your doctor if you now have or if you have ever had allergies, asthma, hay fever, eczema, slow heartbeat, bronchitis, diabetes mellitus, emphysema, heart or blood vessel disease, kidney disease, liver disease, thyroid disease, or poor circulation in the fingers or toes.
- You may want to check your pulse while taking this medication. If your pulse is much slower than your usual rate (or if it is less than 50 beats per minute), check with your doctor. A pulse rate that is too slow may cause circulation problems.
- This medicine may affect your body's response to exercise. Be sure you discuss with your doctor how much exercise is safe for you, taking into account your medical condition.
- It is important that you do not stop taking this medicine unless you first check with your doctor. Some conditions may become worse when the medicine is stopped suddenly, and the danger of a heart attack is increased in some patients. Your doctor may want you to gradually reduce the amount of medicine you take before stopping completely. Make sure that you have enough medicine on hand to last through weekends, vacations, and holidays.
- Before having surgery or any other medical or dental treatment, tell your doctor or dentist that you are taking this medication. Often, this medication will be discontinued 48 hours prior to major surgery.
- This medication can cause dizziness, drowsiness, light-headedness, or decreased alertness. Exercise caution while driving a car or using any potentially dangerous machinery.
- While taking this medicine, do not use any over-the-counter (nonprescription) allergy, asthma, cough, cold, sinus, or diet preparations unless you first check with your pharmacist or doctor. Some of these medicines can result in high blood pressure when combined with timolol.
- Be sure to tell your doctor if you are pregnant. Animal studies have shown that some beta blockers can cause problems in pregnancy when used at very high doses. Adequate studies have not been conducted in humans, but there has been some association between use of beta blockers during pregnancy and low birth weight, as well as breathing problems and slow heart rate in newborn infants. However, other reports have shown no effects on newborn infants. Also, tell your doctor if you are breast-feeding an infant. Small amounts of timolol may pass into breast milk.

---

timolol and hydrochlorothiazide combination

BRAND NAME (Manufacturer)
Timolide (Merck Sharp & Dohme)
TYPE OF DRUG
Beta-adrenergic blocking agent and diuretic
INGREDIENTS
timolol and hydrochlorothiazide
DOSAGE FORM
Tablets (10 mg timolol and 25 mg hydrochlorothiazide)

STORAGE

Timolol and hydrochlorothiazide combination tablets should be stored at room temperature in a tightly closed, light-resistant container.

USES

Timolol and hydrochlorothiazide combination is prescribed to treat high blood pressure. Hydrochlorothiazide is a diuretic, which reduces fluid accumulation in the body by increasing the elimination of salt and water through the kidneys. Timolol belongs to a group of medicines known as beta-adrenergic blocking agents or, more commonly, beta blockers. They work by controlling impulses along certain nerve pathways.

TREATMENT

This medication can be taken with a glass of water, with meals, immediately following meals, or on an empty stomach—depending on your doctor's instructions.

Try to take the medication at the same time(s) each day. Avoid taking a dose after 6:00 P.M.; otherwise, you may have to get up during the night to urinate.

If you miss a dose of this medication, take the missed dose as soon as possible, unless it is almost time for your next dose. In that case, do not take the missed dose at all; just wait until the next scheduled dose. Do not double the dose.

Timolol and hydrochlorothiazide combination does not cure high blood pressure, but it will help to control the condition as long as you continue to take it.

SIDE EFFECTS

Minor. Abdominal pain, constipation, diarrhea, dizziness, drowsiness, dryness of the eyes and skin, headache, heartburn, loss of appetite, or tiredness. These side effects should disappear as your body adjusts to the medication.

If you become extra-sensitive to the cold, be sure to dress warmly during cold weather.

Plain, nonmedicated eye drops (artificial tears) may help to relieve eye dryness.

Sucking on ice chips or chewing sugarless gum helps to relieve mouth and throat dryness.

To relieve constipation, increase the amount of fiber in your diet (fresh fruits and vegetables, salads, bran, and whole-grain breads) and drink more water unless your doctor directs you to do otherwise.

To avoid dizziness or light-headedness when you stand, contract and relax the muscles of your legs for a few moments before rising. Do this by pushing one foot against the floor while raising the other foot slightly, alternating feet so that you are "pumping" your legs in a pedaling motion.

Hydrochlorothiazide can cause increased sensitivity to sunlight. Avoid prolonged exposure to sunlight and sunlamps, wear protective clothing and sunglasses, and use an effective sunscreen.

Major. Tell your doctor about any side effects that are persistent or particularly bothersome. IT IS ESPECIALLY IMPORTANT TO TELL YOUR DOCTOR about blurred vision, chest pain, cold hands or feet (due to decreased blood circulation to skin, fingers, and toes), confusion, decreased sexual ability, depression, difficulty in breathing, dry mouth, fever, hair loss, hallucinations, itching, joint pain, mood changes, muscle pain or cramps, nausea, numbness or tingling in your fingers or toes, palpitations, rapid weight gain (three to five pounds within a week), ringing in the ears, skin rash, sore throat, thirst, unusual bleeding or bruising, vomiting, weakness, or yellowing of the eyes or skin.

INTERACTIONS

This medicine interacts with other types of medications:

1. Indomethacin, aspirin, and other salicylates may decrease the blood-pressure-lowering effects of beta blockers.

2. Concurrent use of timolol and disopyramide or calcium channel blockers (diltiazem, nifedipine, verapamil) can lead to heart failure or very low blood pressure.

3. Side effects can be increased when timolol is taken with cimetidine, clonidine, digoxin, epinephrine, phenylephrine, phenylpropanolamine, phenothiazine tranquilizers, prazosin, reserpine, chlorpromazine, furosemide, hydralazine, oral contraceptives (birth control pills), or monoamine oxidase (MAO) inhibitors. At least 14 days should separate the use of timolol and the use of an MAO inhibitor.

4. Timolol can antagonize (act against) the effects of theophylline, aminophylline, albuterol, isoproterenol, metaproterenol, and terbutaline.

5. Timolol can also interact with insulin and oral antidiabetic agents, raising or lowering blood sugar levels and masking the symptoms of low blood sugar.

6. Alcohol, barbiturates, and rifampin can decrease the blood concentrations of beta blockers, which can result in a decrease of effectiveness.

7. Hydrochlorothiazide can decrease the effectiveness of oral anticoagulants (blood thinners, such as warfarin), antigout medications, and methenamine.

8. Fenfluramine may increase the blood-pressure-lowering effects of this drug, which can be dangerous.

9. Cholestyramine and colestipol can decrease the absorption of hydrochlorothiazide from the gastrointestinal tract. This medication should, therefore, be taken one hour before or four hours after a dose of cholestyramine or colestipol (if you have also been prescribed one of these medications).

10. Hydrochlorothiazide may increase the side effects of amphotericin B, calcium, cortisone and cortisone-like steroids (such as dexamethasone, hydrocortisone, prednisone, and prednisolone), digoxin, digitalis, lithium, quinidine, sulfonamide antibiotics, and vitamin D.

Before starting to take timolol and hydrochlorothiazide combination, BE SURE TO TELL YOUR DOCTOR about any medications you are currently taking, especially any of the medications that are listed above.

WARNINGS

- Tell your doctor about unusual or allergic reactions you have had to any medications, especially to timolol or any other beta blockers (acebutolol, atenolol, betaxolol, carteolol, esmolol, labetalol, metoprolol, nadolol, penbutolol, pindolol, propranolol), to hydrochlorothiazide or other diuretics (such as bendroflumethiazide, benzthiazide, chlorothiazide, chlorthalidone, cyclothiazide, hydroflumethiazide, methyclothiazide, metolazone, polythiazide, quinethazone, trichlormethiazide, and furosemide), or to any other sulfa drug (oral antidiabetic medication, sulfonamide antibiotic).
- Tell your doctor if you now have or if you have ever had asthma, diabetes mellitus, heart disease, gout, kidney disease or problems with urination, liver disease, pancreatitis,

systemic lupus erythematosus, thyroid disease, or poor circulation in the fingers or toes.

• Hydrochlorothiazide can cause potassium loss. Signs of potassium loss include dry mouth, thirst, weakness, muscle pain or cramps, nausea, and vomiting. If you experience any of these symptoms, call your doctor. To help prevent this problem, your doctor may have blood tests performed periodically to monitor your potassium levels. To help avoid potassium loss, take this medication with a glass of fresh or frozen orange juice or cranberry juice, or eat a banana every day. The use of a salt substitute also helps to prevent potassium loss. Do not change your diet, however, until you discuss it with your doctor. Too much potassium may also be dangerous.

• While taking this medication, limit your intake of alcohol in order to prevent dizziness and light-headedness.

• While taking this medication, do not take any over-the-counter (nonprescription) medication for weight control or for allergy, asthma, cough, cold, or sinus problems unless you first check with your doctor.

• To prevent severe water loss (dehydration) while taking this medication, check with your doctor if you have any illness that causes severe or continuous nausea, vomiting, or diarrhea.

• This medication can raise blood sugar levels in diabetic patients. Blood sugar levels should be monitored carefully with blood or urine tests when this medication is being taken.

• You may want to check your pulse while taking this medication. If your pulse is much slower than your usual rate (or if it is less than 50 beats per minute), check with your doctor. A pulse rate that is too slow may cause circulation problems.

• Timolol can affect your body's response to exercise. Make sure you ask your doctor what an appropriate amount of exercise would be for you, taking into account your medical condition.

• Before having surgery or any other medical or dental treatment, tell your doctor or dentist that you are taking this medicine. Often, this medication will be discontinued 48 hours prior to any major surgery.

• This medication can cause dizziness, drowsiness, light-headedness, or decreased alertness. Therefore, you should exercise caution while driving a car or operating potentially dangerous machinery.

• A doctor does not usually prescribe a "fixed-dose" drug like this as the first choice in the treatment of high blood pressure. Usually, the patient first receives each ingredient singly. If there is an adequate response to the fixed dose contained in this product, it can then be substituted. The advantages of a combination product are increased convenience and (often) decreased cost.

• It is important that you do not stop taking this medicine unless you first check with your doctor. Some conditions worsen when this medicine is stopped suddenly, and the danger of a heart attack is increased in some patients. Your doctor may, therefore, want you to gradually reduce the amount of medicine you take before stopping completely. Make sure that you have enough medicine on hand to last through weekends, holidays, and vacations.

• Be sure to tell your doctor if you are pregnant. Animal studies have shown that some beta blockers can cause problems in pregnancy when used at very high doses. Extensive studies have not been conducted in humans, but there has been some association between beta blockers used during pregnancy and low birth weight, as well as breathing problems and slow heart rate in newborn infants. However, other reports have shown no effects on newborn infants. Also, tell your doctor if you are breast-feeding an infant. Although problems in humans have not yet been reported, small amounts of timolol and hydrochlorothiazide may pass into breast milk, so caution is warranted.

Timoptic—see timolol (ophthalmic)

Tipramine—see imipramine

---

tobramycin (ophthalmic)

BRAND NAME (Manufacturer)
Tobrex (Alcon)

TYPE OF DRUG
Ophthalmic antibiotic

INGREDIENT
tobramycin

DOSAGE FORMS
Ophthalmic drops (0.3% tobramycin)
Ophthalmic ointment (0.3% tobramycin)

STORAGE
The ophthalmic solution and ointment should be stored at room temperature in tightly closed containers. Discard any medication that is outdated or no longer needed.

USES

Tobramycin ophthalmic is used for the short-term treatment of bacterial infections of the eyes. Tobramycin is an aminoglycoside antibiotic, which acts to prevent the growth and multiplication of infecting bacteria.

TREATMENT

Wash your hands with soap and water before using this medication. In order to prevent contamination of the medicine, be careful not to touch the tube portion of the dropper and do not let it touch the eye.

Note that the bottle of the eye drops is not completely full—this is to allow control of the number of drops used.

To apply the drops, tilt your head back and pull down the lower eyelid with one hand to make a pouch below the eye. Drop the prescribed amount of medicine into the pouch and slowly close your eyes. Try not to blink. Keep your eyes closed, and place one finger at the corner of the eye next to your nose for a minute or two, applying a slight pressure (this is done to prevent loss of medication through the duct that drains fluid from the surface of the eye into the nose and throat). Then wipe away any excess with a clean tissue. If you think that the medicine did not get into your eye, repeat the process once. If you are using more than one type of eye drop, wait at least five minutes between doses of the two types of medication.

Follow the same general procedure for applying the ointment. Tilt your head back, pull down the lower eyelid, and squeeze the prescribed amount of ointment in a line along the pouch below the eye. Close your eyes, and place your finger at the corner of the eye, near the nose, for a minute or two. Do not rub your eyes. Wipe off excess ointment and the tip of the tube with clean tissues.

Since applying the medication is somewhat difficult to do, you may want someone else to administer the drops or ointment for you.

If you miss a dose of this drug, insert the drops or apply the ointment as soon as possible, unless it is almost time for the next application. In that case, do not use the missed dose at all; just return to your regular dosing schedule.

It is important to continue to take this medication for the entire time prescribed by your doctor, even if the symptoms of infection disappear before the end of that period. If you stop applying the medication too soon, resistant bacteria are given a chance to continue growing, and the infection could recur.

SIDE EFFECTS

Minor. Blurred vision, burning, or stinging. These side effects should disappear as your body adjusts to the drug.

Major. Tell your doctor about any side effects that are persistent or particularly bothersome. IT IS ESPECIALLY IMPORTANT TO TELL YOUR DOCTOR about disturbed or reduced vision; eye pain, itching, or swelling; severe irritation; or rash.

INTERACTIONS

This medication should not interact with other medication as long as it is used according to directions.

WARNINGS

- Tell your doctor about any reactions you have had to drugs, especially to tobramycin or to any other aminoglycoside antibiotic (amikacin, gentamicin, kanamycin, neomycin, netilmicin, paromomycin, streptomycin, viomycin).
- Before starting tobramycin (ophthalmic), tell your doctor if you now have or if you have ever had fungal or viral infections of the eye, kidney disease, or myasthenia gravis.
- If there is no change in your condition two or three days after starting to take this drug, contact your doctor. The drug may not be effective for your infection.
- This medication has been prescribed for your current infection only. A subsequent infection, or one that someone else has, may require a different medicine. You should not give your medicine to other people or use it to treat other infections, unless your doctor specifically directs you to do so.
- In order to allow your eye infection to clear, do not apply makeup to the affected eye.
- Be sure to tell your doctor if you are pregnant. Although tobramycin appears to be safe in humans, extensive studies in pregnant women have not been conducted. Also, tell your doctor if you are breast-feeding an infant. Small amounts of tobramycin may pass into the breast milk.

Tobrex—see tobramycin (ophthalmic)

---

tocainide

BRAND NAME (Manufacturer)
Tonocard (Merck Sharp & Dohme)

TYPE OF DRUG
Antiarrhythmic

INGREDIENT
tocainide

DOSAGE FORM
Tablets (400 mg and 600 mg)

STORAGE
Store at room temperature in a tightly closed container.

USES

Tocainide is used to treat heart arrhythmias. It suppresses irregular heartbeats and helps to achieve a more normal rhythm.

TREATMENT

To decrease stomach irritation, you can take tocainide with a glass of milk or with food (unless your doctor directs you to do otherwise).

Try to take the drug at the same time(s) every day. Tocainide works best when the amount of drug in your bloodstream is kept constant. This medication should, therefore, be taken at evenly spaced intervals day and night. For example, if you are to take tocainide three times per day, the doses should be spaced eight hours apart.

Try not to miss any doses of tocainide. If you do miss a dose, take the missed dose as soon as possible. However, if the next scheduled dose is within four hours (if you are taking tocainide three times daily) or within six hours (if you are taking it twice daily), do not take the missed dose at all; just return to your regular dosing schedule. Do not double the next dose.

SIDE EFFECTS

Minor. Abdominal pain, altered taste, anxiety, constipation, diarrhea, difficulty in swallowing, dizziness, drowsiness, dry mouth, fatigue, headache, heartburn, hot or cold feelings, increased thirst, light-headedness, loss of appetite, nausea, restlessness, sweating, or vomiting. These side effects should disappear as your body adjusts to this medication.

If you feel dizzy or light-headed, sit or lie down for a while; get up slowly from a sitting or reclining position, and be careful on stairs.

If you experience mouth dryness, you might try chewing sugarless gum or sucking on ice chips or a piece of hard candy.

To relieve constipation, increase the amount of fiber in your diet (fresh fruits and vegetables, salads, bran, and whole-grain breads), exercise, and drink more water (unless your doctor directs you to do otherwise).

Major. Tell your doctor about any side effects that are persistent or particularly bothersome. IT IS ESPECIALLY IMPORTANT TO TELL YOUR DOCTOR about chest pain, chills, confusion, coughing, depression, disorientation, earache, fever, hair loss, hallucinations, hearing loss, incoordination, itching, leg cramps, mental changes, mood changes, mouth sores, muscle or joint pain, neck pain, palpitations, rash, ringing in the ears, seizures, shakiness, shortness of breath, sleep disorders, slurred speech, sore throat, tingling in the fingers or toes, unsteadiness, unusual bleeding or bruising, urination problems, visual disturbances, weakness, wheezing, or yellowing of the skin or eyes.

INTERACTIONS

The concurrent use of tocainide and metoprolol can have additive negative effects on the heart.

Before taking tocainide, BE SURE TO TELL YOUR DOCTOR about any medications you are currently taking, especially metoprolol.

WARNINGS

- Be sure to tell your doctor about any unusual or allergic reactions you have had to any medications, especially to tocainide or any other chemically related local anesthetic or antiarrhythmic, such as bupivacaine, dibucaine, etidocaine, lidocaine, mepivacaine, or prilocaine.
- Before starting tocainide, be sure to tell your doctor if you now have or if you have ever had blood disorders, bone marrow disease, heart block, heart failure, kidney disease, or liver disease.
- Before surgery or other medical or dental treatment, tell your doctor or dentist you are taking this drug.
- If this drug makes you dizzy or drowsy, do not take part in any activity that requires alertness, such as driving a car or operating potentially dangerous machinery.
- During the first three months of tocainide therapy, your doctor may schedule periodic blood counts. It is important for you to have these blood tests done to monitor for possible side effects on the bone marrow.
- Tell your doctor if you are pregnant. Studies in pregnant women have not been conducted. However, adverse effects have occurred in the offspring of animals that were given large doses of tocainide. Also, tell your doctor if you are breast-feeding an infant. It is not yet known if tocainide passes into human breast milk.

Tofranil—see imipramine

Tofranil-PM—see imipramine

---

tolazamide

BRAND NAMES (Manufacturers)
tolazamide (various manufacturers)
Tolinase (Upjohn)
TYPE OF DRUG
Oral antidiabetic
INGREDIENT
tolazamide
DOSAGE FORM
Tablets (100 mg, 250 mg, and 500 mg)
STORAGE
This medication should be stored at room temperature in a tightly closed container. Discard any outdated medication.

USES

Tolazamide is used for the treatment of diabetes mellitus (sugar diabetes) that appears in adulthood and cannot be managed by control of diet alone. This type of diabetes is known as non-insulin-dependent diabetes (also called maturity-onset or Type II diabetes). Tolazamide lowers the blood sugar level by increasing the release of insulin from the pancreas.

TREATMENT

In order for this medication to work correctly, it must be taken as directed by your doctor. It is best to take this medicine at the same time each day in order to maintain a constant blood sugar level. It is, therefore, important to try not to miss any doses of tolazamide. If you do miss a dose, take it as soon as possible, unless it is almost time for the next dose. In that case, do not take the missed dose at all; just return to your regular dosing schedule. Do not double the next dose. Tell your doctor if you feel any side effects from missing a dose of this drug.

SIDE EFFECTS

Minor. Diarrhea, headache, heartburn, loss of appetite, nausea, stomach discomfort, stomach pain, or vomiting. These side effects usually disappear as your body adjusts to the drug.

Tolazamide may increase your sensitivity to sunlight. You should, therefore, avoid prolonged exposure to sunlight and sunlamps. Wear protective clothing and sunglasses, and use an effective sunscreen.

Major. Tell your doctor about any side effects that are persistent or particularly bothersome. IT IS ESPECIALLY IMPORTANT TO TELL YOUR DOCTOR about dark urine, fatigue, itching of the skin, light-colored stools, sore throat and fever, unusual bleeding or bruising, or yellowing of the eyes or skin.

INTERACTIONS

Tolazamide interacts with several other types of drugs:

1. Chloramphenicol, guanethidine, fenfluramine, sulfinpyrazone, insulin, monoamine oxidase (MAO) inhibitors, oxyphenbutazone, oxytetracycline, phenylbutazone, probenecid, aspirin or other salicylates, and sulfonamide antibiotics, when combined with tolazamide, can lower blood sugar levels—sometimes to dangerously low levels. At least 14 days should separate the use of this drug and the use of an MAO inhibitor.

2. Thyroid hormones, dextrothyroxine, epinephrine, phenytoin, thiazide diuretics (water pills), and cortisone-like medications (such as dexamethasone, hydrocortisone, and prednisone), combined with tolazamide, can actually increase blood sugar levels—just what you are trying to avoid.

3. Rifampin can decrease the blood concentrations of tolazamide, which can lead to a decrease in its effectiveness.

4. Oral antidiabetic medications can increase the effects of warfarin, which can lead to bleeding complications.

5. Beta-blocking medications (acebutolol, atenolol, betaxolol, carteolol, esmolol, labetalol, metoprolol, nadolol, penbutolol, pindolol, propranolol, timolol) combined with tolazamide can result in either high or low blood sugar levels. Beta blockers can also mask the symptoms of low blood sugar, which can be dangerous.

BE SURE TO TELL YOUR DOCTOR about any medications you are currently taking, especially any of those listed above.

WARNINGS

- It is important to tell your doctor if you have ever had unusual or allergic reactions to tolazamide or to any other sulfa medication (sulfonamide antibiotics, diuretics [water pills], other oral antidiabetics).

• It is also important to tell your doctor if you now have or if you have ever had kidney disease, liver disease, severe infections, or thyroid disease.
• Avoid drinking alcoholic beverages while taking this medication (unless otherwise directed by your doctor). Some patients who take this medicine suffer nausea, vomiting, dizziness, stomach pain, pounding headache, sweating, and redness of the face and skin when they drink alcohol. Also, large amounts of alcohol can lower your blood sugar concentration to a dangerously low level.
• Follow the special diet that your doctor gave you. This is an important part of controlling your blood sugar and is necessary in order for this medicine to work properly.
• Before having surgery or any other medical or dental treatment, be sure to tell your doctor or dentist that you are taking this medicine.
• Test for sugar in your urine as directed by your doctor. It is a convenient way to determine whether your diabetes is being controlled by this medicine.
• Eat or drink something containing sugar right away if you experience any symptoms of hypoglycemia (low blood sugar), such as anxiety, chills, cold sweats, cool or pale skin, drowsiness, excessive hunger, headache, nausea, nervousness, rapid heartbeat, shakiness, or unusual tiredness or weakness. It is important that your family and friends know the symptoms of low blood sugar and what to do if they observe any of these symptoms in you.

Even if the hypoglycemic symptoms seem to disappear after you eat or drink a sugar-containing product, it is important to contact your doctor as soon as possible. The blood-sugar-lowering effects of tolazamide can last for hours, and your symptoms may return during this period. Good sources of sugar are orange juice, corn syrup, honey, sugar cubes, and table sugar. You are at greatest risk of developing low blood sugar if you skip or delay meals, exercise more than usual, are unable to eat because of nausea or vomiting, or drink large amounts of alcohol.
• You may need to be switched to insulin if you suffer diabetic coma, have a severe infection, are scheduled for major surgery, or become pregnant.
• Be sure to tell your doctor if you are pregnant. Your dosing requirements for tolazamide may change during pregnancy. Although extensive studies in humans have not been conducted, adverse effects have been observed in the fetuses of animals that received this type of drug during pregnancy. Also, tell your doctor if you are breast-feeding an infant. Small amounts of tolazamide may pass into breast milk.

---

tolbutamide

BRAND NAMES (Manufacturers)
Oramide (Major)
Orinase (Upjohn)
tolbutamide (various manufacturers)
TYPE OF DRUG
Oral antidiabetic
INGREDIENT
tolbutamide
DOSAGE FORM
Tablets (250 mg and 500 mg)
STORAGE
This medication should be stored at room temperature in a tightly closed container. Discard any outdated medication.

USES

Tolbutamide is used for the treatment of diabetes mellitus (sugar diabetes) that appears in adulthood and cannot be managed by control of diet alone. This type of diabetes is known as non-insulin-dependent diabetes (also called maturity-onset or Type II diabetes). Tolbutamide lowers blood sugar by increasing the release of insulin from the pancreas.

TREATMENT

In order for this medication to work correctly, it must be taken as directed by your doctor. It is best to take this medicine at the same time(s) each day, in order to maintain a constant blood sugar level. It is, therefore, important to try not to miss any doses of tolbutamide. If you do miss a dose, take it as soon as possible, unless it is almost time for the next dose. In that case, do not take the missed dose at all; just return to your regular dosing schedule. Do not double the next dose. Tell your doctor if you feel any side effects from missing a dose of this drug.

SIDE EFFECTS

Minor. Diarrhea, headache, heartburn, loss of appetite, nausea, stomach discomfort, stomach pain, or vomiting. These side effects usually disappear during treatment, as your body adjusts to the medication.

Tolbutamide may increase your sensitivity to sunlight. You should, therefore, avoid prolonged exposure to sunlight and sunlamps. Wear protective clothing and sunglasses, and use an effective sunscreen.

Major. Tell your doctor about any side effects that are persistent or particularly bothersome. IT IS ESPECIALLY IMPORTANT TO TELL YOUR DOCTOR about dark urine, fatigue, itching of the skin, light-colored stools, sore throat and fever, unusual bleeding or bruising, or yellowing of the eyes or skin.

INTERACTIONS

Tolbutamide interacts with a number of other types of drugs:

1. The combination of tolbutamide and chloramphenicol, guanethidine, insulin, fenfluramine, sulfinpyrazone, monoamine oxidase (MAO) inhibitors, oxyphenbutazone, oxytetracycline, phenylbutazone, probenecid, aspirin or other salicylates, or sulfonamide antibiotics can lower blood sugar levels—sometimes to dangerously low levels. At least 14 days should separate the use of this drug and the use of an MAO inhibitor.

2. Thyroid hormones, dextrothyroxine, epinephrine, phenytoin, thiazide diuretics (water pills), and cortisone-like medications (such as dexamethasone, hydrocortisone, and prednisone), combined with tolbutamide, can actually increase blood sugar levels—just what you are trying to avoid.

3. Rifampin can decrease the blood concentrations of tolbutamide, which can lead to a decrease in its effectiveness.

4. Oral antidiabetic medications can increase the effects of blood thinners, such as warfarin, which can lead to bleeding complications.

5. The combination of tolbutamide and beta-blocking medications (acebutolol, atenolol, betaxolol, carteolol, esmolol, labetalol, metoprolol, nadolol, penbutolol, pindolol, propranolol, timolol) can result in either high or low blood sugar levels. Beta blockers can also mask the symptoms of low blood sugar, which can be dangerous.

BE SURE TO TELL YOUR DOCTOR about any medications you are currently taking, especially any of those listed above.

WARNINGS

- It is important to tell your doctor if you have ever had unusual or allergic reactions to tolbutamide or to any other sulfa medication (sulfonamide antibiotics, diuretics [water pills], other oral antidiabetics).
- It is also important to tell your doctor if you now have or if you have ever had kidney disease, liver disease, severe infection, or thyroid disease.
- Avoid drinking alcoholic beverages while taking this medication (unless otherwise directed by your doctor). Some patients who take this medicine suffer nausea, vomiting, dizziness, stomach pain, pounding headache, sweating, and redness of the face and skin when they drink alcohol. Also, large amounts of alcohol can lower your blood sugar concentration to a dangerously low level.
- Follow the special diet that your doctor gave you. This is an important part of controlling your blood sugar levels and is necessary in order for this medicine to work properly.
- Before having surgery or any other medical or dental treatment, be sure to tell your doctor or dentist about this drug.
- Test for sugar in your urine as directed by your doctor. It is a convenient way to determine whether your diabetes is being controlled by this medicine.
- Eat or drink something containing sugar right away if you experience any symptoms of hypoglycemia (low blood sugar), such as anxiety, chills, cold sweats, cool or pale skin, drowsiness, excessive hunger, headache, nausea, nervousness, rapid heartbeat, shakiness, or unusual tiredness or weakness). It is important that your family and friends know the symptoms of low blood sugar and what to do if they observe any of these symptoms in you.

Even if the hypoglycemic symptoms seem to disappear after you eat or drink a sugar-containing product, it is important to contact your doctor as soon as possible. The blood-sugar-lowering effects of tolbutamide can last for hours, and your symptoms may return during this period. Good sources of sugar are orange juice, corn syrup, honey, sugar cubes, and table sugar. You are at greatest risk of developing low blood sugar if you skip or delay meals, exercise more than usual, are unable to eat because of nausea or vomiting, or drink large amounts of alcohol.

- You may need to be switched to insulin if you have a severe infection, are scheduled for major surgery, suffer diabetic coma or become pregnant.
- Be sure to tell your doctor if you are pregnant. Your dosing requirements for tolbutamide may change during pregnancy, or you may be switched to insulin. Although extensive studies in humans have not been conducted, adverse effects have been observed in the fetuses of animals that received the drug tolbutamide during pregnancy. Also, tell your doctor if you are breast-feeding an infant. Since small amounts of tolbutamide may pass into breast milk, cautious use is warranted.

Tolectin—see tolmetin

Tolectin DS—see tolmetin

Tolinase—see tolazamide

---

tolmetin

BRAND NAMES (Manufacturers)
Tolectin (McNeil)
Tolectin DS (McNeil)
TYPE OF DRUG
Nonsteroidal anti-inflammatory analgesic
INGREDIENT
tolmetin
DOSAGE FORMS
Tablets (200 mg)
Capsules (400 mg)
STORAGE
This medication should be stored in tightly closed containers at room temperature away from heat and direct sunlight.

USES

Tolmetin is used to treat the inflammation (pain, swelling, and stiffness) of certain types of arthritis, gout, bursitis, and tendinitis. Tolmetin has been shown to block the production of certain body chemicals that may trigger pain. However, it is not yet fully understood how tolmetin works.

TREATMENT

You should take this medication on an empty stomach 30 to 60 minutes before meals or two hours after meals, so that it gets into your bloodstream quickly. However, to decrease stomach irritation, your doctor may want you to take the medicine with food or antacids.

If you are taking tolmetin to relieve arthritis, you must take it regularly, as directed by your doctor. It may take up to two weeks before you feel the full benefits of this medication. Tolmetin does not cure arthritis, but it will help to control the condition as long as you continue to take it.

It is important to take tolmetin on schedule and not to miss any doses. If you do miss a dose, take it as soon as possible, unless it is almost time for your next dose. In that case, do not take the missed dose at all; just return to your regular dosing schedule. Do not double the next dose.

SIDE EFFECTS

Minor. Bloating, constipation, diarrhea, difficulty in sleeping, dizziness, drowsiness, headache, heartburn, indigestion, light-headedness, loss of appetite, nausea, nervousness, soreness of the mouth, unusual sweating, or vomiting. As your body adjusts to the drug, these side effects should disappear.

To relieve constipation, increase the amount of fiber in your diet (fresh fruits and vegetables, salads, bran, and whole-grain breads), exercise, and drink more water (unless your doctor directs you to do otherwise).

If you become dizzy, sit or lie down for a while; get up slowly from a sitting or reclining position, and be careful on stairs.

Major. Tell your doctor about any side effects that are persistent or particularly bothersome. IT IS ESPECIALLY IMPORTANT TO TELL YOUR DOCTOR about bloody or black, tarry stools; blurred vision; confusion; depression; difficult or painful urination; difficulty in hearing; palpitations; ringing or buzzing in the ears; skin rash, hives, or itching; stomach pain; swelling of the feet; tightness in the chest; unexplained sore throat and fever; unusual bleeding or bruising; unusual fatigue or weakness; unusual weight gain; wheezing or difficulty in breathing; or yellowing of the eyes or skin.

INTERACTIONS

Tolmetin interacts with several types of medications:

1. Anticoagulants (blood thinners, such as warfarin) in combination with tolmetin can lead to an increase in bleeding complications.

2. Aspirin, salicylates, or other anti-inflammatory medications can increase the stomach irritation caused by tolmetin.

3. Probenecid may increase blood levels of tolmetin, which may increase the risk of side effects.

4. The action of beta blockers may be decreased by this drug.

5. This drug can interact with diuretics (water pills).

BE SURE TO TELL YOUR DOCTOR about any medications you are currently taking, especially any listed above.

WARNINGS

• Before you take this medication, it is important to tell your doctor if you have ever had unusual or allergic reactions to tolmetin or any of the other chemically related drugs (including aspirin, other salicylates, diclofenac, diflunisal, fenoprofen, flurbiprofen, ibuprofen, ketoprofen, meclofenamate, mefenamic acid, naproxen, oxyphenbutazone, phenylbutazone, piroxicam, sulindac, or indomethacin).

• Tell your doctor if you have ever had asthma, bleeding problems, colitis, stomach ulcers or other stomach problems, epilepsy, heart disease, high blood pressure, kidney disease, liver disease, mental illness, or Parkinson's disease.

• If this drug makes you dizzy or drowsy, do not take part in any activity that requires alertness, such as driving a car or operating potentially dangerous machinery.

• Because this drug can prolong your bleeding time, it is important to tell your doctor or dentist that you are taking this drug before having surgery or any other medical or dental treatment.

• Stomach problems are more likely to occur if you take aspirin regularly or drink alcohol while being treated with this medication. These should, therefore, be avoided (unless your doctor directs you to do otherwise).

• Be sure to tell your doctor if you are pregnant. The safe use of this medicine in human pregnancy has not been established. Side effects have been observed in the offspring of animals that received this type of medication during pregnancy. If taken late in pregnancy, tolmetin can prolong labor. Also, tell your doctor if you are breast-feeding an infant. Small amounts of tolmetin can pass into breast milk.

Tolu-Sed—see codeine and guaifenesin combination

Tonocard—see tocainide

Torganic-DM—see dextromethorphan and iodinated glycerol combination

Totacillin—see ampicillin

Trandate—see labetalol

Transderm-Nitro—see nitroglycerin (topical)

Transderm-Scop—see scopolamine (transdermal)

Tranxene-SD—see clorazepate

Tranxene T-Tab—see clorazepate

---

trazodone

BRAND NAMES (Manufacturers)
Desyrel (Mead Johnson)
Desyrel Dividose (Mead Johnson)
trazodone (various manufacturers)
TYPE OF DRUG
Antidepressant
INGREDIENT
trazodone
DOSAGE FORM
Tablets (50 mg, 100 mg, and 150 mg)
STORAGE
Trazodone tablets should be stored at room temperature in a tightly closed, light-resistant container.

USES

Trazodone is used to relieve the symptoms of mental depression. It is thought to relieve depression by increasing the concentration of certain chemicals involved with nerve transmission in the brain.

TREATMENT

Trazodone should be taken exactly as your doctor prescribes. It can be taken with water, milk, or food to lessen the chance of stomach irritation (unless your doctor tells you to do otherwise).

If you miss a dose of this medication, take the missed dose as soon as possible, and then return to your regular dosing schedule. If, however, the dose you missed was a once-a-day bedtime dose, do not take that dose in the morning; check with your doctor instead. If the dose is taken in the morning, it may cause some unwanted side effects. Never double the dose.

The benefits of therapy with this medication may not become apparent for two to four weeks.

SIDE EFFECTS

Minor. Blurred vision, constipation, diarrhea, dizziness, drowsiness, dry mouth, gas, headache, heartburn, lightheadedness, nausea, sleep disorders, vomiting, or weight gain or loss. These side effects should disappear as your body adjusts to the medication.

This medication can cause increased sensitivity to sunlight. It is, therefore, important to avoid prolonged exposure to sunlight and sunlamps. Wear protective clothing and sunglasses, and use an effective sunscreen.

Dry mouth can be relieved by chewing sugarless gum or by sucking on ice chips or a piece of hard candy.

To relieve constipation, increase the amount of fiber in your diet (fresh fruits and vegetables, salads, bran, and whole-grain breads), exercise, and drink more water (unless your doctor directs you to do otherwise).

To avoid dizziness and light-headedness when you stand, contract and relax the muscles of your legs for a few moments before rising. Do this by pushing one foot against the floor while raising the other foot slightly, alternating feet so that you are "pumping" your legs in a pedaling motion.

Major. Tell your doctor about any side effects that are persistent or particularly bothersome. IT IS ESPECIALLY IMPORTANT TO TELL YOUR DOCTOR about chest tightness, confusion, difficult or painful urination, hallucinations, loss of coordination, mood changes, muscle aches or pains, palpitations, prolonged or inappropriate erection of the penis, rash, ringing in the ears, shortness of breath, tingling in the fingers or toes, tremors, unusual bleeding or bruising, or unusual tiredness or weakness.

INTERACTIONS

Trazodone interacts with several other types of medications:

1. Extreme drowsiness can occur when trazodone is taken with central nervous system depressants (drugs that slow the activity of the brain and spinal cord), including alcohol, antihistamines, barbiturates, benzodiazepine tranquilizers, muscle relaxants, narcotics, pain medications, phenothiazine tranquilizers, and sleeping medications, or with tricyclic antidepressants.

2. The concurrent use of trazodone and monoamine oxidase (MAO) inhibitors should be avoided because the combination can result in fever, convulsions, or high blood pressure. At least 14 days should separate the use of this drug and the use of an MAO inhibitor.

3. Trazodone may increase the blood levels of digoxin and phenytoin, which can lead to increased side effects.

4. Blood-pressure-lowering effects of antihypertensives may be increased by trazodone, which can be dangerous.

BE SURE TO TELL YOUR DOCTOR about any medications you are currently taking, especially any listed above.

WARNINGS

- Tell your doctor if you have had unusual or allergic reactions to any medications, especially to trazodone.
- Tell your doctor if you have a history of alcoholism or if you ever had electroshock therapy, heart disease, a heart attack, kidney disease, or liver disease.
- If this drug makes you dizzy or drowsy, do not take part in any activity that requires alertness, such as driving a car or operating potentially dangerous machinery.
- Before having surgery or any other medical or dental treatment, be sure to tell your doctor or dentist that you are taking this medication.
- Do not stop taking this drug suddenly. Stopping this medication abruptly may cause nausea, headache, stomach upset, fatigue, or worsening of your condition. Your doctor may, therefore, want to reduce the dosage gradually.
- The effects of this medication may last as long as seven days after you have stopped taking it, so continue to observe all precautions during this period.
- Be sure to tell your doctor if you are pregnant. The safe use of this medication in pregnancy has not been established. Side effects have been observed in the offspring of animals that were given this medication in large doses during pregnancy. Also, tell your doctor if you are breast-feeding an infant. Small amounts of this drug pass into breast milk and may cause unwanted effects, such as irritability or sleeping problems, in nursing infants.

Trendar—see ibuprofen

Trental—see pentoxifylline

---

tretinoin

BRAND NAME (Manufacturer)
Retin-A (Ortho)
TYPE OF DRUG
Acne preparation
INGREDIENT
tretinoin (retinoic acid; vitamin A acid)
DOSAGE FORMS
Cream (0.025%, 0.05%, and 0.1%)
Gel (0.025% and 0.01%, with 90% alcohol)
Liquid (0.05%, with 55% alcohol)
STORAGE
Tretinoin cream, gel, and liquid should be stored at room temperature in tightly closed, light-resistant containers. This medication should never be frozen.

USES

Tretinoin is used topically (on the skin) to treat acne vulgaris. It appears to work by increasing the turnover (death and replacement) of skin cells.

TREATMENT

This product is packaged with instructions for the patient. Read them carefully before applying tretinoin.

Wash your skin with a mild or hypoallergenic soap and warm water. Pat dry with a clean towel. Then wait about 30 minutes before applying tretinoin cream, gel, or liquid. The medication should be applied once a day just before going to bed. Apply it only to the skin where the acne lesions appear, unless you are directed to do otherwise by your doctor. Be sure to cover the entire affected area LIGHTLY. You may use a fingertip, gauze pad, or cotton swab to apply the liquid. To avoid applying too much medication, be careful not to oversaturate the gauze pad or cotton swab. To avoid contamination, use a gauze pad or cotton swab only once and then throw it away.

During the early weeks of treatment with this drug, there may be an apparent increase in skin lesions. This is usually not a reason to discontinue its use. However, your doctor may want to change the concentration of the drug. Benefits may be noted within two to three weeks, although more than six weeks may be required before definite benefits are observed.

If you miss a dose of this medication, apply the missed dose as soon as possible, and then return to your regular dosing schedule. However, if you do not remember until the following day, do not apply the missed dose at all; just return to your regular dosing schedule.

SIDE EFFECTS

Minor. Immediately after applying tretinoin to your skin, you may experience a sensation of warmth or a mild stinging sensation, or your skin may become reddened. After a few days of treatment with this medication, some peeling of the skin is to be expected. You may also find that you have a heightened sensitivity to sunlight, wind, or cold. If this drug does increase your sensitivity to sunlight, avoid prolonged exposure to sunlight and sunlamps. Wear protective clothing, and use an effective sunscreen.

Major. Tell your doctor about any side effects that are persistent or particularly bothersome. IT IS ESPECIALLY IMPORTANT TO TELL YOUR DOCTOR about blistering, crusting, severe redness, severe burning, swelling, or marked darkening or lightening of the skin.

INTERACTIONS

Tretinoin interacts with several other products:

1. Abrasive or medicated soaps or cleaners

2. Other acne preparations (particularly peeling agents containing sulfur, resorcinol, benzoyl peroxide, or salicylic acid)

3. Cosmetics that have a strong drying effect

4. Locally applied products containing high amounts of alcohol, spices, or lime

These products should be used with caution during treatment with tretinoin, since they can increase the irritation caused by this medication.

WARNINGS

- Tell your doctor about unusual or allergic reactions you have had to any medications, especially to tretinoin or vitamin A.
- Before starting to take this medication, be sure to tell your doctor if you have eczema.
- This medication should not be used if you are sunburned; it may increase the irritation.
- Keep tretinoin away from the eyes, the mouth, the creases on either side of the nose, open cuts, and mucous membranes; it can severely irritate these sensitive areas.
- Avoid washing your face too often while using tretinoin. Be sure to use a mild or hypoallergenic soap.
- Normal use of nonmedicated cosmetics is permissible, but the skin should be cleaned thoroughly before tretinoin is applied.
- This medication has been prescribed for your current condition only. Do not give this medication to other people or use it for any other purpose than that prescribed by your doctor.
- Be sure to tell your doctor if you are pregnant. The safe use of this medication in human pregnancy or during breast-feeding has not been established.

Triacet—see triamcinolone (topical)

Triacin-C—see pseudoephedrine, triprolidine, and codeine combination

triamcinolone (systemic)

BRAND NAMES (Manufacturers)
Aristocort (Lederle)
Kenacort (Squibb)
triamcinolone (various manufacturers)

TYPE OF DRUG
Adrenocorticosteroid hormone

INGREDIENT
triamcinolone

DOSAGE FORMS
Tablets (1 mg, 2 mg, 4 mg, and 8 mg)
Oral syrup (2 mg and 4 mg per 5-ml spoonful)

STORAGE
Triamcinolone tablets and oral syrup should be stored at room temperature in tightly closed containers. Discard any outdated medication or any medication that is no longer needed.

USES

Your adrenal glands naturally produce certain cortisone-like chemicals. These chemicals are involved in various processes in the body (such as maintenance of fluid balance, regulation of temperature, and reaction to inflammation). Triamcinolone belongs to a group of drugs known as adrenocorticosteroids (or cortisone-like medications). It is used to treat a variety of disorders, including endocrine and rheumatic disorders; asthma; blood diseases; certain cancers; eye disorders; gastrointestinal disturbances, such as ulcerative colitis; respiratory diseases; and inflammations such as arthritis, dermatitis, and poison ivy. How this drug acts to relieve these disorders is not completely understood.

TREATMENT

In order to prevent stomach irritation, you can take triamcinolone with food or milk (unless your doctor directs you to do otherwise).

To help avoid potassium loss while using this drug, take your dose with a glass of fresh or frozen orange juice, or eat a banana each day. The use of a salt substitute also helps prevent potassium loss. Check with your doctor.

If you are taking only one dose of this medication each day, try to take it before 9:00 A.M. This will mimic the body's normal production of this type of chemical.

The oral syrup form of this medication should be measured carefully with a specially designed 5-ml measuring spoon. An ordinary kitchen teaspoon is not accurate enough.

It is important to try not to miss any doses of triamcinolone. If you do miss a dose of this medication, follow these guidelines:

1. If you are taking it more than once a day, take the missed dose as soon as possible, and then return to your regular dosing schedule. If it is already time for the next dose, double the dose.

2. If you are taking this medication once a day, take the dose you missed as soon as possible, unless you do not remember until the next day. In that case, do not take the missed dose at all; just follow your regular dosing schedule. Do not double the next dose.

3. If you are taking this drug every other day, take it as soon as you remember. If you missed the scheduled dose by a whole day, take it when you remember, and then skip a day before you take the next dose. Do not double the dose.

If you miss more than one dose of triamcinolone, CONTACT YOUR DOCTOR.

SIDE EFFECTS

Minor. Dizziness, false sense of well-being, increased appetite, increased sweating, indigestion, nausea, reddening of the skin on the face, restlessness, sleep disorders, or weight gain. These side effects should disappear as your body adjusts to the medication.

Major. Tell your doctor about any side effects that are persistent or particularly bothersome. IT IS ESPECIALLY IMPORTANT TO TELL YOUR DOCTOR about abdominal enlargement; abdominal pain; acne or other skin problems; back or rib pain; bloody or black, tarry stools; blurred vision; convulsions; difficulty in breathing; eye pain; fatigue; fever and sore throat; filling out of the face; growth impairment (in children); headaches; impaired healing of wounds; increased thirst and urination; menstrual irregularities; mental depression; mood changes; muscle wasting or weakness; nightmares; rapid weight gain (three to five pounds within a week); rash; thinning of the skin; unusual bleeding or bruising; or unusual weakness.

INTERACTIONS

Triamcinolone interacts with several other types of medications:

1. Alcohol, aspirin, and anti-inflammatory medications (such as diflunisal, ibuprofen, indomethacin, ketoprofen, meclofenamate, mefenamic acid, naproxen, piroxicam, sulindac, and tolmetin) aggravate the stomach problems that are common with use of this medication.

2. There may be a change in the dosage requirements of oral anticoagulants, oral antidiabetic drugs, or insulin when this medication is started or stopped.

3. The loss of potassium caused by triamcinolone can lead to serious side effects in individuals taking digoxin.

4. Thiazide diuretics (water pills) can increase the potassium loss caused by triamcinolone.

5. Phenobarbital, phenytoin, rifampin, and ephedrine can increase the elimination of triamcinolone from the body, thereby decreasing its effectiveness.

6. Oral contraceptives (birth control pills) and estrogen-containing drugs may decrease the elimination of this drug from the body, which can lead to an increase in side effects.

7. Triamcinolone can increase the elimination of aspirin and isoniazid from the body, thereby decreasing the effectiveness of these two medications.

8. Cholestyramine and colestipol can chemically bind this medication in the stomach and gastrointestinal tract, preventing its absorption.

BE SURE TO TELL YOUR DOCTOR about any medications you are currently taking, especially any of those listed above.

WARNINGS

• Tell your doctor about unusual or allergic reactions you have had to any medications, especially to triamcinolone or other adrenocorticosteroids (such as betamethasone, cortisone, dexamethasone, hydrocortisone, methylprednisolone, paramethasone, prednisolone, and prednisone).

• Tell your doctor if you now have or if you have ever had bone disease, diabetes mellitus, emotional instability, glaucoma, fungal infections, heart disease, high blood pressure, high cholesterol levels, myasthenia gravis, peptic ulcers, osteoporosis, thyroid disease, tuberculosis, ulcerative colitis, kidney disease, or liver disease.

• If you are using this medication for longer than a week, you may need to receive higher doses if you are subjected to stress, such as serious infections, injury, or surgery. Discuss this with your doctor.

• If you have been taking this drug for more than a week, do not stop taking it suddenly. If it is stopped abruptly, you may experience abdominal or back pain, difficulty in breathing, dizziness, fainting, fever, muscle or joint pain, nausea, vomiting, or extreme weakness. Your doctor may, therefore, want to reduce the dosage gradually. Never increase the dosage or take the drug for longer than the prescribed time, unless you first consult your doctor.

• While you are taking this drug, you should not be vaccinated or immunized. This medication decreases the effectiveness of vaccines and can lead to overwhelming infection if a live-virus vaccine is administered.

• Before having surgery or any other medical or dental treatment, be sure to tell your doctor or dentist that you are taking this medication.

• Because this drug can cause glaucoma and cataracts with long-term use, your doctor may want you to have your eyes examined by an ophthalmologist periodically during treatment.

• If you are taking this medication for prolonged periods, you should wear or carry an identification card or notice stating that you are taking an adrenocorticosteroid.

• This medication can raise blood sugar levels in diabetic patients. Blood sugar levels should, therefore, be monitored carefully with blood or urine tests when this medication is being taken.

• Some of these products contain the color additive FD&C Yellow No. 5 (tartrazine), which can cause allergic-type reactions (wheezing, rash, fainting, difficulty in breathing) in certain susceptible individuals.

• Be sure to tell your doctor if you are pregnant. This drug crosses the placenta, and its safety in human pregnancy is not established. Birth defects have been observed in the offspring of animals given large doses of this type of drug during pregnancy. Also, tell your doctor if you are breast-feeding. Small amounts of this drug pass into breast milk and may cause growth suppression or a decrease in natural adrenocorticosteroid production in the nursing infant.

---

triamcinolone (topical)

BRAND NAMES (Manufacturers)

Aristocort (Lederle)
Aristocort A (Lederle)
Flutex (Syosset)
Kenac (NMC)
Kenalog (Squibb)
Kenalog-H (Squibb)
Triacet (various manufacturers)

triamcinolone acetonide (various manufacturers)
Triderm (Del-Rey)
Trymex (Savage)

TYPE OF DRUG

Adrenocorticosteroid hormone

INGREDIENT

triamcinolone

DOSAGE FORMS

Ointment (0.025%, 0.1%, and 0.5%)
Cream (0.025%, 0.1%, and 0.5%)
Lotion (0.025% and 0.1%)
Aerosol (two seconds of spray delivers approximately 0.2 mg of drug, with 10.3% alcohol)

STORAGE

Triamcinolone ointment, cream, and lotion should be stored at room temperature in tightly closed containers. This medication should never be frozen.

The spray (foam) form of this medication is packed under pressure. It should not be stored near heat or an open flame or in direct sunlight, and the container should never be punctured.

USES

Your adrenal glands naturally produce certain cortisone-like chemicals. These chemicals are involved in various processes in the body (such as maintenance of fluid balance, regulation of temperature, and reaction to inflammation). Triamcinolone belongs to a group of drugs known as adrenocorticosteroids (or cortisone-like medications). It is used to relieve the skin inflammation (redness, swelling, itching, and discomfort) associated with conditions such as dermatitis, eczema, and poison ivy. How this drug acts to relieve these disorders is not completely understood.

TREATMENT

Before applying this medication, wash your hands. Then, unless your doctor gives you different instructions, gently wash the area of the skin where the medication is to be applied. With a clean towel, pat the area almost dry; it should be slightly damp when you put the medicine on.

If you are using the lotion form of this medication, shake it well before pouring out the medicine. The contents tend to settle on the bottom of the bottle, so it is necessary to shake the container to distribute the ingredients evenly and equalize the doses.

Apply a small amount of the medication to the affected area in a thin layer. Do not bandage the area unless your doctor tells you to do so. If you are to apply an occlusive dressing (like kitchen plastic wrap), be sure you understand the instructions. Wash your hands again after application.

If you are using the aerosol spray form of this medication, shake the can in order to disperse the medication evenly. Hold the can upright six to eight inches from the area to be sprayed, and spray the area for one to three seconds. DO NOT SMOKE while you are using the aerosol spray; the contents are under pressure and may explode if exposed to heat or flames.

If you miss a dose of this medication, apply the dose as soon as possible, unless it is almost time for the next application. In that case, do not apply the missed dose; just return to your regular dosing schedule. Do not put twice as much of the medication on your skin at the next application.

SIDE EFFECTS

Minor. Acne, burning sensation, irritation of the affected area, or skin dryness.

If the affected area is extremely dry or scaling, the skin may be moistened by soaking in water or by applying water with a clean cloth before applying the medication. The ointment form is probably better for dry skin.

A mild, temporary stinging sensation may occur after this medication is applied. If this persists, contact your doctor.

Major. Tell your doctor about any side effects that are persistent or particularly bothersome. IT IS ESPECIALLY IMPORTANT TO TELL YOUR DOCTOR about blistering, increased hair growth, itching, loss of skin color, rash, secondary infection in the area being treated, or thinning of the skin with easy bruising.

INTERACTIONS

This medication should not interact with other medications as long as it is used according to the directions given to you by your doctor or pharmacist.

WARNINGS

- Tell your doctor about unusual or allergic reactions you have had to any medications, especially to triamcinolone or other adrenocorticosteroids (such as amcinonide, betamethasone, clocortolone, cortisone, desonide, desoximetasone, dexamethasone, diflorasone, flumethasone, fluocinolone, fluocinonide, fluorometholone, flurandrenolide, halcinonide, hydrocortisone, methylprednisolone, prednisolone, and prednisone).
- Tell your doctor if you now have or if you have ever had blood vessel disease, chicken pox, diabetes mellitus, fungal infection, peptic ulcers, shingles, tuberculosis of the lungs or skin, vaccinia, or any other type of infection, especially at the site currently being treated.
- If irritation develops while using this drug, immediately discontinue its use and notify your doctor.
- This product is not for use in the eyes or on the mucous membranes; contact may result in side effects.
- Do not use this product with an occlusive wrap unless your doctor directs you to do so. Systemic absorption of this drug is increased if extensive areas of the body are treated, particularly if occlusive bandages are used. If it is necessary for you to use this drug under a wrap, follow your doctor's instructions exactly; do not leave the wrap in place longer than specified.
- If you are using this medication on a child's diaper area, do not put tight-fitting diapers or plastic pants on the child. This may lead to increased systemic absorption of the drug and an increase in side effects.
- In order to avoid freezing skin tissue when using the aerosol form of triamcinolone, make sure that you do not spray for more than three seconds, and hold the container at least six inches away from the skin.
- To prevent side effects when using the aerosol form of this medication on the face, cover your eyes, and do not inhale the spray.
- Do not use this medication for longer than the time prescribed by your doctor.
- Be sure to tell your doctor if you are pregnant. If large amounts of triamcinolone are applied for prolonged periods, some of it will be absorbed and may cross the placenta.

Although studies in humans have not been conducted, birth defects have been observed in the offspring of animals that were given large oral doses of this type of drug during pregnancy. Also, tell your doctor if you are breast-feeding an infant. If absorbed through the skin, small amounts of triamcinolone pass into breast milk and may cause growth suppression or a decrease in natural adrenocorticosteroid hormone production in the nursing infant.

triamcinolone acetonide—see triamcinolone (topical)

triamcinolone, neomycin, gramicidin, and nystatin combination (topical)—see triamcinolone, neomycin, nystatin, and gramicidin combination (topical)

triamcinolone, neomycin, nystatin, and gramicidin combination (topical)

BRAND NAMES (Manufacturers)
Myco Triacet (various manufacturers)
triamcinolone, neomycin, gramicidin, and nystatin (various manufacturers)
Tri-Statin (Rugby)
TYPE OF DRUG
Adrenocorticosteroid and anti-infective
INGREDIENTS
triamcinolone, neomycin, nystatin, and gramicidin
DOSAGE FORMS
Cream (0.1% triamcinolone; 2.5 mg neomycin; 100,000 units nystatin; and 0.25 mg gramicidin per gram)
Ointment (0.1% triamcinolone; 2.5 mg neomycin; 100,000 units nystatin; and 0.25 mg gramicidin per gram)
STORAGE
The cream and ointment should be stored at room temperature (never frozen) in tightly closed containers. Discard any outdated medicine or medicine no longer needed.

USES

Your adrenal glands naturally produce certain cortisone-like chemicals. These chemicals are involved in various processes in the body (such as maintenance of fluid balance, regulation of temperature, and reaction to inflammation). Triamcinolone belongs to a group of drugs known as adrenocorticosteroids (or cortisone-like medications). It is used to relieve the skin inflammation (redness, swelling, itching, and discomfort) associated with conditions such as dermatitis, eczema, and poison ivy. How this drug acts to relieve these disorders is not completely understood. Neomycin and gramicidin are antibiotics, which act to prevent the growth and multiplication of infecting bacteria. Nystatin is an anti-infective agent that is active against the fungus *Candida albicans.*

TREATMENT

Before applying this medication, wash your hands. Then, unless your doctor gives you different instructions, gently wash the area of skin where the medication is to be applied. With a clean towel, pat the area almost dry; it should be slightly damp when you put the medication on.

Apply a small amount of this medication to the affected area in a thin layer. Do not bandage the area unless your doctor tells you to do so. If you are to apply an occlusive dressing (like kitchen plastic wrap), be sure you understand the instructions. Wash your hands again after application.

If you miss a dose of this medication, apply the dose as soon as possible, unless it is almost time for the next application. In that case, do not apply the missed dose at all; just return to your regular dosing schedule. Do not put twice as much of the medication on your skin at the next application.

Use this medication for the full length of time prescribed by your doctor; do not take the medication for longer than the prescribed period.

SIDE EFFECTS

Minor. Acne, burning sensation, irritation of the affected area, or skin dryness.

If the affected area is extremely dry or scaling, the skin may be moistened by soaking in water or by applying water with a clean cloth before applying the medication. The ointment form is probably better for dry skin.

A mild, temporary stinging sensation may occur after this medication is applied. If this persists, contact your doctor.

Major. Tell your doctor about any side effects that are persistent or particularly bothersome. IT IS ESPECIALLY IMPORTANT TO TELL YOUR DOCTOR about blistering, increased hair growth, itching, loss of skin color, rash, secondary infection in the area being treated, or thinning of the skin with easy bruising. Also, if your symptoms of infection seem to be getting worse rather than improving, you should contact your doctor.

INTERACTIONS

This medication should not interact with other medications, as long as it is used according to directions.

WARNINGS

- Tell your doctor about unusual or allergic reactions you have had to any medications, especially to triamcinolone or other adrenocorticosteroids (such as amcinonide, betamethasone, clocortolone, cortisone, desonide, desoximetasone, dexamethasone, diflorasone, flumethasone, fluocinolone, fluocinonide, fluorometholone, flurandrenolide, halcinonide, hydrocortisone, methylprednisolone, prednisolone, and prednisone) or to neomycin, nystatin, or gramicidin.
- Tell your doctor if you now have or if you have ever had circulation problems, chicken pox, diabetes mellitus, peptic ulcers, shingles, tuberculosis of the lungs or skin, vaccinia, or viral or fungal infections of the skin in addition to a *Candida* infection.
- If irritation develops while you are using this drug, immediately discontinue its use and notify your doctor.
- Do not use in the eyes; contact may result in side effects.
- This medication should not be used in the external ear canal of people with perforated eardrums.
- Do not use this product with an occlusive wrap unless your doctor directs you to do so. Systemic absorption of this drug is increased when extensive areas of the body are treated, particularly if occlusive bandages are used. If it is necessary for you to use this drug under a wrap, follow your

doctor's instructions exactly, and do not leave the wrap in place longer than specified.

• If you are using this medication on a child's diaper area, do not put tight-fitting diapers or plastic pants on the child. This may lead to increased systemic absorption of the drug and an increase in side effects.

• Be sure to tell your doctor if you are pregnant. If large amounts of this drug are applied for prolonged periods, some of it will be absorbed and may cross the placenta. Although studies in humans have not been conducted, birth defects have been observed in the offspring of animals that were given large oral doses of this type of drug during pregnancy. Also, tell your doctor if you are breast-feeding an infant. If absorbed through the skin, small amounts of this medication pass into breast milk and may cause growth suppression or a decrease in natural adrenocorticosteroid hormone production in the nursing infant.

Triaminic—see phenylpropanolamine and chlorpheniramine combination

Triaminic-12—see phenylpropanolamine and chlorpheniramine combination

---

triamterene

BRAND NAME (Manufacturer)
Dyrenium (Smith Kline & French)
TYPE OF DRUG
Diuretic and antihypertensive
INGREDIENT
triamterene
DOSAGE FORM
Capsules (50 mg and 100 mg)
STORAGE
Triamterene should be stored at room temperature in a tightly closed, light-resistant container.

USES

Triamterene is prescribed to treat high blood pressure. It is also used to reduce fluid accumulation in the body caused by conditions such as heart failure, cirrhosis of the liver, kidney disease, and the long-term use of some medications. Triamterene reduces fluid accumulation by increasing the elimination of salt and water through the kidneys. It may also be used in combination with other diuretics to prevent potassium loss.

TREATMENT

To decrease stomach irritation, you can take this medication with a glass of milk or with a meal (unless your doctor directs you to do otherwise). Try to take it at the same time every day. Avoid taking a dose after 6:00 P.M.; otherwise, you may have to get up during the night to urinate.

If you miss a dose of this medication, take the missed dose as soon as possible, unless it is almost time for the next dose. In that case, do not take the missed dose at all; just wait until the next scheduled dose. Do not double the next dose.

This medication does not cure high blood pressure, but will help control the condition as long as you take it.

SIDE EFFECTS

Minor. Diarrhea, dizziness, drowsiness, dry mouth, headache, increased thirst, increased urination, nausea, tiredness, upset stomach, or vomiting. As your body adjusts to triamterene, these side effects should disappear.

This medication can cause increased sensitivity to sunlight. It is, therefore, important to avoid prolonged exposure to sunlight and sunlamps while you are taking this medication. Wear protective clothing, and use an effective sunscreen.

Triamterene may cause the urine to turn bluish; this is a harmless side effect.

Dry mouth can be relieved by sucking on ice chips or a piece of hard candy or by chewing sugarless gum.

To avoid dizziness or light-headedness when you stand, contract and relax the muscles of your legs for a few moments before rising. Do this by pushing one foot against the floor while raising the other foot slightly, alternating feet so that you are "pumping" your legs in a pedaling motion.

Major. Tell your doctor about any side effects that are persistent or particularly bothersome. IT IS ESPECIALLY IMPORTANT TO TELL YOUR DOCTOR about anxiety; back or flank (side) pain; confusion; cracking at the corners of the mouth; difficulty in breathing; extreme weakness; fever; mouth sores; numbness or tingling in the hands, feet, or lips; painful urination; palpitations; rash; a red or inflamed tongue; sore throat; unusual bleeding or bruising; or unusual tiredness.

INTERACTIONS

Triamterene interacts with several foods and medications:

1. Concurrent use of it with spironolactone, amiloride, potassium salts, low-salt milk, salt substitutes, captopril, enalapril, or laxatives can cause serious side effects from hyperkalemia (high levels of potassium in the blood).

2. Triamterene may decrease the effectiveness of antigout medications, insulin, and oral antidiabetic medications.

3. It may increase the side effects of lithium.

4. Indomethacin may decrease the diuretic effects of triamterene.

Before starting to take triamterene, BE SURE TO TELL YOUR DOCTOR about any medications you are currently taking, especially any of those listed above.

WARNINGS

• Before starting to take triamterene, be sure to tell your doctor if you have ever had unusual or allergic reactions to any medications, especially to triamterene or to any other diuretic.

• Tell your doctor if you now have or if you have ever had kidney disease, kidney stones, urination problems, hyperkalemia, diabetes mellitus, liver disease, acidosis, or gout.

• Triamterene can cause hyperkalemia (high blood levels of potassium). Signs of hyperkalemia include palpitations; confusion; numbness or tingling in the hands, feet, or lips; anxiety; or unusual tiredness or weakness. In order to avoid this problem, do not alter your diet, and do not use salt substitutes unless your doctor tells you to do so.

• Limit your intake of alcoholic beverages while taking this drug to prevent dizziness and light-headedness.

• Do not take any over-the-counter (nonprescription) medication for weight control or for allergy, asthma, cough, cold, or sinus problems unless you first check with your doctor. Some of these products can lead to an increase in blood pressure.

• To prevent severe water loss (dehydration) while taking this medication, check with your doctor if you have any illness that causes severe or continuous nausea, vomiting, or diarrhea.

• If you are taking quinidine (an antiarrhythmia heart medication), it is important to know that triamterene may interfere with the laboratory determination of your blood quinidine concentration. Before you undergo such a test, be sure to tell your doctor that you are also taking the drug triamterene.

• Your doctor may schedule regular office visits to monitor your progress and possibly adjust your dosage.

• Be sure to tell your doctor if you are pregnant. This drug crosses the placenta, and its safety in human pregnancy has not been established. Adverse effects have been reported in the fetuses of animals that received large doses of this drug during pregnancy. Also, tell your doctor if you are breast-feeding an infant. Small amounts of triamterene pass into breast milk.

---

triamterene and hydrochlorothiazide combination

BRAND NAMES (Manufacturers)

Dyazide (Smith Kline & French)
Maxzide (Lederle)
triamterene and hydrochlorothiazide (various manufacturers)

TYPE OF DRUG

Diuretic and antihypertensive

INGREDIENTS

triamterene and hydrochlorothiazide

DOSAGE FORMS

Capsules (50 mg triamterene and 25 mg hydrochlorothiazide) Tablets (75 mg triamterene and 50 mg hydrochlorothiazide)

STORAGE

Triamterene and hydrochlorothiazide combination should be stored at room temperature in a tightly closed, light-resistant container.

USES

Triamterene and hydrochlorothiazide combination is prescribed to treat high blood pressure. It is also used to reduce fluid accumulation in the body caused by conditions such as heart failure, cirrhosis of the liver, kidney disease, and the long-term use of some medications. It reduces fluid accumulation by increasing the elimination of salt and water through the kidneys. Triamterene is combined with hydrochlorothiazide to prevent potassium loss.

TREATMENT

To decrease stomach irritation, you can take this medication with a glass of milk or with a meal (unless your doctor directs you to do otherwise). Try to take it at the same time every day. Avoid taking a dose after 6:00 P.M.; otherwise, you may have to get up during the night to urinate.

If you miss a dose of this medication, take the missed dose as soon as possible, unless it is almost time for the next dose. In that case, do not take the missed dose at all; just wait until the next scheduled dose. Do not double the next dose.

This medication does not cure high blood pressure, but will help control the condition as long as you take it.

SIDE EFFECTS

Minor. Constipation, cramps, diarrhea, dizziness, drowsiness, headache, increased urination, loss of appetite, restlessness, tiredness, or upset stomach. These side effects should disappear as your body adjusts to the medication.

This medication can cause increased sensitivity to sunlight. It is, therefore, important to avoid prolonged exposure to sunlight and sunlamps. Wear protective clothing, and use an effective sunscreen.

Triamterene can cause the urine to turn bluish; this is a harmless side effect.

To relieve constipation, increase the amount of fiber in your diet (fresh fruits and vegetables, salads, bran, and whole-grain breads) and exercise more (unless your doctor directs you to do otherwise).

If you experience dryness of the mouth, you might want to try sucking on ice chips or a piece of hard candy or chewing sugarless gum.

To avoid dizziness or light-headedness when you stand, contract and relax the muscles of your legs for a few moments before rising. Do this by pushing one foot against the floor while raising the other foot slightly, alternating feet so that you are "pumping" your legs in a pedaling motion.

Major. Tell your doctor about any side effects that are persistent or particularly bothersome. IT IS ESPECIALLY IMPORTANT TO TELL YOUR DOCTOR about anxiety; back or flank (side) pain; confusion; cracking at the corners of the mouth; difficulty in urinating; difficulty in breathing; dry mouth; fever; itching; mood changes; mouth sores; muscle cramps or spasms; nausea; painful urination; palpitations; rash; red or inflamed tongue; sore throat; thirst; tingling or numbness in the hands, feet, or lips; unusual bleeding or bruising; unusual tiredness or weakness; vomiting; or yellowing of the eyes or skin.

INTERACTIONS

Triamterene and hydrochlorothiazide combination interacts with several foods and medications:

1. Concurrent use of it with spironolactone, amiloride, potassium salts, low-salt milk, salt substitutes, captopril, enalapril, or laxatives can cause serious side effects from hyperkalemia (high levels of potassium in the blood).

2. This drug may decrease the effectiveness of oral anticoagulants, antigout medications, insulin, oral antidiabetic medicines, and methenamine.

3. Fenfluramine may increase the blood-pressure-lowering effects of this drug (which can be dangerous).

4. Indomethacin may decrease the effectiveness of this medication.

5. Cholestyramine and colestipol can decrease the absorption of this medication from the gastrointestinal tract. Therefore, triamterene and hydrochlorothiazide combination should be taken one hour before or four hours after a dose of cholestyramine or colestipol if one of these medications has also been prescribed.

6. This medication may increase the side effects of amphotericin B, calcium, cortisone and cortisone-like steroids (such as dexamethasone, hydrocortisone, prednisone, and prednisolone), digoxin, digitalis, lithium, quinidine, sulfonamide antibiotics, and vitamin D.

BE SURE TO TELL YOUR DOCTOR about any medications you are currently taking, especially any of those listed above.

WARNINGS

• Tell your doctor about unusual or allergic reactions you have had to any medications, especially to triamterene or hydrochlorothiazide or to any other sulfa drugs, including other diuretics, oral antidiabetic medications, and sulfonamide antibiotics.

• Before you start to take triamterene and hydrochlorothiazide combination, tell your doctor if you now have or if you have ever had kidney disease, kidney stones, problems with urination, diabetes mellitus, gout, liver disease, asthma, acidosis, pancreatic disease, systemic lupus erythematosus, anemia, blood disease, hypercalcemia, or hyperkalemia.

• This drug can occasionally cause potassium loss from the body. Signs of potassium loss include dry mouth, thirst, weakness, muscle pain or cramps, nausea, and vomiting. If you experience any of these symptoms, call your doctor.

• Triamterene can cause hyperkalemia (high levels of potassium in the blood). Signs of hyperkalemia include palpitations; confusion; numbness or tingling in the hands, feet, or lips; anxiety; or unusual tiredness or weakness. In order to avoid this problem, do not alter your diet, and do not use salt substitutes unless you first consult your doctor.

• If you are taking quinidine (an antiarrhythmia heart medication), it is important to know that triamterene may interfere with the laboratory determination of your blood quinidine concentration. Before you undergo such a test, be sure to tell your doctor that you are also taking triamterene and hydrochlorothiazide combination.

• Limit your intake of alcoholic beverages while taking this medication, in order to prevent dizziness and lightheadedness.

• Do not take any over-the-counter (nonprescription) medication for weight control or for allergy, asthma, cough, cold, or sinus problems unless you first check with your doctor. Some of these products can lead to an increase in blood pressure.

• Do not change brands of this medication without consulting your doctor.

• To prevent severe water loss (dehydration) while taking this medication, check with your doctor if you have any illness that causes severe or continuous nausea, vomiting, or diarrhea.

• This medication can raise blood sugar levels in diabetic patients. Therefore, blood sugar should be monitored carefully with blood or urine tests when this medication is being taken.

• A doctor does not usually prescribe a "fixed-dose" drug like this as the first choice in the treatment of high blood pressure. Usually, the patient first receives each ingredient singly. If there is an adequate response to the fixed dose contained in this product, it can then be substituted. The advantages of a combination product are increased convenience and (often) decreased cost.

• Your doctor may schedule regular office visits to monitor your progress and possibly adjust the dosage.

• Be sure to tell your doctor if you are pregnant. This drug crosses the placenta, and its safety in human pregnancy has not been established. Adverse effects have been observed in the fetuses of animals that received large doses of this type of drug during pregnancy. Also, tell your doctor if you are breast-feeding an infant. Small amounts of this drug pass into breast milk.

Triavil—see perphenazine and amitriptyline combination

---

triazolam

BRAND NAME (Manufacturer)
Halcion (Upjohn)
TYPE OF DRUG
Benzodiazepine sedative/hypnotic
INGREDIENT
triazolam
DOSAGE FORM
Tablets (0.125 mg and 0.25 mg)
STORAGE
This medication should be stored at room temperature in a tightly closed, light-resistant container.

USES

Triazolam is prescribed to treat insomnia, including problems with falling asleep, waking during the night, and early morning wakefulness. It is not clear exactly how this medicine works, but it may relieve insomnia by acting as a depressant of the central nervous system (brain and spinal cord).

TREATMENT

This medicine should be taken 30 to 60 minutes before bedtime. It can be taken with a full glass of water or with food if stomach upset occurs. Do not take this medication with a dose of antacids, since they may slow its absorption from the gastrointestinal tract.

If you are taking this medication regularly and you miss a dose, take the missed dose immediately if you remember within an hour. If more than an hour has passed, skip the dose you missed and wait for the next scheduled dose. Do not double the dose.

SIDE EFFECTS

Minor. Bitter taste in mouth, constipation, diarrhea, dizziness, drowsiness (after a night's sleep), dry mouth, excessive salivation, fatigue, flushing, headache, heartburn, loss of appetite, nausea, nervousness, sweating, or vomiting. As your body adjusts to the medication, these should disappear.

To relieve constipation, increase the amount of fiber in your diet (fresh fruits and vegetables, salads, bran, and whole-grain breads), exercise, and drink more water (unless your doctor directs you to do otherwise).

Dry mouth can be relieved by chewing sugarless gum or by sucking on ice chips.

If you feel dizzy, sit or lie down for a while; get up slowly from a sitting or reclining position, and be careful on stairs.

Major. Tell your doctor about any side effects that are persistent or particularly bothersome. IT IS ESPECIALLY IMPORTANT TO TELL YOUR DOCTOR about blurred or double vision, chest pain, depression, difficulty in urinating, fainting, falling, fever, hallucinations, joint pain, mouth sores, nightmares, palpitations, rash, shortness of breath, slurred speech, sore throat, uncoordinated movements, unusual excitement, unusual tiredness, or yellowing of the eyes or skin.

INTERACTIONS

Triazolam interacts with a number of other types of drugs:

1. To prevent oversedation, it should not be taken with alcohol, other sedative drugs, or central nervous system depressants (such as antihistamines, barbiturates, muscle relaxants, pain medicines, narcotics, medicines for seizures, and phenothiazine tranquilizers) or with antidepressants.

2. Triazolam may decrease the effectiveness of carbamazepine, levodopa, and oral anticoagulants (blood thinners, such as warfarin) and may increase the side effects of phenytoin.

3. Disulfiram, oral contraceptives (birth control pills), isoniazid, and cimetidine can increase the blood levels of triazolam, which can lead to toxic effects.

4. Concurrent use of rifampin may decrease the effectiveness of triazolam.

BE SURE TO TELL YOUR DOCTOR about any medications you are currently taking, especially any of those listed above.

WARNINGS

• Tell your doctor about unusual or allergic reactions you have had to any medications, especially to triazolam or other benzodiazepine tranquilizers (such as alprazolam, chlordiazepoxide, clorazepate, diazepam, flurazepam, halazepam, lorazepam, prazepam, and temazepam).

• Tell your doctor if you now have or if you have ever had liver disease, kidney disease, epilepsy, lung disease, myasthenia gravis, porphyria, mental depression, or mental illness.

• This medicine can cause drowsiness. Avoid tasks that require mental alertness, such as driving a car or operating potentially dangerous machinery.

• Triazolam has the potential for abuse and must be used with caution. Tolerance may develop quickly; do not increase the dosage unless you first consult your doctor. It is also important not to stop taking this drug suddenly if you have been taking it in large amounts or if you have used it for several weeks. Your doctor may want to reduce the dosage gradually.

• This is a safe drug when used properly. When it is combined with other sedative drugs or with alcohol, however, serious side effects can develop.

• Be sure to tell your doctor if you are pregnant. This type of medicine may increase the chance of birth defects if it is taken during the first three months of pregnancy. In addition, use of too much of this medicine during the last six months of pregnancy may lead to addiction of the fetus, resulting in withdrawal side effects in the newborn. Also, use of this medicine during the last weeks of pregnancy may cause excessive drowsiness, slowed heartbeat, and breathing difficulties in the infant. Tell your doctor if you are breast-feeding an infant. This medicine can pass into breast milk and cause excessive drowsiness, slowed heartbeat, and breathing difficulties in nursing infants.

Trichlorex—see trichlormethiazide

---

trichlormethiazide

BRAND NAMES (Manufacturers)
Diurese (American Urologicals)
Metahydrin (Merrell Dow)
Naqua (Schering)
Niazide (Major)
Trichlorex (Lannett)
trichlormethiazide (various manufacturers)

TYPE OF DRUG
Diuretic and antihypertensive

INGREDIENT
trichlormethiazide

DOSAGE FORM
Tablets (2 mg and 4 mg)

STORAGE
This medication should be stored at room temperature in a tightly closed container.

USES

Trichlormethiazide is prescribed to treat high blood pressure. It is also used to reduce fluid accumulation in the body caused by conditions such as heart failure, cirrhosis of the liver, and kidney disease and by the long-term use of some medications. This medication reduces fluid accumulation by increasing the elimination of sodium and water through the kidneys.

TREATMENT

To decrease stomach irritation, you can take this medication with a glass of milk or with a meal (unless your doctor directs you to do otherwise). Try to take it at the same time every day. Avoid taking a dose after 6:00 P.M.; otherwise, you may have to get up during the night to urinate.

If you miss a dose of this medication, take the missed dose as soon as possible, unless it is almost time for the next dose. In that case, do not take the missed dose at all; just wait until the next scheduled dose. Do not double the next dose.

This medication does not cure high blood pressure, but will help control the condition as long as you take it.

SIDE EFFECTS

Minor. Constipation, cramps, diarrhea, dizziness, drowsiness, headache, heartburn, loss of appetite, nausea, restlessness, or upset stomach. As your body adjusts to the medication, these side effects should disappear.

This medication can cause increased sensitivity to sunlight. It is, therefore, important to avoid prolonged exposure to sunlight and sunlamps. Wear protective clothing, and use an effective sunscreen.

To avoid dizziness or light-headedness when you stand, contract and relax the muscles of your legs for a few moments before rising. Do this by pushing one foot against the floor while raising the other foot slightly, alternating feet so that you are "pumping" your legs in a pedaling motion.

Major. Tell your doctor about any side effects that are persistent or particularly bothersome. IT IS ESPECIALLY IMPORTANT TO TELL YOUR DOCTOR about blurred vision, confusion, difficulty in breathing, dry mouth, excessive thirst, excessive weakness, fever, itching, joint pain, mood changes, muscle pain or spasms, nausea, palpitations, skin rash, sore throat, tingling in the fingers or toes, vomiting, or yellowing of the eyes or skin.

INTERACTIONS

Trichlormethiazide interacts with other types of medications:

1. It may decrease the effectiveness of oral anticoagulants, antigout medications, insulin, oral antidiabetic medicines, and methenamine.

2. Fenfluramine can increase the blood-pressure-lowering effects of trichlormethiazide (which can be dangerous).

3. Indomethacin can decrease the blood-pressure-lowering effects of trichlormethiazide, thereby counteracting the desired effects.

4. Cholestyramine and colestipol decrease the absorption of this medication from the gastrointestinal tract. Trichlormethiazide should, therefore, be taken one hour before or four hours after a dose of cholestyramine or colestipol if one of these medications has also been prescribed.

5. Trichlormethiazide may increase the side effects of amphotericin B, calcium, cortisone and cortisone-like steroids (such as dexamethasone, hydrocortisone, prednisone, prednisolone), digoxin, digitalis, lithium, quinidine, sulfonamide antibiotics, and vitamin D.

BE SURE TO TELL YOUR DOCTOR about any medications you are currently taking, especially any of those listed above.

WARNINGS

- Tell your doctor about unusual or allergic reactions you have had to any medications, especially to trichlormethiazide or to other sulfa drugs, including other diuretics, oral antidiabetic medications, and sulfonamide antibiotics.
- Before you start taking trichlormethiazide, tell your doctor if you now have or if you have ever had kidney disease or problems with urination, diabetes mellitus, gout, liver disease, asthma, pancreatic disease, or systemic lupus erythematosus.
- Trichlormethiazide can cause potassium loss. Signs of potassium loss include dry mouth, thirst, weakness, muscle pain or cramps, nausea, and vomiting. If you experience any of these symptoms, call your doctor. To help avoid potassium loss, take this drug with a glass of fresh or frozen orange or cranberry juice, or eat a banana every day. The use of a salt substitute also helps to prevent potassium loss. Do not change your diet, however, before discussing it with your doctor; too much potassium can also be dangerous. Your doctor may want to have blood tests performed periodically in order to monitor your potassium levels.
- In order to prevent dizziness and light-headedness, limit your intake of alcoholic beverages while taking this drug.
- Do not take any over-the-counter (nonprescription) medications for weight control or for allergy, asthma, cough, cold, or sinus problems unless directed to do so by your doctor.
- To prevent dehydration (severe water loss) while taking this medication, check with your doctor if you have any illness that causes severe or continuous nausea, vomiting, or diarrhea.
- This medication can raise blood sugar levels in diabetic patients. Therefore, blood sugar should be carefully monitored with blood or urine tests when this medication is being taken.
- Some of these products contain the color additive FD&C Yellow No. 5 (tartrazine), which can cause allergic-type reactions (wheezing, rash, fainting, difficulty in breathing) in certain susceptible individuals.
- The elderly may be more likely to experience dizziness, light-headedness, and too much potassium loss as a result of therapy with this drug.
- Be sure to tell your doctor if you are pregnant. This drug is able to cross the placenta. Safety in human pregnancy has not been established. Adverse effects have been observed in the fetuses of animals that received large doses of this type of drug during pregnancy. Also, tell your doctor if you are breast-feeding an infant. Although problems in humans have not been reported, small amounts of this drug can pass into breast milk, so caution is warranted.

Triderm—see triamcinolone (topical)

Trifed-C—see pseudoephedrine, triprolidine, guaifenesin, and codeine combination

---

trifluoperazine

BRAND NAMES (Manufacturers)

Stelazine (Smith Kline & French)
trifluoperazine (various manufacturers)

TYPE OF DRUG

Phenothiazine tranquilizer

INGREDIENT

trifluoperazine

DOSAGE FORMS

Tablets (1 mg, 2 mg, 5 mg, and 10 mg)
Oral concentrate (10 mg per ml)

STORAGE

The tablet form of this medication should be stored at room temperature in a tightly closed, light-resistant container. The oral concentrate form should be stored in the refrigerator (never frozen) in a tightly closed, light-resistant container. If the oral concentrate turns slightly yellowish, the medicine is still effective and can be used. However, if it changes color markedly or has particles floating in it, it should not be used; instead, it should be discarded down the sink. Discard any outdated medication.

USES

Trifluoperazine is prescribed to treat the symptoms of certain types of mental illness, such as emotional symptoms of psychosis, the manic phase of manic-depressive illness, and severe behavioral problems in children. This medication is thought to relieve the symptoms of mental illness by blocking certain chemicals involved with nerve transmission in the brain.

TREATMENT

In order to avoid stomach irritation, you can take the tablet form of this medication with a meal or with a glass of water or milk (unless your doctor directs you to do otherwise).

The oral concentrate form of this medication should be measured carefully with the dropper provided and then added to four ounces (1/2 cup) or more of water, milk, or a carbonated beverage or to applesauce or pudding immediately prior to administration. Because of a possible loss of effectiveness, the medication should not be diluted with tea, coffee, or apple juice.

Antacids and antidiarrheal medications may decrease the absorption of this medication from the gastrointestinal tract. Therefore, at least one hour should separate doses of one of these medicines and trifluoperazine.

If you miss a dose of this medication, take the missed dose as soon as possible, unless it is almost time for the next dose. In that case, do not take the missed dose at all; just return to your regular dosing schedule. Do not double the next dose (unless your doctor directs you to do so).

The full effects of this medication for the control of emotional or mental symptoms may not become apparent for at least two weeks after you start to take it.

SIDE EFFECTS

Minor. Blurred vision, constipation, decreased sweating, diarrhea, dizziness, drooling, drowsiness, dry mouth, fatigue, jitteriness, menstrual irregularities, nasal congestion, restlessness, vomiting, or weight gain. As your body adjusts to the medication, these side effects should disappear.

This medication can cause increased sensitivity to sunlight. It is, therefore, important to avoid prolonged exposure to sunlight and sunlamps. Wear protective clothing, and use an effective sunscreen.

Trifluoperazine can also cause discoloration of the urine to red, pink, or red-brown. This is a harmless effect.

If you are constipated, increase the amount of fiber in your diet (fresh fruits and vegetables, salads, bran, and whole-grain breads), exercise, and drink more water (unless your doctor directs you to do otherwise).

Chew sugarless gum or suck on ice chips or a piece of hard candy to reduce mouth dryness.

To avoid dizziness or light-headedness when you stand, contract and relax the muscles of your legs for a few moments before rising. Do this by pushing one foot against the floor while raising the other foot slightly, alternating feet so that you are "pumping" your legs in a pedaling motion.

Major. Tell your doctor about any side effects that are persistent or particularly bothersome. IT IS ESPECIALLY IMPORTANT TO TELL YOUR DOCTOR about breast enlargement (in both sexes); chest pain; convulsions; darkened skin; difficulty in swallowing or breathing; fainting; fever; impotence; involuntary movements of the face, mouth, jaw, or tongue; palpitations; rash; sleep disorders; sore throat; suicidal tendencies; tremors; uncoordinated movements; unusual bleeding or bruising; visual disturbances; or yellowing of the eyes or skin.

INTERACTIONS

Trifluoperazine interacts with several other types of drugs:

1. It can cause extreme drowsiness when combined with alcohol or other central nervous system depressants (drugs that slow the activity of the brain and spinal cord), such as barbiturates, benzodiazepine tranquilizers, muscle relaxants, narcotics, and pain medications, or with tricyclic antidepressants.

2. Trifluoperazine can decrease the effectiveness of amphetamines, guanethidine, anticonvulsants, and levodopa.

3. The side effects of epinephrine, monoamine oxidase (MAO) inhibitors, propranolol, phenytoin, and tricyclic antidepressants may be increased by this medication. At least 14 days should separate the use of this drug and the use of an MAO inhibitor.

4. Lithium may increase the side effects and decrease the effectiveness of this medication.

5. Trifluoperazine used with methyldopa may increase blood pressure.

6. False positive pregnancy tests may occur. If you think you may be pregnant, call your doctor.

Before starting to take trifluoperazine, BE SURE TO TELL YOUR DOCTOR about any medications you are currently taking, especially any of those listed above.

WARNINGS

- Tell your doctor about unusual or allergic reactions you have had to any medications, especially to trifluoperazine or other phenothiazine tranquilizers (such as chlorpromazine, fluphenazine, mesoridazine, perphenazine, prochlorperazine, promazine, thioridazine, and triflupromazine) or to loxapine.
- Tell your doctor if you have a history of alcoholism or if you now have or have ever had blood disease, bone marrow disease, brain disease, breast cancer, blockage of the urinary or digestive tract, drug-induced depression, epilepsy, high or low blood pressure, diabetes mellitus, glaucoma, heart or circulatory disease, liver disease, lung disease, Parkinson's disease, peptic ulcers, or an enlarged prostate gland.
- Tell your doctor about any recent exposure to a pesticide or an insecticide. Trifluoperazine may increase the side effects from the exposure.
- To prevent oversedation, avoid drinking alcoholic beverages while taking this medication.
- If this drug makes you dizzy or drowsy, avoid any activity that requires alertness, such as driving a car or operating dangerous machinery. Be careful on stairs, and avoid getting up suddenly from a lying or sitting position.
- Prior to surgery or other medical or dental treatment, tell your doctor or dentist you are taking this drug.
- Some of the side effects caused by this drug can be prevented by taking an antiparkinsonism drug. Discuss this with your doctor.
- This medication can decrease sweating and heat release from the body. You should, therefore, try not to get overheated (avoid exercising strenuously in hot weather, and do not take hot baths, showers, and saunas).
- Do not stop taking this medication suddenly. If the drug is stopped abruptly, you may experience nausea, vomiting, stomach upset, headache, increased heart rate, insomnia, tremors, or a worsening of your condition. Your doctor may want to reduce the dosage gradually.

• If you are planning to have a myelogram or any other procedure in which dye will be injected into your spinal cord, tell your doctor that you are taking this medication.
• Avoid spilling the oral concentrate form of this drug on your skin or clothing; it may cause redness and skin irritation.
• While taking this medication, do not take any over-the-counter (nonprescription) medication for weight control or for cough, cold, allergy, asthma, or sinus problems unless you first check with your doctor. The combination of these medications with trifluoperazine may cause high blood pressure.
• Be sure to tell your doctor if you are pregnant. Small amounts of this medication cross the placenta. Although there are reports of safe use of this drug during pregnancy, there are also reports of liver disease and tremors in newborn infants whose mothers received this medication close to term. Also, tell your doctor if you are breast-feeding an infant. Small amounts of this medication pass into breast milk and may cause unwanted effects in nursing infants.

trifluoperazine hydrochloride—see trifluoperazine

Trihexane—see trihexyphenidyl

Trihexidyl—see trihexyphenidyl

Trihexy—see trihexyphenidyl

---

trihexyphenidyl

BRAND NAMES (Manufacturers)
Artane (Lederle)
Artane Sequels (Lederle)
Trihexane (Rugby)
Trihexidyl (Henry Schein)
Trihexy (Geneva Generics)
trihexyphenidyl hydrochloride (various manufacturers)
TYPE OF DRUG
Antiparkinsonism agent
INGREDIENT
trihexyphenidyl
DOSAGE FORMS
Tablets (2 mg and 5 mg)
Sustained-release capsules (5 mg)
Oral elixir (2 mg per 5-ml spoonful, with 5% alcohol)
STORAGE
Store at room temperature in a tightly closed container. This medication should never be frozen.

USES

Trihexyphenidyl is used to treat the symptoms of Parkinson's disease or to control the side effects of phenothiazine tranquilizers. It is not clearly understood how this medication works, but it is thought to act by balancing certain chemicals in the brain.

TREATMENT

In order to reduce stomach irritation, you should take trihexyphenidyl with food or just after a meal.

Antacids and antidiarrheal medications prevent the absorption of this medication from the gastrointestinal tract, so at least one hour should separate doses of trihexyphenidyl and one of these medicines.

The oral elixir form of this medication should be measured carefully with a specially designed 5-ml measuring spoon. An ordinary kitchen teaspoon is not accurate enough.

The sustained-release capsules should be swallowed whole. Chewing, crushing, or breaking the capsules destroys their sustained-release activity and possibly increases the side effects.

If you miss a dose of this medication, take the missed dose as soon as possible, unless it is within two hours of the next dose of the tablets or oral elixir or within eight hours of the next dose of the sustained-release capsules. In that case, do not take the missed dose at all; just return to your regular dosing schedule. Do not double the next dose.

SIDE EFFECTS

Minor. Bloating; blurred vision; constipation; decreased sweating; dizziness; drowsiness; dry mouth, throat, and nose; false sense of well-being; headache; increased sensitivity of the eyes to light; muscle cramps; nausea; nervousness; and weakness. These side effects should disappear as your body adjusts to the medication.

If you are constipated, increase the amount of fiber in your diet (fresh fruits and vegetables, salads, bran, whole-grain breads), exercise, and drink more water (unless your doctor directs you to do otherwise).

Chew sugarless gum or suck on ice chips or a piece of hard candy to reduce mouth dryness.

Wear sunglasses if you find that your eyes have become sensitive to light.

If you feel dizzy, sit or lie down for a while; get up slowly from a sitting or reclining position, and be careful on stairs.

Major. Tell your doctor about any side effects that are persistent or particularly bothersome. IT IS ESPECIALLY IMPORTANT TO TELL YOUR DOCTOR about confusion, depression, difficulty in urinating, hallucinations, involuntary muscle movements, numbness or tingling of the fingers or toes, palpitations, or unusual excitement.

INTERACTIONS

Trihexyphenidyl interacts with other types of medications:

1. It can cause extreme drowsiness when combined with alcohol or other central nervous system depressants (drugs that slow the activity of the brain and spinal cord), such as antihistamines, barbiturates, benzodiazepine tranquilizers, muscle relaxants, narcotics, and pain medications, or with tricyclic antidepressants.

2. Amantadine, antihistamines, haloperidol, monoamine oxidase (MAO) inhibitors, phenothiazine tranquilizers, procainamide, quinidine, and tricyclic antidepressants can increase the side effects of trihexyphenidyl. At least 14 days should separate the use of this drug and the use of an MAO inhibitor.

3. Trihexyphenidyl can increase the elimination of chlorpromazine from the body and thus decrease its effectiveness.

4. Trihexyphenidyl can decrease the effectiveness of the drug levodopa.

BE SURE TO TELL YOUR DOCTOR about any medications you are currently taking, especially any of the medications that are listed above.

WARNINGS

- Tell your doctor about unusual or allergic reactions you have had to any medications, especially to trihexyphenidyl.
- Tell your doctor if you now have or if you have ever had achalasia, glaucoma, heart disease, myasthenia gravis, blockage of the intestinal or urinary tract, enlarged prostate gland, stomach ulcers, or thyroid disease.
- If this drug makes you dizzy or drowsy, avoid any activity that requires alertness, such as driving a car or operating potentially dangerous machinery. Be careful on stairs, and avoid standing up suddenly.
- This medication can decrease sweating and heat release from the body. You should, therefore, try not to get overheated (avoid exercising strenuously in hot weather, and do not take hot baths, showers, or saunas).
- Your doctor may recommend periodic eye exams to check pressure in your eyes.
- Be sure to tell your doctor if you are pregnant. Although trihexyphenidyl appears to be safe during pregnancy, extensive studies have not been conducted. Also, tell your doctor if you are breast-feeding an infant. Small amounts of this medication may pass into breast milk.

trihexyphenidyl hydrochloride—see trihexyphenidyl

Tri-Hydroserpine—see hydralazine, hydrochlorothiazide, and reserpine combination

Trilafon—see perphenazine

Trilafon Repetabs—see perphenazine

Tri-Levlen—see oral contraceptives

Trimcaps—see phendimetrazine

---

trimethobenzamide

BRAND NAMES (Manufacturers)
Tebamide (G & W)
T-Gen (Goldline)
Tigan (Beecham)
trimethobenzamide (various manufacturers)

TYPE OF DRUG
Antiemetic (antinauseant)

INGREDIENT
trimethobenzamide

DOSAGE FORMS
Capsules (100 mg and 250 mg)
Suppositories (100 mg and 200 mg)

STORAGE
Store at room temperature in a tightly closed container.

USES

This drug is used to control nausea and vomiting. It is thought to act directly on the vomiting center in the brain.

TREATMENT

Trimethobenzamide capsules can be taken with a full glass of water.

The suppository form of this medication should be inserted into the rectum (if the suppository is too soft to insert, run it under cold water or put it in the refrigerator for 30 minutes). To insert it, remove the foil wrapper, moisten the suppository with a little water, and then lie down on your left side with your right knee bent. Push the suppository into your rectum with your finger. Remain lying down for a few minutes. Try to avoid having a bowel movement for an hour or longer after inserting the suppository in order to allow time for the drug to be absorbed.

If you miss a dose of this medication, take the missed dose as soon as possible, unless it is almost time for the next dose. In that case, do not take the missed dose at all; just return to your regular dosing schedule. Do not double the next dose.

SIDE EFFECTS

Minor. Diarrhea, dizziness, drowsiness, headache, or muscle cramps. These side effects should disappear as your body adjusts to the medication.

If you feel dizzy or light-headed, sit or lie down for a while; get up slowly from a sitting or reclining position, and be careful on stairs.

Major. Tell your doctor about any side effects that are persistent or particularly bothersome. IT IS ESPECIALLY IMPORTANT TO TELL YOUR DOCTOR about back pain, blurred vision, convulsions, depression, disorientation, mouth sores, rash, tremors, unusual bleeding or bruising, unusual hand or face movements, or yellowing of the eyes or skin.

INTERACTIONS

Concurrent use of trimethobenzamide with central nervous system depressants (drugs that slow the activity of the brain and spinal cord), such as alcohol, antihistamines, barbiturates, benzodiazepine tranquilizers, muscle relaxants, narcotics, pain medications, phenothiazine tranquilizers, and sleeping medications, or with tricyclic antidepressants can cause extreme drowsiness.

BE SURE TO TELL YOUR DOCTOR about any medications you are currently taking, especially any of those listed above.

WARNINGS

- Tell your doctor about unusual or allergic reactions you have had to any medications, especially to trimethobenzamide (or to benzocaine or other local anesthetics if you are using the suppository form).
- Before starting to take this medication, be sure to tell your doctor if you now have or if you have ever had acute fever, dehydration, electrolyte imbalance, intestinal infection, or viral infections.
- If this drug makes you dizzy or drowsy, do not take part in any activity that requires alertness, such as driving a car or operating potentially dangerous machinery.
- Be sure to tell your doctor if you are pregnant. Safe use in pregnancy has not been established. Extensive studies in pregnant women have not been conducted. Also, tell your doctor if you are breast-feeding an infant. It is not known whether trimethobenzamide passes into breast milk.

trimethoprim

BRAND NAMES (Manufacturers)
Proloprim (Burroughs Wellcome)
trimethoprim (various manufacturers)
Trimpex (Roche)
TYPE OF DRUG
Antibiotic
INGREDIENT
trimethoprim
DOSAGE FORM
Tablets (100 mg and 200 mg)
STORAGE
Trimethoprim tablets should be stored in a dry place at room temperature in a tightly closed, light-resistant container.

USES

This antibiotic is used in the treatment of uncomplicated urinary tract infections. It acts by preventing production of the nutrients that are required for the growth of infecting bacteria. Trimethoprim kills a wide range of bacteria, but it is not effective against viruses or fungi.

TREATMENT

You can take trimethoprim tablets on an empty stomach or, to avoid stomach upset, with food or milk.

This medication works best when the level of the medicine in your urine is kept constant. It is best, therefore, to take the doses at evenly spaced intervals day and night. For example, if you are to take two doses a day, the doses should be spaced 12 hours apart.

If you miss a dose of this medication, take the missed dose immediately. However, if you do not remember to take the missed dose until it is almost time for your next dose, space the missed dose and the following dose ten to 12 hours apart if you are taking one dose a day or five to six hours apart if you are taking two doses a day. Then return to your regular dosing schedule. Try not to skip any doses.

It is important to continue to take this medication for the entire time prescribed by your doctor (usually seven to 14 days), even if the symptoms disappear before the end of that period. If you stop taking the drug too soon, resistant bacteria are given a chance to continue growing, and the infection could recur.

SIDE EFFECTS

Minor. Abdominal pain, diarrhea, headache, loss of appetite, nausea, unusual taste in the mouth, or vomiting. These should disappear as your body adjusts to the drug.
Major. Tell your doctor about any side effects that are persistent or particularly bothersome. IT IS ESPECIALLY IMPORTANT TO TELL YOUR DOCTOR about itching, skin rash, sore throat and fever, swollen or inflamed tongue, unusual bleeding or bruising, unusual fatigue, or unusually pale skin. Also, if your symptoms of infection seem to be getting worse rather than improving, contact your doctor.

INTERACTIONS

Trimethoprim interacts with several other types of drugs:
1. Rifampin can increase the elimination of trimethoprim from the body and thus decrease its antibacterial effectiveness.
2. Concurrent use of trimethoprim with antineoplastic agents (anticancer drugs) can increase the risk of developing blood disorders.
3. Trimethoprim can decrease the elimination of phenytoin from the body and may, therefore, lead to an increase in the risk of side effects.

Before starting to take this medication, BE SURE TO TELL YOUR DOCTOR about any medications you are currently taking, especially any of those listed above.

WARNINGS

- Tell your doctor about unusual or allergic reactions you have had to any medications, especially to trimethoprim.
- Tell your doctor if you now have or if you have ever had megaloblastic anemia (folate-deficiency anemia), kidney disease, or liver disease.
- This medication has been prescribed for your current infection only. Another infection later on, or one that a family member or friend has, may require a different medicine. You should not give your medicine to other people or use it for other infections, unless your doctor specifically directs you to do so.
- If there is no improvement in your condition several days after starting this medication, check with your doctor. Trimethoprim may not be effective against the bacteria causing your infection.
- Before having surgery or any other medical or dental treatment, be sure to tell your doctor or dentist that you are taking this drug.
- Be sure to tell your doctor if you are pregnant. Although there are reports of safe use of trimethoprim during pregnancy, extensive studies in humans have not been conducted. In addition, this medication has been shown to cause birth defects in the offspring of animals that received very large doses of it during pregnancy. Also, tell your doctor if you are breast-feeding an infant. Small amounts of the drug pass into breast milk, and there is a chance that it may cause anemia in the nursing infant.

trimipramine

BRAND NAME (Manufacturer)
Surmontil (Wyeth-Ayerst)
TYPE OF DRUG
Tricyclic antidepressant
INGREDIENT
trimipramine
DOSAGE FORM
Capsules (25 mg, 50 mg, and 100 mg)
STORAGE
This medication should be stored at room temperature in a tightly closed container.

USES

Trimipramine is used to relieve the symptoms of mental depression. This medication belongs to a group of drugs referred to as the tricyclic antidepressants. These medicines are thought to relieve depression by increasing the concentration of certain chemicals necessary for nerve transmission in the brain.

TREATMENT

This medication should be taken exactly as your doctor prescribes. You can take it with water or with food to lessen the chance of stomach irritation, unless your doctor tells you to do otherwise.

If you miss a dose of this medication, take the missed dose as soon as possible, then return to your regular dosing schedule. However, if the dose you missed was a once-a-day bedtime dose, do not take that dose in the morning; check with your doctor instead. If the dose is taken in the morning, it may cause unwanted side effects. Never double the dose.

The effects of therapy with this medication may not become apparent for at least two or three weeks.

SIDE EFFECTS

Minor. Agitation, anxiety, blurred vision, confusion, constipation, cramps, diarrhea, dizziness, drowsiness, dry mouth, fatigue, heartburn, insomnia, loss of appetite, nausea, peculiar tastes in the mouth, restlessness, sweating, vomiting, weakness, or weight gain or loss. As your body adjusts to the medication, these side effects should disappear.

This drug may cause increased sensitivity to sunlight. Avoid prolonged exposure to sunlight and sunlamps, wear protective clothing and sunglasses, and use an effective sunscreen.

Dry mouth can be relieved by chewing sugarless gum or by sucking on ice chips or a piece of hard candy.

To relieve constipation, increase the amount of fiber in your diet (fresh fruits and vegetables, salads, bran, and whole-grain breads), exercise, and drink more water (unless your doctor directs you to do otherwise).

To avoid dizziness or light-headedness when you stand, contract and relax the muscles of your legs for a few moments before rising. Do this by pushing one foot against the floor while raising the other foot slightly, alternating feet so that you are "pumping" your legs in a pedaling motion.

Major. Tell your doctor about any side effects that are persistent or particularly bothersome. IT IS ESPECIALLY IMPORTANT TO TELL YOUR DOCTOR about chest pain, convulsions, difficulty in urinating, enlarged or painful breasts (in both sexes), fainting, fever, hair loss, hallucinations, headaches, impotence, mood changes, mouth sores, nervousness, nightmares, numbness or tingling in the fingers or toes, palpitations, rapid weight gain or loss (three to five pounds within a week), ringing in the ears, seizures, skin rash, sleep disorders, sore throat, tremors, uncoordinated movements or balance problems, unusual bleeding or bruising, or yellowing of the eyes or skin.

INTERACTIONS

Trimipramine interacts with other types of medications:

1. Extreme drowsiness can occur when it is taken with central nervous system depressants (drugs that slow the activity of the brain and spinal cord), including alcohol, antihistamines, barbiturates, benzodiazepine tranquilizers, muscle relaxants, narcotics, pain medications, phenothiazine tranquilizers, and sleeping medications, or with other tricyclic antidepressants.

2. Trimipramine may decrease the effectiveness of antiseizure medications and may block the blood-pressure-lowering effects of clonidine and guanethidine.

3. Oral contraceptives (birth control pills) and estrogen-containing drugs can increase the side effects and reduce the effectiveness of the tricyclic antidepressants (including trimipramine).

4. Tricyclic antidepressants may increase the side effects of thyroid medication and over-the-counter (nonprescription) cough, cold, allergy, asthma, sinus, and diet medications.

5. The concurrent use of tricyclic antidepressants and monoamine oxidase (MAO) inhibitors should be avoided because the combination may result in fever, convulsions, or high blood pressure. At least 14 days should separate the use of this drug and the use of a MAO inhibitor.

Before starting to take trimipramine, BE SURE TO TELL YOUR DOCTOR about any medications you are currently taking, especially any of those listed above.

WARNINGS

- Tell your doctor if you have had unusual or allergic reactions to any medications, especially to trimipramine or other tricyclic antidepressants (such as amitriptyline, imipramine, doxepin, amoxapine, protriptyline, desipramine, maprotiline, and nortriptyline).
- Tell your doctor if you have a history of asthma, high blood pressure, liver or kidney disease, heart disease, heart attack, circulatory disease, stomach problems, intestinal problems, alcoholism, difficulty in urinating, enlarged prostate gland, epilepsy, glaucoma, thyroid disease, or mental illness or have ever received electroshock therapy.
- If this drug makes you dizzy or drowsy, do not take part in any activity that requires alertness, such as driving a car or operating potentially dangerous machinery.
- Before having surgery or any other medical or dental treatment, be sure to tell your doctor or dentist that you are taking this medication.
- Do not stop taking this drug suddenly. Stopping it abruptly can cause nausea, headache, stomach upset, fatigue, or a worsening of your condition. Your doctor may want to reduce the dosage gradually to prevent or minimize this reaction.
- The effects of this medication may last as long as seven days after you have stopped taking it, so continue to observe all precautions during that period.
- Be sure to tell your doctor if you are pregnant. The use of this medication in human pregnancy has not been established. Studies have shown side effects in the offspring of animals that were given large doses of this medication during pregnancy. Also, tell your doctor if you are breast-feeding an infant. Small amounts of this drug can pass into breast milk and may cause unwanted effects, such as irritability or sleeping problems, in nursing infants.

Trimox—see amoxicillin

Trimpex—see trimethoprim

Trimstat—see phendimetrazine

Trimtabs—see phendimetrazine

Trinalin Repetabs—see pseudoephedrine and azatadine combination

Trind—see phenylpropanolamine and chlorpheniramine combination

Tri-Norinyl—see oral contraceptives

Triphasil-21—see oral contraceptives

Tri-Phen-Chlor—see phenylpropanolamine, phenylephrine, chlorpheniramine, and phenyltoloxamine combination

Triphenyl—see phenylpropanolamine and chlorpheniramine combination

Triple Antibiotic—see hydrocortisone, polymyxin B, neomycin, and bacitracin combination (ophthalmic)

Triple-Gen—see hydrocortisone, polymyxin B, neomycin, and bacitracin combination (ophthalmic)

Triple Sulfa (systemic)—see sulfonamide antibiotics (oral)

Triple Sulfa (vaginal)—see sulfathiazole, sulfacetamide, and sulfabenzamide combination

Triple-Vita-Flor—see vitamins A, D, and C with fluoride

Tri-Statin—see triamcinolone, neomycin, nystatin, and gramicidin combination (topical)

Tri-Vi-Flor—see vitamins A, D, and C with fluoride

Tri-Vitamin with Fluoride Drops—see vitamins A, D, and C with fluoride

Truphylline—see aminophylline

Trymegen—see chlorpheniramine

Trymex—see triamcinolone (topical)

Trysul—see sulfathiazole, sulfacetamide, and sulfabenzamide combination

Tussadon—see phenylpropanolamine and caramiphen combination

Tussafed—see pseudoephedrine, carbinoxamine, and dextromethorphan combination

Tuss-Allergine Modified T.D.—see phenylpropanolamine and caramiphen combination

Tuss-Genade Modified Capsules—see phenylpropanolamine and caramiphen combination

Tusside—see dextromethorphan and iodinated glycerol combination

Tussi-Organidin—see codeine and iodinated glycerol

Tussi-Organidin DM—see dextromethorphan and iodinated glycerol combination

Tussi-R-Gen—see codeine and iodinated glycerol

Tussi-R-Gen DM—see dextromethorphan and iodinated glycerol combination

Tussogest—see phenylpropanolamine and caramiphen combination

Tuss-Ornade—see phenylpropanolamine and caramiphen combination

Tusstat—see diphenhydramine

Twilite—see diphenhydramine

Tylenol with Codeine—see acetaminophen and codeine combination

Tylox—see acetaminophen and oxycodone combination

Ty-tabs—see acetaminophen and codeine combination

Ultracef—see cefadroxil

Unipen—see nafcillin

Uniphyl—see theophylline

Unipres—see hydralazine, hydrochlorothiazide, and reserpine combination

Unisom Nighttime Sleep Aid—see diphenhydramine

Urabeth—see bethanechol

Urecholine—see bethanechol

Urex—see methenamine

Uri-Tet—see oxytetracycline

Urobak—see sulfonamide antibiotics (oral)

Urodine—see phenazopyridine

Urogesic—see phenazopyridine

Uticillin VK—see penicillin VK

Utimox—see amoxicillin

Valisone—see betamethasone valerate (topical)

Valisone Reduced Strength—see betamethasone valerate (topical)

Valium—see diazepam

valproic acid

BRAND NAMES (Manufacturers)
Depakene (Abbott)
Depakote* (Abbott)
Myproic acid (My-K Labs)
valproic acid (various manufacturers)
*Note: Divalproex sodium, sold under the brand name Depakote, is chemically and therapeutically similar to valproic acid. It has been formulated as an enteric-coated tablet in order to prolong its effects and to decrease stomach irritation.
TYPE OF DRUG
Anticonvulsant
INGREDIENT
valproic acid
DOSAGE FORMS
Capsules (250 mg)
Enteric-coated tablets (125 mg, 250 mg, and 500 mg)
Oral syrup (250 mg per 5-ml spoonful)
STORAGE
Valproic acid should be stored at room temperature in tightly closed containers. This medication should never be frozen.

USES

Valproic acid is used to treat various seizure disorders. It prevents seizures or convulsions by increasing concentrations of a certain chemical (gamma-aminobutyric acid) in the brain.

TREATMENT

In order to avoid stomach irritation, you should take valproic acid with food or milk (unless your doctor directs you to do otherwise).

The capsules or enteric-coated tablets should be swallowed whole. Chewing or opening the capsules before swallowing releases their contents, which may cause irritation of the mouth and throat.

Each dose of valproic acid oral syrup should be measured carefully with a specially designed 5-ml measuring spoon. An ordinary kitchen teaspoon is not accurate enough to ensure that you receive the proper dose.

Valproic acid works best when the level of medication in the bloodstream is kept constant. It is best, therefore, to take the doses at evenly spaced intervals day and night. For example, if you are to take four doses a day, the doses should be spaced six hours apart.

It is important to try not to miss any doses of this medication. If you do miss a dose and remember within six hours, take the missed dose immediately. If more than six hours has passed, do not take the missed dose at all; just return to your regular dosing schedule. Do not double the next dose of this medication. If you miss two or more consecutive doses of valproic acid, contact your doctor as soon as possible for further instructions.

SIDE EFFECTS

Minor. Constipation, diarrhea, dizziness, drowsiness, hair loss, headache, increased or decreased appetite, insomnia, nausea, stomach upset, vomiting, or weight gain or loss. These side effects should disappear as your body adjusts to the medication.

To relieve constipation, increase the amount of fiber in your diet (fresh fruits and vegetables, salads, bran, and whole-grain breads), exercise, and drink more water (unless your doctor directs you to do otherwise).

If you feel dizzy, sit or lie down for a while; get up slowly from a sitting or reclining position, and be careful on stairs.
Major. Tell your doctor about any side effects that are persistent or particularly bothersome. IT IS ESPECIALLY IMPORTANT TO TELL YOUR DOCTOR about blurred vision, cramps, depression, facial edema (swelling), loss of coordination, menstrual disorders, mental disorders, skin rash, tremors, unusual bleeding or bruising, weakness, or yellowing of the eyes or skin.

INTERACTIONS

Valproic acid interacts with several other types of drugs:
1. Concurrent use of it with other central nervous system depressants (drugs that slow the activity of the brain and spinal cord), such as alcohol, antihistamines, barbiturates, muscle relaxants, narcotics, pain medications, phenothiazine tranquilizers, and sleeping medications, or with tricyclic antidepressants can lead to extreme drowsiness.
2. Valproic acid can lead to bleeding complications when combined with oral anticoagulants (blood thinners, such as warfarin), aspirin, dipyridamole, or sulfinpyrazone.
3. Valproic acid can increase the blood levels and side effects of phenobarbital and primidone.
4. The combination of valproic acid and clonazepam or phenytoin can lead to an increase in seizure activity.
5. Aspirin may interfere with the metabolism of valproic acid, which may result in increased toxicity and increased side effects.

BE SURE TO TELL YOUR DOCTOR about any medications you are currently taking, especially any listed above.

WARNINGS

- Tell your doctor about unusual or allergic reactions you have had to any medications, especially to valproic acid, sodium valproate, or divalproex sodium.
- Before starting to take this medication, be sure to tell your doctor if you now have or if you have ever had blood disorders, kidney disease, or liver disease.
- If this drug makes you dizzy or drowsy, do not take part in any activity that requires alertness, such as driving a car or operating potentially dangerous machinery.
- Before having surgery or any other medical or dental treatment, be sure to tell your doctor or dentist that you are taking this medication.
- Do not stop taking this medication unless you first check with your doctor. Stopping the drug abruptly may lead to a worsening of your condition. Your doctor may want to reduce your dosage gradually or start you on another medication when valproic acid is discontinued. Make sure you have enough medication on hand to last through weekends, holidays, and vacations.
- Diabetic patients should know that valproic acid can interfere with urine tests for ketones. You should, therefore, check with your doctor before adjusting your insulin dose to determine if changes are necessary.
- Be sure to tell your doctor if you are pregnant. Valproic acid has been shown to cause birth defects in the offspring of animals that received large doses of the drug during preg-

nancy. It has also been associated with spinal cord birth defects in humans when used during the first three months of pregnancy. The risks and benefits of treatment should be discussed with your doctor. Also, tell your doctor if you are breast-feeding an infant. Small amounts of valproic acid pass into breast milk.

Valrelease—see diazepam

Vamate—see hydroxyzine

Vasotec—see enalapril

Vazepam—see diazepam

V-Cillin K—see penicillin VK

Veetids—see penicillin VK

Velosef—see cephradine

Velosulin—see insulin

Veltane—see brompheniramine

Veltap Elixir—see phenylpropanolamine, phenylephrine, and brompheniramine combination

Ventolin—see albuterol

---

verapamil

BRAND NAMES (Manufacturers)
Calan (Searle)
Calan SR (Searle)
Isoptin (Knoll)
Isoptin SR (Knoll)
verapamil (various manufacturers)
TYPE OF DRUG
Antianginal (calcium channel blocker) and antihypertensive
INGREDIENT
verapamil
DOSAGE FORMS
Tablets (40 mg, 80 mg, and 120 mg)
Sustained-release tablets (180 mg and 240 mg)
STORAGE
Store at room temperature in a tightly closed container.

USES

Verapamil is used to treat angina pectoris (chest pain) and high blood pressure. It belongs to a group of drugs known as calcium channel blockers. It is not clearly understood how verapamil works, but it is thought to increase the blood supply to the heart. It is also a vasodilator that relaxes the muscle tissue of the blood vessels, thereby lowering blood pressure.

TREATMENT

Verapamil can be taken either on an empty stomach or with meals, as directed by your doctor or pharmacist. The sustained-release tablets should not be crushed or chewed, but swallowed whole.

If you miss a dose of this medication, take the missed dose as soon as possible, unless it is almost time for the next dose. In that case, do not take the missed dose at all; just return to your regular dosing schedule. Do not double the next dose.

This medication does not cure high blood pressure, but it will help to control the condition as long as you continue to take it.

SIDE EFFECTS

Minor. Abdominal pain, blurred vision, constipation, dizziness, headache, muscle cramps, nausea, sleeplessness, or sweating. These side effects should disappear as your body adjusts to the medication.

To relieve constipation, increase the amount of fiber in your diet (fresh fruits and vegetables, salads, bran, and whole-grain breads), and drink more water (unless your doctor directs you to do otherwise).

Major. Tell your doctor about any side effects that are persistent or particularly bothersome. IT IS ESPECIALLY IMPORTANT TO TELL YOUR DOCTOR about changes in menstruation, confusion, depression, fainting, fatigue, hair loss, itching, loss of balance, palpitations, rapid weight gain (three to five pounds within a week), shortness of breath, swelling of the hands or feet, tremors, or unusual weakness.

INTERACTIONS

This medication interacts with a number of other types of medications:

1. The concurrent use of alcohol, quinidine, or prazosin and verapamil can cause a severe drop in blood pressure and result in fainting.

2. Beta blockers (acebutolol, atenolol, betaxolol, carteolol, esmolol, labetalol, metoprolol, nadolol, penbutolol, pindolol, propranolol, timolol) and digoxin should be used cautiously with verapamil, because side effects to the heart may be increased.

3. Disopyramide should not be taken within 48 hours of verapamil; the combination could lead to heart failure.

4. Cimetidine can decrease the elimination of verapamil from the body, which can lead to an increased risk of side effects.

5. Sulfinpyrazone and rifampin can increase the elimination of verapamil from the body, which can lead to a decrease in its effectiveness.

6. Verapamil can cause an increase in the effects of the drug theophylltine.

BE SURE TO TELL YOUR DOCTOR about any medications you are currently taking, especially any of those listed above.

WARNINGS

- Tell your doctor about unusual or allergic reactions you have had to any medications, especially to verapamil.
- Before starting therapy with this medication, be sure that you inform your doctor if you have ever had any type of heart disease, kidney disease, liver disease, low blood pressure, or a slowed heartbeat.
- Your doctor may want you to check your pulse regularly while you are taking this medication. If your heart rate drops below 50 beats per minute, contact your doctor.

• Verapamil is not effective for an attack of chest pain that has already started; it is used to prevent attacks.
• Do not stop taking this drug without first consulting your doctor. Stopping abruptly may lead to a worsening of your chest pain. Your doctor may, therefore, want to reduce your dosage gradually or have you switch to another medication when verapamil is discontinued.
• In order to prevent dizziness or fainting while taking this medication, try not to stand for long periods of time, avoid drinking alcoholic beverages, and try not to become overheated (avoid exercising strenuously in hot weather, and do not take hot baths, showers, and saunas).
• Be sure to tell your doctor if you are pregnant. Extensive studies in pregnant women have not been conducted. Also, tell your doctor if you are breast-feeding an infant. Small amounts of verapamil pass into breast milk.

Vibramycin Hyclate—see doxycycline

Vibra Tabs—see doxycycline

Vicodin—see acetaminophen and hydrocodone combination

Vi-Daylin F—see vitamins, multiple, with fluoride

Vi-Daylin F ADC Drops—see vitamins A, D, and C with fluoride

Viodo HC—see hydrocortisone and iodochlorhydroxyquin combination (topical)

Vioform-Hydrocortisone—see hydrocortisone and iodochlorhydroxyquin combination (topical)

Viokase—see pancrelipase

Virilon—see methyltestosterone

Visken—see pindolol

Vistaril—see hydroxyzine

vitamin D—see ergocalciferol (vitamin D)

---

vitamin K

BRAND NAMES (Manufacturers)
Mephyton (Merck Sharp & Dohme)
Synkayvite (Roche)
TYPE OF DRUG
vitamin K supplement
INGREDIENTS
menadione, menadiol sodium diphosphate, or phytonadione
DOSAGE FORM
Tablets (5 mg)
STORAGE
Vitamin K tablets should be stored at room temperature in a tightly closed, light-resistant container.

USES

Vitamin K is required by the body to produce the blood clots that are necessary for wound healing and the day-to-day repair of body tissues. Normally, bacteria present in the gastrointestinal tract produce large quantities of the vitamin, which is then absorbed into the bloodstream. Some vitamin K is also absorbed directly from the foods we eat (leafy green vegetables, meats, and dairy products). This medication is used as a supplement for those patients who cannot, for various reasons (for example, gastrointestinal bypass surgery, malnutrition, antibiotic therapy), absorb sufficient vitamin K from their gastrointestinal tracts. This supplement, therefore, prevents the blood clotting disorders that would result from vitamin K deficiency.

TREATMENT

Vitamin K can be taken either on an empty stomach or, to avoid stomach irritation, with food or milk (unless your doctor directs you to do otherwise).

If you miss a dose of this medication, take the missed dose as soon as possible, unless it is almost time for the next dose. In that case, do not take the missed dose of the medication at all; just return to your regular dosing schedule. Do not double the next dose of medication. Be sure to tell your doctor about any missed doses.

SIDE EFFECTS

Minor. Alterations in taste, headache, nausea, stomach upset, or vomiting. These side effects should disappear as your body adjusts to the medication.
Major. Tell your doctor about any side effects that are persistent or particularly bothersome. IT IS ESPECIALLY IMPORTANT TO TELL YOUR DOCTOR about itching, shortness of breath, or skin rash.

INTERACTIONS

Vitamin K interacts with a number of other types of medications:
1. Antibiotics, quinine, quinidine, aspirin, oral antidiabetic medications, cholestyramine, colestipol, and mineral oil can increase the dosage requirements of vitamin K.
2. Vitamin K can reduce the effectiveness of oral anticoagulants (blood thinners, such as warfarin).

BE SURE TO TELL YOUR DOCTOR about any medications you are currently taking, especially any of those listed above.

WARNINGS

• Be sure to tell your doctor about any unusual or allergic reactions you have had to any medication, especially to vitamin K supplements.
• Before starting to take this medication, be sure to tell your doctor if you now have or if you have ever had glucose-6-phosphate dehydrogenase (G6PD) deficiency or liver disease.
• Before having surgery or any other medical or dental treatment, be sure to tell your doctor or dentist that you are taking this medication.
• Be sure to tell your doctor if you are pregnant. Extensive studies in humans have not been conducted. Also, tell your doctor if you are breast-feeding an infant. It is not known whether vitamin K passes into breast milk.

vitamins A, D, and C with fluoride

BRAND NAMES (Manufacturers)
Triple-Vita-Flor (P.B.I)
Tri-Vi-Flor (Mead Johnson)
Tri-Vitamin with Fluoride Drops (Rugby)
Vi-Daylin F ADC Drops (Ross)
TYPE OF DRUG
Multivitamin and fluoride supplement
INGREDIENTS
vitamin A, vitamin D, vitamin C, and fluoride
DOSAGE FORMS
Chewable tablets (2,500 IU [international units] vitamin A; 400 IU vitamin D; 60 mg vitamin C; and 1 mg fluoride)
Oral drops (1,500 IU vitamin A; 400 IU vitamin D; 35 mg vitamin C; and 0.25 mg or 0.5 mg fluoride per ml)
STORAGE
The chewable tablets should be stored at room temperature in a tightly closed, light-resistant container. The oral drops should be stored at room temperature in the original plastic container (glass containers interact with and destroy the fluoride in the solution). A slight darkening in the color of the drops does not indicate a loss in potency of the vitamins or fluoride; the solution can still be used safely. This medication should never be frozen.

USES

Multivitamins with fluoride are used to protect against tooth decay and vitamin deficiencies in children. Fluoride has been found to be helpful in preventing cavities.

TREATMENT

The tablets should be chewed or crushed before being swallowed. To provide maximum protection, the tablets should be given at bedtime after the teeth have been brushed. To allow the fluoride to work on the teeth, nothing should be eaten for at least 15 minutes after chewing the tablets.

The oral drop form of this multivitamin and fluoride supplement can be taken directly or can be mixed with juice or foods. The dose should be measured carefully with the dropper provided.

Milk prevents the absorption of fluoride from the gastrointestinal tract. Therefore, this product should not be taken with milk or other dairy products.

If your child misses a dose of this medication, administer the missed dose as soon as possible, unless it is almost time for the next dose. In that case, do not give the missed dose at all; just return to the child's regular dosing schedule. Do not double the next dose.

SIDE EFFECTS

Minor. This product seldom causes side effects, but can occasionally cause constipation, diarrhea, drowsiness, fatigue, loss of appetite, nausea, vomiting, and weakness. These side effects should disappear as the body adjusts to the medication.

To relieve constipation, increase the amount of fiber in your child's diet (fresh fruits and vegetables, salads, bran, and whole-grain breads) and encourage the child to drink more water (unless your doctor directs you to do otherwise).

Major. Tell your doctor about any side effects that are persistent or particularly bothersome. IT IS ESPECIALLY IMPORTANT TO TELL YOUR DOCTOR about bloody or black, tarry stools; difficulty in swallowing; discoloration of the teeth; excessive drooling; excitation; mouth sores; rash; stomach cramps; or tremors.

INTERACTIONS

This product should not interact with other medications if it is used according to directions.

WARNINGS

- Tell your doctor about unusual or allergic reactions your child has had to any medications, especially to vitamins or to fluoride.
- Tell your doctor if your child now has or has ever had bone, heart, kidney, or thyroid disease.
- The chewable tablets should not be used if the fluoride content of your drinking water is 0.7 part per million or more. The oral drops should not be used by children less than two years of age in areas where the drinking water contains 0.3 part per million or more of fluoride. If you are unsure of the fluoride content of your drinking water, ask your doctor or call the county health department.
- Vitamins with fluoride are often prescribed for infants who are not being given any source of fluorinated water. Once your infant is given fluorinated water consistently, ask your doctor if you should continue this medication.
- You should NEVER refer to this medication as "candy" or "candy-flavored vitamins." Your child may take you literally and swallow too many.

---

vitamins, multiple, with fluoride

BRAND NAMES (Manufacturers)
Florvite (Everett)
Multi-Vita Drops with Fluoride (P.B.I)
Poly-Vi-Flor (Mead Johnson)
Polyvitamins with Fluoride Drops (Rugby)
Polyvite with Fluoride Drops (Geneva Generics)
Vi-Daylin F (Ross)
TYPE OF DRUG
Multivitamin and fluoride supplement
INGREDIENTS
vitamins A, D, E, C, B_6, B_{12}, folic acid, riboflavin, niacin, fluoride, and thiamine
DOSAGE FORMS
Chewable tablets (2,500 IU [international units] vitamin A; 400 IU vitamin D; 15 IU vitamin E; 60 mg vitamin C; 0.3 mg folic acid; 1.0 mg thiamine; 1.2 mg riboflavin; 13.5 mg niacin; 1.0 mg vitamin B_6; 4.5 mcg vitamin B_{12}; and 0.5 mg or 1.0 mg fluoride)
Oral drops (1,500 IU vitamin A; 400 IU vitamin D; 4.1 or 5 IU vitamin E; 35 mg vitamin C; 0.5 mg thiamine; 0.6 mg riboflavin; 8 mg niacin; 0.4 mg vitamin B_6; 2 mcg vitamin B_{12}; and 0.25 mg or 0.5 mg fluoride per ml)
STORAGE
The chewable tablets should be stored at room temperature

in a tightly closed, light-resistant container. The oral drops should be stored at room temperature in the original plastic container (glass containers interact with and destroy the fluoride in the solution). A slight darkening in the color of the drops does not indicate a loss in potency of the vitamins or fluoride; the solution can still be used safely. This medication should never be frozen.

USES

Multivitamins with fluoride are used to protect against tooth decay and vitamin deficiencies in children. Fluoride has been found to be helpful in preventing cavities.

TREATMENT

The tablets should be either chewed or crushed before being swallowed. To provide maximum protection, the tablets should be given at bedtime after the teeth have been brushed. Nothing should be eaten for at least 15 minutes after chewing the tablets to allow the fluoride to work on the teeth.

The oral drop form of this medication can be taken directly, or can be mixed with juice or foods. The dose should be measured carefully with the dropper provided.

Milk prevents the absorption of fluoride from the gastrointestinal tract. Therefore, this product should not be taken with milk or other dairy products.

If your child misses a dose, administer the missed dose as soon as possible, unless it is almost time for the next dose. In that case, do not give the missed dose at all; just return to the child's regular dosing schedule. Do not double the next dose.

SIDE EFFECTS

Minor. Occasionally, this product causes constipation, diarrhea, drowsiness, fatigue, loss of appetite, nausea, vomiting, or weakness. These side effects should disappear as the body adjusts to the medication.

To relieve constipation, increase the amount of fiber in your child's diet (fresh fruits and vegetables, salads, bran, and whole-grain breads) and encourage your child to drink more water (unless your doctor directs you to do otherwise).

Major. Tell your doctor about any side effects that are persistent or particularly bothersome. IT IS ESPECIALLY IMPORTANT TO TELL YOUR DOCTOR about bloody or black, tarry stools; difficulty in swallowing; discoloration of the teeth; excessive drooling; excitation; mouth sores; rash; stomach cramps; or tremors.

INTERACTIONS

This product should not interact with other medications if it is used according to directions.

WARNINGS

- Tell your doctor about unusual or allergic reactions your child has had to any medications, especially to vitamins or to fluoride.
- Tell your doctor if your child now has or has ever had bone, heart, kidney, or thyroid disease.
- The chewable tablets should not be used if the fluoride content of your drinking water is 0.7 part per million or more. The oral drops should not be used by children less than two years of age in areas where the drinking water contains 0.3 part per million or more of fluoride. If you are unsure of the fluoride content of your drinking water, ask your doctor or call the county health department.
- Vitamins with fluoride are often prescribed for infants who are not being given any source of fluorinated water. Once your infant is given fluorinated water consistently, ask you doctor if you should continue this medication.
- NEVER call this medication "candy" or "candy-flavored vitamins." Your child may take you literally and swallow too many.

---

vitamins, prenatal

BRAND NAME (Manufacturer)

StuartNatal 1 + 1 (Stuart)

TYPE OF DRUG

Multivitamin and mineral supplement

INGREDIENTS

calcium, iron, folic acid, zinc, copper, niacin, riboflavin, thiamine, and vitamins A, D, E, B_6, B_{12}, and C

DOSAGE FORM

Tablets (200 mg calcium; 65 mg iron; 1.0 mg folic acid; 4,000 IU [international units] vitamin A; 400 IU vitamin D; 11 IU vitamin E; 1.5 mg thiamine; 3 mg riboflavin; 20 mg niacin; 10 mg vitamin B_6; 12 mcg vitamin B_{12}; 120 mg vitamin C; 25 mg zinc; 2 mg copper)

STORAGE

These tablets should be stored at room temperature in a tightly closed, light-resistant container.

USES

This product is a multivitamin and mineral supplement for use during pregnancy and nursing.

TREATMENT

In order to avoid stomach irritation, you can take this product with food or with a full glass of water or milk.

If you miss a dose of this medication, take the missed dose as soon as possible, unless it is almost time for the next dose. In that case, do not take the missed dose at all; just return to your regular dosing schedule. Do not double the next dose.

SIDE EFFECTS

Minor. Constipation, diarrhea, nausea, stomach upset, or vomiting. These side effects should disappear as your body adjusts to the medication.

To relieve constipation, increase the amount of fiber in your diet (fresh fruits and vegetables, salads, bran, and whole-grain breads), exercise, and drink more water (unless your doctor directs you to do otherwise).

Black stools are a normal consequence of iron therapy and do not indicate a problem.

Major. Tell your doctor about any side effects that are persistent or particularly bothersome. IT IS ESPECIALLY IMPORTANT TO TELL YOUR DOCTOR about bloody or tarry stools or severe abdominal pain.

INTERACTIONS

This product should not interact with other medications if it is used according to directions.

WARNINGS

• Tell your doctor about unusual or allergic reactions you have had to any medications, especially to any vitamins, minerals, or iron.

• Be sure to tell your doctor if you have ever had bone disease, liver disease, kidney disease, or stomach ulcers.

• Because this product may mask the symptoms of pernicious anemia, it should be used only under a doctor's supervision.

Vivactil—see protriptylline

Vivox—see doxycycline

Voltaren—see diclofenac

Vytone—see hydrocortisone and iodochlorhydroxyquin combination (topical)

---

warfarin

BRAND NAMES (Manufacturers)
Coumadin (DuPont)
Panwarfin (Abbott)
Sofarin (Lemmon)
warfarin sodium (various manufacturers)

TYPE OF DRUG
Anticoagulant

INGREDIENT
warfarin

DOSAGE FORM
Tablets (2 mg, 2.5 mg, 5 mg, 7.5 mg, and 10 mg)

STORAGE
Warfarin should be stored at room temperature in a tightly closed, light-resistant container.

USES

Warfarin is used to prevent blood clot formation. It acts by decreasing the production of blood clotting substances by the liver.

TREATMENT

You can take warfarin with a full glass of water. In order to become accustomed to taking this medication, try to take it at the same time each day.

If you miss a dose of this medication, take the missed dose as soon as possible, unless it is almost time for the next dose. In that case, do not take the missed dose at all; just return to your regular dosing schedule. Do not double the next dose. If you miss more than two doses in a row of this medication, contact your doctor.

SIDE EFFECTS

Minor. Blurred vision, cramps, decreased appetite, diarrhea, or nausea. These side effects should disappear as your body adjusts to the medication. Warfarin may produce a red-orange discoloration of urine.

Major. Tell your doctor about any side effects that are persistent or particularly bothersome. IT IS ESPECIALLY IMPORTANT TO TELL YOUR DOCTOR about bloody or black, tarry stools; blood in sputum; fever; heavy bleeding from cuts; internal bleeding (signs of internal bleeding include abdominal pain or swelling and vomiting of blood or material that resembles coffee grounds); loss of hair; mouth sores; nosebleeds; nausea; rash; red urine; severe bruising; severe headache; swelling of joints; unusually heavy menstrual bleeding; or yellowing of the eyes or skin.

INTERACTIONS

Warfarin interacts with several other types of drugs:

1. Alcohol, allopurinol, amiodarone, anabolic steroids, antibiotics, chloral hydrate, chloramphenicol, chlorpropamide, cimetidine, clofibrate, danazol, disulfiram, erythromycin, glucagon, isoniazid, ketoconazole, methyldopa, methylphenidate, metronidazole, monoamine oxidase (MAO) inhibitors, nalidixic acid, phenylbutazone, propoxyphene, quinidine, quinine, salicylates, sulfamethoxazole and trimethoprim combination, sulfinpyrazone, sulfonamides, sulindac, tetracycline, thyroid hormones, tolbutamide, and triclofos can increase the effects of warfarin, which can be dangerous.

2. Azathioprine, barbiturates, carbamazepine, cholestyramine, colestipol, estrogens, ethchlorvynol, glutethimide, griseofulvin, oral contraceptives (birth control pills), phenytoin, propylthiouracil, rifampin, sucralfate, and vitamin K can decrease the effectiveness of warfarin.

3. Adrenocorticosteroids (cortisone-like medications), anticancer drugs, aspirin, diflunisal, dipyridamole, fenoprofen, ibuprofen, indomethacin, oxyphenbutazone, phenylbutazone, potassium, quinidine, quinine, and salicylates can increase the bleeding complications of warfarin.

4. Warfarin can increase the side effects of oral antidiabetic agents and phenytoin.

5. Diuretics (water pills) may either increase the effects or decrease the effectiveness of warfarin. Ask your doctor about concurrent use of diuretics and warfarin.

Before starting to take warfarin, BE SURE TO TELL YOUR DOCTOR about any medications you are currently taking, especially any of those listed above.

WARNINGS

• Tell your doctor about unusual or allergic reactions you have had to any medications, especially to warfarin.

• Before starting to take this medication, BE SURE TO TELL YOUR DOCTOR if you now have or if you have ever had any condition for which bleeding is an added risk—an aneurysm, blood disorders, cancer, diabetes mellitus, congestive heart failure, edema, endocarditis, high blood pressure, indwelling catheters, intestinal infections, kidney or liver disease, malnutrition, menstrual difficulties, pericarditis, surgery, thyroid disease, tuberculosis, ulcers, vasculitis, or wounds and injuries.

• Before having surgery or any other medical or dental treatment, BE SURE TO TELL YOUR DOCTOR OR DENTIST THAT YOU ARE TAKING WARFARIN.

• Do not take any aspirin-containing products or any over-the-counter products while you are on warfarin, unless you first check with your doctor. Aspirin can increase the risk of bleeding complications from warfarin.

• Avoid any activity, such as a contact sport, that might lead to physical injury. Tell your doctor about any fall or blow that occurs. Warfarin can cause HEAVY bleeding from cuts.

• Use an electric razor for shaving to reduce the risk of cutting yourself, and be careful while brushing your teeth.
• Since factors such as travel, diet, the environment, and your health can affect your body's response to warfarin, your dosage level should be carefully monitored.
• Do not stop taking warfarin unless you first consult your doctor. If you stop taking this drug abruptly, you may experience blood clotting. Your doctor may, therefore, want to reduce your dosage gradually.
• Do not change brands of this medication without consulting your doctor.
• Some of these products contain the color additive FD&C Yellow No. 5 (tartrazine), which can cause allergic-type reactions (rash, shortness of breath, fainting) in certain susceptible individuals.
• Be sure to tell your doctor if you are pregnant. Warfarin has been associated with birth defects and bleeding complications in fetuses. Also, tell your doctor if you are breastfeeding an infant. Small amounts of warfarin pass into breast milk.

Weh-less—see phendimetrazine

Wehvert—see meclizine

Weightrol—see phendimetrazine

Wellbutrin—see bupropion

Westcort—see hydrocortisone (topical)

Wigraine—see ergotamine and caffeine combination

Wigrettes—see ergotamine

Wilpowr—see phentermine

Wyamycin E—see erythromycin

Wyamycin S—see erythromycin

Wygesic—see acetaminophen and propoxyphene combination

Wymox—see amoxicillin

Wytensin—see guanabenz

Xanax—see alprazolam

Yutopar—see ritodrine

Zantac—see ranitidine

Zarontin—see ethosuximide

Zaroxolyn—see metolazone

Zebrax—see chlordiazepoxide and clidinium combination

Zestril—see lisinopril

ZORprin—see aspirin

Zovirax—see acyclovir

Zurinol—see allopurinol

Zydone—see acetaminophen and hydrocodone combination

Zyloprim—see allopurinol

Canadian Brand Names

Following is a list of commonly prescribed Canadian brand-name medications and their manufacturers. Also listed are the profile names under which you can find information about each brand-name drug. Please note that in Canada **acetaminophen** is known as **paracetamol, albuterol** is known as **salbutamol, metaproterenol** is known as **orciprenaline,** and **meperidine** is known as **pethidine.**

BRAND NAME (Manufacturer)	Profile
Acet-Am® (Organon)	**theophylline**
Acetazolam® (ICN)	**acetazolamide**
Alloprin® (ICN)	**allopurinol**
Amersol® (Horner)	**ibuprofen**
Ampicin® (Bristol)	**ampicillin**
Ampilean® (Organon)	**ampicillin**
Ansaid® (Upjohn)	**flurbiprofen**
Antazone® (ICN)	**sulfinpyrazone**
Anturan® (Geigy)	**sulfinpyrazone**
Aparkane® (ICN)	**trihexyphenidyl**
Apo-Ampi® (Apotex)	**ampicillin**
Apo-Pen-VK® (Apotex)	**penicillin VK**
Athrombin-K® (Purdue Frederick)	**warfarin**
Bactopen® (Beecham)	**cloxacillin**
Bensylate® (ICN)	**benztropine**
Bentylol® (Merrell)	**dicyclomine**
Benuryl® (ICN)	**probenecid**
Betaloc® (Astra)	**metoprolol**
Bonamine® (Pfizer)	**meclizine**
Canesten® (Miles)	**clotrimazole (vaginal)**
Carbolith® (ICN)	**lithium**
Ceporex® (Glaxo)	**cephalexin**
Chlorpromanyl® (Technilab)	**chlorpromazine**
Claripex® (ICN)	**clofibrate**
Clavulin® (Beecham)	**amoxicillin and clavulanic acid combination**
Corium® (ICN)	**chlordiazepoxide and clidinium combination**
Coronex® (Ayerst)	**isosorbide dinitrate**
Corophyllin® (Beecham)	**aminophylline**
Cytotec® (Searle)	**misoprostol**
Dalacin C® (Upjohn)	**clindamycin (systemic)**
Depen® (Horner)	**penicillamine**
Detensol® (Desbergers)	**propranolol**
Dimelor® (Lilly)	**acetohexamide**
Diuchlor H® (Medic)	**hydrochlorothiazide**
Dixarit® (Boehringer Ingelheim)	**clonidine**
Dopamet® (ICN)	**methyldopa**
Eltroxin® (Glaxo)	**levothyroxine**
Emex® (Beecham)	**metoclopramide**
E-Pam® (ICN)	**diazepam**
Erythromid® (Abbott)	**erythromycin**
Euglucon® (Boehringer Mannheim)	**glyburide**
Fivent® (Fisons)	**cromolyn sodium (inhalation)**
Froben® (Organon)	**flurbiprofen**
Hibidel 1:2000 (Ayerst)	**chlorhexidine gluconate**
Hibitane® Gluconate 20% (Ayerst)	**chlorhexidine gluconate**

…D NAME (Manufacturer)	Profile
…ane® Skin Cleanser 2% and …% (Ayerst)	chlorhexidine gluconate
…ip-Rex® (Riker)	methenamine
Hismanal® (Janssen)	astemizole
Impril® (ICN)	imipramine
Indocid® (MSD)	indomethacin
Intrabutazone® (Organon)	phenylbutazone
Kwellada® (R & C)	lindane
Largactil® (Rhône-Poulenc)	chlorpromazine
Lenoltec with codeine No. 4® (Technilab)	acetaminophen and codeine combination
Levate® (ICN)	amitriptyline
Lidemol® (Syntex)	fluocinonide (topical)
Lithane® (Pfizer)	lithium
Lithizine® (Maney)	lithium
Loxapac® (Lederle)	loxapine
Maxeran® (Nordic)	metoclopramide
Mazepine® (ICN)	carbamazepine
Medilium® (Medic)	chlordiazepoxide
Megacillin® (Frosst)	penicillin G
Meval® (Medic)	diazepam
Minestrin 1/20® (P.D.)	oral contraceptives
Min-Ovral® (Wyeth)	oral contraceptives
Mobenol® (Horner)	tolbutamide
Moduret® (MSD)	amiloride and hydrochlorothiazide combination
Myclo® (Boehringer Ingelheim)	clotrimazole (topical), clotrimazole (vaginal)
Nadopen-V® (Nadeau)	penicillin VK
Natrimax® (Trianon)	hydrochlorothiazide
Naxen® (SynCare)	naproxen
Neo-Codema® (Neolab)	hydrochlorothiazide

BRAND NAME (Manufacturer)	Profile
Neo-Metric® (Neolab)	metronidazole
Nephronex® (Cortunon)	nitrofurantoin
Nobesine® (Rougier)	diethylpropion
Novamoxin® (Novopharm)	amoxicillin
Novobutamide® (Novopharm)	tolbutamide
Novobutazone® (Novopharm)	phenylbutazone
Novocimetine® (Novopharm)	cimetidine
Novocloxin® (Novopharm)	cloxacillin
Novodipam® (Novopharm)	diazepam
Novodoparil® (Novopharm)	methyldopa and hydrochlorothiazide combination
Novofibrate® (Novopharm)	clofibrate
Novoflupam® (Novopharm)	flurazepam
Novoflurazine® (Novopharm)	trifluoperazine
Novofuran® (Novopharm)	nitrofurantoin
Novohexidyl® (Novopharm)	trihexyphenidyl
Novohydrazide® (Novopharm)	hydrochlorothiazide
Novolexin® (Novopharm)	cephalexin
Novomedopa® (Novopharm)	methyldopa
Novomethacin® (Novopharm)	indomethacin
Novonaprox® (Novopharm)	naproxen
Novonidazole® (Novopharm)	metronidazole
Novopen G® (Novopharm)	penicillin G
Novopen-VK® (Novopharm)	penicillin VK
Novopoxide® (Novopharm)	chlordiazepoxide
Novopramine® (Novopharm)	imipramine
Novopranol® (Novopharm)	propranolol
Novoprofen® (Novopharm)	ibuprofen
Novopropamide® (Novopharm)	chlorpropamide
Novopropoxyn® (Novopharm)	propoxyphene
Novopurol® (Novopharm)	allopurinol
Novopyrazone® (Novopharm)	sulfinpyrazone

BRAND NAME (Manufacturer)	Profile
Novoridazine® (Novopharm)	**thioridazine**
Novosemide® (Novopharm)	**furosemide**
Novosorbide® (Novopharm)	**isosorbide dinitrate**
Novospiroton® (Novopharm)	**spironolactone**
Novospirozine® (Novopharm)	**spironolactone and hydrochlorothiazide combination**
Novotetra® (Novopharm)	**tetracycline**
Novothalidone® (Novopharm)	**chlorthalidone**
Novotriamzide® (Novopharm)	**triamterene and hydrochlorothiazide combination**
Novotrimel® (Novopharm)	**sulfamethoxazole and trimethoprim combination**
Novotriptyn® (Novopharm)	**amitriptyline**
Nyaderm® (TARO)	**nystatin**
Orbenin® (Ayerst)	**cloxacillin**
Oxpam® (ICN)	**oxazepam**
Oxycocet® (Technilab)	**acetaminophen and oxycodone combination**
Oxycodan® (Technilab)	**aspirin and oxycodone combination**
Penbritin® (Ayerst)	**ampicillin**
Peptol® (Horner)	**cimetidine**
Peridol® (Technilab)	**haloperidol**
Pertofrane® (Geigy)	**desipramine**
Phenazo® (ICN)	**phenazopyridine**
Ponderal® (Servier)	**fenfluramine**
Proavil® (Pro Doc)	**perphenazine and amitriptyline combination**
Procytox® (Horner)	**cyclophosphamide**
Purinol® (Horner)	**allopurinol**
PVF® (Frosst)	**penicillin VK**
Reserfia® (Medic)	**reserpine**

BRAND NAME (Manufacturer)	Profile
Rival® (Riva)	**diazepam**
Rivotril® (Roche)	**clonazepam**
Rofact® (ICN)	**rifampin**
Rogaine™ Topical Solution (Upjohn)	**minoxidil (topical)**
Roubac® (Rougier)	**sulfamethoxazole and trimethoprim combination**
Rouhex®-G 2% and 4% (Rougier)	**chlorhexidine**
Rounox with Codeine® (Rougier)	**acetaminophen and codeine combination**
Rynacrom® (Fisons)	**cromolyn sodium (nasal)**
Rhythmodan® (Roussel)	**disopyramide**
Salazopyrin® (Pharmacia)	**sulfasalazine**
Solazine® (Horner)	**trifluoperazine**
Solium® (Horner)	**chlordiazepoxide**
Somnol® (Horner)	**flurazepam**
Som-Pam® (ICN)	**flurazepam**
Stemetil® (May & Baker)	**prochlorperazine**
Stieva-A® (Stiefel)	**tretinoin**
Sulcrate® (Nordic)	**sucralfate**
Tecnal® (Technilab)	**aspirin, caffeine, and butalbital combination**
Terfluzine® (ICN)	**trifluoperazine**
Transderm-V (Ciba-Geigy)	**scopolamine (transdermal)**
Triadapin® (Fisons)	**doxepin**
Uridon® (ICN)	**chlorthalidone**
Uritol® (Horner)	**furosemide**
Urozide® (ICN)	**hydrochlorothiazide**
Vivol® (Horner)	**diazepam**
Voltaren® (Geigy)	**diclofenac (sodium)**
Warfilone® (Frosst)	**warfarin**
Winpred® (ICN)	**prednisone (systemic)**

Over-the-Counter Drug Guide

As the title of this book would indicate, the majority of drugs that we have listed can be acquired by prescription only. However, there are certain types of drugs, such as non-narcotic pain relievers or antihistamine preparations, that are also available over-the-counter—in other words, you can purchase them without a prescription.

For your convenience, we have also listed some of the most popular over-the-counter drugs in this edition. You will find these drugs in our non-prescription drug guide below.

Index

On the following pages, you will find an alphabetical listing of the brand-name drugs discussed in this book. When you turn to the page number of the drug you are looking for, its name will appear beneath the bold-faced heading BRAND NAME(S) (Manufacturer[s]). Information about your drug can then be found on that page or the pages that follow.

For your convenience, some popularly prescribed generic medications have also been listed in this index. The names of these generic medications are lower-cased in print.

A

B

C

D

E

F

M

N

Q

R

S

T

U

V

W

X

Y

Z